Biological Mechanisms of Tooth Movement

Biological Mechanisms of Tooth Movement

Edited by

Vinod Krishnan
Sri Sankara Dental College
Thiruvananthapuram, Kerala, India

Anne Marie Kuijpers-Jagtman
University Medical Center Groningen
The Netherlands

University of Bern
Switzerland

Universitas Indonesia
Jakarta, Indonesia

and

Ze'ev Davidovitch
Harvard University
Cambridge, Massachusetts, USA

Third Edition

WILEY Blackwell

This edition first published 2021
© 2021 John Wiley & Sons Ltd

Edition History
1e 2008 John Wiley & Sons Ltd.; 2e 2015 John Wiley & Sons Ltd.

All rights reserved. No part of this publication may be reproduced, stored in a retrieval system, or transmitted, in any form or by any means, electronic, mechanical, photocopying, recording or otherwise, except as permitted by law. Advice on how to obtain permission to reuse material from this title is available at http://www.wiley.com/go/permissions.

The right of Vinod Krishnan, Anne Marie Kuijpers-Jagtman, and Ze'ev Davidovitch to be identified as the authors of the editorial material in this work has been asserted in accordance with law.

Registered Offices
John Wiley & Sons, Inc., 111 River Street, Hoboken, NJ 07030, USA
John Wiley & Sons Ltd, The Atrium, Southern Gate, Chichester, West Sussex, PO19 8SQ, UK

Editorial Office
9600 Garsington Road, Oxford, OX4 2DQ, UK

For details of our global editorial offices, customer services, and more information about Wiley products visit us at www.wiley.com. Wiley also publishes its books in a variety of electronic formats and by print-on-demand. Some content that appears in standard print versions of this book may not be available in other formats.

Limit of Liability/Disclaimer of Warranty
The contents of this work are intended to further general scientific research, understanding, and discussion only and are not intended and should not be relied upon as recommending or promoting scientific method, diagnosis, or treatment by physicians for any particular patient. In view of ongoing research, equipment modifications, changes in governmental regulations, and the constant flow of information relating to the use of medicines, equipment, and devices, the reader is urged to review and evaluate the information provided in the package insert or instructions for each medicine, equipment, or device for, among other things, any changes in the instructions or indication of usage and for added warnings and precautions. While the publisher and authors have used their best efforts in preparing this work, they make no representations or warranties with respect to the accuracy or completeness of the contents of this work and specifically disclaim all warranties, including without limitation any implied warranties of merchantability or fitness for a particular purpose. No warranty may be created or extended by sales representatives, written sales materials or promotional statements for this work. The fact that an organization, website, or product is referred to in this work as a citation and/or potential source of further information does not mean that the publisher and authors endorse the information or services the organization, website, or product may provide or recommendations it may make. This work is sold with the understanding that the publisher is not engaged in rendering professional services. The advice and strategies contained herein may not be suitable for your situation. You should consult with a specialist where appropriate. Further, readers should be aware that websites listed in this work may have changed or disappeared between when this work was written and when it is read. Neither the publisher nor authors shall be liable for any loss of profit or any other commercial damages, including but not limited to special, incidental, consequential, or other damages.

Library of Congress Cataloging-in-Publication Data

Names: Krishnan, Vinod, editor. | Kuijpers-Jagtman, Anne Marie, 1949– editor.
 Davidovitch, Ze'ev editor.
Title: Biological mechanisms of tooth movement / edited by Vinod Krishnan,
 Anne Marie Kuijpers-Jagtman, Ze'ev Davidovitch.
Description: Third edition. | Hoboken, NJ : Wiley-Blackwell, 2021. |
 Includes bibliographical references and index.
Identifiers: LCCN 2021001141 (print) | LCCN 2021001142 (ebook) |
 ISBN 9781119608936 (cloth) | ISBN 9781119608943 (adobe pdf) |
 ISBN 9781119608929 (epub)
Subjects: MESH: Tooth Movement Techniques
Classification: LCC QP88.6 (print) | LCC QP88.6 (ebook) | NLM WU 400 |
 DDC 612.3/11–dc23
LC record available at https://lccn.loc.gov/2021001141
LC ebook record available at https://lccn.loc.gov/2021001142

Cover Design: Wiley
Cover Image: Vinod Krishnan, Jaap C. Maltha, Raffaele Spena and Carlalberta Verna

Set in 9/11pt Minion by SPi Global, Pondicherry, India

Printed in Singapore

M099676_250221

My ever inspiring family, especially my parents, brother, wife, and kids (Jithu and Malu) who supported me throughout this project.

All my teachers, colleagues, and students who made me think about the science behind orthodontic tooth movement.

Vinod Krishnan

My colleagues and friends who inspired me the most along my journey into the biological background of orthodontics, Jaap Maltha and Birte Melsen.

Anne Marie Kuijpers-Jagtman

My wife, Galia, for her enduring support throughout the preparation of this volume.

The people who shared their knowledge and guidance with me along the path of explorations: Ino Sciaky, Edith Kaye, Leif Johanesen, Coenraad F.A, Moorrees, Vince De Angelis, Gunnar Gustafson, Joe Shanfeld, and Ed Korostoff.

Ze'ev Davidovitch

Contents

Contributors, viii

Preface to the First Edition, x

Preface to the Second Edition, xi

Preface to the Third Edition, xii

Part 1: Evolution of Biological Concepts, 1

1. Biological Basis of Orthodontic Tooth Movement: A Historical Perspective, 3
   Vinod Krishnan and Ze'ev Davidovitch

2. Biology of Orthodontic Tooth Movement: The Evolution of Hypotheses and Concepts, 16
   Vinod Krishnan and Ze'ev Davidovitch

Part 2: Mechanics Meets Biology, 33

3. Cellular and Molecular Biology of Orthodontic Tooth Movement, 35
   Jaap C. Maltha, Vinod Krishnan, and Anne Marie Kuijpers-Jagtman

4. Inflammatory Response in the Periodontal Ligament and Dental Pulp During Orthodontic Tooth Movement, 49
   Masaru Yamaguchi and Gustavo Pompermaier Garlet

5. The Effects of Mechanical Loading on Hard and Soft Tissues and Cells, 68
   Itzhak Binderman, Nasser Gadban, and Avinoam Yaffe

6. Biological Aspects of Bone Growth and Metabolism in Orthodontics, 77
   James K. Hartsfield, Jr., Priyanka Gudsoorkar, Lorri A. Morford, and W. Eugene Roberts, Jr.

7. Mechanical Load, Sex Hormones, and Bone Modeling, 100
   Sara H. Windahl and Ulf H. Lerner

8. Biological Reactions to Temporary Anchorage Devices, 117
   Gang Wu, Jiangyue Wang, Ding Bai, Jing Guo, Haikun Hu, and Vincent Everts

9. Tissue Reaction to Orthodontic Force Systems. Are we in Control?, 129
   Birte Melsen, Michel Dalstra, and Paolo M. Cattaneo

Part 3: Inflammation and Orthodontics, 139

10. The Influence of Orthodontic Treatment on Oral Microbiology, 141
    Alessandra Lucchese and Lars Bondemark

11. Markers of Paradental Tissue Remodeling in the Gingival Crevicular Fluid and Saliva of Orthodontic Patients, 159
    Taylor E. Glovsky and Laura R. Iwasaki

Part 4: Personalized Diagnosis and Treatment, 169

12. Genetic Influences on Orthodontic Tooth Movement, 171
    Margarita Zeichner-David

13. Precision Orthodontics: Limitations and Possibilities in Practice, 189
    James K. Hartsfield, Jr., Priyanka Gudsoorkar, and Lorri A. Morford

14. The Effect of Drugs, Hormones, and Diet on Orthodontic Tooth Movement, 199
    Vinod Krishnan, James J. Zahrowski, and Ze'ev Davidovitch

Part 5: Rapid Orthodontics, 217

15. Biological Orthodontics: Methods to Accelerate or Decelerate Orthodontic Tooth Movement, 219
    Vinod Krishnan, Ze'ev Davidovitch, and Anne Marie Kuijpers-Jagtman

16. Surgically Assisted Tooth Movement: Biological Application, 238
    Carlalberta Verna, Raffaele Spena, Michel Dalstra, Paolo M. Cattaneo, and Judith V. Ball

17. Precision Accelerated Orthodontics: How Micro-osteoperforations and Vibration Trigger Inflammation to Optimize Tooth Movement, 265
    Mani Alikhani, Jeanne M. Nervina, and Christina C. Teixeira

Part 6: Long-term Effects of Tooth-moving Forces, 277

18. Mechanical and Biological Determinants of Iatrogenic Injuries in Orthodontics, 279
    Vinod Krishnan, Ambili Renjithkumar, and Ze'ev Davidovitch

19. The Biological Background of Relapse of Orthodontic Tooth Movement, 297
    Jaap C. Maltha, Vaska Vandevska-Radunovic, and Anne Marie Kuijpers-Jagtman

Part 7: Tooth-movement Research, 309

20. Planning and Executing Tooth-movement Research, 311
    Vinod Krishnan, Ze'ev Davidovitch, and Rajesh Ramachandran

21. Controversies and Research Directions in Tooth-movement Research, 327
    Vinod Krishnan, Anne Marie Kuijpers-Jagtman, and Ze'ev Davidovitch

Index, 343

Contributors

Mani Alikhani, DMD, MS, PhD, Ortho Cert
Lecturer, Advanced Graduate Education Program in Orthodontics,
Department of Developmental Biology,
Harvard School of Dental Medicine,
Boston, MA, USA
and
Professor and Dean,
Consortium for Translational Orthodontic Research Academy,
Hoboken, NJ, USA

Ding Bai, DDS, PhD
Professor, Department of Orthodontics and Pediatric Dentistry,
West China School of Stomatology,
Sichuan University,
Chengdu, Sichuan Province, People's Republic of China

Judith V. Ball, BChD, FDSRCPS, DOrth, MOrth, MSc (Lon)
Senior Teaching Assistant, Department of Paediatric Oral Heath and Orthodontics,
University Centre for Dental Medicine UZB,
University of Basel,
Basel, Switzerland

Itzhak Binderman, DMD
Professor, Department of Oral Biology,
The Maurice and Gabriela Goldschleger School of Dental Medicine,
Tel Aviv University,
Tel Aviv, Israel

Lars Bondemark, DDS, Odont Dr (PhD)
Professor Emeritus,
Department of Orthodontics, Faculty of Odontology,
Malmö University,
Malmö, Sweden

Paolo M. Cattaneo, Engineer, PhD
Associate Professor,
Department of Dentistry and Oral Health,
Section of Orthodontics,
Institute of Odontology and Oral Health,
University of Aarhus,
Aarhus C, Denmark
and
Adjunct Associate Professor, University of Southern Denmark,
Odense, Denmark
and
Associate Professor,
Melbourne Dental School,
The University of Melbourne, Australia

Michel Dalstra, Engineer, PhD
Associate Professor,
Department of Dentistry and Oral Health,
Section of Orthodontics,
Institute of Odontology and Oral Health,
University of Aarhus, Aarhus C, Denmark
and
Senior Lecturer, Department of Pediatric Oral Health and Orthodontics
University Centre for Dental Medicine in Basel UZB,
University of Basel, Basel, Switzerland

Ze'ev Davidovitch, DMD, Cert. Ortho
Harvard University,
Cambridge, Massachusetts, USA

Vincent Everts, PhD
Professor Emeritus, Department of Oral Cell Biology,
Academic Centre for Dentistry Amsterdam (ACTA),
University of Amsterdam and Vrije Universiteit Amsterdam, The Netherlands

Nasser Gadban, DMD, PhD
Private Practice,
Acco, Israel

Taylor E. Glovsky, BS
DMD Candidate 2023
Oregon Health & Science University School of Dentistry, Portland, OR, USA

Priyanka Gudsoorkar, BDS
Volunteer Assistant Professor,
Department of Oral Health Science,
University of Kentucky College of Dentistry,
Lexington, KY, USA

Jing Guo, DDS, PhD
Orthodontist, DenCos,
Hoofddorp, The Netherlands

James K. Hartsfield, Jr., DMD, PhD
E. Preston Hicks Professor of Orthodontics and Oral Health Research, Department of Oral Health Science,
University of Kentucky College of Dentistry,
Lexington, KY, USA
and
Adjunct Professor of Medical and Molecular Genetics,
Department of Medical and Molecular Genetics,
Indiana University School of Medicine,
Indianapolis, IN, USA
and
Clinical Professor of Orthodontics,
College of Dentistry,
University of Illinois at Chicago,
Chicago, IL, USA
and
Clinical Professor, Division of Oral Development and Behavioural Sciences,
University of Western Australia Dental School,
Perth, Western Australia, Australia
and
Visiting Professor, Department of Developmental Biology, Harvard School of Dental Medicine,
Boston, MA, USA

Haikun Hu, DDS, PhD
Assistant Professor
Department of Jinjiang Clinic,
West China Hospital of Stomatology,
Sichuan University, Chengdu, Sichuan Province,
People's Republic of China

Laura R. Iwasaki, DDS, MSc, PhD, CDABO
Chair and Professor, Department of Orthodontics,
Oregon Health & Science University School of Dentistry,
Portland, OR, USA

Vinod Krishnan, BDS, MDS, M.Orth RCS, FDS RCS, PhD
Professor of Orthodontics,
Sri Sankara Dental College,
Varkala, Thiruvananthapuram, Kerala, India

Anne Marie Kuijpers-Jagtman, DDS, PhD, FDSRCS Eng
Researcher, University of Groningen,
University Medical Center Groningen,
Department of Orthodontics,
Groningen, The Netherlands
and
Adjunct Professor, Department of Orthodontics and Dentofacial Orthopedics, University of Bern,
Bern, Switzerland
and
Adjunct Professor, Faculty of Dentistry,
Universitas Indonesia,
Jakarta, Indonesia

Ulf H. Lerner, DDS, PhD
Senior Professor, Centre for Bone and Arthritis Research at Institute of Medicine,
Sahlgrenska Academy at University of Gothenburg,
Gothenburg, Sweden
and
Professor of Oral Cell Biology, Department of Molecular Periodontology,
Faculty of Medicine, Umeå University,
Umeå, Sweden

Alessandra Lucchese, DDS, MS Orth, PhD
Professor of Orthodontics,
Department of Orthodontics,
Vita Salute San Raffaele University,
Milan, Italy
and
Unit of Orthodontics, Division of Dentistry,
IRCCS San Raffaele Scientific Institute,
Milan, Italy

Jaap C. Maltha, PhD
Emeritus Associate Professor of Orthodontics,
Department of Dentistry -
Orthodontics and Craniofacial Biology,
Radboud University Medical Center,
Nijmegen, The Netherlands

Birte Melsen, DDS Dr. Odont.
Adjunct Professor, Department of Orthodontics,
University of Western Australia.
Perth, Australia
and
Visiting Professor,
New York University College of Dentistry,
New York, NY, USA

Lorri A. Morford, PhD
Assistant Professor of Craniofacial Genetics, Division of Orthodontics,
Department of Oral Health Science,
University of Kentucky College of Dentistry,
Lexington, KY, USA

Jeanne M. Nervina, DMD, PhD, Ortho Cert
Professor and Program Director, Consortium for Translational Orthodontic Research Academy,
Hoboken, NJ, USA

Gustavo Pompermaier Garlet, DDS, PhD
Professor, Department of Biological Sciences,
Sao Paulo University, School of Dentistry,
FOB/USP, Bauru, Brazil

Rajesh Ramachandran, MSc
Director, Biogenix Research Center,
Thiruvananthapuram, Kerala, India

Ambili Renjithkumar, BDS, MDS, FDS RCS (Glas), PhD
Professor, Department of Peridontics,
PMS College of Dental Sciences and Research,
Thirivananthapuram, Kerala, India

W. Eugene Roberts, Jr., DDS, PhD
Professor Emeritus, Department of Orthodontics and Oral Facial Genetics,
Indiana University School of Medicine,
Indianapolis, IN, USA

Raffaele Spena, DDS, MS
Adjunct Professor, Department of Orthodontics,
University of Ferrara,
Ferrara, Italy
and
Private Practice, Naples, Italy

Cristina C. Teixeira, DMD MS, PhD, Ortho Cert
Associate Professor, Department of Orthodontics,
New York University College of Dentistry,
New York, NY, USA

Vaska Vandevska-Radunovic, DDS, MSc, Dr. Odont
Professor of Orthodontics,
Department of Orthodontics,
Institute of Clinical Dentistry, University of Oslo,
Oslo, Norway

Carlalberta Verna, DDS, PhD
Professor and Head, Department of Pediatric Oral Heath and Orthodontics,
University Centre for Dental Medicine UZB,
University of Basel,
Basel, Switzerland

Jiangyue Wang, DDS
PhD Candidate, Department of Orthodontics and Pediatric Dentistry,
West China School of Stomatology,
Sichuan University,
Chengdu, Sichuan Province, People's Republic of China

Sara H. Windahl, PhD
Lecturer, Department of Laboratory Medicine, Division of Pathology, Karolinska Institutet, Huddinge, Sweden

Gang Wu, DDS, MD, PhD
Assistant Professor, Department of Oral Implantology and Prosthetic Dentistry,
Academic Centre for Dentistry Amsterdam (ACTA),
University of Amsterdam and Vrije Universiteit
Amsterdam, The Netherlands

Avinoam Yaffe, DMD
Professor, Department of Prosthodontics,
Hebrew University – Hadassah School of Dental Medicine,
Jerusalem, Israel

Masaru Yamaguchi, DDS, PhD
Associate Professor, Department of Orthodontics,
Nihon University School of Dentistry at Matsudo,
Chiba, Japan

James J. Zahrowski, DMD, MS, PharmD
Diplomate of American Board of Orthodontics,
13372 Newport Avenue, Suite E,
Tustin, CA, USA

Margarita Zeichner-David, PhD
Clinical Professor, Division of Biomedical Sciences,
Herman Ostrow School of Dentistry of USC,
Los Angeles, CA, USA

Preface to the First Edition

The first international conference on the biology of tooth movement was held in November 1986 at the University of Connecticut, under the leadership of Louis A. Norton and Charles J. Burstone. In the Foreword to the book that emanated from that conference, Coenraad F.A. Moorrees, to whom the first edition of this book is dedicated, wrote:

> Notwithstanding continued progress from numerous histologic and biochemical studies describing tissue behavior after force application, the key question on the biology of tooth movement remains unresolved: namely, how force application evokes molecular response in the cells of the periodontal membrane. Only when this fundamental question in bone physiology is better understood can appliances for optimal tooth movement in orthodontics be achieved.

In the two decades that have passed since that conclusion, scientists worldwide seem to have followed the direction pointed out by Professor Moorrees. Basic research pertaining to the response of tissues and cells to mechanical loading has grown broader and deeper. The emphasis at the end of the first decade of the twenty-first century is on molecular biology and molecular genetics. Genes are being identified which seem to play important roles in the response of paradental cells and tissues to orthodontic forces, and a growing number of signal molecules that modulate this process have been elucidated. These findings now enable clinicians to utilize some of these molecules as markers of processes associated with tooth movement, such as inflammation and root resorption.

This unrelenting increase of knowledge in basic science has not yet resulted in the development of orthodontic appliances that can be tailored to fit the biological peculiarities of individual patients. But with the growing understanding of the nature of various common diseases, such as diabetes, asthma, arthritis, obesity, and various cardiovascular diseases, it is now possible to assess their potential effects on orthodontic tooth movement, clinically and molecularly. The time seems to be approaching when the nature of optimal orthodontics will be fully exposed as a consequence of the increasing widening of the highway connecting clinical and basic sciences.

The goal of this book is to inform orthodontic students as well as practitioners on the known details of the biological aspects of tooth movement. We hope that this information will enhance their ability to render excellent treatment to all of their patients, young and old. Moreover, we hope that this compendium will convince readers that the dentofacial complex is an integral part of the complete human body, and as such, and like any other region of the body, is prone to be influenced by many factors, genetic or environmental.

Vinod Krishnan
Ze'ev Davidovitch
Editors

Preface to the Second Edition

Basic biologic research in orthodontics has witnessed rapid growth since the publication of the first edition of *Biological Mechanisms of Tooth Movement*. This research not only identified biologic factors associated with tooth movement and its iatrogenic reactions but has expanded even deeper into exploration at the molecular and genomic levels, to generate new knowledge that can be used in clinical settings.

The concept of personalized or individualized medicine is rapidly gaining a hold in medicine as may be seen from the global annual conferences on this subject. In medicine, at this time, the focus is on the personal determinants of cancer and diabetes. Efforts to adapt this concept to all of medicine are gaining momentum. Dentistry is no exception, and orthodontics is potentially the pioneer in this regard. Orthodontists have long been customizing their diagnoses and treatment plans according to the physical characteristics of their patients but now we are entering a period when it would be possible to evaluate the biological features of each patient, by measuring specific tissue markers in fluids, such as saliva and gingival crevicular fluid. The task of establishing reliable tests for the identification of the sought-for markers may not be imminent because of the complexity and variability of the individual genomics but investigations of this pathway have already begun.

The role of basic biologic research has frequently been portrayed as the identification of factors and processes that participate in clinical functions, and test the validity of any hypothesis regarding the efficacy and safety of new and old clinical methods. The specialty of orthodontics has benefitted from this relentless flow of new information, derived from a plethora of publications in numerous scientific periodicals, which focused on mechanism of mechanotransduction, the birth, life and death of the osteoclast, the molecular genetics of bone modeling and remodeling, and the effects of hormones and drugs on soft and mineralized connective tissues. This ongoing growth in information is already affecting clinical orthodontics. One major concept gaining support is the proven ability of bone and periodontal fibroblastic cells to respond simultaneously to more than one signaling factor. Evidence in support of this principle has already led to the application, in addition to orthodontic force, of surgical procedures, vibrations, laser radiation, electricity, and vitamin D3. All of these factors have displayed an ability to enhance the velocity and reduce the duration of tooth movement. The orthodontist now has at his/her disposal a choice of methods, invasive and noninvasive, local and systemic, that can augment the pace of tissue changes that facilitate tooth movement. These mechanisms act on the tissue and cellular levels, and can be manipulated based on increasing knowledge derived from worldwide laboratory experiments and clinical trials, all of which elevate the clinical potential of orthodontics to attain positive results, with a long-range stability, and with a low risk for undesirable side effects.

We are pleased to present this second edition of *Biological Mechanisms of Tooth Movement*, in which we have assembled chapters about topics closely related to the *basic biologic aspects of orthodontics*, which affect the movement of teeth during orthodontic treatment. It updates most of the subjects addressed in the first edition, and includes new topics, such as the search for efficient methods to accelerate tooth movement.

We would like to thank all our contributors who have demonstrated dedication to this project. We would also like to express our sincere appreciation to the book reviewers, who critically analyzed the first edition of the book and let us know its shortcomings so that the second edition is made much stronger. We express our gratitude to our publisher, Wiley-Blackwell, especially Sophia Joyce, Hayley Wood, Jessica Evans, Sara Crowley-Vigneau, and Katrina Hulme-Cross, who helped us complete the project successfully. We would also like to thank the support staff, Jayavel Radhakrishnan, David Michael and all others, who worked tirelessly to facilitate this publication.

As we have stated in the preface to the first edition of this book, "*we really* hope that this compendium will convince the readers that the dentofacial complex is an integral part of the complete human body, and as such, is prone to be influenced by any factor, genetic or environmental, like any other region of the body." Orthodontic academicians and clinicians increasingly recognize this principle and try to treat patients as humans, not merely as typodonts. We hope that this book will assist all orthodontists in this effort.

Vinod Krishnan
Ze'ev Davidovitch
Editors

Preface to the Third Edition

Oral health, as defined by the FDI World Dental Federation, is multifaceted and includes the ability to speak, smile, smell, taste, touch, chew, swallow, and convey a range of emotions through facial expressions with confidence and without pain, discomfort, or disease of the craniofacial complex. Oral health has a close relationship with the general health of an individual and dental treatment contributes to the overall wellbeing of the individual, which is a well-established fact that remains undiminished. The definition from the FDI implicates that malocclusion is not only an aesthetic problem, and states that orthodontic treatment can prevent and intercept further oral diseases and improve quality of life. To effect this, and to reach the stated goal together with our patients, we need to have a broad knowledge ranging from basic science to psychology, or stated in another way, from molecule to man.

Orthodontic tooth movement is the outcome of subjecting teeth to a wide variety of mechanical forces, for long periods of time. This movement is totally dependent upon stimulation and activity of cells near the affected dental roots. Investigations of these cellular responses focus on molecular events on the nuclear, cytoplasmic, and plasma membrane levels. We are very pleased to discover that our initial effort to organize all research related to tooth movement 'under one roof' and the subsequent second edition of *Biological Mechanisms of Tooth Movement* has made its mark among researchers, academicians, residents, and clinicians, equally. It stimulated basic science research in orthodontics, leading to the creation of a strong scientific foundation for the specialty. A sizeable body of new information related to the biology of orthodontic tooth movement has emerged since the publication of the second edition of this book by Wiley-Blackwell in 2015. Since then, reports on studies about the molecular biology of bone metabolism, root resorption, and relapse of orthodontic treatment outcomes have appeared in orthodontic literature. With Professor Anne Marie Kuijpers-Jagtman joining the team, who has contributed extensively to tooth movement research and its clinical translation, we are sure that the third edition will be a 'reading and learning treat' to all those who embrace it.

We have made the utmost effort updating the contents of this third edition and organizing it into specific areas, with the aim of highlighting the recent findings emanating from basic research, and bring them to the attention of clinicians specializing in moving teeth to new positions, effectively and comfortably. This edition presents four new chapters (tissue reactions, periodontal microbiology, surgically assisted tooth movement, as well as micro-osteo perforations) and extensive revision of existing ones, especially the third chapter on mechanisms of tooth movement with orthodontic force application.

We would like to thank all our contributors, who are experts in their research area and have demonstrated dedication to this project. We would also like to express our sincere appreciation to the book reviewers, who analyzed critically the first and second editions of the book, which helped us to improve this edition. We express our gratitude to our publisher, John Wiley & Sons, especially Loan Nguyen, Tanya McMullin, Susan Engelken, Jayadivya Saiprasad, Bhavya Boopathi and to our copy-editor Jane Grisdale who helped us complete the project successfully. We would also like to thank the supporting staff who worked hard to facilitate this publication.

The third edition of the book is aimed at the same audience as the first and second edition – clinicians, academicians, and researchers in the field of orthodontics and allied specialties such as periodontists, bone biologists, and also basic science researchers. The book is also indispensable for postgraduates in orthodontics, not only to understand *how* but also *why* teeth can be moved. Our main goal is to decipher the minute details of the investigations on cellular responses, focusing on molecular events on the nuclear, cytoplasmic, and plasma membrane levels, and its cross-interactions leading to tissue level changes. We attempt to provide clinically plausible translational data which lead to practising a better, biologically oriented orthodontic treatment. We really hope that the educated clinicians who follow these developments can collect pieces of the unfolding puzzle, and relate them to individual patients, leading to a 'biologic-friendly orthodontics.'

Vinod Krishnan
Anne Marie Kuijpers-Jagtman
Ze'ev Davidovitch
Editors

PART 1

Evolution of Biological Concepts

CHAPTER 1
Biological Basis of Orthodontic Tooth Movement: A Historical Perspective

Vinod Krishnan and Ze'ev Davidovitch

> **Summary**
>
> For millennia, we were unable to understand why teeth can be moved by finger pressure, as advocated by Celsus around the dawn of the Common Era, but it was working. Indeed, our ancestors were keenly aware of malocclusions, and the ability to push teeth around by mechanical force. The modern era in dentistry began in 1728 with the publication of the first comprehensive book on dentistry by Fauchard. He described a procedure of "instant orthodontics," whereby he aligned ectopically erupted incisors by bending the alveolar bone. A century-and-a-half later, in 1888, Farrar tried to explain why teeth might be moved when subjected to mechanical loads. His explanation was that the teeth move either because the orthodontic forces bend the alveolar bone, or they resorb it. The bone resorption idea of Farrar was proven by Sandstedt in 1901 and 1904, with the publication of the first report on the histology of orthodontic tooth movement. Histology remained the main orthodontic research tool until and beyond the middle of the twentieth century. At that time medical basic research began evolving at an increasing pace, and newly developed research methods were being adapted by investigators in the various fields of dentistry, including orthodontics; Farrar's assumption that orthodontic forces bend the alveolar bone was proven to be correct, and the race was on to unravel the mystery of the biology of tooth movement. During the second half of the twentieth century, tissues and cells were challenged and studied *in vitro* and *in vivo* following exposure to mechanical loads. The main fields of research that have been plowed by these investigations include histochemistry, immunohistochemistry, immunology, cellular biology, molecular biology, and molecular genetics. From this broad research effort it has been concluded that teeth can be moved because cells around their roots are enticed by the mechanical force to remodel the tissues around them. This conclusion has opened the door for quests aimed at discovering means to recruit the involved paradental cells to function in a manner that would result in increased tooth movement velocity. The means tried in these investigations have been pharmaceutical, physical, and surgical. In all these categories, experimental outcomes proved that the common denominator, the cell, is indeed very sensitive to most stimuli, physical and chemical. Hence, the way ahead for orthodontic biological researchers is clear. It is a two-lane highway, consisting of a continuous stream of basic experiments aiming at uncovering additional secrets of tissue and cellular biology, alongside a lane of trials exploring means to improve the quality of orthodontic care. Gazing toward the horizon, these two lanes seem to merge.
>
> Biological research has exposed differences between individuals based on molecular outlines and entities. In people who possess similar facial features and malocclusions, this variability, which should be reflected in the diagnosis, may require the crafting of treatment plans that address the individual molecular peculiarities. These differences may be due to genetic and/or environmental factors and should be addressed by a personalized orthodontic treatment plan, adapted to the biological profile and needs of each individual patient.

Introduction

Orthodontics, the first specialty of dentistry, has evolved and progressed from its inception to the present time, and the credits for this evolution belong to pioneers, who aimed at improving their clinical capabilities. The evolution of clinical orthodontics is rooted in strong foundations, based on scientific studies and mechanical principles. However, as the specialty began prospering, interest in its association with biological facts began to decline. For a while, orthodontics was taught predominantly as a mechanical endeavor. It can be taught in a short course lasting a few days, usually without any associated clinical exposure. However, recent advancements in medicine have provided orthodontic researchers with investigative tools that enable them to pave new roads toward the target of personalized orthodontics, adapted to the biological profile and needs of each individual patient.

The unfolding of science behind the biology of orthodontic tooth movement (OTM) has been slow and tedious. Our ancestors, as far back as the dawn of history, in all civilizations, cultures, and nations, were interested in images of bodies and faces, covered or exposed. Their artists painted these images on cave walls, cathedral ceilings,

---

Biological Mechanisms of Tooth Movement, Third Edition. Edited by Vinod Krishnan, Anne Marie Kuijpers-Jagtman and Ze'ev Davidovitch.
© 2021 John Wiley & Sons Ltd. Published 2021 by John Wiley & Sons Ltd.

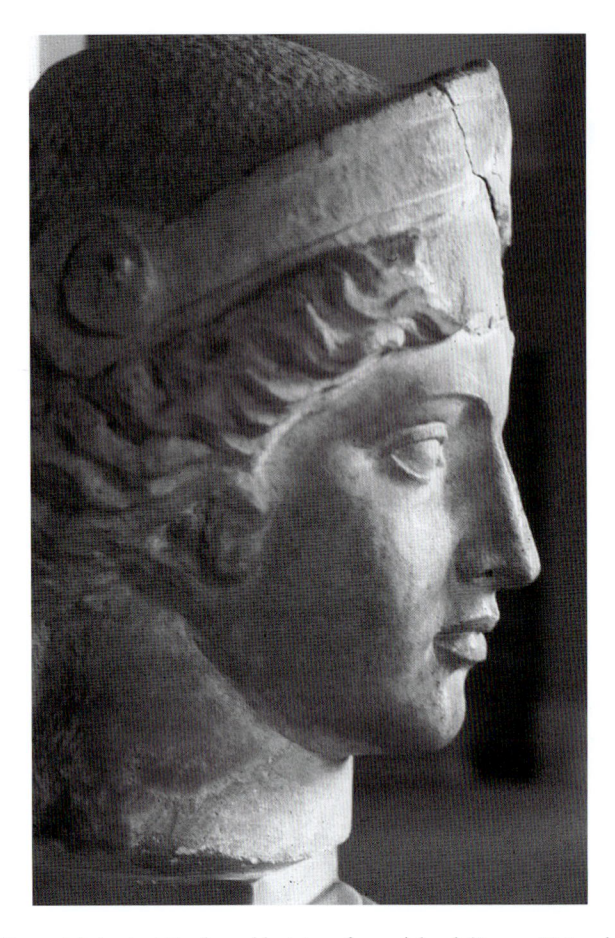

Figure 1.1 Ancient Greek marble statue of a man's head. (Source: National Museum of Greece, Athens.)

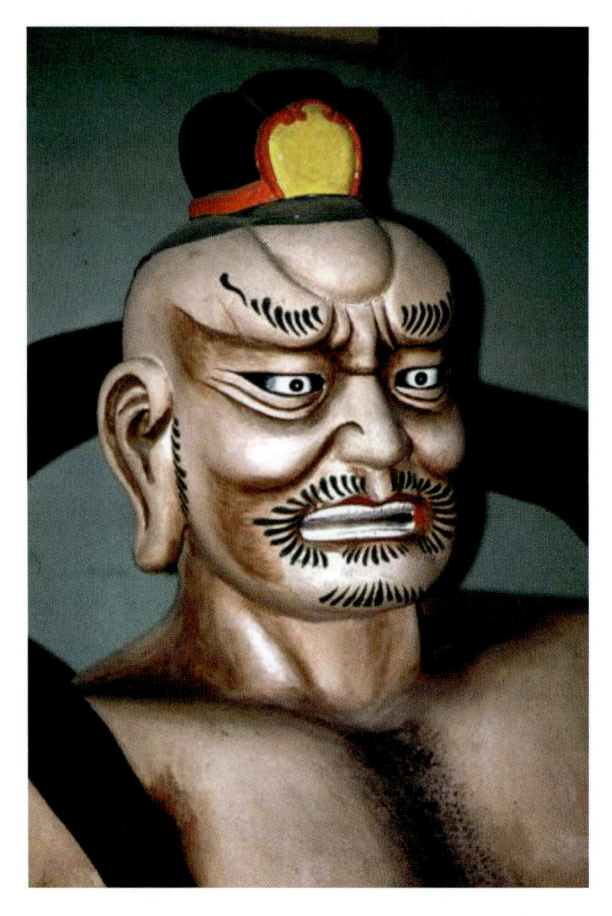

Figure 1.2 Contemporary bust sculpture of a shrine guardian, Seoul, Korea.

and on canvas pieces that were hung in private homes. They also created a huge array of sculptures as monuments, religious fixtures, or outdoor decorations. These works of art reflected images of faces that were carved and crafted along guidelines unique for each tribal, ethnic, and cultural group. Figure 1.1 presents a profile view of a marble statue of a man's head, found in an archeological dig in Greece. Typically, the facial profile is divided into three equal parts (upper, middle, and lower), and the outline of the nose is continuous with the forehead. Figure 1.2 shows a contemporary sculpture of a shrine guardian in Korea. The features are exaggerated, but the facial proportions are similar to those of the ancient Greek statue. Some artists, like Picasso, attracted attention by intentionally distorting well established facial features. Frequently, facial features in old and contemporary paintings and sculptures express a variety of emotions, ranging from love to fear, and a wide array of shapes, from the ideal to the grotesque.

The importance of possessing a full complement of teeth was very evident in ancient times as evidenced by the complimentary words of Solomon to the queen of Sheba "Thy teeth are like a flock of sheep that are even shorn, which came up from the washing" (Song of Solomon 4:2). Even the first code of Roman law, written in 450 BCE, specifies the importance of teeth by incorporating penalties for the master or his agent if they dare to pull out the teeth of slaves or freemen. If this happens, the law stated that the slave is eligible for immediate freedom. The prose and poetry of the Greek and Roman era portrays numerous references to teeth, smiling faces, and the importance of having a regular arrangement of teeth, indicating a desire to correct dental irregularities. There was an emphasis on a correct relationship between the dental arches, and its importance in defining female beauty, and a correct enunciation in oratory. With attention focusing on correction of dental irregularities, orthodontia in that era was already divided into biological and mechanical fields, and it was assumed that a successful practitioner should have clear idea of both. The first orthodontic investigators adopted the biological knowledge of the day and concluded that success or failure in the treatment of malocclusions depends on these fields. The superstructure of orthodontics is built upon this fundamental relationship.

Naturally, therefore, orthodontic research has followed closely the scientific footsteps imprinted by biologists and physicians. Present day orthodontists are aware of scientific advances in material and biological sciences, that gradually move us all closer to an era of personalized medicine and dentistry, in which a high degree of diagnostic accuracy and therapeutic excellence is required.

Orthodontic treatment in the ancient world, the Middle Ages, and through the Renaissance period: Mechanics, but few biological considerations

Archeological evidence from all continents and many countries, including written documents, reveal that our forefathers were aware of the presence of teeth in the mouth, and of various associated health problems. These early Earth dwellers confronted diseases like caries and periodontitis with a variety of medications, ranging from prayers to extractions, and fabrication of dentifrice pastes. Gold inlays and incisor decorations were discovered in South America, and gold crowns and bridges, still attached to the teeth, were discovered in pre-Roman era Etruscan graves (Weinberger, 1926). All these findings bear witness to the awareness of our ancestors to oral health issues.

Recognition of malocclusions and individual variability in facial morphology and function were first noted in Ancient Greece. Hippocrates of Cos (460–377 BCE), who is the founder of Greek medicine, instituted for the first time a careful, systematic, and thorough examination of the patient. His writings are the first known literature pertaining to the teeth. He discussed the timing of shedding of primary teeth and stated that "teeth that come forth after these grow old with the person, unless disease destroys them." He also commented that the teeth are important in processing nutrition, and the production of sound. Hippocrates, like other well-educated people of his time, was keenly aware of the variability in the shapes of the human craniofacial complex. He stated that "among those individuals whose heads are long-shaped, some have thick necks, strong limbs and bones; others have highly arched palates, their teeth are disposed irregularly, crowding one on the other, and they are afflicted by headaches and otorrhea" (Weinberger, 1926). This statement is apparently the first written description of a human malocclusion. Interestingly, Hippocrates saw here a direct connection between the malocclusion and other craniofacial pathologies.

A prominent Roman physician, Celsus (25 BCE–50 CE; Figure 1.3), was apparently the first to recommend the use of mechanical force to evoke tooth movement. In his Book VII, Chapter XII entitled "Operations requisite in the mouth," he wrote: "If a permanent tooth happens to grow in children before the deciduous one has fallen out, that which should have dropped must be scrapped round and pulled out; that which is growing in place of former must be pushed into its proper place with the finger every day, till it comes to its own size." Celsus was also the first to recommend the use of a file in the mouth, mainly for the treatment of carious teeth (Weinberger, 1926). Another Roman dentist, Plinius Secundus (23–79), expressed opposition to the extraction of teeth for the correction of malocclusions, and advocated filing elongated teeth "to bring them into proper alignment." Plinius was evidently the first to recommend using files to address the vertical dimension of malocclusion, and this method had been widely used until the nineteenth century (Weinberger, 1926).

There were few, if any, known advances in the fields of medicine, dentistry, and orthodontics from the first to the eighteenth centuries, with the exception of Galen (131–201), who established experimental medicine, and defined anatomy as the basis of medicine. He devoted chapters to teeth, and, like Celsus, a century earlier, advocated the use of finger pressure to align malposed teeth. Galen advocated the same method to that of Celsus through his writings in 180 CE, which stated that a tooth that projects beyond its neighbors should be filed off to reduce the irregularity (Caster, 1934). Another exception was Vesalius (1514–1564), whose dissections produced the first illustrated and precise book on human anatomy.

For reasons connected with the church, Galen and his writings monopolized medicine for more than a thousand years. However, there were minor advancements in European medicine during that protracted era and advancements evidenced by writings of Muslim physicians from Arabia, Spain, Egypt, and Persia.

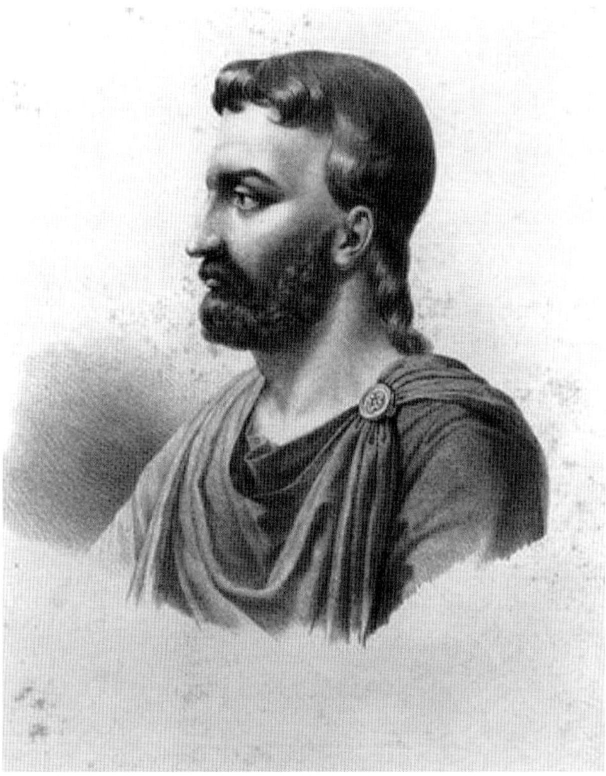

Orthodontic treatment during the Industrial Revolution: Emergence of identification of biological factors

The writings of authors in the Middle Ages were mainly repetitions of what already existed, and there were no new references to mechanical principles for correcting dental irregularities. It was Pierre Fauchard (1678–1761), the father of dentistry and orthodontics (Figure 1.4), who organized previous knowledge and opinions, and provided an extensive discussion on the rationale for numerous clinical procedures (Wahl, 2005a). His book titled *Le chirurgien dentiste (The Surgeon-Dentist)* was published in two editions, the first in 1728 and the second in 1746. The second edition described a few orthodontic cases (Volume II, Chapter VIII) along with an extensive description of appliances and mechanical principles. This book is considered to be dentistry's first scientific publication. Fauchard also advocated keeping young patients under observation and removing long-retained deciduous teeth to prevent irregularity in the permanent dentition. He also stated that blows and violent efforts may increase the chances of developing an irregular tooth arrangement and reported that the greatest incidence of these mishaps occur in the incisor and canine regions. Most of the appliances he fabricated were made of gold or silver and were designed according to the patient's needs, marking the beginning of "customized orthodontic appliances" (Figure 1.5). The orthodontic appliance described by Fauchard used silk or silver ligatures to move malposed teeth to new positions, and "pelican" pliers for instant alignment of incisors, facilitated by bending of the alveolar bone. After placing teeth in position with pelican forceps, he retained them with silver ligatures or lead plates adjusted on either side, over

Figure 1.3 Aulus Cornelius Celsus (25 BCE–50 CE). (Picture courtesy: http://www.general-anaesthesia.com/.)

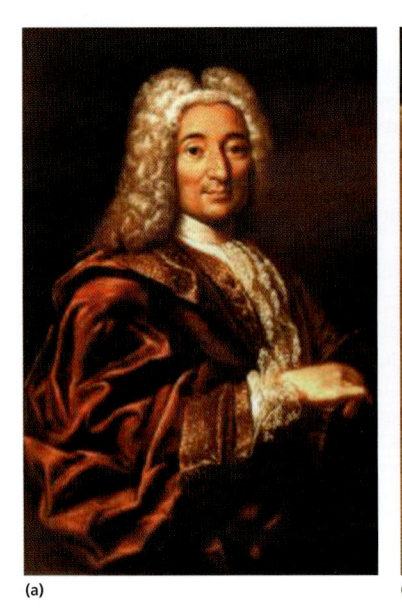

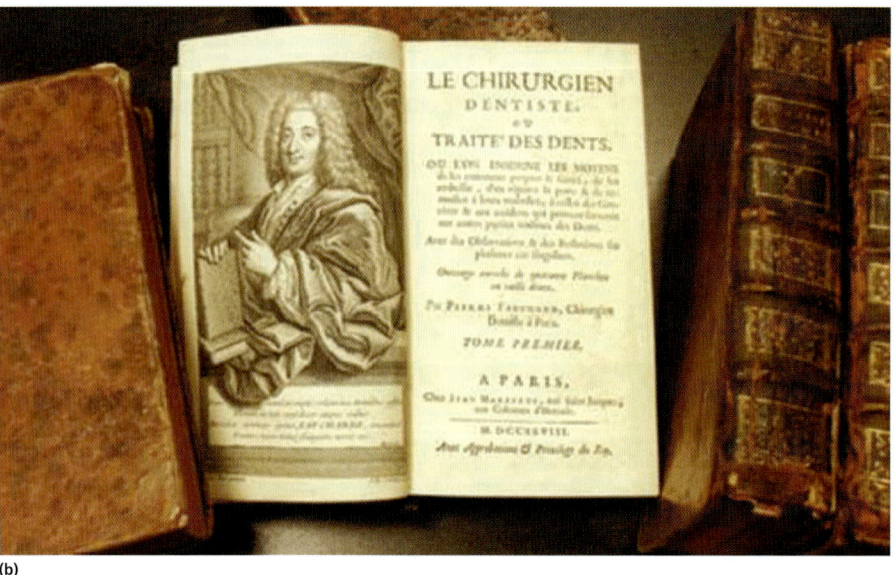

Figure 1.4 (a) Pierre Fauchard (1678–1761), the father of dentistry and orthodontics. (Source: Vasconcellos Vilella, 2007.) (b) His book titled *Le chirurgien dentiste (The Surgeon-Dentist)*. (Source: Picture courtesy: Andrew I. Spielman.)

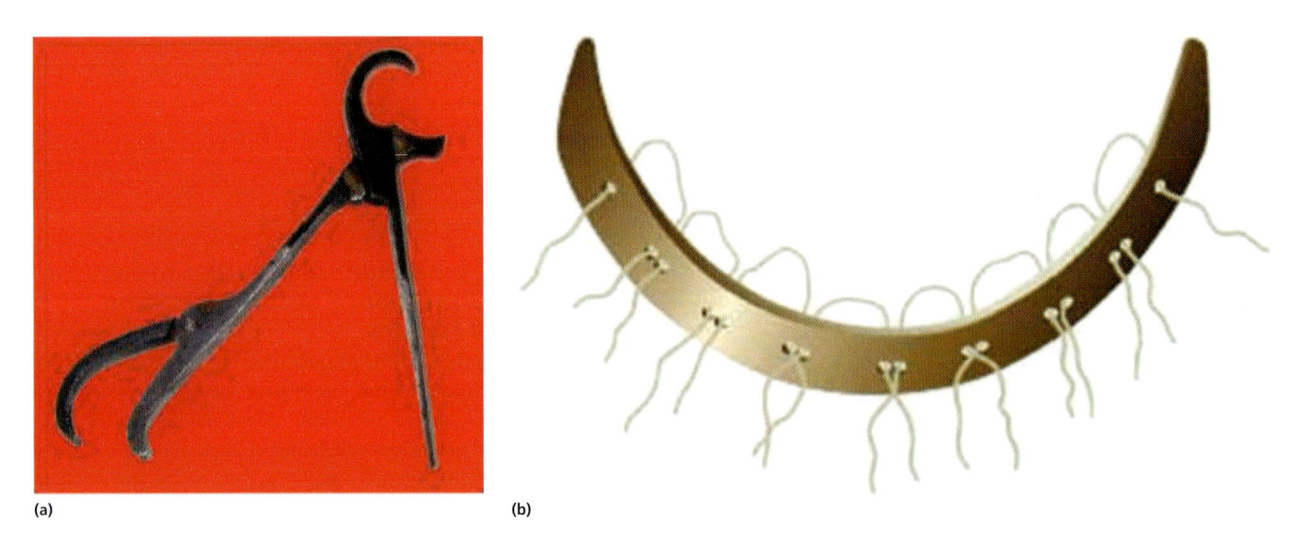

Figure 1.5 (a) Dental pelican forceps (resembling a pelican's beak). (Source: Courtesy of Alex Peck Medical Antiques.) (b) Bandeau–the appliance devised by Pierre Fauchard. (Source: Vasconcellos Vilella, 2007.)

which linen was placed and sewed into position with needle and thread, between interproximal spaces and over the occlusal surfaces of the teeth. This device, named bandeau, marked the beginning of the era of modern orthodontic appliances and their utilization in treating malocclusions (Asbell, 1990).

John Hunter (1728–1793), in 1778, in his book titled *A Practical Treatise on the Diseases of the Teeth,* stated that teeth might be moved by applied force, because "bone moves out of the way of pressure." This book, along with his previously published book, titled *The Natural History of Human Teeth,* marked the beginning of a new era in the practice of dentistry in England (Wahl, 2005a). Hunter recognized the best time to carry out orthodontic treatment to be the youthful period, in which the jaws have an adaptive disposition. In 1815, Delabarre reported that orthodontic forces cause pain and swelling of paradental tissues, two cardinal signs of inflammation.

Up to 1841, about a century after Fauchard had written a chapter about orthodontics, there was no single book devoted entirely to orthodontics alone, but in 1841, Schange published a book solely confined to orthodontics (Wahl, 2005a), which served as a stimulus for conducting investigations in this defined clinical field. Moreover, this book initiated the notion that orthodontics is a unique dental specialty. Schange described the tooth-eruption process, causes of irregularities, their prevention, and classified defects of conformation. In treating irregularities, Schange took a different view from Fauchard, who had advocated the use of radical procedures. He warned practitioners of the attendant danger to the tooth when these procedures were performed and favored application of delicate forces in a continuous manner, hence being the first to favor light orthodontic forces. He recommended silk ligatures to apply light forces, and gold for constructing bands and plates, and recognized the importance of retaining teeth after OTM.

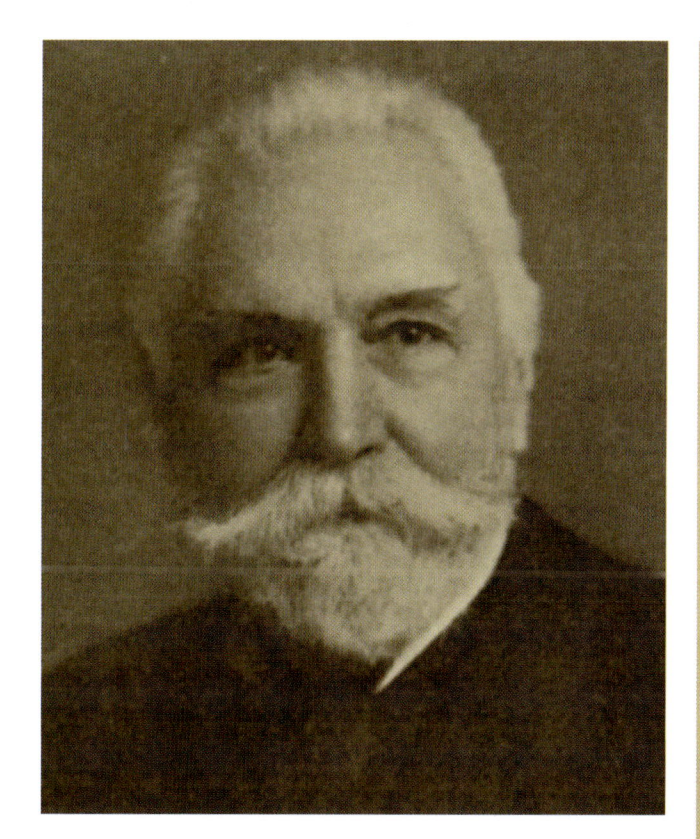

Figure 1.6 Norman William Kingsley (1829–1913). (Source: Dr Sheldon Peck, University of North Carolina at Chapel Hill. Reproduced with permission of Dr Sheldon Peck.)

Samuel Fitch's book titled *A System of Dental Surgery*, published in 1835, marked the beginning of a new era in the practice of dentistry in America. He drew attention to the mobility of teeth within the alveolar process during OTM and characterized the growth period as the time for attaining best results of treatment. Norman Kingsley's treatise on "oral deformities" (1880) had an immediate impact, by placing orthodontics as a specialty, which requires more than general information to solve many of the problems its practitioners face. The book emphasized the importance of basic biology and mechanical principles while studying orthodontia as a science. While describing structural changes due to tooth-moving forces, Kingsley (Figure 1.6) stated that "the physiological fact being that bone will yield or become absorbed under some influences, and also be reproduced … and in moving teeth, the power used creates a pressure which produces absorption." He also stated that "the function of absorption and reproduction may or may not go coincidentally, simultaneously and with equal rapidity."

The article published in *Dental Cosmos* by John Nutting Farrar in 1887 titled "An enquiry into physiological and pathological changes in animal tissues in regulating teeth" stated that "in regulating teeth, the traction must be intermittent and must not exceed certain limits." He also stated that the system of moving teeth with rubber elastic is unscientific, leads to pain and inflammation, and is dangerous to future usefulness of the teeth. He tried to describe optimal rate of tooth movement as 1/240 inch twice daily, in the morning and the evening, and stated that at this rate, tooth movement will not produce any pain or nervous exhaustion. He stated further that the tissue changes with this procedure are physiological, but if the rate exceeds this range, the tissue reactions will become pathological.

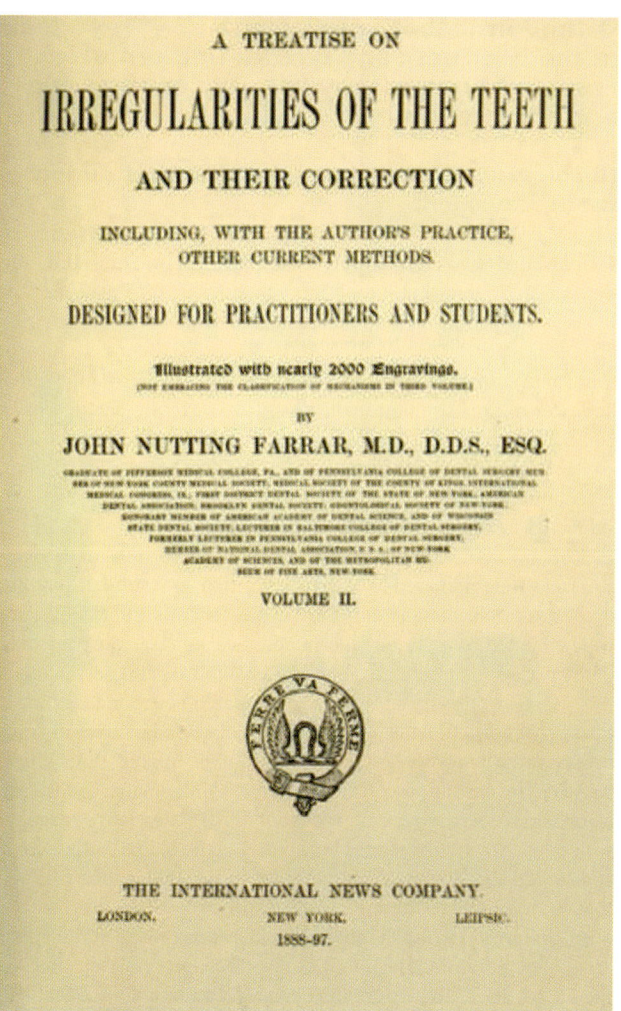

Figure 1.7 The front page of the book *A Treatise on the Irregularities of the Teeth and their Correction* by John Nutting Farrar. (Source: Picture courtesy: https://openlibrary.org.)

His work, which appeared as a series of articles in *Dental Cosmos* from 1876 to 1887, was summed up in his book titled *A Treatise on Irregularities of The Teeth and Thier Correction* published in 1888 (Figure 1.7). In this book he devoted a large section to fundamental principles behind orthodontic mechanics and to the use of various mechanical devices (Asbell, 1998). Farrar, the "Father of American Orthodontics," was credited with developing the hypothesis that rated intermittent forces as best for carrying out OTM which led to the introduction of a screw device for controlled delivery of such forces. A remarkable statement by Farrar was that OTM is facilitated by bending or resorption of the alveolar bone, or both. His publications endowed him as the founder of "scientific orthodontics" (Wahl, 2005b).

Eugene Talbot, in his book titled *Irregularities of Teeth and their Treatment* (1888) rightly mentioned that "without the knowledge of etiology, no one can successfully correct the deformities as is evident in the many failures by men who profess to make this a specialty." He argued that every case of malocclusion is different, making it difficult to classify, and proposed customizing appliances suited for each patient. He was the first to use X rays as a diagnostic aid in orthodontics, to identify abnormal and broken roots, locate third molars, and expose absorption of roots and alveolar process due to OTM.

Orthodontic tooth movement in the twentieth and twenty-first centuries: From light microscopy to tissue engineering and stem cells

Histological studies of paradental tissues during tooth movement

Chappin Harris, in 1839, published a book titled *The Dental Art*, which stated that OTM in the socket depends on resorption and deposition of bone, but it took more than 60 years to have the first histological picture of this phenomenon, which was provided by Carl Sandstedt (Figure 1.8). Sandstedt's experimental studies of tooth movements in dogs were first published in German in 1901, and later in English (Sandstedt, 1904, 1905). His systematic way of conducting experiments was evident from the incorporation of a control group from the same litter as his two experimental dogs. A sectional fixed appliance was inserted in the upper jaw, which was subjected to repeated activations for palatal tipping of the upper incisors over a three-week period. Histological sections of the incisor areas were prepared to assess tissue changes. In order to document positional changes of the teeth, plaster casts and radiographs were obtained. With these experiments, he could observe stretching of the periodontal ligament (PDL) in tension sites and narrowing of this tissue in pressure sites. He demonstrated new bone formation in areas of tension, while resorption was observed in areas of compression. In the compressed periodontium, he initially saw signs of necrosis (hyalinization), and described it as "an obviously degenerated product, a hyaline transformation of the connective tissue, in which regenerative processes take place … the old mortified tissue is resorbed and substituted by granulation tissue." He further noted that "at the limit of the hyaline zone, the alveolar wall presents a deep, undermining notch filled by proliferating cells as in resorptive areas." Furthermore, "the intensive resorptive process even attacked the incisor itself deeply into the dentine," and he assumed that this process is a common secondary effect of OTM. Figure 1.9 is a photograph of a cross section of a premolar root, showing areas of necrosis in the PDL, as well as multiple osteoclasts in Howship's lacunae at the PDL–alveolar bone interface. These cells were, in Sandsted's opinion, the main cells responsible for force-induced tooth movement (Persson, 2005; Bister and Meikle, 2013).

He ended his landmark article by proposing a role for bone bending in the tooth movement process in line with the thinking provided by Kingsley and Farrar.

In 1911/1912, Oppenheim reported that tooth-moving forces caused complete transformation (remodeling) of the entire alveolar process, indicating that orthodontic force effects spread beyond the limits of the PDL. E.H. Angle, the father of modern orthodontics, invited Oppenheim to lecture to his students, who accepted Oppenheim's hypothesis enthusiastically. Oppenheim, the proponent of "the law of bone transformation," rejected both the pressure/tension hypothesis supported by the histological evidence of Sandstedt, and the theory of bone bending hypothesis advanced by Kingsley and Farrar, based on the elastic properties of bone. Oppenheim's experiments were conducted on mandibular deciduous incisors of baboons (the number of animals he used and the appliances he used remain ambiguous) and suggested that only very light forces evoke the required tissue responses. He stated that an increase in the force levels will produce occlusion of the vascular supply, as well as damage to the PDL and the other supporting tissues, and that the tooth will act as a one-armed lever when light forces were applied, and like a two-armed lever during the application of heavy forces. He also demonstrated how alveolar bone is restored structurally and functionally during the retention period (Noyes, 1945). As a proponent of bone transformation and Wolff's law, Oppenheim received acceptance from Angle, as it supported his thoughts in the matter. Oppenheim was also supported by Noyes, one of Angle's followers and an established histologist.

Oppenheim's research highlighted common concepts, shared by orthodontists and orthopedists, who were convinced that both specialties should be based upon a thorough knowledge of bone biology, particularly in relation to mechanical forces and their cellular reactions. However, it became evident that in orthodontics the PDL, in addition to bone, is a key tissue with regards to OTM.

Working on *Macacus rhesus* monkeys in 1926, Johnson, Appleton, and Rittershofer reported the first experiment where they recorded the relationship between the magnitude of the applied force and the distance in which it was active. In 1930, Grubrich reported surface

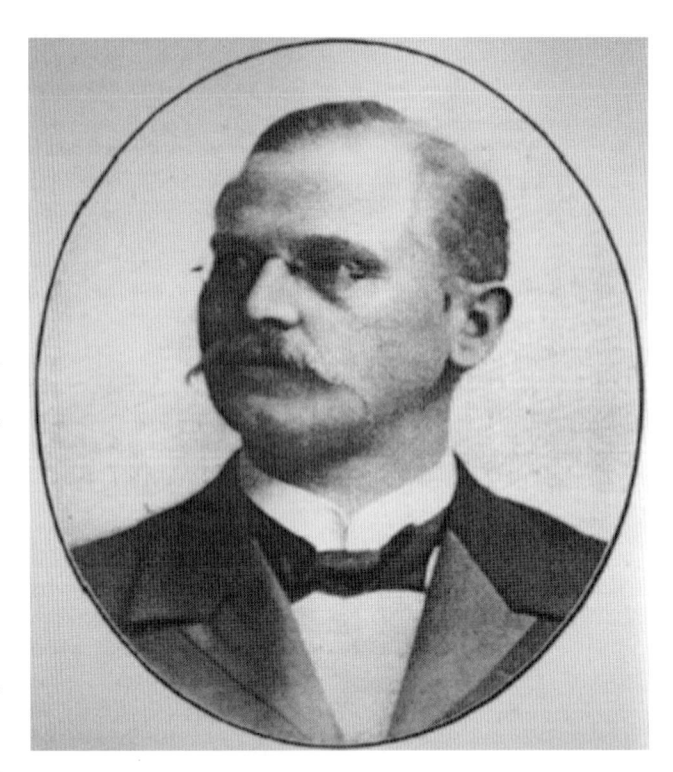

Figure 1.8 Carl Sandstedt (1860–1904), the father of biology of orthodontic tooth movement.

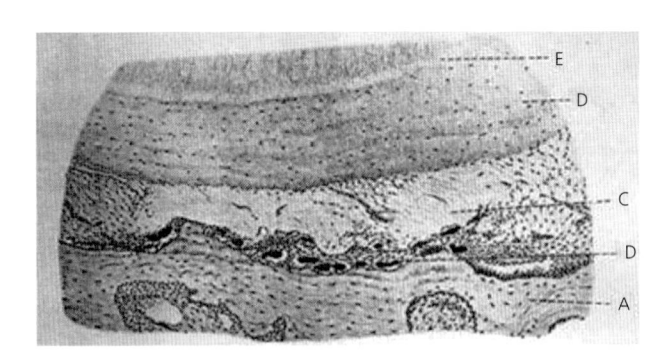

Figure 1.9 A figure from Carl Sandstedt's historical article in 1904, presenting a histological picture of a dog premolar in cross section, showing the site of PDL compression, including an osteoclastic front and necrotic (hyalinized) areas.

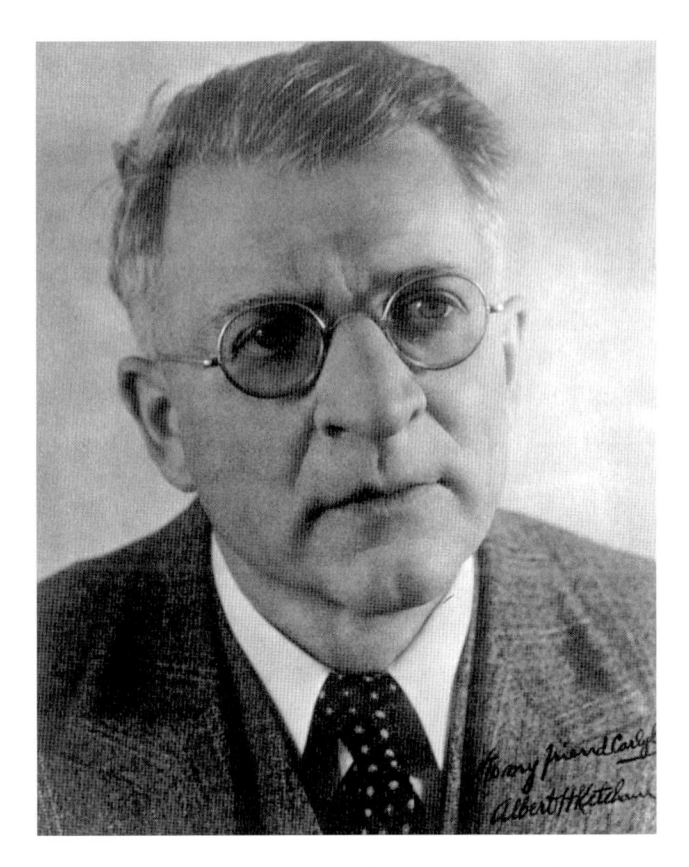

Figure 1.10 Albert Ketcham (1870–1935), who presented the first radiographic evidence of root resorption. He was also instrumental in forming the American Board of Orthodontics. (Source: Siersma, 2015. Reproduced with permission of Elsevier.)

resorptions in teeth subjected to orthodontic forces, a finding confirmed by Gruber in 1931. Even before these histological observations of surface changes were reported, Ketcham (Figure 1.10) (1927, 1929) presented, radiographic evidence that root resorption may result from the application of faulty mechanics and the existence of some unknown systemic factors. Schwarz (1932) conducted extensive experiments on premolars in dogs, using known force levels for each tooth. The effects of orthodontic force magnitude on the dog's paradental tissue responses were examined with light microscopy. Schwarz classified orthodontic forces into four degrees of biological efficiency:
- below threshold stimulus;
- most favorable – about 20 g/cm² of root surface, where no injury to the PDL is observed;
- medium strength, which stops the PDL blood flow, but with no crushing of tissues;
- very high forces, capable of crushing the tissues, causing irreparable damage.

He concluded that an optimal force is smaller in magnitude than that capable of occluding PDL capillaries. Occlusion of these blood vessels, he reasoned, would lead to necrosis of surrounding tissues, which would be harmful, and would slow down the velocity of tooth movement.

The proposed optimal orthodontic force concept by Schwartz was supported by Reitan (Figure 1.11), who conducted thorough histological examinations of paradental tissues incidental to tooth movement. Reitan's studies were conducted on a variety of species, including rodents, canines, primates, and humans, and the results

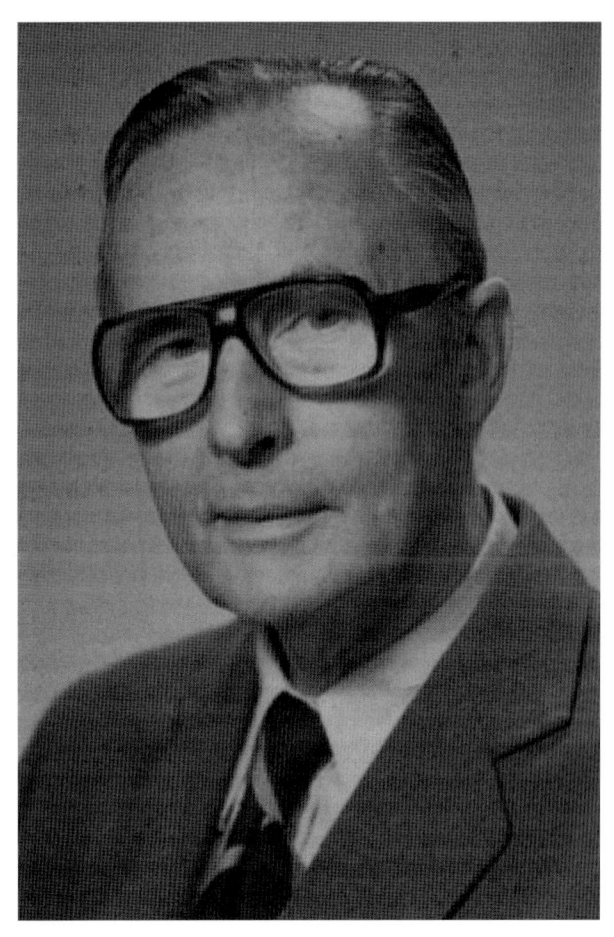

Figure 1.11 Kaare Reitan (1903–2000), who conducted thorough histological examinations of paradental tissues.

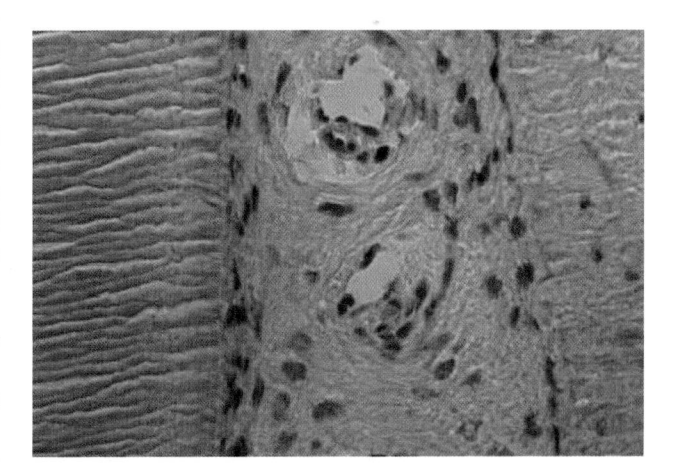

Figure 1.12 A 6 μm sagittal section of a frozen, unfixed, nondemineralized cat maxillary canine, stained with hematoxylin and eosin. This canine was not treated orthodontically (control). The PDL is situated between the canine root (left) and the alveolar bone (right). Most cells appear to have an ovoid shape.

were published during the period from the 1940s to the 1970s. Figure 1.12 displays the appearance of an unstressed PDL of a cat maxillary canine. The cells are equally distributed along the ligament, surrounding small blood vessels. Both the alveolar bone and the canine appear intact. In contrast, the compressed PDL of a

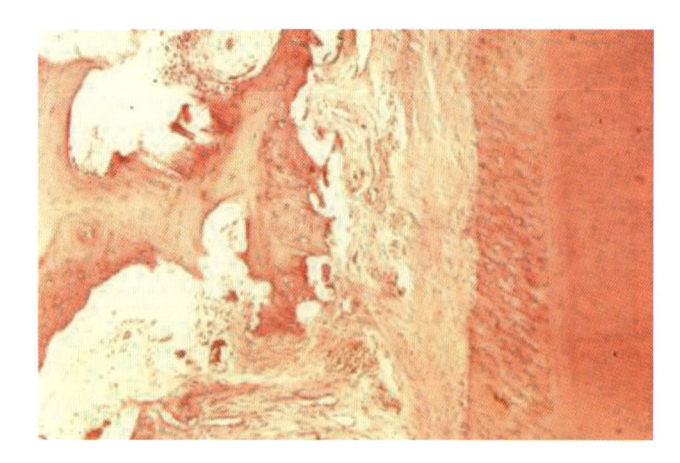

Figure 1.13 A 6 μm sagittal section of a cat maxillary canine, after 28 days of application of 80 g force. The maxilla was fixed and demineralized. The canine root (right) appears to be intact, but the adjacent alveolar bone is undergoing extensive resorption, and the compressed, hyalinized PDL is being invaded by cells from neighboring viable tissues (fibroblasts and immune cells). H & E staining.

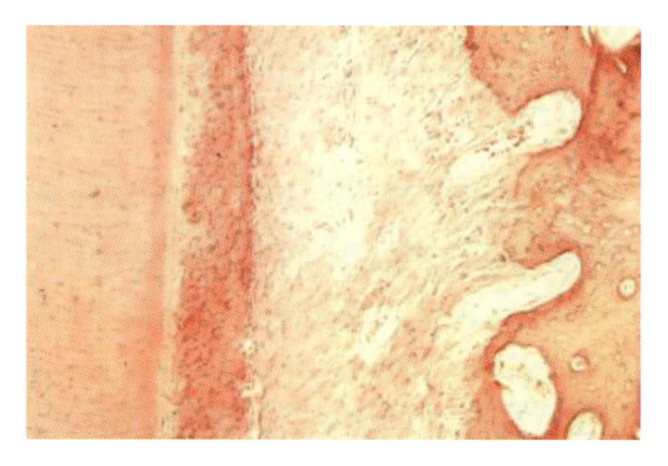

Figure 1.14 The mesial (PDL tension) side of the tooth shown in Figure 1.13. Here, new trabeculae protrude from the alveolar bone surface, apparently growing towards the distal-moving root. H & E staining.

cat maxillary canine that had been tipped distally for 28 days, with an 80 g force (Figure 1.13), appears very stormy. The PDL near the root is necrotic, but the alveolar bone and PDL at the edge of the hyalinized zone are being invaded by cells that appear to remove the necrotic tissue, as evidenced by a large area where undermining resorption has taken place. Figure 1.14 shows the mesial side of the same root, where tension prevails in the PDL. Here the cells appear busy producing new trabeculae arising from the alveolar bone surface, in an effort to keep pace with the moving root. To achieve this type of tissue and cellular responses to orthodontic loads, Reitan favored the use of light intermittent forces, because they cause minimal amounts of tissue damage and cell death. He noted that the nature of tissue response differs from species to species, reducing the value of extrapolations.

With experiments on human teeth, Reitan observed that tissue reactions can vary, depending upon the type of force application, the nature of the mechanical design, and the physiological constrains of the individual patient. He observed the appearance of hyalinized areas in the compressed PDL almost immediately after continuous force application and the removal of those hyalinized areas after 2–4 weeks. Furthermore, Reitan reported that in dogs, the PDL of rotated incisors assumes a normal appearance after 28 days of retention, while the supracrestal collagen fibers remain stretched even after a retention period of 232 days. Consequently, he recommended severing the latter fibers surgically. He also called attention to the role of factors such as gender, age, and type of alveolar bone, in determining the nature of the clinical response to orthodontic forces. He also reported that 50 g of force is ideal for movement of human premolars, resulting from direct resorption of the alveolar bone.

Another outlook on differential orthodontic forces was proposed by Storey (1973). Based upon experiments in rodents, he classified orthodontic forces as being bioelastic, bioplastic, and biodisruptive, moving from light to heavy. He also reported that in all categories, some tissue damage must occur in order to promote a cellular response, and that inflammation starts in paradental tissues right after the application of orthodontic forces.

Continuing the legacy of Sandstedt, Kvam and Rygh studied cellular reactions in the compression side of the PDL. Rygh (1974, 1976) reported on ultrastructural changes in blood vessels in both human and rat material as packing of erythrocytes in dilated blood vessels within 30 minutes, fragmentation of erythrocytes after 2–3 hours, and disintegration of blood vessel walls and extravasation of their contents after 1–7 days. He also observed necrotic changes in PDL fibroblasts, including dilatation of the endoplasmic reticulum and mitochondrial swelling within 30 minutes, followed by rupture of the cell membrane and nuclear fragmentation after 2 hours; cellular and nuclear fragments remained within hyalinized zones for several days. Root resorption associated with the removal of the hyalinized tissue was reported by Kvam and Rygh. This occurrence was confirmed by a scanning electron microscopic study of premolar root surfaces after application of a 50 g force in a lateral direction (Kvam, 1972). Using transmission electron microscopy (TEM), the participation of blood-borne cells in the remodeling of the mechanically stressed PDL was confirmed by Rygh and Selvig (1973), and Rygh (1974, 1976). In rodents, they detected macrophages at the edge of the hyalinized zone, invading the necrotic PDL, phagocytizing its cellular debris and strained matrix.

After direct measurements of teeth subjected to intrusive forces, Bien (1966) hypothesized that there are three distinct but interacting fluid systems involved in the response of the PDL to mechanical loading: the fluids in the vascular network, in the cells and fibers, and the interstitial fluid. Mechanical loading moves fluids into the vascular reservoir of the marrow space through the many minute perforations in the tooth alveolar wall. The hydrodynamic damping coefficient (Figure 1.15) is time dependent, and therefore the damping rate is determined by the size and number of these perforations. As a momentary effect, the fluid that is trapped between the tooth and the socket tends to move to the boundaries of the film at the neck of the tooth and the apex, while acting to cushion the load and is referred to as the "squeeze film effect". As the squeeze film is depleted, the second damping effect occurs after exhaustion of the extracellular fluid, and the ordinarily slack fibers tighten. When a tooth is intruded, the randomly oriented periodontal fibers, which crisscross the blood vessels, tighten, then compress and constrict the vessels that run between them, causing stenosis and ballooning of the blood vessels, creating a back pressure. Thus, high hydrodynamic pressure heads can be created suddenly in the vessels above the stenosis. At the stenosis, a drop of pressure would occur in the vessel in accordance with Bernoulli's principle that the pressure in the region of the constriction will be less than elsewhere in the system. Bien also differentiated the varied responses obtained

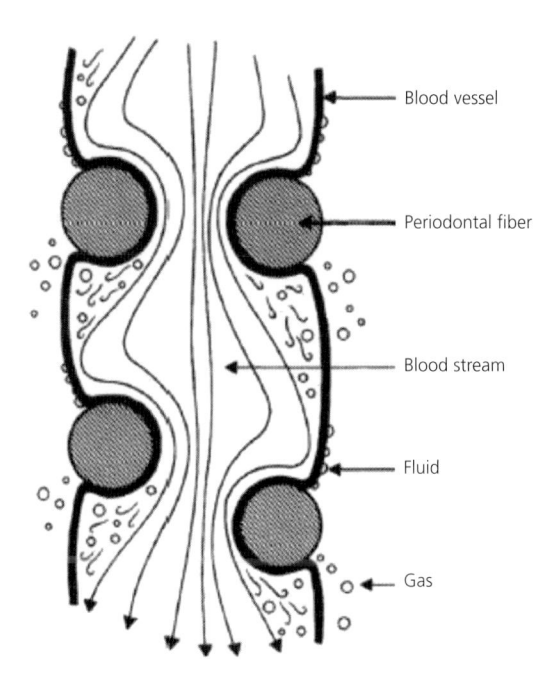

Figure 1.15 The constriction of a blood vessel by the periodontal fibers. The flow of blood in the vessels is occluded by the entwining periodontal fibers. Below the stenosis, the pressure drop gives rise to the formation of minute gas bubbles, which can diffuse through the vessel walls. Above the stenosis, fluid diffuses through the walls of the cirsoid aneurysms formed by the build-up of pressure. (Source: Bien, 1966. Reproduced with permission of SAGE Publications.)

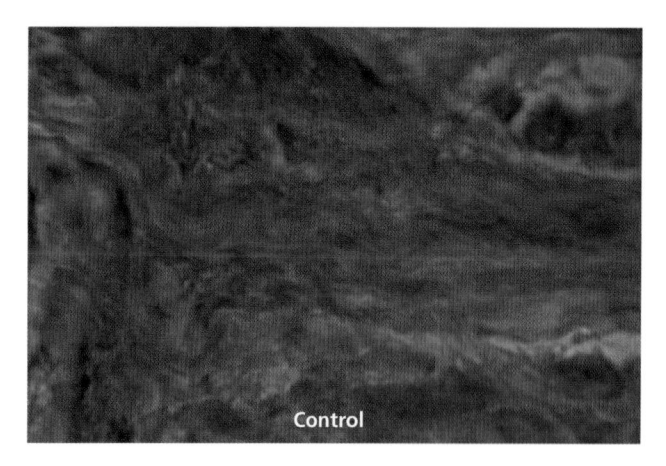

Figure 1.16 A 6 μm sagittal section of a cat maxilla, unfixed and nondemineralized, stained immunohistochemically for PGE_2. This section shows the PDL-alveolar bone interface near one canine that received no orthodontic force (control). PDL and alveolar bone surface cells are stained lightly for PGE_2.

from momentary forces of mastication from that of prolonged forces applied in orthodontic mechanics and suggested that biting forces in the range of 1500 g/cm² will not crush the PDL or produce bone responses.

Pointing out a conceptual flaw in the pressure tension hypothesis proposed by Schwarz (1932), Baumrind (1969) concluded from an experiment on rodents that the PDL is a continuous hydrodynamic system, and any force applied to it will be transmitted equally to all regions, in accordance with Pascal's law. He stated that OTM cannot be considered as a PDL phenomenon alone, but that bending of the alveolar bone, PDL, and tooth is also essential. This report renewed interest in the role of bone bending in OTM, as reflected by Picton (1965) and Grimm (1972). The measurement of stress-generated electrical signals from dog mandibles after mechanical force application by Gillooly et al. (1968), and measurements of electrical potentials, revealed that increasing bone concavity is associated with electronegativity and bone formation, whereas increasing convexity is associated with electropositivity and bone resorption (Bassett and Becker, 1962). These findings led Zengo et al. (1973) to suggest that electrical potentials are responsible for bone formation as well as resorption after orthodontic force application. This hypothesis gained initial wide attention but its importance diminished subsequently, along with the expansion of new knowledge about cell–cell and cell–matrix interactions, and the role of a variety of molecules, such as cytokines and growth factors in the cellular response to physical stimuli, like mechanical forces, heat, light, and electrical currents.

Histochemical evaluation of the tissue response to applied mechanical loads

Identification of cellular and matrix changes in paradental tissues following the application of orthodontic forces led to histochemical studies aimed at elucidating enzymes that might participate in this remodeling process. In 1983, Lilja, Lindskog, and Hammarström reported on the detection of various enzymes in mechanically strained paradental tissues of rodents, including acid and alkaline phosphatases, β-galactosidase, aryl transferase, and prostaglandin synthetase. Meikle et al. (1989) stretched rabbit coronal sutures *in vitro,* and recorded increases in the tissue concentrations of metalloproteinases, such as collagenase and elastase, and a concomitant decrease in the levels of tissue inhibitors of this class of enzymes. Davidovitch et al. (1976, 1978, 1980a, b, c, 1992, 1996) used immunohistochemistry to identify a variety of first and second messengers in cats' mechanically stressed paradental tissues *in vivo*. These molecules included cyclic nucleotides, prostaglandins, neurotransmitters, cytokines, and growth factors. Computer-aided measurements of cellular staining intensities revealed that paradental cells are very sensitive to the application of orthodontic forces, that this cellular response begins as soon as the tissues develop strain, and that these reactions encompass cells of the dental pulp, PDL, and alveolar bone marrow cavities. Figure 1.16 shows a cat maxillary canine section, stained immunohistochemically for prostaglandin E_2 (PGE_2), a 20-carbon essential fatty acid, produced by many cell types and acting as a paracrine and autocrine. This canine was not treated orthodontically (control). The PDL and alveolar bone surface cells are stained lightly for PGE_2. In contrast, 24 hours after the application of force to the other maxillary canine, the stretched cells (Figure 1.17) stain intensely for PGE_2. The staining intensity is indicative of the cellular concentration of the antigen in question. In the case of PGE_2, it is evident that orthodontic force stimulates the target cells to produce higher levels than usual of PGE_2. Likewise, these forces increase significantly the cellular concentrations of cyclic AMP, an intracellular second messenger (Figures 1.18–1.20), and of the cytokine interleukin-1β (IL-1β), an inflammatory mediator, and a potent stimulator of bone resorption (Figures 1.21 and 1.22).

The era of cellular and molecular biology as major determinants of orthodontic treatment

A review of bone cell biology as related to OTM identified the osteoblasts as the cells that control both the resorptive and formative phases of the remodeling cycle (Sandy et al. 1993). A decade after this publication, Pavlin et al. (2001) and Gluhak-Heinrich et al. (2003)

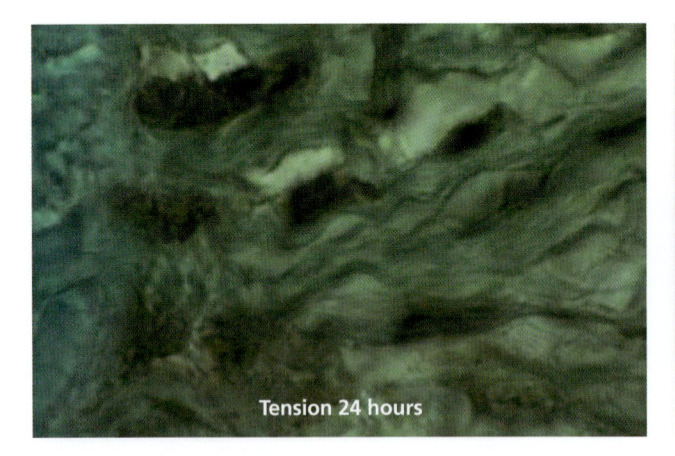

Figure 1.17 A 6 μm sagittal section of the same maxilla shown in Figure 1.16, but derived from the other canine that had been tipped distally for 24 hours by a coil spring generating 80 g of force. The PDL and alveolar bone-surface cell in the site of PDL tension are stained intensely for PGE_2.

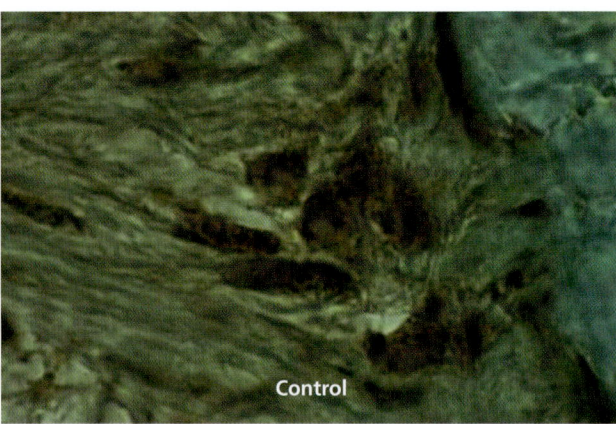

Figure 1.18 Immunohistochemical staining for cyclic AMP in a 6 μm sagittal section of a cat maxillary canine untreated by orthodontic forces (control). The PDL and alveolar bone surface cells stain mildly for this cyclic nucleotide.

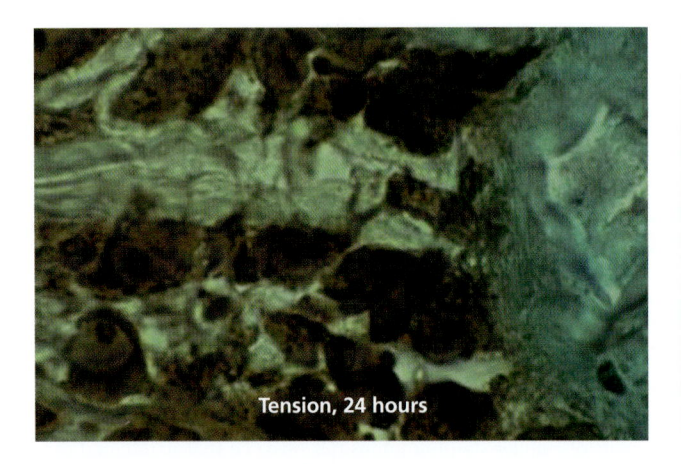

Figure 1.19 Staining for cyclic AMP in a 6 μm sagittal section of a cat maxillary canine subjected for 24 hours to a distalizing force of 80 g. This section, which shows the PDL tension zone, was obtained from the antimere of the control tooth shown in Figure 1.18. The PDL and bone surface cells are stained intensely for cyclic AMP, particularly the nucleoli.

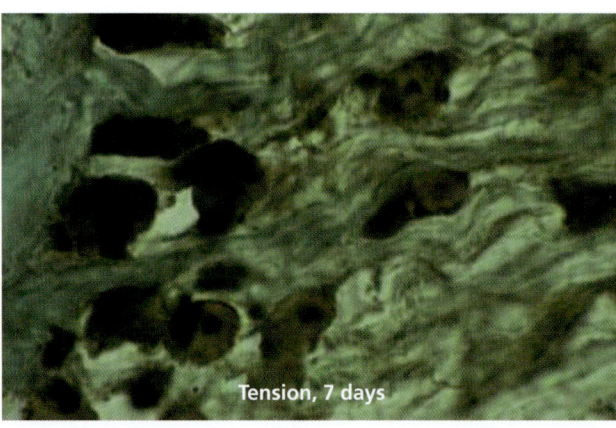

Figure 1.20 Staining for cyclic AMP in the tension zone of the PDL after 7 days of treatment. The active osteoblasts are predominantly round, while the adjacent PDL cells are elongated. All cells are intensely stained for cAMP.

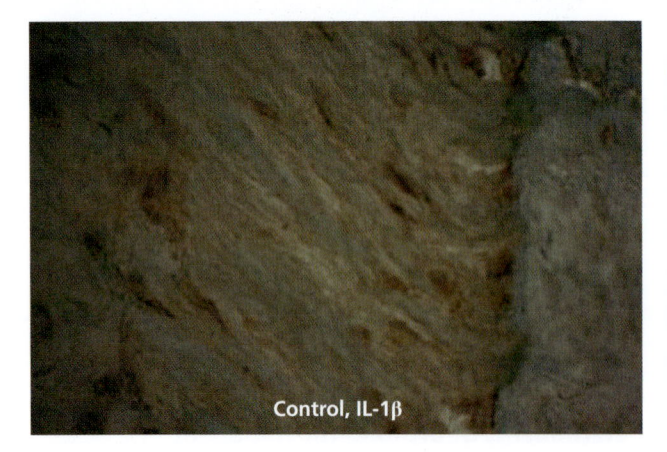

Figure 1.21 Immunohistochemical staining for IL-1β in PDL and alveolar bone cells near a cat maxillary canine untreated by orthodontic forces (control). The PDL and alveolar bone surface cells are stained lightly for IL-1β.

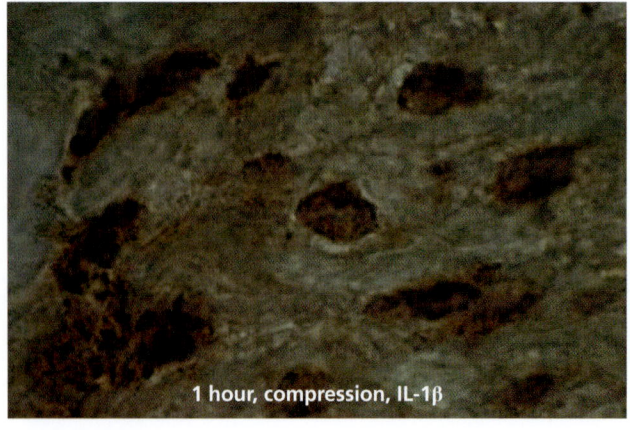

Figure 1.22 Staining for IL-1β in PDL and alveolar bone surface cells after 1 hour of compression resulting from the application of an 80 g distalizing force to the antimere of the tooth shown in Figure 1.21. The cells stain intensely for IL-1β in the PDL compression zone, and some have a round shape, perhaps signifying detachment from the extracellular matrix. × 840.

highlighted the importance of osteocytes in the bone remodeling process. They showed that the expression of dentine matrix protein-1 mRNA in osteocytes of the alveolar bone increased twofold as early as 6 hours after loading, at both sites of formation and resorption. Receptor studies have proven that these cells are targets for resorptive agents in bone, as well as for mechanical loads. Their response is reflected in fluctuations of prostaglandins, cyclic nucleotides, and inositol phosphates. It was, therefore, postulated that mechanically induced changes in cell shape produce a range of effects, mediated by adhesion molecules (integrins) and the cytoskeleton. In this fashion, mechanical forces can reach the cell nucleus directly, circumventing the dependence on enzymatic cascades in the cell membrane and the cytoplasm.

Efforts to identify specific molecules involved in tissue remodeling during OTM have unveiled numerous components of the cell nucleus, cytoplasm, and plasma membrane that seem to affect stimulus-cell interactions. These interactions, as well as those between adjacent cells, seem to determine the nature and the extent of the cellular response to applied mechanical forces. The receptor activator of nuclear factor kappa B ligand (RANKL) and its decoy receptor, osteoprotegerin (OPG) were found to play important roles in the regulation of bone metabolism. Essentially, RANKL promotes osteoclastogenesis, while OPG inhibits this effect. The expression of RANKL and OPG in human PDL cells was measured by Zhang et al. (2004). The cells were cultured for 6 days in the presence or absence of vitamin D_3, a hormone that evokes bone resorption. The expression of mRNA for both molecules was assessed by RT-PCR, while the level of secreted OPG in the culture medium was measured by ELISA. It was found that both molecules were expressed in PDL cells, and that vitamin D_3 downregulated the expression of OPG and upregulated the expression of RANKL. These results suggest that these molecules play key roles in regulating bone metabolism. The response of human PDL and osteoblast-like cells to incubation for 48 hours with PGE_2 revealed that both cell types were stimulated to express RANKL, but that the bone cells were significantly more productive in this respect. When the cells were co-cultured with osteoclast-like cells, the osteoblasts evoked osteoclastogenesis significantly greater than the PDL cells (Mayahara et al., 2012). Recent studies in this regard have confirmed the same in human volunteers (Otero et al., 2016) and were even able to establish a clear role between RANKL production and the root resorption process associated with OTM (Yamaguchi, 2009).

The abovementioned studies illuminate information on the biological aspects of OTM but many gaps still remain. Tooth movement is primarily a process dependent upon the reaction of cells to applied mechanical loads. It is by no means a simple response, but rather a complex reaction. Components of this reaction have been identified in experiments on isolated cells *in vitro*. However, in this environment the explanted cells are detached from the rest of the organism and are not exposed to signals prevailing in intact animals. In contrast, in orthodontic patients the same cell types are exposed to a plethora of signal molecules derived from endocrine glands, migratory immune cells, and ingested food and drugs. A review of pertinent literature published between 1953 and 2007 by Bartzela et al. (2010) revealed details on the effects and side-effects of commonly used medications on tooth movement. Nonsteroidal anti-inflammatory drugs and estrogen were found to decrease OTM, whereas corticosteroids, PTH, and thyroxin seem to accelerate it. However, the individual responses to these medications may differ significantly from patient to patient, and such differences may have profound effects on treatment duration and outcomes.

This fact implies that an orthodontic diagnosis should include information about the overall biological status of each patient, not merely a description of the malocclusion and the adjacent craniofacial hard and soft tissues. Moreover, periodic assessments of specific biological signal molecules in body fluids, especially in the gingival crevicular fluid and saliva, may be useful for the prediction of the duration and outcome of orthodontic treatment. The ever-growing flow of basic information into the orthodontic domain promotes the adoption of the concept of "personalized medicine" (Kornman and Duff, 2012). The main investigative tool in this regard is molecular genetics, which has been used successfully in oncology in the search for faulty genes, responsible for the initiation, growth, and dissemination of a variety of tumors. This approach is growing in significance in medicine and is beginning to occur in dentistry. Orthodontics, where genetics plays a major role in determining the morphology and physiology of the orofacial region, is a natural candidate to use this rapidly expanding body of basic information in order to formulate treatment plans that fit closely the biological features of each individual patient.

Conclusions and the road ahead

Orthodontics started with the use of a finger or a piece of wood to apply pressure to crowns of malposed teeth. The success of those manipulations proved convincingly that mechanical force is an effective means to correct malocclusions. Until the early years of the twentieth century, understanding the reasons why teeth move when subjected to mechanical forces was only a guess, based on reason and empirical clinical observations. Farrar hypothesized in 1888 that teeth are moved orthodontically due to resorption of the dental alveolar socket and/or bending of the alveolar bone. Both hypotheses were proven to be correct during the twentieth century, as orthodontic research has spread into increasingly fundamental levels of biological basic research. The rationale for these basic investigations was the wish to unveil the mechanism of translation of mechanical signals into biological/clinical responses; the etiology of iatrogenic effects resulting from OTM; and to discover efficient means to shorten significantly the duration of OTM. Many details on the behavior of cells involved in OTM have emerged from those investigations but, despite this progress, the final answer to the above issues remains elusive.

At present, molecular biology and molecular genetics remain at the cutting edge of orthodontic research. Multiple genes that may be involved in the cellular response to mechanical loads have been identified (Reyna et al., 2006), and genes associated with orthodontic-induced root resorption (Abass and Hartsfield, 2006). The role played by specific genes in OTM was revealed by Kanzaki et al. (2004), who reported that a transfer of an OPG gene into the PDL in rats inhibits OTM by inhibiting RANKL-mediated osteoclastogenesis. According to Franceschi (2005), future efforts in dental research will include genetic engineering, focusing on bone regeneration. Recently, Zhao et al. (2012), through experiments in male Wistar rats, reported inhibition of relapse with local OPG gene transfer through the inhibition of osteoclastogenesis.

The body of knowledge that has evolved from multilevel orthodontic research supports the notion that the patient's biology is an integral part of orthodontic diagnosis, treatment planning, and treatment. Therefore, orthodontic appliances and procedures should be designed to address the patient's malocclusion in light of his/her biological profile, in much the same fashion as is done by medical specialists in other fields of medicine. As outlined by Jheon et al. (2017), analyses of genetic and molecular factors may soon uncover indicators predicting slow tooth movement, increased predisposition to root resorption, and accelerated late stage skeletal growth. Patients will be provided with customized appliances printed through the treatment stages, as per the devised virtual plan. In addition, specific biologic/pharmacologic agents based on patients' molecular and genetic background will be delivered to enhance treatment efficiency and outcomes.

Orthodontics started in ancient times by pushing malposed teeth with a finger for a few minutes a day, but today we know that the reason teeth can be moved is because cells respond to changes in their physical and chemical environment. Research will continue to unravel new details of this process, and the beneficiaries will be all people seeking and receiving orthodontic care.

References

Abass, S. K. and Hartsfield, J. K. Jr. (2006) Genetic studies in root resorption and orthodontia, in *Biological Mechanisms of Tooth Eruption, Resorption, and Movement* (eds Z. Davidovitch, J. Mah, and S. Suthanarak). Harvard Society for the Advancement of Orthodontics, Boston, pp. 39–46.

Asbell, M. B. (1990) A brief history of orthodontics. *American Journal of Orthodontics and Dentofacial Orthopedics* **98**(2), 176–183.

Asbell M. B. (1998) John Nutting Farrar 1839–1913. *American Journal of Orthodontics and Dentofacial Orthopedics* **114**, 602.

Bartzela, T., Turp, J. C., Motschall, E. and Maltha, J. C. (2010) Medication effects on the rate of orthodontic tooth movement: A systematic literature review. *American Journal of Orthodontics and Orofacial Orthopedics* **135**, 16–26.

Bassett, C. A. L. and Becker, R. O. (1962) Generation of electrical potentials in bone in response to mechanical stress. *Science* **137**, 1063–1064.

Baumrind, S. (1969) A reconsideration of the propriety of the "pressure-tension" hypothesis. *American Journal of Orthodontics* **55**, 12–22.

Bien, S. M. (1966) Hydrodynamic damping of tooth movement. *Journal of Dental Research* **45**, 907–914.

Bister, D. and Meikle, M. C. (2013) Re-examination of "Einige Beiträge zur Theorie der Zahnregulierung" (Some contributions to the theory of the regulation of teeth) published in 1904–1905 by Carl Sandstedt. *European Journal of Orthodontics* **35**, 160–168.

Caster, F. M. (1934) A historical sketch of orthodontia. *Dental Cosmos* **76**(1), 110–135.

Davidovitch, Z., Finkelson, M. D., Steigman, S. et al. (1980c) Electric currents, bone remodeling, and orthodontic tooth movement. II. Increase in rate of tooth movement and periodontal cyclic nucleotide levels by combined force and electric current. *American Journal of Orthodontics* **77**, 33–47.

Davidovitch, Z., Gogen, M. H., Okamoto, Y. and Shanfeld, J. L. (1992) Neurotransmitters and cytokines as regulators of bone remodeling, in *Bone Biodynamics in Orthodontic and Orthopedic Treatment* (eds D. S. Carlson and S. A. Goldstein). University of Michigan Press, Ann Arbor, MI, pp. 141–162.

Davidovitch, Z., Korostoff, E., Finkelson, M. D. et al. (1980a) Effect of electric currents on gingival cyclic nucleotides in vivo. *Journal of Periodontal Research* **15**, 353–362.

Davidovitch, Z., Montgomery, P. C., Eckerdal, O. and Gustafson, G. T. (1976) Demonstration of cyclic AMP in bone cells by immuno-histochemical methods. *Calcified Tissue Research* **19**, 317–329.

Davidovitch, Z., Montgomery, P. C., Yost, R. W. and Shanfeld, J. L. (1978) Immunohistochemical localization of cyclic nucleotides in the periodontium: Mechanically-stressed osteoblasts in vivo. *The Anatomical Record* **192**, 351–361.

Davidovitch, Z., Okamoto, Y., Gogen, H. et al. (1996) Orthodontic forces stimulate alveolar bone marrow cells. In: *Biological Mechanisms of Tooth Movement and Craniofacial Adaptation* (eds Z. Davidovitch and L. A. Norton). Harvard Society for the Advancement of Orthodontics, Boston, pp. 255–270.

Davidovitch, Z., Steigman, S., Finkelson, M. D. et al. (1980b) Immunohistochemical evidence that electric currents increase periosteal cell cyclic nucleotide levels in feline alveolar bone in vivo. *Archives of Oral Biology* **25**, 321–327.

Fauchard, P. (1728) *Le chirurgien dentiste ou traite des dents* (trans. Lilian Lindsay). Butterworth, London.

Franceschi, R. T. (2005) Biological approaches to bone regeneration by gene therapy. *Journal of Dental Research* **84**, 1093–1103.

Gillooly, C. J., Hosley, R. T., Mathews, J. R. and Jewett, D. L. (1968) Electrical potentials recorded from mandibular alveolar bone as a result of forces applied to the tooth. *American Journal of Orthodontics* **54**, 649–654.

Gluhak-Heinrich, J., Ye, L., Bonewald, L. F. et al. (2003) Mechanical loading stimulates dentin matrix protein 1 (DMP1) expression in osteocytes in vivo. *Journal of Bone and Mineral Research* **18**, 807–817.

Grimm, F. M. (1972) Bone bending, a feature of orthodontic tooth movement. *American Journal of Orthodontics* **62**, 384–393.

Jheon, A. H., Oberoi, S., Solem, R. C. and Kapila, S. (2017). Moving towards precision orthodontics: An evolving paradigm shift in the planning and delivery of customized orthodontic therapy. *Orthodontics & Craniofacial Research* **20**, 106–113.

Kanzaki, H., Chiba, M., Takahashi, I. et al. (2004) Local OPG gene transfer to periodontal tissue inhibits orthodontic tooth movement. *Journal of Dental Research* **83**, 920–925.

Ketcham, A. H. (1927) A preliminary report of an investigation of apical root resorption of permanent teeth. *International Journal of Orthodontia, Oral Surgery and Radiography* **13**(2), 97–127.

Ketcham, A. H. (1929) A progress report of an investigation of apical root resorption of vital permanent teeth. *International Journal of Orthodontia, Oral Surgery and Radiography* **15**(4), 310–328.

Kingsley, N. W. (1880) *A Treatise on Oral Deformities*, Birmingham, Alabama.

Kornman, K. S. and Duff, G. W. (2012) Personalized medicine: will dentistry ride the wave or watch from the beach? *Journal of Dental Research* **91**(suppl.), 8S–11S.

Kvam E. (1972) Scanning electron microscopy of tissue changes on the pressure surface of human premolars following tooth movement. *Scandinavian Journal of Dental Research* **80**, 357–368.

Lilja, E., Lindskog, S. and Hammarström, I. (1983) Histochemistry of enzymes associated with tissue degradation incident to orthodontic tooth movement. *American Journal of Orthodontics* **83**, 62–75.

Mayahara, K., Yamaguchi, A., Takenouchi, H. et al. (2012) Osteoblasts stimulate osteoclastogenesis via RANKL expression more strongly than periodontal ligament cells do in response to PGE(2). *Archives of Oral Biology* **57**(10), 1377–1384.

Meikle, M. C., Heath, J. K., Atkinson, S. J. et al. (1989) Molecular biology of stressed connective tissues at sutures and hard tissues in vitro, in *The Biology of Tooth Movement* (eds L. A. Norton and C. J. Burstone). CRC Press, Boca Raton, FL, pp. 71–86.

Noyes, F. B. (1945) The contribution of Albin Oppenheim to orthodontia. *The Angle Orthodontist* **15**, 47–51.

Oppenheim, A. (1911/1912) Tissue changes, particularly of the bone, incident to tooth movement. *American Journal of Orthodontics* **3**, 113–132.

Otero, L., García, D. A. and Wilches-Buitrago, L. (2016). Expression and presence of OPG and RANKL mRNA and protein in human periodontal ligament with orthodontic force. *Gene Regulation and Systems Biology* **10**, 15–20.

Pavlin, D., Zadro, R. and Gluhak-Heinrich, J. (2001) Temporal pattern of osteoblast associated genes during mechanically induced osteogenesis in vivo: early responses of osteocalcin and type I collagen. *Connective Tissue Research* **42**, 135–148.

Persson, M. (2005) A100th anniversary: Sandstedt's experiments on tissue changes during tooth movement. *Journal of Orthodontics* **32**, 27–28.

Picton, D. C. A. (1965) On the part played by the socket in tooth support. *Archives of Oral Biology* **10**, 945–955.

Reitan, K. (1957) Some factors determining the evaluation of forces in orthodontics. *American Journal of Orthodontics* **43**, 32–45.

Reitan, K. (1958) Experiments of rotation of teeth and their subsequent retention. *Transactions of the European Orthodontic Society* **34**, 124–138.

Reitan, K. (1961) Behavior of Malassez' epithelial rests during orthodontic tooth movement. *Acta Odontologica Scandinavia* **19**, 443–468.

Reitan, K. and Kvam, E. (1971) Comparative behavior of human and animal tissue during experimental tooth movement. *The Angle Orthodontist* **41**, 1–14.

Reyna, J., Beom-Moon, H. and Maung, V. (2006) Gene expression induced by orthodontic tooth movement and/or root resorption, in *Biological Mechanisms of Tooth Eruption, Resorption, and Movement* (eds Z. Davidovitch, J. Mah and S. Suthanarak). Harvard Society for the Advancement of Orthodontics, Boston, pp. 47–76.

Rygh, P. (1974) Elimination of hyalinized periodontal tissues associated with orthodontic tooth movement. *Scandinavian Journal of Dental Research* **82**, 57–73.

Rygh, P. (1976) Ultrastructural changes in tension zone of rat molar periodontium incident to orthodontic tooth movement. *American Journal of Orthodontics* **70**, 269–281.

Rygh, P. and Selvig, K. A. (1973) Erythrocytic crystallization in rat molar periodontium incident to tooth movement. *Scandinavian Journal of Dental Research* **81**, 62–73.

Sandstedt, C. (1901) *Någrabidrag till tandregleringensteori*. Kungl. Boktryckeriet, Stockholm.

Sandstedt, C. (1904) Einige Beiträge zur Theorie der Zahnregulierung. *Nordisk Tandläkare Tidskrift* **5**, 236–256.

Sandstedt, C. (1905) Einige Beiträge zur Theorie der Zahnregulierung. *Nordisk Tandläkare Tidskrift* **6**, 1–25, 141–168.

Sandy, J. R., Farndale, R. W. and Meikle, M. C. (1993) Recent advances in understanding mechanically induced bone remodeling and their relevance to orthodontic theory and practice. *American Journal of Orthodontics and Dentofacial Orthopedics* **103**, 212–222.

Schwarz, A. M. (1932) Tissue changes incidental to orthodontic tooth movement. *International Journal of Orthodontia, Oral Surgery and Radiography* **18**(4), 331–352.

Storey, E. (1973) The nature of tooth movement. *American Journal of Orthodontics* **63**(3), 292–314.

Vasconcellos Vilella, O. D. (2007) Development of orthodontics in Brazil and in the world. *Revista Dental Press de Ortodontia e Ortopedia Facial* **12**(6), 131–156. https://dx.doi.org/10.1590/S1415-54192007000600013 ((accessed August 25, 2019).).

Wahl, N. (2005a) Orthodontics in 3 millennia. Chapter 1: Antiquity to the mid-19th century. *American Journal of Orthodontics and Dentofacial Orthopedics* **127**, 255–259.

Wahl, N. (2005b) Orthodontics in 3 millennia. Chapter 2: Entering the modern era. *American Journal of Orthodontics and Dentofacial Orthopedics* **127**, 510–515.

Weinberger, B. W. (1926) *Orthodontics: A Historical Review of its Origin and Evolution*. C. V. Mosby, St. Louis, MO.

Yamaguchi, M. (2009). RANK/RANKL/OPG during orthodontic tooth movement. *Orthodontics & Craniofacial Research* **12**(2), 113–119.

Zengo, A. N., Pawluk, R. J. and Bassett, C. A. L. (1973) Stress-induced bioelectric potentials in the dentoalveolar complex. *American Journal of Orthodontics* **64**, 17–27.

Zhang, D., Yang, Y. Q., Li, X. T. and Fu, M. K. (2004) The expression of osteoprotegerin and the receptor activator of nuclear factor kappa B ligand in human periodontal ligament cells cultured with and without 1α, 25–dihydroxyvitamin D3. *Archives of Oral Biology* **49**, 71–76.

Zhao, N., Lin, J., Kanzaki, H. et al. (2012). Local osteoprotegerin gene transfer inhibits relapse of orthodontic tooth movement. *American Journal of Orthodontics and Dentofacial Orthopedics* **141**(1), 30–40.

CHAPTER 2
Biology of Orthodontic Tooth Movement: The Evolution of Hypotheses and Concepts

Vinod Krishnan and Ze'ev Davidovitch

> **Summary**
>
> Orthodontic treatment has been practiced for 2000–3000 years, but the last century-and-a-half has witnessed major advances in the accumulation of meaningful biological information, which facilitates the formulation of hypotheses that help in the design, explanation, and improvement of clinical procedures. These hypotheses focus on the biological nature of the physical and biochemical events, which occur in teeth and their surrounding tissues following the administration of mechanical forces. Among the chief hypotheses are those related to creation of tissue strain and electrical signals that stimulate the cells in the regions affected by these forces. These studies revealed extensive cellular activities in the mechanically stressed periodontal ligament, involving neurons, immune cells, fibroblasts, endothelial cells, osteoblasts, osteoclasts, osteocytes, and endosteal cells. Moreover, mechanical stresses were found to alter the structural properties of tissues at the cellular, molecular, and genetic levels. The rapid reactions occurring at the initial stage of mechanotherapy, and slower adaptive changes at the later stages of treatment, have attracted increasing attention. This chapter addresses the evolutionary traits of the development of concepts pertaining to the biology of orthodontic tooth movement.

Introduction

Orthodontic tooth movement (OTM) is facilitated by remodeling of the dental and paradental tissues which, when exposed to varying degrees of magnitude, frequency, and duration of mechanical loading, express extensive physical and chemical changes that differ from the processes of physiological dental drift, or tooth eruption. In OTM, a tooth moves as a result of mechanical forces derived from external devices, while forces leading to mesial migration of teeth are derived from the individual's own musculature, and tooth eruption results from complex interactions between dental and paradental cells. The common denominator of all these phenomena is the generation of mechanical forces, either physiologically or therapeutically. OTM resembles tooth eruption because both processes depend on remodeling of the periodontal ligament (PDL) and the alveolar bone, but the two processes present different models of bone remodeling (Davidovitch, 1991; Wise and King, 2008). The status of bone metabolism determines the specific characteristics of tissue remodeling associated with tooth eruption and OTM. In both cases mechanical forces are applied to the teeth, which are transmitted through the PDL to the alveolar bone, followed by an instantaneous cellular reaction. The details of this reaction have been the main target of investigation since the end of the nineteenth century.

However, since orthodontic forces are usually greater than the forces of eruption, the tissue reaction during OTM may include iatrogenic injury to teeth and their surrounding tissues. OTM can occur rapidly or slowly, depending on the physical characteristics of the applied force, and the size and biological response of the PDL. Typically, when a tooth is tipped by mechanical forces, the root movement within the PDL develops areas of compression and of tension. When optimal forces are applied, alveolar bone resorption occurs in PDL compression sites, while new bone apposition takes place on the alveolar bone surfaces facing the stretched PDL (Sandstedt, 1904, 1905; Oppenheim, 1911; Schwarz, 1932). However, when the applied force exceeds a threshold, cells in the compressed PDL may die, and the orientation of the collagenous PDL fibers may change from horizontal to vertical. This change in PDL fiber orientation causes the necrotic area to appear opaque in the microscope, resembling the appearance of hyaline cartilage (Reitan, 1960). Tooth movement will resume only after these hyalinized tissues and the adjacent alveolar bone are removed by invading cells from the adjacent viable PDL or alveolar bone marrow spaces. Some of these cells coalesce to form multinucleated osteoclasts, targeting the alveolar bone, while macrophages that are attracted to the site remove the necrotic PDL, thus enabling the tooth to move.

Biological Mechanisms of Tooth Movement, Third Edition. Edited by Vinod Krishnan, Anne Marie Kuijpers-Jagtman and Ze'ev Davidovitch.
© 2021 John Wiley & Sons Ltd. Published 2021 by John Wiley & Sons Ltd.

During OTM, cellular activities in sites of PDL tension are meant to narrow the widened space created by the movement of the dental root away from the alveolar bone. This stretching of the PDL affects both the cells and their extracellular matrix (ECM). The stretched cells detach themselves from their surrounding ECM, then reattach, and engage in a variety of functions commensurate with returning the width of the PDL to its original dimensions. These functions include proliferation, differentiation, synthesis and secretion of autocrine and paracrine molecules, and new ECM components. Some of these components are mineralizable and will eventually become the new layer of bone that covers the alveolar surface that faces the stretched PDL. The new bone first appears as fingerlike projections, which grow along the stretched PDL fibers, perpendicular to the surface of the old alveolar bone. The force-induced strains alter the PDL's nervous network, vascularity, and blood flow, resulting in local synthesis and/or release of various key molecules, such as vasoactive neurotransmitters, cytokines, growth factors, colony-stimulating factors, and arachidonic acid metabolites. These molecules evoke a plethora of cellular responses by many cell types in and around teeth, providing a favorable microenvironment for tissue deposition or resorption (Davidovitch, 1991; Krishnan and Davidovitch, 2006).

The studies performed in the early years of the twentieth century were mainly directed towards analyzing the histological changes in paradental tissues following short-term and long-term OTM. Those studies revealed extensive cellular activities in the mechanically stressed PDL, involving neurons, immune cells, fibroblasts, endothelial cells, osteoblasts, osteoclasts, osteocytes, and endosteal cells. Moreover, mechanical stresses were found to alter the structural properties of tissues at the cellular, molecular, and genetic levels. The rapid reactions occurring at the initial stage of mechanotherapy, and slower adaptive changes at the later stages of treatment, have attracted increasing attention. This chapter addresses the evolutionary traits of the development of concepts pertaining to the biology of OTM.

Hypotheses about the biological nature of OTM: The conceptual evolution

OTM is the result of a biological response to interference in the physiological equilibrium of the dentofacial complex by an externally applied force (Proffit, 2013). The biological foundation of force-induced tooth movement, along with some concepts related to it, has been extensively investigated since the onset of the twentieth century. From the classic reports by Sandstedt in 1904 (Figure 2.1), the race was set for exploring the biological foundations of OTM, using histology, radiology, and clinical observations as the main investigative tools. A list of the then prevailing hypotheses aimed at explaining the biological reasons for OTM is presented below:

- The old pressure hypothesis of Schwalbe–Flourens, which postulated that pressure moves teeth, preceded the concept that alveolar bone resorption takes place on one side of the dental root, while deposition occurs on the opposite side, until the pressure is eliminated. Hecht (1900), Sandstedt (1904), Pfaff (1906), and Angle (1907) supported this hypothesis (Oppenheim, 1911).
- Based on his vast clinical experience, Kingsley (1881) stated that slow OTM is associated with favorable tissue-remodeling changes (resorption and deposition of alveolar bone), while quick movements displace the entire bony lamellae along with the teeth, while retaining their functional and structural integrity. He attributed these features to the elasticity, compressibility, and flexibility of bone tissue. This report is one of the first written explanations for the biological basis of OTM, although it is not frequently cited (Oppenheim, 1911).

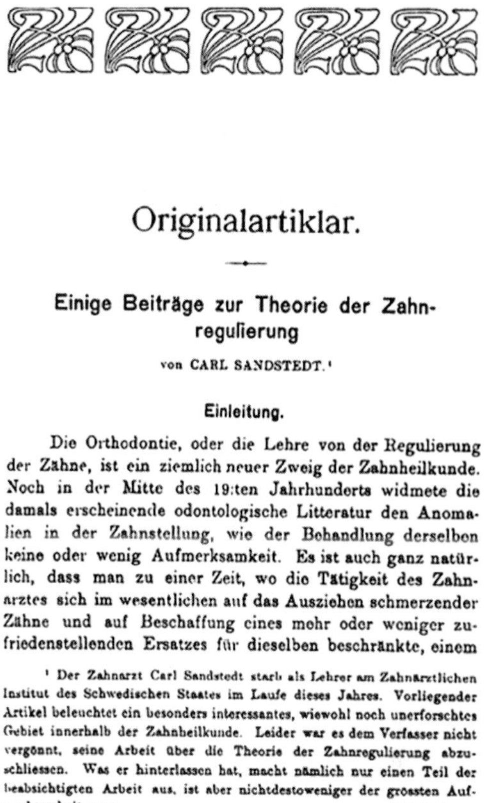

Originalartiklar.

Einige Beiträge zur Theorie der Zahnregulierung

von CARL SANDSTEDT.[1]

Einleitung.

Die Orthodontie, oder die Lehre von der Regulierung der Zähne, ist ein ziemlich neuer Zweig der Zahnheilkunde. Noch in der Mitte des 19:ten Jahrhunderts widmete die damals erscheinende odontologische Litteratur den Anomalien in der Zahnstellung, wie der Behandlung derselben keine oder wenig Aufmerksamkeit. Es ist auch ganz natürlich, dass man zu einer Zeit, wo die Tätigkeit des Zahnarztes sich im wesentlichen auf das Ausziehen schmerzender Zähne und auf Beschaffung eines mehr oder weniger zufriedenstellenden Ersatzes für dieselben beschränkte, einem

[1] Der Zahnarzt Carl Sandstedt starb als Lehrer am Zahnärztlichen Institut des Schwedischen Staates im Laufe dieses Jahres. Vorliegender Artikel beleuchtet ein besonders interessantes, wiewohl noch unerforschtes Gebiet innerhalb der Zahnheilkunde. Leider war es dem Verfasser nicht vergönnt, seine Arbeit über die Theorie der Zahnregulierung abzuschliessen. Was er hinterlassen hat, macht nämlich nur einen Teil der beabsichtigten Arbeit aus, ist aber nichtdestoweniger der grössten Aufmerksamkeit wert. *Die Red.*

Figure 2.1 Page 1 from Sandstedt's original article on histological studies of tooth movement published in 1904. (Source: Sandstedt, 1904, 1905.)

Walkhoff's hypothesis on the biology of OTM

Soon after Kingsley's contribution, Walkhoff (1890) stated that "movement of a tooth consists in the creation of different tensions in the bony tissue, its consolidation in the compensation of these tensions." Walkhoff's hypothesis was largely based on the elasticity, flexibility, and compressibility of bone, and the transposition of the histological elements (such as the PDL). He also stated that alveolar bone, after all the remodeling changes, maintains its thickness, due to transformation or apposition of bone during the consolidating (retentive) period (Walkhoff, 1891). He emphasized the importance of retention, stating that "osteoid tissue has nothing to do with tooth movement. If we were to remove the retaining devices already after a few weeks from corrected protruding front teeth like from a fractured bone after the formation of a callus, we had only to deal with failures." The propositions by Walkhoff were based solely on his clinical observations and practical knowledge but lacked the backing of histological evidence.

In 1900, Hecht described a cartilaginous transformation of the bone and rupture of bony spicules surrounding teeth during OTM. He interpreted this situation as an indication of severe changes and leaned upon Schwalbe–Flourens' pressure hypothesis (Oppenheim, 1911) to substantiate his interpretation. However, Oppenheim argued against this viewpoint, stating that the severe changes, which Hecht had observed, might have been the result of the application of excessive force (Oppenheim, 1911). In any case, Hecht did not support his assumptions with any histological evidence.

Histological examination of paradental tissues during OTM was reported for the first time by Sandstedt (1904), who tipped teeth uncontrollably in dogs, and later studied their tissues by light microscopy (Figures 2.2–2.5). In these sections he observed areas of

18 Biological Mechanisms of Tooth Movement

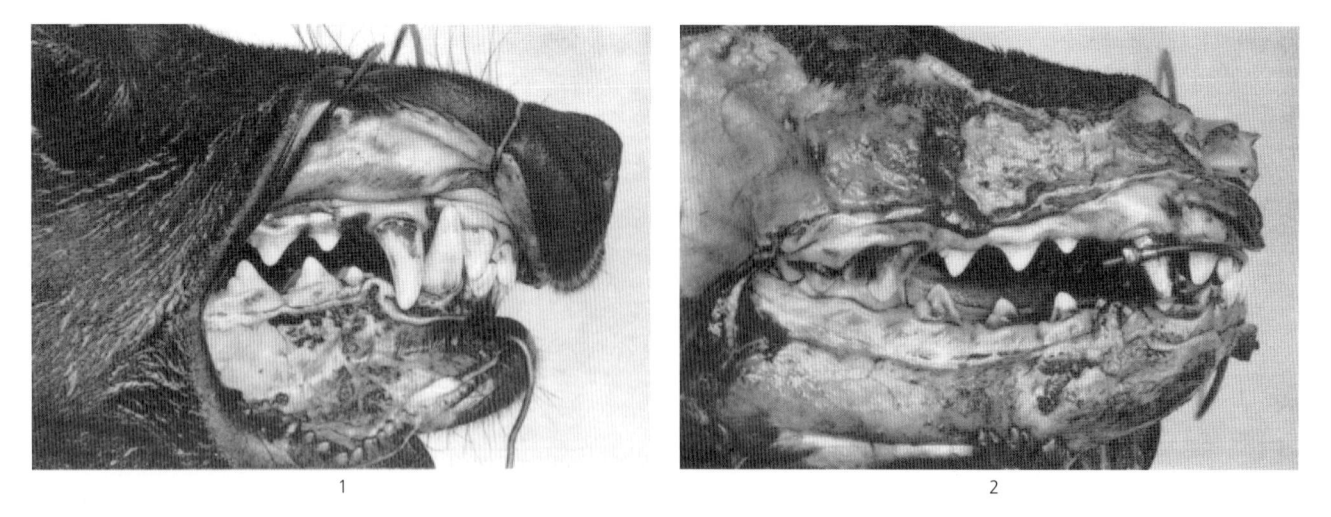

Figure 2.2 Plate I from Sandstedt's original article showing photographs of the control (1) and experimental (2) dogs at sacrifice. The mandibular canines were removed to allow the movement of the maxillary teeth. The appliance consisted of an archwire inserted into tubes attached to bands on the upper canines; distal to the tubes was a screw mechanism, which, when tightened, moved the incisors lingually and the canines mesially. (Source: Sandstedt, 1904, 1905).

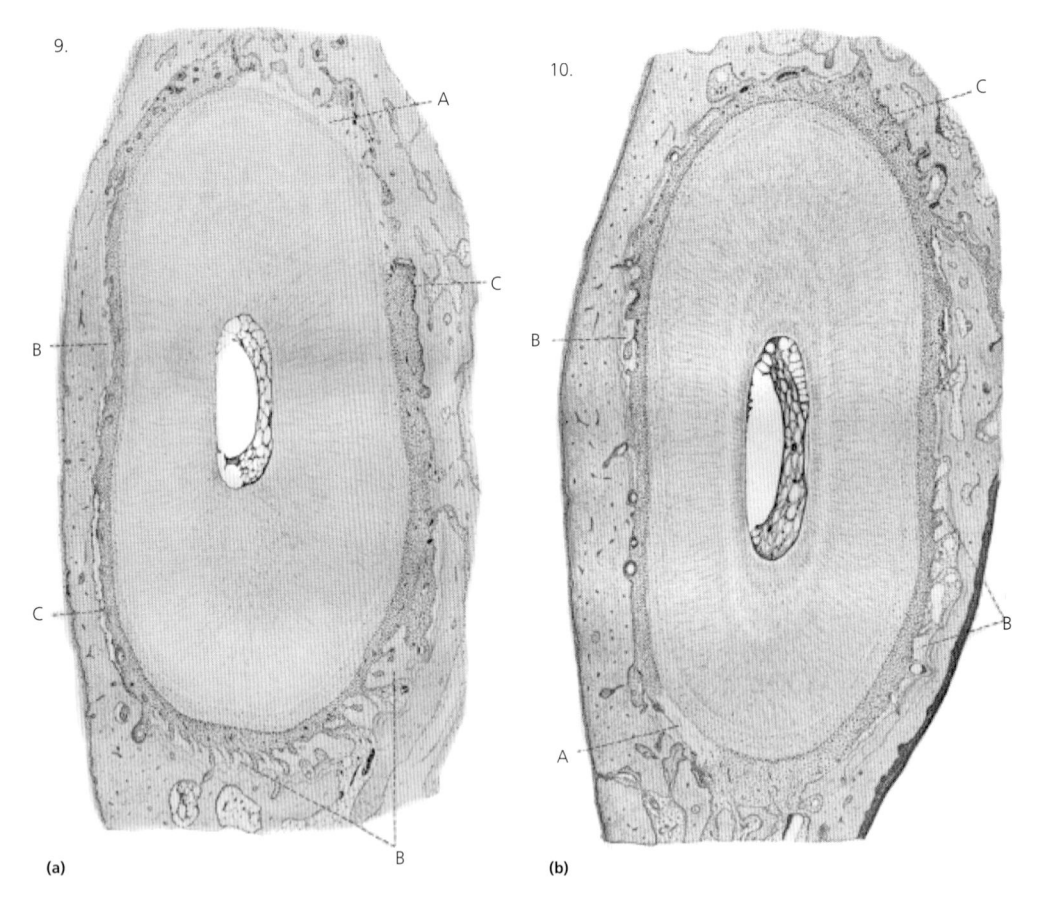

Figure 2.3 Plate III from Sandstedt's original article showing horizontal sections through the right maxillary canine; the direction of movement is towards the top. (Source: Sandstedt, 1904, 1905.). (a) (Sandstedt's Figure 9.) A section cut in close proximity to the alveolar rim. A. At the site of presumptive compression, the PDL shows the glassy appearance characteristic of hyalinization, with osteoclasts undermining the adjacent alveolar wall. B. On the buccal side of the root, a thin layer of lighter staining new bone is demarcated from the old bone by a von Ebner (reversal) line. At the bottom, new bone takes the form of lighter staining bony trabeculae of woven bone orientated in the direction of pull. C. On the right side, osteoclasts are resorbing the alveolar wall; on the left, the detachment of the PDL from the bone is the result of a tear during sectioning. (Source: Sandstedt, 1904, 1905.).
(b) (Sandstedt's Figure 10) A section through the middle third of the same tooth (in dogs, the pulp canal expands towards the middle third of the root before narrowing towards the apex). General remodeling activity at the bone–PDL interface is seen but evidence of the accelerated bone formation and resorption is absent. This area corresponds to the center of rotation of the tooth. (Source: Sandstedt, 1904, 1905.)

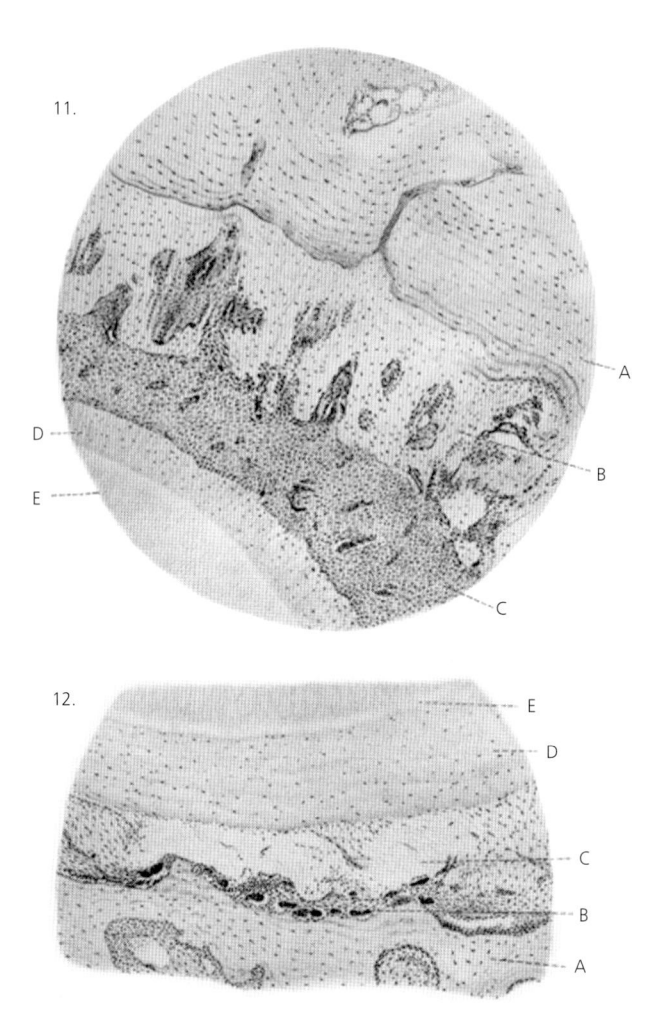

Figure 2.4 Plate IV A from Sandstedt's original article. These sections show at a higher power the cellular and tissue changes in the PDL and alveolar bone at sites of presumptive tension and compression. Sandstedt's Figure 11: tension in the PDL. A. Bone of the original alveolar wall. B. Newly laid-down woven bone with vascular spaces clearly demarcated from the older lamellar bone. C. Highly vascular PDL. D. Cementum. E. Dentine. Sandstedt's Figure 12: compression in the PDL. A. Bone of the original alveolar wall. B. Numerous dark-staining osteoclasts lining the bone surface. C. The PDL in which the fibrillar structure has been lost and replaced by a glassy homogeneous or hyalinized tissue. D. Cementum. E. Dentine. (Source: Sandstedt, 1904, 1905.)

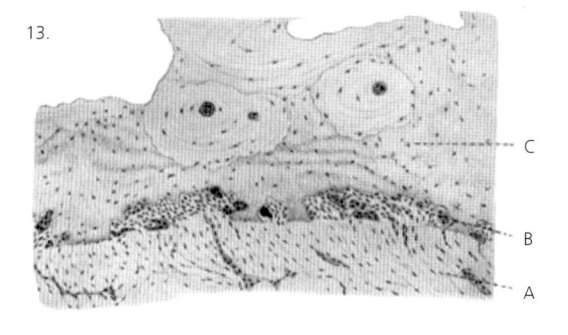

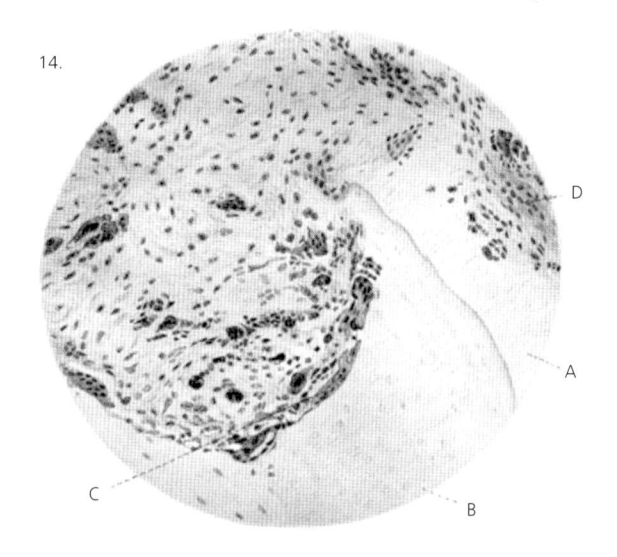

Figure 2.5 Plate IV B from Sandstedt's original article. Sandstedt's Figure 13: direct resorption. A. PDL at a compression site showing its normal fibrillar appearance. B. Numerous multinucleate osteoclasts in Howship's lacunae are resorbing the surface of the bone. C. Cortical bone of the alveolus; two Haversian systems or secondary osteones are clearly visible. Sandstedt's Figure 14. A. Hyalinized PDL. B. Although one cannot be absolutely sure, this section was likely to have been included to represent resorption of the root cementum at C by multinucleate giant cells. D. Unaffected periodontal ligament cells. (Source: Sandstedt, 1904, 1905.)

pressure and tension in the PDL, and necrosis or hyalinization zones in the PDL at sites of great compression. Oppenheim (1911), while trying to duplicate those experiments, could not find any thrombosis in vessels or hyalinization in the PDL. He speculated that the lack of necrosis in his own experiment might have been due to the use of light force, in contrast to the heavy forces used by Sandstedt.

Edward H. Angle, the father of modern orthodontics and follower of Wolff's law of bone adaptation to mechanical stress, was a proponent of the bone-bending concept. He stated that the degree of bending of the alveolar bone is determined by the magnitude of the applied force, the age of the patient, and the direction of force application (Angle, 1907; Oppenheim, 1911). He advocated the bone remodeling hypothesis and suggested that resorption is seen in areas of pressure and traction, while deposition/apposition is for filling up of hollow areas created with this act. His writings were also in favor of the pressure hypothesis.

Oppenheim's transformation hypothesis

Oppenheim (1911) conducted OTM on a juvenile baboon, wherein he performed all sorts of tooth movements (labial, lingual, intrusion, extrusion, and rotation), with a split mouth design (where one side of the dental arch is operated upon, while the other side serves as control). He processed the jaw tissues histologically, and concluded that

> The bony tissue, be it compact or cancelleous, reacts to pressure by a transformation of its entire architecture; this takes place by resorption of the bone present and deposition of new bony tissue; both processes occur simultaneously. Deposition finally preponderates over resorption. The newly formed bony spicules are arranged in the direction of the pressure [Figure 2.6]. Increased pull has similarly resulted in addition of new bony tissue as a result, and simultaneous orientation of the spicules thereof in the direction of the pull [Figure 2.7]. The entire transformation of the architecture and the orientation of the newly formed spongy bone spicules always occur so characteristically and lawfully, that we can say by the histological preparations in what manner the movements were accomplished. This characteristic transformation results only upon the application of very slight, physiological-like influences. Should the force be too strong, the result will be such serious injuries to the periosteum, due to the disturbances in circulation, that there will be no typical reaction of the bony cells.

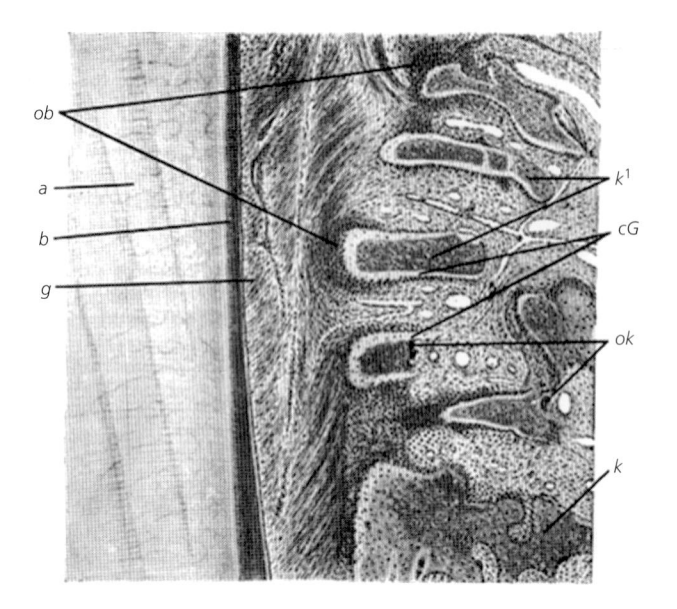

Figure 2.6 Histologic section from the original article by Oppenheim (1911). Lingual movement; lingual side of the PDL, where it forms compression. The individual newly formed bone spicules (k^1) have arranged themselves in the direction of the force, perpendicular to the long axis of the tooth. The ends of the spicules directed toward the tooth: the ends subjected directly to the pressure show broad, uncalcified zones (cG), which are surrounded by densely arranged rows of osteoblasts (ob). At the ends of the spicules directed from the tooth, occasionally numerous osteoclasts are seen. a, dentine; b, cementum; g, PDL; ok, osteoclasts; nearer to the apex of the root old unchanged bone (k). (Source: Oppenheim, 1911. Reproduced with permission of Oxford University Press.)

Oppenheim substantiated his findings by drawing support from Wolff's law, and his investigations could not find any injury in the PDL. He concluded that, in OTM, all mechanical forces applied to a tooth are absorbed by the PDL, and at times he could observe a hypertrophy to withstand the increased demand placed upon it. Unlike Sandstedt, Oppenheim reported on seeing no hyalinization or undermining resorption in his experimental material. He further wrote that "The vitality of the periosteum suffers no injury during the application of "physiological forces," even on compression of the PDL to a third of its original thickness. It may be exposed to slight hemorrhages, to occasional constriction in the lumen, or disappearance of the vessels, but the staining ability of the cell nuclei is retained, and no disintegration can be demonstrated by any photographs.

The pressure–tension hypothesis

Schwarz (1932), working along the same lines as both Sandstedt and Oppenheim, formulated the "pressure–tension hypothesis" of OTM. It is postulated that in sites of compression in the PDL, it displays disorganization and diminution of fiber production. Here, cell replication decreases, seemingly as a result of vascular constriction. In contrast, in PDL tension sites, stimulation produced by stretching of fiber bundles results in an increase in cell replication. Schwarz detailed the concept further by correlating the tissue response to the magnitude of the applied force with the capillary blood pressure and categorized it as four degrees of biologic effect:

- *First degree of biologic effect.* The force is of such a short duration or so slight that no reaction whatsoever is caused in the periodontium.
- *Second degree of biologic effect* (Figure 2.8). The force is gentle, speaking biologically; it remains below the pressure in the blood capillaries, i.e., less than 20–26 g for 1 cm² of root surface, but it is nevertheless sufficient to cause resorption in the alveolar bone at the regions of pressure in the PDL. After the force ceases there will be anatomic and functional resolution of integrity of the PDL and alveolar bone without resorption of dental roots.
- *Third degree of biologic effect* (Figure 2.9). The force is fairly strong; sustaining increased pressure in the blood capillaries of the compressed PDL. At these areas, suffocation of the strangled PDL develops, followed by resorption of the necrotic tissue, including the dental root surfaces. This resorption takes an impetuous course and attacks also those parts of the surface of the root, the vitality of which may be injured by the pressure. After the force ceases, there will be anatomic and functional resolution of integrity of the PDL and alveolar bone, with resorption of roots frequently progressing into the dentin.
- *Fourth degree of biologic effect* (Figure 2.10). The force is strong, squeezing the strangled PDL, and the tooth touches the bone after the soft tissues are crushed. Alveolar bone resorption occurs in the periphery of the hyalinized PDL zones, as well as in bone marrow cavities near the compressed PDL. However, this situation is associated with a high risk of severe alveolar bone and root resorption, and damage to tissues of the dental pulp. In some cases, ankylosis of the tooth with the alveolar bone may occur.

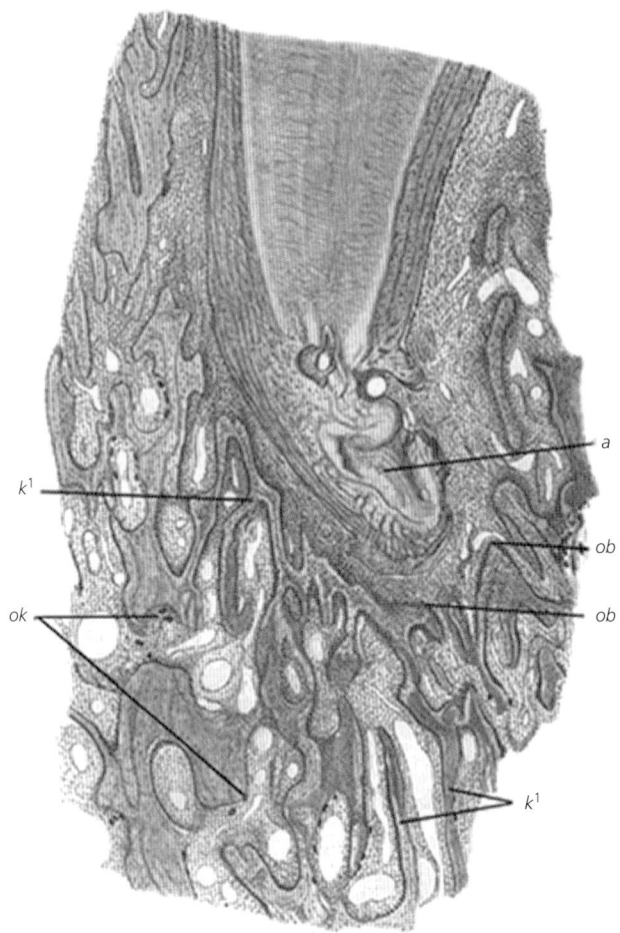

Figure 2.7 Elongation from the original article by Oppenheim (2011). Apex of the root (a). The spongy bone spicules at the root apex appear as long, thin, buttresses, stretching from the depth toward the root apex (k^1), their tops and sides being enclosed by narrow uncalcified zones and strong layers of osteoblasts (ob). ok, osteoclasts. (Source: Oppenheim, 1911. Reproduced with permission of Oxford University Press.)

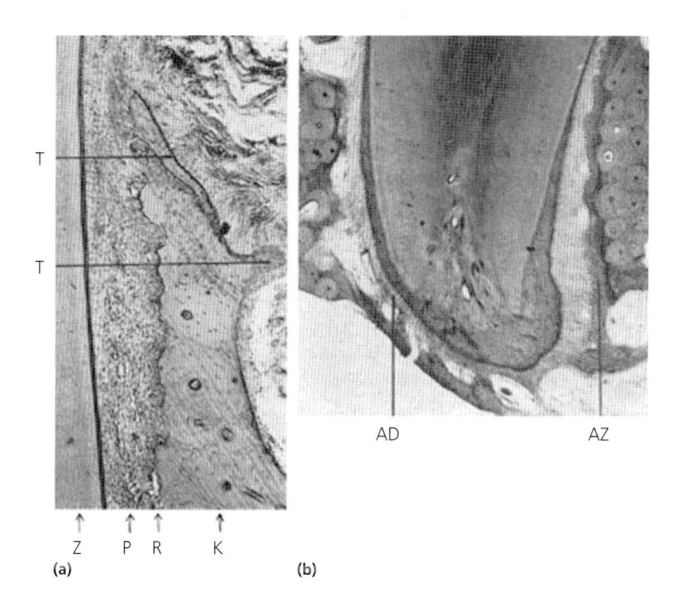

Figure 2.8 Second degree of biologic effect seen on the (a) marginal side of PDL pressure side of tooth movement as portrayed in Schwarz (1932). Z, tooth; P, periodontium; R, line or resorption; K, old alveolar bone; T, newly formed bone on the outer periosteal surface of the alveolar bone. (b) Apex of the tooth shown. AZ, apical side of pull with newly formed bones; AD, apical side of PDL pressure. (Source: Schwarz, 1932. Reproduced with permission of Elsevier.)

Schwarz concluded "that the most favorable treatment is that which works with forces not greater than the pressure of blood capillaries." He identified this pressure as 15–20 mmHg in man and most mammals, and calculated the optimal force level to be 20–26 g to 1 cm² of root surface area, suggesting that these limits of pressure are critical, capable of generating a continuous resorption of alveolar bone in areas of pressure in the PDL. Schwarz postulated further that the width changes in the PDL alter the cell population and increases cellular activity. There is an apparent disruption of collagen fibers in the PDL, with evidence of cell and tissue damage. If one exceeds this pressure, compression could cause tissue necrosis through "suffocation of the strangulated periodontium." Application of even greater force levels will result in obliteration of blood vessels, followed by cell death in the ischemic area, which will lead to alteration in the orientation of PDL fibers from horizontal to vertical. This change in orientation will appear as glassy in nature, when observed through the light microscope and is labeled as hyalinization. There will be hyperemia in the area surrounding the necrotic area, which produces tenderness to the tooth. This hyperemia is considered to be essential to the resolution of the problem and speeding up the recovery phenomenon. The resolution of the problem starts when cellular elements such as macrophages, foreign body giant cells, and osteoclasts from adjacent undamaged areas invade the necrotic tissue (Figure 2.10). These cells also resorb the underside of bone immediately adjacent

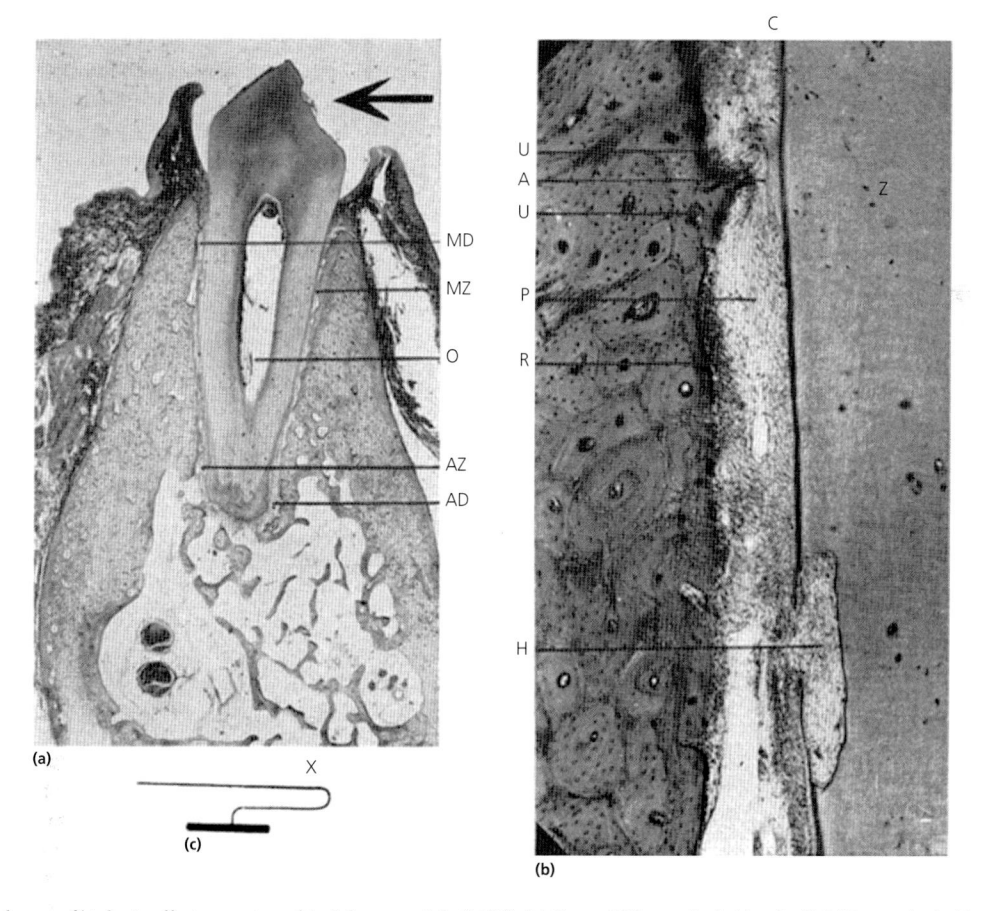

Figure 2.9 Third degree of biologic effect as portrayed in Schwarz article (1932). (a) Shows MZ, marginal side of pull; MD, marginal side of pressure; 0, tilt axis; AZ, apical side of pull; AD, apical side of pressure. (b) Marginal side of pressure, greatly enlarged: Z, tooth (dentine); C, cementum; H, resorption cavity reaching far into the dentine; P, periodontium; R, line of resorption on the alveolar wall, densely covered by osteoblasts; early stages of regeneration; A, compressed area of the periodontium, no nuclei of cells; U, signs of undermining resorption. (c) Sketch of the spring. The point of application on the tooth is shown at X. (Source: Schwarz, 1932. Reproduced with permission of Elsevier.)

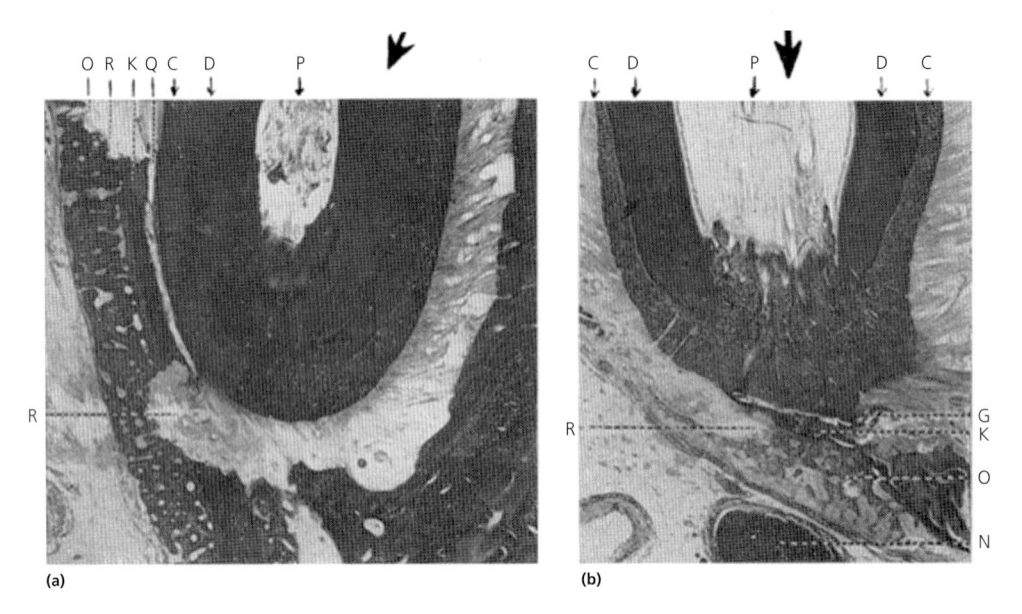

Figure 2.10 Fourth degree of biologic effect as portrayed in Schwarz article (1932) depicting osteophytes on the outer surface in the apical region. (a) The influence created by strong force applied in the direction of the arrow: P, pulp; D, dentine; C, cementum; K, old alveolar bone; O, osteophytes; Q, region of compression of the periodontium; R, region of resorption stretching over the newly formed osteophytes. (b) The osteophytes, O, were formed in the lumen of the canalis mandibulae (N, nervus mandibularis). At the region of compression, the old alveolar bone, K, is removed by undermining resorption, R. The young osteophytes were also attacked by the latter. Arrow and also P, C and D as in (a). (Source: Schwarz, 1932. Reproduced with permission of Elsevier.)

to the necrotic PDL area and remove it together with the necrotic tissue (Schwarz, 1932).

Through his writings, Schwarz tried to indicate the methodological differences between the approaches made by Sandstedt and Oppenheim (Figure 2.11), and concluded that Oppenheim had euthanized his experimental animals several days after the appliance had been last activated, and Schwarz attributed this fact to the reason why Oppenheim saw only normal adaptation phenomena. Moreover, Oppenheim ignored the acute phase reactions and focused only on the stage of regeneration after the force had been exhausted. It seems more likely that what Oppenheim was describing was the response of cells of the periosteal and endosteal bone surfaces to the bending of the labial alveolar bone plate (Meikle, 2006).

Following Schwarz's publication, Oppenheim performed additional studies on tissue reactions in mature monkeys (*Macaca rhesus*) to applications of light and heavy forces (Oppenheim, 1944). He concluded that with light forces, osteoclasts are mobilized at a very fast pace and attack bone by a uniform superficial lacunar resorption. These cells, called "primary osteoclasts," stayed active in the site for almost 4 days (Figure 2.12). In contrast, the use of heavy forces resulted in crushing of the PDL, with a cutoff in all its nutritional supplies, resulting in undermining resorption. The direction of bone resorption comes from unintended sources, with an inflow of osteoclasts from adjacent unaffected areas. These osteoclasts, called "secondary osteoclasts," persist until the crushed PDL, bone, and cementum are removed (Figure 2.12). Oppenheim further examined the hemorrhage formed by crushed blood vessels and found that the impaired nourishment along with encroachment of osteophytes and toxins from decomposed red blood cells lead to mobilization of osteoclasts from far off sites, called "tertiary osteoclasts" (Figures 2.13 and 2.14). All these cells were observed by application of higher amounts of force (240–360 g) to teeth. With these findings, Oppenheim advocated the use of intermittent forces, consisting of force application for a short period (1 day) followed by a rest period

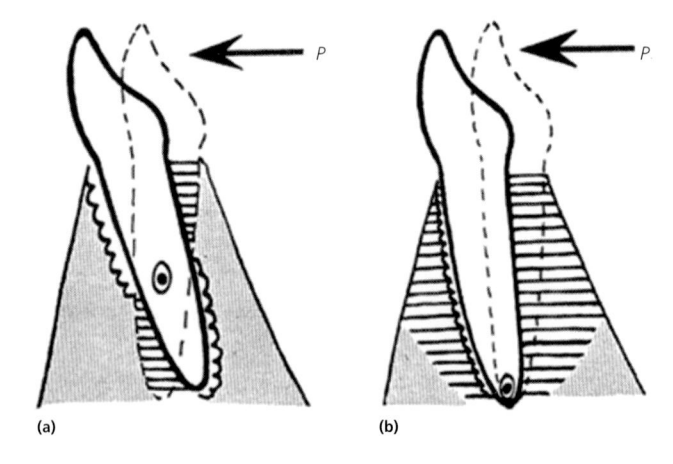

Figure 2.11 Comparative diagram of the theories put forward by Sandstedt (1904) and Oppenheim (1911) as drawn by Schwarz (1932). In (a), which depicts the theory of pressure (Sandstedt), the tooth moved by the force, P, tilts around an axis, O, lying a little apically from the center of the root. By this means two regions of pressure and pull arise, lying diametrically opposite. In the regions of pressure in the PDL, the old alveolar bone is resorbed (jagged line) and in the regions of pull, new bone is added (horizontal shading). Gray shading, alveolar bone without transformation. (b) This depicts the theory of transformation (Oppenheim, 1911, 1944). There is only one side of pressure and one side of pull. On both sides the alveolar bone opens into a transitional spongy bone, whose elements are arranged vertically to the surface of the tooth (horizontal shading). On the side of pressure, this newly formed transitional bone is resorbed (jagged line). On the side of pull, new bone is added. Gray shading indicates the old untransformed alveolar bone at a greater distance from the moved tooth, (Source: Schwarz, 1932. Reproduced with permission of Elsevier.)

of longer duration (3 or 4 days). He considered this formula to be a biologic approach, but was later disproved by the evolution of mechanical devices of greater potential. He concluded that primary osteoclasts are the type, which is of great help to the orthodontist, and that only light forces can induce their production in abundance.

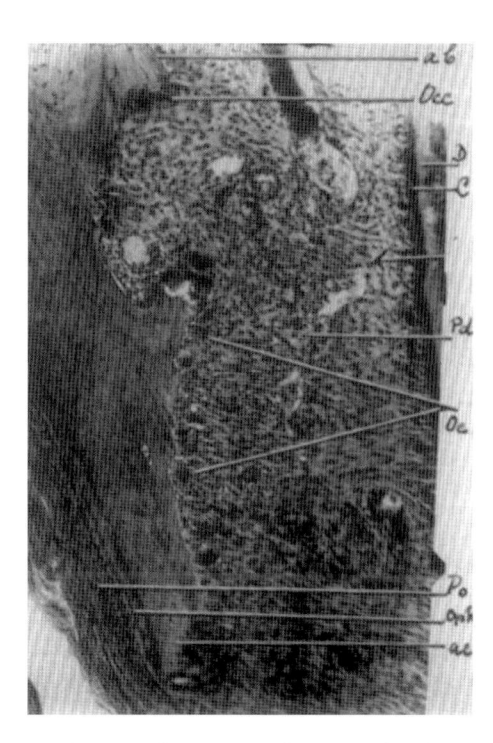

Figure 2.12 Higher magnification image from Oppenheim's article (1944) showing labial alveolar crest. The aplastic zone facing the periodontium has for the greatest part disappeared, as has the crest itself. Where some aplastic bone is still present (ab), the secondary osteoclasts (Occ) are still at work removing it. No osteoclastic activity whatsoever is found at the periosteal smooth bone surface. The still remaining but decreased pressure caused the appearance of primary osteoclasts (Oc) and will be present for 2 days after force discontinuation. D, dentine; C, cementum; Pd, periodontal membrane; Po, formation of smooth periosteal bone surface; Opk, scarce osteophyte. ac, acellular cementum. (Source: Oppenheim, 1944. Reproduced with permission of Elsevier.)

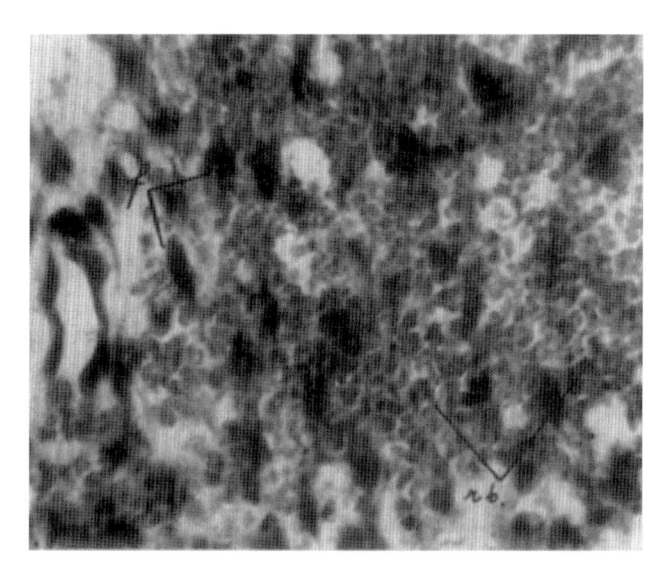

Figure 2.13 Higher magnification image of hemorrhage as portrayed in Oppenheim (1944). (Source: Oppenheim, 1944. Reproduced with permission of Elsevier.)

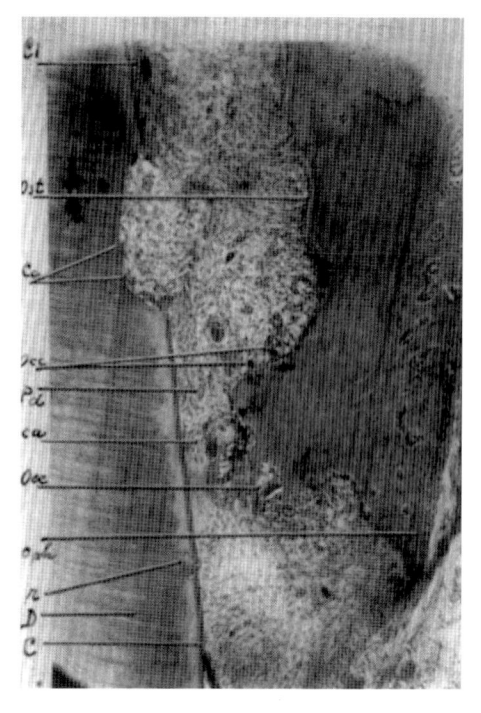

Figure 2.14 Hyalinization reaction as portrayed in Oppenheim (1944). The osteocytes are mostly normal; the osteophytic bone formation (Oph) is quite poor; no sign of any periosteal osteoclastic activity was found. The cementum within the compression area is aplastic, and again displays its signs of vitality (cementoblasts, cementoid seam) above the compression area (C). Within this area, we see a cementum resorption with cementoclasts (Cc) still present 4 days after force discontinuation. A proof that the lowering of the crest has really taken place is found in the presence of another small cementum resorption (r) in a region opposite which bone is no longer present. The larger resorption, though not deep, is already quite extended buccolingually. Above the crest we find the effect of the relapse movement of 4 days, the formation of an osteoid seam (Ost). C, Aplastic cementum; D, dentine; Pd, periodontal membrane; ca, crushed periodontal tissue with hyaline degeneration and debris; Occ, secondary osteoclasts: Oph, osteophytic apposition; r, small cementum resorption: cc, greater cementum resorption with cementoclasts still present; Ost, osteoid. (Source: Oppenheim, 1944. Reproduced with permission of Elsevier.)

In short, all three major researchers (Sandstedt, 1904, 1905; Oppenheim, 1911, 1944; Schwarz, 1932) exploring tissue reactions during OTM, agreed that there is a creation of pressure and tension sites in the PDL during OTM. Furthermore, it appears that cell replication is decreased in pressure sites owing to a decrease in vascular supply, whereas it is increased in tension sites due to PDL fiber stretching.

Reitan (1957, 1960), in his classic papers on histological changes during OTM, reported that hyalinization refers to cell-free areas within the PDL, in which the normal tissue architecture and staining characteristics of collagen in the processed histological material have been lost (Figures 2.15 and 2.16). He observed that:

- hyalinization occurred within the PDL following the application of even minimal force, meant to bring about a tipping movement;
- a greater degree of hyalinization occurred following application of force, if a tooth had a short root;
- during tooth translation, very little hyalinization was observed.

Reitan (1960) concluded that the tissue changes observed were those of degeneration related to force per unit area, and that attempts should be made to minimize these changes.

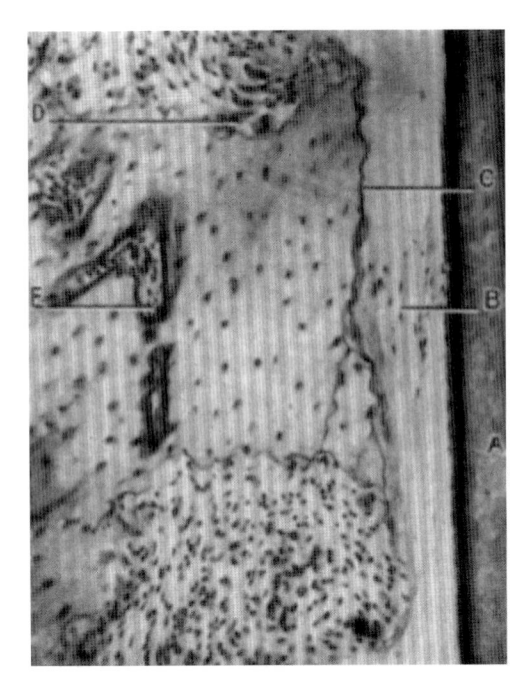

Figure 2.15 Cell free areas as shown by Reitan (1960). The figure shows pressure in the PDL during tooth movement, where cells gradually disappear in a circumscribed area. A, Root surface: B, compressed cell free fibers; C, border line between bone and hyalinized tissue: D, undermining bone resorption; E, small marrow space in dense, compact lamina dura. (Source: Reitan, 1960. Reproduced with permission of Elsevier.)

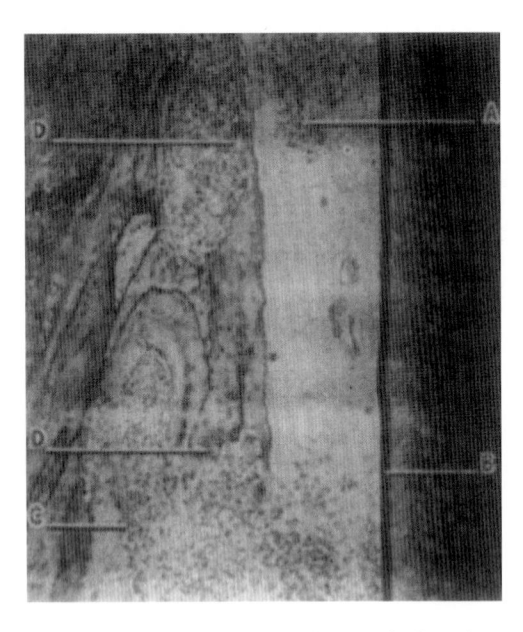

Figure 2.16 (A) Formation of cells and capillaries in hyalinized tissue after the force was released as shown by Reitan (1960). B, Root surface; C, direct resorption; D, undermining resorption. (Source: Reitan, 1960. Reproduced with permission of Elsevier.)

The fluid dynamic hypothesis

Bien (1966), through his research on the effect of intrusive forces on mandibular incisors, recorded an oscillation of the force inside the dental socket, and named it the hydraulic damping effect. He identified three distinct but interactive fluid systems present in paradental tissues: the vascular system, interstitial fluids, and cellular fluids. All

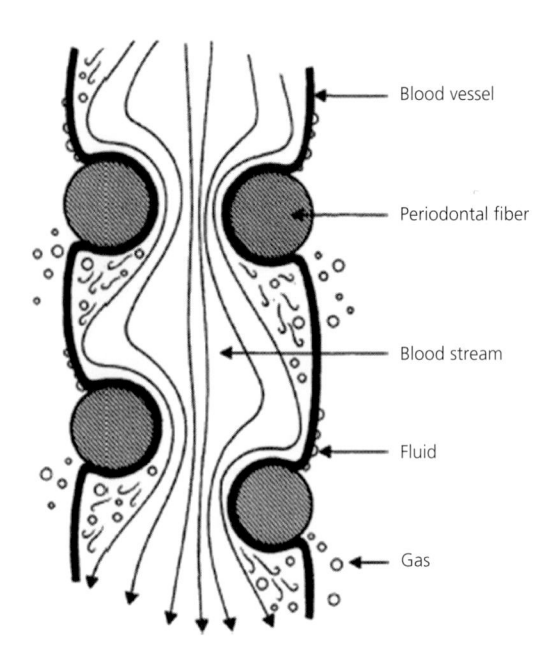

Figure 2.17 The constriction of a blood vessel by the periodontal fibers. The flow of blood in the vessels is occluded by the entwining periodontal fibers. Below the stenosis, the pressure drop gives rise to the formation of minute gas bubbles, which can diffuse through the vessel walls. Above the stenosis, fluid diffuses through the walls of the cirsoid aneurysms formed by the build-up of pressure. (Source: Bien, 1966. Reproduced with permission of SAGE Publications.)

three are presumably involved in damping oscillations of the tooth. He used Reynold's numbers to measure tooth oscillation and concluded that the low Reynold's number observed for the tooth subjected to oscillations is due to predominance of viscous forces acting within the system. He observed an escape of extracellular fluids from the PDL to the marrow spaces through the minute perforations in the alveolar wall (Figure 2.17). This phenomenon, occurring in the first stage of OTM, when PDL fibers are slack, depends mainly on size and number of alveolar bone perforations. The slack fibers become tightened once the extracellular fluids are exhausted. Owing to the presence of interstitial fluid or ground substance throughout the PDL, and the fact that the PDL is extremely thin, when compared with the sizes of the dental root and alveolus, he related the behavior of the PDL to that of the "squeeze film effect" proposed by Hays (1961). The presence of this film enables the tooth to withstand the heavy forces applied as part of orthodontic treatment or masticatory efforts. Masticatory forces, which are momentary in nature, will displace the fluid in the PDL space to its boundaries of the squeeze film (towards the apex and cervical areas of the dental root). Once the force is released, replenishment of fluid occurs through recirculation of interstitial fluid and diffusion through capillary walls, restoring the equilibrium. Likewise, a similar chain of events may occur following the application of low, sustained orthodontic forces.

With application of high sustained forces, as was the practice in the early era of orthodontics, capillary pressure will not be sufficient enough to counteract the effect and thus to replenish the fluid back to equilibrium. In this stage, the randomly running PDL fibers, which crisscross the blood vessels, tighten-up, leading to compression, constriction of blood vessels, and leading to stenosis. This constriction point creates ballooning of the vessel wall above it, creating hydrodynamic pressure heads. Drawing support from Bernoulli's principle, Bien explained the creation of a pressure drop in areas of stenosed

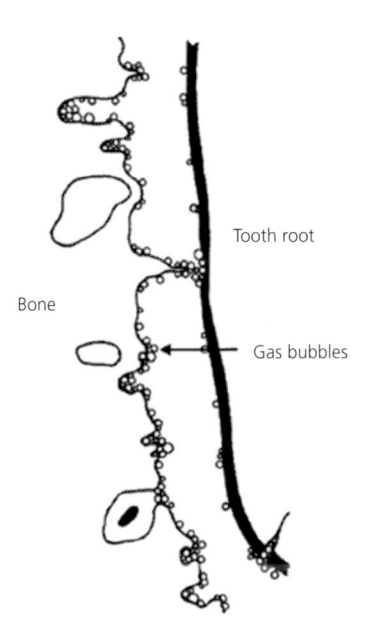

Figure 2.18 The lodgment of minute gas bubbles at small radii of curvature. The minute bubbles of gas, which diffuse through the blood vessel walls below the stenosis, lodge against the solid boundaries of tooth root and bone. Since there are many more areas of small radii of curvature in the bone, a greater number of gas bubbles may accumulate on the bone surface rather than on the root surface. (Source: Bien, 1966. Reproduced with permission of SAGE Publications.)

blood vessels, leading to gas formation and sub-atmospheric pressure. The gas bubbles formed might escape out of the capillaries and become lodged between bone spicules to create a favorable area for bone resorption. Bien attributed the large vacuoles seen in histologic sections of bone to be the escaped gas bubbles lodged there (Figure 2.18). Furthermore, he associated the lack of cementum resorption with its smooth nature, containing fewer small radii of curvature, producing unfavorable areas for gas lodgment.

The bone-bending hypothesis

Baumrind (1969) explored the assumption that orthodontic forces bend the alveolar bone. He measured changes in PDL cell dimensions, metabolic activity, and fiber synthesis with the help of radio-isotopes (tritiated thymine, uridine, and proline). While discussing the findings of his research, he highlighted a conceptual flaw in Schwarz's pressure–tension hypothesis. He described the PDL as a continuous hydrostatic system, which, in accordance with Pascal's law, dictates that force applied to this system is distributed equally to all regions of the PDL. He emphasized that the presence of fibers in the PDL does not modify the operation of this law, because of the concomitant existence of a continuous body of liquefied ground substance. He recognized that only part of the PDL, where differential pressures exist, as mentioned in the pressure–tension hypothesis, can be developed, is actually solid, i.e., bone, tooth, and discrete solid fractures of the PDL.

Kingsley (1881) and Farrar (1888) were the first to be credited for proposing the concept of bone bending as being an integral part of OTM. Farrar wrote in favor of this hypothesis: "Teeth move by one of two kinds of tissue changes in the alveolus … by the reduction of the alveolus through what is called absorption on one side of the tooth, followed by the growth of new supporting tissue on the other and by bending of the alveolar bone." Kingsley and Farrar increased the force levels to such an extent that visible bending of alveolar bone could be observed, but several authors who followed this approach complained that their patients had experienced alveolar fractures. Because of this problem, and the influence of Oppenheim and his lectures in the Angle School, the pressure–tension hypothesis was uplifted, while the bone-bending hypothesis was abandoned. Baumrind criticized the application of excessive forces for bone bending by describing them as "practical excesses of Kingsley and Farrar rather than theoretical misconceptions they had." He revived the legacy of bone bending by basing it on Hook's law (any solid body subjected to a load within its elastic limit will, if maintained in a static position, deform to a degree proportional to the magnitude of the applied force), the physical law of elasticity, which is fundamental to solid-state mechanics, and stated that "alveolar bone does indeed deflect under mechanical loading and these can be produced by forces lower than those required to produce consequential changes in the PDL width."

Proposing the bone-bending hypothesis, Baumrind (1969) stated that "when orthodontic appliances are placed, forces delivered to the tooth are transmitted to all the tissues in the region of force application. In accordance with universally operating physical laws, each of the three types of structure in the area (tooth, PDL, and bone) is deformed. The amount of deformation produced in each material by a given force is a function of the elastic properties of that material. The elastic properties of the tooth itself have not been studied. Of the other two materials, I contend that the bone deforms far more readily than PDL." When bone is held under mechanical forces, the remodeling and reorganization process is accelerated not only in the lamina dura, but also on the surface of every trabeculum within the corpus of the bone. The force/stress directed to the teeth will be dissipated by the development of stress lines in the deflected bone and becomes a major stimulus for altered biological activity, which in turn brings about adaptive changes. Baumrind claimed that his proposed hypothesis was complying with the basic rules of Wolff's law, as outlined by D'Arcy Thompson (1917), that strains are induced in bone by deflective forces within the elastic limit, and the tissue turnover and renewal are active so that bone can reorganize to accommodate the applied stress. In accordance with this theory, he could explain the phenomena behind

- Relative slowness of en-mass movements, and relative rapidity in the alignment of crowded anterior teeth.
- The rapidity in which teeth can be moved into an extraction site.
- The appearance of an axis of rotation beyond the apex of the incisors. The logic of the pressure–tension hypothesis makes it mandatory to have the axis between the apex and the alveolar crest.
- The relative rapidity of tooth movement in children.

Baumrind also challenged the existence of the fluid dynamic hypothesis of Bien by stating that "there is simply no objective evidence for theories which postulate 'squeezing out' of tissue fluids from the PDL on the 'pressure' side. In any event, the PDL is a continuous system, so that if fluid were to be 'squeezed out' in one region it would have to be 'squeezed out' in all regions."

The apposition and resorption of bone in response to its bending by orthodontic forces is evidently an attractive hypothesis, but it seems to contradict the current orthopedic dogma (Melsen, 1999), which states that "any mechanical compression stimulates bone formation and tension stimulates resorption." Epker and Frost (1965) described the change in shape of the alveolar bone circumference resulting from stretching of the PDL fibers. This fiber stretching decreases the radius of the alveolar wall, i.e., bending of bone in the tension zone, where apposition of bone takes place. They attributed this response to a regional acceleratory phenomenon (RAP). Frost (1983) demonstrated that regional noxious stimuli of sufficient magnitude result in markedly accelerated reorganizing activity of osseous and soft tissues. It is a burst of localized remodeling process, which speeds up the healing potential, especially following the surgical wounding of cortical bone. Accordingly, any regional noxious stimulus of sufficient magnitude can evoke RAP. The extent of the affected region and intensity of the response vary directly with the magnitude and nature of the stimulus.

Experimenting with dog mandibles *in vitro* and *in vivo*, Zengo *et al.* (1973) demonstrated that orthodontic canine tipping bends the alveolar bone, creating on it concave and convex surfaces identical to those generated in bent long bones. In areas of PDL tension, the interfacing bone surface assumes a concave configuration in which the molecules are compressed, whereas in zones of compressed PDL the adjacent alveolar bone surface becomes convex (Figure 2.19). Hence, there is no contradiction between the response of alveolar bone and other parts of the skeleton to mechanical loading. The confusion in this regard has resulted from the usage of the same descriptions for different tissues. While orthodontic "tension" refers to the PDL, an orthopedist may declare the area as being under "compression," because the bone near the stretched PDL has become concave.

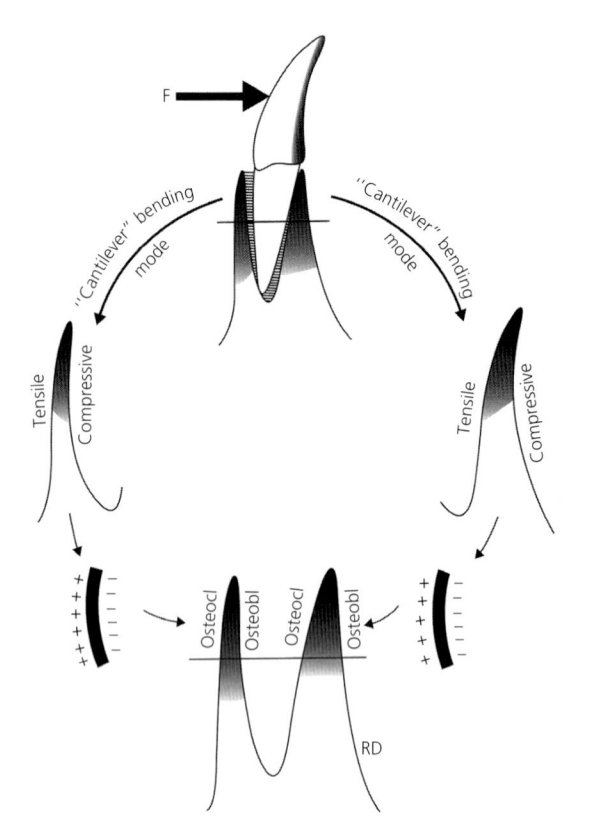

Figure 2.19 Behavior of bone during orthodontic tooth movement. The net force, compression, and tension applied by the "leading" edge of the tooth deforms the alveolar bone convexly toward the root. At the "trailing" edge, the periodontal fibers distort the alveolar bone, producing concavity toward the root. Areas that have been described as characterized by osteoblastic activity were electronegative and, conversely, areas of positivity of electrical neutrality were observed in regions characterized by osteoclasia. (Source: Zengo *et al.*, 1973. Reproduced with permission of Elsevier.)

Bioelectric signals in orthodontic tooth movement

In 1957, Fukada and Yasuda published the results of their systematic investigation on dry specimens cut from human and bovine long bones, in an article titled "On the piezoelectric effect of bone," which credited them with the discovery of the existence of piezoelectricity in bone. They demonstrated that dry bone under proper load application generates surface charges, called piezoelectric currents. They established that the piezoelectric effect appears only when shearing force is applied to the collagen fibers in the bone, which are highly oriented, to make them slip past each other. There exist two types of piezoelectric effects – positive and negative. The former is due to strains generated within the crystal lattice of a material, leading to the production of a potential difference across the faces of that crystal and the latter, when an electric charge is passed across a molecule or crystal and leads to an inherent strain within that molecule (Isaacs, 1987). Both effects involve the organic molecules of collagen and the inorganic crystals of hydroxyapatite (McDonald, 1993). Bassett and Becker (1962) extended that research and discovered that the charges emanating from the bone surface at the time of bending are proportional to the internal strains engendered by the bending. They also showed that the polarization sign always depended upon the type of stress – there was a positive sign where there is tension and a negative sign where there is compression. These experiments were further developed by Shamos *et al.* (1963) and Shamos and Lavine (1964), who reported finding this phenomenon in a number of different bones, in different anatomical sites and species. They suggested that local electric fields resulting from these surface changes influence the deposition of ions and polarizable molecules.

The first observations of the piezoelectric phenomenon in wet and living bone was made by Bassett (1968), and this finding has contributed to the working hypothesis that piezoelectricity leads to a physical explanation of Wolff's law. Following this discovery, the universal existence of piezoelectricity in biological tissues was demonstrated by Fukada and Hara (1969) through their experiments on trachea, aorta, intestines, ligaments, and venous vessels. Marino and Becker (1975) reported on the piezoelectric characteristics of collagen, and concluded that these effects originate in tropocollagen molecules, or in molecules no larger than 50 Å in diameter. However, the hypothesis claiming that piezoelectricity is a major determinant of bone remodeling is weakened by the following:

- The generated electric potential is dependent on a strain gradient, and this was not taken into account when the hypothesis was proposed. Bone always experiences nonhomogeneous deformation because of its centro-symmetric nature, and because it can produce electrical polarization proportional to the strain gradient.
- The modulus of elasticity (E) of cortical bone under physiologic conditions is frequency dependent. Hence, bone cannot be considered as an elastic-plastic material.
- End-for-end rotation of the sample in cantilever bending mode does not change the sign of generated potential as would be expected from classical piezoelectric material.

Proffit (2013) outlined two unusual properties of piezoelectricity, which do not seem to correlate well with OTM:

- A quick decay rate, where the electron transfer from one area to another following force application reverts back when the force is removed, which does not or should not happen once orthodontic treatment is over.
- Production of an equivalent signal in the opposite direction upon force removal.

Anderson and Erikkson (1968) challenged the piezoelectric hypothesis and reported that although dry collagen is strongly piezoelectric, full hydrated collagen is not, because of the structured water it contains. They argued that bone is a tissue with high symmetry, as the hydroxyapatite it contains is centrosymmetric in nature, and not piezoelectric. Follow-up experiments conducted by these investigators (1970), using a similar apparatus to the one used by Fukada and Yasuda in 1957, proved that the piezoelectric coefficients varied with the state of hydration of bone, and that the variation decreased as the specimens were dried by evaporation. The loss of piezoelectricity in fully hydrated tendon collagen was explained as attainment of more symmetrical, nonpiezoelectric structure by absorption of water. Instead, the electrical signals generated when stress is applied to fully wet collagen are actually streaming potentials.

The electrokinetic phenomenon known as streaming potential or streaming current was described by many authors, like Glasstone, Overbeek, and Kortum (Gross and Williams, 1982). Anderson and Eriksson (1968) reintroduced the concept against the theoretical faults of the piezoelectric effect, and reported it to be present in bone as it is a porous tissue containing a fluid phase and calcified matrix (which is composed of inorganic (mainly hydroxyapatite) and organic (collagen) contents). Further, the porosity of bone contains membrane-lined capillary vessels helping in the transportation of nutrition to the inside of bone. There exists a compartmental model for the bone fluid system whereby extracellular fluid in the calcified matrix is separated from membrane-lined vascular channels. When the bone is mechanically stressed, as part of different loading conditions, or therapeutically induced as in orthodontic treatment, remodeling changes are initiated by the bioelectric potentials generated from inside of the bone. The presence of bioelectric potentials in bone matrix, which also contains extracellular ionic fluid, will generate a charge separation at the matrix–fluid interface. There will be attraction of opposite-charged molecules at the matrix–fluid interface and repelling of similar charged molecules away from this interface. When the fluid is forced through a bone plug, the ionic charges in the fluid phase near the fluid–matrix interface are carried towards the low pressure end, which is otherwise known as Poiseuille flow. This flow constitutes the streaming current and accumulation of charges set up as an electrical field. This field will result in generation of conduction currents which flow in opposite directions through the bulk of liquid in the porous structure of bone. In steady state the conduction current is equal to the streaming current. The resulting electrostatic potential difference between these two sides of bone plug is known as streaming potential (Figure 2.20) (Walsh and Guzelsu, 1993). Briefly, streaming potential is the electric potential developed between two components by an electrolyte flowing between the solid surfaces. The movement of the electrostatic double layer at the fluid bone interface, created through the net surface charge gained by the bone surface in contact with an ionic fluid, generates this effect (Anderson and Eriksson, 1968). In bone, streaming potentials can be observed in vascular channels, Haversian systems, canaliculi, and microporosities of the structure due to blood flow and interstitial fluid movement. Neutrality is restored following equilibration of ion distribution.

Zeta potential, the common link among different electrokinetic potentials and the one used to allow comparison of different measuring techniques, is defined as average potential difference between the bulk and surface of shear. Surface of shear is an imaginary surface present in the area adjacent to electrically charged bone matrix,

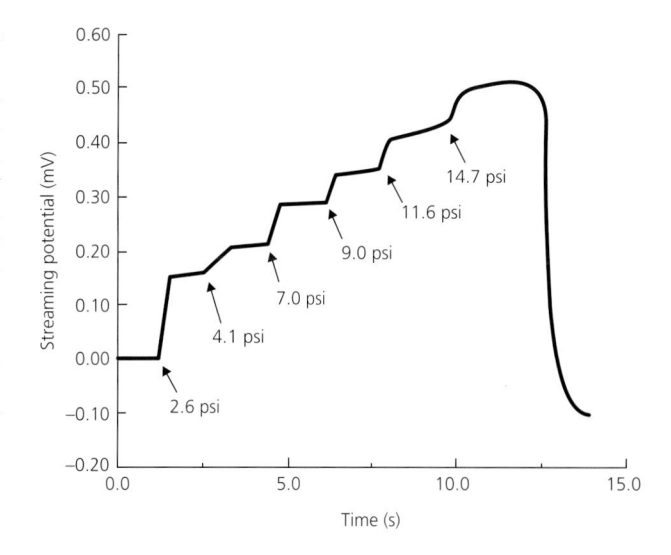

Figure 2.20 Results of a typical intact bone-streaming potential (mV) in pH 7.3, 0.145 M ionic strength buffer (physiologic conditions) versus time at various pressures (kPa). The arrows indicate when an increase in pressure (nitrogen gas) was placed on the sample. Streaming potential magnitude increased with an increase in pressure and a stable streaming potential was obtained. A positive streaming potential versus pressure response corresponds to a negative zeta potential and an exposed organic interface. Streaming potentials were consistently positive throughout all pressure levels in 0.145–0.6 M NaCl. (Source: Walsh and Guzelsu, 1993. Reproduced with permission of Elsevier.)

where the ions and fluid molecules remain stationary. The role of zeta potential is to separate the movement of ions bound to the solid surface from other ions that show normal viscous behavior under mechanical force application (Lech and Iwaniec, 2010). Zeta potential can be calculated from streaming potential experiments by knowing the applied pressure difference across the sample and generated streaming potentials (Hunter, 1981). Fluid conductivity and fluid viscosity determines the stress-generated potentials in fluid-filled bone, and it is possible to calculate the potential generated by the distortion of a fluid by the formula (McDonald, 1993):

$$V = \frac{z\varepsilon\delta P}{4\pi n\sigma}$$

where z is the zeta potential; V is the magnitude of the potential; δP is the pressure difference that forces the liquid through the channel; ε is the dielectric constant of the liquid; n is the viscosity of the liquid; σ is the specific conductance.

Scientists working in this field have concluded that piezoelectricity and streaming potentials are two coexisting phenomena and both play an important role in stress information transmission. They combined both phenomena as a bioelectric hypothesis, which states that structural alterations throughout the bone are conducted and/or triggered by ionic charge differences (Masella and Chung, 2008). Stress-generated electric potentials were first reported in dog mandibles and teeth by Cochran, Pawluk and Bassett (1968). They postulated that these stress-induced bioelectric potentials play a major role in regulating the orientation and functional demands of bone per se. Zengo et al. (1973) measured the electric potential in mechanically stressed dog alveolar bone during in vivo and in vitro experiments. They have demonstrated that the concave side of orthodontically treated bone is electronegative and favors osteoblastic activity, whereas the areas of positivity or electrical neutrality,

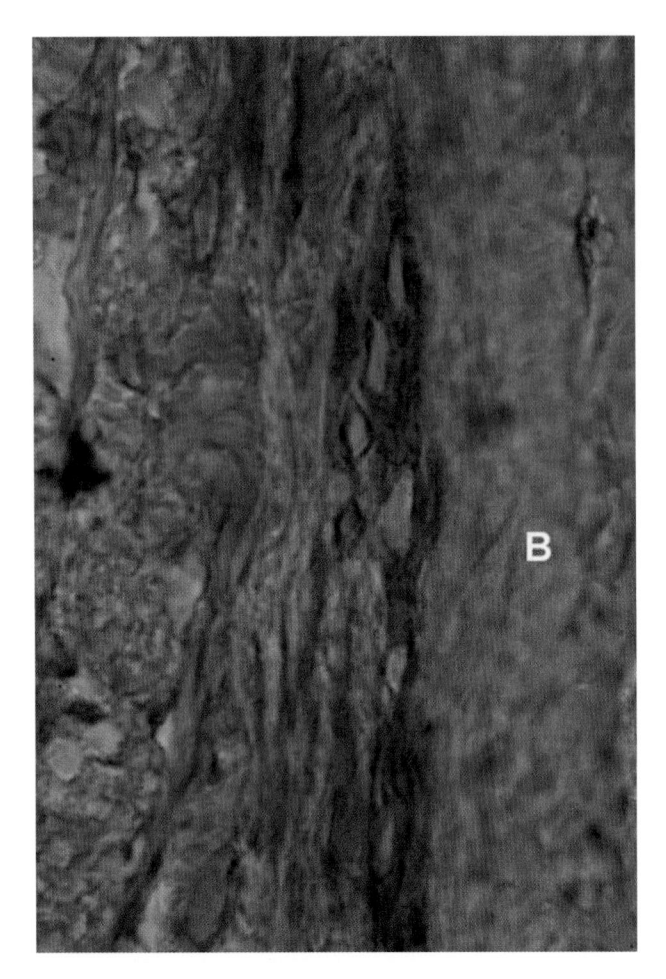

Figure 2.21 Transverse section, 6 μm thick, of a 1-year-old female cat's mandible, after a 7-day exposure to sham electrodes (control). Shown is the buccal periosteum of the second premolar opposite the sham cathode, stained immunohistochemically for cAMP. B, Alveolar bone. The bone surface lining cells are flat, and most stain lightly for cAMP.

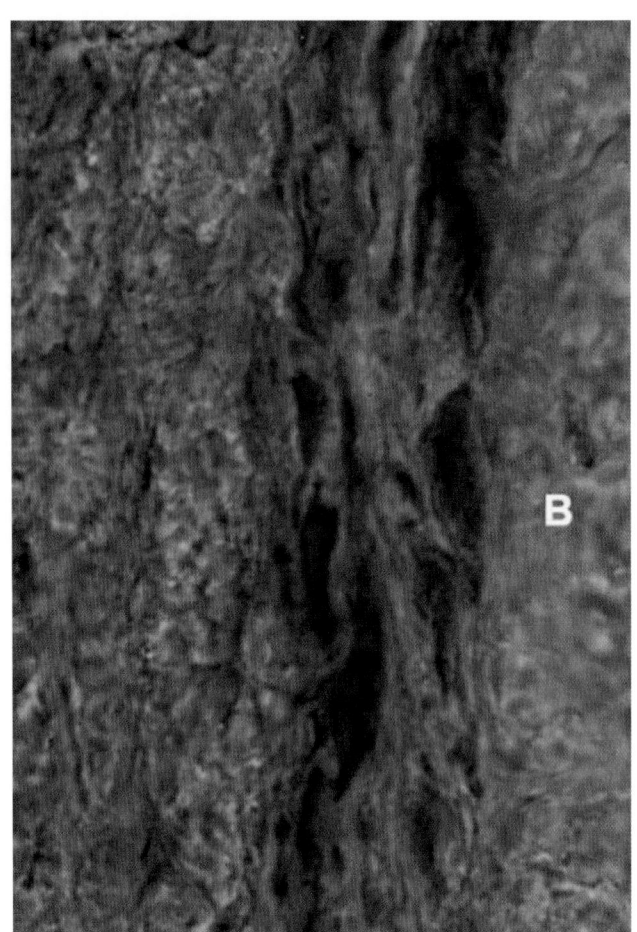

Figure 2.22 Transverse section, 6 μm thick, of a 1-year-old female cat's mandible (the same animal as shown in Figure 2.21), after exposure for 7 days to a constant application of a 20 μA direct current to the gingival mucosa, noninvasively. Shown are the tissues near the stainless-steel cathode, stained immunohistochemically for cAMP. B, Alveolar bone. Compared with the cells shown in Figure 2.21, the bone surface lining cells near the cathode are larger and more darkly stained for cAMP.

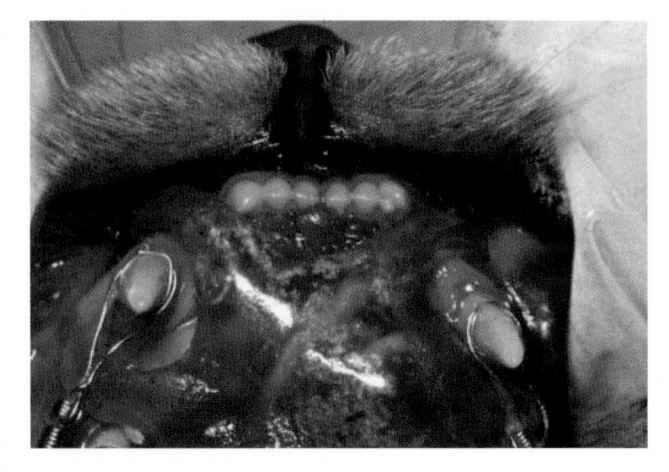

Figure 2.23 Constant direct current, 20 μA, noninvasively, to the gingival and oral mucosa labial to the left maxillary canine in a cat. The right canine (control) received the same electrodes, but without electrical current. Both canines were moved distally by an 80 g tipping force. The right canine, which had been subjected only to mechanical force, moved distally a smaller distance than the left canine, which had been administered a combination of mechanical force and electrical current.

i.e., convex surfaces, showed elevated osteoclastic activity (Figure 2.19). Shapiro, Roeber, and Klempner (1979) suggested that application of piezoelectric charges as pulses of force to the teeth can accelerate the osteogenic response. Based on their experiment in one patient, with application of 8 ounces of force, they reported increase in the rate of movement of maxillary second molar with less pain perception than that of the control teeth.

It has been proposed by Davidovitch et al. (1980a, b) that a physical relationship exists between mechanical and electrical perturbation of bone. Their experiments in female cats with administration of exogenous electrical currents in conjunction with orthodontic forces demonstrated enhanced cellular activities in the PDL and alveolar bone, as well as rapid tooth movement (Figures 2.21–2.23). Taken together, these findings led to the suggestion that bioelectric responses (piezoelectricity and streaming potentials) propagated by bone bending incident to orthodontic force application, might act as pivotal cellular first messengers.

Borgens (1984) investigated this phenomenon in bone fracture sites by inducing electric current for healing purposes. His experiments did not disclose any correlation with what had been proposed as piezoelectric effects and showed that the dispersion of current as it enters the lesion is unpredictable. He attributed this finding to the complexity of distribution of mineralized and non‐mineralized matrices. However, he observed generation of endogenous ionic currents evoked in intact and damaged mouse bones, and classified these currents as stress‐generated potentials or streaming potentials, rather than piezoelectric currents. In contrast to piezoelectric spikes, the streaming potentials were having long decay periods. This finding led him to hypothesize that the mechanically stressed bone cells themselves, not the matrix, are the source of the electric current. His hypothesis received support from Pollack et al. (1984), who proposed a mechanism by which force‐evoked electric potentials may reach the surface of bone cells. Accordingly, an electric double layer surrounds bone, where electric charges flow in coordination with stress‐related fluid flow. These stress‐generated potentials may affect the charge of cell membranes, and of macromolecules present in the neighborhood. Davidovitch et al. (1980a, b) suggested that piezoelectric potentials result from distortion of fixed structures of the periodontium, such as collagen, hydroxyapatite, or bone cells' surface. In hydrated tissues, however, streaming potentials (the electrokinetic effects that arise when an electrical double layer overlying a charged surface is displaced) predominate as the interstitial fluid moves. They further reported that mechanical perturbations of the order of about 1 min/day are apparently sufficient to cause an osteogenic response (Figure 2.24), perhaps due to matrix proteoglycan related strain memory.

The major criticism faced by both the piezoelectric as well as the streaming potentials theories was due to the highly conductive nature of the vascular system, periosteum, and tissue fluids. They often tend to drain away the change in potential difference. Researchers failed to establish whether the generated strain‐induced potentials were actual players in cellular remodelling or irrelevant by‐products of bone deformation. McDonald (1993) argued against the role of electrical signals in bone remodeling by stating that

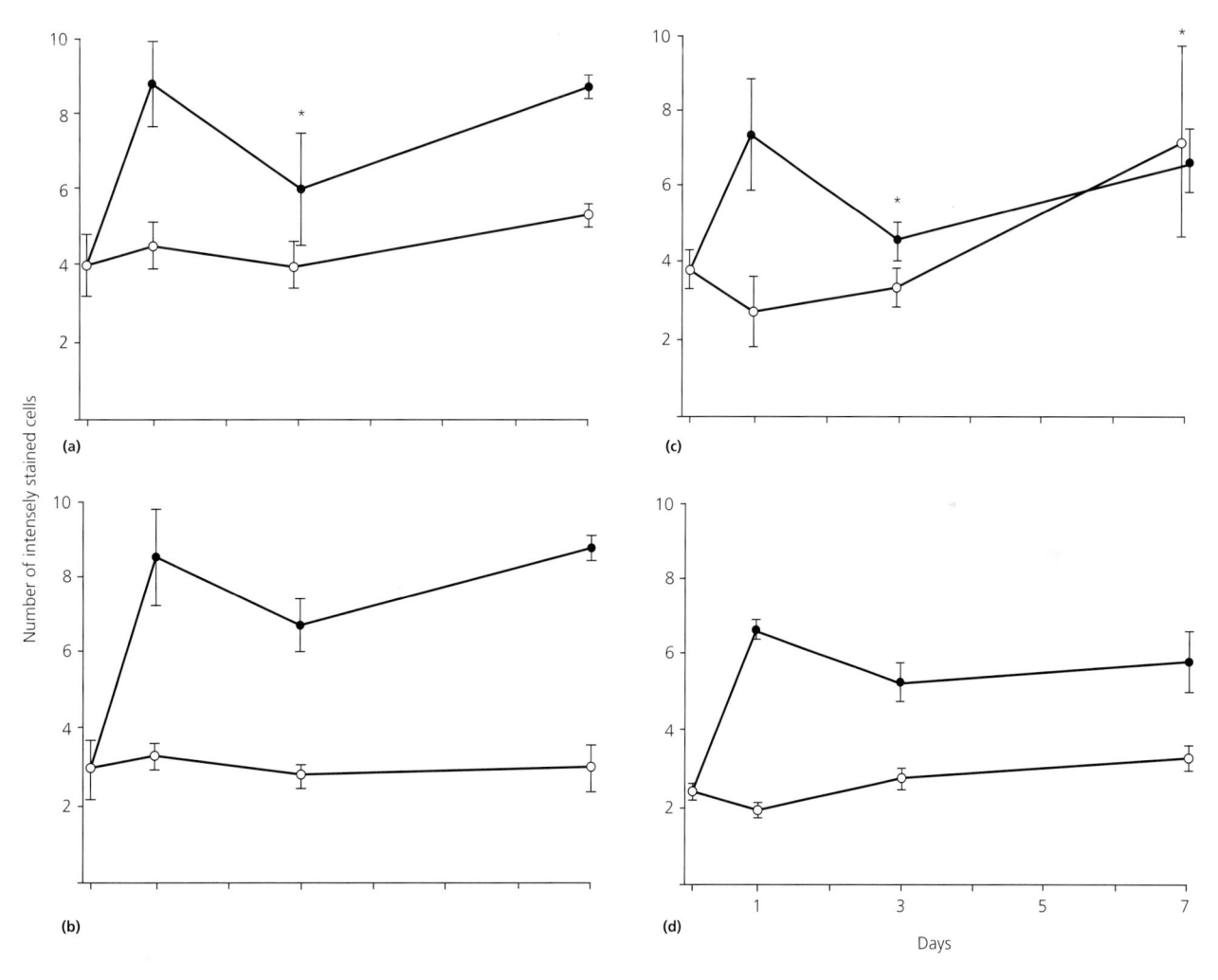

Figure 2.24 The number of alveolar bone osteoblasts bordering the PDL (±SEM) near cat maxillary canines, intensely stained for cAMP or cGMP following an electric stimulation. Cells were counted along a 0.1 mm surface opposite each electrode. Open circles, Control sites. Solid circles, Electrically treated sites. (a) Osteoblasts near cathode stained for cAMP. (b) Osteoblasts near anode, stained for cAMP. (c) Osteoblasts near cathode, stained for cGMP. (d) Osteoblasts near anode, stained for cGMP. Time periods when differences in number of cells intensely stained for cAMP and cGMP between electrically treated and control sites were not significant: cAMP near the cathode at day 3; cGMP at days 3 and 7 near the cathode. At the other time periods near the cathode and at all time periods near the anode, the differences between the treated and control sites were statistically significant ($P < 0.01$). It should be noted that all the bone surface cells are labeled as "osteoblasts," although it is quite possible that some cells near the anode are stimulated by the electric currents to resorb bone rather than to participate in the synthesis and mineralization of new bone matrix. However, the authors did not detect typical osteoclastic lacunae at the alveolar socket wall near the anode and thus defined all bone surface cells as osteoblasts. (Source: Davidovitch, 1980a. Reproduced with permission of Elsevier.)

"surface potential differences are very small compared to the potential differences generated with muscle activity." He concluded that the knowledge of action of electrical signaling inside the cells is inadequate and warrants further research into cellular behavior in response to applied mechanical forces.

It is evident from the ongoing discussion that neither of these hypotheses could provide conclusive evidence on the detailed nature of the biological mechanism of OTM. Histological, histochemical, and immunohistochemical studies performed in the twentieth century, as well as early in the twenty‑first century, have demonstrated that multiple phenomena, both physical and chemical, are involved in the process of tooth movement. When mechanical forces are applied, cells, as well as the ECM of the PDL and alveolar bone, respond concomitantly, resulting in tissue remodeling activities. During early phases of tooth movement, PDL fluids are shifted, producing cell and matrix distortions as well as interactions between these tissue elements. In response to these physicochemical events and interactions, cytokines, growth factors, colony stimulating factors, and vasoactive neurotransmitters are released, initiating and sustaining the remodeling activity, which facilitates the movement of teeth. A detailed discussion on these molecules along with the mechanisms of their operation is provided in Chapter 3.

Concluding remarks

Our ancestors noticed, two or three millennia ago, that malposed teeth can be straightened by the application of mechanical force to the crowns of those teeth. With the passage of time, a large variety of devices had been designed in order to correct malocclusions, and were usually claimed to be superior to other appliances aiming at the same targets. The inability to determine which of those gadgets would be best for clinical use was limited by the paucity of biological information that could support most of the claims made by their inventors. However, there was a breakthrough with the introduction of histology into orthodontics at the start of the twentieth century. The visualization of the response of tissues and cells to mechanical forces opened the gate to thoughtful proposals of hypotheses, to explain the reason for tooth movement. The two prevailing dogmas during the following decades were the "pressure–tension" and the "bone‑bending" hypotheses. Other hypotheses stemming from these two focused on the roles of the dynamics of tissue fluids and evoked electric potentials in the strained tissues in OTM. Altogether, each of these hypotheses improves our understanding of the fundamental principles of OTM. Additional building blocks to assist in crafting a unified theory based on biological evidence have been derived from research at the cellular and molecular levels, which is reviewed in the next chapter.

References

Anderson, J. C. and Eriksson, C. (1968) Electrical properties of wet collagen. *Nature* **218**, 166–168.
Anderson, J. C. and Eriksson, C. (1970) Piezoelectric properties of dry and wet bone. *Nature* **227**, 491–492.
Angle, E. H. (1907) *Treatment of Malocclusion of the Teeth: Angle's System*, 7th edn, White Dental Manufacturing Co., Philadelphia.
Basset, C. A. L. (1968) Biologic significance of piezoelectricity. *Calcified Tissue Research* **1**, 252–272.
Basset, C. A. L. and Becker, R. O. (1962) Generation of electric potentials by bone in response to mechanical stress. *Science* **137**, 1063–1065.
Baumrind, S. (1969) A reconsideration of the property of the pressure tension hypothesis. *American Journal of Orthodontics* **55**, 12–22.
Bien, S. M. (1966) Hydrodynamic damping of tooth movement. *Journal of Dental Research* **44**(3), 907–914.
Borgens, R. B. (1984) Endogenous ionic currents traverse intact and damaged bone. *Science* **225**, 478–482.
Cochran, G. V. B., Pawluk, R. J. and Bassett, C. A. L. (1968) Electromechanical characteristics of bone under physiologic moisture conditions. *Clinical Orthopedics* **58**, 249–270.
Davidovitch, Z. (1991) Tooth movement. *Critical Reviews in Oral Biology and Medicine*, **2**, 411–450.
Davidovitch, Z., Finkelson, M.D., Steigman, S. et al. (1980a) Electric currents, bone remodeling and orthodontic tooth movement. I—The effect of electric currents on periodontal nucleotides. *American Journal of Orthodontics* **77**, 14–32.
Davidovitch, Z., Finkelson, M. D., Steigman, S. Et al. (1980b) Electric currents, bone remodeling and orthodontic tooth movement. II—Increase in rate of tooth movement and periodontal cyclic nucleotide levels by combined force and electric current. *American Journal of Orthodontics* **77**, 33–47.
Epker, B. N. and Frost, H. M. (1965) Correlation of bone resorption and formation with the physical behavior of loaded bone. *Journal of Dental Research* **44**, 33–41.
Farrar, J. N. (1888) *Irregularities of the Teeth and Their Correction*, DeVinne Press, New York, Vol. **1**, Chapter 62, p. 658.
Frost, H. M. (1983) The regional acceleratory phenomenon: a review. *Henry Ford Hospital Medical Journal* **31**, 3–9.
Fukada, E. and Hara, A. (1969) Piezoelectric effects in blood vessel walls. *Journal of Physics Society of Japan* **26**, 777–780.
Fukada, E. and Yasuda, I. (1957) On the piezoelectric effect on bone. *Journal of Physics Society of Japan* **12**, 1158–1162.
Gross, D. and Williams, W. S. (1982) Streaming potential and the electromechanical response of physiologically‑moist bone. *Journal of Biomechanics* **15**(4), 277–295.
Hays, D. F. (1961) Squeeze films, a finite bearing with a fluctuating load. *Transactions of the American Society of Mechanical Engineering Series D* **83**, 579–588.
Hecht, H. (1900) Über die Vorgänge, die sich bei der künstlichen regulierung der Zähne in dem Alveolarfortsatz abspielen. *Korrenspondenzblatt für Zahnarzte.*
Hunter, R. J. (1981) *Zeta Potential in Colloid Science*, Academic Press, New York, NY.
Isaacs, A. (1987) *Concise Science Dictionary*, Oxford University Press, Oxford.
Kingsley, N. W. (1881) Die Anomalien der Zahnstellung und Defecte des Gaumens, A. Felix, Leipzig.
Krishnan, V. and Davidovitch, Z. (2006) The cellular, molecular and tissue level reactions to orthodontic force. *American Journal of Orthodontics and Dentofacial Orthopedics* **129**, e1–32.
Lech, L. and Iwaniec, M. (2010) The Meaning of the Piezoelectric Effect and Streaming Potential in Bone Remodeling. Twenty‑Fourth Symposium on Vibrations in Physical Systems, Poznan–Bedlewo, May 12–15.
Marino, A. A. and Becker, R. O. (1975) Piezoelectricity in hydrated bone and tendon. *Nature* **253**, 627–628.
Masella, R. S. and Chung, P. L. (2008) Thinking beyond the wire: Emerging biologic relationships in orthodontics and periodontology. *Seminars in Orthodontics* **14**, 290–304.
McDonald, F. (1993) Electrical effects at the bone surface. *European Journal of Orthodontics* **15**(3), 175–183.
Meikle, M. C. (2006) The tissue, cellular and molecular regulation of orthodontic tooth movement: 100 years after Carl Sandstedt. *European Journal of Orthodontics* **28**, 221–240.
Melsen, B. (1999) Biological reaction of alveolar bone to orthodontic tooth movement. *The Angle Orthodontist* **69**, 151–158.
Oppenheim, A. (1911) Tissue changes, particularly of the bone, incident to tooth movement. *Transactions of the European Orthodontic Society* 303–359. [Reprinted (2007) *European Journal of Orthodontics* **29**, i2–i15.]
Oppenheim, A. (1944) A possibility for physiologic tooth movement. *American Journal of Orthodontics and Oral Surgery* **30**(6), 277–328.
Pfaff, W. (1906) *Lehrbuch des Orthodontie*, Zentralstelle für Zahnhygiene, Dresden.
Pollack, S. R., Salzstein, R. and Pienkowski, D. (1984) The electric double layer in bone and its influence on stress generated potentials. *Calcified Tissue International* **36**, 577–581.
Proffit, W. R. (2013) Biological basis of orthodontic therapy, in *Contemporary Orthodontics* (ed. W. R. Proffit), 5th edn. Elsevier Mosby, St. Louis, MO, pp. 278–311.
Reitan, K. (1957) Some factors determining the evaluation of force in orthodontics. *American Journal of Orthodontics* **44**, 32–45.
Reitan, K. (1960) Tissue behavior during orthodontic tooth movement. *American Journal of Orthodontics* **46**, 881–890.
Sandstedt, C. (1904) Einige Beiträge zur Theorie der Zahnregulierung. *Nordisk Tandläkare Tidskrift* **5**, 236–256.
Sandstedt, C. (1905) Einige Beiträge zur Theorie der Zahnregulierung. *Nordisk Tandläkare Tidskrift* **6**, 1–25, 141–168.

Schwarz, A. M. (1932) Tissue changes incidental to orthodontic tooth movement. *International Journal of Orthodontia, Oral Surgery and Radiography* **18**(4), 331–352.

Shamos, M. H. and Lavine, L. S. (1964) Physical basis for bioelectric effect in mineralized tissues. *Clinical Orthopedics and Related Research* **35**, 177–188.

Shamos, M. H., Lavine, L. S. and Shamos, M. I. (1963) Piezoelectric effects in bone. *Nature* **197**, 81.

Shapiro, E., Roeber, F. W. and Klempner, L. S. (1979). Orthodontic movement using pulsating force-induced piezoelectricity. *American Journal of Orthodontics* **76**(1), 59–66.

Thompson, D'Arcy W. (1917). *On Growth and Form*, Cambridge University Press, Cambridge (Dover reprint).

Walkhoff, O. (1890) Über die Veränderungen der Gewebe, insbesonder des Knochengewebes beim Richten der Zähne. Deutsche Monatsschrift für Zahnheilkunde.

Walkhoff, O. (1891) *Die Unregelmässigkeiten in den Zahnstellungen und ihre Behandlung*, Felix, Leipzig.

Walsh, W. R. and Guzelsu, N. (1993) Ion concentration effects on bone streaming potentials and zeta potentials. *Biomaterials* **14**, 331–336.

Wise, G. E. and King, G. J. (2008) Mechanisms of tooth eruption and orthodontic tooth movement. *Journal of Dental Research* **87**(5), 414–434.

Zengo, A. N., Pawluk, R. J. and Bassett, C. A. (1973) Stress induced bioelectric potentials in the dentoalveolar complex. *American Journal of Orthodontics* **64**, 17–27.

PART 2

Mechanics Meets Biology

CHAPTER 3
Cellular and Molecular Biology of Orthodontic Tooth Movement

Jaap C. Maltha, Vinod Krishnan, and Anne Marie Kuijpers-Jagtman

Summary

Orthodontic tooth movement is the result of a goal-oriented application of an external force to a complex biological system. For a proper understanding of the processes underlying this complicated system, knowledge of its constituents is necessary. Therefore, this chapter begins with a description of the morphology and physical characteristics of fiber systems and the ground substance of the extracellular matrix, and a description of the different cell types involved in the synthesis and turnover of this matrix. Also, the biomechanical characteristics of the periodontal ligament are described.

Orthodontic tooth movement is a result of mutual interactions between cells and between cells and the extracellular matrix. General systems of cell–cell and cell–matrix interactions are described in detail. Tooth movement and the different phases that can be distinguished in this process are explained. Each phase is characterized by specific cell biological regulatory systems. Particular attention will be given to the linear phase in which a mechanosensory system is responsible for a cascade of events that ultimately leads to bone resorption at the leading side and bone deposition at the trailing side of the moving tooth.

Introduction

Orthodontic tooth movement (OTM) is the result of externally applied forces on a complex biological system that contains the alveolar bone, the periodontal ligament (PDL), the tooth, and the gingiva. Under physiologic conditions, this complex is adapting to ever changing mechanical conditions due to chewing, swallowing, and muscle activities in and around the oral cavity. The application of orthodontic forces leads to a cascade of reactions in the extracellular matrix (ECM) and the cells in the dento-alveolar complex.

In orthodontics, the fields of biology and mechanics are intertwined, and research keeps unfolding the details of this relationship. The chief questions are about the nature of the biological response of a living organism to applied mechanical forces, and what the features of an optimal force are, for each individual patient. Basic research, at the cellular and molecular levels, has revealed meaningful information about the mechanism of mechanotransduction, and about the signaling systems controlling the interactions between cells during periods of tissue remodeling. This chapter reviews details of the biological responses of paradental tissues and cells to applications of mechanical forces *in vitro* and *in vivo*.

Entities important for tooth movement – the players in the game

Extracellular matrix

The PDL, the root cementum, and the alveolar bone consist, like all connective tissues, of cells and ECM of which the principal component is formed by fibers, embedded in a gel-like ground substance (Kerrigan et al., 2000; Nanci and Bosshardt, 2006).

The most predominant type of fiber in the alveolar bone, the PDL, and the root cementum is collagen type I, which is mainly present as strong extracellular fibers (Figure 3.1A). This protein is synthetized by fibroblasts starting with the intracellular synthesis of triple helices called procollagen, containing two type-α1 and one type-α2 "pre-procollagen" peptide chains. Procollagen is secreted by exocytosis. Outside the cell, procollagen is assembled into collagen fibrils and subsequently, by crosslinking, into collagen fibers. These fibers have a very well organized and complex internal structure that resembles a hawser. This structure results in flexible fibers with a great tensile strength (Kerrigan et al., 2000; Wenger et al., 2007; Dean, 2017).

Biological Mechanisms of Tooth Movement, Third Edition. Edited by Vinod Krishnan, Anne Marie Kuijpers-Jagtman and Ze'ev Davidovitch.
© 2021 John Wiley & Sons Ltd. Published 2021 by John Wiley & Sons Ltd.

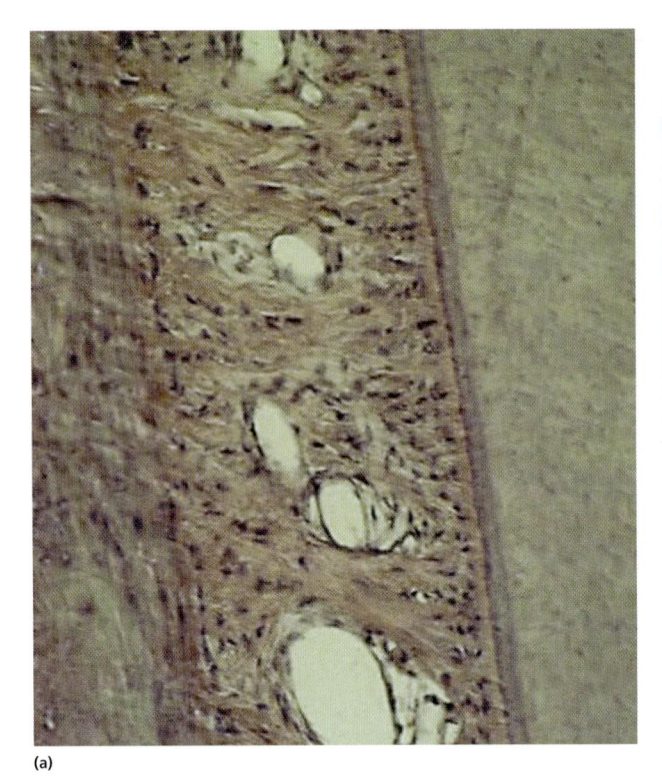

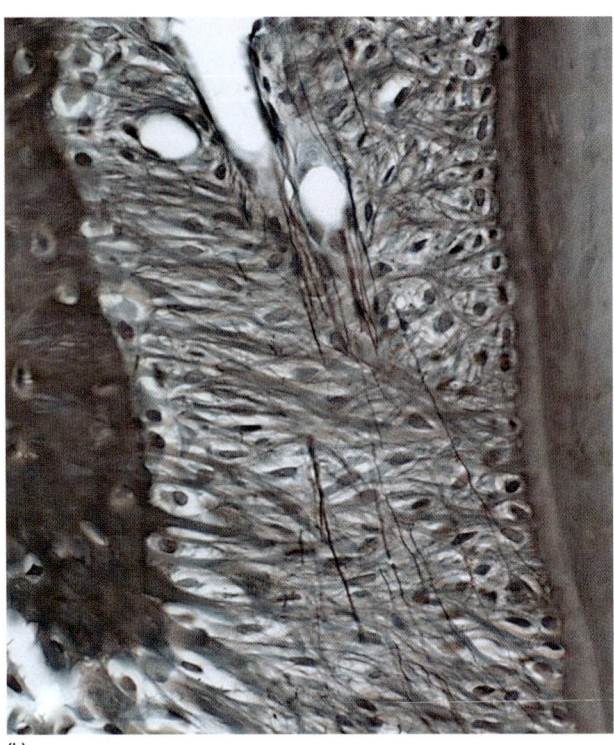

Figure 3.1 Photomicrographs of the normal PDL in a dog, showing the main orientation of the collagen fibers (A, H & E staining) and the oxytalan fibers (B, Oxone-Halmi Aldehyde Fuchsin staining). (Source: Jaap Maltha.)

A second type of fiber in the PDL is the oxytalan fiber (Figure 3.1B). This type of fiber belongs to the elastic fiber family, which consists of elastic, elaunin, and oxytalan fibers. The elastic and elaunin fibers mainly contain elastin and fibrillins, while the oxytalan fibers lack elastin and only contain fibrillin-1 and fibrillin-2. These glycoproteins are synthetized in fibroblasts and polymerize after exocytosis, and, through lateral association and the incorporation of other components, they form microfibrils. Individual microfibrils again associate with one another to form microfibril bundles, the oxytalan fibers (Marson et al., 2005; Hubmacher et al., 2006; Kielty, 2006; Strydom et al., 2012).

The ground substance is primarily composed of water and large organic molecules, such as glycosaminoglycans (GAGs), including hyaluronic acid, heparan sulfate, dermatan sulfate, and chondroitin sulfate. Most of the GAGs are bound to proteins and then called proteoglycans. They are able to bind a considerable amount of water, giving the ground substance a gel-like texture (Nanci and Bosshardt, 2006; Bergomi et al., 2010; Ortun-Terrazas et al., 2018).

In the PDL, but also in all other connective tissues, the fibrous components are embedded in the "ground substance", a network of proteoglycans, such as heparan sulfate, dermatan sulfate, and chondroitin sulfate, consisting of a core protein covalently bound to GAG chains. These GAGs can form large complexes when hundreds of GAG molecules become noncovalently attached to a single long polysaccharide molecule, such as hyaluronic acid. Under physiological conditions, GAGs have a strong water-binding capacity as the GAG chains are negatively charged due to the presence of sulfate and uronic acid groups (Nanci and Bosshardt, 2006; Bergomi et al., 2010; Ortun-Terrazas et al., 2018). They form an amorphous gel-like structure, of which the stiffness depends on the amount of bound water. Apart from the bound water, also free water is present in the ground substance. The viscoelastic characteristics recorded for the PDL essentially result from interactions between unbound fluid and the compressible visco-elastic porous matrix that makes up the bulk of the ground substance. Proteoglycans of the ground substance also bind to fibrous matrix proteins, such as collagen and oxytalan (Svensson et al., 2001). Together, these components form the ECM, which acts as a substrate for PDL cells and allows them to migrate and to communicate with each other (Kerrigan et al., 2000; Waddington and Embery, 2001; Nanci and Bosshardt, 2006; Dean, 2017; Listik et al., 2019).

Finally, the PDL contains extensive vascular and neural systems. The blood vessels originate from three sources: apical vessels, which branch from vessels that supply the pulp; perforating vessels, which originate from the lamina and perforate the cribriform plate in the socket wall; and the gingival vessels, which come from the gingival tissue. Blood vessels in PDL may help in mechanical suspension and support of the tooth and supply surrounding PDL. These vessels transport blood cells, nutrients, and oxygen to the tissues of the PDL and remove waste and carbon dioxide (Lee et al., 1991; Selliseth and Selvig, 1994; Dean, 2017)

The neural system in the PDL contains free and specialized nerve endings. Free nerve endings are nociceptive and are present along the whole length of the tooth. The specialized nerve endings are divided in Ruffini-like endings, coiled nerve endings, spindle-shaped nerve endings, and expanded nerve endings. The Ruffini-like endings are mainly present near the root apex and secrete various neuropeptides, such as calcitonin gene-related peptide (CGRP) and substance P. The coiled type endings are mainly located in the mid-region of the PDL. Both act as mechanoreceptors and as fast acting nociceptors (Maeda et al., 1990; Davidovitch, 1991; Maeda et al., 1999; Krishnan and Davidovitch, 2006; Yamaguchi et al., 2012 Dean, 2017)

Cells

The fibroblast is the major cell type in all connective tissues, including the PDL. Fibroblasts differentiate from mesenchymal stem cells and are responsible for the synthesis and secretion of all the elements of the ECM, collagen and oxytalan fibers, and proteoglycans. Furthermore, fibroblasts synthesize and secrete a wide variety of regulatory molecules that act as local signals for the adaptation of the tissue to changing conditions (Lekic and McCulloch, 1996; Jiang et al., 2016).

Osteoblasts are large cells (20–30 μm), in the form of a polyhedron, with a basophilic cytoplasm, and with a substantial rough endoplasmic reticulum and Golgi apparatus. They originate from the mesenchymal stem cells of the bone marrow, endosteum, periosteum, and perivascular pericytes (Fernández-Tresguerres-Hernández-Gil et al., 2006a). They differ from fibroblasts because they can express RUNX2, which is essential for the differentiation of mature osteoblasts. RUNX2 is the first transcription factor that is upregulated in pre-osteoblasts and it is downregulated again in mature osteoblasts (Li et al., 2018). The osteoblasts synthesize and secrete the collagen and noncollagen proteins, such as osteocalcin and osteopontin, that form the organic bone matrix or osteoid material. Furthermore, they express alkaline phosphatase (ALP), which is essential for the mineralization of the osteoid (Lerner et al., 2019). Osteoblasts also produce and secrete hydroxyapatite into the osteoid, forming the strong and well-organized mineralized matrix of the bone (Hasegawa, 2018). Part of the osteoblasts are buried in the bone matrix as osteocytes, maintaining contact with each other and osteoblasts through extended cellular processes that lie in narrow canals within the bone matrix, the canaliculi (Figure 3.2).

Although osteocytes are relatively inert cells, they are capable of transmission of signals over long distances through the canalicular network (Lerner, 2012). They are considered to be mechanosensory cells that play an important role in the regulation of the activity of osteoblasts and osteoclasts (Burger and Klein-Nulend, 1999; Klein-Nulend et al., 2013; Tresguerres et al., 2020) (Figure 3.3).

Osteoclasts are multinucleated cells that are derived from hemopoietic stem cells, and more specifically from extravasated monocytes that can differentiate into macrophages and through fusion into osteoclasts. They are responsible for the resorption of bone. The formation of an effective seal around the resorption compartment is essential, because it enables the formation of an isolated compartment between the bone and the cell, called Howship's lacuna. The cell membrane of the Howship's lacuna becomes highly invaginated and forms the so-called ruffled border, allowing massive secretory and endocytotic activity. This enables the vesicular transcytosis of the mineral and degraded collagen from the ruffled border to the free membrane of the cell, and its release into the extracellular compartment (Roodman, 1993; Duong et al., 2000; Fernández-Tresguerres-Hernández-Gil et al., 2006b; Takahashi

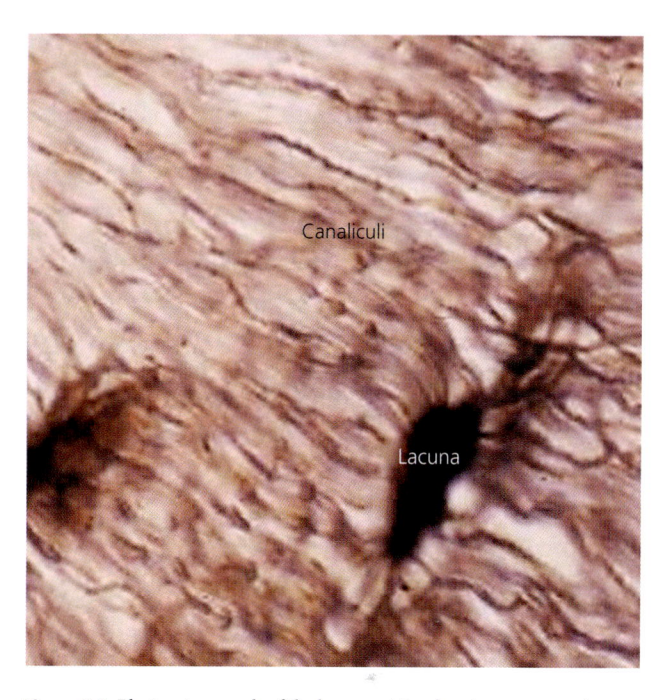

Figure 3.2 Photomicrograph of the bone matrix, showing osteocyte lacuna and lacuna–canalicular network. (Source: Jaap Maltha.)

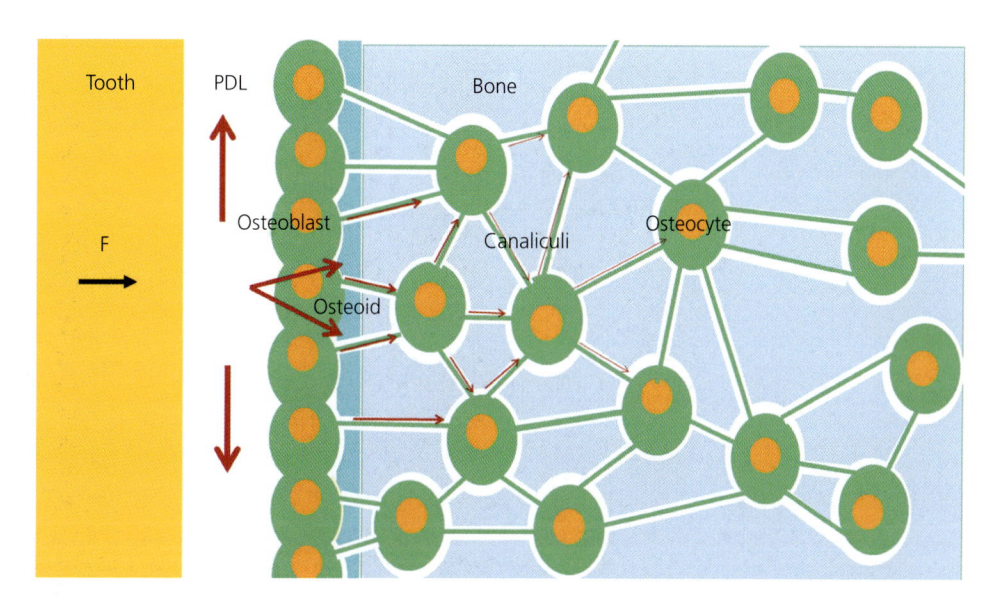

Figure 3.3 Fluid flow (arrows) after the application of an orthodontic force (F). Apart from a very rapid redistribution of fluid within the PDL, a limited fluid flow in the lacuna-canalicular system leads to shear stress as a message for the mechanosensory system. (Source: Jaap Maltha.)

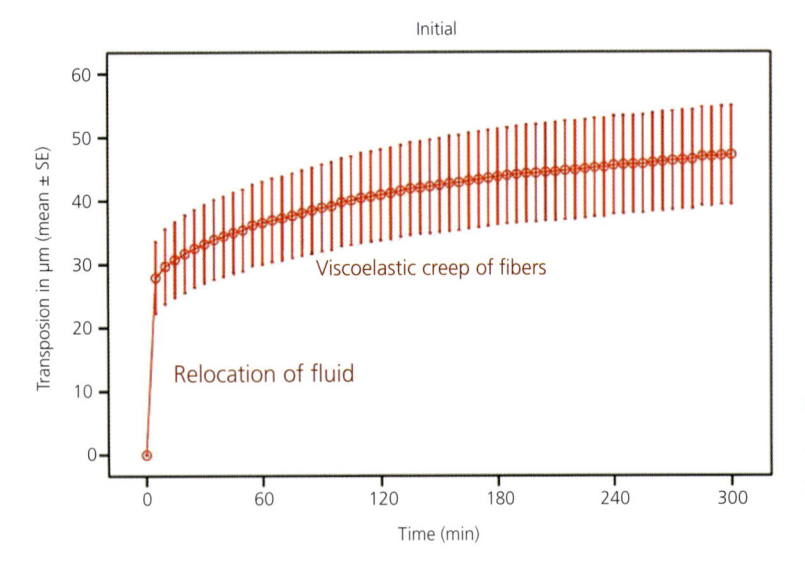

Figure 3.4 The transposition of a dog premolar during the first 5 hours after the application of an orthodontic force. Two phases can be recognized: an initial phase lasting only a few seconds with a very rapid tooth movement, and a second phase in which the rate of tooth movement gradually decreases until it stabilizes. (Source: Jaap Maltha.)

et al., 2007). For an elaborate overview on the concerted interplay between osteoblasts, osteocytes, and osteoclasts see Lerner (2012) and Chapter 4 of this book.

In addition, cementoblasts are part of the PDL and are derived from the mesenchymal dental follicle. They cover the root surface and are responsible for cementogenesis, through processes more or less comparable with osteogenesis. Some cementoblasts are buried in the cementum matrix to form cementocytes, especially in the more apical areas of the root. Similarly to osteocytes, they show thin cell processes in the ECM. However, they are far less extensive than in bone and do not form an intercellular network (Nanci and Bosshardt, 2006; Yamamoto et al., 2016).

Macrophages are a type of white blood cells that have the same origin as osteoclasts, namely extravasated monocytes. They are essential as phagocytes in defense against pathogenic microorganisms, in clearance of dead or senescent cells, and in removal of cell debris. Furthermore, they promote homeostasis through their trophic, regulatory, and repair functions (Gordon and Martinez-Pomares, 2017; Gordon and Plüddemann, 2017)

Biomechanical characteristics of the PDL

Orthodontic forces are applied in an environment where the mechanical properties depend on the material properties, sizes, and shapes of the constituent entities within the dento-alveolar units (Viecilli et al., 2008, 2013). The initial effect of the application of an orthodontic force is deformation or strain in the PDL and, to a lesser extent, the alveolar bone. This deformation depends on the biomechanical characteristics of the PDL, which in turn are dependent on the constituents of the extracellular compartment, i.e. fluid, fibers, and ground substance. This complicates mechanical behavior. In most biomechanical literature on the PDL a linear elastic behavior is assumed, which is an oversimplification of the real situation.

Experimental studies have described the time-dependent behavior of the PDL in the first period after orthodontic force application (van Driel et al., 2000; Jónsdóttir et al., 2006; Bergomi et al., 2010). Two subperiods can be recognized: the first lasts for only a few seconds when a rapid transposition within the socket indicates a redistribution of free-floating fluid; the second lasts for about 5 hours and shows a decelerating transposition, indicating viscoelastic behavior of the ECM of the PDL, with the collagen fibers leading to fiber-reinforced properties (Jónsdóttir et al., 2006; Jonsdottir et al., 2012) (Figure 3.4).

Therefore, the most likely model for the biomechanical properties of the normal PDL would be a biphasic poroviscoelastic fiber-reinforced material (van Driel et al., 2000; Wang et al., 2012; Ortún-Terrazas et al., 2018; Uhlir et al., 2017; Wu et al., 2019).

However, a serious drawback of all the literature pertaining to the mechanical properties of the PDL is that it is exclusively based on the normal state. The dramatic changes in the structure and composition of the PDL during OTM have never been taken into account.

General regulatory mechanisms

Cell–cell interactions

Cell–cell interactions allow cells to communicate with each other in response to changes in their microenvironment. These interactions can be stable through intercellular junctions, such as tight junctions, desmosomes, and gap junctions. They can also be variable, through the binding of soluble proteins secreted by one cell to receptor proteins on another cell. Such interactions allow cells to communicate with adjacent cells (autocrine actions), nearby cells (paracrine actions) (Tse and Wong, 2019), and even distant cells via the vascular system (endocrine actions). The latter actions are dealing with hormonal regulation.

For OTM, autocrine and paracrine interactions are essential. Secreted regulatory factors can bind to specific receptors on the target cell. These receptors are transmembrane structures containing proteins, carbohydrates, and lipids that project into the extracellular compartment. The binding of the signaling molecule to the receptor induces conformational changes in the receptor which, in turn, elicits a response in the corresponding cell. These responses include changes in cytoskeletal structure and subsequently change gene expression (McGeachie and Tennant, 1997; Meikle, 2006; Jiang et al., 2015).

Two groups of local regulatory proteins are distinguished, namely growth factors and cytokines. The growth factors mainly affect cellular growth, proliferation, differentiation, and maturation, while the cytokines are primarily associated with hematopoietic and immunological processes. The latter can act as proinflammatory or as anti-inflammatory mediators, and they can enhance cellular immune and antibody responses. The distinction between growth factors and cytokines is not very strict, since some cytokines can also act as growth factors and stimulate or inhibit cell growth and differentiation.

Growth factors and cytokines are grouped in several families. The most important factors involved in bone remodeling and thus in OTM belong to the transforming growth factor-β (TGFβ) super family including TGFβs and bone morphogenetic proteins (BMPs), epidermal growth factors (EGF) including EGF and transforming growth factor-α (TGFα), fibroblast growth factors (FGFs), insulin-like growth factors (IGFs), vascular endothelial growth factors (VEGFs), tumor necrosis factors (TNFs), and colony-stimulating factors (CSFs) (Roodman, 1993; McGeachie and Tennant, 1997; Hadjidakis and Androulakis, 2006; Jiang et al., 2015).

Another group of local regulatory molecules consists of the eicosanoids. They synthetize from arachidonic acid that is released from cell membranes through phospholipase A2. Free arachidonic acid can be converted to bioactive eicosanoids through the so-called arachidonic cascade, chains of enzymatic reactions, resulting in different subgroups of signaling molecules such as prostacyclines, thromboxanes, lipoxanes, and leukotrienes. For OTM, the most important subgroup is formed by the prostaglandins, which are formed through the activity of cyclooxygenases (COX1 and COX2) and prostaglandin synthase (Harizi et al., 2008; Xia et al., 2016; Vansant et al., 2018). Prostaglandins are synthesized within a large variety of cells. After exocytose they can bind to prostaglandin receptors on different target cells, in which a wide variety of effects can be induced (Binderman et al., 1988; Mundy, 1993; Hadjidakis and Androulakis, 2006)

Cell–matrix interactions

The ECM provides a scaffold for cell adhesion, which can occur in two ways: by hemidesmosomes, connecting the ECM to intermediate filaments such as keratin, and by focal adhesions, connecting the ECM to actin filaments within the cell. The latter is the most important for OTM. In both types of adhesion, specific cellular adhesion molecules known as integrins are essential (Barczyk et al., 2013; Walko et al., 2015).

Integrins are transmembrane proteins formed as heterodimers of specific α and β transmembrane proteins that bind cells to ECM structures (Figure 3.5). Integrins can contain many combinations of 18 different α subunits and eight β subunits. For example, osteoblasts have mainly α2β1 integrins, and osteoclasts have mainly αVβ3 integrins (Duong et al., 2000).

Integrins act as receptors for ECM glycoproteins such as fibronectin, vitronectin, and proteins such as collagen and laminin, which contain the amino acid sequence arginine, glycine, aspartate (RGD motif). They can also bind to integrins on the surface of other cells (Duong et al., 2000; Kechagia et al., 2019)

Intracellularly, integrins induce the formation of focal adhesion complexes which consist of the intracellular part of the integrins, focal adhesion kinase, which triggers intracellular mechanotransduction, by activating downstream mechanotransducers and many cytoplasmic proteins, such as tallin, vinculin, paxillin, and alpha-actinin (Figure 3.6)

The focal adhesion complex binds the integrin to actin filaments, the most important constituent of the cytoskeleton (Meikle, 2006;

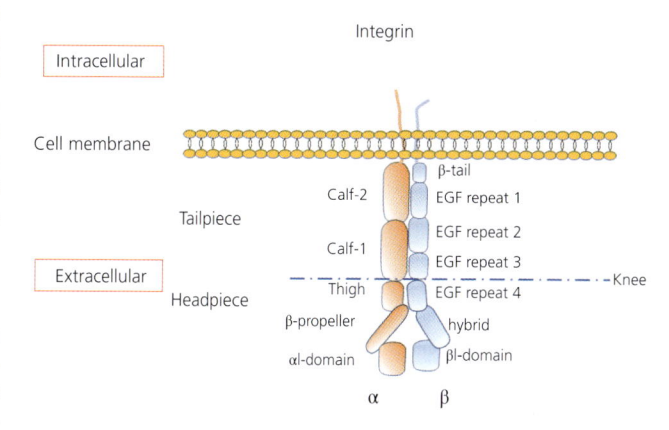

Figure 3.5 Integrin and its subunits. (Source: Jaap Maltha.)

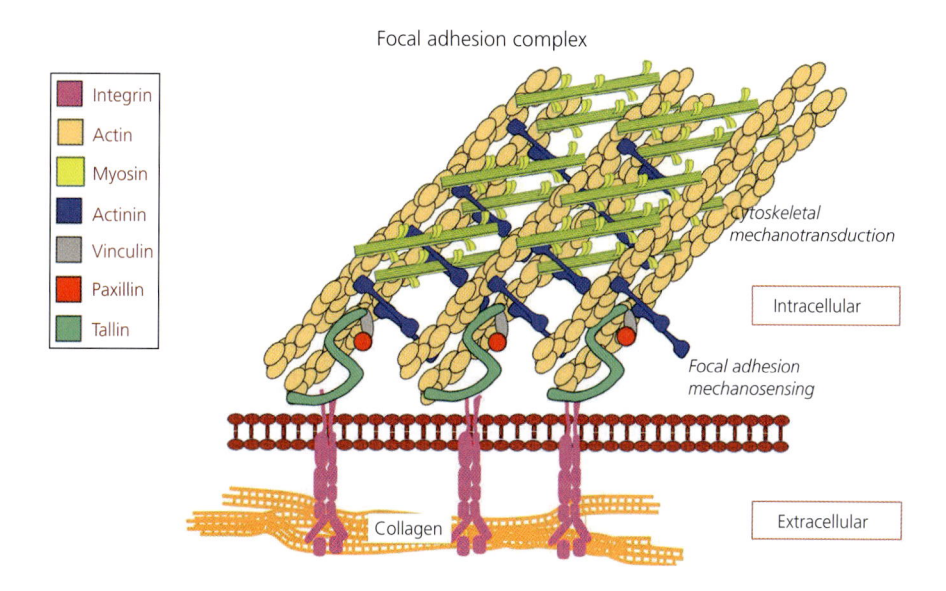

Figure 3.6 The focal adhesion complex. (Source: Jaap Maltha.)

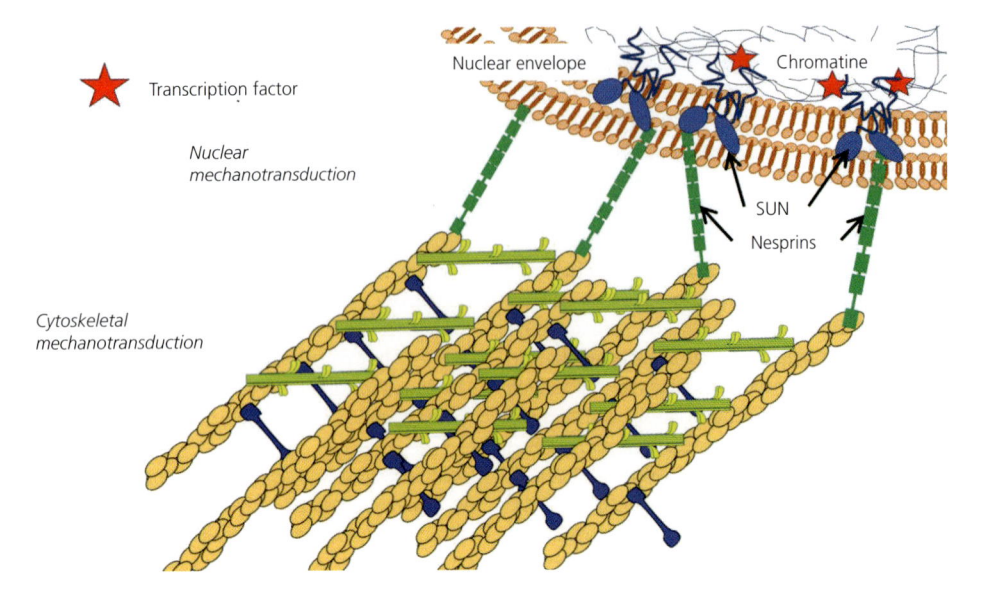

Figure 3.7 The nucleus-related part of the cytoskeleton. (Source: Jaap Maltha.)

Martino *et al.*, 2018). Focal adhesions as well as the cytoskeleton are constantly remodeled under the influence of the ECM: proteins associate and disassociate with it continually as signals are transmitted to other parts of the cell. Furthermore, the cytoskeleton can contract by F-actin sliding on the motor protein myosin II. These processes are responsible for cell deformation and cell migration (Burridge and Chrzanowska-Wodnicka, 1996). Gradients of different environmental cues, such as diffusible ligands (chemotaxis), substrate-bound ligands in the ECM (haptotaxis), or ECM rigidity (durotaxis) dictate the direction of migration (Kechagia *et al.*, 2019).

It is essential that the composition and the distribution of the focal adhesions within a cell change to allow its migration. Initially, new focal adhesion complexes and cytoskeletal structures are formed at cellular protrusions, the lamellipodia. They mature and remain stationary with respect to the ECM through integrins. The cell uses this as an anchor on which it can push or pull itself over the ECM. At the same time, focal adhesion complexes at the trailing edge are disassembled, together with the cytoskeletal structures, allowing cell migration along the ECM (Martino *et al.*, 2018; Kechagia *et al.*, 2019).

Furthermore, the cytoskeleton is linked to the nuclear envelope by SUN and nesprin proteins. They transfer mechanical stimuli from the cytoskeleton to the nucleus where mechanosensitive transcription factors activate mechanosensitive genes (Feller *et al.*, 2015; Martino *et al.*, 2018) (Figure 3.7).

Effects of orthodontic force application

Phases of OTM

In 1962, Burstone suggested that, if the rates of OTM were plotted against time, there would be three phases of OTM: the initial phase, a lag phase, and a post-lag phase. The initial phase is characterized by a period of very rapid movement, which occurs immediately after application of force to the tooth. This rate is attributed to the displacement of the tooth within the PDL space and bending of the alveolar bone. This phase is followed by a lag period, when no or low rates of tooth displacement occur. This lag results from hyalinization of the PDL in areas of compression. No further tooth movement will occur until cells complete the

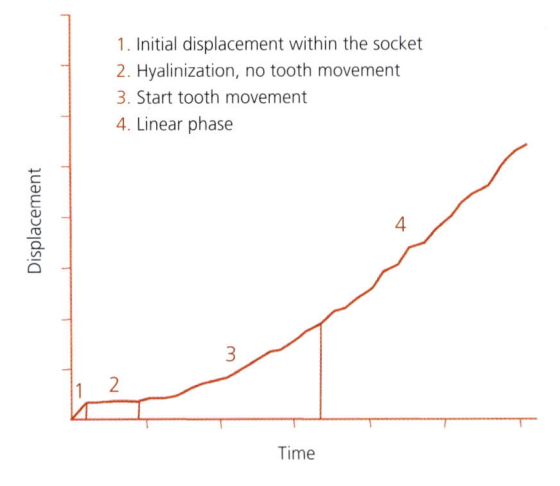

Figure 3.8 General time–displacement curve of OTM. (Source: Jaap Maltha.)

removal of all necrotic tissues. During the third phase, the rate of movement gradually or suddenly increases. Experiments by Hixon and co-workers (Hixon *et al.*, 1969, 1970) revealed two phases in OTM: an initial mechanical displacement, and a delayed metabolic response.

More recently, a new time–displacement model for OTM was proposed (van Leeuwen *et al.*, 1999; Von Böhl, *et al.*, 2004b) (Figure 3.8). These studies, performed on beagle dogs, divided the curve of tooth movement into four phases.

The first phase lasts 24 hours to 2 days and represents the initial movement of the tooth inside its bony socket, causing structural changes in the ECM. In this initial phase, the ECM is compressed in the direction of the tooth movement, leading to a temporal increase in tissue pressure, constriction of blood vessels, and deformation of nerves. In many cases this results in an anoxic situation leading to local tissue necrosis, called hyalinization (Figure 3.9).

At the trailing side of the tooth (formerly incorrectly called the tension side), the periodontal space is widened, which leads to a temporal decrease in tissue pressure, and a widening of the blood vessels (von Böhl and Kuijpers-Jagtman, 2009).

The initial phase is, in most cases, followed by a second phase, where there is an arrest in tooth movement lasting for approximately 20–30 days. As long as the hyalinized tissue remains, tooth movement is prevented, as direct bone resorption is not possible, because osteoclasts cannot differentiate within the necrotic areas of the PDL. Actual OTM, the third phase, begins with an increasing rate only after the complete removal of the hyalinized tissue.

In the fourth phase, tooth movement takes place at a constant rate, as long as the force is exerted and no obstacles are encountered.

This is the linear phase. In this phase, alveolar bone is resorbed at the leading side of the root (formerly incorrectly called the pressure side) (Figure 3.10), and bone deposition is found at the trailing side (Pilon, Kuijpers-Jagtman, and Maltha, 1996; van Leeuwen et al., 1999) (Figure 3.11).

In fact, this pattern of OTM concurs with the three phases described by Burstone (van Leeuwen et al., 1999; Von Böhl et al., 2004a, 2004b).

If the force application is discontinued because the tooth is in its desired position, the tooth tends to move in the opposite direction. This process is called relapse and can be prevented by stabilizing the tooth in its position by a retention appliance (van Leeuwen et al., 2003; Littlewood et al., 2017).

Cell biological processes during initial phase and hyalinization

The initial phase is completely determined by the biophysical properties of the PDL (van Driel et al., 2000; Jónsdóttir et al., 2006). In the first few seconds the tooth moves at a rate of approximately 10 µm/s, in the subsequent 20 seconds at a rate of approximately 1 µm/s, and thereafter at 0.1 µm/s or less. It stabilizes within 5 hours. In the initial few seconds the movement is determined by a rapid reallocation of fluid, and the remaining movement indicates the viscoelastic behavior of the ECM of the PDL (van Driel et al., 2000; Jonsdottir et al., 2006, 2012) (Figure 3.4).

As a result, blood vessels in the PDL are occluded, causing hypoxic conditions. This causes local cell death through the loss of cell membrane integrity and an uncontrolled release of organelles and debris into the ECM, with cell-free areas as a result.

The necrotizing tissues initiate an inflammatory response through the action of inflammatory mediators such as interleukin-1β (IL-1β) and PGE2 in the surrounding tissue, which attract leukocytes and nearby phagocytes, such as macrophages and foreign body giant cells. These cells eliminate the dead cells and debris by phagocytosis (Murdoch et al., 2004). Also, the ECM changes by protein denaturation. This means that the secondary and tertiary structures of the collagen type I fibers, for example, are lost but their

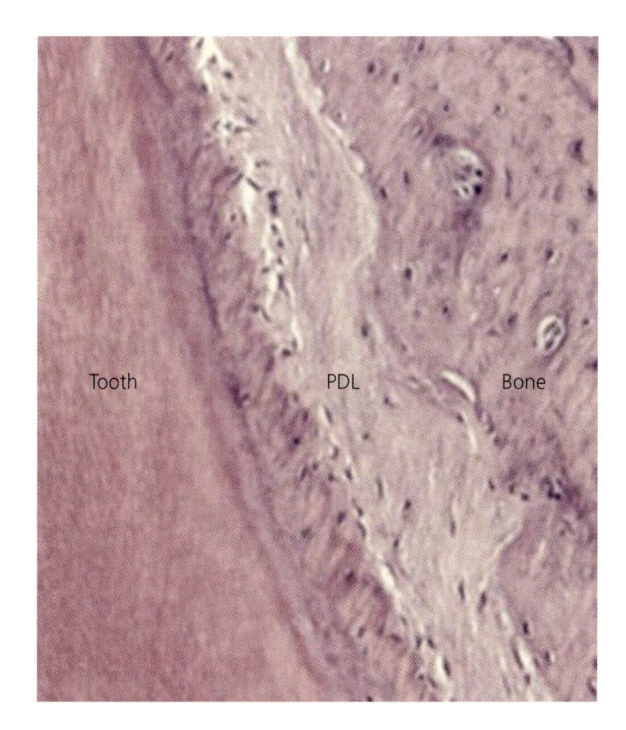

Figure 3.9 Photomicrograph of the PDL after orthodontic force application for 36 hours on a rat molar. The internal structure of the PDL is almost completely lost due to hyalinization. (Source: Jaap Maltha.)

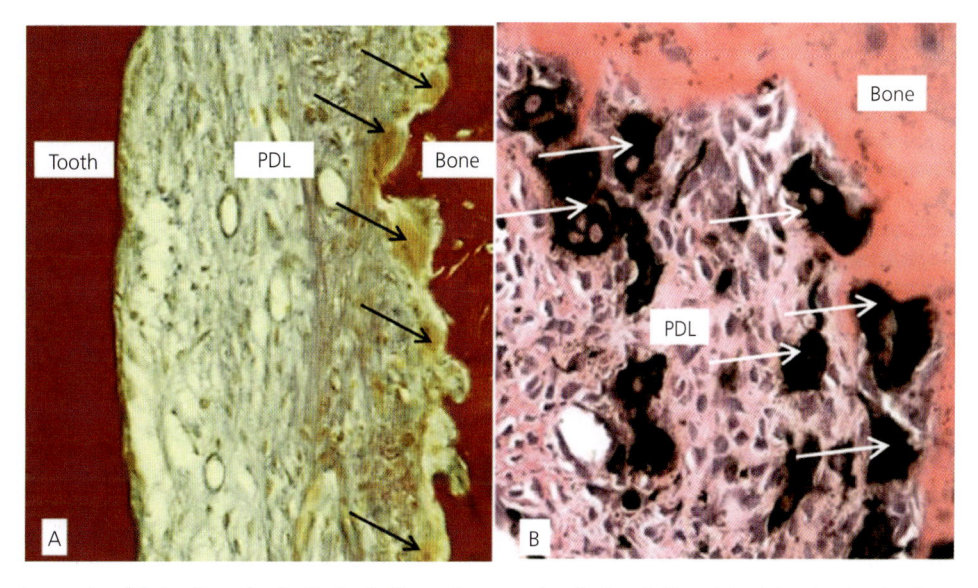

Figure 3.10 Photomicrographs of the leading side of orthodontically moving premolar of a dog. A. Herovici staining showing the absence of type I collagen fibers and their replacement by type III collagen. B. ED1 staining, specific for osteoclast cytoplasm. Arrows indicate osteoclasts. (Source: Japp Maltha.)

42 Biological Mechanisms of Tooth Movement

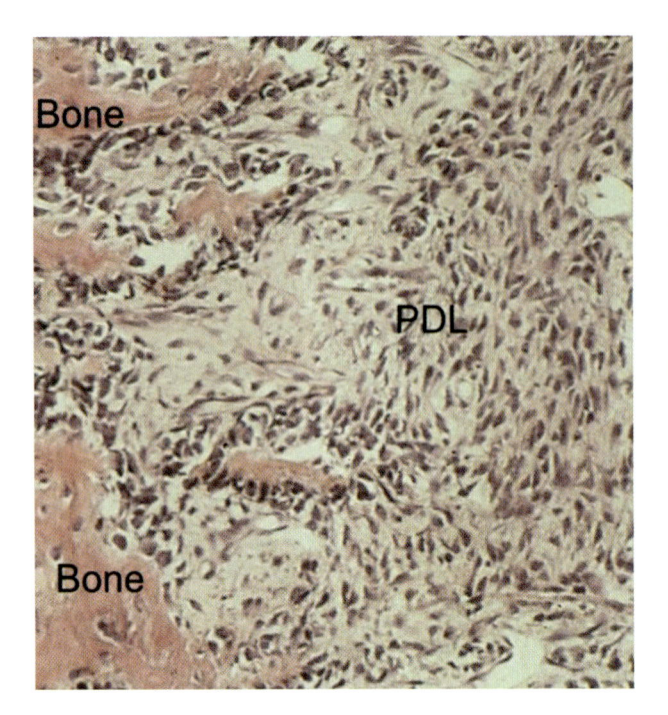

Figure 3.11 Photomicrograph of the trailing side of orthodontically moving premolar of a dog. The bone surface is covered with active osteoblasts indicating rapid bone deposition. H & E staining. (Source: Jaap Maltha.)

primary structures remain. Therefore, the proteins can no longer perform their function, and a gelatinous (gel-like, hyaline) substance is formed. This process in called hyalinization and is mediated by enzymes from the matrix metalloproteinase family (MMP-1, MMP-8, MMP-13). Furthermore, osteoclasts migrate to the area from nearby marrow spaces, after having resorbed the bone immediately adjacent to the necrotic PDL area, in a process known as undermining resorption (Krishnan and Davidovitch, 2006; von Böhl and Kuijpers-Jagtman, 2009), This process is enabled by the mechanosensory action of the lacuna–canalicular system in the alveolar bone. OTM becomes only possible after all necrotic tissue has been removed. Because it is almost impossible to avoid blood vessel occlusion completely, hyalinization, and the subsequent interruption of tooth movement, is a very common process.

The inflammatory processes related to orthodontic force application are described in detail in Chapter 4 of this book.

At the trailing side of the tooth, the very fast initial movement of the tooth leads to a rapid influx of fluid in the first few seconds. In the subsequent hours, widening of the blood vessels and tensioning of the collagenous fibers are seen. During the hyalinization phase, the situation at the trailing side remains stable.

Cell biological processes during real tooth movement

At the leading side of the tooth, removal of the necrotic tissue is accompanied by an influx of differentiating fibroblasts, which secrete new ECM (Figure 3.12). This migration is probably stimulated by

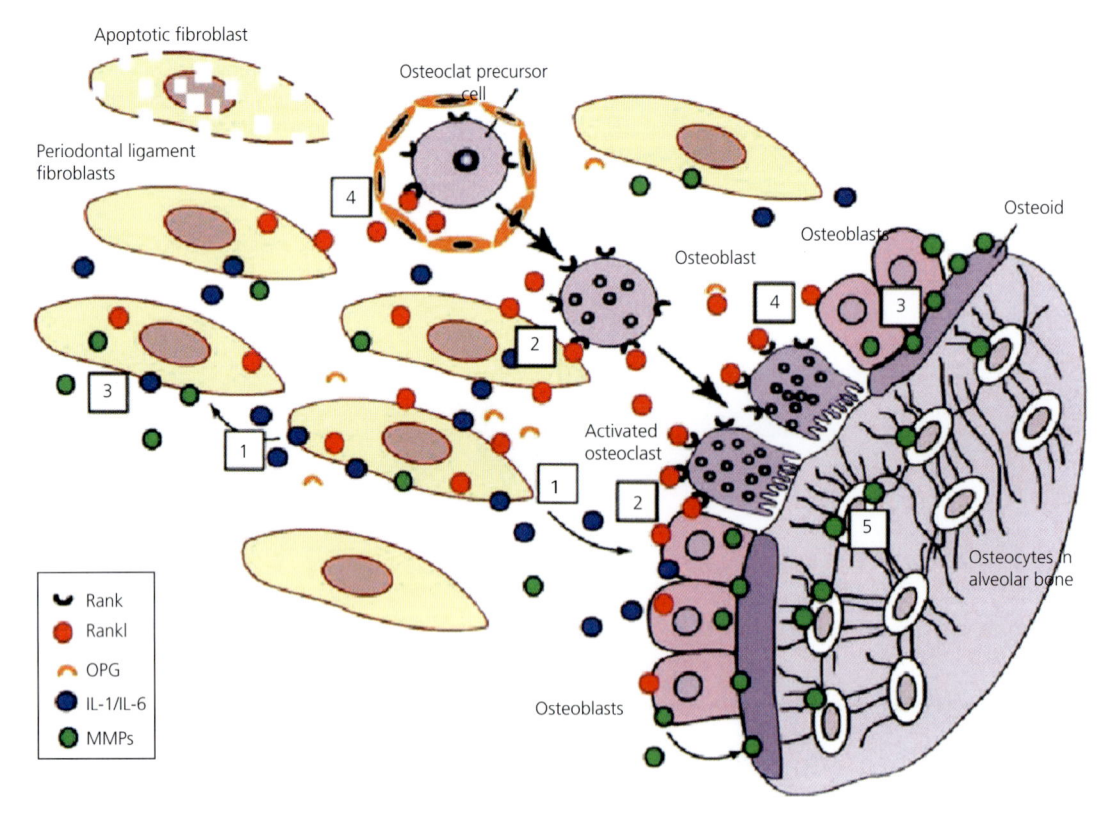

Figure 3.12 Summary of the remodeling processes at the leading side. Fibroblasts (1) under compressive strain secrete IL-1 and IL-6 which under these conditions upregulate the expression of the ligand for the receptor activator of nuclear factor kappa-B (RANKL) (2) and MMPs (3) The MMPs degrade the ECM of the PDL and the osteoid (4), and RANKL stimulates the differentiation and activation of osteoclasts (5). (Source Meikle, 2006. Reproduced with permission of Oxford University Press.)

periostin, an ECM protein that is expressed in periodontal tissues subjected to continuous mechanical stress (Cobo et al., 2016).

In contrast to the normal PDL, the newly formed ECM contains mainly collagen type III instead of collagen type I. Similarly to collagen type I, type III collagen is a fibrillar collagen. It is a homotrimer containing three α1(III) chains forming a triple helix. It is rapidly produced by young fibroblasts and other mesenchymal cells in granulation tissue, and in other areas where rapid tissue formation is essential.

Simultaneously, capillaries, that are quickly recruited through endothelial cell proliferation, capillary enlargement, and elongation, restore the vasculature of the PDL. This process is mediated through VEGFs, which are synthesized and secreted by a variety of cells, such as mast cells, macrophages, and fibroblasts. Binding of circulating VEGF to VEGF receptors on endothelial cells triggers the pathway leading to angiogenesis (Salomão et al., 2014; Tsuge et al., 2016; Militi et al., 2019).

At the trailing side of the tooth, the proinflammatory cytokine IL-1β and pentraxin- related protein (PTX3) are secreted shortly after force application by mononuclear phagocytes, fibroblasts, and endothelial cells throughout the PDL. PTX3 is involved in tissue remodeling and repair in sterile conditions (Tsuge et al., 2016).

After the hyalinized tissue is completely removed, the tooth is again surrounded by a vital PDL. At the leading side of the tooth, the PDL contains mainly collagen type III, and at the trailing side it contains newly formed collagen type I as well as type III collagen. The orthodontic force induces negative strain at the leading side, and positive strain at the trailing side. This results in strain of the periodontal fibroblasts. The integrins by which they are attached to the ECM can act as force transducers or "strain gauges" (Chiquet et al., 2003; Chiquet et al., 2007). Furthermore, fluid flow in the PDL, and also within the canalicular network in the alveolar bone, is induced. In addition, this fluid flow induces strain in the cell membranes, not only of the fibroblasts, but also of the osteoblasts and the osteocytes. The osteocytes within the canaliculi of the alveolar bone are important mechanosensors and transducers of applied mechanical strain. Together with osteoblasts and periodontal fibroblasts they contribute to the activation of cells by integrin-mediated strain transmission to the cytoskeleton and the subsequent induction of the expression of a variety of growth factors and cytokines (Klein-Nulend et al., 2013; Tresguerres et al., 2020). These factors, such as FGF, IGF-1, IL-1α, IL-1β, IL-6, and TNFα mediate the differentiation of precursors into osteoblasts and osteoclasts (Eriksen, 2010; Vansant et al., 2018).

For OTM, resorption of the alveolar bone by osteoclasts at the leading side of the tooth is essential. These cells are derived from myeloid precursors that have differentiated into monocytes and subsequently into osteoclast precursors through macrophage colony-stimulating factor (M-CSF). Their further differentiation is dependent on the ligand for the receptor activator of nuclear factor kappa-B (RANKL) that is secreted by fibroblasts and osteoblasts. RANKL binds to RANK, expressed on the osteoclast precursors that subsequently become mononuclear osteoclasts, characterized by the expression of tartrate resistant acid phosphatase (TRAP). After fusion, these cells become multinuclear osteoclasts (Suda et al., 1999; Yamaguchi, 2009; Vansant et al., 2018). The differentiation of osteoclasts is counteracted by osteoprotegerin (OPG). This is a soluble decoy receptor for RANKL. This means that binding of OPG to RANKL inhibits the binding of RANKL to RANK on the osteoclast precursors and thus hampers both the further differentiation and the functioning of osteoclasts. Interestingly, strain affects both the secretion of RANKL and the secretion of OPG (Figure 3.13).

At the leading side of the tooth the negative strain stimulates the secretion of RANKL, but decreases the secretion of OPG, and thus the differentiation and functioning of osteoclasts are stimulated. On the other hand, in the areas with positive strain, the trailing side of the tooth, RANKL as well as OPG are upregulated, but OPG is more upregulated than RANKL, and thus osteoclast differentiation is prevented (Hadjidakis and Androulakis, 2006; Yamaguchi, 2009; Vansant et al., 2018).

For the functioning of osteoclasts, they should be attached to mineralized bone matrix through αVβ3 integrin. This is only possible when the osteoblasts, as well as the osteoid, the nonmineralized bone matrix covering the surface of the alveolar bone, are removed (Duong et al., 2000; Takahashi et al., 2007; Eriksen, 2010). The ECM of the osteoid is degraded through the action of MMPs, more specifically the collagenases MMP1, MMP8, MMP13, and MMP14 (Tokuhara et al., 2019). These enzymes are synthetized and secreted as pro-enzymes by a variety of cell types, including lymphocytes and granulocytes, but in particular by activated macrophages. They are activated by proteolytic cleavage and regulated by a family of inhibitors called the tissue inhibitors of matrix metalloproteinases (TIMPs). The MMP activity is thus dependent on the balance between production and activation of MMPs and the local levels of TIMPs (Snoek-van Beurden and Von den Hoff, 2005; Verstappen and Von den Hoff, 2006; Tokuhara et al., 2019). The osteoblasts disappear by apoptosis (programmed cell death), induced by binding of TNF-α (that is secreted by activated macrophages, fibroblasts, and osteoblasts, in an autocrine way) to its receptors TNFR1 and TNFR2 on osteoblasts and the subsequent activation of the caspase pathway (Hill et al., 1997; Jilka et al., 1998; Hock et al., 2001).

The combined osteoblast apoptosis and ECM degradation leads to areas of exposure of mineralized bone matrix, which can serve as landing sites for osteoclasts. The osteoclasts move to the landing

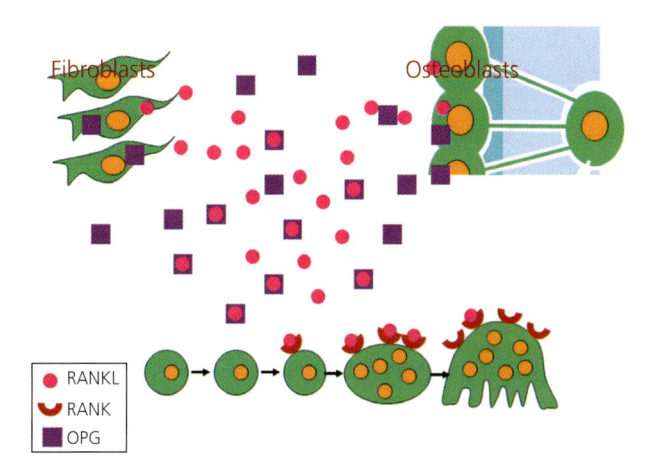

Figure 3.13 The RANK/RANKL/OPG system. The RANKL that is secreted by fibroblasts and osteoblasts binds to RANK, expressed on the osteoclast precursors. The latter subsequently become mononuclear osteoclasts. After fusion, these cells become multinuclear osteoclasts. However, fibroblasts and osteoblasts also can secrete osteoprotegerin (OPG), a soluble factor that also binds to RANKL, thereby hampering the differentiation of osteoclasts. (Source: Jaap Maltha.)

sites by chemotaxis, and attach to the bone by αVβ3 integrins, connecting the osteoclast to RGD peptides in the bone matrix (Takahashi *et al.*, 2007; Lerner *et al.*, 2019). Upon adhesion to bone, osteoclasts polarize and reorganize their cytoskeleton to generate a ring-like F-actin-rich structure, the sealing zone, that isolates the Howship's lacuna from the surroundings. Inside the sealing zone, the ruffled border is formed. The isolated area becomes acidic through an H⁺-ATPase-mediated proton pump. This favors the dissolution of bone minerals. In addition, the lysosomal enzyme cathepsin K, a cysteine proteinase with a pH optimum of 4.5, and matrix metalloproteinases, especially MMP-9 (pH optimum = 7.4) are secreted into Howship's lacunae to degrade the organic bone matrix (Teitelbaum, 2000) (Figure 3.14).

At the trailing side of the moving tooth, the PDL is widened, accompanied with a positive strain in the ECM and an acute inflammatory reaction (Figure 3.15). This results in an increase in IL-1β,

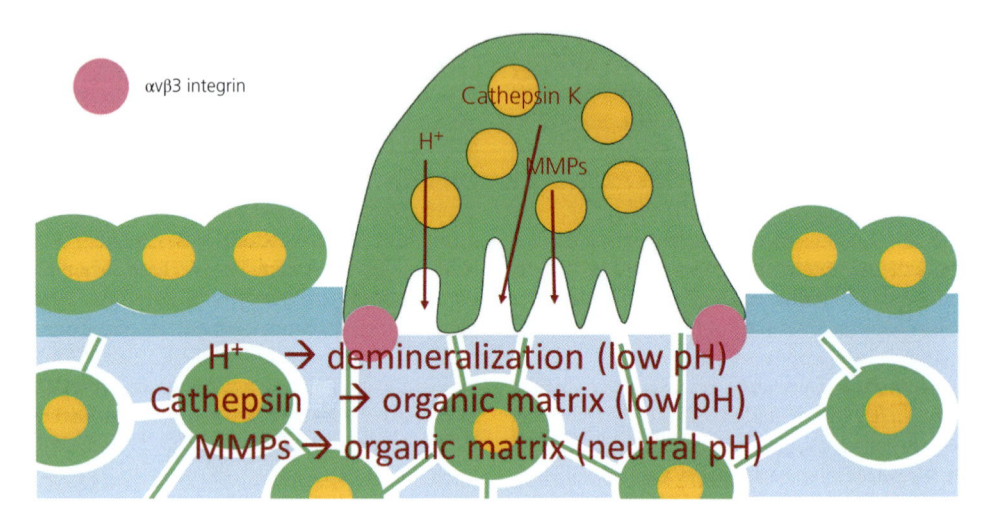

Figure 3.14 An active osteoclast. (Source: Jaap Maltha.)

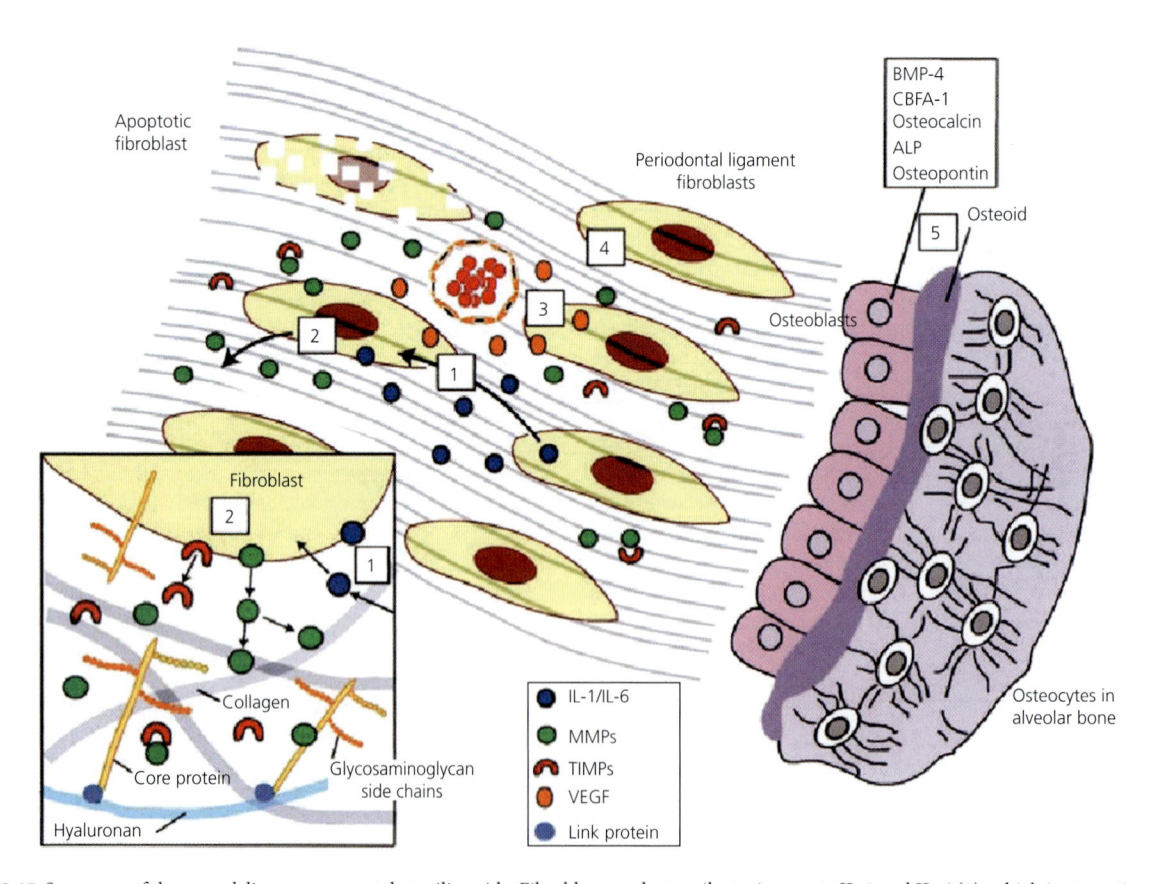

Figure 3.15 Summary of the remodeling processes at the trailing side. Fibroblasts under tensile strain secrete IL-1 and IL-6 (1), which in turn stimulate MMPs and inhibit TIMPs (2). Fibroblasts also secrete VEGF that stimulates angiogenesis (3). These actions result together in anabolic activities of fibroblasts (4) and osteoblasts (5). (Source Meikle, 2006. Reproduced with permission of Oxford University Press.)

IL-10, PGE2, and TGF-β expression (Tsuge et al., 2016; Li et al., 2018), and subsequently in an increase in OPG and a decrease in RANKL secretion by the osteoblasts and periodontal fibroblast (Li et al., 2018).

Furthermore, the number of fibroblasts increases, and the secretion of collagen type I and collagen type III, as well as the formation of new Sharpey's fibers, is stimulated. Simultaneously with the deposition of the Sharpey's fibers, osteoblasts deposit new bone matrix on the adjacent alveolar bone socket wall, anchoring the Sharpey's fibers in the bone matrix (Garant and Cho, 1979; Militi et al., 2019). On the other hand, the expression of MMPs is downregulated and the expression of TIMPs is upregulated, and thus ECM breakdown is inhibited.

Finally, FGF-2 and VEGF, growth factors involved in the development of vascular elements, are upregulated (Chen et al., 2014; Salomão et al., 2014; Li et al., 2018; Militi et al., 2019).

The cumulative result is that at the trailing side osteoclast differentiation is prevented, the formation of new ECM and bone deposition is stimulated, and adaptation of the vascular system to the new situation is induced.

Cell biological processes during relapse and retention

It is generally accepted that if the orthodontic appliance is removed, the teeth tend to revert back in the direction of their original position by a process called relapse. This starts almost immediately after removal of the appliance and the rate of the relapse decreases over time. This process can be described as a logarithmic decay curve, with a half-life time (T½) of approximately 1–11 days and stabilization after approximately 10 weeks (Maltha and Von den Hoff, 2017).

The classic theory is that relapse is caused by the relaxation of stretched fibers in the PDL and/or the supra-alveolar region (Littlewood et al., 2017). However, recent studies have shown that the turnover rate of the collagen fibers in the normal PDL and the supra-alveolar region is very high. Their T½ varies between 3 and 10 days, which means for example that after about 3 months only 0.2% of the original fibers still remain (Henneman et al., 2012). Furthermore, within a few days after the start of the active treatment, the structure of the PDL at the leading side is completely remodeled, while at the trailing side, part of the original fibers are embedded in the alveolar bone, and newly synthetized collagen fibers bridge the gap to the moving tooth (Von Böhl et al., 2004a; Nakamura et al., 2008; Tsuge et al., 2016).

This indicates that the classic theory should be rejected. It is more likely that the relapse is initiated by the changes in the mechanical conditions in the PDL due to the abolition of the external force. This leads to changes in the stress and strain distribution in the PDL, which in turn will induce changes in the synthesis and release of molecules that modulate the differentiation, proliferation, and activation of cells in the PDL, the alveolar bone, and the cementum.

At the leading side of the relapsing tooth, the sign of the strain has changed from positive to negative, and at the trailing side the opposite has happened. Consequently, the signaling and the cellular response in the PDL, the cementum, and the alveolar bone change to the opposite. This strongly indicates that the same processes as found during active tooth displacement now will take place at the opposite side of the tooth (Franzen et al., 2013).

Indeed, histological studies have shown that during the very start of relapse, in some instances the PDL at the leading side is hyalinized. After the hyalinized tissue is removed, or directly after the start of the relapse in cases in which no hyalinization had developed, the normal structure of the PDL is completely lost through the upregulation of the MMPs by its inducer (EMMPRIN) (Xia et al., 2019). It is replaced by loose connective tissue in which collagen type I is absent, and collagen type III fibers parallel to the root surface not connecting the tooth to the alveolar bone. Osteoclasts differentiate in this area and start alveolar bone resorption. This osteoclastogenesis and alveolar bone resorption is probably correlated with the expression of EMMPRIN and its association with RANKL and VEGF expression (Xia et al., 2019). At the trailing side of the relapsing tooth, the PDL contains newly formed collagen type I as well as type III collagen, osteoclasts are no longer present, and osteoblasts differentiate and secrete bone tissue (Yoshida et al., 1999).

In Chapter 19 of this book, the histological changes during relapse are described in more detail and compared with the histological changes during active OTM.

Unfortunately, very little research has been performed on the cell and molecular biology aspects of relapse. Franzen and co-workers (2013) found that during active tooth movement gene expression of OCN, Coll-I, and ALP decreased at the leading side, and that they tended to increase again while the molars relapsed. The reverse was seen for the genes of RANKL and TRAP. Their expression increased at the leading side during active tooth movement and returned to control levels during relapse

Although the literature on this topic is sparse, the available data suggest that changes in the mechanical circumstances in the PDL, due to the abolition of the external orthodontic forces, result in similar biological reactions as when an orthodontic appliance is activated. This means that teeth do not have "a tendency to move back towards the original malocclusion", as stated in many textbooks, but that they react to changes in local mechanical conditions.

Conclusions

Orthodontic movement of teeth to a new position in the dental arch is the result of a highly complex biological process in response to the applied force. The PDL and the alveolar bone with their different cell types and ECM play a dominant role in activating the tissue response to enable movement. Many molecules have been implicated in this response, but a well-integrated model representing a unified scheme is still incomplete.

The most recent model is given in the systematic review by Vansant et al. (2018) on the expression of biological mediators during OTM which is based on the model by Henneman et al. (2008) (Figure 3.16). Future research will fill in the gaps of knowledge that still exist. Every patient differs biologically and with increasing knowledge of the biological processes involved in OTM we may be able to design a personalized approach for each individual patient based on his or her biological profile. This will hopefully make the process of OTM more efficient than the standard approach we offer our patients today.

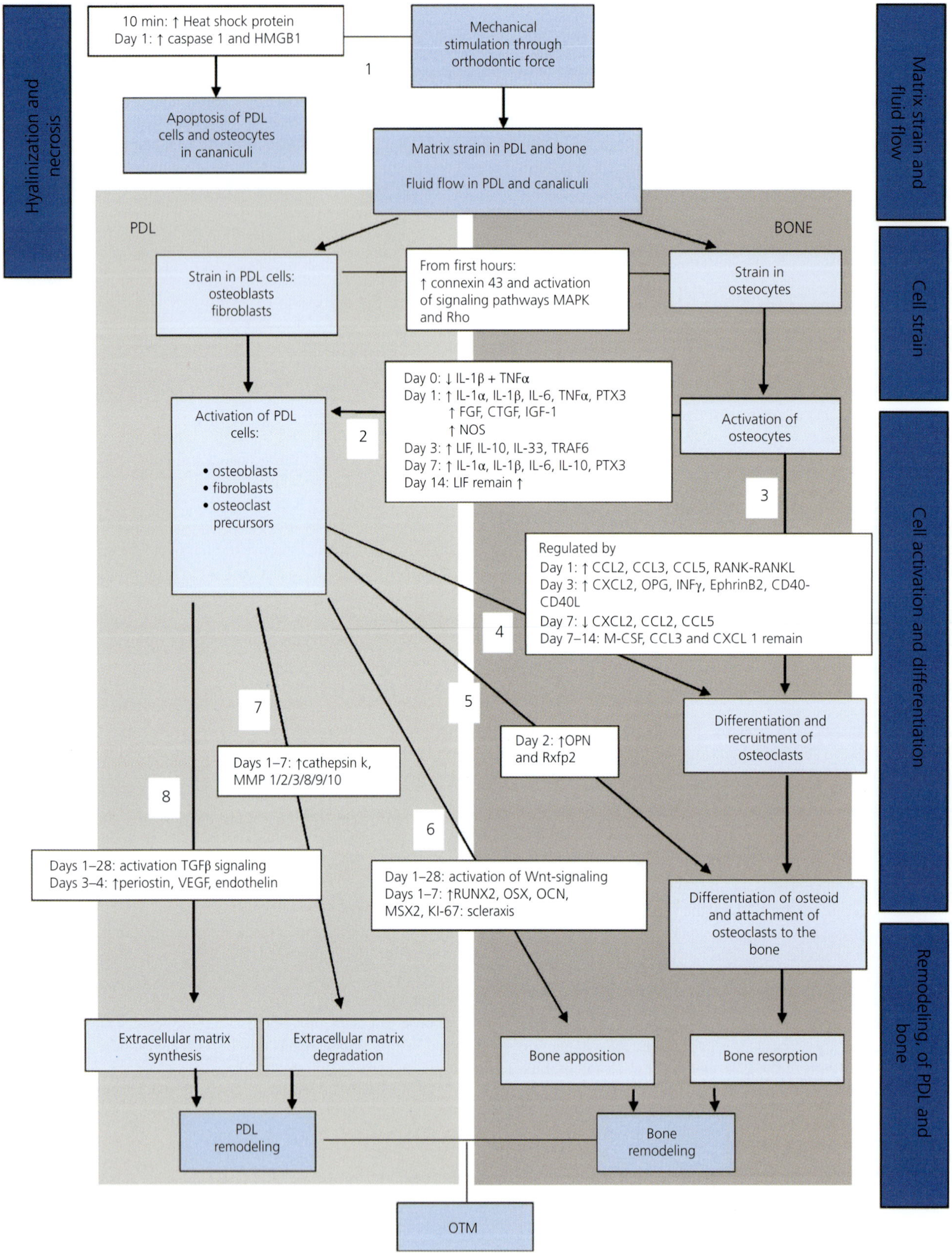

46 Biological Mechanisms of Tooth Movement

Figure 3.16 Theoretical model of orthodontic tooth movement (OTM) based on the model by Henneman et al. (2008). (Source: Vansant et al., 2018. Reproduced with permission of Elsevier.)

References

Barczyk, M., Bolstad, A. I. and Gullberg, D. (2013) Role of integrins in the periodontal ligament: organizers and facilitators. *Periodontology 2000* **63**(1), 29–47. doi:10.1111/prd.12027.

Bergomi, M., Cugnoni, J., Botsis, J. et al. (2010) The role of the fluid phase in the viscous response of bovine periodontal ligament. *Journal of Biomechanics* **43**(6), 1146–1152. doi:10.1016/j.jbiomech.2009.12.020.

Binderman, I., Zor, U., Kaye, A. M. et al. (1988) The transduction of mechanical force into biochemical events in bone cells may involve activation of phospholipase A2. *Calcified Tissue International* **42**(4), 261–266. doi:10.1007/bf02553753.

Burger, E. H. and Klein-Nulend, J. (1999) Mechanotransduction in bone – role of the lacuno-canalicular network. *The FASEB Journal* **13**(Suppl.), S101–112.

Burridge, K. and Chrzanowska-Wodnicka, M. (1996) Focal adhesions, contractility and signaling. *Annual Review of Cell and Developmental Biology* **12**, 463–518. doi:10.1146/annurev.cellbio.12.1.463.

Burstone, C. J. (1962) The biomechanics of tooth movement, in *Vistas in Orthodontics* (eds B. S. Kraus and R. A. Riedel). Lee & Febiger, Philadelphia, PA, pp. 197–213.

Chen, X., Li, N., LeleYang, Liu, J. et al. (2014) Expression of collagen I, collagen III and MMP-1 on the tension side of distracted tooth using periodontal ligament distraction osteogenesis in beagle dogs. *Archives of Oral Biology* **59**(11), 1217–1225. doi:10.1016/j.archoralbio.2014.07.011.

Chiquet, M., Renedo, A. S., Huber, F. and Flück, M. (2003) How do fibroblasts translate mechanical signals into changes in extracellular matrix production? *Matrix Biology* **22**(1), 73–80. doi:10.1016/s0945-053x(03)00004-0.

Chiquet, M., Tunç-Civelek, V. and Sarasa-Renedo, A. (2007) Gene regulation by mechanotransduction in fibroblasts. *Applied Physiology, Nutrition and Metabolism* **32**(5), 967–973. doi:10.1139/h07-053.

Cobo, T., Viloria, C. G., Solares, L. et al. (2016) Role of periostin in adhesion and migration of bone remodeling cells. *PLoS One* **11**(1), e0147837. doi:10.1371/journal.pone.0147837.

Davidovitch, Z. (1991) Tooth movement. *Critical Reviews in Oral Biology and Medicine* **2**, 411–450.

Dean R. (2017) The periodontal ligament: development, anatomy and function. *Oral Health and Dental Management* **16**(6), 1–7.

Duong, L. T., Lakkakorpi, P., Nakamura, I. and Rodan, G. A. (2000) Integrins and signaling in osteoclast function. *Matrix Biology* **19**(2), 97–105. doi:10.1016/s0945-053x(00)00051-2.

Eriksen, E. F. (2010) Cellular mechanisms of bone remodeling. *Reviews in Endocrine and Metabolic Disorders* **11**(4), 219–227. doi:10.1007/s11154-010-9153-1.

Feller, L., Khammissa, R. A., Schechter, I. et al. (2015) periodontal biological events associated with orthodontic tooth movement: the biomechanics of the cytoskeleton and the extracellular matrix. *Scientific World Journal* 894123. doi:10.1155/2015/894123.

Fernández-Tresguerres-Hernández-Gil, I., Alobera-Gracia, M. A., del-Canto-Pingarrón, M. and Blanco-Jerez, L. (2006a) Physiological bases of bone regeneration I. Histology and physiology of bone tissue. *Medicina Oral Patologia Oral y Cirugia Bucal* **11**(1), E47–51.

Fernández-Tresguerres-Hernández-Gil, I., Alobera-Gracia, M. A., del-Canto-Pingarrón, M. and Blanco-Jerez, L. (2006b) Physiological bases of bone regeneration II. The remodeling process. *Medicina Oral Patologia Oral y Cirugia Bucal* **11**(2), E151–157.

Franzen, T. J., Brudvik, P. and Vandevska-Radunovic, V. (2013) Periodontal tissue reaction during orthodontic relapse in rat molars. *European Journal of Orthodontics* **35**(2), 152–159. doi:10.1093/ejo/cjr127.

Garant, P. R. and Cho, M. I. (1979) Autoradiographic evidence of the coordination of the genesis of Sharpey's fibers with new bone formation in the periodontium of the mouse. *Journal of Periodontal Research* **14**(2), 107–114. doi:10.1111/j.1600-0765.1979.tb00779.x.

Gordon, S. and Martinez-Pomares, L. (2017) Physiological roles of macrophages. *Pflugers Archiv* **469**(3–4), 365–374. doi:10.1007/s00424-017-1945-7.

Gordon, S. and Plüddemann, A. (2017) Tissue macrophages: heterogeneity and functions. *BMC Biology* **15**(1), 53. doi:10.1186/s12915-017-0392-4.

Hadjidakis, D. J. and Androulakis, II. (2006) Bone remodeling. *Annals of the New York Academy of Sciences* **1092**, 385–396. doi:10.1196/annals.1365.035.

Harizi, H., Corcuff, J.-B. and Gualde, N. (2008) Arachidonic-acid-derived eicosanoids: roles in biology and immunopathology. *Trends in Molecular Medicine* **14**(10), 461–469. doi:10.1016/j.molmed.2008.08.005.

Hasegawa, T. (2018) Ultrastructure and biological function of matrix vesicles in bone mineralization. *Histochemistry and Cell Biology* **149**(4), 289–304. doi:10.1007/s00418-018-1646-0.

Henneman, S., Von den Hoff, J. W., and Maltha, J. C. (2008). Mechanobiology of tooth movement. *European Journal of Orthodontics* **30**, 299–306. doi.org/10.1093/ejo/cjn020

Henneman, S., Reijers, R. R., Maltha, J. C. and Von den Hoff, J. W. (2012) Local variations in turnover of periodontal collagen fibers in rats. *Journal of Periodontal Research* **47**(3), 383–388. doi:10.1111/j.1600-0765.2011.01444.x.

Hill, P. A., Tumber, A. and Meikle, M. C. (1997) Multiple extracellular signals promote osteoblast survival and apoptosis. *Endocrinology* **138**(9), 3849–3858. doi:10.1210/endo.138.9.5370.

Hixon, E. H., Aasen, T. O., Clark, R. A. et al. (1970) On force and tooth movement. *American Journal of Orthodontics* **57**(5), 476–478. doi:10.1016/0002-9416(70)90166-1.

Hixon, E. H., Atikian, H., Callow, G. E. et al. (1969) Optimal force, differential force and anchorage. *American Journal of Orthodontics* **55**(5), 437–457. doi:10.1016/0002-9416(69)90083-9.

Hock, J. M., Krishnan, V., Onyia, J. E. et al. (2001) Osteoblast apoptosis and bone turnover. *Journal of Bone and Mineral Research* **16**(6), 975–984. doi:10.1359/jbmr.2001.16.6.975.

Hubmacher, D., Tiedemann, K., and Reinhardt, D. P. (2006) Fibrillins: from biogenesis of microfibrils to signaling functions. *Current Topics in Developmental Biology* **75**, 93–123.

Jiang, C., Li, Z., Quan, H. et al. (2015) Osteoimmunology in orthodontic tooth movement. *Oral Diseases* **21**(6), 694–704. doi:10.1111/odi.12273.

Jiang, N., Guo, W., Chen, M. et al. (2016) Periodontal ligament and alveolar bone in health and adaptation: tooth movement. *Frontiers of Oral Biology* **18**, 1–8. doi:10.1159/000351894.

Jilka, R. L., Weinstein, R. S., Bellido, T. et al. (1998) Osteoblast programmed cell death (apoptosis): modulation by growth factors and cytokines. *Journal of Bone and Mineral Research* **13**(5), 793–802. doi:10.1359/jbmr.1998.13.5.793.

Jonsdottir, S. H., Giesen, E. B. and Maltha, J. C. (2012) The biomechanical behaviour of the hyalinized periodontal ligament in dogs during experimental orthodontic tooth movement. *European Journal of Orthodontics* **34**(5), 542–546. doi:10.1093/ejo/cjq186.

Jónsdóttir, S. H., Giesen, E. B. and Maltha, J. C. (2006) Biomechanical behaviour of the periodontal ligament of the beagle dog during the first 5 hours of orthodontic force application. *European Journal of Orthodontics* **28**(6), 547–552. doi:10.1093/ejo/cjl050.

Kechagia, J. Z., Ivaska, J. and Roca-Cusachs, P. (2019) Integrins as biomechanical sensors of the microenvironment. *Nature Reviews Molecular Cell Biology* **20**(8), 457–473. doi:10.1038/s41580-019-0134-2.

Kerrigan, J. J., Mansell, J. P. and Sandy, J. R. (2000) Matrix turnover. *Journal of Orthodontics* **27**, 227–233.

Kielty, C.M. (2006) Elastic fibres in health and disease. *Expert Reviews in Molecular Medicine* **8**(19), 1-23. doi: 10.1017/S146239940600007X.

Klein-Nulend, J., Bakker, A. D., Bacabac, R. G. et al. (2013) Mechanosensation and transduction in osteocytes. *Bone* **54**(2), 182–190. doi:10.1016/j.bone.2012.10.013.

Krishnan, V. and Davidovitch, Z. (2006) Cellular, molecular and tissue-level reactions to orthodontic force. *American Journal of Orthodontics and Dentofacial Orthopedics* **129**(4), 469.e461-432. doi:10.1016/j.ajodo.2005.10.007.

Lee, D., Sims, M. R., Dreyer, C. W., & Sampson, W. J. (1991) A scanning electron microscope study of microcorrosion casts of the microvasculature of the marmoset palate, gingiva and periodontal ligament. *Archives of Oral Biology* **36**, 211–220.

Lekic, P. and McCulloch, C. A. (1996) Periodontal ligament cell population: the central role of fibroblasts in creating a unique tissue. *Anatomical Record* **245**(2), 327–341. doi:10.1002/(sici)1097-0185(199606)245:2<327::Aid-ar15>3.0.Co;2-r.

Lerner, U. H. (2012) Osteoblasts, osteoclasts and osteocytes: Unveiling their intimate-associated responses to appplied orthodontic forces. *Seminars in Orthodontics* **18**, 237–248.

Lerner, U. H., Kindstedt, E. and Lundberg, P. (2019) The critical interplay between bone resorbing and bone forming cells. *Journal of Clinical Periodontology* **46**(Suppl 21.), 33–51. doi:10.1111/jcpe.13051.

Li, Y., Jacox, L. A., Little, S. H. and Ko, C. C. (2018) Orthodontic tooth movement: The biology and clinical implications. *Kaohsiung Journal of Medical Science* **34**(4), 207–214. doi:10.1016/j.kjms.2018.01.007.

Listik, E., Azevedo Marques Gaschler, J., Matias, M., et al. (2019) Proteoglycans and dental biology: the first review. *Carbohydrate Polymers* **225**, 115199.

Littlewood, S. J., Kandasamy, S. and Huang, G. (2017) Retention and relapse in clinical practice. *Australian Dental Journal* **62**(Suppl. 1), 51–57. doi:10.1111/adj.12475.

Maeda, T., Kannari, K., Sato, O. and Iwanaga, T. (1990) Nerve terminals in human periodontal ligament as demonstrated by immunohistochemistry for neurofilament protein (NFP) and S-100 protein. *Archives of Histology and Cytology* **53**, 259–265.

Maeda, T., Ochi, K., Nakakura-Ohshima, K. et al. (1999) The Ruffini ending as the primary mechanoreceptor in the periodontal ligament: its morphology, cytochemical features, regeneration, and development. *Critical Reviews in Oral Biology and Medicine* **10**, 307–327.

Maltha, J. C. and Von den Hoff, J. W. (2017) Biological basis for orthdontic relapse, in *Stabiity, Retention and Relapse in Orthodontics* (eds C. Katsaros and T. Eliades). Quinessence, Berlin. Pp. 15–28.

Marson, A., Rock, M. J., Cain, S. A. et al. (2005) Homotypic fibrillin-1 interactions in microfibril assembly. *The Journal of Biological Chemistry* **280**, 5013–5021.

Martino, F., Perestrelo, A. R., Vinarský, V. et al. (2018) Cellular mechanotransduction: from tension to function. *Frontiers in Physiology* **9**, 824. doi:10.3389/fphys.2018.00824.

McGeachie, J. and Tennant, M. (1997) Growth factors and their implications for clinicians: a brief review. *Australian Dental Journal* **42**(6), 375–380. doi:10.1111/j.1834-7819.1997.tb06081.x.

Meikle, M. C. (2006) The tissue, cellular and molecular regulation of orthodontic tooth movement: 100 years after Carl Sandstedt. *European Journal of Orthodontics* **28**(3), 221–240. doi:10.1093/ejo/cjl001.

Militi, A., Cutroneo, G., Favaloro, A. et al. (2019) An immunofluorescence study on VEGF and extracellular matrix proteins in human periodontal ligament during tooth movement. *Heliyon* **5**(10), e02572. doi:10.1016/j.heliyon.2019.e02572.

Mundy, G. R. (1993) Cytokines and growth factors in the regulation of bone remodeling. *Journal of Bone and Mineral Research* **8**(Suppl. 2), S505–S510. doi:10.1002/jbmr.5650081315.

Murdoch, C., Giannoudis, A. and Lewis, C. E. (2004) Mechanisms regulating the recruitment of macrophages into hypoxic areas of tumors and other ischemic tissues. *Blood* **104**(8), 2224–2234. doi:10.1182/blood-2004-03-1109.

Nakamura, Y., Noda, K., Shimoda, S. et al. (2008) Time-lapse observation of rat periodontal ligament during function and tooth movement, using microcomputed tomography. *European Journal of Orthodontics* **30**(3), 320–326. doi:10.1093/ejo/cjm133.

Nanci, A. and Bosshardt, D. D. (2006) Structure of periodontal tissues in health and disease. *Periodontology 2000* **40**, 11–28. doi:10.1111/j.1600-0757.2005.00141.x.

Ortún-Terrazas, J., Cegoñino, J., Santana-Penín, U. et al. (2018) Approach towards the porous fibrous structure of the periodontal ligament using micro-computerized tomography and finite element analysis. *Journal of the Mechanical Behaviour of Biomedical Materials* **79**, 135–149. doi:10.1016/j.jmbbm.2017.12.022.

Pilon, J. J., Kuijpers-Jagtman, A. M. and Maltha, J. C. (1996) Magnitude of orthodontic forces and rate of bodily tooth movement. An experimental study. *American Journal of Orthodontics and Dentofacial Orthopedics* **110**(1), 16–23. doi:10.1016/s0889-5406(96)70082-3.

Roodman, G. D. (1993) Role of cytokines in the regulation of bone resorption. *Calcified Tissue International* **53**(Suppl. 1), S94–98. doi:10.1007/bf01673412.

Salomão, M. F., Reis, S. R., Vale, V. L. et al. (2014) Immunolocalization of FGF-2 and VEGF in rat periodontal ligament during experimental tooth movement. *Dental Press Journal of Orthodontics* **19**(3), 67–74. doi:10.1590/2176-9451.19.3.067-074.oar.

Selliseth, N. J. and Selvig, K. A. (1994) The vasculature of the periodontal ligament: a scanning electron microscopic study using corrosion casts in the rat. *Journal of Periodontology* **65**, 1079–1087.

Snoek-van Beurden, P. A. M. and Von den Hoff, J. W. (2005) Zymographic techniques for the analysis of matrix metalloproteinases and their inhibitors. *BioTechniques* **38**(1), 73–83. doi:10.2144/05381RV01.

Strydom, H., Maltha, J. C., Kuijpers-Jagtman, A. M. and Von den Hoff, J. W. (2012) The oxytalan fibre network in the periodontium and its possible mechanical function. *Archives of Oral Biology* **57**, 1003–1011.

Suda, T., Takahashi, N., Udagawa, N. et al. (1999) Modulation of osteoclast differentiation and function by the new members of the tumor necrosis factor receptor and ligand families. *Endocrine Reviews* **20**(3), 345–357. doi:10.1210/edrv.20.3.0367.

Svensson, L., Oldberg, A., & Heinegård, D. (2001) Collagen binding proteins. *Osteoarthritis and Cartilage* **9** Suppl A, S23–S28.

Takahashi, N., Ejiri, S., Yanagisawa, S. and Ozawa, H. (2007) Regulation of osteoclast polarization. *Odontology* **95**(1), 1–9. doi:10.1007/s10266-007-0071-y.

Teitelbaum, S. L. (2000) Bone resorption by osteoclasts. *Science* **289**(5484), 1504–1508. doi:10.1126/science.289.5484.1504.

Tokuhara, C. K., Santesso, M. R., Oliveira, G. S. N. et al. (2019) Updating the role of matrix metalloproteinases in mineralized tissue and related diseases. *Journal of Applied Oral Science* **27**, e20180596. doi:10.1590/1678-7757-2018-0596.

Tresguerres, F. G. F., Torres, J., López-Quiles, J. et al. (2020) The osteocyte: A multifunctional cell within the bone. *Annals of Anatomy* **227**, 151422. doi:10.1016/j.aanat.2019.151422.

Tse, L. H. and Wong, Y. H. (2019) GPCRs in Autocrine and Paracrine Regulations. *Frontiers in Endocrinology* **10**, 428. doi:10.3389/fendo.2019.00428.

Tsuge, A., Noda, K. and Nakamura, Y. (2016) Early tissue reaction in the tension zone of PDL during orthodontic tooth movement. *Archives of Oral Biology* **65**, 17–25. doi:10.1016/j.archoralbio.2016.01.007.

Uhlir, R., Mayo, V., Lin, P. H. et al. (2017) Biomechanical characterization of the periodontal ligament: Orthodontic tooth movement. *The Angle Orthodontist* **87**(2), 183–192. doi:10.2319/092615-651.1.

van Driel, W. D., van Leeuwen, E. J., Von den Hoff, J. W. et al. (2000) Time-dependent mechanical behaviour of the periodontal ligament. *Proceedings of the Institute of Mechanical Engineers H* **214**(5), 497–504. doi:10.1243/0954411001535525.

van Leeuwen, E. J., Maltha, J. C. and Kuijpers-Jagtman, A. M. (1999) Tooth movement with light continuous and discontinuous forces in beagle dogs. *European Journal of Oral Sciences* **107**(6), 468–474. doi:10.1046/j.0909-8836.1999.eos107608.x.

van Leeuwen, E. J., Maltha, J. C., Kuijpers-Jagtman, A. M. and van 't Hof, M. A. (2003) The effect of retention on orthodontic relapse after the use of small continuous or discontinuous forces. An experimental study in beagle dogs. *European Journal of Oral Sciences* **111**(2), 111–116. doi:10.1034/j.1600-0722.2003.00024.x.

Vansant, L., Cadenas De Llano-Pérula, M., Verdonck, A. and Willems, G. (2018) Expression of biological mediators during orthodontic tooth movement: A systematic review. *Archives of Oral Biology* **95**, 170–186. doi:10.1016/j.archoralbio.2018.08.003.

Verstappen, J. and Von den Hoff, J. W. (2006) Tissue inhibitors of metalloproteinases (TIMPs): their biological functions and involvement in oral disease. *Journal of Dental Research* **85**(12), 1074–1084. doi:10.1177/154405910608501202.

Viecilli, R. F., Kar-Kuri, M. H., Varriale, J. et al. (2013) Effects of initial stresses and time on orthodontic external root resorption. *Journal of Dental Research* **92**(4), 346–351. doi:10.1177/0022034513480794.

Viecilli, R. F., Katona, T. R., Chen, J. et al. (2008) Three-dimensional mechanical environment of orthodontic tooth movement and root resorption. *American Journal of Orthodontics and Dentofacial Orthopedics* **133**(6), 791.e711–726. doi:10.1016/j.ajodo.2007.11.023.

Von Böhl, M. and Kuijpers-Jagtman, A. M. (2009) Hyalinization during orthodontic tooth movement: a systematic review on tissue reactions. *European Journal of Orthodontics* **31**(1), 30–36. doi:10.1093/ejo/cjn080.

Von Böhl, M., Maltha, J., Von den Hoff, H. and Kuijpers-Jagtman, A. M. (2004a) Changes in the periodontal ligament after experimental tooth movement using high and low continuous forces in beagle dogs. *The Angle Orthodontists* **74**(1), 16–25. doi:10.1043/0003-3219(2004)074<0016:Citpla>2.0.Co;2.

Von Böhl, M., Maltha, J. C., Von Den Hoff, J. W. and Kuijpers-Jagtman, A. M. (2004b) Focal hyalinization during experimental tooth movement in beagle dogs. *American Journal of Orthodontics and Dentofacial Orthopedics* **125**(5), 615–623. doi:10.1016/j.ajodo.2003.08.023.

Waddington, R. J. and Embery, G. (2001) Proteoglycans and orthodontic tooth movement. *Journal of Orthodontics* **28**, 281–290.

Walko, G., Castañón, M. J. and Wiche, G. (2015) Molecular architecture and function of the hemidesmosome. *Cell and Tissue Research* **360**(3), 529–544. doi:10.1007/s00441-015-2216-6.

Wang, C. Y., Su, M. Z., Chang, H. H. et al. (2012) Tension-compression viscoelastic behaviors of the periodontal ligament. *Journal of the Formosan Medical Association* **111**(9), 471–481. doi:10.1016/j.jfma.2011.06.009.

Wenger, M. P., Bozec, L., Horton, M. A. and Mesquida, P. (2007) Mechanical properties of collagen fibrils. *Biophysical Journal* **93**, 1255–1263.

Wu, B., Zhao, S., Shi, H. et al. (2019) Viscoelastic properties of human periodontal ligament: effects of the loading frequency and location. *The Angle Orthodontist* **89**(3), 480–487. doi:10.2319/062818-481.1.

Xia, L., Li, H., Wang, S., Al-Balaa, M. et al. (2019) The expression of extracellular matrix metalloproteinase inducer (EMMPRIN) in the compression area during orthodontic relapse. *European Journal of Orthodontics* **42**(Suppl. 1). doi:10.1093/ejo/cjz046.

Xiao, W., Wang, Y., Pacios, S. et al. (2016) Cellular and molecular aspects of bone remodeling. *Frontiers of Oral Biology* **18**, 9–16. doi:10.1159/000351895.

Yamaguchi, M. (2009) RANK/RANKL/OPG during orthodontic tooth movement. *Orthodontics and Craniofacial Research* **12**(2), 113–119. doi:10.1111/j.1601-6343.2009.01444.x.

Yamaguchi M., Nakajima R. and Kasai K. (2012) Mechanoreceptors, nociceptors, and orthodontic tooth movement. *Seminars in Orthodontics* **18**(4), 249–256. doi.org/10.1053/j.sodo.2012.06.003.

Yamamoto, T., Hasegawa, T., Yamamoto, T. et al. (2016) Histology of human cementum: Its structure, function and development. *Japanese Dental Science Review* **52**(3), 63–74. doi:10.1016/j.jdsr.2016.04.002.

Yoshida, Y., Sasaki, T., Yokoya, K. et al. (1999) Cellular roles in relapse processes of experimentally-moved rat molars. *Journal of Electron Microscopy* **48**(2), 147–157. doi:10.1093/oxfordjournals.jmicro.a023661.

CHAPTER 4
Inflammatory Response in the Periodontal Ligament and Dental Pulp During Orthodontic Tooth Movement

Masaru Yamaguchi and Gustavo Pompermaier Garlet

Summary

Orthodontic tooth movement is induced by mechanical stimuli and facilitated by remodeling of the periodontal ligament and alveolar bone. A precondition for these remodeling activities, and ultimately for tooth displacement, is the occurrence of an inflammatory process in the periodontium and dental pulp, in response to the mechanical damage caused by orthodontic forces. Recent data suggests that cellular/tissue stress or damage-related products, such as damage-associated molecular pattern molecules, can trigger an aseptic inflammatory response. Vascular and cellular changes were the first events to be recognized and described, and a number of inflammatory mediators of immune and neural origin, such as cytokines, growth factors, and neuropeptides have been demonstrated in the periodontal supporting tissues. Their increased levels during orthodontic tooth movement have led to the assumption that a network of interactions between cells producing these substances (i.e., nerve, immune, and endocrine system cells), regulate the biological responses that occur following the application of orthodontic forces.

Peripheral nerve fibers and neurotransmitters are also involved in the inflammatory process and bone remodeling as evidenced by the presence of neurogenic inflammation-related substances such as calcitonin gene regulated peptide and substance P, leading to increased vasodilation, increased microvasculature permeability, production of exudate, and increased proliferation of endothelial cells and fibroblasts. Inflammatory mediators of immunological origin, such as prostaglandins, interleukins (ILs; IL-1, IL-6, IL-17) as well as cytokines of the tumor necrosis factor α superfamily, which includes the RANK/RANKL/osteoprotegerin system, are also described in the periodontal ligament and dental pulp in increased levels after orthodontic force application. Considering the importance of RANK, RANKL, and osteoprotegerin in physiological osteoclast formation, it is reasonable to propose that the RANKL/RANK/osteoprotegerin system plays an important role in orthodontic tooth movement. This chapter reviews current knowledge regarding the role of inflammation in the periodontal tissue reactions in response to orthodontic forces.

Introduction

Orthodontic tooth movement (OTM) is induced by mechanical stimuli and facilitated by remodeling of the periodontal ligament (PDL) and alveolar bone. A precondition for these remodeling activities, and ultimately for tooth displacement, is the occurrence of an aseptic inflammatory process. Vascular and cellular changes were the first events to be recognized and described, and a number of inflammatory mediators, including cytokines and neuropeptides, have been demonstrated in periodontal supporting tissues. Their increased levels during OTM have led to the assumption that interactions between cells producing these substances, such as nerve, immune, and endocrine system cells, regulate the biological responses that occur following the application of orthodontic forces (Krishnan and Davidovitch, 2006a).

Mechanical stress evokes biochemical responses and structural changes in a variety of cell types *in vivo* and *in vitro*. The overall objective of many investigations has been to further the understanding of the mechanisms involved in converting molecular and/or mechanical stress to the cellular responses that result in tooth movement. The recent advances in the understanding of the mechanisms underlying so-called aseptic inflammation, mediated by tissue damage products collectively denominated damage associated molecular pattern proteins (DAMPs), have provided a rationale for inflammatory response triggering after orthodontic force-induced mechanical stress/damage (Chen and Nunez, 2010). In sites at which inflammation and tissue destruction have occurred, cells may communicate with one another through the interaction of cytokines and other related molecules. Thus it is important to elucidate completely the complex cytokine cascade flow associated with inflammation-mediated tissue destruction at the molecular level (Davidovitch *et al.*, 1988), as well as the intricate molecular network where the simultaneous action and presence of several mediators

---

Biological Mechanisms of Tooth Movement, Third Edition. Edited by Vinod Krishnan, Anne Marie Kuijpers-Jagtman and Ze'ev Davidovitch.
© 2021 John Wiley & Sons Ltd. Published 2021 by John Wiley & Sons Ltd.

can determine the outcome of the response to the orthodontic force. This chapter reviews current evidence regarding the role of inflammation in the periodontal tissue reactions in response to orthodontic force application.

Inflammation during tooth movement

Inflammation characteristically displays the clinical signs of redness, heat, swelling, pain, and associated loss of function. It may be caused by a number of factors, including bacterial infection, or chemical or mechanical irritation. Histological examination reveals that acute inflammation is characterized by vasodilatation and is accompanied by increased permeability of the microvasculature. This increased permeability, with additional signals that confer chemotaxis specificity (provided by a class of chemotactic cytokines, collectively called chemokines), allows the migration of cellular components of blood from the lumen of the vessels into the extracellular spaces within the surrounding tissue. Once in the tissue, the cells follow a chemotactic gradient generated by the interaction of chemokines with the extracellular matrix, directing their migratory process. The migration of the leukocytes from the blood vessel lumen is also accompanied by secretion of exudates from the capillaries. There are a number of biochemical substances known to mediate cell migration-associated changes, such as histamine, leukotrienes, prostaglandins, cytokines, and chemokines.

An inflammatory response is essential in the remodeling of alveolar bone and PDL during OTM. Researchers have been able to demonstrate histological and vascular changes in the PDL, as well as in the alveolar bone following inflammation associated with orthodontic force application (Table 4.1) (Storey, 1973; Kvinnsland et al., 1989). Biological factors, such as different classes of cytokines, chemokines, neurotransmitters, and genes implicated in the process and its associated increase in periodontal tissues of mechanically stressed teeth have been identified (Vandevska-Radunovic, 1999). At this point, it is didactically possible to consider some of these molecules as the molecular triggers of host response (i.e., the first mediators produced in response to mechanical stimulation/damage of cells and tissues), which will subsequently lead to the development of a cascade pathway, mediated by effector molecules (also called first messengers). The first messengers will continue, sustain and/or amplify the inflammatory response by means of second messengers' activation, which will ultimately be responsible for the cellular/tissue response and/or outcome. Recent evidence points to endogenous molecules, collectively named DAMPs, as the potential molecular triggers of the inflammatory process after orthodontic force application. In this context, both mechanical distortion of PDL cells and blood flow alterations subsequent to orthodontic force application could trigger DAMPs release, which in turn would elicit the subsequent first to second messengers cascade that ultimately leads to inflammation development.

Proinflammatory cytokines, such as interleukin-1 (IL-1) and tumor necrosis factor-α (TNF-α), have been shown to be involved in the cascade pathways to elicit acute and chronic inflammation. These cytokines are also involved in bone remodeling (Davidovitch et al., 1988). Literature regarding this suggests that peripheral nerve fibers and neurotransmitters are involved with the inflammatory process and bone remodeling. Mediating substances in neurogenic inflammation such as calcitonin gene-related peptide (CGRP) and substance P (SP), have also been proposed to be involved with many inflammatory processes like vasodilatation, increased microvascular permeability, production of exudate, and increased proliferation of endothelial cells and fibroblasts (Vandevska-Radunovic, 1999).

Different types of neurotransmitters have also been shown to contribute either directly or indirectly to the regulation of osteoblasts and osteoclasts. These neurotransmitters include: CGRP, SP, vasoactive intestinal polypeptide (VIP) and nitric oxide. The various neurotransmitters are synthesized within the ganglion sensory cells before being distributed throughout the central and peripheral nervous system. Release of these neurotransmitter substances is stimulated by the activation of mechanoreceptors or nociceptors (Nicolay et al., 1990). These neurotransmitters then help in generating cyclic adenosine 3´,5´-monophosphate (cAMP) and inositol triphosphate (IP3), which act as second messengers within the cells (Sandy et al., 1993). The intracellular second-messenger molecules transmit their signals to the nucleus via a series of enzymatic reactions. The stimulated nucleus synthesizes the immediate early genes (IEG), depending on the differing signals received. These IEGs have been identified as c-fos, c-jun and egr-1. The IEGs are eventually translated into activator protein-1 (AP-1), which is a transcription factor that modulates the activity of the gene to which it binds, the effect of which is to produce proliferation or differentiation of the cells (Dolce et al., 2002).

Increased blood vessel dilation and permeability are necessary components of the inflammatory process and are therefore involved with bone remodeling. Migration and chemotaxis of leukocytes extravasated from the blood vessel lumens are also necessary processes in bone remodeling (Davidovitch et al., 1988). The converse is also true. Any inhibition of leukotriene or prostaglandin synthesis will inhibit inflammation and bone remodeling. Monocytes, lymphocytes, and mast cells have been shown to express neuropeptide

Table 4.1 Difference in response of PDL and alveolar bone to light and heavy forces.

Time	Light pressure	Heavy pressure
< 1 s	PDL fluid compressible, alveolar bone bending leading to release of signals. (Piezoelectric and streaming potentials.)	PDL fluid compressible, alveolar bone bending leading to release of signals. (Piezoelectric and streaming potentials.)
1–2 s	PDL fluid expressed and tooth movement occurs utilizing PDL space.	PDL fluid expressed and tooth movement occurs utilizing PDL space.
3–5 s	PDL cells and fibers are mechanically distorted. Blood vessels will become partially compressed on pressure side and dilated on tension side.	PDL blood vessels on pressure side become occluded.
Minutes	Blood flow is altered leading to changes in PO_2 (partial pressure of oxygen). Release of first messengers (prostaglandins and cytokines).	Blood flow cut off due to excessive pressure.
Hours	Metabolic changes, enzyme release, release of second messengers leading to rapid cellular activity.	The compressed area shows signs of cell death (necrosis and hyalinization).
Approx. 4 hours	Increase in level of second messengers (cAMP and others). Increased cellular differentiation within PDL.	Cellular differentiation occurs in adjacent unaffected areas. Beginning of undermining resorption.
Approx. 2 days	Tooth movement begins as bone remodeling progresses.	Continuing undermining resorption.
7–14 days		Undermining resorption removes lamina dura adjacent to PDL and tooth movement occurs.

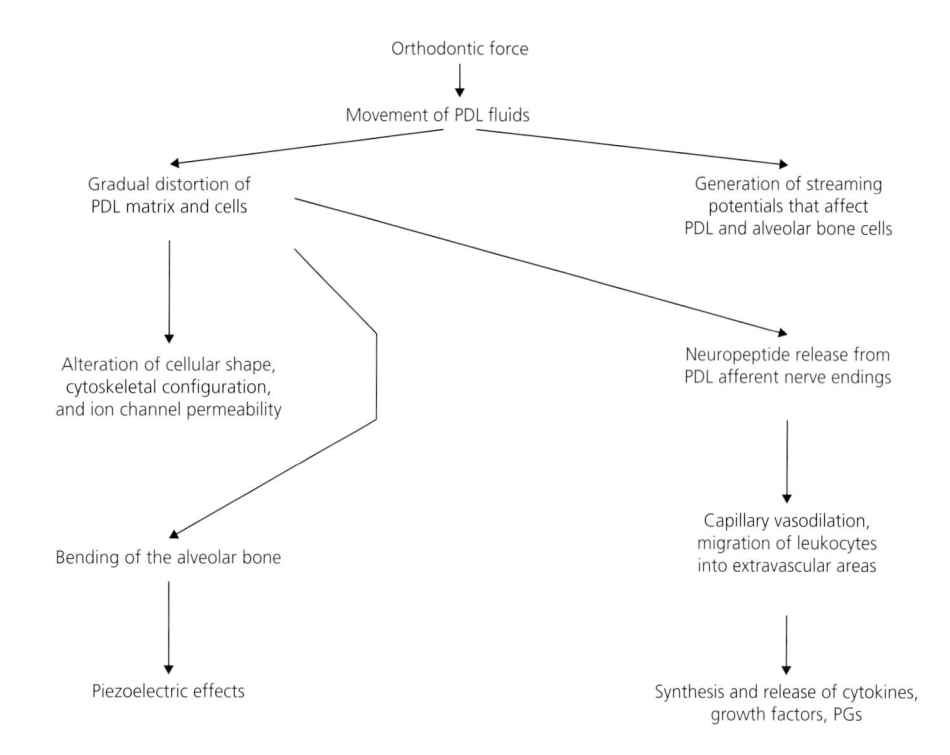

Figure 4.1 Initial effects of orthodontic forces on paradental tissues.

receptors on their cell surfaces, and therefore it has been postulated that CGRP and SP may have a direct influence on the inflammatory process. With this evidence in hand, the peripheral nervous system has been proposed to act as a link between physical stimuli and biological responses in tooth movement.

The hypothesis proposed by Davidovitch et al. (1988) suggests that the mechanical stress, which distorts the cells and matrix of the paradental tissues, imparts strain to the nerve fibers in these tissues, leading to the release of vasoactive peptides from the nerve endings. As previously mentioned, this hypothesis is also supported by the recent discovery of the role of DAMPs in the genesis of inflammation in response to tissue stress or damage (Chen and Nunez, 2010), which can comprise mechanical distortion and hypoxia resulting from orthodontic force application. The vasodilatation produced leads to plasma exudate formation, and migration of leukocytes out of the capillaries. In parallel, inflammatory mediators are essential to generate the local signals that confer specificity to the diapedesis and chemotaxis processes. The leukocytes that then occupy the extravascular space in the involved tissues release cytokines and growth factors to stimulate PDL and bone remodeling (Figure 4.1).

Inflammatory mediators in OTM

The transduction of mechanical forces to the cells triggers a biological response that has been described as an aseptic inflammation because it is mediated by a variety of inflammatory cytokines and does not represent a pathological condition. In contrast to chronic inflammatory responses, in which persistent stimuli sustain a long-lasting inflammatory response and result in tissue damage, the expression of inflammatory mediators after orthodontic force application is transitory and essential for orthodontic movement, as anti-inflammatory drugs are capable of blocking tooth movement. The concept of aseptic inflammation was recently strengthened by discovery of the DAMPs system, where endogenous molecules are able to trigger inflammatory response by cellular stress or damage through the binding of toll-like receptors (TLRs) and nod-like

Table 4.2 Inflammatory factors from PDL in response to OTM.

In vitro studies (stimulated by mechanical stress)	In vivo studies
Prostaglandin E_2 (PGE_2)	Prostaglandin E_2 (PGE_2)
cAMP	cAMP, cGMP
IL-1β	IL-1α
IL-6	IL-6
	TNF-α
RANKL	RANKL
MMP-1, 2	MMP-1, 2, 3, 8, 9, and 13
	CGRP and SP

receptors (NLRs) (Chen and Nunez, 2010). This tissue response initially involves vascular changes, followed by the synthesis of prostaglandins, cytokines, and growth factors. Finally, such mediators are believed to activate tissue remodeling, characterized by selective bone resorption or deposition in compression and tension regions of the PDL, respectively (Garlet et al., 2007). Various inflammatory mediators, identified to date, associated with OTM, are summarized in Table 4.2.

DAMPs

Inflammation is usually defined as a complex biological response to harmful stimuli aimed to protect or to restore the homeostasis of a given organism. Considering that the inflammatory process is generally associated with infectious conditions, the term aseptic (or sterile) inflammation was created to describe specifically the responses generated by trauma, damaged cells, or irritants in the absence of any microorganisms. Indeed, the recent discovery of the DAMPs system rejuvenated the concept of aseptic inflammation, which has gained increasing attention from the scientific community in recent times (Chen and Nunez, 2010; McDonald et al., 2010). The DAMPs comprise a series of endogenous molecules (previously called "danger patterns," "alarmins," or "endokines") released upon cellular stress, injury, or tissue damage and are capable of triggering an inflammatory response and mediate tissue repair (Chen and Nunez, 2010). DAMPs' effects are mediated by their binding to pattern recognition receptors (PRRs), such as the TLRs or NLRs. While the PRRs were originally identified as responsible for the microbial detection, the discovery of DAMPs/PRRs binding provided a key molecular basis to understand the trigger behind aseptic inflammatory response (Chen and Nunez, 2010; McDonald et al., 2010).

As examples among DAMPS studied so far, HMGB1 (high mobility group box 1) and HSPs (heat shock proteins) have been identified in tissues after orthodontic force stimulation. HMGB1 is a protein present in the nucleus of all mammalian cells, responsible for structural and transcriptional activities, but HMGB1 is released upon cellular stress/damage by almost all nucleated cells (Goodwin and Johns, 1977; Bonaldi et al., 2002). It was recently demonstrated that HMGB1 is released by PDL fibroblasts in vivo during orthodontic movement (Wolf et al., 2013). Once secreted, HMGB1 can trigger the production of inflammatory and osteoclastogenic cytokines by PDL cells (Kim et al., 2010), and mediate their proliferation and migration (Chitanuwat et al., 2013). In addition to HMGB1, the HSPs comprise another class of DAMPS, possibly related to inflammation associated with the OTM. It was demonstrated that HSPA1A and HSPB1 are upregulated in PDL at an early stage of tooth movement (Arai et al., 2010; Baba et al., 2011). Like HMGB1, HSPs can act as a trigger for inflammatory reaction to orthodontic forces during the early stages of tooth movement. Accordingly, unpublished data from our group (Garlet laboratory) demonstrate that HMGB1 and HSP levels are upregulated even before the increase in first-messengers expression (i.e., IL1beta and TNF-alpha), reinforcing its potential role as trigger of the inflammatory reaction. Accordingly, recent studies demonstrate that the application of orthodontic forces upregulates HMGB1 expression in rat periodontal tissue in a time- and force-dependent manner (Wolf et al., 2014a, b; Zou et al., 2019). It is also important to mention that both HMGB1 and HSPs are produced in response to hypoxia (Oettgen, 1990; Hendrick and Hartl, 1993), a condition characteristically present in the PDL area during orthodontic movement. Therefore, DAMPs are potentially the trigger of the inflammatory reaction in response to orthodontic forces, as well in the subsequent reparative events that lead to tissue remodeling. It is also important to consider that DAMPs can act as triggers and regulators of inflammatory response. Recent studies demonstrate that HSP production by PDL cells, triggered by mechanical loading, can dampen the subsequent inflammatory response, suggesting the existence of auto-regulatory mechanisms that limits the inflammatory process (Marciniak et al., 2019; Wolf et al., 2016). Importantly, DAMPs (such as HMGB1) can also exert direct anabolic effects on PDL cells, suggesting that its involvement in OTM can be extended beyond its proinflammatory properties (Wolf et al., 2014a, b).

Prostaglandins

Prostaglandins (PGs), products of arachidonic acid metabolism, are local, hormone-like chemical agents produced by mammalian cells including osteoblasts that are synthesized within seconds following cell injury. One of the derivatives of the arachidonic acid cascade, PGE_2, acts as a vasodilator by causing increases in vascular permeability and chemotactic properties, and also stimulates the formation of osteoclasts and an increase in bone resorption. The cyclooxygenase (COX) family of enzymes consists of two proteins that convert arachidonic acid, a 20-carbon polyunsaturated fatty acid comprising a portion of the plasma membrane phospholipids of most cells, to PGs. The constitutive isoform (COX-1) is found in nearly all tissues and is tissue protective. In contrast, COX-2, the inducible isoform of COX, appears to be limited in basal conditions within most tissues, while de novo synthesis is activated by cytokines, bacterial lipopolysaccharides, or growth factors, to produce PGs in large quantities in inflammatory processes. There are several lines of evidence showing that COX is also closely associated with periodontitis, and that PGs are mediators of gingival inflammation and alveolar bone resorption (Offenbacher et al., 1993).

With the help of in vivo studies, an injection of biochemical agents such as PG has been suggested as one effective method that significantly increases OTM (Yamasaki et al., 1980; Yamasaki, 1983). The mechanism of action of PGE_2 can be explained by the pressure–tension theory of tooth movement, which assumes chemical signals to be cell stimulants that lead to tooth movement (Rygh, 1989). According to this theory, pressure causes changes in the PDL blood circulation and the resultant release of chemical mediators. Inflammatory mediators may act in concert and produce synergistic potentiation of prostanoid formation in cells of the human PDL (Ransjo et al., 1998). There is evidence that PG is released when cells are mechanically deformed (Rodan et al., 1975). Indeed, in vitro studies have shown that the expression and production of PGE_2 is promoted by mechanical stimulation of the PDL (Yamaguchi et al., 1994). COX-2 is induced in PDL cells by cyclic mechanical stimulation and is responsible for the augmentation of PGE_2 production in vitro (Shimizu et al., 1998). Furthermore, PGE_2 plays an important role as a mediator of bone remodeling under mechanical forces (Yamasaki et al., 1982). Saito et al. (1991) reported that there is a local increase in PGs in the PDL and alveolar bone during orthodontic treatment, while other studies have demonstrated an arrest in tooth movement in experimental animals when nonsteroidal anti-inflammatory drugs were administered (Chumbley and Tuncay, 1986). Indomethacin, a specific inhibitor of prostaglandin synthesis, reduced the rate of OTM (Yamasaki et al., 1980). Further, when PGE_1 was administered locally or systemically to rats as an adjunct to orthodontic force, accelerated bone resorption and tooth movement were observed (Yamasaki et al., 1984).

Interestingly, HMGB1 can trigger PG synthesis (Leclerc et al., 2013), suggesting that an inducer-first messenger (PG) cascade can take place in the development of an inflammatory reaction to orthodontic forces. Also, DAMP-induced PG can modulate cytokines, demonstrating the existence of complex regulatory networks involving different classes of mediators in the response to orthodontic forces (Prockop and Oh, 2012). Therefore, it may be concluded that PGs play an important role in OTM.

The second-messenger system

According to Krishnan and Davidovitch (2006a), while paradental tissues become progressively strained by applied forces, their cells are continuously subjected to other first messengers, derived from cells of the immune and nervous systems. The binding of these signal molecules to cell membrane receptors leads to enzymatic conversion of cytoplasmic ATP and GTP into adenosine 3′,5′-monophosphate (cyclic AMP [cAMP]), and guanosine 3′,5′-monophosphate (cyclic GMP [cGMP]), respectively. These latter molecules are known as intracellular second messengers. Immunohistochemical staining during OTM in cats showed high concentrations of these molecules in the strained paradental tissues (Davidovitch et al., 1988).

Internal cellular signaling systems are those that translate many external stimuli into a narrow range of internal signals or second messengers (Sandy *et al.*, 1993). Cyclic AMP and cGMP are two second messengers associated with bone remodeling. Bone cells, in response to hormonal and mechanical stimuli, produce cAMP *in vivo* and *in vitro*. Alterations in cAMP levels have been associated with synthesis of polyamines, nucleic acids, and proteins, and with secretion of cellular products. The action of cAMP is mediated through phosphorylation of specific substrate proteins by its dependent protein kinases. In contrast to this role, cGMP is considered an intracellular regulator of both endocrine and nonendocrine mechanisms (Davidovitch, 1995). The action of cGMP is mediated through specific substrate proteins by cGMP-dependent protein kinases. This signaling molecule plays a key role in the synthesis of nucleic acids and proteins, as well as secretion of cellular products.

According to Meikle (2006), the second messenger system classically associated with mechanical force transduction is cAMP. The first evidence for the involvement of the cAMP pathway in mechanical signal transduction was provided independently by Rodan *et al.* (1975), and by Davidovitch and Shanfeld (1975). Rodan *et al.* (1975) showed that a compressive force of $60\,g/cm^2$ applied to 16-day-old chick tibia *in vitro* inhibited the accumulation of cAMP in the epiphyses, as well as in cells isolated from the proliferative zone of the growth plate. The effect was mediated by an enhanced uptake of Ca^{2+} which inhibited membrane-associated adenyl cyclase activity.

Davidovitch and Shanfeld (1975) sampled alveolar bone from compression and tension sites surrounding orthodontically tipped canines in cats. They found that cAMP levels initially decreased, followed by an increase after 1–2 days, which remained elevated to the end of the experimental period of 28 days. They suggested that the initial decrease at the compression sites was due to necrosis of PDL cells, and at the tension sites to a rapid increase in the cell population; the elevation in cAMP observed 2 weeks after the initiation of treatment was probably a reflection of increased bone remodeling activity. Subsequently, Davidovitch *et al.* (1976), in a study on the cellular localization of cAMP in the same model, found an increase in the number of cAMP-positive cells in areas of the PDL where bone resorption or deposition subsequently occurred. Osteocytes in the adjacent alveolar bone, however, appeared to be relatively unaffected by the mechanical force.

Cytokines

Cytokines are proteins that act as signals between the cells of the immune system. These molecules are produced during the activation of immune cells and usually act locally, although some act systemically with overlapping functions. Depending on the major outcomes driven by different cytokines, they can be didactically grouped into subfamilies such as interleukins (the broader group comprising pleiotropic cytokines initially nominated as the mediators of the communication "between leukocytes"), TNF superfamily (comprising TNF-α and the RANK/RANKL/OPG [receptor activator of nuclear factor kappa B ligand/osteoprotegerin] system, the major regulators of the osteoclastogenesis process), chemokines (cytokines with primary chemotactic function), and growth factors (cytokines having prominent actions in proliferative and differentiation processes).

Previous studies have implicated the involvement of different classes of cytokines in bone remodeling *in vitro* and *in vivo*. These cytokines are considered as key mediators involved in a variety of immune and acute-phase inflammatory response activities. The role of the immune system in the regulation of bone remodeling through cytokine production by inflammatory cells that have migrated from dilated PDL capillaries after the application of orthodontic forces is well established (Davidovitch *et al.*, 1988).

Interleukins

IL-1 exists in two forms, α and β, of which IL-1β is the form mainly involved in bone metabolism, stimulation of bone resorption, and inhibition of bone formation. IL-1β also plays a central role in the inflammatory process. The staining of feline PDL cells for IL-1β showed the presence of bound signal complexes in the plasma membrane, which was expected as it is known that receptors for IL-1β are present on fibroblasts (Dinarello and Savage, 1989). The response of gingival fibroblasts to IL-1 might represent a mechanism for amplification of gingival inflammation. Further, IL-1β may act synergistically with TNF-α as a powerful inducer of IL-6. Recent studies have described positive correlations between IL-1β gingival crevicular fluid (GCF) levels and the rate of OTM, derived from low-level laser therapy application (Varella *et al.*, 2018; Fernandes et al., 2019).

IL-6, a multifunctional cytokine previously referred to as B cell stimulatory factor 2, hepatocyte stimulating factor, or interferon-$α_2$, is produced by both lymphoid and nonlymphoid cells. This cytokine can apparently induce osteoclastic bone resorption through an effect on osteoclastogenesis. The levels of IL-1β and IL-6 were significantly higher in inflamed gingivae, when compared with non-inflamed gingival tissues in young adults. The finding that there is an elevation in levels of IL-1α and β, and IL-6 in the PDL and alveolar bone (Figure 4.2) following mechanical force application was demonstrated through *in vivo* studies (Davidovitch *et al.*, 1988; Alhashimi *et al.*, 2001; Bletsa *et al.*, 2006) and *in vitro* studies (Saito *et al.*, 1991; Shimizu *et al.*, 1994; Yamamoto *et al.*, 2006). In a general context, IL-1β and IL-6 are associated with inflammatory reaction development and the subsequent osteoclastogenesis, and possibly operate in a cooperative way in order to promote tooth movement. Accordingly, the IL-1Ra, a naturally occurring IL-1 antagonist, was demonstrated to downregulate OTM in mice (Salla *et al.*, 2012). As described for IL-1, recent studies have shown positive correlations between IL-6 GCF levels and the rate of OTM associated with photobiomodulation (Fernandes *et al.*, 2019).

IL-17 is an inflammatory cytokine that is produced exclusively by activated T cells (Th17 cells) (Yao *et al.*, 1995). IL-17 has been shown to be an important mediator of autoimmune diseases, including rheumatoid arthritis (Kotake *et al.*, 1999), multiple sclerosis (Ishizu *et al.*, 2005; Lock *et al.*, 2002), and allergic airway inflammation (Molet *et al.*, 2001). Recently, IL-17 has been reported to induce osteoclastogenesis directly from monocytes alone (Yago *et al.*, 2009). In addition, IL-17 induces RANKL production by osteoblasts, and was shown to be related to bone destruction in periodontitis (Kotake *et al.*, 1999; Johnson *et al.*, 2004). Moreover, it has been shown that compressive force stimulates the expression of the IL-17 genes and their receptors in MC3T3-E1 cells, and also results in the induction of osteoclastogenesis (Zhang *et al.*, 2010). Further, the immunoreactivity for Th17, IL-17, IL-17R, and IL-6 was detected in PDL tissues subjected to orthodontic force on day 7 (Hayashi *et al.*, 2012). Yamada *et al.* (2013) reported that the immunoreactivities for TRAP, IL-17, IL-6, and RANKL in the atopic dermatitis group were found to be significantly increased. The secretion of IL-17, IL-6, and RANKL, and the mRNA levels of IL-6 and RANKL in the atopic dermatitis patients were increased compared with those in healthy individuals when subjected to orthodontic force application. These cytokines may therefore also contribute to alveolar bone remodeling during OTM.

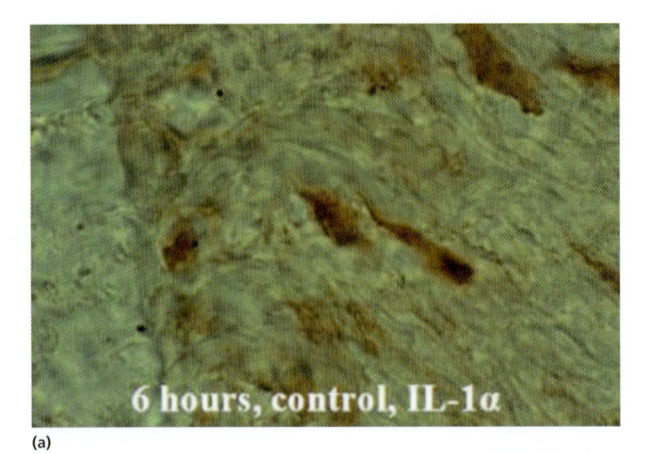

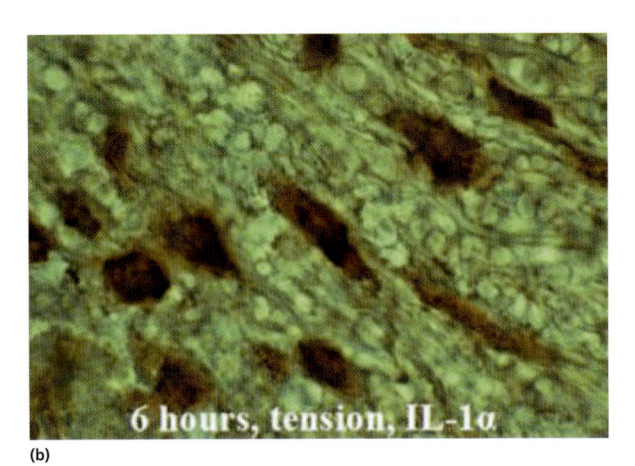

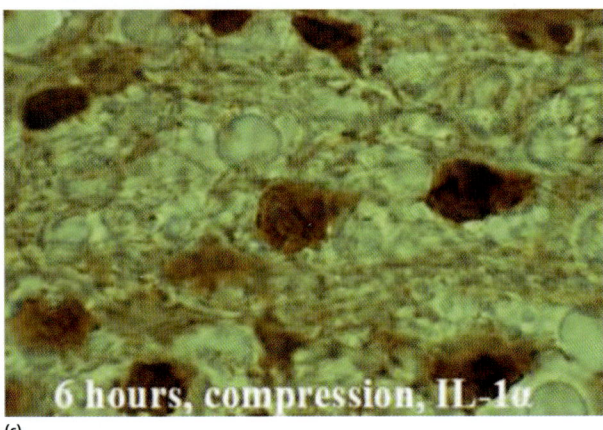

Figure 4.2 Immunohistochemical localization of the cytokine IL-1α in a 6 μm sagittal section of a maxillary canine from a 1-year-old male cat. (a) This section was obtained from a maxillary canine that had not been subjected to orthodontic force (control). A few PDL fibroblasts are stained lightly (brown) for IL-1α. Light staining intensity is suggestive of a low cellular concentration of the cytokine. (b) This tooth was subjected to 80 g of translatory force for 6 hours. The cells in this photograph are located in the tension zone, and are stained intensely for the cytokine, indicative of high cellular concentrations, compared with the control. Many of the cells appear elongated due to stretching. The round-shaped cells may have already detached themselves from the stretched extracellular matrix. (c) The cells in the photographs belong to the compression zone. They are stained intensely for IL-1α. The shape of most cells is round, either because of a reduction in available space due to pressure, or because of cell detachment from the surrounding matrix. (Source: Courtesy Dr. Ze'ev Davidovitch.)

While some cytokines have been positively associated with the inflammatory reaction and bone resorption occurring during OTMs, others have been described as presenting an inverse effect. The expression of anti-inflammatory cytokine, IL-10, is significantly higher on the tension side than the compression side (Garlet et al., 2007). Accordingly, it was demonstrated that tensile strain induces IL-10 synthesis in PDL (Long et al., 2001). In this context, IL-10 is supposed to counteract the effect of inflammatory cytokines during the tooth-movement process and contribute to bone formation in PDL tension areas. Indeed, previous studies demonstrate an important role for IL-10 in bone metabolism *in vivo*, as IL-10-deficient mice present an increased inflammatory responsiveness, decreased osteoblast generation and bone formation (Claudino et al., 2010). These findings suggest that both pro- and anti-inflammatory interleukins play an important role in mechanical-force-induced OTM.

TNF and the RANK/RANKL/OPG system

TNF-α is a proinflammatory cytokine that is often overexpressed in a number of disease states such as sepsis syndrome, rheumatoid arthritis, inflammatory bowel disease, and periodontitis. The human polymorphonuclear leukocytes derived from alveolar bone can spontaneously produce IL-1α, IL-1β and TNF-α in the site of inflammation, and likely initiate inflammation and regulate augmentation of bone resorption *in vivo*. *In vivo* studies demonstrated that TNF-α was expressed in the PDL and alveolar bone during OTM (Bletsa et al., 2006; Garlet et al., 2007). Indeed, TNF-α present a central role in tooth movement process, since TNF receptor type 1 deficient mice present a significant decrease in tooth movement in response to orthodontic force (Andrade et al., 2007).

Other cytokines of the TNF-α family, namely the cytokines of the RANKL/RANK/OPG system, play a critical role in inducing bone remodeling. The TNF-related ligand RANKL and its two receptors RANK and OPG, have been shown to be involved in this remodeling process (Alhashimi et al., 2001). RANKL is a downstream regulator of osteoclast formation and activation, through which many hormones and cytokines produce their osteoresorptive effect. In the bone system, RANKL is expressed on the osteoblast cell lineage and it exerts its effect by binding to the RANK receptor on osteoclast lineage cells. This binding leads to rapid differentiation of hematopoietic osteoclast precursors to mature osteoclasts. OPG is a decoy receptor produced by osteoblastic cells, which compete with RANK for RANKL binding. The biological effects of OPG on bone cells include inhibition of terminal stages of osteoclast differentiation, suppression of activation of matrix osteoclasts, and induction of apoptosis. Thus, bone remodeling is controlled by a balance between RANK–RANKL binding and OPG production (Theoleyre et al., 2004).

Kanzaki et al. (2002) demonstrated that compressive forces up-regulated RANKL expression and induction of COX-2 in human PDL cells in vitro. Aihara et al. (2005) also showed the presence of RANKL in periodontal tissues during experimental tooth movement of rat molars. The number and distribution patterns of RANKL and RANK-expressing osteoclasts change when excessive orthodontic force is applied to periodontal tissues. Interestingly, different patterns of RANKL/OPG expression are present in PDL tension and compression sites of teeth submitted to orthodontic forces, being the differential balance that is supposed to determine the tissue response outcome (Menezes et al., 2008). Accordingly, compression force significantly increased RANKL and decreased OPG secretion in human PDL cells in a time- and force-magnitude-dependent manner (Nishijima et al., 2006; Yamaguchi et al., 2006). Accordingly, Kanzaki et al. (2004, 2006) demonstrated that transfer of the RANKL gene to the periodontal tissue activated osteoclastogenesis and accelerated the amount of experimental tooth movement in rats. In contrast, OPG gene transfer inhibited RANKL-mediated osteoclastogenesis, and inhibited experimental tooth movement. While the exact source(s) of RANKL in PDL area remains to be determined, it was recently demonstrated that deletion in PDL and bone lining cells blocks OTM (Yang et al., 2018). Additionally, mice specifically lacking RANKL in osteocytes present a reduction of OTM (Shoji-Matsunaga et al., 2017), suggesting that multiple cellular sources may account for the RANKL production in response to orthodontic forces. Interestingly, a recent study demonstrates that an injectable Poly (lactic acid-co-glycolic acid: PLGA) formulation containing RANKL, which is able to sustain RANKL for more than 30 days, accelerates OTM in rats (Chang et al., 2019), suggesting a potential translational application. The higher force magnitudes did not increase RANKL expression or osteoclasts counts or amount of tooth movement. This suggests that after a certain magnitude of force, there is a saturation in the biological response, which does not support the concept of higher forces application to accelerate the rate of tooth movement (Alikhani et al., 2015).

It is also important to consider that RANKL and OPG expression may be decisively modulated by cytokines. Indeed, it was previously demonstrated that higher TNF-α expression on the compression side possibly drives the upregulation of RANKL; higher levels of IL-10 are supposed to increase OPG expression on the tension side (Garlet et al., 2007). Recent studies point to sclerostin as an additional important regulator of RANKL along OTM (Odagaki et al., 2018; Ohori et al., 2019), reinforcing the complexity of the RANK system regulation. It is therefore suggested that the RANKL–RANK system is directly involved in regulation of OTM (Figure 4.3).

CD40, another member of the TNF superfamily, is a cell surface receptor seen in a variety of inflammatory and resident cells. Cellular responses mediated by CD40 are triggered by its counter receptor CD40L, which also belongs to the TNF gene family. It was found that CD40–CD40L interaction appears to be an active process during OTM, and that orthodontic force induces T-cell activation (Hayashi et al., 2012). Such activation might be involved in the induction of inflammatory mediators and subsequent bone remodeling (Alhashimi et al., 2004). Indeed, it has been suggested that OPG exists in both membrane-bound and soluble forms and that its expression is up-regulated by CD40 stimulation.

The chemokine system

Collectively, chemokines are defined as small proteins of the cytokine family that have a broad range of activities involved in the recruitment and function of specific populations of leukocytes at the site of inflammation. Chemokine messages are decoded by specific chemokine receptors, which, once activated, regulate cytoskeletal rearrangement, integrin-dependent adhesion, and the binding and detachment of cells from their substrate. Chemokines target all types of leukocytes and are being considered as major regulators of inflammatory processes (Silva et al., 2007). Chemokines have been identified as essential signals for the trafficking of osteoblast and osteoclast precursors, and also for the development, activity and survival of bone cells (Silva et al., 2007).

Regarding OTM, mechanical loading triggers the expression of several chemokines, which in turn create microenvironments that direct inflammatory cell migration and can influence bone formation and resorption processes. The chemokines CCL2, CCL3, CCL5, and CXCL2, which present a marked inflammatory character, were found to be highly expressed during orthodontic movement, mainly in the PDL pressure zone (Alhashimi et al., 1999; Garlet et al., 2008), which is characterized by the predominance of bone resorptive activity. Accordingly, the expression of CCL2 and CCL5 was found to be upregulated during orthodontic force application in mice PDL as being associated with the presence of TRAP positive cells (Andrade et al., 2007; Madureira et al., 2012).

Experimental studies demonstrate a pivotal role for the chemokine system in the orthodontic movement, since CCL3 deficient mice showed impairment in the amount of tooth movement and a reduced number of TRAP-positive osteoclasts after mechanical loading (Taddei et al., 2013). It was also demonstrated that the proinflammatory and osteoclastogenic role of CCL3 is dependent on its binding to the receptor CCR1, in theory, expressed by cells of monocytic lineage and consequently potential preosteoclasts (Taddei et al., 2013). Interestingly, other chemokine receptors characteristically expressed by cells of the monocytic lineage, such as CCR2 and CCR5, are described as playing distinct roles in the OTM process. CCR2, specifically the CCR2-CCL2 axis, is positively associated with osteoclast recruitment, bone resorption, and OTM (Taddei et al., 2012). On the other hand, the chemokine receptor CCR5 is described as a downregulator of alveolar bone resorption during orthodontic movement (Andrade et al., 2009). In this setting, a linear relation between the force and the level of CCL2 and CCL5 was shown, while higher force magnitudes did not increase the expression of such chemokines (Alikhani et al., 2015). Recently, ACKR2, a decoy receptor for CC chemokines, was demonstrated to function as a regulator of mechanically induced bone remodeling by affecting the differentiation and activity of bone cells and the availability of CC chemokines, such as CCL2 and CCL3, in the periodontal microenvironment (Lima et al., 2017). Collectively, such data suggests that different subpopulations of the monocytic lineage may be attracted to the PDL area by different chemokines, and subsequently present opposing roles in the determination of tooth movement outcome.

It is also important to consider that chemokine expression in the PDL environment can also impact soft tissue remodeling and bone formation associated with the tooth movement process. The chemokine CXCL12 was described to be highly expressed in both

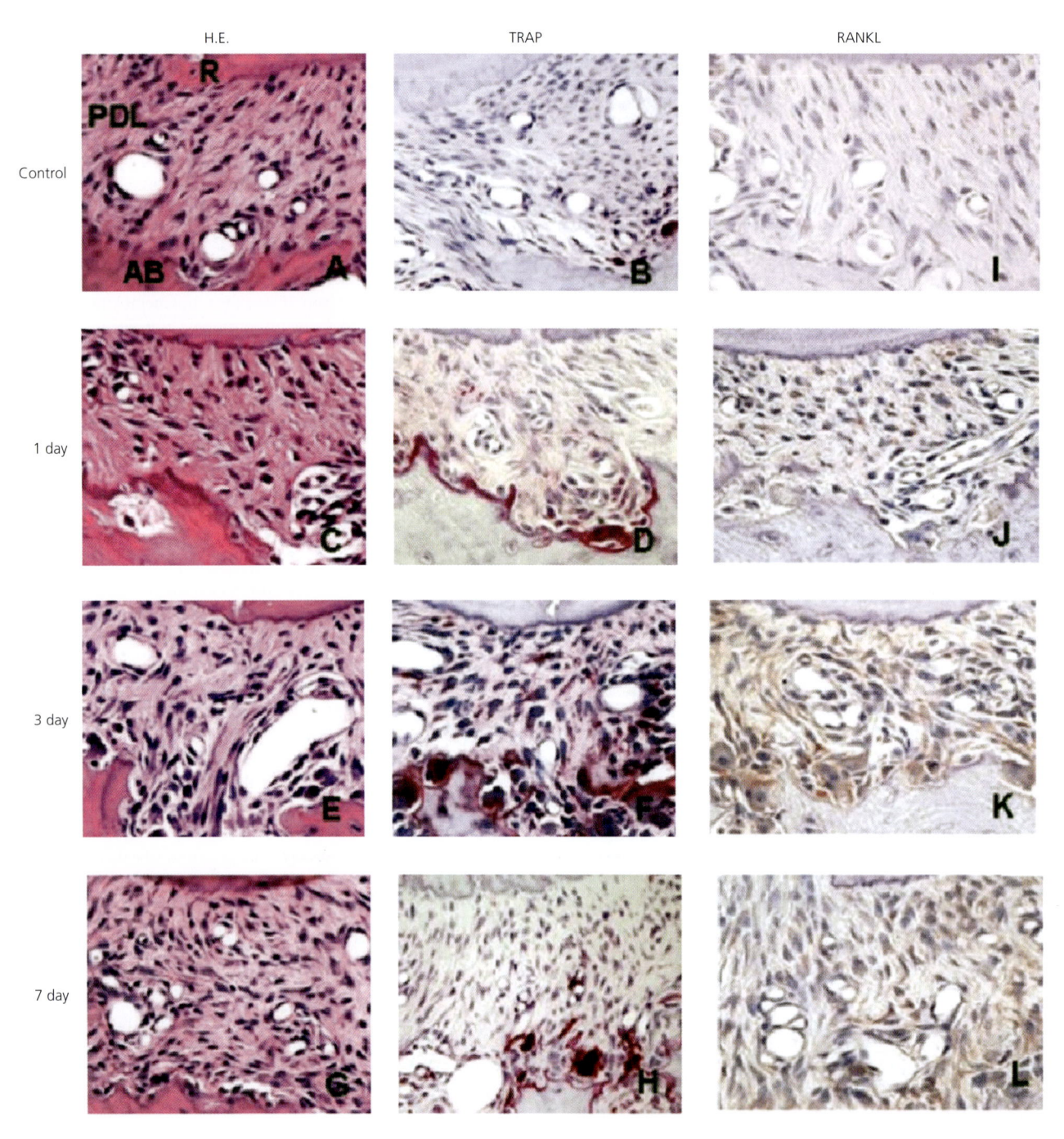

Figure 4.3 Immunohistochemical staining for RANKL in PDL after 7 days during tooth movement. Rat PDL specimens were composed of relatively dense connective tissue fibers and fibroblasts that regularly ran in a horizontal direction from the root cementum toward the alveolar bone. Blood capillaries were mainly recognized near the alveolar bone in the PDL. The alveolar bone and root surface were relatively smooth, but only a few mononuclear and multinucleate osteoclasts and resorption lacunae were rarely observed on the alveolar bone surface (A). Some of these mononuclear and multinucleate osteoclasts were positive to TRAP (B). On 1 day after tooth movement, the arrangement of the fibers and fibroblasts become coarse and irregular, and blood capillaries were pressured (C). Resorption lacunae with a few TRAP-positive multinucleate osteoclasts were observed on the surface of the alveolar bone and root (D). Three days after tooth movement, the PDL was composed of coarse arrangement of fibers and expanded blood capillaries (E). Many resorption lacunae with TRAP-positive multinucleate osteoclasts appeared on the alveolar bone surface, while in the fibers of the PDL, many mononuclear TRAP-positive cells were present (F). Seven days after tooth movement, fibroblasts in the PDL were increased (G). Further, on the surface of the alveolar bone, bone resorption lacunae with multinucleate TRAP-positive osteoclasts were recognized. Mononuclear TRAP-positive cells were decreased in comparison with these 3 days after the movement (H). The immunoreactivity of RANKL was weakly localized in cytoplasm of some fibroblasts and pericytes near the alveolar bone surface (I). One day after tooth movement, RANKL positive fibroblasts in the PDL and osteoblasts at the bone surface were increased (J). Three days after tooth movement, many RANKL positive osteoclasts and fibroblasts were observed. The immunoreactivity to RANKL of the fibroblasts become more strong (K). Seven days after movement, the immunoreactivity of RANKL was observed in the fibroblasts and osteoclasts on the alveolar bone surface, but the degree was decreased (L).

pressure and tension areas of mechanically challenged PDL (Garlet et al., 2008). Such chemokine is described as significantly inducing proliferation, migration, and collagen type I expression in PDL stem cells and osteoblasts (Lisignoli et al., 2006; Du et al., 2012), suggesting an anabolic role in the tooth-movement process. The involvement of CXCL12 in OTM is reinforced by the interruption of experimental tooth movement in rats by AMD3100, an antagonist of the CXCL12 receptor, named CXCR4 (Hatano et al., 2018). Similarly, CCR5 is supposed to contribute to bone formation in response to orthodontic forces, since RUNX2 and osteocalcin levels are decreased in CCR5 deficient mice (Andrade et al., 2009).

Finally, cross regulation between cytokines and chemokines has been demonstrated in the OTM context (Andrade et al., 2009), reinforcing the existence of a complex regulatory network involved in the determination of tissue response to orthodontic forces.

Growth factors

Growth factors are usually described as molecules with the ability to stimulate or enhance cellular growth, proliferation, and differentiation; and consequently, capable of regulating a variety of cellular processes involved in development, maintenance of tissue homeostasis, and wound healing. Different types of mediators can fit in the growth factor description, including a series of cytokines, TGF-β being the prototypic example.

TGF-β is a pleiotropic cytokine that can regulate cell growth, differentiation, and matrix production. Generally, TGF-β has an anabolic nature, increasing the proliferation and chemotaxis of PDL cells, and upregulating the expression of COL-I (Matsuda et al., 1992; Sporn and Roberts, 1993; Chang et al., 2002). TGF-β also presents anabolic properties on bone tissue, recruiting osteoblast precursors and inducing their differentiation, and enhancing the production of bone matrix proteins (Kanaan and Kanaan, 2006). TGF-β expression was found to be increased during OTM, being observed in osteoblasts in the tension zone, and in bone-resorbing osteoclasts in the compression zone (Kobayashi et al., 2000; Dudic et al., 2006), which suggests a broad role for this cytokine in the tooth movement process (Garlet et al., 2007). Barbieri et al. (2013) reported a significant increase in TGF-β in GCF during OTM at the pressure side. A recent study investigated the potential application of platelet-rich plasma, characteristically rich in growth factors such as TGF-β, in experimental OTM in rats. However, no significant effects were observed (Akbulut et al., 2019), suggesting that the endogenous levels of molecules may be sufficient to promote an effective tooth movement.

Matrix metalloproteinases (MMPs)

These agents are zinc-ion-dependent proteolytic enzymes, produced by a wide variety of cells during developmental processes, inflammatory diseases, degenerative articular diseases, tumor invasion, and wound healing. These enzymes are classified into several subgroups, i.e., collagenases (MMP-1, 8, and 13), gelatinases (MMP-2 and 9), stromelysins, membrane-type MMPs, and other subfamilies. Most of the MMPs are produced as pro-enzymes, cleaved at the specific site to become a mature form, and then secreted and activated in the presence of zinc and calcium ions. The activation of MMPs is also regulated by a group of endogenous proteins named tissue inhibitors of metalloproteinases (TIMPs), which are each capable of inhibiting almost every member of the MMP family in a nonspecific way. The MMPs/TIMPs ratio is supposed to determine the turnover rate of periodontal tissues, and consequently to influence the outcome of OTM (Garlet et al., 2007).

In vivo studies demonstrated that MMP-1, 2, 3, 8, 9, and 13 were expressed in the PDL and alveolar bone during OTM (Takahashi et al., 2003, 2006; Garlet et al., 2007; Leonardi et al., 2007). Further, in vitro studies also demonstrated that the expression of MMP-1 and MMP-2 mRNA in human PDL cells was detected after exposure to mechanical stress (He et al., 2004; Redlich et al., 2004). When MMPs and TIMPs were investigated simultaneously in PDL under orthodontic forces, higher MMP-1 levels were found in the compression than in the tension side, while TIMP-1 levels were upregulated in the tension area (Garlet et al., 2007), suggesting that there exists a differential pattern of expression providing distinct microenvironments favorable for extracellular matrix synthesis or degradation. The role of the MMP system in the regulation of OTM was experimentally confirmed, since the inhibition of MMPs activity with chemically modified tetracyclines, or by anti-inflammatory or immunosuppressive drugs (such as potassium diclofenac and dexamethasone), inhibited experimental tooth movement in rats (Bildt et al., 2007; Molina Da Silva et al., 2017).

Neuropeptides

According to Lundy and Linden (2004) it is generally accepted that the nervous system contributes to the pathophysiology of peripheral inflammation, and a neurogenic component has been implicated in many inflammatory diseases including periodontitis. Neurogenic inflammation should be regarded as a protective mechanism, which forms the first line of defense and protects tissue integrity. Sensory neuropeptides play important roles in neurogenic inflammation, including vasodilatation, plasma extravasation, and recruitment of immune cells. However, a more extensive function for neuropeptides in the regulation of immune cell activity has also been proposed. During inflammation, there is a sprouting of peptidergic peripheral fibers and increased neuropeptide content.

Substance P and neurokinin A

SP and neurokinin A (NKA) are members of the tachykinin (tachyswift) neuropeptide family, and as such evoke rapid responses upon release. They exert a wide variety of biological actions and are intimately linked with neurogenic inflammation. The intensity of neurogenic inflammation has been shown to have a dose-dependent relationship with the levels of SP and/or NKA. SP causes vasodilatation by acting directly on smooth-muscle cells and indirectly by stimulating histamine release from mast cells in a concentration-dependent manner. Increased microvascular permeability, edema formation, and subsequent plasma protein extravasation are prominent peripheral effects of the tachykinins, underlying their powerful proinflammatory properties. The SP-induced contraction of endothelial cells and subsequent plasma extravasation allow substances such as bradykinin and histamine to gain access to the site of injury and to afferent nerve terminals. SP also interacts with other neurotransmitters: indeed, the characteristic edema formation mediated by SP has been shown to be modulated by nitrous oxide (Hughes et al., 1990). Lee et al. (2007), who outlined the mechanism of action of SP on OTM, demonstrated increased expression of the chemokine C–C ligand (CCL) 20 mRNA, CCL20 protein, and heme oxygenase (HO)-1 in a dose- and time-dependent manner. SP is also responsible for initiating phosphorylation of IkappaB, degradation of IkappaB, and activation of nuclear factor (NF)-kappaB. This reaction confirms the role of SP, along with other immunoregulators, in inducing HO-1, and the inflammatory mediator macrophage inflammatory protein (MIP)-3 alpha/CCL20 in PDL cells in the development of inflammation associated with OTM.

Calcitonin gene-related peptide

CGRP is widely distributed throughout the central and peripheral nervous systems and is found at particularly high levels in sensory nerves. CGRP has potent vasodilator activity and is frequently co-localized with SP. Bone tissue contains CGRP-immunoreactive nerve fibers, whose increased concentrations during bone development and regeneration suggest that they are directly involved in the local regulation of bone remodeling. Further evidence shows that CGRP, which is derived from alternative splicing of calcitonin gene mRNA, plays a role in bone metabolism. It inhibits osteoclastic bone resorption by directly blocking osteoclast activation, or by indirectly regulating the osteoblast release of cytokines such as interleukin-1 and TNF-α, which can affect osteoclast function.

Villa et al. (2006) reported that CGRP influences the process of mechanically induced bone remodeling through its pro-osteoclastogenic effect on the OPG/RANK/RANKL triad. Through this mechanism, it reduces OPG release and expression by hOB (human osteoblast-like cells). Their results also demonstrated that the cAMP/PKA pathway is involved in the CGRP inhibition of OPG mRNA and protein secretion by hOB, and that this effect favors osteoclastogenesis. CGRP could thus modulate the balance between osteoblast and osteoclast activity, participating in the fine-tuning of all of the bone remodeling phases necessary for the subsequent anabolic effect.

Vasoactive intestinal polypeptide

VIP is another neuropeptide with immunosuppressive properties. VIP is one of a group of regulatory molecules termed macrophage-deactivating factors that are believed to prevent the excessive production of proinflammatory cytokines. Since the mid-1990s, VIP has been identified as an important immunomodulatory peptide, capable of regulating the production of both pro- and anti-inflammatory mediators. Interestingly, VIP can also counteract the inflammatory effects of DAMPs, suggesting that neural–immunological regulatory pathways can operate in the regulation of force-induced OTM (Chorny and Delgado, 2008).

Neuropeptide Y

Neuropeptide Y (NPY) is a potent vasoconstrictor and amplifies the postsynaptic effects of other vasoconstrictors such as noradrenaline. The vasoconstrictor activities of NPY *in vivo* are mediated principally by the NPY Y1 receptor. In addition, NPY has potent angiogenic properties.

Neuropeptides and OTM: A synthesis

Norevall et al. (1995) observed that the expression of CGRP and SP increases in the PDL in response to buccally directed OTM of the upper first molar in the rat. Further, their continuous observations suggest that VIP and NPY, in contrast to the main sensory neuropeptides, CGRP and SP, are not involved in the tissue processes that occur in the remodeling of PDL and alveolar bone during OTM. In relation to tooth movement, Kvinnsland and Kvinnsland (1990) localized CGRP in the pulp and PDL of rats receiving orthodontic forces to maxillary molars for five days. In unstressed teeth, CGRP immunoreactivity was localized primarily in pulp and PDL nerves surrounding blood vessels. In moving teeth, the number of CGRP-containing nerves in both pulp and PDL increased, and their staining intensified, particularly in PDL tension sites. In these areas, dark "spots," which were probably fibroblasts that have bound CGRP released from stressed sensory nerve endings, were observed (Figure 4.4). The experimental tooth movement induces dynamic changes in density and distribution of periodontal as well as pulpal nerve fibers, indicating their involvement in both early stages of PDL remodeling and, later, in its regenerative processes, generally occurring in concert with modulation of blood vessels (Vandevska-Radunovic et al., 1997). The study by Kato et al. (1996) suggested that the neurofilament protein (NFP)-, CGRP-, VIP- and NPY-containing nerve fibers in the PDL play important roles in the modulation of pain, tissue remodeling, and blood flow regulation during tooth movement.

Activation of inflammation, apoptosis, and cell cycles of PDL in OTM

Funakoshi et al. (2013) reported increased numbers of TUNEL- and caspase 8-positive PDL cells at day 5 after the application of an orthodontic force in rat OTM experiments. They also reported that application of a compressive force to human PDL cells induced G1 arrest and caspase 8 protein production in human PDL cells. McCulloch et al. (1989) and Kobayashi et al. (1999) reported that cell death by apoptosis occurred following cell proliferation in response to mechanical stress. Mabuchi et al. (2002) reported that the ratios of cell proliferation and cell death were closely related to the regeneration and reconstruction of PDL in response to orthodontic force. Therefore, the rate of tooth movement may be involved in the ratios of cell proliferation and cell death of PDL cells. Furthermore, TNF-α plays a significant role in the control of proliferation, differentiation, and apoptosis. TNF-α has been shown to trigger apoptosis in osteoblast and PDL cells. Sugimori et al. (2018) concluded that micro-osteoperforations may accelerate tooth movement through activation of cell proliferation and apoptosis of PDL cells.

These present and previous findings suggest that activation of inflammation, apoptosis, and cell cycles of PDL may potentially increase the rate of tooth movement.

Response of the dental pulp to mechanical forces

The dental pulp is a highly vascularized tissue situated in an inextensible environment surrounded by rigid dentin walls. The pulp vascular system is not only responsible for nutrient supply but also contributes actively to the pulp inflammatory response and subsequent regeneration (Rombouts et al., 2017).

Periodontal and pulpal blood flow increased by rat experimental tooth movement (Kvinnsland et al., 1989) and humans (Sabuncuoglu and Ersahan, 2015). Furthermore, the expression of HIF-1α and VEGF was enhanced by mechanical force. HIF-1α and VEGF may play an important role in retaining the homeostasis of dental pulp during OTM (Wei et al., 2015)

Römer et al. (2014) showed the induction of hypoxia in dental pulp after OTM. The induction of oxidative stress in human dental pulp cells showed up-regulation of the proinflammatory and angiogenic genes Cox-2, VEGF, IL-6, and IL-8. It suggests that OTM affects dental pulp circulation by hypoxia, which leads to an inflammatory response inside treated teeth.

Recent studies reported that an orthodontic force mediated the IL-17 level in the dental pulp microenvironment (Yu et al., 2016). Therefore, pulp tissue may be expected to undergo a remodeling process after tooth movement.

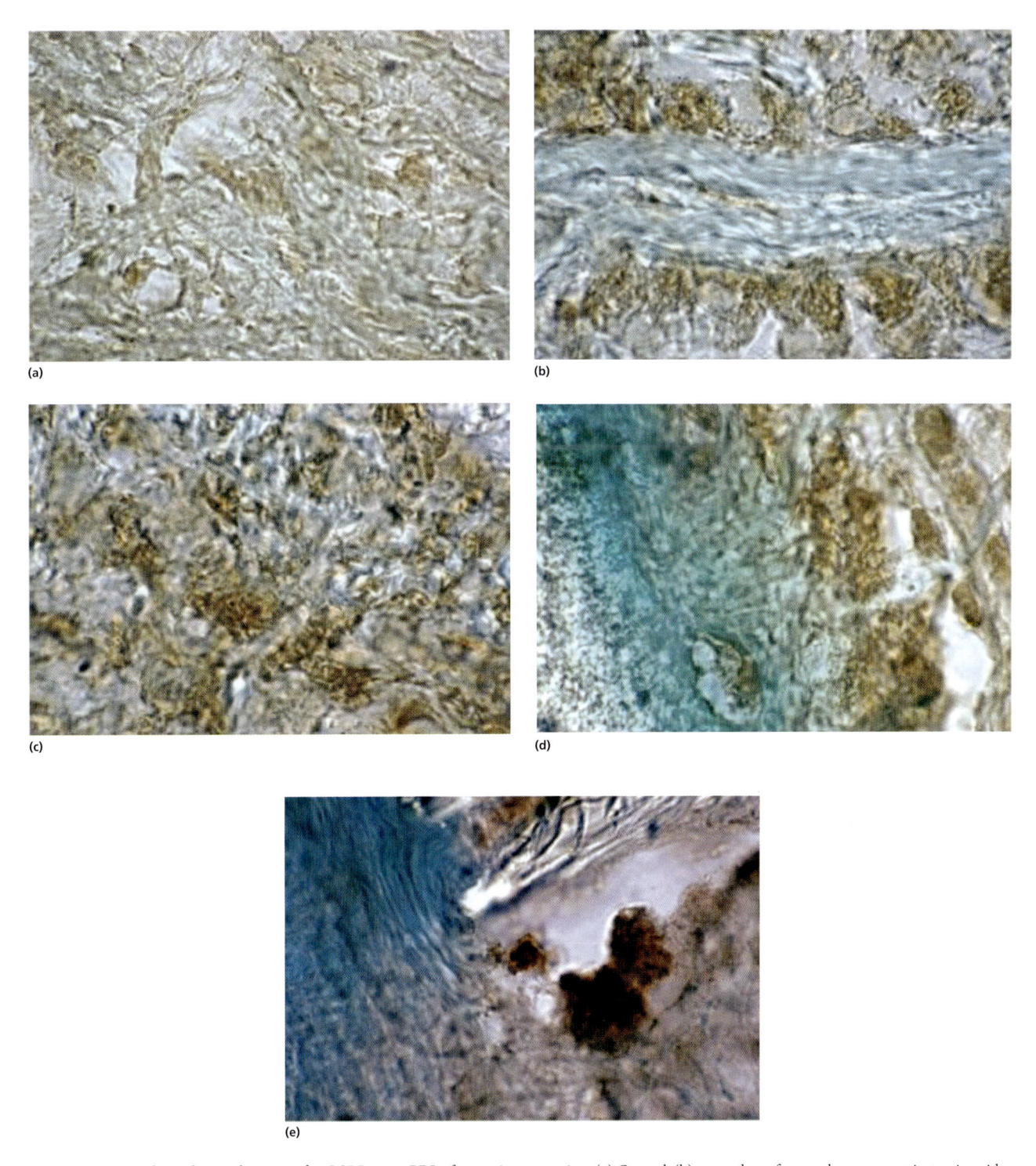

Figure 4.4 Immunohistochemical staining for CGRP in cat PDL after canine retraction. (a) Control; (b) seven days after tooth movement in tension side; (c) seven days after tooth movement in compression side; (d) 28 days after tooth movement in tension side; (e) 28 hours after tooth movement in compression side. (Source: Courtesy of Dr. Ze'ev Davidovitch.)

Neuropeptide response in dental pulp to orthodontic force

The innervation of the dental pulp includes sensory nerve fibers, which may also subserve dentinal fluid dynamics and regulate pulpal blood flow, providing reflexes to preserve dental tissues and promote wound healing. The main neuropeptides associated with these functions include SP, CGRP, and NKA, which are abundant in the pulp and periodontium (Kim, 1990; Ohkubo et al., 1993). Release of these neuropeptides after stimulation of sensory nerve fibers induces vasodilatation and increases vascular permeability, a condition referred to as neurogenic inflammation (Fristad et al., 1997). It is concluded that the stimulation of sensitive teeth may induce pulpal changes such as induction of neurogenic inflammation and alteration of pulpal blood flow.

The morphology and distribution of CGRP and SP through immunoreactive nerves have been shown to change their pattern as a result of local pulp trauma, indicating their role in the inflammatory process in connection with tissue injury and repair. The expressions of SP, CGRP, and NKA in inflamed human dental pulp tissue are significantly higher compared with healthy pulp. In addition, it was observed that the expression of CGRP and/or SP increases in the dental pulp in response to orthodontic treatment in rats, cats, and humans (Parris et al., 1989; Kvinnsland and Kvinnsland, 1990; Norevall et al., 1998). Another report suggested that these neuropeptides might be involved in inflammation of the dental pulp at the time of OTM (Norevall et al., 1995). Previous immunohistochemical studies demonstrated that MMP-1, 3, 8, 9, and tissue-type plasminogen activator expressions were significantly higher in the inflamed pulps than in clinically healthy pulps. These mediators may play an important role in the pathogenesis of pulpal inflammation.

Yamaguchi et al. (2004) reported that SP and CGRP stimulated the production of IL-1β, IL-6, and TNF-α in human dental pulp fibroblasts (HDPF) in vitro. Moreover, Kojima et al. (2006) reported that SP significantly stimulated the production of PGE_2 and RANKL by HDPF cells, and the increase of RANKL caused by SP stimulation in HDPF cells were partially mediated by PGE_2. Shimizu et al. (2013) demonstrated that the immunoreactivity for Th17, IL-17, IL-17R, IL-6 and KC (IL-8 related protein in rodents) in the atopic dermatitis group was found to be increased in the dental pulp tissue subjected to the orthodontic force on day 9. The atopic dermatitis patients increased the release of IL-6 and IL-8 from human dental pulp cells. Taken together, these findings and our results suggest that HDPF may be actively involved in the progress of inflammation in the pulp tissue during OTM.

Vasodilatation and angiogenesis response to orthodontic forces

Blood flowing through the tooth is confronted with a unique environment. The dental pulp is encased within a rigid, noncompliant shell and its survival is dependent on the blood vessels that access the interior of the tooth through the apical foramen. As a consequence of these unusual environmental constraints, changes in pulpal blood flow or vascular tissue pressure can have serious implications for the health of the dental pulp (Kim, 1990).

The changes occurring in respiration in the dental pulp tissue while it is being subjected to orthodontic force have been reported (Hamersky et al., 1980). Kvinnsland et al. (1989) described a detectable increase in the pulpal blood flow in rats caused by an orthodontic appliance. Rana et al. (2001) found apoptosis in dental pulp tissues of rats undergoing orthodontic stress, whereas Derringer et al. (1996) observed an increase in angiogenesis in human dental pulp tissue following orthodontic force application. Further, aspartate aminotransferase, a cytoplasmic enzyme that is released extracellularly upon cell death, was elevated in the pulp of orthodontically treated teeth (Perinetti et al., 2004). The role of the vascular system and blood circulation incident to OTM has been studied by several investigators. It was concluded that orthodontic force might stimulate vasodilatation in dental pulp tissues (Yamaguchi and Kasai, 2007). The processes that occur in the dental pulp, which were explored in in vivo and in vitro studies, are summarized in Table 4.3.

Pain during OTM

OTM causes inflammatory reactions in the periodontium and dental pulp, which will stimulate release of various biochemical

Table 4.3 Inflammatory responses in dental pulp in response to orthodontic force application.

In vitro studies (stimulated by substance P)	In vivo studies
Prostaglandin E_2 (PGE_2)	CGRP and SP
IL-1α and β	Blood flow
IL-6	Apoptosis
TNF-α	Angiogenesis
RANKL	Aspartate amino transferase activity

mediators. The perception of orthodontic pain is the result of a hyperalgesic response elicited by these mediators. Periodontal pain is caused by a process involving the development of pressure, ischemia, inflammation, and edema. Burstone (1964) identified both immediate and delayed pain responses, which begin a few hours after the application of an orthodontic force and last for approximately 5 days (Scheurer et al., 1996). Krukemeyer et al. (2009) concluded from a survey conducted on 118 patients that 58.5% indicated that they experienced pain for a few days after their appointment, out of which only 26.5% of the patients used pain medication immediately following and 1 day after the last appointment.

Painful sensations result, in part, from the stretching and distortion of tissues by the mechanical loads (Stephenson, 1992), as well as from interactions of multiple inflammatory mediators with local pain receptors (Davies and MacIntyre, 1992). According to a review by Krishnan (2007), the perception of orthodontic pain is due to the changes in blood flow caused by the appliances, correlated with the release and presence of various substances, such as SP, histamine, enkephalin, dopamine, serotonin, glycine, glutamate, gamma-aminobutyric acid, PGs, leukotrienes, and cytokines (Yamasaki et al., 1984; Davidovitch et al., 1988; Davidovitch, 1991; Alhashimi et al., 2001).

Processing of complex information arising from mechanical force application induces recruitment of neurons, which act by way of chemical mediators as modulators of the effector response to the stimulus. The neurogenic inflammation, which evolves following activation of an orthodontic appliance, starts with the release of neuropeptides from strained afferent nerve endings in and around the treated teeth, as well as in the central nervous system. The simultaneous release of neuropeptides, peripherally and centrally, elicits a painful response (Vandevska-Radunovic, 1999). Kato et al. (1996) examined the distribution of nerve fibers containing NFP, CGRP, VIP, and NPY in the PDL of the rat first molar after mechanical force application. They observed an increase in the number of NFP- and CGRP-containing nerve fibers at both the stretched and the compressed sides of the PDL after 3 days of force application, which returned to normal after 14 days. They concluded that NFP-, CGRP-, VIP-, and NPY-containing nerve fibers play an important role in blood flow regulation, tissue remodeling, and modulation of pain perception during tooth movement. This finding was in accordance with earlier reports. Norevall et al. (1995) also agreed about the role of CGRP and SP in tooth movement but contradicted the role of other neuropeptides such as VIP and NPY.

It is imperative that pain control be considered an important aspect of orthodontic mechanotherapy, and that the administration of nonsteroidal anti-inflammatory drugs (NSAIDs) remains the preferred method for pain control during orthodontic treatment. NSAIDs have been used for the relief of orthodontic pain for decades (Krishnan and Davidovitch, 2006b; Angelopoulou et al., 2012). It has been well documented that the synthesis of prostaglandin is mediated by COX enzymes and NSAIDs inhibit the activity of COX enzymes. Therefore, NSAIDs could relieve orthodontic pain by inhibiting the release of prostaglandin (Shenoy et al., 2013). The major concern regarding NSAIDs is the interference with the inflammatory process associated with tooth movement. NSAIDs intake may induce a decrease in levels of prostaglandin, and as a result may inhibit osteoclasts and reduce the rate of tooth movement (Arias and Marquez-Orozco, 2006). Therefore, their effects on the rate of tooth movement need to be validated in future studies (Long et al., 2016).

Currently, several treatment modalities have been applied for the relief of orthodontic pain, such as mechanical and behavioural approaches, and low-level laser therapy (Long et al., 2016). Mechanical approaches have been proposed to relieve orthodontic pain including vibration, chewing gums, biting wafers, and acupuncture. The proposed mechanism for vibration, chewing gum, and biting wafers lies in the fact that mechanical stimuli activate mechanoreceptors that transmit tactile signals while suppressing the transmission of painful signals (Guyton and Hall, 2000). However, its mechanism remains large unknown.

Behavioural approaches that are applied to relieve orthodontic pain include cognitive behavioral therapy (CBT), physical activity, and music therapy. CBT, a form of psychotherapy, uses several treatment sessions to correct the patient's negative attitude and decrease their anxiety. As a result, orthodontic pain is relieved in clinical practice (Wang et al., 2015). Music therapy and physical activity distract patient's attention via the insular cortex-mediated neural pathway (Xu et al., 2013; Sandhu and Sandhu 2015). However, the mechanisms are not convincing.

Low-level laser therapy has been extensively applied for pain relief in both medical and dental practice (Huang et al., 2015; Landucci et al., 2016). A large body of evidence has confirmed the effectiveness of low-level laser therapy in alleviating orthodontic pain (Tortamano et al., 2009; Artés-Ribas et al., 2013; Eslamian et al., 2014). PGE_2 and IL-1β production in stretched human PDL cells was inhibited by laser irradiation *in vitro* (Shimizu et al., 1995). Therefore, it is concluded that low-energy laser irradiation may be useful in reducing the levels of inflammation and pain, as well as decreasing orthodontic treatment time by accelerating the pace of tooth movement, without causing any side effects.

Root resorption and inflammation

Many orthodontists consider external apical root resorption (EARR) to be an unavoidable pathologic consequence of OTM. However, an opposing view is presented in Chapter 17, which describes means to avoid this destructive side effect of orthodontic treatment altogether. The common approach to EARR is to visualize it as an iatrogenic disorder that occurs, unpredictably, after orthodontic treatment, whereby the resorbed apical root portion is replaced with normal bone. This undesirable side effect is described as being the outcome of a sterile, complex inflammatory process that involves various disparate components including mechanical forces, tooth roots, bone, cells, surrounding matrix, and certain known biological messengers (Brezniak and Wasserstein, 2002). Killiany (1999) reported that EARR of >3 mm occurs at a frequency of 30% of a patient population, while 5% of treated individuals were found to have >5 mm of root resorption. Harris et al. (1997, 2001) reported that the sum of the effects of the patients' sex, age, severity of the malocclusion, and the kind of mechanics used accounts for little of the overall variation in EARR. Orthodontic force applications induce a local process that includes all of the characteristics of inflammation (redness, heat, swelling, pain, and reduced function). This inflammation, which is an essential feature of tooth movement, is actually the fundamental component behind the root-resorption process (Bosshardt et al., 1998).

The process of resorption requires specific interactions between various inflammatory cells and hard tissues, whether bone, cementum, or dentine. It is a multistep process. The underlying cellular processes involved in root resorption are thought to be similar if not identical to those that occur during bone resorption, which allow the expected and nonpathological tissue changes that result in the effective tooth movement in response to orthodontic forces (Pierce et al., 1991). Multinucleated clast cells are formed as a result of cellular injuries to bone, cementum, or dentine (Boyde et al., 1984). The progenitor cells arrive at the resorption site via the bloodstream as mononuclear cells, derived from hemopoietic precursors in the spleen or bone marrow, which fuse prior to getting involved in the resorptive process. Its pathogenesis has been assumed to be the removal of necrotic tissue from areas of the PDL that have been compressed by an orthodontic load. It is believed that PGs are involved in root resorption (Seifi et al., 2003), and that inflammatory cytokines and chemokines can play a role in this process (Yamaguchi et al., 2008; Asano et al., 2011; Curl and Sampson, 2011; Diercke et al., 2012). While specific data regarding the molecular basis of root resorption is relatively scarce, at this point it is possible to consider that similar mechanisms seems to operate in the "constructive" inflammation that mediates tooth movement, and in the "destructive" inflammation that results in root resorption. However, it is still unclear if differences in the intensity of the inflammatory process could explain the constructive/destructive dichotomy. Low et al. (2005) reported that RANK and OPG regulated the root resorption process. Yamaguchi et al. (2006) reported that the compressed PDL cells obtained from patients with severe EARR produce a large amount of RANKL and up-regulate osteoclastogenesis. It was recently demonstrated that IL-1β and compressive forces lead to a significant induction of RANKL-expression in cementoblasts, suggesting that the activation of this specific cell type could direct the resorptive response to the apex area (Diercke et al., 2012). Furthermore, exposure to excessive orthodontic force by the PDL of rats produced IL-6, IL-8, IL-17 in resorbed root, and these cytokines may be associated with the deterioration of root resorption (Asano et al., 2011; Hayashi et al., 2012; Yamada et al., 2013).

There have been some reports that systemic forms of chronic inflammation may exacerbate the inflammatory response during OTM, and thus predispose the teeth to increased root resorption. McNab et al. (1999) found that asthmatic patients, both well controlled with medication as well as nonmedicated individuals, have an increased incidence of orthodontically induced EARR in their maxillary molars. This observation was supported by other researchers (Owman-Moll and Kurol, 2000), and it is also supported by the comorbidity concept, which states that a pre-existing inflammatory condition may modify the response to a subsequent stimulus. In this context, the response to the secondary stimulus is clearly exacerbated, and can result in the development of a pathological reaction, which would not take place without the primed inflammatory status (Trombone et al., 2010; Queiroz-Junior et al., 2011; Claudino et al., 2012). Translating such a concept to the OTM scenario, if such chronic inflammation does indeed exacerbate the underlying inflammation in OTM, then, logically, elimination of the chronic inflammation should reduce the increased incidence of root resorption. Accordingly, it has been reported that prednisolone treatment (as used in the treatment and prevention of asthma) leads to significantly less root resorption during OTM (Ong et al., 2000).

Root resorption is believed to be related initially to the force magnitude, and light forces have long been recommended for minimizing this adverse outcome. However, recent reports indicate that force magnitude may not be the most decisive etiologic factor responsible for root resorption, and that the severity of this condition is highly related to the regimen of force application. In this regard, intermittent forces cause less severe root resorption than continuously applied forces (Acar et al., 1999; Maltha et al., 2004).

A search for risk factors affiliated with the development of EARR during orthodontic treatment has led to the suggestion that individual susceptibility, genetics, and systemic factors may be significant modulators of this process. Current research on orthodontic root resorption is directed toward identifying genes involved in the process, their chromosome loci, and their possible clinical significance. Al-Qawasmi et al. (2003) firstly reported evidences of linkage disequilibrium of IL-1β polymorphism in allele 1 and EARR. Subsequently, other groups replicated the possible association of IL-1β genetic variants with the root-resorption process (Bastos Lages et al., 2009; Urban and Mincik, 2010; Iglesias-Linares et al., 2012), and also suggested the involvement of polymorphisms in other genes, such as the vitamin D receptor (Fontana et al., 2012). Experimental data from inbred mouse strains reinforce the hypothesis that the genetic background presents a significant impact in experimentally induced root resorption (Al-Qawasmi et al., 2006). Recent studies reported the extent of genetic influence in the root resorption process in humans. In their review on cellular and molecular pathways in the external root resorption process, Iglesias-Linares and Hartsfield (2017) described clast cell adhesion and the specific role of α/β integrin, osteopontin, and related extracellular matrix proteins, as well as clast cell fusion and activation by the RANKL/OPG and ATP-P2RX7-IL-1 pathway. On the other hand, the meta-analysis by Nowrin et al. (2018) showed that the IL-1β polymorphism is not associated with a predisposition to external apical root resorption. Further research is needed about the extent of genetic influence in the root resorption process.

From the above, root resorption may be regulated by genetic factors and inflammatory cytokines. The role of cytokines as well as neuropeptides, released in response to orthodontic force application, in producing root resorption is outlined in Figure 4.5.

Root resorption in the cementum

Cementum contains 65% inorganic material and 12% water on a wet-weight basis. By volume, inorganic material comprises approximately 45%, organic material 33%, and water 22%. Cementum is less densely mineralized than dentine and enamel, contains no blood vessels, and does not undergo physiological remodelling (Selving et al., 1962; Neiders et al., 1972; Cohen et al., 1992). The chemical composition of cementum may vary by individual, and morphologically, cementum is classified as both cellular and acellular (Foster, 2017).

Chutimanutskul et al. (2005) examined the physical properties of the cementum on the buccal and lingual surfaces of the roots at the cervical third, middle third, and apical third. The authors reported a decreasing gradient in the hardness and elastic modulus of cementum in both surface groups, from the cervical to apical thirds. Apical cementum is predominately cellular, less densely mineralized, and has lower hardness and elastic modulus values than the more densely mineralized acellular cementum found in the middle and cervical thirds of the root (Foster, 2017) . Therefore, the hardness and elastic modulus of cementum depend on the direction of the structural arrangement and the mineral content of the cementum (Henry and Weinmann, 1951; Jones and Boyde, 1972; Rex et al., 2005). Several studies have reported that the hardness of mineralized tissues was positively correlated with the extent of mineralization (Brear et al., 1990; Mahoney et al., 2000; Malek et al., 2001). Some have suggested that the mineral content of cementum might influence the resistance or susceptibility to root resorption.

Yamaguchi et al. (2016) examined whether there was individual variation in the Vickers hardness value of the cementum at the surface of the crown and root at three locations (cervical third, middle third, and apical third) of human first premolar teeth. The results of the study demonstrated that the hardness of the cementum decreased from the cervical to apical regions of the root surfaces. Furthermore, individual variations were observed in the hardness of the cementum, and the Vickers hardness value of the hard group was approximately two times higher than that of the soft group.

Yao-Umezawa et al. (2017) investigated whether individual variation in the hardness and chemical composition of the root apex of the cementum affects the degree of root resorption. In a pit formation assay, the resorbed area in the soft group showed a greater increase than the moderate and hard groups. A correlation was noted between the Vickers hardness and the resorbed area of the cementum in the apical cementum. The Ca/P ratio of the cementum in the soft and moderate groups showed greater decreases than the hard group. A correlation was noted between the Vickers hardness and the Ca/P ratio of the cementum in the apical cementum. These results suggested that the hardness and Ca/P ratio of the cementum may be factors in the occurrence of root resorption caused by orthodontic forces. Furthermore, Iglesias-Linares and Hartsfield (2017) suggested regulatory mechanisms of root resorption repair by cementum at the proteomic and transcriptomic levels.

Conclusions

Tooth movement by orthodontic force application is characterized by remodeling changes in dental and paradental tissues, including the dental pulp, PDL, alveolar bone, and gingiva. Studies during the early years of the twentieth century attempted mainly to analyze the histological changes in paradental tissues during and after tooth movement. Those studies have demonstrated that OTM causes inflammatory reactions in the periodontium and dental pulp. These reactions stimulate the release of various biochemical signals and mediators, causing alveolar bone remodeling and pain.

Although the orthodontic patient may feel periodic discomfort during treatment, the inflammation occurring along the entire duration of treatment is a crucial phenomenon because it is stationed in the heart of the remodeling process that facilitates tooth movement. Therefore, the control of inflammation and the efficiency of OTM are closely intertwined. Continuous unfolding of this intimate association will yield new information, which should enable orthodontists to provide ever improving treatment to their patients, based upon the acquisition of personal biological data of high diagnostic value. This approach to diagnosis and treatment planning draws its power from an increasing reliance upon meaningful personal information about ingredients and functions of cells affiliated with the nervous, skeletal, immune vascular, and endocrine systems. Such biological data, if included in the orthodontic diagnosis, should enable the orthodontist to tailor the treatment plan to fit the patient's biological profile and minimize the risk of causing iatrogenic damage, such as root resorption.

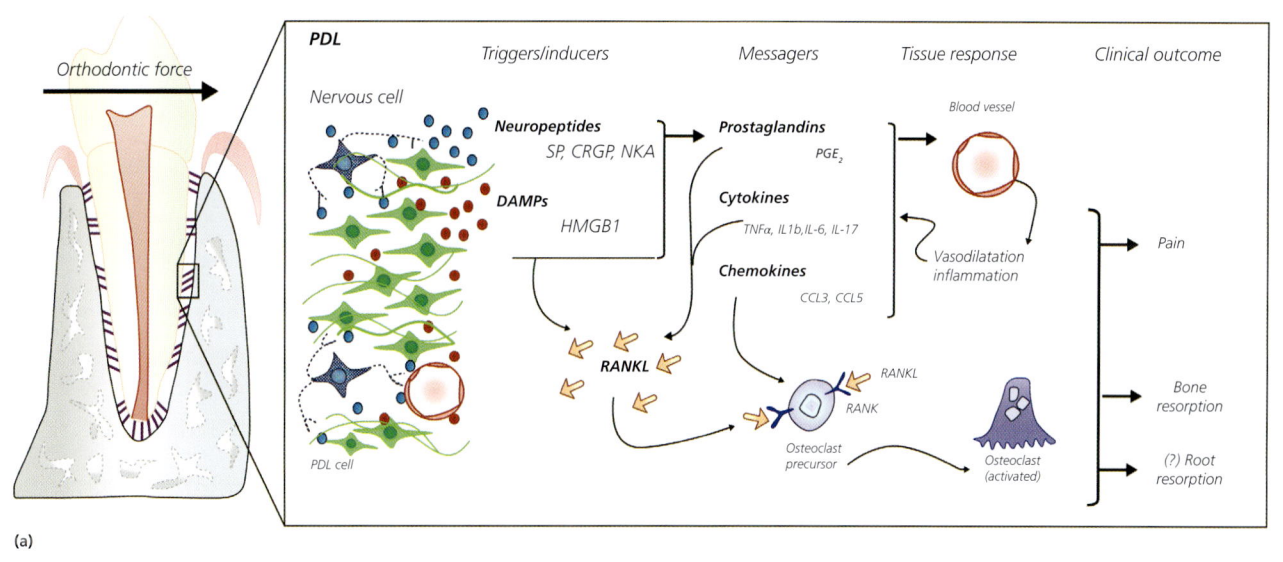

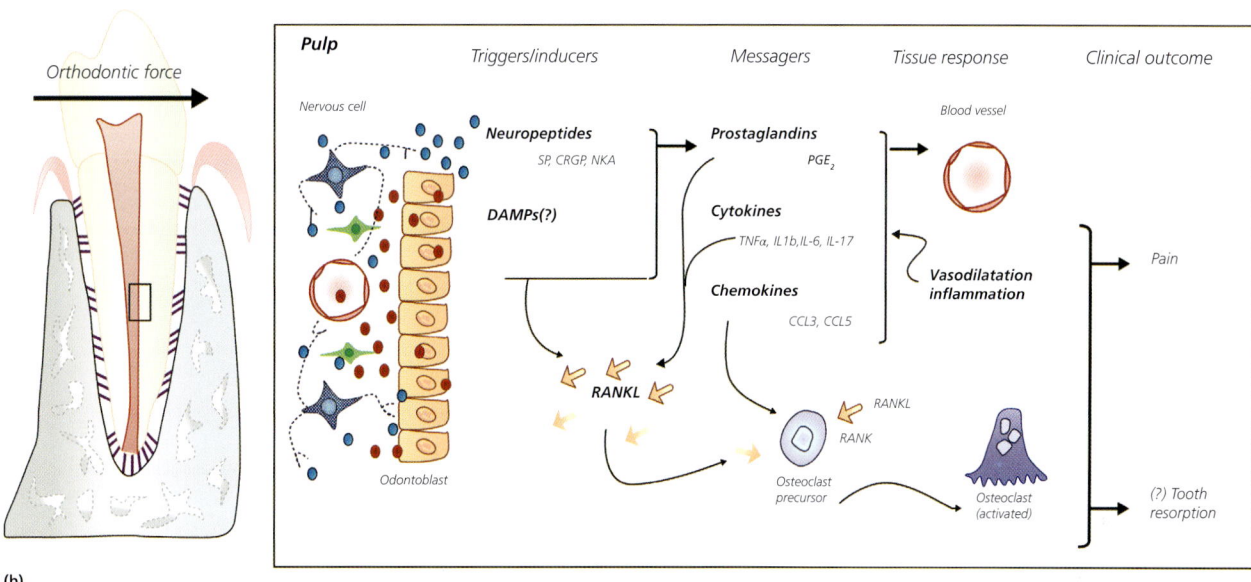

Figure 4.5 (a) Schematic presentation of inflammation in the PDL cells resulting in cytokine release leading to pain, bone resorption, and possible root resorption. (b) Schematic presentation of inflammation of the dental pulp cells resulting in neuropeptide release leading to pain and possible tooth resorption.

References

Acar, A., Canyürek, U., Kocaaga, M. and Erverdi, N. (1999) Continuous vs. discontinuous force application and root resorption. *The Angle Orthodontist* **69**, 159–163.

Aihara, N., Otsuka, A., Yamaguchi, M. et al. (2005) Localization of RANKL and cathepsin K, B, and L in rat periodontal tissues during experimental tooth movement. *Orthodontic Waves* **64**, 107–113.

Akbulut S., Yagci A., Yay A.H. and Yalcin B. (2019) Experimental investigation of effects of platelet-rich plasma on early phases of orthodontic tooth movement. *American Journal of Orthodontic and Dentofacial Orthopedics* **155**, 71–79. doi: 10.1016/j.ajodo.2018.03.015.

Alhashimi, N., Frithiof, L., Brudvik, P. and Bakhiet, M. (1999) Chemokines are upregulated during orthodontic tooth movement. *Journal of Interferon and Cytokine Research* **19**(9), 1047–1052.

Alhashimi, N., Frithiof, L., Brudvik, P. and Bakhiet, M. (2001) Orthodontic tooth movement and de novo synthesis of proinflammatory cytokines. *American Journal of Orthodontics and Dentofacial Orthopedics* **119**, 307–312.

Alhashimi, N., Frithiof, L., Brudvik, P. and Bakhiet, M. (2004) CD 40-CD 40L expression during orthodontic tooth movement in rats. *The Angle Orthodontist* **74**, 100–105.

Alikhani M., Alyami B., Lee I. S. et al. (2015) Saturation of the biological response to orthodontic forces and its effect on the rate of tooth movement. *Orthodontics and Craniofacial Research* **18**(Suppl 1), 8–17. doi: 10.1111/ocr.12090.

Al-Qawasmi, R. A., Hartsfield, J. K. Jr, Everett, E. T. et al. (2003) Genetic predisposition to external apical root resorption in orthodontic patients: linkage of chromosome-18 marker. *Journal of Dental Research* **82**, 356–360.

Al-Qawasmi, R. A., Hartsfield, J. K. Jr, Everett, E. T. et al. (2006) Root resorption associated with orthodontic force in inbred mice: genetic contributions. *European Journal of Orthodontics* **28**(1), 13–19.

Andrade, I. Jr, Silva, T. A., Silva, G. A. et al. (2007) The role of tumor necrosis factor receptor type 1 in orthodontic tooth movement. *Journal of Dental Research* **86**, 1089–1094.

Andrade, I. Jr, Taddei, S. R., Garlet, G. P. et al. (2009) CCR5 down-regulates osteoclast function in orthodontic tooth movement. *Journal of Dental Research* **88**, 1037–1041.

Angelopoulou, M. V., Vlachou, V. and Halazonetis, D. J. (2012) Pharmacological management of pain during orthodontic treatment: a meta-analysis. *Orthodontics and Craniofacial Research* **15**, 71–83.

Arai, C., Nomura, Y., Ishikawa, M. et al. (2010) HSPA1A is upregulated in periodontal ligament at early stage of tooth movement in rats. *Histochemistry and Cell Biology* **134**, 337–343.

Arias, O. R. and Marquez-Orozco, M. C. (2006) Asprin, acetaminophen, and ibuprofen: their effects on orthodontic tooth movement. *American Journal of Orthodontics and Dentofacial Orthopedics* **130**, 364–370.

Artés-Ribas, M., Arnabat-Dominguez, J. and Puigdollers, A. (2013) Analgesic effect of a low-level laser therapy (830 Nm) in early orthodontic treatment. *Lasers in Medical Science* **28**, 335–341.

Asano, M., Yamaguchi, M., Nakajima, R. et al. (2011) IL-8 and MCP-1 induced by excessive orthodontic force mediates odontoclastogenesis in periodontal tissues. *Oral Diseases* **17**, 489–498.

Baba, S., Kuroda, N., Arai, C. et al. (2011) Immunocompetent cells and cytokine expression in the rat periodontal ligament at the initial stage of orthodontic tooth movement. *Archives of Oral Biology* **56**, 466–473.

Barbieri, G., Solano, P., Alarcón, J.A. et al. (2013) Biochemical markers of bone metabolism in gingival crevicular fluid during early orthodontic tooth movement. *The Angle Orthodontist* **83**, 63–69.

Bastos Lages, E. M., Drummond, A. F., Pretti, H. et al. (2009) Association of functional gene polymorphism IL-1beta in patients with external apical root resorption. *American Journal of Orthodontics and Dentofacial Orthopedics* **136**, 542–546.

Bildt, M. M., Henneman, S., Maltha, J. C. et al. (2007) CMT-3 inhibits orthodontic tooth displacement in the rat. *Archives of Oral Biology* **52**, 571–578.

Bletsa, A., Berggreen, E. and Brudvik, P. (2006) Interleukin-1alpha and tumor necrosis factor-alpha expression during the early phases of orthodontic tooth movement in rats. *European Journal of Oral Sciences* **114**, 423–429.

Bonaldi, T., Langst, G., Strohner, R. et al. (2002) The DNA chaperone HMGB1 facilitates ACF/CHRAC-dependent nucleosome sliding. *EMBO Journal* **21**, 6865–6873.

Bosshardt, D. D., Masseredjian, V. and Nanci, A. (1998) Root resorption and tissue repair in orthodontically treated human premolars, in *Biological Mechanisms of Tooth Eruption, Resorption and Replacement by Implants* (eds Z. Davidovitch and J. Mar). Harvard Society for the Advancement of Orthodontics, Boston, MA, pp. 425–437.

Boyde, A., Ali, N. N. and Jones, S. J. (1984) Resorption of dentine by isolated osteoclasts in vitro. *British Dental Journal* **156**, 216–220.

Brezniak, N. and Wasserstein, A. (2002) Orthodontically induced inflammatory root resorption. Part II: The clinical aspects. *The Angle Orthodontist* **72**,180–184.

Brear, K., Currey, J. D., Pond, C.M. and Ramsay, M. A. (1990) The mechanical properties of the dentine and cement of the tusk of the narwhal Monodon monoceros compared with those of other mineralized tissues. *Archives of Oral Biology* **35**, 615–621.

Burstone, C. (1964) Biomechanics of tooth movement, in *Vistas in Orthodontics* (eds. B. S. Kraus, R. A. Riedel). Lea & Febiger, Philadelphia, PA, pp. 197–213.

Chang J. H., Chen P. J., Arul M. R. et al. (2019) Injectable RANKL sustained release formulations to accelerate orthodontic tooth movement. *European Journal Orthodontics* **31**. pii: cjz027. doi: 10.1093/ejo/cjz027.

Chang, Y.C., Yang, S. F., Lai, C. C. et al. (2002) Regulation of matrix metalloproteinase production by cytokines, pharmacological agents and periodontal pathogens in human periodontal ligament fibroblast cultures. *Journal of Periodontal Research* **37**, 196–203.

Chen, G. Y. and Nunez, G. (2010) Sterile inflammation: sensing and reacting to damage. *Nature Reviews Immunology* **10**, 826–837.

Chitanuwat, A., Laosrisin, N. and Dhanesuan, N. (2013) Role of HMGB1 in proliferation and migration of human gingival and periodontal ligament fibroblasts. *Journal of Oral Science* **55**, 45–50.

Chorny, A. and Delgado, M. (2008) Neuropeptides rescue mice from lethal sepsis by down-regulating secretion of the late-acting inflammatory mediator high mobility group box 1. *American Journal of Pathology* **172**, 1297–1307.

Chumbley, A. B. and Tuncay, O. C. (1986) The effect of indomethacin (an aspirin-like drug) on the rate of orthodontic tooth movement. *American Journal of Orthodontics* **89**, 312–314.

Chutimanutskul W., Darendeliler M. A. et al. (2005) Physical properties of human premolar cementum: hardness and elasticity. *Australian Orthodontic Journal* **21**, 117–121

Claudino, M., Garlet, T. P., Cardoso, C. R. et al. (2010) Down-regulation of expression of osteoblast and osteocyte markers in periodontal tissues associated with the spontaneous alveolar bone loss of interleukin-10 knockout mice. *European Journal of Oral Sciences* **118**, 19–28.

Claudino, M., Gennaro, G., Cestari, T. M. et al. (2012) Spontaneous periodontitis development in diabetic rats involves an unrestricted expression of inflammatory cytokines and tissue destructive factors in the absence of major changes in commensal oral microbiota. *Experimental Diabetes Research* **2012**, 356841.

Cohen, M., Garnick, J. J., Ringle, R.D. et al. (1992) Calcium and phosphorus content of roots exposed to the oral environment. *Journal of Clinical Periodontology* **19**, 268–273.

Curl, L. and Sampson, W. (2011) The presence of TNF-alpha and TNFR1 in aseptic root resorption. A preliminary study. *Australian Orthodontic Journal* **27**, 102–109.

Davidovitch, Z. (1991) Tooth movement. *Critical Reviews in Oral Biology and Medicine* **2**, 411–450.

Davidovitch, Z. (1995) Cell biology associated with orthodontic tooth movement, in *The Periodontal Ligament in Health and Disease* (eds. B. B. Berkovitz, B. J. Moxham and H. N. Newman). Mosby, St. Louis, MO, pp. 259–277.

Davidovitch, Z. and Shanfield, J. L. (1975) Cyclic AMP levels in alveolar bone of orthodontically treated cats. *Archives of Oral Biology* **20**, 567–574.

Davidovitch, Z., Montgomery, P. C., Gustafson, G. T. and Eckerdal, O. (1976) Cellular localization of cyclic AMP in periodontal tissues during experimental tooth movement in cats. *Calcified Tissue Research* **19**, 317–329.

Davidovitch, Z., Nicolay, O. F., Ngan, P. W. and Shanfeld, J. L. (1988) Neurotransmitters, cytokines, and the control of alveolar bone remodeling in orthodontics. *Dental Clinics of North America* **32**, 411–435.

Davies, P. and MacIntyre, D. E. (1992) Prostaglandin and inflammation, in *Inflammation: Basic Principles and Clinical Correlates*, 2nd edn (eds J. I. Gallin, I. M. Goldstein and R. Synderman). Raven Press, New York, pp. 123–138.

Derringer, K. A., Jaggers, D. C. and Linden, R. W. (1996) Angiogenesis in human dental pulp following orthodontic tooth movement. *Journal of Dental Research* **75**, 1761–1766.

Diercke, K., Kohl, A., Lux, C. J. and Erber, R. (2012) IL-1beta and compressive forces lead to a significant induction of RANKL-expression in primary human cementoblasts. *Journal of Orofacial Orthopedics* **73**, 397–412.

Dinarello, C. A. and Savage, N. (1989) Interleukin-1 and its receptor. *Critical Reviews in Immunology* **9**, 1–20.

Dolce, C., Maloney, J. S. and Wheeler, T. T. (2002) Current concepts in the biology of orthodontic tooth movement. *Seminars in Orthodontics* **8**, 6–12.

Du, L., Yang, P. and Ge, S. (2012) Stromal cell-derived factor-1 significantly induces proliferation, migration, and collagen type I expression in a human periodontal ligament stem cell subpopulation. *Journal of Periodontology* **83**, 379–388.

Dudic, A., Kiliaridis, S., Mombelli, A. and Giannopoulou, C. (2006) Composition changes in gingival crevicular fluid during orthodontic tooth movement: comparisons between tension and compression sides. *European Journal of Oral Sciences* **114**, 416–422.

Eslamian, L., Borzabadi-Farahani, A., Hassanzadeh-Azhiri, A. et al. (2014) The effect of 810-nm low-level laser therapy on pain caused by orthodontic elastomeric separators. *Lasers in Medical Science* **29**, 559–564.

Fernandes, M. R. U., Suzuki, S. S., Suzuki, H. et al. (2019) Photobiomodulation increases intrusion tooth movement and modulates IL-6, IL-8 and IL-1β expression during orthodontically bone remodeling. *Journal of Biophotonics* **19**, e201800311. doi: 10.1002/jbio.201800311.

Foster B.L. (2017) On the discovery of cementum. *Journal of Periodontal Research* **52**, 666–685.

Fontana, M. L., De Souza, C. M., Bernardino, J. F. et al. (2012) Association analysis of clinical aspects and vitamin D receptor gene polymorphism with external apical root resorption in orthodontic patients. *American Journal of Orthodontics and Dentofacial Orthopedics* **142**, 339–347.

Fristad, I., Kvinnsland, I. H., Jonsson, R. and Heyeraas, K. J. (1997) Effect of intermittent long-lasting electrical tooth stimulation on pulpal blood flow and immunocompetent cells: A hemodynamic and immunohistochemical study in young rat molars. *Experimental Neurology* **146**, 230–239.

Funakoshi, M., Yamaguchi, M., Asano, M. et al. (2013) Effect of compression force on apoptosis in human periodontal ligament cells. *Journal of Hard Tissue Biology* **22**, 41–50.

Garlet, T. P., Coelho, U., Repeke, C. E. et al. (2008) Differential expression of osteoblast and osteoclast chemmoatractants in compression and tension sides during orthodontic movement. *Cytokine* **42**, 330–335.

Garlet, T. P., Coelho, U., Silva, J. S. and Garlet, G.P. (2007) Cytokine expression pattern in compression and tension sides of the periodontal ligament during orthodontic tooth movement in humans. *European Journal of Oral Sciences* **115**, 355–362.

Goodwin, G. H. and Johns, E. W. (1977) The isolation and purification of the high mobility group (HMG) nonhistone chromosomal proteins. *Methods in Cell Biology* **16**, 257–267.

Guyton, A. C. and Hall, J.E. (2000) *Somatic sensations: II pain, headache, and thermal sensations, in Textbook of Medical Physiology*, 10th edn. Elsevier Sciences, Singapore.

Hamersky, P., Weimar, A. and Taintor, J. (1980) The effect of orthodontic force application on the pulpal tissue respiration rate in the human premolar. *American Journal of Orthodontics* **77**, 368–378.

Harris, E. F., Boggan, B. W. and Wheeler, D. A. (2001) Apical root resorption in patients treated with comprehensive orthodontics. *Journal of the Tennessee Dental Association* **81**, 30–33.

Harris, E. F., Kineret, S. E. and Tolley, E. A. (1997) A heritable component for external apical root resorption in patients treated orthodontically. *American Journal of Orthodontics and Dentofacial Orthopedics* **111**, 301–309.

Hatano, K., Ishida, Y., Yamaguchi, H. et al. (2018) The chemokine receptor type 4 antagonist, AMD3100, interrupts experimental tooth movement in rats. *Archives of Oral Biology* **86**, 35–39.

Hayashi, N., Yamaguchi, M., Nakajima, R. et al. (2012) T-helper 17 cells mediate the osteo/odontoclastogenesis induced by excessive orthodontic forces. *Oral Diseases* **18**, 375–388.

He, Y., Macarak, E. J., Korostoff, J. M. and Howard, P. S. (2004) Compression and tension: differential effects on matrix accumulation by periodontal ligament fibroblasts in vitro. *Connective Tissue Research* **45**, 28–39.

Hendrick, J. P. and Hartl, F. U. (1993) Molecular chaperone functions of heat-shock proteins. *Annual Review of Biochemistry* **62**, 349–384.

Henry, J. L. and Weinmann, J. P. (1951) The pattern of resorption and repair of human cementum. *Journal of the American Dental Association* **42**, 270–290.

Huang, Z., Ma, J., Chen, J. et al. (2015) The effectiveness of low-level laser therapy for nonspecific chronic low back pain: a systematic review and meta-analysis. *Arthritis Research and Therapy* **17**, 360.

Hughes, S. R., Williams, T. J. and Brain, S. D. (1990) Evidence that endogenous nitric oxide modulates oedema formation induced by substance P. *European Journal of Pharmacology* **191**, 481–484.

Iglesias-Linares, A., Yanez-Vico, R. M., Ballesta, S. et al. (2012) Interleukin 1 gene cluster SNPs (rs1800587, rs1143634) influences post-orthodontic root resorption in endodontic and their contralateral vital control teeth differently. *International Endodontic Journal* **45**, 1018–1026.

Iglesias-Linares, A. and Hartsfield, J.K. Jr. (2017) Cellular and molecular pathways leading to external root resorption. *Journal of Dental Research* **96**, 145–152.

Ishizu, T., Osoegawa, M., Mei, F. J. et al. (2005) Intrathecal activation of the IL-17/IL-8 axis in opticospinal multiple sclerosis. *Brain* **128**, 988–1002.

Johnson, R. B., Wood, N. and Serio, F. G. (2004) Interleukin-11 and IL-17 and the pathogenesis of periodontal disease. *Journal of Periodontology* **75**, 37–43.

Jones, S. J. and Boyde, A. (1972) A study of human root cementum surfaces as prepared for and examined in the scanning electron microscope. *Zeitschrift für Zellforschung und mikroskopische Anatomie* **130**, 318–337.

Kanaan, R. A. and Kanaan, L. A. (2006) Transforming growth factor beta1, bone connection. *Medical Science Monitor* **12**, RA164–169.

Kanzaki, H., Chiba, M., Arai, K. et al. (2006) Local RANKL gene transfer to the periodontal tissue accelerates orthodontic tooth movement. *Gene Therapy* **13**, 678–685.

Kanzaki, H., Chiba, M., Shimizu, Y. and Mitani, H. (2002) Periodontal ligament cells under mechanical stress induce osteoclastogenesis by receptor activator of nuclear factor kappaB ligand up-regulation via prostaglandin E2 synthesis. *Journal of Bone and Mineral Research* **17**, 210–220.

Kanzaki, H., Chiba, M., Takahashi, I. et al. (2004) Local OPG gene transfer to periodontal tissue inhibits orthodontic tooth movement. *Journal of Dental Research* **83**, 920–925.

Kato, J., Wakisaka, S. and Kurisu, K. (1996) Immunohistochemical changes in the distribution of nerve fibers in the periodontal ligament during experimental tooth movement of the rat molar. *Acta Anatomica*, **157**, 53–62.

Killiany, D. M. (1999) Root resorption caused by orthodontic treatment: an evidence-based review of literature. *Seminars in Orthodontics* **5**, 128–133.

Kim, S. (1990) Neurovascular interactions in the dental pulp in health and inflammation. *Journal of Endodontics* **16**, 48–53.

Kim, Y. S., Lee, Y. M., Park, J. S. et al. (2010) SIRT1 modulates high-mobility group box 1-induced osteoclastogenic cytokines in human periodontal ligament cells. *Journal of Cellular Biochemistry* **111**, 1310–1320.

Kobayashi, E.T., Hashimoto, F., Kobayashi, Y. et al. (1999) Force-induced rapid changes in cell fate at midpalatal suture cartilage of growing rats. *Journal of Dental Research* **78**, 1495–1504.

Kobayashi, Y., Hashimoto, F., Miyamoto, H. et al. (2000) Force-induced osteoclast apoptosis in vivo is accompanied by elevation in transforming growth factor beta and osteoprotegerin expression. *Journal of Bone and Mineral Research* **15**, 1924–1934.

Kojima, T., Yamaguchi, M. and Kasai, K. (2006) Substance P stimulates release of RANKL via COX-2 expression in human dental pulp cells. *Inflammation Research* **55**, 78–84.

Kotake, S., Udagawa, N., Takahashi, K. et al. (1999) IL-17 in synovial fluids from patients with rheumatoid arthritis is a potent stimulator of osteoclastogenesis. *Journal of Clinical Investigation* **103**, 1345–1352.

Krishnan, V. (2007) Orthodontic pain: from causes to management – a review. *European Journal of Orthodontics* **29**, 170–179.

Krishnan, V. and Davidovitch, Z. (2006a) Cellular, molecular, and tissue-level reactions to orthodontic force. *American Journal of Orthodontics and Dentofacial Orthopedics* **129**, 469.e1–32.

Krishnan, V. and Davidovitch, Z. (2006b) The effect of drugs on orthodontic tooth movement. *Orthodontics and Craniofacial Research* **9**, 163–171.

Krukemeyer, A. M., Arruda, A. O. and Inglehart, M. R. (2009) Pain and orthodontic treatment. *The Angle Orthodontist* **79**, 1175–1181.

Kvinnsland, I. and Kvinnsland, S. (1990) Changes in CGRP-immunoreactive nerve fibres during experimental tooth movement in rats. *European Journal of Orthodontics* **12**, 320–329.

Kvinnsland, S., Heyeraas, K. and Ofjord, E. S. (1989) Effect of experimental tooth movement on periodontal and pulpal blood flow. *European Journal of Orthodontics* **11**, 200–205.

Landucci, A., Wosny, A.C., Uetanabaro, L.C. et al. (2016) Efficacy of a single dose of low-level laser therapy in reducing pain, swelling, and trismus following third molar extraction surgery. *International Journal of Oral Maxillofacial Surgery* **45**, 392–398.

Leclerc, P., Wahamaa, H., Idborg, H. et al. (2013) IL-1beta/HMGB1 complexes promote the PGE2 biosynthesis pathway in synovial fibroblasts. *Scandinavian Journal of Immunology* **77**, 350–360.

Lee, S. K., Pi, S. H., Kim, S. H. et al. (2007) Substance P regulates macrophage inflammatory protein 3 alpha/chemokine C-C ligand 20 (CCL20) with heme oxygenase-1 in human periodontal ligament cells. *Clinical and Experimental Immunology* **150**, 567–575.

Leonardi, R., Talic, N. F. and Loreto, C. (2007) MMP-13 (collagenase 3) immunolocalisation during initial orthodontic tooth movement in rats. *Acta Histochemica* **109**, 215–220.

Lima, I.L.A., Silva, J.M.D., Rodrigues, L.F.D. et al. (2017) Contribution of atypical chemokine receptor 2/ackr2 in bone remodeling. *Bone* **101**, 113–122.

Lisignoli, G., Toneguzzi, S., Piacentini, A. et al. (2006) CXCL12 (SDF-1) and CXCL13 (BCA-1) chemokines significantly induce proliferation and collagen type I expression in osteoblasts from osteoarthritis patients. *Journal of Cellular Physiology* **206**, 78–85.

Lock, C., Hermans, G., Pedotti, R. et al. (2002) Gene-microarray analysis of multiple sclerosis lesions yields new targets validated in autoimmune encephalomyelitis. *Nature Medicine* **8**, 500–508.

Long, P., Hu, J., Piesco, N. et al. (2001) Low magnitude of tensile strain inhibits IL-1beta-dependent induction of pro-inflammatory cytokines and induces synthesis of IL-10 in human periodontal ligament cells in vitro. *Journal of Dental Research* **80**, 1416–1420.

Long, H., Wang, Y., Jian, F. et al. (2016) Current advances in orthodontic pain. *International Journal of Oral Science* **8**, 67–75.

Low, E., Zoellner, H., Kharbanda, O. P. and Darendeliler MA (2005) Expression of mRNA for osteoprotegerin and receptor activator of nuclear factor kappa beta ligand (RANKL) during root resorption induced by the application of heavy orthodontic forces on rat molars. *American Journal of Orthodontics and Dentofacial Orthopedics* **128**, 497–503.

Lundy, F. T. and Linden, G. J. (2004) Neuropeptides and neurogenic mechanisms in oral and periodontal inflammation. *Critical Reviews in Oral Biology and Medicine* **15**, 82–98.

Mabuchi, R., Matsuzaka, K. and Shimono, M. (2002) Cell proliferation and cell death in periodontal ligaments during orthodontic tooth movement. *Journal of Periodontal Research* **37**, 118–124.

Madureira, D. F., Taddei, S. A., Abreu, M. H. et al. (2012) Kinetics of interleukin-6 and chemokine ligands 2 and 3 expression of periodontal tissues during orthodontic tooth movement. *American Journal of Orthodontics and Dentofacial Orthopedics* **142**, 494–500.

Mahoney, E., Holt, A., Swain, M. et al. (2000) The hardness and modulus of elasticity of primary molar teeth: an ultra-micro-indentation study. *Journal of Dentistry* **28**, 589–594.

Malek, S., Darendeliler, M. A., Swain, M. V. and Kilpatrick, N. (2001) Physical properties of root cementum: Part I. A new method for 3-dimensional evaluation. *American Journal of Orthodontics and Dentofacial Orthopedics* **120**, 198–208.

Maltha, J. C., van Leeuwen, E. J., Dijkman, G. E. and Kuijpers-Jagtman, A. M. (2004) Incidence and severity of root resorption in orthodontically moved premolars in dogs. *Orthodontics and Craniofacial Research* **7**, 115–121.

Marciniak, J., Lossdörfer, S., Kirschneck, C. et al. (2019) Heat shock protein 70 dampens the inflammatory response of human PDL cells to mechanical loading in vitro. *Journal of Periodontal Research* **13**. doi: 10.1111/jre.12648.

Matsuda, N., Lin, W. L., Kumar, N. M. et al. (1992) Mitogenic, chemotactic, and synthetic responses of rat periodontal ligament fibroblastic cells to polypeptide growth factors in vitro. *Journal of Periodontology* **63**, 515–525.

McCulloch, C. A., Barghava, U. and Melcher, A. H. (1989) Cell death and the regulation of populations of cells in the periodontal ligament. *Cell and Tissue Research* **255**, 129–138.

McDonald, B., Pittman, K., Menezes, G. B. et al. (2010) Intravascular danger signals guide neutrophils to sites of sterile inflammation. *Science* **330**, 362–366.

McNab, S., Battistutta, D., Taverne, A. and Symons, A. L. (1999) External apical root resorption of posterior teeth in asthmatics after orthodontic treatment. *American Journal of Orthodontics and Dentofacial Orthopedics* **116**, 545–551.

Meikle, M. C. (2006) The tissue, cellular, and molecular regulation of orthodontic tooth movement: 100 years after Carl Sandstedt. *European Journal of Orthodontics* **28**, 221–240.

Menezes, R., Garlet, T. P., Letra, A. et al. (2008) Differential patterns of receptor activator of nuclear factor kappa B ligand/osteoprotegerin expression in human periapical granulomas: possible association with progressive or stable nature of the lesions. *Journal of Endodontics* **34**, 932–938.

Molet, S., Hamid, Q., Davoine, F. et al. (2001) IL-17 is increased in asthmatic airways and induces human bronchial fibroblasts to produce cytokines. *Journal of Allergy and Clinical Immunology* **108**, 430–438.

Molina Da Silva, G. P., Tanaka, O. M., Campos Navarro, D.F. *et al.* (2017) The effect of potassium diclofenac and dexamethasone on MMP-1 gene transcript levels during experimental tooth movement in rats. *Orthodontics and Craniofacial Research* **20**, 30–34.

Nicolay, O. F., Davidovitch, Z., Shanfeld, J. L. and Alley, K. (1990) Substance P immunoreactivity in periodontal tissues during orthodontic tooth movement. *Bone and Mineral* **11**, 19–29.

Neiders, M. E., Eick, J.D., Miller, W.A. and Leitner, J. W. (1972) Electron probe microanalysis of cementum and underlying dentin in young permanent teeth. *Journal of Dental Research* **51**, 122–130.

Nishijima, Y., Yamaguchi, M., Kojima, T. *et al.* (2006) Levels of RANKL and OPG in gingival crevicular fluid during orthodontic tooth movement and effect of compression force on releases from periodontal ligament cells *in vitro*. *Orthodontics and Craniofacial Research* **9**, 63–70.

Norevall, L. I., Forsgren, S. and Matsson, L. (1995) Expression of neuropeptides (CGRP, substance P) during and after orthodontic tooth movement in the rat. *European Journal of Orthodontics* **17**, 311–325.

Norevall, L. I., Matsson, L. and Forsgren, S. (1998) Main sensory neuropeptides, but not VIP and NPY, are involved in bone remodeling during orthodontic tooth movement in the rat. *Annals of the New York Academy of Sciences* **865**, 353–359.

Nowrin, S. A., Jaafar, S., Rahman. N. *et al.* (2018) Association between genetic polymorphisms and external apical root resorption: A systematic review and meta-analysis. *Korean Journal of Orthodontics* **48**, 395–404.

Odagaki, N., Ishihara, Y. and Wang, Z *et al.* (2018) Role of osteocyte-PDL crosstalk in tooth movement via SOST/sclerostin. *Journal of Dental Research* **97**, 1374–1382.

Oettgen, H. F. (1990) Biological agents in cancer therapy: cytokines, monoclonal antibodies and vaccines. *Journal of Cancer Research and Clinical Oncology* **116**, 116–119.

Offenbacher, S., Heasman, P. A. and Collins, J. G. (1993) Modulation of host PGE2 secretion as a determinant of periodontal disease expression. *Journal of Periodontology* **64**, 432–444.

Ohkubo, T., Shibata, M., Yamada, Y. *et al.* (1993) Role of substance P. in neurogenic inflammation in the rat incisor pulp and the lower lip. *Archives of Oral Biology* **38**, 151–158.

Ohori, F., Kitaura, H., Marahleh, A. *et al.* (2019) Effect of TNF-α-induced sclerostin on osteocytes during orthodontic tooth movement. *Journal of Immunology Research* **24**, 2019:9716758. doi: 10.1155/2019/9716758.

Ong, C. K., Walsh, L. J., Harbrow, D. *et al.* (2000) Orthodontic tooth movement in the prednisolone-treated rat. *The Angle Orthodontist* **70**, 118–125.

Owman-Moll, P. and Kurol, J. (2000) Root resorption after orthodontic treatment in high- and low-risk patients: analysis of allergy as a possible predisposing factor. *European Journal of Orthodontics* **22**, 657–663.

Parris, W. G., Tanzer, F. S., Fridland, G. H. *et al.* (1989) Effects of orthodontic force on methionine enkephalin and substance P concentrations in human pulpal tissue. *American Journal of Orthodontics and Dentofacial Orthopedics* **95**, 479–489.

Perinetti, G., Varvara, G., Festa, F. and Esposito, P. (2004) Aspartate aminotransferase activity in pulp of orthodontically treated teeth. *American Journal of Orthodontics and Dentofacial Orthopedics,* **125**, 88–92.

Pierce, A.M., Lindskog, S. and Hammarstrom, L. (1991) Osteoclasts: structure and function. *Electron Microscopy Reviews* **4**, 1–45.

Prockop, D. J. and Oh, J. Y. (2012) Mesenchymal stem/stromal cells (MSCs): role as guardians of inflammation. *Molecular Therapy* **20**, 14–20.

Queiroz-Junior, C. M., Madeira, M. F., Coelho, F. M. *et al.* (2011) Experimental arthritis triggers periodontal disease in mice: involvement of TNF-alpha and the oral microbiota. *Journal of Immunology* **187**, 3821–3830.

Rana, M. W., Pothisiri, V., Killiany, D. M. and Xu, X. M. (2001) Detection of apoptosis during orthodontic tooth movement in rats. *American Journal of Orthodontics and Dentofacial Orthopedics* **119**, 516–521.

Ransjo, M., Marklund, M., Persson, M. and Lerner, U. H. (1998) Synergistic interactions of bradykinin, thrombin, interleukin 1 and tumor necrosis factor on prostanoid biosynthesis in human periodontal-ligament cells. *Archives of Oral Biology* **43**, 253–260.

Redlich, M., Roos, H., Reichenberg, E. *et al.* (2004) The effect of centrifugal force on mRNA levels of collagenase, collagen type-I, tissue inhibitors of metalloproteinases and beta-actin in cultured human periodontal ligament fibroblasts. *Journal of Periodontal Research* **39**, 27–32.

Rex, T., Kharbanda, O. P., Petocz, P. and Darendeliler, M.A. (2005). Physical properties of root cementum: Part 4. Quantitative analysis of the mineral composition of human premolar cementum. *American Journal of Orthodontics and Dentofacial Orthopedics* **127**, 177–185.

Rodan, G. A., Bouret, L. A., Harvey, A. and Mensi, T. (1975) Cyclic AMP and cyclic GMP: mediators of the mechanical effects of bone remodeling. *Science* **189**, 467–471.

Rombouts, C., Giraud, T., Jeanneau, C. and About, I. (2017) Pulp vascularization during tooth development, regeneration, and therapy. *Journal of Dental Research* **96**, 137–144.

Römer, P., Wolf, M., Fanghänel, J. *et al.* (2014) Cellular response to orthodontically-induced short-term hypoxia in dental pulp cells. *Cell and Tissue Research* **355**, 173–180.

Rygh, P. (1989) The periodontal ligament under stress, in *The Biology of Tooth Movement* (eds. L. A. Norton and C. J. Burstone). CRC Press, Boca Raton, FL, pp. 9–28.

Sabuncuoglu, F.A., Ersahan, S. (2015) Comparative evaluation of pulpal blood flow during incisor intrusion. *Australian Orthodontic Journal* **31**, 171–177.

Saito, M., Saito, S., Ngan, P. W. *et al.* (1991) Interleukin 1 beta and prostaglandin E are involved in the response of periodontal cells to mechanical stress in vivo and in vitro. *American Journal of Orthodontics and Dentofacial Orthopedics* **99**, 226–240.

Salla, J. T., Taddei, S. R., Queiroz-Junior, C. M. *et al.* (2012) The effect of IL-1 receptor antagonist on orthodontic tooth movement in mice. *Archives of Oral Biology* **57**, 519–524.

Sandhu, S. S. and Sandhu, J. (2015) Effect of physical activity level on orthodontic pain perception and analgesic consumption in adolescents. *American Journal of Orthodontics and Dentofacial Orthopedics* **148**, 617–627.

Sandy, J. R., Farndale, R. W. and Meikle, M. C. (1993) Recent advances in understanding mechanically induced bone remodeling and their relevance to orthodontic theory and practice. *American Journal of Orthodontics and Dentofacial Orthopedics* **103**, 212–222.

Scheurer, P. A., Firestone, A. R. and Burgin, W. B. (1996) Perception of pain as a result of orthodontic treatment with fixed appliances. *European Journal of Orthodontics* **18**, 349–357.

Seifi, M., Eslami, B. and Saffar, A. S. (2003) The effect of prostaglandin E2 and calcium gluconate on orthodontic tooth movement and root resorption in rats. *European Journal of Orthodontics* **25**, 199–204.

Selving, K. A. and Selving, S. K. (1962) Mineral content of human and seal cementum. *Journal of Dental Research* **41**, 624–632.

Shenoy, N., Shetty, S., Ahmed, J. and Shenoy, K. A. (2013) The pain management in orthodontics. *Journal of Clinical and Diagnostic Research* **7**, 1258–1260.

Shimizu, N., Yamaguchi, M., Fujita, S. *et al.* (2013) Interleukin-17/T-helper 17 cells in an atopic dermatitis mouse model aggravate orthodontic root resorption in dental pulp. *European Journal of Oral Sciences* **121**, 101–110.

Shimizu, N., Ozawa, Y., Yamaguchi, M. *et al.* (1998) Induction of COX-2 expression by mechanical tension force in human periodontal ligament cells. *Journal of Periodontology* **69**, 670–677.

Shimizu, N., Yamaguchi, M., Goseki, T. *et al.* (1994) Cyclic-tension force stimulates interleukin-1 beta production by human periodontal ligament cells. *Journal of Periodontal Research* **29**, 328–333.

Shimizu, N., Yamaguchi, M., Goseki, T. *et al.* (1995) Inhibition of prostaglandin E2 and interleukin 1-beta production by low-power laser irradiation in stretched human periodontal ligament cells. *Journal of Dental Research* **74**, 1382–1388.

Shoji-Matsunaga, A., Ono, T., Hayashi, M. *et al.* (2017) Osteocyte regulation of orthodontic force-mediated tooth movement via RANKL expression. *Scientific Reports* **7**(1):8753. doi: 10.1038/s41598-017-09326-7.

Silva, T. A., Garlet, G. P., Fukada, S. Y. *et al.* (2007) Chemokines in oral inflammatory diseases: apical periodontitis and periodontal disease. *Journal of Dental Research* **86**, 306–319.

Sporn, M. B. and Roberts, A. B. (1993) A major advance in the use of growth factors to enhance wound healing. *Journal of Clinical Investigation* **92**, 2565–2566.

Stephenson, T. J. (1992) Inflammation, in *General and Systematic Pathology* (ed. J. C. E. Underwood). Churchill Livingstone, London, pp. 177–200.

Storey, E. (1973) The nature of tooth movement. *American Journal of Orthodontics* **63**, 292–314.

Sugimori, T., Yamaguchi, M., Shimizu, M. *et al.* (2018). Micro-osteoperforations accelerate orthodontic tooth movement by stimulating periodontal ligament cell cycles. *American Journal of Orthodontics and Dentofacial Orthopedics* **154**, 788–796.

Taddei, S. R., Andrade, I. Jr, Queiroz-Junior, C. M. *et al.* (2012) Role of CCR2 in orthodontic tooth movement. *American Journal of Orthodontics and Dentofacial Orthopedics* **141**, 153–160.

Taddei, S. R., Queiroz, C. M. Jr, Moura, A. P. *et al.* (2013) The effect of CCL3 and CCR1 in bone remodeling induced by mechanical loading during orthodontic tooth movement in mice. *Bone* **52**, 259–267.

Takahashi, I., Nishimura, M., Onodera, K. *et al.* (2003) Expression of MMP-8 and MMP-13 genes in the periodontal ligament during tooth movement in rats. *Journal of Dental Research* **82**, 646–651.

Takahashi, I., Onodera, K., Nishimura, M. *et al.* (2006) Expression of genes for gelatinases and tissue inhibitors of metalloproteinases in periodontal tissues during orthodontic tooth movement. *Journal of Molecular Histology* **37**, 333–342.

Theoleyre, S., Wittrant, Y., Tat, S. K. *et al.* (2004) The molecular triad OPG/RANK/RANKL: involvement in the orchestration of pathophysiological bone remodeling. *Cytokine and Growth Factor Reviews* **15**, 457–475

Tortamano, A., Lenzi, D.C., Haddad, A.C. et al. (2009) Low-level laser therapy for pain caused by 27 placement of the first orthodontic archwire: a randomized clinical trial. *American Journal of Orthodontics and Dentofacial Orthopedics* **136**, 662–667.

Trombone, A. P., Claudino, M., Colavite, P. et al. (2010) Periodontitis and arthritis interaction in mice involves a shared hyper-inflammatory genotype and functional immunological interferences. *Genes and Immunity* **11**, 479–489.

Urban, D. and Mincik, J. (2010) Monozygotic twins with idiopathic internal root resorption: A case report. *Australian Endodontic Journal* **36**, 79–82.

Vandevska-Radunovic, V. (1999) Neural modulation of inflammatory reactions in dental tissues incident to orthodontic tooth movement. A review of the literature. *European Journal of Orthodontics* **21**, 231–247.

Vandevska-Radunovic, V., Kvinnsland, S. and Kvinnsland, I. H. (1997) Effect of experimental tooth movement on nerve fibres immunoreactive to calcitonin gene-related peptide, protein gene product 9.5, and blood vessel density and distribution in rats. *European Journal of Orthodontics* **19**, 517–529.

Varella, A. M., Revankar, A. V. and Patil, A.K. (2018) Low-level laser therapy increases interleukin-1β in gingival crevicular fluid and enhances the rate of orthodontic tooth movement. *American Journal of Orthodontics and Dentofacial Orthopedics* **154**, 535–544.e5. doi: 10.1016/j.ajodo.2018.01.012.

Villa, I., Mrak, E., Rubinacci, A. et al. (2006) CGRP inhibits osteoprotegerin production in human osteoblast-like cells via cAMP/PKA-dependent pathway. *American Journal of Physiology and Cell Physiology* **291**, C529–37.

Wang, J., Wu, D., Shen, T. et al. (2015) Cognitive behavioral therapy eases orthodontic pain: EEG states and functional connectivity analysis. *Oral Diseases* **21**, 572–582.

Wei, F., Yang, S., Xu, H. et al. (2015) Expression and function of hypoxia inducible factor-1α and vascular endothelial growth factor in pulp tissue of teeth under orthodontic movement. *Mediators of Inflammation* **2015**:215761. doi: 10.1155/2015/215761.

Wolf, M., Lossdörfer, S., Küpper, K. and Jäger A. (2014a) Regulation of high mobility group box protein 1 expression following mechanical loading by orthodontic forces in vitro and in vivo. *European Journal of Orthodontics* **36**, 624–631.

Wolf, M., Lossdörfer, S., Römer, P. et al. (2014b) Anabolic properties of high mobility group box protein-1 in human periodontal ligament cells in vitro. *Mediators of Inflammation* **2014**:347585. doi: 10.1155/2014/347585.

Wolf, M., Lossdörfer, S., Römer, P. et al. (2016) Short-term heat pre-treatment modulates the release of HMGB1 and pro-inflammatory cytokines in hPDL cells following mechanical loading and affects monocyte behavior. *Clinical Oral Investigation* **20**, 923–931. doi: 10.1007/s00784-015-1580-7.

Wolf, M., Lossdorfer, S., Abuduwali, N. Jager, A. (2013) Potential role of high mobility group box protein 1 and intermittent PTH (1-34) in periodontal tissue repair following orthodontic tooth movement in rats. *Clinical Oral Investigations* **17**, 989–997.

Xu, X., Zhang, L., Jiang, Y. et al. (2013) [Clinical research of music in relieving orthodontic pain.] *Hua Xi Kou Qiang Yi, Xue, Za Zhi* **3**, 365–368. (Chinese)

Yago, T., Nanke, Y., Ichikawa, N. et al. (2009) IL-17 induces osteoclastogenesis from human monocytes alone in the absence of osteoblasts, which is potently inhibited by anti-TNF-α antibody: a novel mechanism of osteoclastogenesis by IL-17. *Journal of Cellular Biochemistry* **108**, 947–955.

Yamada, K., Yamaguchi, M., Asano, M. et al. (2013) Th17-cells in atopic dermatitis stimulate orthodontic root resorption. *Oral Diseases* **19**, 683–693.

Yamaguchi, M. and Kasai, K. (2007) The effect of orthodontic mechanics on the dental pulp. *Seminars in Orthodontics* **13**, 272–280.

Yamaguchi, M., Aihara, N. and Kojima, T. (2006) RANKL increase in compressed periodontal ligament cells from root resorption. *Journal of Dental Research* **85**, 751–756.

Yamaguchi, M., Kojima, T., Kanekawa, M. et al. (2004) Neuropeptides stimulate production of interleukin-1 beta, interleukin-6, and tumor necrosis factor-alpha in human dental pulp cells. *Inflammation Research* **5**, 199–204.

Yamaguchi, M., Shimizu, N., Goseki, T. et al. (1994) Effect of different magnitudes of tension force on prostaglandin E2 production by human periodontal ligament cells. *Archives of Oral Biology* **39**, 877–884.

Yamaguchi, M., Ukai, T., Kaneko, T. et al. (2008) T cells are able to promote lipopolysaccharide-induced bone resorption in mice in the absence of B cells. *Journal of Periodontal Research* **43**, 549–555.

Yamaguchi, M., Yao-Umezawa, E., Tanimoto, Y. et al. (2016) Individual variations in the hardness and elastic modulus of the human cementum. *Journal of Hard Tissue Biology* **25**(4), 345–350.

Yamamoto, T., Kita, M., Kimura, I. et al. (2006) Mechanical stress induces expression of cytokines in human periodontal ligament cells. *Oral Diseases* **12**, 171–175.

Yamasaki, K. (1983) The role of cyclic AMP, calcium, and prostaglandins in the induction of osteoclastic bone resorption associated with experimental tooth movement. *Journal of Dental Research* **62**, 877–881.

Yamasaki, K., Miura, F. and Suda, T. (1980) Prostaglandin as a mediator of bone resorption induced by experimental tooth movement in rats. *Journal of Dental Research* **59**, 1635–1642.

Yamasaki, K., Shibata, Y. and Fukuhara, T. (1982) The effect of prostaglandins on experimental tooth movement in monkeys (Macaca fuscata). *Journal of Dental Research* **61**, 1444–1446.

Yamasaki, K., Shibata, Y., Imai, S. et al. (1984) Clinical application of prostaglandin E1 (PGE1) upon orthodontic tooth movement. *American Journal of Orthodontics* **85**, 508–518.

Yang, C. Y., Jeon, H. H., Alshabab, A. et al. (2018) RANKL deletion in periodontal ligament and bone lining cells blocks orthodontic tooth movement. *International Journal of Oral Science* **10**(1), 3. doi: 10.1038/s41368-017-0004-8.

Yao, Z., Painter, S. L., Fanslow, W. C. et al. (1995) Human IL-17: a novel cytokine derived from T cells. *Journal of Immunology* **155**, 5483–5486.

Yao-Umezawa, E., Yamaguchi, M., Shimizu, M. et al. (2017) Relationship between root resorption and individual variation in the calcium/phosphorous ratio of cementum. *American Journal of Orthodontics and Dentofacial Orthopedics* **152**, 465–470.

Yu, W., Zhang, Y., Jiang, C. et al. (2016) Orthodontic treatment mediates dental pulp microenvironment via IL17A. *Archives of Oral Biology* **66**, 22–29.

Zhang, F., Wang, C. L., Koyama, Y. et al. (2010) Compressive force stimulates the gene expression of IL-17s and their receptor in MC3T3-E1 cells. *Connective Tissue Research* **51**, 359–369.

Zou, Y., Xu, L. and Lin, H. (2019) Stress overload-induced periodontal remodeling coupled with changes in high mobility group protein B1 during tooth movement: an in-vivo study. *European Journal of Oral Science* **127**, 396–407.

CHAPTER 5
The Effects of Mechanical Loading on Hard and Soft Tissues and Cells

Itzhak Binderman, Nasser Gadban, and Avinoam Yaffe

Summary

Tooth movement is expressed during eruption and orthodontic treatment. It is important to note that, in normal dentition, teeth are attached to each other mechanically by bundles of collagen fibers. In addition, each tooth is attached to marginal gingival epithelial cells and gingival fibroblasts. Since the gingival and the periodontal ligament fibroblasts are aligned along the extracellular matrix fibers, mainly collagen fibers, they create physiological strains upon the tooth surfaces, in the matrix, on bone surfaces, and in the epithelium, through attachment to the basal membrane. Similar strains develop between the cells as well. Also, external forces are applied when teeth of the opposite jaws occlude during oral functions. On the other hand, external forces of different magnitudes and durations can be applied by various orthodontic appliances. Such forces change the distribution of strains in the tissues, increasing strain in certain regions and lowering it in others. When applied stresses reach certain magnitudes and frequencies, the engendered strains are transduced into cellular biochemical and molecular activities, aimed at reaching a new equilibrium. Increased strains transmitted into bone induce cell proliferation, osteoblast differentiation and, finally, bone formation. However, lowering of physiological strains results in osteoclastic bone resorption. Reduced physiological strains in the marginal gingival fibroblasts activates molecular up-regulation of ATP purinoreceptors. Extracellular ATP, through activation of purinoreceptors, initiates a cascade of signals, probably through Ca+2 fluxes, which propagate to the alveolar bone surface, stimulating its remodeling.

Introduction

Tooth movement is a physiologic process that occurs throughout the development of human dentition, and it continues throughout lifetime, albeit at a slower rate. The movement pattern of the permanent dentition is primarily established by the genetic programs of development, being influenced by changes in their environment.

Orthodontists have used this natural phenomenon by superimposing an external artificial force system to align teeth into esthetic and functional positions. The orthodontic appliances and procedures were developed in conformance with Wolff 's law – that remodeling of bone and surrounding tissues is an adaptive biological response to such external forces. In fact, surgeons sometimes use mechanical forces as therapeutics, such as when traction forces are used to accelerate bone healing during distraction osteogenesis. In recent years, conventional orthodontic appliances combined with surgical elevation, labially and lingually, of mucoperiosteum flaps accelerated tooth movement and post-treatment stability of the dentition. However, in this procedure, only sparse details are known about how these physical and surgical interventions influence cellular and tissue functions. The question of how force application evokes molecular response in cells and tissues, particularly in and around teeth, remains only partially answered. To explain mechanoregulation, we should adopt the notion that a hierarchy of tiers of systems within systems exists, combining various tissues like gingival epithelium and connective tissue, bone and periodontal ligament (PDL), including vascular endothelium and nerves. These tissues, in turn, are composed of groups of living cells held together by an extracellular matrix (ECM). We must also identify the mechanosensor apparatus in the cells, and the path by which mechanical forces are transmitted across these structural tissues, namely: marginal gingiva, PDL, cementum, and alveolar bone, which are physically interconnected. Thus, forces that are applied to specific tissues would be distributed to individual cells via their adhesions to ECM that link cells and tissues throughout the organ. In fact, cell-generated tensional forces directly regulate the shape and function of essentially all cell types. In this chapter we shall analyze and discuss these issues based on past and recent findings.

Biological Mechanisms of Tooth Movement, Third Edition. Edited by Vinod Krishnan, Anne Marie Kuijpers-Jagtman and Ze'ev Davidovitch.
© 2021 John Wiley & Sons Ltd. Published 2021 by John Wiley & Sons Ltd.

Mechanobiology

In biology and medicine we tend to focus on the importance of genes and chemical factors for control of tissue physiology and the development of diseases, whereas we commonly ignore physical factors. Gravitational force plays a central role in vertebrate development and evolution. Under the influence of an external gravitational field, both mineralized and non-mineralized vertebrate tissues exhibit internal tensile forces that serve to preserve a synthetic phenotype in the resident cell population. These gravitational forces are balanced by tensional forces developed by the cell cytoskeleton (mainly actin), which are resisted by external adhesions to the ECM and neighboring cells, and by other cytoplasmic filaments (microtubules), that resist inward-directed tensional forces, termed "tensegrity" (Ingber, 2003). The cell mechanical behavior and structure depict the cell as a pre-stressed tensegrity structure (Ingber, 1997). Gravitational forces acting on mammalian tissues cause the net muscle forces required for locomotion to be higher on earth than on a body subjected to a microgravitational field.

As body mass increases during development, the musculoskeleton must be able to adapt by increasing the size of its functional units. Although it is common knowledge that mechanical forces are critical regulators in biology, serving as important regulators at the cell and molecular levels, they are equally potent as chemical cues. Thus, mechanical forces required to do the work (mechanical energy) of locomotion, must be sensed by cells and converted into chemical energy (synthesis of new tissue). Forces that are applied to individual tissues would be distributed to individual cells via their adhesion to the ECM, that link cells and tissues throughout the body. The ECMs are multicomponent matrices that transduce internal and external mechanical signals into changes in tissue structure and function through a process termed mechanochemical transduction. Application of additional external forces alters the balance between the external gravitational force and internal forces acting on resident cells, leading to changes in the expression of genes and production of proteins, which may ultimately alter the exact structure and function of the ECM (Silver and Siperko, 2003). Changes in the equilibrium between internal and external forces acting on ECMs, and changes in mechanochemical transduction processes at the cellular level, appear to be important mechanisms by which mammals adjust their needs to store, transmit, and dissipate the energy required during development and bodily movements.

Mechanotransduction in bone tissue

Muscular and gravitational forces determine the mass and distribution of bone tissue. Wolff's law, which states that bone remodels along lines of stress, was published in 1892. The experimental studies of Glucksmann (1942) demonstrated that static mechanical perturbation of bone and cartilage *in vitro*, devoid of blood supply, was able to mimic in principle the *in vivo* effects of mechanical stress. The process by which cells sense and respond to mechanical signals is mediated by the ECM, transmembrane integrin receptors, cytoskeletal structures, and associated signaling molecules (Wang *et al.*, 1993). Rodan *et al.* (1975) applied hydrostatic pressure to isolated cells from chick long bone rudiments and found changes in cyclic AMP (cAMP) levels similar to those found in response to hormones. Our group has demonstrated that by mechanical deformation of culture dishes in which periosteum cells were grown, after 5 minutes the cells synthesized significant amounts of prostaglandins (PGE_2), followed by transient increases in cAMP and the accumulation of Ca^{+2} (Harell *et al.*, 1977; Somjen *et al.*, 1980; Binderman *et al.*, 1984). We have reported that such static mechanical perturbation stimulated phospholipase A_2 activity, an enzyme that releases arachidonic acid from membrane phospholipids, the substrate for synthesis of prostanoids (Binderman *et al.*, 1988). Several reports confirmed these findings through *in vivo* and *in vitro* studies (see review by Turner and Robling, 2004).

Bone cells are highly responsive to mechanical stimuli but the critical components in the load profile are still unclear. Whether different components such as fluid shear, tension, or compression may affect cells differently is also not known. Although both tissue strain and fluid shear stress cause cell deformation, these stimuli might excite different signaling pathways related to bone growth and remodeling (Klein-Nulend *et al.*, 2005). It is currently believed that mechanical adaptation is governed by the osteocytes, which respond to a loading-induced flow of interstitial fluid through the lacuno-canalicular network, by producing signaling molecules ((Klein-Nulend et al., 2013). An optimal bone architecture and density may thus not only be determined by the intensity and spatial distribution of mechanical stimuli but also by the mechano-responsiveness of osteocytes. While osteocytes are the sensor cells and signal changes in mechanical loads, the osteoclasts are the effector cells.

Mechanical loading through exercise builds bone strength, and this effect is most pronounced during skeletal growth and development. The mechanosensors within bone direct osteogenesis to where it is most needed to improve bone strength. It is common knowledge that mechanical forces are critical regulators in biology. Mechanical stresses resulting in tissue deformation can be concentrated in certain regions in tissues like muscle attachment sites, ligaments, blood vessels, and bone matrix. Tissue deformation involves the resident cells within and on matrix surfaces, enticing them to detect the structural change, and respond very efficiently. In fact, tissue deformation produces straining on one side and at the same time cells detect lowering of strains on the compression side. It thus seems that cells are sensitive to increases in matrix and intercellular strains, or to abrupt lowering of cellular strains.

Thus, bending of tibia produces larger strains on the periosteal surface than on the endosteal surface, simply due to the mechanics of bending. Woven bone is formed on the periosteal surface, while lamellar bone is laid down on the endosteal surface. The dissimilar biological situations at these two bone surfaces may be important in causing such distinctly different responses (Turner *et al.*, 1994). Rubin and Lanyon (1985) assumed that a threshold of 0.1% strain would have to be exceeded to become anabolic, while strains below this level of deformation would be considered insufficient for retaining tissue morphology, and thus would be permissive to catabolism. Frost (1987) suggested that bone adapts to increased loading after a minimum effective strain threshold has been reached. However, Rubin *et al.* (2001) found that vibratory mechanical signals that generate matrix deformations of less than 0.001% strain, depended on the frequency at which they were applied, with the greatest response arising within the range of 20–100 Hz, have significant anabolic effect on bone. Moreover, they found that bone formation is dependent on the applied frequency but not on the strain magnitude, suggesting a different activation of cell mechanosensors.

A range of tissues have the capacity to adapt to mechanical challenges, an attribute presumed to be regulated through deformation of the cell and/or surrounding matrix. In contrast, extremely small oscillatory accelerations, applied as unconstrained motion and inducing negligible deformation, serve as an anabolic stimulus to osteoblasts, *in vivo*. The means by which such low-level mechanical signals can be anabolic to a tissue such as bone is not clear. Given that deformations by this oscillatory energy may be too small to be recognized by cells, by products of matrix deformation, such as fluid flow induced shear stresses, streaming potentials, fluid drag on pericellular processes, or enhanced nutrient transport, may contribute to a cell's responsiveness to mechanical signals. Yet, even these alternative pathways are dependent on matrix deformation and, therefore, will be very small in magnitude during low-level mechanical stimulation. Indeed, a mechanism that would allow a cell to sense mechanical signals directly without reliance on matrix strain would obviate the need for compensatory tissue-level amplification mechanisms, reduce complexity in the system, and may provide cells with mechanical information without the potential for damaging the surrounding tissue (Garman *et al.*, 2007).

Mechanosensing is postulated to involve many different cellular and extracellular components. Mechanical forces cause direct stretching of protein–cell surface integrin binding sites that occur on all eukaryotic cells. Stress-induced conformational changes in the ECM may alter integrin structure and lead to activation of several secondary messenger pathways within the cell. Activation of these pathways leads to altered regulation of genes that synthesize and catabolize ECM proteins, as well as to alterations in cell division. Another aspect by which mechanical signals are transduced involves deformation of gap junctions containing calcium-sensitive stretch receptors. Once activated, these channels trigger second messenger activation through pathways similar to those involved in integrin-dependent activation and allow cell-to-cell communications between cells with similar and different phenotypes.

Another process by which mechanochemical transduction occurs is through the activation of ion channels in the cell membrane. Mechanical forces have been shown to alter cell membrane ion channel permeability associated with Ca^{+2} and other ion fluxes. In addition, the application of mechanical forces to cells leads to the activation of growth factor and hormone receptors even in the absence of ligand binding. These are some of the mechanisms that have evolved in vertebrates by which cells respond to changes in external forces that lead to changes in tissue structure and function. Many *in vivo* and *in vitro* reports suggested that the mechanism by which mechanical forces are translated into biochemical events in connective tissue cells is by increased secretion of prostaglandins, elevation of cyclic nucleotides, and by changes in fluid flow and streaming potentials of the connective tissues cells' environment (Pollack *et al.*, 1984).

Biological processes involved in bone mechanotransduction are still poorly understood, yet several pathways are emerging from current research. These pathways include ion channels in the cell membrane, ATP signaling, and second messengers such as prostaglandins and nitric oxide. Specific targets of mechanical loading include the L-type calcium channel, a gadolinium-sensitive stretch activated channel, P2Y2 and P2X7 purinergic receptors, EP2 and EP4 prostanoid receptors, and the parathyroid hormone (PTH) receptor (see review by Turner, 2002; Chukkapalli & Lele, 2018).

Mechanotransduction in periodontal tissues

The human dentition is constantly under physiological forces of tooth eruption and mechanical loading of the occluding teeth. The former is the result of strains developing in the periodontium environment and the latter is the result of normal function of muscles attached to the jaws. The normal function of our dentition depends on complex hierarchical structures, which are composed of bone, muscle, connective tissue, vascular endothelium, nerve, and epithelium. These tissues, in turn, are composed of groups of living cells held together by an ECM, and attached to each other, creating mechanical and molecular communications. To understand how individual cells experience mechanical forces we, therefore, must identify the path by which these stresses are transmitted through tissues of different strength and density, and finally across the cell membrane. The PDL plays a pivotal role in mediating between the alveolar bone and the root surface cellular network during physiological, iatrogenic, and therapeutic tooth movement. The PDL cells have the capacity to regulate the tissue remodeling processes, synthesize and resorb the matrices of alveolar bone, cementum, and the PDL itself. Unlike bone and PDL, which regain their original structure after removal of an applied mechanical force, the marginal gingiva tissue does not regain its pretreatment structure, possibly being associated with slow remodeling changes during and after application of orthodontic forces (Redlich *et al.*, 2001). The process by which cells sense and respond to mechanical signals, mechanotransduction, is mediated by the ECM, transmembrane integrin receptors, cytoskeletal structures and associated signaling molecules. It means that mechanical loads are transmitted across structural elements that are physically interconnected (Figure 5.1).

Clinicians are always looking for effective orthodontic force systems that produce optimal biological responses. Generally, we wish to attain an optimal biological response while applying minimal orthodontic forces for the shortest periods possible. It will, therefore, be appropriate to define the features of the forces that will activate mechanosensors in the relevant tissues to evoke controlled, local remodeling of PDL and alveolar bone tissues, facilitating optimal tooth alignment. A significant component of orthodontic tooth movement (OTM) involves bone remodeling and growth alteration by the application of mechanical forces. Teeth and bones, both hard tissues, are thus stressed by orthodontic forces, leading to a comprehensive remodeling of bone, PDL, periosteum, cementum, and sutures. The changes within the periodontium are well documented and demonstrate the adaptability of the PDL and the surrounding bone. Since OTM is performed via bone resorption and apposition, factors influencing these processes may enhance it.

Orthodontic forces together with bioelectric changes, local hormones, and a variety of drugs act as first messengers to promote production of intracellular second messengers, such as Ca^{2+}, cGMP, or cAMP. Davidovitch and Shanfeld (1975) applied orthodontic forces to cat maxillary canines for periods of time ranging from 1 hour to 4 weeks, and observed significant elevations in the concentrations of cAMP in the PDL and alveolar bone in both sites of compression and tension. Moreover, addition of PTH increased significantly cAMP in paradental cells, above the levels measured when only orthodontic force was applied. They also observed increased levels of the proinflammatory, vasoactive neurotransmitter, substance P, in the cat mechanically stressed PDL. The results of those *in vivo* experiments, as well as a series of *in vitro* studies, illuminated several factors derived from the nervous, vascular, and immune systems in the strained tissues, which might be correlated with the elevated levels of the cellular second messengers (Davidovitch *et al.*, 1989; Mikuni-Takagaki, 1999). Thus, it is reasonable to suggest that alterations in second messenger formation can affect the velocity of OTM. Another factor that may play a crucial role in OTM is nitric oxide, a molecule that modulates both bone resorption and formation, and thus can facilitate these processes during orthodontic force application (Shirazi *et al.*, 2002;

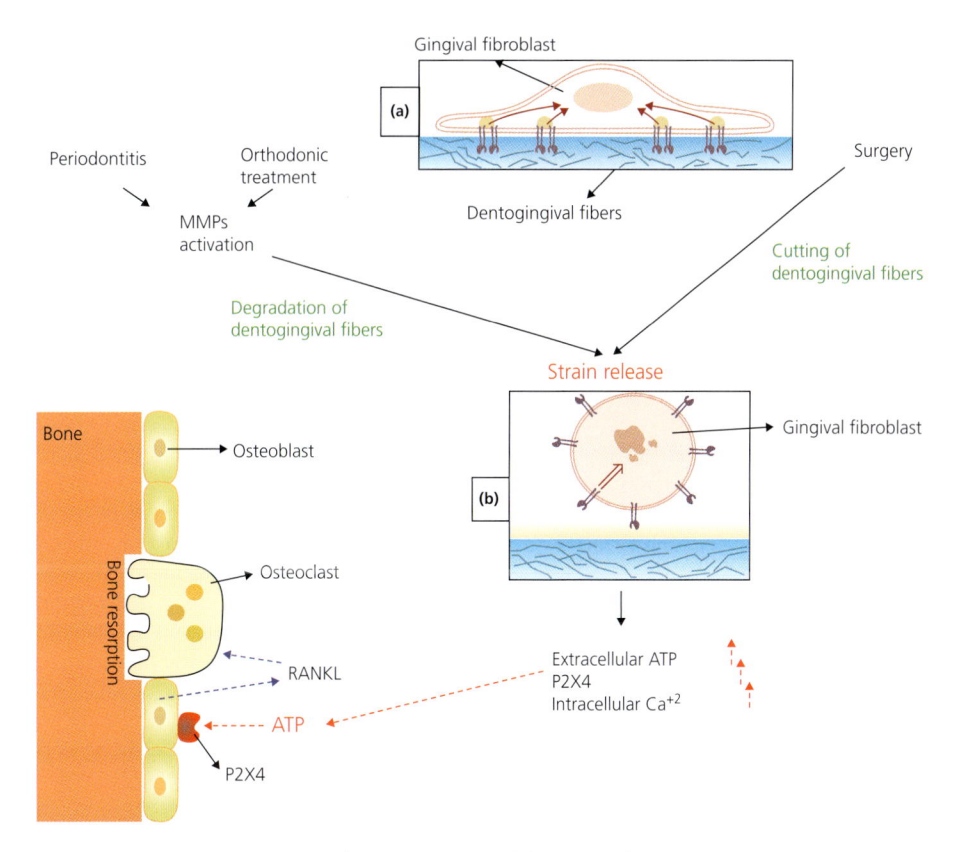

Figure 5.1 The cellular and molecular pathways, starting with strain relaxation of the gingival fibroblasts, resulting in activation of osteoclasts to resorb alveolar bone. (a) A physiologically normal strained gingival fibroblast attached to the ECM by integrins. (b) A rounded and detached fibroblast after lowering of the physiological strain. Lowering of the physiological strain occurs in PDL compression sites during OTM, or as a result of MMPs activity. Fiberotomy surgery or mucoperiosteum flap also lower the strain. The abrupt change in gingival bone surface, which causes a change in fibroblast shape, stimulates release of ATP and upregulation of purinoreceptor (P2X4 in rats). Ca^{+2} is influxed into the cells, and the signal is propagated to the alveolar bone activating osteoblasts to secrete RANKL (receptor activator of nuclear factor kappa B ligand), which affects osteoclast activity.

Baloul, 2016). These investigators hypothesized that a treatment regimen that combines mechanical force with the local application of another agent capable of enhancing tissue remodeling may lead to decreased root resorption of teeth undergoing OTM.

The role of marginal gingiva in orthodontic tooth movement

Moving a tooth requires coordinated bone remodeling and regeneration processes while maintaining its periodontal attachment, including attachment of the marginal gingiva to the dental roots. It is also apparent that tooth movement is enhanced by procedures that elevate the remodeling of alveolar bone, and periodontal and gingival fibrous tissues (Wilcko et al., 2003). When the process of tooth movement is completed, the new architecture of the dentition and its surrounding tissues is stabilized and maintained by retention procedures. Finally, the tendency of teeth to return to their original position, known as relapse, occurs, while being mostly unpredictable and unavoidable. Interestingly, orthodontic relapse may continue for many years after the retention period. It was, therefore, advocated to use permanent retention wherever possible.

Several authors have proposed to perform surgical fiberotomy as an adjunct to retention in an effort to reduce the extent of relapse (Redlich et al., 1999). Wilcko et al. (2003) have demonstrated that rapid OTM can be achieved following a surgical procedure, which includes elevation of a full mucoperiosteum flap, a limited selective labial and lingual alveolar decortication, and alveolar bone augmentation. This method has been described as accelerated osteogenic orthodontics, based on the hypothesis that rapid tooth movement is associated with increased local bone turnover, also known as "regional acceleratory phenomenon" (RAP) (Frost, 1989; Yaffe et al., 1994). Support for this concept is derived from studies reporting that a transient burst of osteoclastic alveolar bone and soft tissues remodeling is attained even by only elevating a full thickness flap, but without surgical wounding of the cortical bone (Grevstad, 1993; Yaffe et al., 1995; Kaynak et al., 2000; Binderman et al., 2001). Moreover, we have demonstrated that surgical sectioning and separation of the gingiva from the dental root surfaces, and disruption of the dento-gingival fibers, rather than separation of the mucoperiosteum from the bone, is a major trigger for alveolar bone remodeling (Figures 5.1 and 5.2). It seems, therefore, that the intact continuity of fibers that attach chemically and mechanically the marginal gingiva to the root surface and its aligned strained cellular network is the main sensor system that protects the normal structure of the PDL and alveolar bone. We found that disrupting surgically or chemically (enzymatically, by matrix metalloproteinases, MMPs) this strained fibrous network causes an abrupt lowering of strains in the marginal gingiva. The cells usually round up, and facilitate both the formation and activation of osteoclasts, resulting in alveolar bone resorption (Binderman et al., 2001). The local fibroblasts are sensing the detachment of the fibers and the lowering of strains, signaling the initiation of alveolar bone resorption.

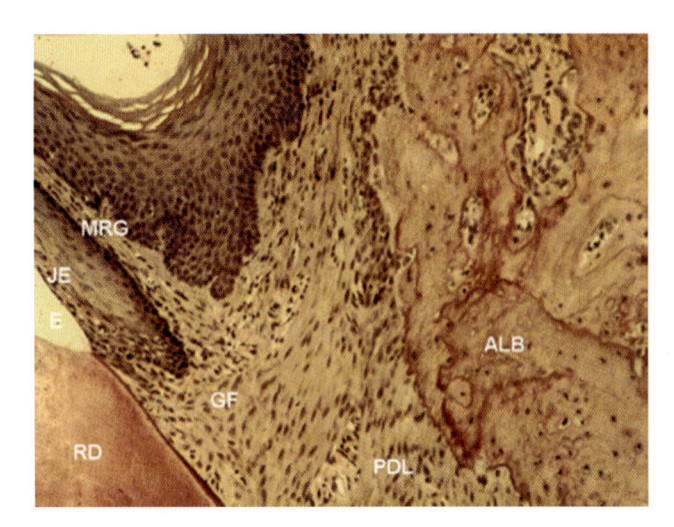

Figure 5.2 A longitudinal section of the cervical part of the tooth presenting normal periodontal structures of a rat molar, including cementum, PDL, alveolar bone (ALB), marginal gingiva (MRG), marginal gingival fibroblasts (GF) along Sharpey fibers and junctional epithelium. E, enamel; RD, root dentine; JE, junctional epithelium.

Therefore, we propose that effective tooth movement and even reduction of orthodontic relapse may depend on our understanding of the major role of the marginal gingival cells in controlling the architecture of the dentition. Figure 5.1 describes the cellular and molecular pathway by which the marginal gingiva controls the architectural pattern of the dentition.

The cells that ultimately form or resorb bone may not necessarily be those that transduce signals in response to the applied mechanical loads. In cells sensitive to mechanical loads, mechanotransduction may involve signaling through mechanically activated ion channels in the cell membrane, focal adhesions of the cytoskeleton, or a G protein coupled mechanoreceptor.

Marginal gingiva is the mechanosensor of the periodontium

The marginal gingiva is the frontier where bacteria and trauma are sustained. This tissue is lining the alveolar bone and attaches to the root cementum. The connective tissue of the marginal gingiva is also traversed by many blood vessels, nerves, and elastin fibers. The marginal gingiva is covered by epithelium, which communicates with the connective tissue through the basal membrane and is attached to the cervical region of the enamel, defined there as junctional epithelium (Figure 5.2). The marginal gingival fibroblasts are attached chemically to the acellular cementum on the cervical part of the root surface, creating a strong cell attachment to the tooth. We propose that this cell attachment to the root surfaces at one end, and to the gingival fibrous matrix at the other end, strongly suggests that this tissue plays an important role in controlling the architecture of the dentition.

During root formation and tooth eruption, epithelial–mesenchymal interactions produce a very complex pattern of tissues, namely marginal gingiva, cementum, PDL, and alveolar bone. Developmentally, the marginal gingiva is created and formed during tooth eruption, while the cementum, PDL, and alveolar bone are created during root development, being integrated at their interfaces (Figure 5.2). Normally, in the erupted tooth, bundles of collagen fibers (Sharpey fibers) run from the cementum of the cervical part of the root toward the papilla, toward the periosteum that is lining the alveolar bone, and toward the adjacent teeth. The fibroblasts and collagen fibers, which extend from the cementum, create a very intimate physical and strong chemical attachment between the cells and the cementum surface, as well as a tight contact of the cell surface to the fibers. The intimate contact of this fibrous tissue – which emerges from the root cementum – with neighboring teeth, as well as with the periosteum and the basal membrane of the oral epithelium, enables it to be an excellent transmitter of mechanical stimuli.

Yamamoto et al. (1998) described in detail the unique cell-matrix relationship at the root cervical cementum. They characterized "finger like projections," which extend from the cementum-facing ends of the collagen fibers toward the cementum surface. Gingival fibroblasts in that area exhibit motility and contractile properties, features characteristic of smooth muscle cells, having substantial amounts of intracellular actomyosin microfilaments, connecting with the ECM via transmembrane integrins. Many authors consider these cells to be myofibroblasts. It is, therefore, evident that this gingival structure is most important in establishing and in stabilizing the architectural pattern of the dentition, altogether creating an efficient communicative system.

The structure and shape of gingival and PDL fibroblasts are determined by their internal molecular framework, or lattice, which is composed of three different types of cytoskeletal molecular structures. The internal cell cytoskeleton is an interconnected network of microfilaments, microtubules, and intermediate filaments, which links the nucleus to cell surface adhesion receptors, forming the shape, mechanical properties, and behavior of these cells. Beside the intermediate filaments, which provide a stable three-dimensional cell shape, like in epithelial cells, the microfilaments and microtubules can remodel themselves. The microfilaments remodel by polymerization of G-actin into F-actin, and by depolymerization in an energy-dependent mechanism. Similarly, the microtubules, using tubulin monomers to polymerize, create a very versatile structure which is able to locomote molecules and efficiently change the cell shape. This functional structure is guiding the framework changes in the cell, thus creating intracellular tractional forces.

To understand how individual cells experience mechanical forces, we must identify the path by which these stresses are transmitted through ECM and across the cell surface. Since the microfilaments adhere chemically to proteins in the cell membrane and to proteins in the nuclear membrane, they are able mechanically to transmit traction forces from inside the cell through cadherins to neighbor cells, and through integrins to the ECM. These tensional forces are resisted and balanced by external adhesions through integrins to the ECM, by cadherins to neighboring cells, and by other molecular filaments like microtubules that locally resist inward-directed tensional forces inside the cytoskeleton (Galbraith and Scheetz, 1998). This physiological pre-existing tensile stress (pre-stress) in the cell, known as "tensegrity" is pivotal for normal function of tissues and organs, and can at times govern the response to the mechanical stimulus (Ingber, 2003). Most of the cells require this attachment and subsequent spreading on the ECM substrate for proper growth, function, and even survival. Without it, they often die by undergoing apoptosis (programmed cell death). This dependence on substrate attachment is known as anchorage dependence. Ingber (2003) suggested that each cell has the ability to create intracellular traction forces by chemical connectivity and interactions between cytoskeleton, integrin, and ECM.

Strains that have been measured in different tissues *in vivo* vary widely, depending mostly on the rigidity of the ECM. Because individual cells apply tractional forces on their adhesions, they spread on rigid surfaces (like on bundles of collagen fibers), whereas they retract and round up on flexible ECMs. Thus, the physicality of the ECM substrate and degree of cell distortion govern cell behavior, regardless of the presence of hormones, cytokines, or soluble regulatory factors. Local alterations in ECM structure produced by MMPs (like in periodontitis), surgery, or by deprivation of strains (like in orthodontics), are associated with immediate changes in cytoskeletal mechanics, which evoke molecular changes in the cells, leading to specific responses, signaling pathways toward alteration of cellular and tissue functions. It is important to note that the chemical and mechanical information is running all the way to nuclear proteins. Changes in ECM mechanics will not transfer forces equally to all points on the surface of neighboring adherent cells. Rather, a tug on the ECM will be felt by the cell through its focal adhesions and, hence, through its transmembrane integrin receptors that link to the cytoskeleton. It is therefore proposed that, by disrupting the chemico-physical connectivity of the marginal gingiva from the dental root, the intracellular tensile forces of the gingival fibroblasts are abruptly lowered, thus changing the balanced physiological strains that had existed in the cells, immediately affecting their shape. In response, molecular changes occur, which activate the propagation of intercellular messages that start the remodeling process of the gingival tissue and the neighboring alveolar bone. Hence, we propose that marginal gingival fibroblasts are the mechanosensors that recognize and respond to changes in physical stimuli.

Mechanical loads are transmitted across structural tissue elements, which are physically interconnected. Several studies (Yaffe *et al.*, 1995, 2003; Kaynak *et al.*, 2000; Binderman *et al.*, 2001) have demonstrated that surgical detachment of the marginal gingiva close to the cervical cementum of rat mandibular molars is a distinct stimulus for alveolar bone resorption, starting on the periodontal aspects of the socket. Interestingly, Grevstad (1993) reported earlier that while a similar mucoperiosteum flap surgical procedure resulted in alveolar bone resorption, a gingivectomy surgical procedure discarding the detached marginal gingiva including cells, prevented alveolar bone resorption. We have confirmed these findings by demonstrating that discarding the marginal gingiva, including the cells, during surgical elevation of the mucoperiosteum prevented alveolar bone resorption and bone loss. We have also demonstrated that alveolar bone resorption commences only when the surgery is performed by coronal approach, in contrast to an apical surgical approach (Binderman *et al.*, 2001). It seems that the separation of the gingiva from the tooth and disruption of the dentogingival fibers, rather than separation of the mucoperiosteum from the alveolar bone, is the major trigger for alveolar bone resorption (Binderman *et al.*, 2002). These experiments strongly support the notion that by disrupting the fibrous tissue, the local fibroblasts of the free marginal gingiva are undergoing an abrupt change of shape, due to lowering of traction strains between the cells and the ECM. Another study (Kozlovsky *et al.*, 1988) showed that eruptive tooth movements result in a coronal alveolar bone growth, while supracrestal fiberotomy has a negative effect on alveolar bone growth.

Clinical data imply that alveolar bone resorption in patients with periodontal disease commences when degradation of fibrous tissue in the marginal gingiva is progressing. Seguier *et al.* (2000) found that in patients with periodontitis, the amount of collagen disrupted fibers was much higher than in gingivitis or in healthy gingiva, suggesting that enzymatic degradation of marginal gingival fibers induces alveolar bone resorption. It seems that surgical disruption or enzymatic degradation of collagen fibrous tissue of the marginal gingiva, immediately lowering the tensile strains of the marginal gingiva fibroblasts, is the main trigger for alveolar bone remodeling. Melsen (1999) proposed that alveolar bone resorption at PDL compression sites during OTM happens, at least partially, due to the lowering of the normal tensile strains. Once lowering of intercellular and intercell-ECM strains occur, a specific molecular signaling is initiating a cascade of pathways leading to alveolar bone resorption. Redlich *et al.* (1996) reported that after gingival fiberotomy during rotational tooth movement, most fibers resumed the appearance of the organized pattern of large fiber bundles, similar to those seen in control teeth.

It is apparent that tooth movement is enhanced by procedures that elevate the remodeling of alveolar bone, and of periodontal and gingival fibrous tissues (Binderman *et al.*, 2010). The periodontally accelerated osteogenic orthodontics (PAOO), which involves full-thickness labial and lingual mucoperiosteal flaps accompanied by surgical scarring of cortical bone (corticotomy), evokes a burst of extensive bone remodeling. The authors suggest that the RAP is the major stimulus for alveolar bone remodeling, enabling the PAOO (Sebaoun *et al.*, 2008). In contrast, we propose that detachment of the bulk of dentogingival and interdental fibers from the coronal part of root surfaces by itself should suffice to stimulate alveolar bone resorption, mainly on its PDL surfaces, leading to widening of the PDL space, which can greatly contribute to accelerated osteogenic orthodontics. Nobuto *et al.* (2003) showed that when a mucoperiosteum flap is elevated, the PDL vascular plexus is severed from the vascular plexus of the gingiva, and many osteoclasts are observed, especially around the alveolar crest close to openings of Volkmann canals 5 days after surgery. They proposed that increased alveolar bone resorption on its periodontal aspect due to newly formed vessels is most probably responsible for the expanded PDL width (Nobuto *et al.*, 2003).

It our studies fiberotomy is sufficient to accelerate tooth movement and minimize relapse, in a rat model (Young *et al.*, 2013). It should be noted that in fiberotomy surgery where dento-gingival, dento-periosteal, and interdental fibers were disrupted, the tooth movement was significantly accelerated, but not when apical elevation of a mucoperiosteum flap was performed (Young *et al.*, 2013). It is well accepted that during tooth eruption the alveolar bone that envelops the roots is embedded in the basal bone. The buccal plates are mostly alveolar bone since teeth erupt in a buccal direction. We suggest that the resorption following fiberotomy is specifically accelerating remodeling of the alveolar bone envelope, while the resorption on the buccal plate following apical flap surgery and corticotomy has a RAP nature.

The genetic positioning of teeth in the dental arch during the development of occlusion and their interdental strained fibrous and cellular connectivity, establishes a "positional physical memory of the dentition" (PPMD) (Binderman *et al.*, 2010). During fiberotomy, the loss of interdental physical connectivity results in a transient loss of PPMD, thus allowing effective rapid change in alignment of teeth, achieving a new stable position, without undergoing relapse.

Collectively, the findings suggest that the osteoclastic activity that resorbs the periodontal surface of the alveolar bone in response to fiberotomy is the key in accelerating the kinetics of tooth movement, during activation of the orthodontic appliance.

Furthermore, we have observed that during surgical disruption of marginal gingiva from its anchorage to a dental root, release of adenosine-5′-triphosphate (ATP) from the gingival cells occurs, and a specific P2X4 purinoreceptor is upregulated in the gingival fibroblasts (Binderman et al., 2007). This finding led us to envision the communication between spatially distant cellular compartments, membrane, cytoskeleton, and cell nucleus, as a bidirectional flow of information, based on subtle multilevel structural and biochemical equilibrium.

ATP-purinoreceptors are mechanosensors in marginal gingiva

The ATP molecule is an abundant and most important intracellular source for inorganic phosphate, being critical for energy-dependent chemical interactions and phosphorylation activities. In contrast, the extracellular ATP molecule is a messenger in neural and non-neural tissues, where it activates several cell-surface-purinoreceptor subtypes, including G-protein-coupled receptors and ligand-gated ion channels (Burnstock, 1997; Buckley et al., 2002). It is now well established that purinoreceptors are subdivided into ligand-gated ion channel P2X receptors, of which there are seven subtypes ($P2X_{1-7}$), and eight (currently known) G protein-coupled P2Y receptors ($P2Y_{1,2,4,6,11-14}$). ATP is released from cells when they are damaged, and in response to mechanical stress or biological activation (McNeil, 1993; Burnstock, 1997; Loomis et al., 2003). When released to the extracellular environment, the ATP molecule can activate ATP ionic ligand-gated channels, termed P2X receptors, which have been characterized on smooth muscle cells and autonomic and sensory neurons, where they mediate membrane depolarization and increased Ca^{+2} entry into cells (Yu and Ferrier, 1994; Jorgensen et al., 2002). It was demonstrated that paracrine action of ATP on P2X receptors was responsible for the rapid flow of calcium inside cells, through ionic ligand-gated channels. Thus, intercellular calcium waves of increases in intracellular calcium concentrations in single cells, subsequently propagating to adjacent cells, can be a possible mechanism for the coupling of bone formation to bone resorption (Hoebertz et al., 2000; Jorgensen et al., 2002). This event might be the mechanism by which mechanical stimuli are translated into biological signals in bone cells, and propagated through the network of skeletal cells. Moreover, the calcium signals can be propagated not only among osteoblasts but also between osteoblasts and osteoclasts, in response to mechanical stimulation. Our studies have revealed that disruption of the marginal gingiva from its tooth anchorage lowers the tractional forces of gingival fibroblasts, triggering a signal that propagates to the alveolar bone surface, resulting in bone resorption. Several reports showed that extracellular ATP can activate purinoreceptors in macrophages, stimulating their differentiation into osteoclasts (Naemsch et al., 1999). Connexins form gap junction channels that provide a hydrophilic path between cell interiors. Hemichannels, which are nonselective conduits to the extracellular environment, are probably another ATP-release system caused by mechanical stimulation, suggesting that they are mechanosensitive, like in the ocular lens (Bao et al., 2004). Moreover, ATP and ADP can activate osteoclasts and inhibit osteoblasts to form bone (see review by Hoebertz et al., 2003). However, the extracellular ATP can be easily hydrolyzed via ectonucleotidase activity. In our study (Binderman et al., 2007), inhibitors of purinoreceptors like Coomassie Blue R and G, when applied locally at the site of surgery of marginal gingiva, reduced alveolar bone loss significantly (Jiang et al., 2000). Our experiments also demonstrated that a local application of apyrase, which degrades extracellular ATP at the site of surgery, significantly reduced alveolar bone resorption. It seems that controlling locally the level of extracellular ATP and its receptors in the marginal gingival environment will effectively reduce alveolar bone loss after periodontal surgery.

Intracellular Ca^{+2} is an early response second messenger that plays an important role in a number of intracellular signaling pathways and is typically observed to increase dramatically within seconds of stimulation. As a second messenger, Ca^{+2} transduces extracellular changes to the cell interior, and potentially to the genome, and is important in the regulation of a variety of cellular functions. Thus, understanding the molecular mechanisms of fluid-induced Ca^{+2} mobilization is a very important step elucidating mechanotransduction pathways in osteoblastic cells. It is well documented that extracellular nucleotides such as ATP and UTP induce a broad spectrum of cell responses, including Ca^{+2} mobilization. It is also recognized that extracellular nucleotides act as important signaling molecules for cell–cell communication among bone cells (Jorgensen et al., 2002), and in bone remodeling (Dixon and Sims, 2000). Therefore, these molecules are considered to be potential candidates responsible for fluid flow induced Ca^{+2} mobilization in bone cells. Oscillatory fluid flow regulates steady state osteopontin mRNA levels in a manner dependent on Ca^{+2} mobilization.

Remodeling occurs at discrete sites in bones. The focal nature of remodeling indicates that this process is sensitive to local stimuli, including mechanical strain. In addition, systemic factors, in particular PTH, are known to increase the rate of activation. Thus, remodeling at foci involves the combined action of systemic factors and local cues. Bowler et al. (2001) suggested that the local stimulus obtained from extracellular nucleotides, like ATP, UTP, and ADP, activates P2X and P2Y receptors, which sensitizes osteoblasts and osteoclasts. Bone cells release ATP into the extracellular environment and the release is enhanced by mechanical strain and regulatory factors. Li et al. (2005) showed that ATP signaling through P2X7R is necessary for mechanically induced release of prostaglandins (PGs) by bone cells, and subsequent osteogenesis. Release of ATP by the primary calvarial osteoblasts occurred within 1 minute of the onset of fluid shear stress. It increased PGE_2 release by WT cells but did not alter PGE_2 release by KO cells (knock out mice for P2X7R).

In bone, the purinergic P2X7 ion channel receptor is expressed on both cells of the stromal lineage such as the bone-forming osteoblasts and the mechano-sensing osteocytes and on cells belonging to the immune-related monocyte–macrophage lineage, the bone resorbing osteoclasts. Recent studies have demonstrated that the receptor plays important roles in the anabolic responses to mechanical loading on bone and, together with the pannexin1 hemi-channel, in the process of initiating bone remodeling in response to microdamage (Jørgensen, 2018). Pannexin1 is a hemi-channel that serves as a release channel for several molecules, including ATP. It has also been proposed to be part of the pore-forming unit together with P2X7R. In macrophages, ATP-induced activation of the P2X7R leads to pannexin1 dependent IL-1β secretion (Pelegrin and Surprenant, 2006). Also, pannexin1 is expressed on both osteoblasts and osteocytes, though the exact roles of the hemi-channel in bone have not yet been elucidated in detail. Thus, mechanical loading and cell damage seems to be able to create relatively high extracellular ATP concentrations which are necessary to activate the receptor. Using an *in vivo* model of osteocytic cells, the authors demonstrate colocalization of pannexin1, P2X7R, and T-type calcium channels with specialized, mechanosensing β3 integrins (Cabahug-Zuckerman, et al., 2018).

Conclusions

The PDL mediates between the alveolar bone and the root surface cellular network during physiological, iatrogenic, and therapeutic tooth movement. The PDL cells regulate tissue remodeling processes, synthesize, and resorb the matrices of alveolar bone, cementum, and the PDL itself. However, it is evident that marginal gingiva has a pivotal role in controlling the architecture of the dentition in the periodontium. Surgical disruption, or enzymatic degradation of collagen fibrous tissue (Sharpey fibers) of the marginal gingiva, immediately lowering the tensile strains of the marginal gingival fibroblasts, is the main trigger for alveolar bone remodeling. The process by which cells sense and respond to mechanical signals is mediated by ECM, transmembrane integrin receptors, cytoskeletal structures, and associated signaling molecules. Many *in vivo* and *in vitro* reports suggested that the mechanism by which mechanical forces are translated into biochemical events in connective tissue cells is by increased secretion of prostaglandins, elevation of cyclic nucleotides, and by changes in fluid flow and streaming potentials of the connective tissues cells' environment, resulting in bone remodeling. We found that local release of ATP by gingival fibroblasts and up-regulation of P2X4 receptors in these cells, increasing calcium influx, is a major signal that propagates to the alveolar bone surface, activating osteoclastic bone resorption. It seems that controlling locally the level of extracellular ATP and its receptors, in the marginal gingival environment, will effectively control alveolar bone remodeling. It should be noted that combined action of systemic factors and local cues may become an effective and accelerated treatment in orthodontics. In addition, a treatment regimen that combines mechanical force with the separation of the gingival fibers from the root is capable of enhancing tissue remodeling and may lead to decreased root resorption of teeth undergoing OTM.

Acknowledgement

We would like to thank Dr. Lital Young and Dr. Hila Bahar for their significant contributions to the earlier versions of this chapter in the first and second editions of this book.

References

Baloul, S. S. (2016) Osteoclastogenesis and osteogenesis during tooth movement. *Frontiers in Oral Biology* **18**, 75–79.

Bao, L., Sachs, F. and Dahl G. (2004) Connexins are mechanosensitive. *American Journal of Cell Physiology* **287**, C1389–C1395.

Binderman, I., Adut, M., Zohar, R. et al. (2001) Alveolar bone resorption following coronal versus apical approach in a mucoperiosteal flap surgery procedure, in the rat mandible. *Journal of Periodontology* **72**, 1348–1353.

Binderman, I., Bahar, H., Jacob-Hirsch, J. et al. (2007) P2x4 is upregulated in gingival fibroblasts after periodontal surgery. *Journal of Dental Research* **86**, 181–185.

Binderman, I., Bahar, H. and Yaffe, A. (2002) Strain relaxation of fibroblasts in the marginal periodontium is the common trigger for alveolar bone resorption: A novel hypothesis. *Journal of Periodontology* **73**, 1210–1215.

Binderman, I., Gadban, N., Bahar, H. et al. (2010) Commentary on: Periodontally accelerated osteogenic orthodontics (PAOO)—a clinical dilemma. *International Orthodontics* **8**, 268–277.

Binderman, I., Shimshoni, Z. and Somjen, D. (1984) Biochemical pathways involved in the translation of physical stimulus into biological message. *Calcified Tissue International* **36**(Suppl. 1), S82–85.

Binderman, I., Zor, U., Kaye, A. M. et al. (1988) The transduction of mechanical force into biochemical events in bone cells involve activation of phospholipase A2. *Calcified Tissue International* **42**, 261–267.

Bowler, W. G., Buckley, K. A., Gartland, A. et al. (2001) Extracellular nucleotide signaling: A mechanism for integrating local and systemic responses in the activation of bone remodeling. *Bone* **28**, 507–512.

Buckley, K. A., Hipskind, R. A., Gartland, A. et al. (2002) Adenosine triphosphate stimulates human osteoclast activity via upregulation of osteoblast-expressed receptor activator of nuclear factor-kB ligand. *Bone* **31**, 582–590.

Burnstock, G. (1997) The past, present and future of purine nucleotides as signalling molecules. *Neuropharmacology* **36**, 1127–1139.

Cabahug-Zuckerman, P., Stout, R.F. Jr., Majeska, R.J. et al. (2018) Potential role for a specialized beta3 integrin-based structure on osteocyte processes in bone mechanosensation. *Journal of Orthopedic Research* **36**, 642–652.

Chukkapalli, S. S. and Lele, T.P. (2018) Periodontal cell mechanotransduction. *Open Biology* **8**, 180053.

Davidovitch, Z., Nicolay, O., Alley, K. et al. (1989) First and second messenger interactions in stressed connective tissues in vivo, in *The Biology of Tooth Movement* (eds. L. A. Norton and C. J. Burstone). CRC Press, Boca Raton, FL, pp. 97–131.

Davidovitch, Z. and Shanfeld, J. L. (1975) Cyclic AMP levels in alveolar bone of orthodontically-treated cats. *Archives of Oral Biology* **20**, 567–574.

Dixon, S. J., Sims, S. M. (2000) P2 purinergic receptors on osteoblasts and osteoclasts. Potential targets for drug development. *Drug Development Research* **49**, 187–200.

Frost, H. M. (1987) Bone "mass" and the "mechanostat": A proposal. *The Anatomical Record* **219**, 1–9.

Frost, H. M. (1989) The biology of fracture healing. *An overview for clinicians. Clinical Orthopedics and Related Research* **248**, 283–293.

Galbraith, C. G. and Sheetz, M. P. (1998) Forces on adhesive contacts affect cell function. *Current Opinion in Cell Biology* **10**, 566–571.

Garman, R., Rubin, C. and Judex, S. (2007) Small oscillatory accelerations, independent of matrix deformations, increase of osteoblast activity and enhance bone morphology. *Plos One* **2**, e653.

Glucksmann, A. (1942) The role of mechanical stresses in bone formation in vitro. *Journal of Anatomy* **76**, 231–239.

Grevstad, H. J. (1993) Doxycycline prevents root resorption and alveolar bone loss in rats after periodontal surgery. *Scandinavian Journal of Dental Research* **101**, 287–291.

Harell, A., Dekel, S. and Binderman, I. (1977) Biochemical effects of mechanical stress on cultured bone cells. *Calcified Tissues Research (Suppl.)* **22**, 202–209.

Hoebertz, A., Arnett, T. R. and Burnstock, G. (2003) Regulation of bone resorption and formation by purines and pyrimidines. *Trends in Pharmacoogical Sciences* **24**, 290–297.

Hoebertz, A., Townsend-Nicholson, A., Glass, R. et al. (2000) Expression of P2 receptors in bone and cultured bone cells. *Bone* **27**, 503–510.

Ingber, D. E. (1997) Tensegrity: the architectural basis of cellular mechanotransduction. *Annual Review of Physiology* **59**, 575–599.

Ingber, D. E. (2003) Mechanobiology and diseases of mechanotransduction. *Review. Annals of Medicine* **35**, 564–577.

Jiang, L. H., Mackenzie, A. B., North, R. A. and Surprenant, A. (2000) Brilliant blue G selectively blocks ATP-gated rat P2X(7) receptors. *Molecular Pharmacology* **58**, 82–88.

Jorgensen, N. R., Henriksen, Z., Sorensen, O. H. et al. (2002) Intercellular calcium signaling occurs between human osteoblasts and osteoclasts and requires activation of osteoclast P2X7 receptors. *Journal of Biological Chemistry* **277**, 7574–7580.

Jørgensen, N.R. (2018). The purinergic P2X7 ion channel receptor—a 'repair' receptor in bone. *Current Opinion in Immunology* **52**, 32–38.

Kaynak, D., Meffert, R., Gunhan, M. et al. (2000) A histopathological investigation on effects of the bisphosphonate alendronate on resorptive phase following mucoperiosteal flap surgery in the mandible of rats. *Journal of Periodontology* **71**, 790–796.

Klein-Nulend, J., Bacabac, R. G. and Mullender, M. G. (2005) Mechanobiology of bone tissue. *Pathological Biology* **53**, 576–580.

Klein-Nulend, J., Bakker, A. D. & Bacabac, R. G. et al. (2013) Mechanosensation and transduction in osteocytes. *Bone* **54**, 182–190.

Kozlovsky, A., Tal, H. and Lieberman, M. (1988) Forced eruption combined with gingival fiberotomy. A technique for clinical crown lengthening. *Journal of Clinical Periodontology* **15**(9), 534–538.

Li, J., Liu D., Hua, H. Z. et al. (2005) The $P2X_7$ nucleotide receptor mediates skeletal mechanotransduction. *Journal of Biological Chemistry* **280**, 42952–42959.

Loomis, W. H., Namiki, S., Ostrom, R. S. et al. (2003) Hypertonic stress increases T cell interleukin-2 expression through a mechanism that involves ATP release, P2 receptor, and P38 MAPK activation. *Journal of Biological Chemistry* **278**, 4590–4596.

McNeil, P. L. (1993) Cellular and molecular adaptations to injurious mechanical stress. *Trends in Cell Biology* **3**, 302–307.

Melsen, B. (1999) Biological reaction of alveolar bone to orthodontic tooth movement. *The Angle Orthodontist* **69**, 151–158.

Mikuni-Takagaki, Y. (1999) Mechanical responses and signal transduction pathways in stretched osteocytes. *Journal of Mineral Metabolism* **17**, 57–60.

Naemsch, L. N., Weidema, A. F., Sims, S. M. *et al.* (1999) P2X4 purinoreceptors mediate an ATP-activated, non selective cation current in rabbit osteoclasts. *Journal of Cell Science* **112**, 4425–4435.

Nobuto, T., Imai, H., Suwa, F. *et al.* (2003) Microvascular response in the periodontal ligament following mucoperiosteal flap surgery. *Journal of Periodontology* **74**, 521–528.

Pelegrin, P. and Surprenant, A. (2006). Pannexin-1 mediates large pore formation and interleukin 1-b release by the ATP-gated P2X7 receptor. *EMBO Journal* **25**, 5071–5082.

Pollack, S. R., Salzstein, R. and Peinkowski, D. (1984) The electric double layer in bone and its influence on stress generated potentials. *Calcified Tissue International* **36**, S77–S83.

Redlich, M., Rahamim, E., Gaft, A. and Shoshan, S. (1996) The response of supraalveolar gingival collagen to orthodontic rotation movement in dogs. *American Journal of Orthodontics and Dentofacial Orthopedics* **110**, 247–255.

Redlich, M., Reichenberg, E., Harari, D. *et al.* (2001) The effect of mechanical force on mRNA levels of collagenase, collagen type I, and tissue inhibitors of metalloproteinases in gingivae of dogs. *Journal of Dental Research* **80**(12), 2080–2084.

Redlich, M., Shoshan, S. and Palmon A. (1999) Gingival response to orthodontic force. *American Journal of Orthodontics and Dentofacial Orthopedics* **116**, 152–158.

Rodan, G. A., Bourret, L. A., Harvey, A. and Mensi, T. (1975) Cyclic AMP and cyclic GMP: mediators of the mechanical effects on bone remodeling. *Science* **189**(4201), 467–469.

Rubin, C. and Lanyon, L. E. (1985) Regulation of bone mass by mechanical strain magnitude. *Calcified Tissue International* **37**, 411–417.

Rubin, C., Turner, A. S., Bain, S. *et al.* (2001) Anabolism: Low mechanical signals strengthen long bones. *Nature* **412**, 603–604.

Sebaoun, J. D., Kantarci, A., Turner, J. W. *et al.* (2008) Modeling of trabecular bone and lamina dura following selective alveolar decortication in rats. *Journal of Periodontology* **79**, 1679–1688.

Seguier, S., Godeau, G. and Brousse, N. (2000) Collagen fibers and inflammatory cells in healthy and diseased human gingival tissues: A comparative and quantitative study by immunohistochemistry and automated image analysis. *Journal of Periodontology* **71**, 1079–1085.

Shirazi, M., Nilforoushan, D., Alghasi, H. and Dehpour, A. R. (2002) The role of nitric oxide in orthodontic tooth movement in rats. *The Angle Orthodontist* **72**, 211–215.

Silver, F. H. and Siperko, L. M. (2003) Mechanosensing and mechanochemical transduction: how is mechanical energy sensed and converted into chemical energy in an extracellular matrix? *Critical Reviews in Biomedical Engineering* **31**, 255–331.

Somjen, D., Binderman, I., Berger, E. and Harell, A. (1980) Bone remodeling induced by physical stress is prostaglandin E2 mediated. *Biochimica et Biophysica Acta* **627**, 91–100.

Turner, C. H. (2002) Mechanotransduction in skeletal cells (invited review). *Current Opinion in Orthopedics* **13**, 363–367.

Turner, C. H., Forwood, M. R., Rho, J. Y. and Yoshikawa, T. (1994) Mechanical loading thresholds for lamellar and woven bone formation. *Journal of Bone and Mineral Research* **9**, 87–97.

Turner, C. H. and Robling, A. G. (2004) Exercise as anabolic stimulus for bone. *Current Pharmaceutical Design* **10**, 2629–2641.

Wang, N., Butler, J. P. and Ingber, D. E. (1993) Mechanotransduction across the cell surface and through the cytoskeleton. *Science* **260**, 1124–1127.

Wilcko, W. M., Ferguson, D. J., Bouquot, J. E. and Wilcko, T. (2003) Rapid orthodontic decrowding with alveolar augmentation: Case report. *World Journal of Orthodontics* **4**, 197–205.

Wolff, J. (1892) *Das Gesetz der Transformation der Knochen*. Hirschwald, Berlin.

Yaffe, A., Fine, N., Alt, I. and Binderman, I. (1995) Effect of bisphosphonate on alveolar bone resorption following mucoperiosteal flap surgery in the mandible of rats. *Journal of Periodontology* **66**, 999–1003.

Yaffe, A., Fine, N. and Binderman, I. (1994) Regional accelerated phenomenon (RAP) in the mandible following mucoperiosteal flap surgery. *Journal of Periodontology* **65**, 79–83.

Yaffe, A., Herman, A., Bahar, H. and Binderman, I. (2003) Combined local application of tetracycline and bisphosphonate bone resorption in rats. *Journal of Periodontology* **74**, 1038–1042.

Yamamoto, T., Domon, T., Takahashi, S. *et al.* (1998) The structure and function of periodontal ligament cells in acellular cementum in rat molars. *Annals of Anatomy* **180**, 519–522.

Young, L., Binderman, I., Yaffe, A. *et al.* (2013) Fiberotomy enhances orthodontic tooth movement and diminishes relapse in a rat model. *Orthodontic and Craniofacial Research* **16**, 161–168.

Yu, H. and Ferrier, J. (1994) Mechanisms of ATP-induced Ca+2 signaling in osteoclasts. *Cellular Signaling* **6**, 905–914.

CHAPTER 6
Biological Aspects of Bone Growth and Metabolism in Orthodontics

James K. Hartsfield, Jr., Priyanka Gudsoorkar, Lorri A. Morford, and W. Eugene Roberts, Jr.

Summary

Understanding the mechanisms of bone growth and craniofacial development, as well as recognizing the processes of bone modeling versus remodeling, are key to the practice of orthodontics and dentofacial orthopedics. Although bone manipulation is important to most aspects of dentistry, orthodontists are craniofacial bone specialists. As such, a thorough understanding of these principles and their application to the individual patient will not only aid in generating an esthetically appealing result and stable clinical outcome, but also may enhance the success of a multidisciplinary case. This chapter reviews the basic concepts of bone growth and development with references for further reading. Fundamental to understanding these concepts is the section on bone formation that describes both endochondral bone formation and intramembranous bone formation in detail. The focus then shifts into a discussion of the primary growth centers and sites within the facial bones and introduces the concepts of bone modeling and remodeling. Unfortunately, dental professionals have often used the terms "modeling" and "remodeling" with a different meaning than typically employed by other professionals in medical research and clinical practice. Hence, a discussion of the terms modeling (changes in the shape, size, or position of bone) and remodeling (bone turnover) has been included. In the second half of the chapter, genetic mechanisms for the adaptation of bone to environmental factors are reviewed through a discussion of the importance of vascular invasion, inflammatory response, and cellular agents in bone growth and development. More detail on the understanding of remodeling, the coupling of bone formation to resorption in bone remodeling, and metabolic control of bone remodeling are then discussed. Of interest to the orthodontist are the mechanical aspects of bone modeling, cortical bone remodeling, and trabecular bone remodeling. The section which follows highlights elements of growth and development of facial bones, including temporomandibular joint development and mature temporomandibular joint adaptation that are of importance in gnathology. The relationship of tooth movement, bone modeling and external apical root resorption concurrent with orthodontia are pertinent to the orthodontist and are reviewed at the end of the chapter, as is the topic of dental facial orthopedics and bone modeling because of its importance in any discussion of functional appliances.

Introduction

Bone is a complex tissue that grows, develops, and responds to the surrounding environment. Among its many roles in the body, bone serves to support and maintain the body's structure and organization, it serves as a reservoir of minerals, and it functions as a key site for the generation of immune cells. Craniofacial bones not only serve to maintain shape and organization of the face, but they also protect the brain, support the dentition, and facilitate mastication.

The proper application of orthodontic force to move teeth safely requires a solid understanding of bone growth and development, as well as bone modeling and remodeling. As such, orthodontists learn to recognize the strengths and/or limitations that they may face with each clinical case by gathering important pretreatment information such as estimates of the remaining growth potential of a patient's bone, as well as its volume, thickness, quality, and overall health. An orthodontic treatment plan, including appliance selection and the timing of its use, is often influenced by one or all of these bone-related factors.

In addition, it is understood that the application of excessive or prolonged force on the teeth and the surrounding bone can lead to undesirable orthodontic results and possibly place the patient at risk of developing some forms of irreversible damage (e.g., severe external apical root resorption [EARR]). This chapter begins with a description of the key features of early bone growth and development and is designed to emphasize many of the bone-related processes that are central to the practice of orthodontics.

Biological Mechanisms of Tooth Movement, Third Edition. Edited by Vinod Krishnan, Anne Marie Kuijpers-Jagtman and Ze'ev Davidovitch.
© 2021 John Wiley & Sons Ltd. Published 2021 by John Wiley & Sons Ltd.

Basic concepts of bone growth and development

The neural crest/neural plate is a transient structure that extends along the rostro-caudal axis of developing vertebrate embryos. A primary role is to produce ectomesenchyme that will form the facial structures that are the entrance to the airway and alimentary canal (Stocum and Roberts, 2018). Following gastrulation, which is involved in formation of three basic germ layers – ectoderm, mesoderm and endoderm – the primary embryonic induction initiates neurulation. The notochord and adjacent mesoderm interact with the overlying dorsal ectoderm, which thickens and rises above the surface, forming neural plate. The neural crest establishes itself during the final stages of the process of neurulation. Neural crest cells are defined as a transient population of embryonic pluripotent cells that originate from the dorsal aspect of the neural tube and migrate through the trunk and head in vertebrates to form a diverse set of cell types. The neural crest is divided into four functional domains:

- cranial neural crest (CNC) – giving rise to various structures that develop from the transition of the cells into craniofacial ectomesenchyme that differentiates into various cranial ganglia and craniofacial cartilages and bones;
- trunk neural crest – giving rise to pigment synthesizing melanocytes and dorsal root ganglia containing sensory neurons;
- vagal and sacral neural crest – giving rise to intestinal parasympathetic ganglia;
- cardiac neural crest – giving rise to melanocytes, neurons, and connective tissue of some of the branchial arches, and to some structures of the heart, including the septum.

Our main concern is with the CNC, which plays a significant role in development of craniofacial structures with its contribution to skeletal, muscular, neural, and vascular elements.

Before the migration can commence, the cells must undergo an event known as epithelial to mesenchymal transformation, resulting in ectomesenchyme. Epithelial cells are characterized by their arrangement in a single layer of cells with clearly defined apical and basal sides whereas mesenchymal cells are characterized by their arrangement and less uniform shape (Bronner-Fraser, 1993; Hunt et al., 1998; Cobourne, 2000).

During craniofacial development, neural crest cells especially CNC cells migrate ventrolaterally as they populate the branchial arches. Cell labeling studies have demonstrated the formation of CNC cells from rhombomeres 1–4, which are also involved in formation of posterior midbrain and anterior hind brain. These cells migrate into the first branchial arch and thereafter reside within maxillary and mandibular prominences. The migration of these rhombencephalic crest cells may be regulated by growth factor signaling pathways and their downstream transcription factors before they become committed to different cell types (Noden, 1983; Le Douarin et al., 1994; Chai et al., 2000). In early embryonic development it appears that the CNC cells use a similar patterning plan as the developing nervous system, whereby a grid-like system of positional cues is created by gradients of morphogens affecting homeobox-containing transcription factors (Gilbert, 2000; Santagati and Rijli, 2003). Various growth (such as TGF-β) and transcription factors (such as *Msx1* and *Msx2* in a mouse model) have been implicated during the specification and fate determination of neural crest cells. In particular, the presence of TGF-β subtypes is obvious in mesenchyme during critical epithelial–mesenchymal interactions related to the formation of tooth organ and Meckel's cartilage during mandibular morphogenesis (Chai et al., 1999). The initial distribution of cartilage and bone occurs

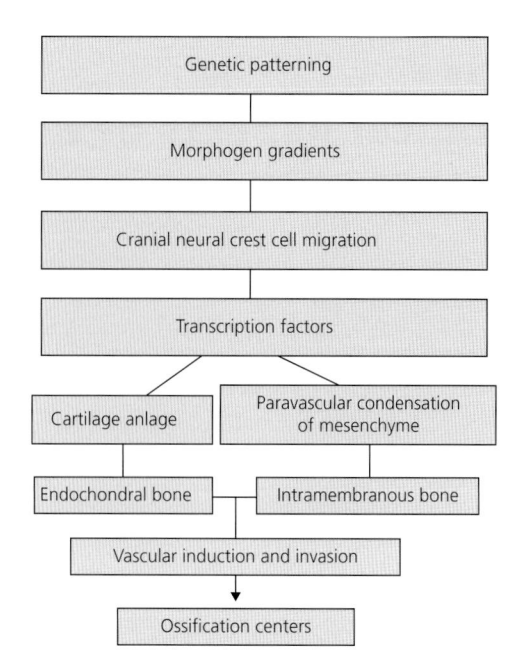

Figure 6.1 Genetic patterning to produce craniofacial ossification centers involves cranial neural crest cell migration along morphogen gradients, followed by formation of cartilaginous or intramembranous structures, which are then targets for vascular invasion to form specific bones. (Source: Roberts and Hartsfield, 2004. Reproduced with permission of Elsevier.)

during the genetic patterning of the skeletal system in two fundamental ways: endochondral and intramembranous bone formation (Figure. 6.1).

It appears that the neurovascular distribution controls the patterning of ossification and subsequent response to mechanical loading of both endochondral and intramembranous bone. In a series of *in situ* hybridization studies it had been shown that several nerve growth factors and high affinity receptors are expressed during the development of craniofacial skeletal tissues (Yamashiro et al., 2001c, 2002). Furthermore, it has been demonstrated that intact nerves are important for a normal response to mechanical loading, such as experimental tooth movement (Yamashiro et al., 2000a, 2000b, 2001a, 2001b). A nociceptive mechanism in the trigeminal nerve is associated with the inflammatory response to mechanical stimulation of the periodontal ligament (PDL) (Yamashiro et al., 1997; Yamashiro et al., 1998; Fujiyoshi et al., 2000).

Bone formation

The developmental events and mechanism of response to the mechanical stimuli are important to the understanding of fundamental differences between bone formed through endochondral (Figure 6.2) and intramembranous ossification (Figure 6.3). However, this distinction is sometimes blurred, such as when the bilateral intramembranous ossification centers of the maxilla and mandible grow toward the midline and form synchondroses in the posterior palate and mid symphysis.

Endochondral bone formation

Two types of cartilage, hyaline cartilage and fibrocartilage, are associated with bone growth, fracture healing, and functional articular surfaces. The cellular source for these tissues is undifferentiated mesenchymal cells, which differentiate into chondrocytes. In the

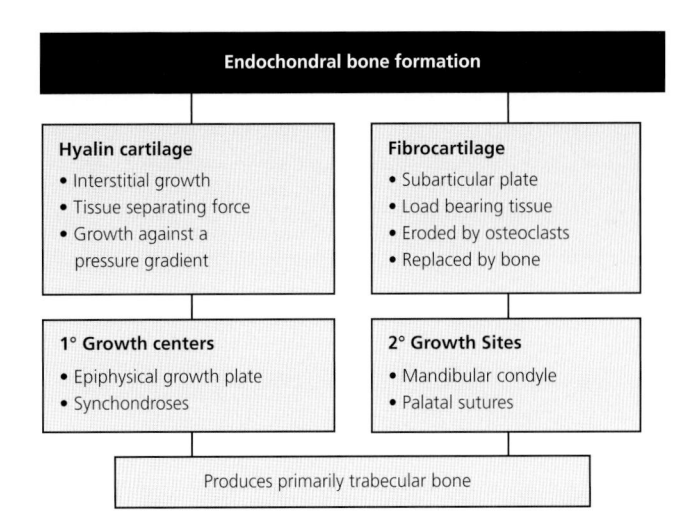

Figure 6.2 Endochondral bone formation via hyaline cartilage is associated with primary growth centers such as growth plates and synchondroses. Fibrocartilage is the precursor for secondary growth sites such as the mandibular condyle and early postnatal growth of palatal sutures. Because of the vascular invasion process, endochondral ossification results in a characteristic patterning of trabecular bone. (Source: Roberts and Hartsfield, 2004. Reproduced with permission of Elsevier.)

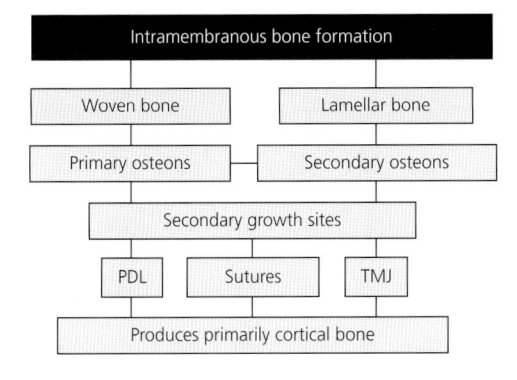

Figure 6.3 Intramembranous bone formation produces a woven or lamellar structure depending on the rate of apposition. Woven bone is compacted with lamellar bone to form primary osteons. Circumferential lamellae are remodeled to secondary osteons. All intramembranous bone formation is associated with secondary growth sites, such as the PDL, sutures, and the TMJ. Intramembranous bone formation produces primarily cortical bone. (Source: Roberts and Hartsfield, 2004. Reproduced with permission of Elsevier.)

process of endochondral bone formation, chondrocytes undergo well-organized and controlled phases of proliferation, hypertrophic differentiation, death, blood vessel invasion, and finally replacement of cartilage with bone. A characteristic of endochondral ossification in areas of growth that have intrinsic tissue separating capability (growth centers) is the formation of round proliferative chondrocytes in columnar layers as they synthesize type II collagen. In areas such as the mandibular condyles that grow in response to growth in other areas or tissue (growth sites), the chondrocytes do not form columnar layers. As the chondrocytes undergo hypertrophy, they begin to predominantly express type X collagen and mineralize the surrounding matrix. The mineralized matrix is progressively resorbed by osteoclasts, while osteoblasts begin to deposit osteoid, which is then mineralized to facilitate the

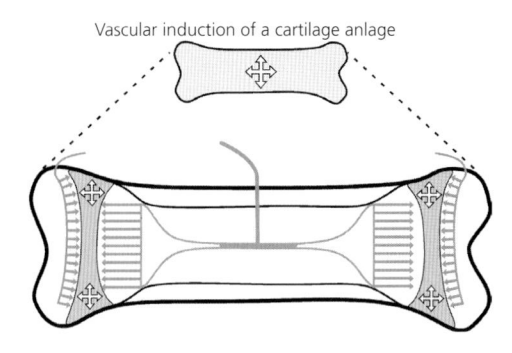

Figure 6.4 Vascular invasion of the cartilage anlage for a long bone occurs at the mid-diaphyseal and epiphyseal regions. Endochondral ossification from two directions results in remnants of the cartilage anlage forming growth plates, which are primary growth centers that can grow against a pressure gradient. (Source: Roberts and Hartsfield, 2004. Reproduced with permission of Elsevier.)

replacement of cartilage by bone (Chen and Carter, 2005; Provot and Schipani, 2005).

The initial osseous structure resulting from the mineralization of either hyaline or fibrocartilage is cancellous or trabecular bone because the cartilage cells die following hypertrophy and the intercellular substance mineralizes. In the primary spongiosa of long bones, mineralized hyaline cartilage serves as a substrate for woven bone apposition. On the other hand, mineralized fibrocartilage in the metaphysis of the mandibular condyle is eroded by osteoclasts and replaced by lamellar bone apposition. In the metaphysis of both the mandibular condyle and long bones, the initial cancellous bone is remodeled to lamellar trabeculae that are aligned along the line of stress. This reflects Wolff's law, i.e., every change in the form and function of bone or of their function alone is followed by certain definite changes in their internal architecture, and equally definite alteration in their external conformation, in accordance with mathematical laws (Frost, 1994). Peripheral cancellous bone in subperiosteal areas condenses and remodels to cortical bone, while the primary and secondary spongiosa beneath the epiphyseal growth plate is the initial pattern of the trabecular bone of the metaphysis (Figure 6.4).

Hypertrophic chondrocytes express the vascular endothelial growth factor (VEGF), which guides the path of vascular invasion for endochondral bone formation (Kornak and Mundlos, 2003). Ossification centers occur at genetically defined positions in the cartilage anlage, which correspond to the points of vascular invasion (Figure 6.4). In brief, endochondral bone formation in the metaphysis produces primarily trabecular bone. The vascular invasion and bone remodeling on the diaphyseal surface of the growth plate is the mechanism for patterning the trabeculae. A similar trabecular structure is produced in the epiphysis of long bones and in the head of the mandibular condyle.

The molecular mechanism for developmental regulation of the growth plate is controlled by a complex interaction of local and systemic factors. The local mediators include bone morphogenetic proteins (BMPs), Wingless-related integration site proteins (WNTs), fibroblast growth factors (FGFs), hedgehog proteins, parathyroid hormone-related protein (PTHrP), insulin-like growth factors (IGFs), and retinoids. Systemic factors that help control the growth of long bones are growth hormone, thyroid hormone, estrogen, androgen, vitamin D, and glucocorticoids (Kronenberg, 2003). In general, the genetic influence on a primary growth center, like the epiphyseal growth plate, is well defined.

Examples of the complexity of genetic influences in skeletal development include the more than 24 genes associated with craniosynostosis (Lattanzi et al., 2017). In addition, genetic variants of pathological significance in the fibroblast growth factor 2 (*FGFR2*) gene can be associated with more than one phenotype including Crouzon, Pfeiffer, Jackson-Weiss, and Apert syndromes (Mulvihill, 1995; Meyers et al., 1996; Oldridge et al., 1999). Genetic variants of pathological significance in the *FGFR3* gene can be associated with other craniosynostosis syndromes such as Crouzon syndrome with acanthosis nigricans and Muenke syndrome, and also with conditions with varying severity of short-limbed dwarfism that include craniofacial affects (e.g., achondroplasia, and thanatophoric dysplasia types I and II) (Wilcox et al., 1998; Vajo et al., 2000).

Since genetic variants of pathological significance in different areas of the same gene, or even the same variant in a gene, can have markedly different effects on skeletal growth and development, it is not surprising that genetic variations may have variably subtle or profound effects. Animal and human studies are exploring these genetic variations that affect proteins including skeletal muscle, transcription factors, growth factors, bone and cartilage formation, extracellular matrix and connective tissue, and membrane receptor and intracellular signaling and their effect on or association with jaw growth (Kluemper et al., 2019; Manocha et al., 2019; Hartsfield et al., 2013). This is a fertile area for clinically relevant research, including the analysis of genetic polymorphisms associated with response to early maxillary protraction and subsequent growth in skeletal Class III patients, and variance of mandibular growth and the response to functional appliances in skeletal Class II patients (Hartsfield, 2015; Hartsfield Jr. et al., 2017).

Intramembranous bone formation

In contrast to the cartilage precursor in endochondral ossification, intramembranous ossification occurs without a cartilaginous precursor. Mesenchymal cells initially differentiate to preosteoblasts in intramembranous bone formation (as opposed to chondrocytes in endochondral ossification), which later differentiate to osteoblasts. The osteoblasts deposit osteoid, which then mineralizes. As ossification progresses, some osteoblasts are enclosed within the mineralized bone tissue and become osteocytes. If this process occurs on the surfaces of existing bone, it is also referred to as appositional ossification.

As with endochondral bone formation where the mechanical environment can influence chondrocyte mitosis, extracellular matrix production, hypertrophy, mineralization, and vascularization, the mechanical environment can also regulate osteoblast differentiation and activity during intramembranous ossification. A key component to understanding the interaction of environmental (mechanical) and biological (genetic) factors is that genetic differences among individuals strongly determine responsivity to environmental factors, including mechanical force (Chen and Carter, 2005). Epigenetic factors (modifiers of gene expression and therefore protein production that may be heritable) are also important in bone formation and may explain some variation in mandibular morphology in response to food consistency, and be a mechanism to modulate bone formation and influence bone healing (Mavropoulos et al., 2004; Renaud et al., 2010; Rubin et al., 2018; Chen et al., 2019).

The formation of the flat bones (face, cranium, sternum, and scapula) is initiated as intramembranous condensations of mesenchyme adjacent to blood vessels (Stocum and Roberts, 2018). In animal models, expression of SRY-Box Transcription Factor-5 (*Sox5*), *Sox6*, and *Sox9* is critical to the process of cell stickiness and adhesion (Kornak and Mundlos, 2003). The RUNX Family Transcription Factor 2 (*Runx2*) controls postnatal bone formation by regulating osteoblast differentiation (Karsenty, 2003). In humans, haploinsufficiency of *RUNX2* causes cleidocranial dysplasia, in which the skull bones are hypomineralized with very large sutural spaces, short stature, hypoplasia or agenesis of the clavicles, other skeletal effects, supernumerary teeth, and a lack of eruption of some teeth (Mundlos et al., 1997).

In the previous sentences the gene name was written as *Runx2* and *RUNX2*. It is customary, but not necessary, that the names of genes be italicized. It is standard that all the letters in human genes are capitalized, while the genes of other species such as mice are capitalized followed by lower case letters. Many genes have different names in the literature since they may have been named differently initially by different investigators, and or had the name changed to better fit within some organizational nomenclature or gene family. For example, the gene for cleidocranial dysplasia was named *CBFA1* at the time of discovery but is now called *RUNX2* following the Human Genome Organization (HUGO) Gene Nomenclature Committee website (http://www.genenames.org). This is a good source to find aliases for the same gene, and to also determine which name the committee recommends for use (Braschi et al., 2018). In addition, the USA National Center for Biotechnology Information (NCBI) is an extensive resource on biotechnology. Databases and other resources including PubMed, Nucleotide and Protein Sequences, Genomes, Taxonomy, and others may be found at the NCBI website (https://www.ncbi.nlm.nih.gov/).

The center of ossification appears to be initiated in areas where growth factors are secreted lateral to neurovascular bundles (Stocum and Roberts, 2018). As evidenced by the high degree of vascularity and lack of a cartilage precursor, the intramembranous mechanism is the prototype for subperiosteal bone formation. Depending on the apposition rate, the bone formed may be of the woven or lamellar type. Woven bone is formed rapidly (up to ~100 μm/day) and has a poorly organized matrix. Lamellar bone is formed slowly (≤1 μm/day) and has a highly organized matrix. Primary osteons are formed by laying down a perivascular lattice of woven bone, which is then compacted in the direction of the central vessel with lamellar bone. Secondary osteons are composed entirely of lamellar bone (Figure 6.5) (Roberts, 2000a).

Intramembranous bone formation cannot grow against a pressure gradient because it is dependent upon patent blood vessels along the bone surface. This is the osteogenic mechanism of secondary growth sites such as the PDL, sutures, and the temporomandibular joint (TMJ) (Figure 6.3). In contrast to the production of primarily trabecular bone at endochondral growth centers, intramembranous bone formation at secondary growth sites is cortical bone: circumferential lamellae or primary osteons (Roberts, 2000a).

Primary growth centers and sites in facial bones

The primary anlage for the long bones and most secondary growth cartilages is composed of hyaline cartilage. They are primary growth centers in the late prenatal and early postnatal periods. Some sites like the epiphyseal growth plates and cranial base synchondroses retain primary growth capability until skeletal maturity. Primary growth centers are defined as tissues capable of: (i) interstitial growth, (ii) generating tissue-separating force, and (iii) growing against a pressure gradient. The epiphyseal growth plates are the primary growth centers of the axial and appendicular skeleton.

Since fibrocartilage fails to generate tissue-separating force, it is a morphological feature of secondary growth sites such as the man-

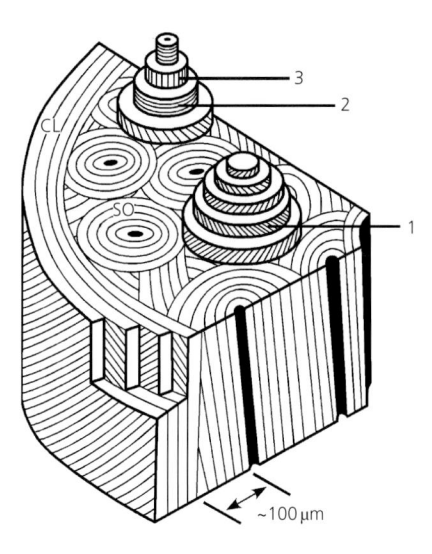

Figure 6.5 A wedge of a cortical bone that is growing to the left demonstrates the morphology of circumferential lamellae (CL) and secondary osteons (SO). Depending on the mechanical loading at the time the matrix is formed, bone lamellae may have a collagen orientation that is an alternating bias (1) or alternating horizontal (2) and vertical (3) orientations. (Source: Roberts and Hartsfield, 2004. Reproduced with permission of Elsevier.)

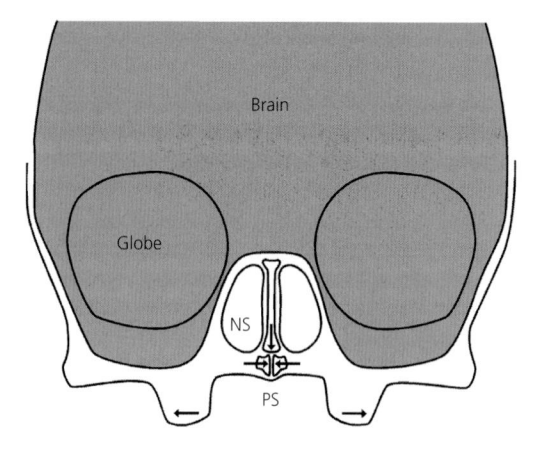

Figure 6.6 The early postnatal growth of the maxillary complex up until the time that the primary first molars come into occlusion. Two primary growth centers are involved: (1) cartilaginous nasal septum (NS), and (2) palatal synchondrosis (PS). Growth of the NS and PS results in vertical displacement and an increase in width, respectively. (Source: Roberts and Hartsfield, 2004. Reproduced with permission of Elsevier.)

dibular condyle and palatal suture (Stocum and Roberts, 2018). Fibrocartilage is a load-bearing articular tissue that should not be confused with the primary growth centers, which are composed of hyaline cartilage (Figure 6.2). Fibrocartilage has no inherent growth potential. It is produced by mechanically stressed periosteum. The articular surfaces of the mandibular condyle and fossa are covered with periosteum, which differentiates into a subarticular layer of fibrocartilage that can mineralize to form bone (Roberts and Stocum, 2018; Stocum and Roberts, 2018).

In addition to the cartilaginous cranial base, the principal primary growth centers of the craniofacial complex during the prenatal period are the brain, eyes (globes), nasal septum, and palatal synchondrosis (Figure 6.6). The body of the maxilla is formed by intramembranous ossification of bilateral plates of bone. As the palatal shelves reorient and grow toward the midline, the soft tissue is invaded by intramembranous bone (Hughes *et al.*, 1967). As the palatal bones grow toward the midline, the intervening mesenchymal cells form a synchondrosis that drives maxillary growth in width, until a functional occlusion is established (Bloore *et al.*, 1969; Griffiths *et al.*, 1967; Hughes *et al.*, 1967). Prenatally, anterior and inferior displacement of the maxilla is driven by the nasal septum (Furstman *et al.*, 1971).

Sometime after birth, much of the nasal septum ossifies and the maxillary midline synchondrosis converts itself to a suture. Thus, prenatal and early postnatal maxillary growth is driven by primary cartilaginous growth centers, but after an occlusion is established, functionally driven secondary growth sites take over. Figure 6.7 is an enlarged view of the maxillary complex demonstrating the direction of growth during the prenatal period for the nasal septum and posterior palatal synchondrosis. Before the onset of postnatal function and alveolar process development, the nasal septum, palatal synchondrosis, and tooth buds are the skeletal growth centers for development of the maxilla in width, length, and depth. Postnatally, the cartilaginous growth centers disappear as a functional occlusion is established and the skeletal growth of the maxilla depends on secondary bone apposition in the maxillary sutures and development

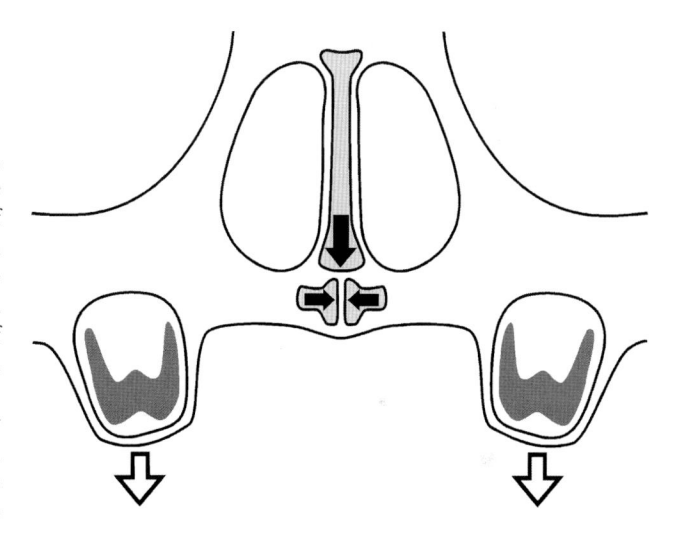

Figure 6.7 An enlarged drawing demonstrates the primary growth mechanism of the maxillary complex before eruption of the deciduous molars. Once the molars are in occlusion, the primary growth centers revert to secondary growth sites that respond to functional loading. (Source: Roberts and Hartsfield, 2004. Reproduced with permission of Elsevier.)

of the dentition. Normal masticatory loading is important for optimal growth of the maxilla and mandible (Ito *et al.*, 1988).

Meckel's cartilage provides embryonic support for the musculoskeletal structures of the lower face, but it is not a direct endochondral precursor for the mandible. As the developing face rapidly increases in width, the body of the mandible is formed lateral to Meckel's cartilage (Stocum and Roberts, 2018). Ossification of the mandible begins as bilateral plates of intramembranous bone are deposited near the junction of the mental and inferior alveolar nerves. The mandible must grow and develop against pressure gradients generated by attachment of the powerful muscles of mastication. Muscles grow in length by an adaptive (secondary) mechanism, which means that the origin and insertion of a muscle must be separated by growth at primary growth centers or by displacement between articulating bones.

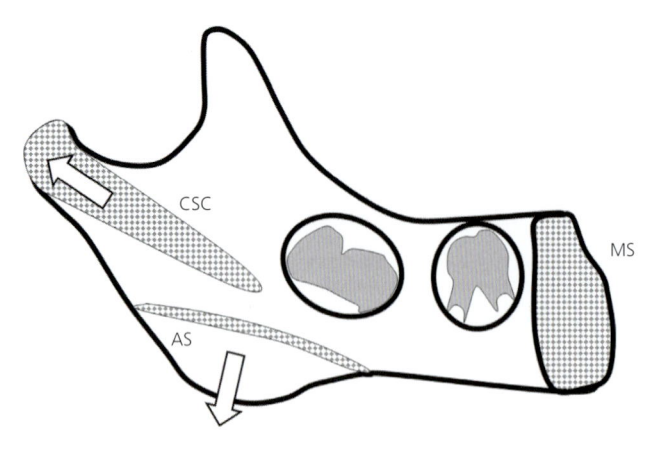

Figure 6.8 After the body of the mandible forms by the intramembranous mechanism, late prenatal and early postnatal growth involves three principal primary growth centers: (1) condylar secondary cartilage (CSC), (2) angular synchondrosis (AS), and (3) mandibular midline synchondrosis (MS). These primary growth centers grow against pressure gradients until masticatory function is established. At that point, the AS and MS fuse and the mandibular condyle reverts to a secondary growth site. (Source: Roberts and Hartsfield, 2004. Reproduced with permission of Elsevier.)

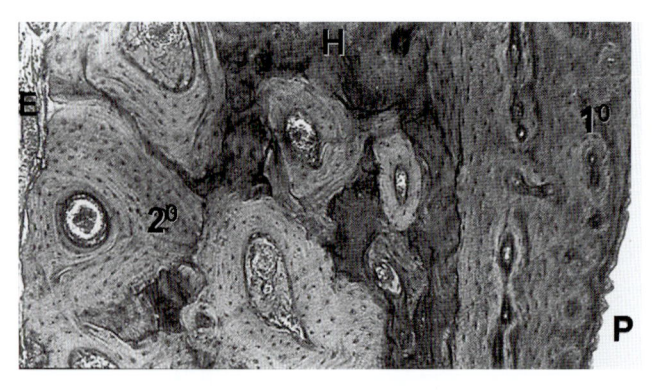

Figure 6.9 A photomicrograph of a cross-section through the mandible of a monkey demonstrates primary (1°) and secondary (2°) bone. The three envelopes of cortical bone originally described by Frost are: endosteal (E), Haversian (H), and periosteal (P). The endosteal surface is strongly influenced by the metabolic factors of the marrow while the other envelopes respond primarily to mechanical loading. (Source: Roberts et al., 2006. Reproduced with permission of Elsevier.)

Since intramembranous bone formation cannot occur against a pressure gradient, three secondary cartilages form during the prenatal period to promote mandibular development: (i) midline synchondrosis, (ii) angular synchondrosis, and (iii) condylar cartilage (Figure 6.8). As the bilateral plates of bone grow toward the midline, the mandibular symphyseal synchondrosis (MS) is formed. It is a primary growth center that is responsible for prenatal growth of the mandible in width. The angular synchondrosis (AS) is formed to grow against the pressure gradient of the developing masseter and inferior pterygoid muscles. The condylar secondary cartilage (CSC) provides for sagittal and vertical growth of the mandible prenatally (Stocum and Roberts, 2018). All of the secondary cartilages, which serve as primary growth centers prenatally, ossify or evolve into secondary growth sites shortly after birth, when function assumes the primary role in effecting mandibular growth (Ishii-Suzuki et al., 1999; Zhao and Westphal, 2002; Rabie et al., 2003; Roberts and Hartsfield, 2004; Marcucio et al., 2015).

Bone modeling and remodeling

Since the dawn of microscopy, bone histologists have been aware that there was a mechanism for physiologic replacement of mature cortical bone (Figure 6.9) (Havers, 1691; Hunter, 1778). Because of the scalloped resorption arrest lines on the periphery of secondary osteons, it was hypothesized that osteoclasts created resorption cavities within cortical bone and osteoblasts filled them with new lamellar bone. The recognition of secondary osteons by the early English histologist Clopton Havers (b.1657–d.1702) is the source of the term "Haversian Systems" (Goldberg, 1982).

Although more recent histologists have been able to resolve greater detail in demineralized and ground sections of bone, there was no real progress in recognizing the dynamic nature of bone turnover for more than two centuries. In the second edition of *Bone and Bones*, Weinmann and Sicher (1955) made an early attempt to segregate the physiologic processes of cortical bone modeling and remodeling. The terms "modeling formation" and "modeling resorption" were used for the bone surface sculpting mechanisms

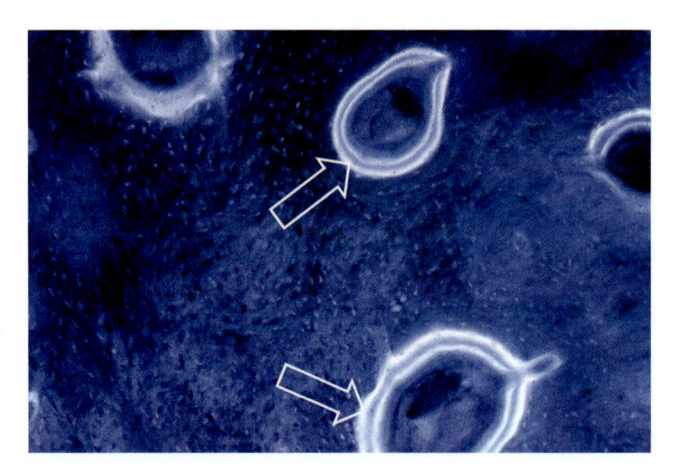

Figure 6.10 The concentric pairs of bright lines (arrows) are double tetracycline labels marking secondary osteons in cortical bone of an adult dog. There was a 7-day interval between the two injected doses of tetracycline (10 mg/kg of body weight). The fluorescent lines are permanent time markers of bone formation that remain *in situ* until the bone tissue is resorbed. (Source: Roberts et al., 2006. Reproduced with permission of Elsevier.)

essential for growth, development, and functional adaptation. In addition, they recognized the "internal reconstruction" of cortical bone, but like other scientists of the time, failed to appreciate its physiologic significance.

The modern physiologic concept of bone remodeling (turnover) is largely attributed to Frost (Frost et al., 1961). In the early 1960s, he developed the dynamic histomorphometric method of using tetracycline labels in humans to define bone physiologic mechanisms *in vivo* (Figure 6.10). With this dynamic kinetic marker, Frost and his followers deciphered the dynamics of bone physiology and concluded that bone surface changes were physiologically distinct from internal turnover events and had different control mechanisms. With respect to the use of the terms "modeling" and "remodeling," Frost followed the lead of Weinmann and Sicher. Modeling is the sculpting mechanism that uses the raw material of bone growth to shape structures, under the combined influence of developmental programs and mechanical loading.

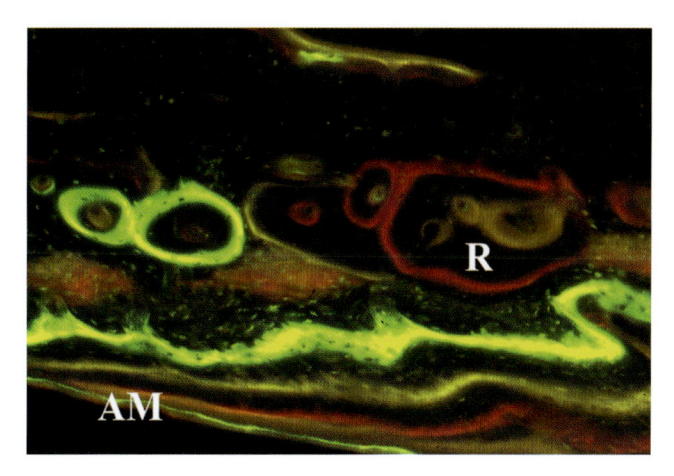

Figure 6.11 A series of multifluorochome labels at 7-day intervals in rabbit bone shows the morphological pattern of subperiosteal apposition (yellow, gold, and orange labels) in the lower third of the photomicrograph. This process is anabolic modeling (AM). Concentric bone labels in the center of the illustration demonstrate the front of remodeling (R) that follows primary cortical bone formation. Subperiosteal bone apposition (modeling followed by remodeling) is progressing in an inferior direction. (Source: Roberts et al., 2006. Reproduced with permission of Elsevier.)

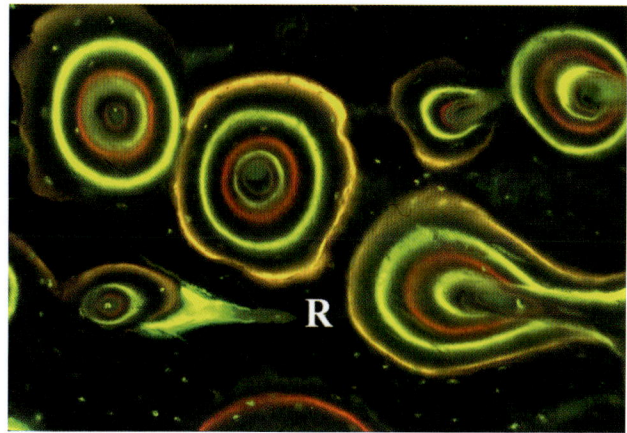

Figure 6.12 A series of multiple fluorochrome labels at 2-week intervals demonstrate intense remodeling activity in cortical bone of a young adult dog (R). The concentric colored lines mark the respective mineralization front at the time each label was injected. (Source: Roberts et al., 2006. Reproduced with permission of Elsevier.)

Remodeling is the mechanism for lifelong skeletal turnover and maintenance with a specific, coupled turnover sequence (A → R → F) of cell activation (A), resorption (R) of a cavity, and replacement by formation (F) of new bone. Frost also pioneered the concept of the regional acceleratory phenomenon ("RAP"). This is a complex reaction of soft and hard tissues to diverse noxious stimuli, including damage to bone. When this phenomenon is activated, the healing process is locally accelerated for a limited duration, which in bone results in a transient decrease in bone density (Frost, 1983).

Two essential technologies were critical for the development of the modern principles of bone physiology: the bone labels of Harold Frost (Frost et al., 1961) and the undemineralized thin sectioning method of Jim Arnold (Arnold, 1951). These methods continue to be used for many important basic science experiments and were essential technologies for the development of clinical bone histomorphometry (Jee, 2005). The latter is a widely used method for diagnosing and monitoring the treatment of metabolic bone disease (Recker, 1983; Parfitt et al., 1987). It is important for orthodontists to understand both methods to deliver appropriate care for patients with insipient or frank metabolic bone disease.

The combined techniques of undemineralized sections and intravital bone labels have been widely exploited to explore and define the mechanisms of skeletal adaptation to mechanical loads and metabolic demands. From a series of animal experiments (Figures 6.11 and 6.12), and clinical studies of normal and diseased bone, it was possible to formulate the biodynamic concepts of bone modeling and remodeling. Figure 6.13 is an illustration of a cross-section of a long bone drifting in space. Longitudinal sections of cortical bone have revealed the A → R → F sequence of cutting/filling cones responsible for replacing old bone with new secondary osteons (Figure 6.14) (Roberts, 1984). The overall concept of bone adaptation associated with the drift of a long bone (Figure 6.13) is quite similar to alveolar process adaptation during tooth movement (Figure 6.15) (Roberts, 2005). During the modeling process, apposition along bone surfaces can produce lamellar, woven, or composite bone depending on the rate of bone formation (Storey, 1972; Roberts et al., 2004). However, normal remodeling processes produce only lamellar bone at an appositional rate of ~0.6–1.0 μm/day (Figures 6.10 and 6.12).

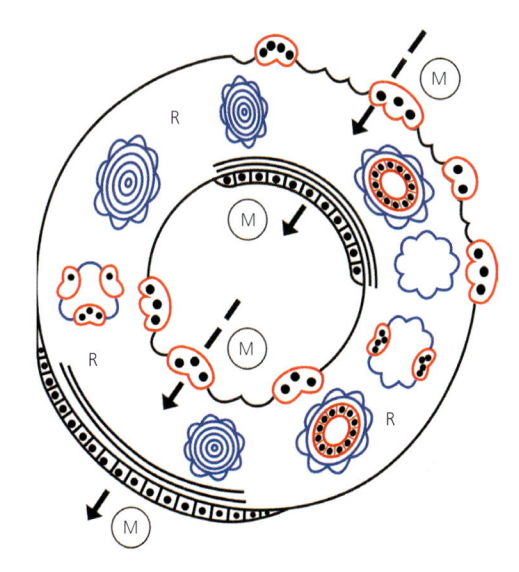

Figure 6.13 The integration of anabolic and catabolic modeling (M) activity along bone surfaces with internal remodeling (turnover, R) to produce new secondary osteons. (Source: Adapted from Roberts et al., 1989.)

In brief, modeling changes the shape, size, and/or position of bones in response to mechanical loading and/or wounding. On the other hand, remodeling is turnover of bone that is related to bone maturation, skeletal maintenance, and mineral metabolism. Remodeling *per se* does not change the overall shape or size of a bone (Figures 6.11 and 6.13). Because the definitions were based on kinetic data, which has been confirmed by multiple species in many laboratories around the world, Frost's terms for bone "modeling" and "remodeling" were ultimately accepted as the gold standard in anatomy, physiology, and biomechanics (Bouvier and Hylander, 1981; Burr et al., 1989; Bidez and Misch, 1992; Boyde et al., 1992; Bagge, 2000).

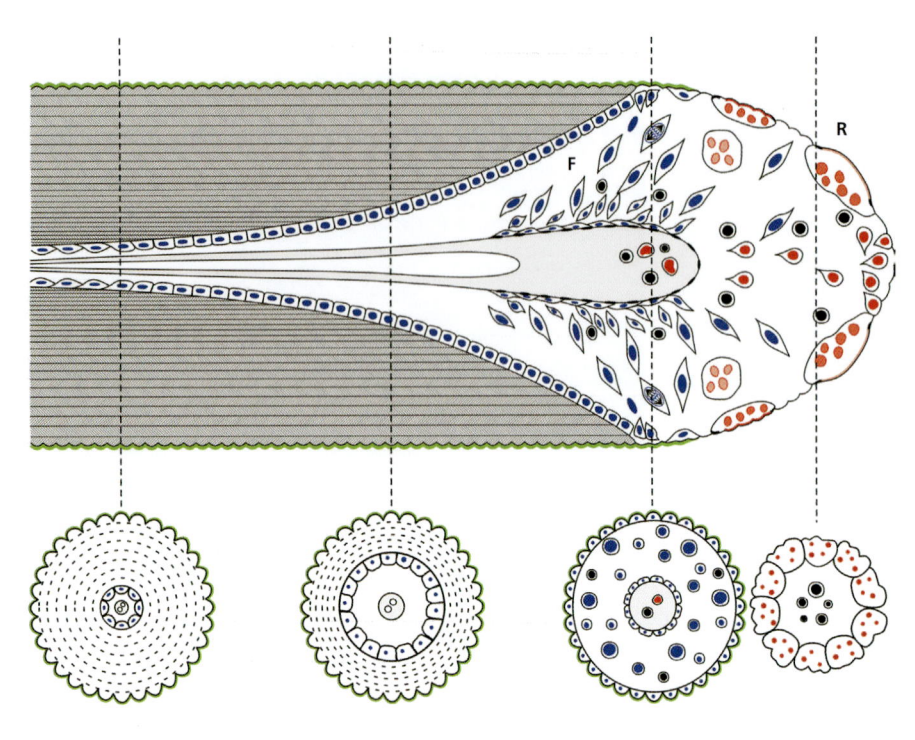

Figure 6.14 A longitudinal section through a cutting/filling cone in cortical bone (moving to the right) illustrates the perivascular cellular activity associated with the coupled resorption (R) and formation (F) responses. Four cross-sections of the evolving secondary osteons are shown below. The progression of resorption to form a cavity within cortical bone, to refilling it with lamellar bone, is shown from left to right. T lymphocytes are black, the osteoclast cell line is red, and the osteoblastic line is blue. See text for details. (Source: Roberts *et al.*, 2006. Reproduced with permission of Elsevier.)

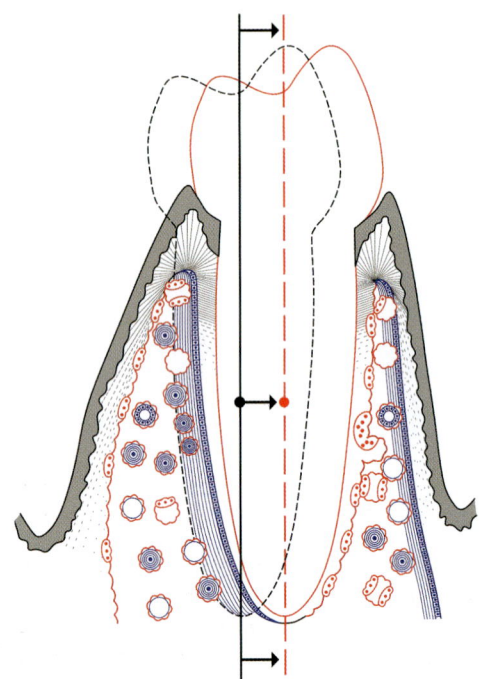

Figure 6.15 The bone physiology associated with translation of a tooth. Note that there is a coordinated bone modeling and remodeling response leading and trailing the moving tooth. This mechanism allows a tooth to move relative to basilar bone while maintaining a normal functional relationship with its periodontium. Osteoclastic and osteoblastic activities are in red and blue, respectively. (Source: Roberts *et al.*, 2006. Reproduced with permission of Elsevier.)

human skulls of different ages and mapped areas of bone surface patterns of resorption and formation to explain the surface anabolic and catabolic mechanisms for facial growth and development (Enlow, 1962; Enlow and Bang, 1965). He chose to use the word "remodeling" as an anatomical term to describe the bone sculpting process of growth and development. However, this is what others were calling the process of bone modeling. Enlow's concept of bone surface "remodeling" was very important for understanding the surface sculpting and drift mechanisms of facial growth and development. Unfortunately, orthodontic investigators have tended to embrace the term "remodeling" to describe bone surface change, and have essentially ignored internal turnover mechanisms (Storey, 1972; Isaacson *et al.*, 1976; Baumrind *et al.*, 1997). Because bone modeling and remodeling are independent processes under different control mechanisms, it is very important for orthodontists to use the correct terminology to avoid scientific confusion and barriers to scientific exchange with other biomedical disciplines (Roberts *et al.*, 2006).

Genetic mechanisms for environment adaptation

Bone form and function are regulated by an interaction of genetic, environmental, and epigenetic factors. In addition to determining the patterning of the sites of ossification, genetic factors influence skeletal morphology by three interactive cellular mechanisms: (i) vascular invasion, (ii) mechanically induced inflammation, and (iii) localized secretion of cellular control agents (Figure 6.16). These fundamental interactive processes direct the bone modeling and remodeling aspects of biomechanics. Catabolic modeling removes bone adjacent to the necrotic, compressed regions of the PDL via undermining resorption. Anabolic modeling is the formation of primary cortical bone in areas where the PDL is widened. Remodeling is the process of vascular invasion that replaces primary bone with secondary lamellar bone. The latter is the principal osseous tissue of the mature alveolar process. In addition to these

However, in the current orthodontics literature, there continues to be substantial confusion regarding usage of the term "remodeling." This semantics problem arises from Enlow's concept of bone surface "remodeling." In the early 1960s, Enlow sectioned dry

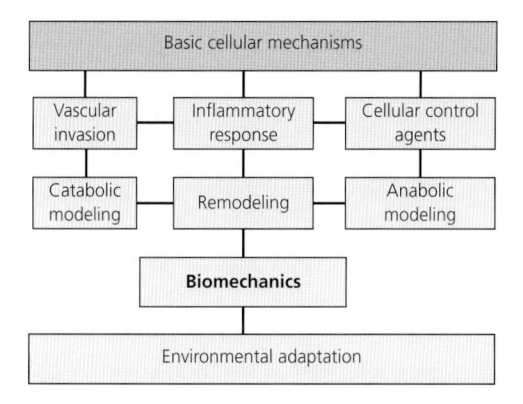

Figure 6.16 With respect to environmental adaptation of bone, the basic cellular mechanisms are vascular invasion, inflammatory response, and production of cellular control agents (cytokines, and so on). These cellular mechanisms are the basis of the cellular adaptive processes of bone: catabolic modeling, remodeling, and anabolic modeling. Environmental adaptation of the skeleton is driven by biomechanics, which are the inherent response thresholds to mechanical loading. (Source: Roberts and Hartsfield, 2004. Reproduced with permission of Elsevier.)

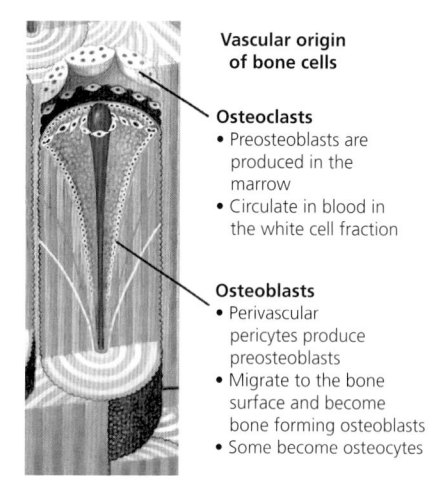

Figure 6.17 The vascular origin of bone cells. Note that osteoclasts are derived from circulating preosteoclasts while the origin of osteoblasts is from perivascular proliferation of osteogenic precursor cells (pericytes). (Source: Roberts and Hartsfield, 2004. Reproduced with permission of Elsevier.)

cellular mechanisms, variations in muscle fibers and therefore muscle activity that are associated with genetic variation also influence skeletal morphology (Rowlerson et al., 2005; Raoul et al., 2011; Huh et al., 2013; Sciote et al., 2013; Desh et al., 2014; Zebrick et al., 2014). An appreciation of the potential and limitation of the skeletal system for mechanical manipulation is essential to understanding bone-related response and anomalies, and devising appropriate therapy directed at the improvement of a malocclusion.

Genetic determinants of overall craniofacial growth

The craniofacial phenotype is determined during early embryogenesis and impacts the early stages of facial development (Sperber et al., 2010). Studies have shown that bone formation in the facial region is a series of complex interactions that involves many factors such as FGFs, sonic hedgehog proteins, BMPs, homeobox genes, and local retinoic acid gradients (Marcucio et al., 2015). For example, the homeobox genes play a significant role in determining the identity and position of the various structures along the craniocaudal axis. The homeobox genes control the morphogenetic process by regulating the synthesis of specific transcription factors (Zhao and Westphal, 2002).

Common orthodontic clinic scenarios like condylar growth, orthodontic tooth movement (OTM), mandibular propulsion, etc. are affected by postnatal craniofacial growth. Genetic variation along with environmental variation, especially as it may then affect epigenetic influence on gene expression, are fundamental factors in the complex development of facial growth. Propulsion of the mandible in animal models changes the biophysical environment of the condylar cartilage. For example, rat studies have demonstrated an increase in expression of SRY-Box Transcription Factor-9 (*Sox9*) following mandibular advancement (Rabie et al., 2003), reflecting that this transcription factor is involved in endochondral ossification. Mandibular advancement also shows an increased expression of PTHrP that coincides with maturation of chondrocytes (Ishii-Suzuki et al., 1999). However, although animal studies looking at changes in gene and protein expression show the response to the mandibular advancement, they do not necessarily indicate the genes involved in causing mandibular prognathism in humans (Kluemper et al., 2019). This may reflect the difference in a secondary response to mandibular propulsion and what leads to primary mandibular prognathism.

Vascular invasion

Vascularity is a prerequisite for new bone formation because perivascular pericytes are the precursors of osteoblasts. Vascular invasion is the common denominator for initiation of bone formation in cartilage anlagen, callus ossification during wound healing, cortical bone remodeling, and endochondral bone formation of growth plates and synchondroses. Thus, all new bone formation requires vascularity, which is often initiated by some form of vascular invasion into soft or cartilaginous connective tissue. Adequate vascularity is also a prerequisite for bone maintenance and adaptation because it provides both nutrition for vital osseous tissue and new bone cells. As illustrated in Figure 6.17, osteoblasts and osteocytes are derived from perivascular pericytes while the osteoclast precursors circulate in the blood and pass through the blood vessel wall to enter the tissue.

Vascular invasion is a basic mechanism for responding to skeletal wounding or applied mechanical loads, both physiological and/or therapeutic (Chang et al., 1996; Chang et al., 1997). In concert with the inflammatory response and localized cellular control agents, bone adapts to environmental challenges by surface modeling (including catabolic and anabolic) and internal remodeling (Figure 6.16).

From a clinical perspective, the most critical aspect for generating and maintaining new bone is the preservation of the blood supply. Surgical and nonsurgical techniques, which promote vascular invasion to promote healing and adaptation to loading, are far more important than attempting to achieve a favorable response by the pharmacological application of growth factors. Regarding skeletal manipulation, there is no substitute for good surgical and dentoalveolar orthopedic technique.

VEGF plays a crucial role in osteogenesis. VEGF is the regulator of the process of neovascularization into the hypertrophic cartilage matrix of the condyle. The VEGF also stimulates secretion of growth factors and cytokines thereby participating in the osteogenic cycle (Yang et al., 2012). Various studies compared and identified mandibular positioning solicited cellular responses that led to significant increase in the invasion of new blood vessels into the condyle when compared with natural growth. The highest levels of expression of VEGF in response to forward mandibular positioning in the condyle preceded the highest level of bone formation induced by mandibular protrusion (Rabie et al., 2003).

Inflammatory response

Inflammation is usually associated with pathology. However, the inflammatory response is also a physiologic mechanism for adapting to mechanical overload (Viecilli et al., 2013; Roberts et al., 2015). Hypertrophy is a response to mechanical overload that may generate substantial internal damage such as EARR (Viecilli et al., 2013). The pain response limits function during the period of hypertrophic adaptation. Limited function diminishes additional damage while bones and muscle fibers increase in diameter to adapt to the new set of loading conditions. Otherwise, the continuing overload during the healing and adaptation period could result in severe tissue damage and loss of structural integrity (fractures, muscle tears, and so on). Thus, inflammation is a fundamental physiologic mechanism for influencing musculoskeletal form and function mediated by genetic factors (Roberts et al., 2015). Similar to overload hypertrophy of the musculoskeletal system, tooth movement is an inflammatory osseous adaptation that is accompanied by varying levels of sensitivity. Expression of the *c-Fos* gene in the trigeminal nerve and forebrain is involved in the inflammatory mechanism of tooth movement (Yamashiro et al., 1997, 1998; Fujiyoshi et al., 2000). An interesting study suggests activation of the extracellular signal-regulated protein kinase (ERK) signaling cascade following noxious mechanical pressure on the teeth regulates Fos expression in neurons and may thereby contribute to pain associated with orthodontic treatment (Hasegawa et al., 2012).

Numerous inflammatory cytokines have been implicated in tooth movement and skeletal modeling, including interleukin (IL)-1, IL-2, IL-3, IL-6, IL-8, tumor necrosis factor alpha (TNFα), gamma interferon (IFNγ), and osteoclast differentiation factor (ODF). One of the inflammatory cytokines that appears to have a direct role in the dentoalveolar response to orthodontic loads is IL-1. IL-1 has two forms, α and β, which code by different genes. It has been reported that these interleukins have similar biologic actions, including attracting leukocytes and stimulating fibroblasts, endothelial cells, osteoclasts, and osteoblasts to promote bone resorption and inhibit bone formation (Sabatini et al., 1988).

In brief, the skeletal physiologic response to applied loads ("biomechanics") is an inflammatory mechanism similar to wound healing. Nerve fibers in the PDL respond to tooth movement. Therefore, musculoskeletal adaptation, such as tooth movement and physical training (hypertrophic conditioning), is painful to some degree because the reaction is an inflammation-mediated form of bone adaptation mediated by inflammatory cytokines (Fujiyoshi et al., 2000; Yamashiro et al., 2000a, 2000b; Deguchi et al., 2003). The nociceptive response may play a key role in limiting masticatory function as the occlusion adapts to changes in position of the teeth (Roberts and Hartsfield, 2004).

Cellular agents

In addition to inflammatory cytokines, other types of cellular control agents modulating the bone modeling and remodeling are growth factors, specific cell differentiation mediators such as the receptor activator of nuclear factor kappa-B/receptor activator of nuclear factor kappa-B/ligand osteoprotegerin (RANK/RANKL/OPG) system (Khosla, 2001). There are five principal types of growth factors involved in the OTM and alveolar bone modeling: (i) transforming growth factor (TGFβ), which includes TGFβ1, activins, inhibins, and BMPs; (ii) FGFs and (iii) IGFs, which function in a similar way; (iv) growth factors for mesenchymal cells, in the form of platelet-derived growth factor (PDGF); and (v) connective tissue growth factor (CTGF) (Krishnan and Davidovitch, 2006).

The RANK/RANKL/OPG system plays a role in bone remodeling and orthodontic induced osteoclasis (Khosla, 2001; Boyle et al., 2003; Zelzer and Olsen, 2003). Osteoclast differentiation and activation is controlled by a group of genes related to tumor necrosis factor (TNF) and its receptor (TNFR); OPG, RANK, and RANKL. Colony stimulating factor 1 (CSF-1) induces differentiation of hematopoietic precursor cells, resulting in osteoclast precursors with the receptors referred to as RANK. Local bone related cells of osteoblast lineage secrete RANKL, which binds with RANK on the preosteoclast cell surface, and signals the development of a functional osteoclast. As a feedback control, the same regulatory cells produce OPG, which can bind RANKL, and thereby down regulates osteoclast activation (Figure 6.18).

OPG is a soluble receptor that acts as a bone protector. It is also known as osteoclast inhibitor factor (OCIF). OPG protects bone from excessive resorption by binding to RANKL and preventing it from binding to RANK. Therefore, the relative concentration of RANKL and OPG in bone is a major determinant of bone mass and strength. The RANKL–OPG complex counterbalances the effect of the RANKL–RANK complex, thus playing the most important role in bone homeostasis (Boyce and Xing, 2008). Interestingly, both previous and more recent studies have also indicated that the molecular mechanism of vitamin E is as a bone-protecting agent. This was confirmed in a study which demonstrated that vitamin E plays a pivotal role in the modulation of RANK/RANKL/OPG, NF-κB, mitogen-activated protein kinase (MAPK), and oxidative stress signaling (Wong et al., 2019).

As an example of how manipulation of the balance within the RANK/RANKL/OPG system can affect tooth movement, it was demonstrated that experimental tooth movement could be inhibited when functional copies of the OPG gene were transferred by injection into the periodontal tissue of male Wistar rats and increased the local production of OPG (Kanzaki et al., 2004). Another study investigated the effect of local injection of RANKL protein on experimental tooth movement and subsequent alveolar bone remodeling in mice. This study concluded local RANKL injection leads to increased osteoclastic activity. It thereby facilitates tooth movement and alveolar bone formation (Li et al., 2019).

In addition to functioning as an inflammatory cytokine, IL-1β can stimulate bone resorption *in vitro* and *in vivo* by affecting all stages of osteoclast development (Boyce et al., 1989; Pfeilschifter et al., 1989). In a study combining mechanics and biology of bone and tooth movement, stress, average relative amounts of IL-1β and its receptor antagonist (IL-1RA) in gingival crevicular fluid during tooth movement, and IL-1 gene cluster polymorphisms, were found to be important variables for the prediction of tooth translation velocity and rate of bone modeling in healthy patients (Iwasaki et al., 2006).

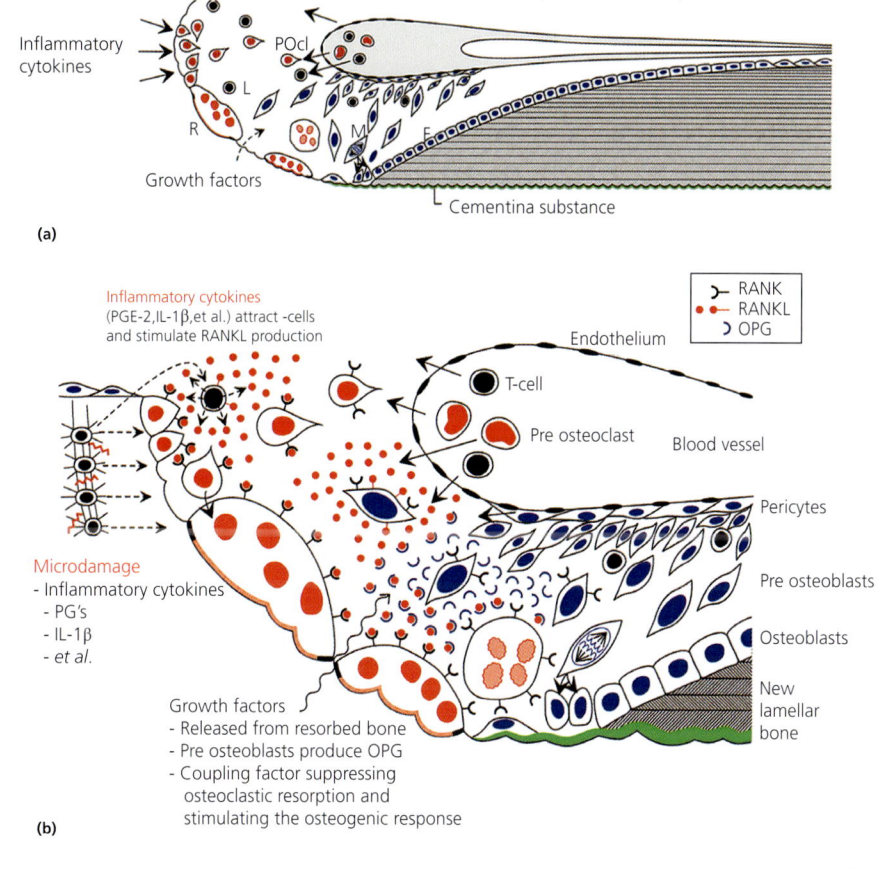

Figure 6.18 (a) A hemisection of a cutting/filling cone moving to the left demonstrates the intravascular and perivascular mechanisms for coupling bone resorption (R) to formation (F) during the remodeling process. Lymphocytes (L) are attracted from the circulation by inflammatory cytokines. They help recruit preosteoclasts (POcl) from the circulation. See text for details. (b) A magnified view of the head of a hemicutting/filling cone illustrates the proposed mechanism for coupling bone resorption to formation via the genetic RANK/RANKL/OPG mechanism. The cutting head is stimulated by inflammatory cytokines produced by osteocytes in damaged bone (left). Growth factors from resorbed bone (bottom) stimulate production of preosteoblasts, which produce RANKL. Preosteoclasts have RANK receptors that are bound and activated by RANKL. The RANKL--RANK interaction between osteoblast/stromal cells and osteoclast precursors is diminished and therefore to some degree regulated by preosteoblasts releasing osteoprotegerin (OPG). RANKL can bind to OPG instead of RANK, thus inhibiting the differentiation of the osteoclast precursor into a mature osteoclast. Relatively flat mononuclear cells (bottom center) form cementing substance to form a resorption arrest line. Osteoblasts (bottom right) produce new lamellar bone to fill the resorption cavity. (Source: Roberts *et al.*, 2006. Reproduced with permission of Elsevier.)

Factors influencing bone remodeling and modeling

Coupling of bone formation to resorption in bone remodeling

One of the most distinctive features of bone remodeling of both cortical and trabecular bone is the precise coupling of bone resorption and formation. The A → R → F process is similar for all types of bone remodeling. The current proposed mechanism for controlling the initiation and coupling of the remodeling process is illustrated in Figure 6.18. The following sequence is hypothesized:
1. Bone and possibly dentin microdamage leads to release of inflammatory cytokines (prostaglandins, IL-1β, and others) and exposure of mineralized collagen to extracellular fluid.
2. This results in osteoblasts producing RANKL.
3. Preosteoclasts from circulating blood have RANK receptors, which are activated by the RANKL to form activated osteoclasts.
4. As bone is resorbed, growth factors are released that stimulate osteoblasts to produce OPG (a decoy receptor that binds RANKL and diminishes osteoclast differentiation), which then retract from the bone surface.
5. Mononuclear cells move in and coat the scalloped resorbed surface with cementing substance (green).
6. Perivascular osteogenic cells migrate through the low cell density zone and differentiate to preosteoblasts (Roberts *et al.*, 1987a), which then divide and form two osteoblasts each (Roberts *et al.*, 1982; Roberts and Morey, 1985).
7. Osteoblasts form new bone, filling the resorption cavity and completing the turnover process.

Metabolic control of bone remodeling

Because of the essential life support function of calcium homeostasis, it has long been proposed that the initiation of a bone remodeling event (A in the ARF sequence) is primarily under metabolic control. There is vast literature supporting the concept that trabecular bone remodeling is an important aspect of calcium homeostasis (Epker, 1967; Frost, 1969; High *et al.*, 1981; Eriksen *et al.*, 1986; Minaire, 1989; Frost, 1991; Robey *et al.*, 1993; Frost, 1998; Holick, 1998; Eriksen *et al.*, 1999; Li *et al.*, 2001; Manolagas et al., 2002; Parfitt, 2003; Hofbauer and Schoppet, 2004; van't Hof et al., 2004). Roberts and coworkers (Roberts et al., 1987a, 1987b, 1991, 1992; Roberts, 1994, Becker et al., 1997; Roberts, 1997; Roberts and Hartsfield, 1997; Roberts, 2000b, 2000a, 2005) have reviewed the bone metabolism literature from an orthodontics and implant perspective.

Remodeling of trabecular bone serves as a flexible source of metabolic calcium for mineral homeostasis. Once the trabecular pattern matures, bone remodeling (coupled turnover) responds to both metabolic and mechanical control. On the other hand, cortical bone remodeling and EARR are related primarily to mechanical loading (Verna and Melsen, 2003). All remodeling activity plays a role in calcium metabolism: the balance of bone resorption and formation at any point in time controls the net balance of ionic calcium released into the extracellular fluid. In effect, metabolically controlled trabecular bone remodeling is a buffer system, which is up- or down regulated by the endocrine system, notably via parathyroid hormone (PTH) and calcitonin.

Mechanical control of bone remodeling

Mechanical loading and initiation of microdamage are important for controlling remodeling of both cortical and trabecular bone. Although mechanical strain itself was long thought to be the direct stimulus controlling remodeling, strain may simply be the force driving fluid shifts within the bone (Owan et al., 1997; You et al., 2000). Osteocytes are considered as key players in the process of bone mechanotransduction. The fluid shifts create shear within the lacuno-canalicular system of bone. The fluid flow around osteocytes probably provides the signal directing the remodeling process (Pavalko et al., 2003).

The initiation of microdamage in bone is another stimulus for remodeling (Burr, 2002; Martin, 2002; Parfitt, 2002). Mori and Burr (Mori and Burr, 1993) demonstrated that there is a cause and effect relationship between damage initiation and the induction of remodeling. Subsequently, Bentolila and coworkers (Bentolila et al., 1998) induced remodeling in rat cortical bone, which normally does not undergo remodeling, by creating microdamage through cyclic loading of the forelimb. The initiation of remodeling probably occurs through a sequence of events that includes osteocyte apoptosis in damaged regions (Verborgt et al., 2000). The process of cell death through apoptosis appears to be permissive in allowing the recruitment of osteoclasts that then initiate the resorptive process. An apoptotic cycle of osteocytes signal neighboring viable osteocytes to synthesize cytokines like RANKL and VEGF, which recruit osteoclasts to remove the dead cells and initiate the remodeling of the surrounding matrix (Jilka et al., 2013).

Regarding tooth movement, the relationship of microdamage to remodeling is unclear. Verna and coworkers (Verna et al., 2004) noticed an increased number of cracks in alveolar bone one day after initiation of orthodontic force in pigs. However, cracks were not visible 2–15 days after initiation of tooth movement. Frost's hypothesis (Frost, 1994) that microdamage initiates bone remodeling under physiologic conditions is a popular concept, but there has been no clear demonstration of the mechanism, at least with respect to stomatognathic function and tooth movement.

Orthodontics is an ideal model for resolving the relationship between induced microdamage and a physiologic remodeling response. As previously hypothesized from human specimens (Roberts et al., 1981; Roberts, 1994), orthodontics in dogs generates a generalized increase in the incidence of bone remodeling following 4 weeks of continuous loading (Deguchi et al., 2003). It is tempting to speculate that the response is mediated by a transient increase in microdamage of the bone supporting orthodontically loaded teeth, but further studies are needed to confirm or reject the hypothesis (Roberts et al., 2006).

Mechanical aspects of bone modeling

Bone modeling is the biomechanically controlled, physiologic mechanism for skeletal adaptation to functional loads. Lifelong modeling, both subperiosteal adaptation and mini modeling of cancellous bone, maintains skeletal mass at the minimum necessary to sustain metabolic and structural function. Unlike with remodeling, bone modeling is an uncoupled process, meaning anabolic and catabolic sites are controlled by the different functional loading on bone independently.

Physical activity results in site-specific bone modeling (Nevill et al., 2003). Thus, the mass and architecture of most bones is controlled by the loading history. Peak strains delivered at a high rate (impact loading) is more effective than a slowly applied load in eliciting an anabolic response (Mosley and Lanyon, 1998). In orthodontics, static loads are superimposed on function to produce a net dynamic load that dictates the osseous response that permits tooth movement (Roberts, 1984). The mechanical influence of functional loading on bone modeling has been demonstrated by a positive correlation of muscle mass to bone density in "*GDF8*" (myostatin gene) knockout mice. Growth Differentiation Factor 8 (*GDF8*) was the previous gene symbol and name for myostatin (now abbreviated *MSTN* in humans and *Mstn* in mice) and is a member of the transforming growth factor-beta (TGF-β) superfamily of secreted growth and differentiation factors. Myostatin functions as a negative regulator of skeletal muscle growth. Myostatin knockout mice have approximately twice the skeletal muscle mass of normal mice and skeletal density increases accordingly (Hamrick, 2003).

Strain is defined as deformation per unit length. It is a dimensionless parameter that is expressed as percentage strain (10^{-2} strain) or microstrain (10^{-6} strain). Frost's mechanostat (Frost, 1987, 1990) is a practical means for conveying the complex concepts of bone biomechanics. Bone modeling activity is controlled by the peak strain of dynamic loading (Figure 6.19). For instance, when a bone of 100 mm in length is elongated by 2 mm, the associated strain is expressed as 2% strain, 0.02 strain, or 20,000 microstrain. The ultimate strength of bone is ~ 25,000 microstrain. The normal physiologic range of bone loading is ~ 200–2,500 microstrain. Thus, under physiologic conditions, dynamic bone loading is less than 10% of its ultimate strength. When the peak strain exceeds 2,500 microstrain, subperiosteal hypertrophy builds bone mass to reduce surface strain. If bone is repetitively loaded at ~ 4,000 microstrain, fatigue damage accumulates more rapidly than it can be repaired, and the bone is at risk for stress fracture. However, when repetitively loaded in the physiologic range (~200–2,500 microstrain), bone mass remains constant and its structural integrity is maintained by remodeling to repair accumulated fatigue damage (Figure 6.19) (Burr, 1993).

Bone mass is maintained at a minimum consistency with dynamic functional loading. The size and shape of bones are controlled by surface strain, which is the mechanism for maintaining the shape of a bone as it increases in size. Bone modeling activity is driven by dynamic loads above and below the normal physiologic range. Sensitive biomechanical feedback of anabolic and catabolic modeling is the mechanism of growth, adaptation, and atrophy of the skeletal system. Dynamic peak strain to maintain bone mass is site and species specific; for example, an experimentally determined

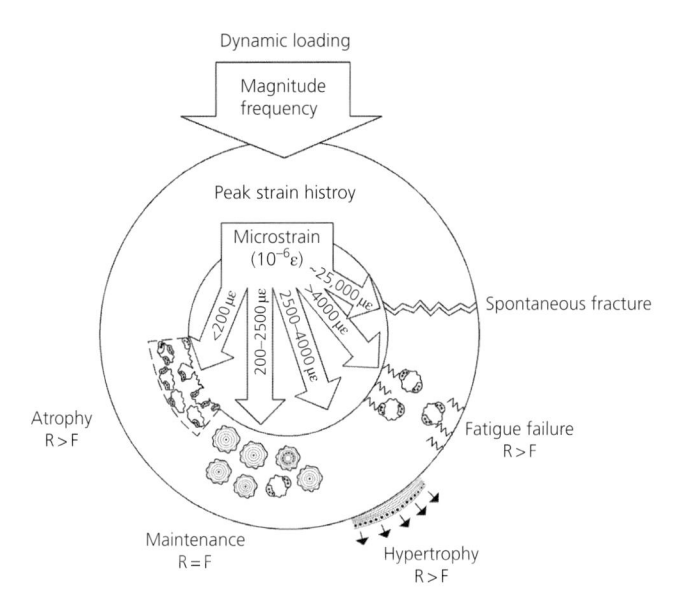

Figure 6.19 Frost's mechanostat shows the relationship of dynamic loading and peak strain history to: atrophy, physiologic maintenance, hypertrophy, fatigue failure, and spontaneous fracture. R= resorption; F = formation. (Source: Roberts and Hartsfield, 2004. Reproduced with permission of Elsevier.)

atrophic threshold of ~ 70 microstrain is representative (Qin et al., 1998). At relatively low peak strains of, say, ~ 50–200 microstrain, resorption along bone surfaces is deemed disuse atrophy. Bone formation is a surface hypertrophy that is driven by dynamic loads exceeding 2,500 microstrain. Disuse atrophy and overload hypertrophy are the means for sculpting bones and adapting their mass and orientation to optimally support functional loading.

Dentofacial orthopedics and orthodontics is the superimposition of constant, intermittent, or interrupted loads on function. Therapeutic loading changes the physiologic equilibrium of dynamic loading. The skeletal system adapts to the new loading conditions by localized sites of bone atrophy and hypertrophy, which changes a bone's form until optimal peak strain levels are restored (Weinstein, 1967). The new equilibrium is maintained until loading conditions trigger further bone modeling events. In brief, bone modeling is a mechanically mediated mechanism for skeletal adaptation to applied loads, both physiologic and therapeutic (Frost, 1990; Roberts, 2000a, 2000b). Mechanically induced anabolic bone modeling is mediated in part by prostaglandins (Miller and Marks, 1993), which are powerful anabolic agents (Jee et al., 1990). Systemic administration of prostaglandin E$_2$ (PGE$_2$) results in a generalized anabolic modeling response (Yao et al., 1999). On the other hand, nitric oxide (NO) is a mechanically induced mediator of catabolic modeling (Nomura and Takano-Yamamoto, 2000).

Fluid flow that arises from the functional loading of osseous tissue has long been proposed as the critical regulator of skeletal mass and morphology. Mechanically generated fluid flow plays a regulatory role in the bone modeling process (Qin et al., 2003). It has been hypothesized that fluid flow in bone generates streaming potentials that help control bone modeling and remodeling (MacGinitie et al., 1994; Duncan and Turner, 1995). However, the generation of streaming potentials is inconsistent in living bone preparations (Beck et al., 2002). In addition, the molecular mechanisms, known to control bone modeling (NO, PGE2), are not responsive to streaming potentials.

On the contrary, both NO and PGE$_2$ are induced directly by shear stress. Although they have enjoyed considerable theoretical support, no bioelectric signals (piezoelectricity or streaming potentials) have been shown to play a role in controlling bone physiology (Bakker et al., 2001). Indeed, bioelectric signals are a favorite of theoretical bone biologists, but there is no evidence that they play a physiologic role. It is more likely that the change in bioelectric activity is caused by the intense cellular activity of bone adaptation, not causing it. Mechanical stimulation of bone has been associated with apoptosis (cell death) of osteocytes. If the necrotic process is associated with accumulation of bone microdamage, it may help attract osteoclasts for destruction of overloaded cortical bone (Noble et al., 2003).

An important clinical aspect of mechanically mediated bone modeling is the alteration of functional loads on the jaws, following orthognathic surgery. Calculating TMJ loading during the power stroke in rabbits provides a realistic clinical simulation. Changing the mandibular form can produce torques on the TMJ greater than previously predicted. These results suggest that altered patterns of postoperative bone modeling may be significant factors in assessing the long-term outcomes of orthognathic surgical procedures (Widmer et al., 2002; Roberts et al., 2004).

Bone modeling/remodeling, tooth movement, and external apical root resorption

Histologic sectioning of dental roots routinely shows resorption lacunae in the cementum, presumably due to masticatory forces on the teeth. These histologic lacunae have been referred to as root resorption, and usually are repaired with secondary cementum. The resorption lacunae increase in number and depth with application of orthodontic force and increased strain on dental roots. Less than 10 kPa of stress in the PDL, which is less than the 16 kPa of stress required to occlude vascularity, is associated with increased inflammation and lateral root resorption (Viecilli et al., 2013; Roberts et al., 2015). If the resorption process exceeds cemental repair capability and underlying dentin is exposed, then an increased number of clastic cells are attracted, leading to enough destruction to be observable on standard diagnostic radiographs (Hartsfield, 2009). Along with force placed on the teeth, differing alveolar bone densities and bone modeling/remodeling processes affect the strain on the dental root, thus influencing the OTM process and the increased occurrence of EARR as a deleterious secondary effect (Al-Qawasmi et al., 2003; Iglesias-Linares et al., 2016).

Since alveolar bone modeling/remodeling is the rate limiting factor in OTM, a smaller bone modeling/remodeling rate will correspond with slower tooth movement. However, if orthodontic force is continuing to be applied, a smaller bone modeling/remodeling rate will lead to a prolonged strain upon the root, which could lead to increased microdamage of the cementum and increased resorption of the root. During most OTM, the rate of cemental lacunae reception and repair is enough to protect the root even while the adjacent alveolar bone is being resorbed due to fatigue failure. However, at some point this protective mechanism of the cementum becomes insufficient and destruction of the root occurs.

Macrophages play a critical role in this differentiation of cemental resorption and repair. Two distinct *in vitro* phenotypes are described: classically activated macrophages (M1), or "killer" macrophages, and alternatively activated macrophages (M2), or "healer" macrophages (Novak and Koh, 2013). A remarkable plasticity can be observed in the switch from M1 to M2 polarization states depending on the different conditions in the cellular microenvironment (He et al., 2015), which allows them to mediate inflammation and tissue homeostasis. In this respect, increased numbers of the M1 versus M2 cell type is likely to be associated with root resorption (increased M1:M2 ratio). The severity of root resorption was less when a decrease in the ratio of M1:M2 macrophages was detected in an animal model (He et al., 2015).

OTM depends directly on the coordinated activity of osteoblasts, osteocytes, and osteoclasts. EARR is root resorption that can be seen on standard diagnostic radiographs caused by undesirable activity of osteoclastic cells on the root surface. This hypothesis is worthy of investigation relative to the undermining resorption mechanism of tooth movement. Localized fatigue damage, associated with production of the inflammatory cytokine IL-1β, has been implicated in the initial resorptive response to orthodontics (Al-Qawasmi et al., 2003). Osteocytes are activated in bone adjacent to compressed PDL (Terai et al., 1999; Yamashiro et al., 2000b), but the mechanism of IL-1β induction is still unknown. Specific signaling pathways are associated with compression and tension due to orthodontic loading (Huang et al., 2014). Localized hypoxia develops as a reaction to orthodontic loading which alters blood flow in the PDL either by tension or stretch. While the PDL reacts to this as depicting an aseptic inflammatory response, the synergistic effect of bone remodeling is observed. It is of special interest to orthodontists that a fabricated modulation of sustained release injectable RANKL is effective in accelerating OTM (Chang et al., 2019). The formulation acts through biologically effective reactions like increasing osteoclast-mediated alveolar resorption. This could theoretically effectively shorten treatment time but needs to be clinically evaluated in controlled studies.

Cortical bone remodeling

Cortical bone remodeling in man requires about 29 days (~1 month) to create a resorption cavity that is approximately 200–250 μm in diameter and 134 days (~4 months) to refill it (Eriksen et al., 1986). In a similar study on human trabecular bone, the overall duration of sigma (duration of the entire A → R → F process, which is also deemed the remodeling period) was found to be 151 days (Eriksen et al., 1985). In cortical bone from iliac crest specimens, the formation phase was about a month longer than for trabecular bone (Brockstedt et al., 1996). However, from a volumetric perspective there is slight difference in the turnover kinetics for cortical and trabecular bone. Although bone formation occurs for a longer period in forming a secondary osteon, the rate of apposition progressively decreases. During the additional month of formation for cortical bone remodeling, the appositional rate is very slow as evidenced by periodic, single tetracycline labels. In general, the duration of the remodeling cycle is inversely related to the size of the animal (Roberts, 1988). The reversal phase involves cessation of osteoclastic resorption and initiation of the formation of cement substance on the previously resorbing surface. The cement substance is formed by mononuclear cells of unknown origin, but they are likely to be lining cells (Everts et al., 2002), related to fibroblasts or osteoblasts (Figure 6.18a). Once the cement line is formed, osteoblasts lay down new bone to fill the resorption cavity (Parfitt, 1976). An important scientific question is the mechanism for coordination of the osteoblastic and osteoclastic cell activity. It is presently proposed that the RANK/RANKL/OPG genetic mechanism is the means for controlling the coupling of sequential resorption and formation processes of bone remodeling (Roberts et al., 2006).

Trabecular bone remodeling

The trabecular bone remodeling mechanism, "multicellular unit," is essentially a hemi cutting/filling cone. The A → R → F process is similar to the cutting/filling cones of cortical bone remodeling (Figures 6.14 and 6.18). A schematic drawing (Figure 6.20a) of adult trabecular bone illustrates the pattern of turnover associated with continuous remodeling to support calcium homeostasis. A magnified remodeling site is shown in Figure 6.20b.

Figure 6.21 illustrates the bone labeling that occurs in the trabeculae of rat vertebrae. This is a remodeling process because the new bone is laid down on a scalloped resorption reversal line. The latter is the principal distinction between micro-modeling and remodeling. Remodeling of trabecular bone is under mechanical and hormonal control. Corticosteroids have long been associated with metaphyseal growth (Shaw and Lacey, 1975) and osteopenia of trabecular bone (Jee et al., 1966). Although the catabolic effect of PTH has been known for decades, its anabolic effect has been exploited more recently (Jerome et al., 2001; Seeman and Delmas, 2001; Roberts et al., 2006).

Growth and development of facial bones

Prenatal and early postnatal development of the craniofacial structures is largely under genetic control and is mediated by primary

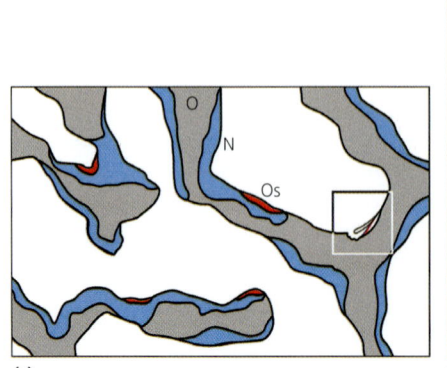

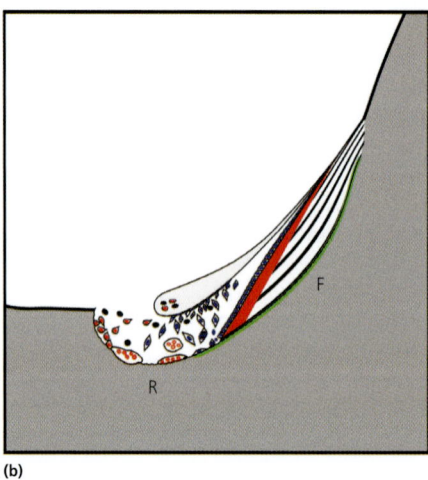

Figure 6.20 (a) A Trabecular bone remodeling over a 1-year interval shows the pattern of new bone formation (N) relative to old bone (O) and osteoid seams (Os). The box marks an area of active trabecular resorption, which is magnified in (b). (b) A detailed drawing of an active remodeling site (a) shows a hemicutting/filling cone with a similar perivascular array of resorptive (R) and formative (F) cells as shown for cortical bone remodeling. The osteoclastic and osteoblastic cell lines are red and blue, respectively. An unmineralized osteoid seam (solid red line) marks the bone forming surface. (Source: Roberts et al., 2006. Reproduced with permission of Elsevier.)

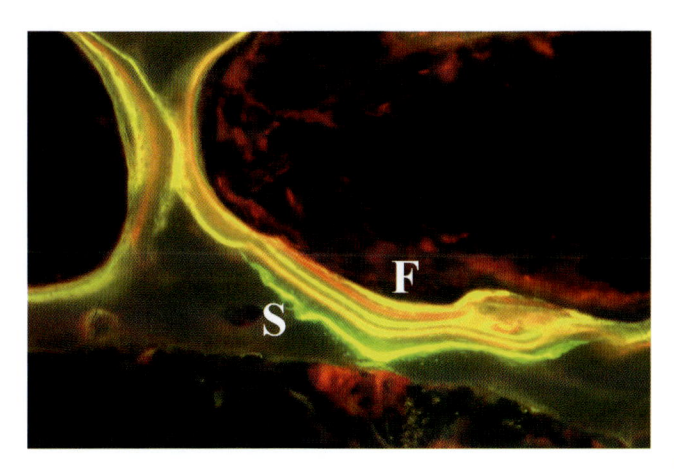

Figure 6.21 Trabecular bone remodeling in the vertebrae in a rat: multiple fluorochrome labels demonstrate bone formation (F) over a scalloped resorption arrest line (S). (Source: Roberts et al., 2006. Reproduced with permission of Elsevier.)

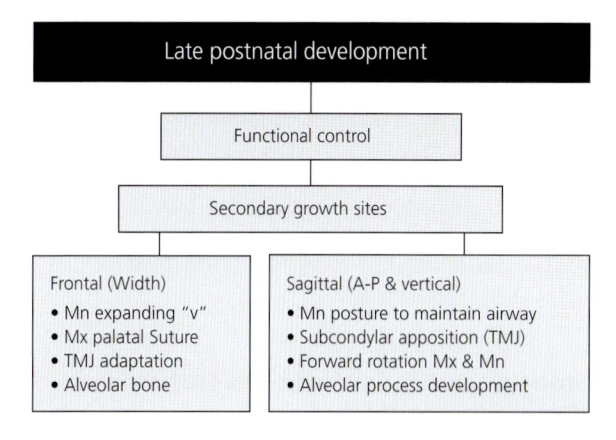

Figure 6.23 Late postnatal development of the face is under functional influence via secondary growth sites. This mechanism supports growth in the transverse, anterior--posterior, and vertical dimensions (Mn = mandibular, Mx = maxillary). (Source: Roberts and Hartsfield, 2004. Reproduced with permission of Elsevier.)

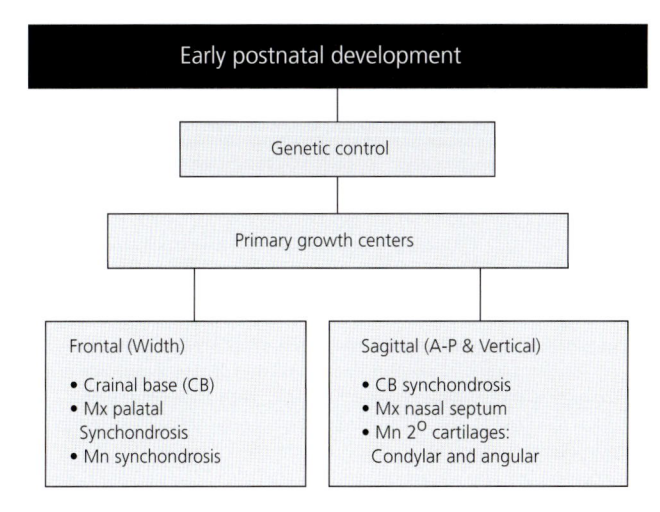

Figure 6.22 Early postnatal development of the craniofacial complex involves genetically controlled primary growth centers that contribute to growth in width, depth, and length of the face (Mn = mandibular, Mx = maxillary). (Source: Roberts and Hartsfield, 2004. Reproduced with permission of Elsevier.)

growth centers (Figure 6.22). In the frontal dimension, width of the face increases by interstitial growth of cartilage. The principal structures serving as primary growth centers are the cranial base, maxillary palatal (posterior) synchondrosis, and the mandibular midline (symphyseal) synchondrosis (Bloore et al., 1969; Schacter et al., 1969). In the prenatal period, the sagittal dimension is affected by both anterior-posterior and vertical growth. The principal primary growth centers in the sagittal plane are the cranial base synchondroses (spheno-ethmoidal and spheno-occipital), maxillary nasal septum, and mandibular secondary cartilages. Growth of the condylar secondary cartilage displaces the mandible away from the cranium, stretching muscles, which then grow in length by secondary intention (Barnett et al., 1980; Ashmore and Summers, 1981). Once occlusion is established, postnatal growth and development of the face shifts to predominately functional influence and is mediated by secondary growth sites (Figure 6.23). In the frontal dimension, growth in the width of the face involves the expanding "V" of mandibular growth, the maxillary palatal suture, TMJ adaptation, and development of the alveolar process. As the maxillary teeth erupt in an occlusal and buccal direction, the attached gingiva and supracrestal fibers induce bone hypertrophy to maintain the same level of osseous support relative to the epithelial attachment. Following birth, growth and development in the sagittal plane results in increased dimensions in the anterior-posterior and vertical directions. The functionally related growth mechanism is secondary to a more downward and forward posturing of the mandible to maintain the airway. The distracted mandibular condyle grows in length by subarticular proliferation in the TMJ. Studies associating genetic variation with growth trends in the sagittal and especially the vertical dimension have found a number of genes or candidate genes by association coding for skeletal muscle, growth factors, bone, cartilage, extracellular matrix/connective tissue, transcription factors and membrane receptor–intracellular signaling, and other proteins. These are associated with facial growth as a complex trait, or an autosomal dominant trait with incomplete penetrance in some cases of skeletal Class III with variable expressivity, and the possible effect of secondary genetic and epigenetic factors (Rowlerson et al., 2005; Raoul et al., 2011; Huh et al., 2013; Sciote et al., 2012; Sciote et al., 2013; Zebrick et al., 2014; da Fontoura et al., 2015; Cruz et al., 2017; Arun et al., 2016; Claes et al., 2018; Kluemper et al., 2019; Cunha et al., 2019).

The condyle, which is an anatomically significant component of the TMJ, also a major growth site of mandible, grows by proliferation of articular periosteum on the articular surface, which differentiates into a subarticular layer of fibrocartilage that participates in endochondral bone formation. The condylar cartilage has a multidirectional growth potential and remodeling capacity throughout life, even after episodes of degeneration (Roberts and Stocum, 2018). Mandibular asymmetry is one of the most common craniofacial malformations besides cleft lip and cleft palate (Pirttiniemi et al., 2009). The etiology of these are heterogeneous including trauma (Gilhuus-Moe, 1971; Lund, 1974; Proffit et al., 1980), developmental anomalies such as hemifacial microsomia (Hartsfield, 2007), and variation in muscle fiber type variance from one side to the other (Raoul et al., 2011). In addition, abnormal bone formation is one of the most established causes of mandibular asymmetry (Vasconcelos et al., 2012). Orthodontic treatment is not a suitable option in severe cases of asymmetry and distraction osteogenesis; surgical corrections including orthognathic surgeries are sometimes not a viable option in children or might have associated disadvantages. However, even degenerated mandibular condyles in adults can be orthopedically lengthened up to a centimeter by differential distraction via asymmetric adjustment of an interocclusal orthotic (Roberts and Stocum, 2018). Research focuses on PTH as it has both catabolic and anabolic effects on bone formation depending on its mode of administration (Qin et al., 2004). It is currently hypothesized that early treatment of mandibular asymmetry could utilize the approach of intraarticular injection of PTH in the TMJ for both children and adults (Wan and Li, 2010).

Temporomandibular joint development and mature adaptation

To understand the osseous physiology of the TMJ, it is important to appreciate its development (Figure 6.24). Prenatally, condylar secondary cartilages grow out from the intramembranous body of the mandible bilaterally. These primary growth centers grow against the pressure gradient generated by the developing pterygoid-masseteric sling of masticatory muscles. Periodic contraction and relaxation of the masticatory and suprahyoid muscles rotates the developing condyle and moves it anteriorly and posteriorly. Pressure against the temporal bone and the wide range of repetitive motion induces the formation of the temporal fossa. The interarticular meniscus is formed from interposed connective tissue. As the TMJ develops into a functioning joint, the meniscus and the articulating surfaces of the condyle and fossa are composed of dense fibrous connective tissue. Similar to other joints, the TMJ is enclosed in a capsule that is lubricated with synovial fluid (Okeson, 2003).

Postnatally, the TMJ becomes a secondary growth site with two articular surfaces that can adapt to changing environmental conditions (Pancherz et al., 1998). The temporal fossa can change position by apposition of cortical bone (Voudouris et al., 2003a, 2003b), which is an example of anabolic modeling. The mandibular condyle changes its shape and length by subarticular proliferation of connective tissue cells that differentiate into fibrocartilage. The fibrocartilage is eroded by osteoclasts at the metaphyseal surface and replaced by lamellar trabecular bone. This process is similar to the ossification that occurs beneath the articulating cartilage of the epiphysis of long bones. There are no primary and secondary spongiosa in contrast to metaphyseal growth plates in long bones. As demonstrated in Figures 6.25 and 6.26, both articulating surfaces of the mature TMJ have the unique adaptive capability.

What distinguishes the TMJ from other joints of the body is the articular layer of dense fibrous connective tissue with a subcondylar zone of proliferating connective tissue cells (Okeson, 2003). In the fossa, the articular surface is analogous to the fibrous and cambium layer of the periosteum, which has a full range of bone modeling capabilities. In the condyle, beneath the proliferative zone, is a layer

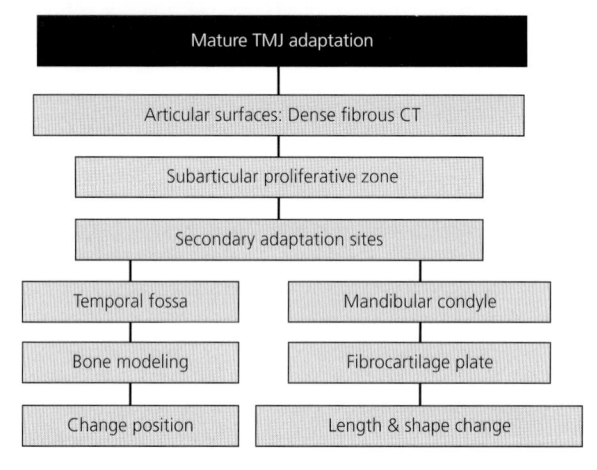

Figure 6.25 Continuous osseous adaptation of the TMJ occurs over a lifetime by a mechanism that is similar to the periosteum covering other bones. Healthy articular surfaces are covered with a layer of dense fibrous tissue ("fibrous layer of the periosteum"), and the subarticular proliferative zone is akin to the cambium (osteogenic) layer of the periosteum. The temporal fossa can change position via bone modeling. The mandibular condyle changes in length and shape by modeling and adaptation of the subarticular plate and its supporting fibrocartilage (CT, connective tissue). (Source: Roberts and Hartsfield, 2004. Reproduced with permission of Elsevier.)

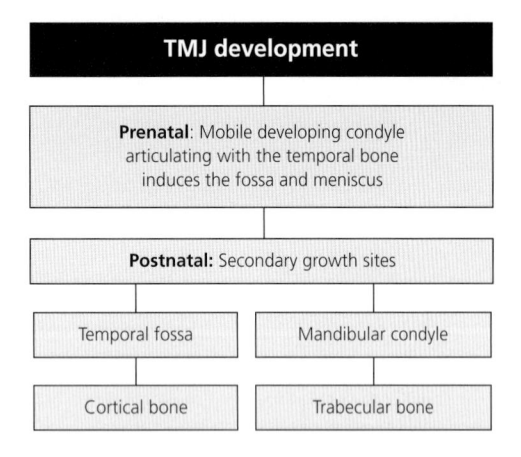

Figure 6.24 TMJ development in the prenatal period involves the primary growth mechanism of the condylar secondary cartilage. The motion of the developing condyle articulating with the temporal bone induces development of the fossa and meniscus. Postnatally, the secondary growth sites of the TMJ are the temporal fossa and the mandibular condyle, which model into cortical and trabecular bone, respectively. (Source: Roberts and Hartsfield, 2004. Reproduced with permission of Elsevier.)

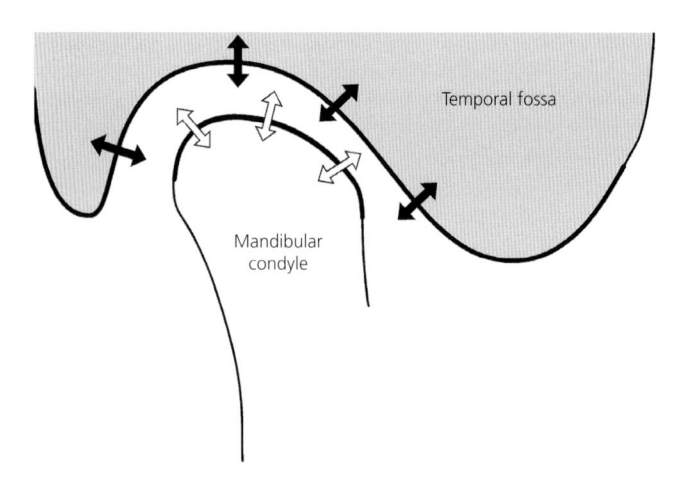

Figure 6.26 The mandibular condyle and the temporal fossa of the TMJ can change position by anabolic and catabolic modeling. Unlike other joints in the body, a healthy TMJ retains the ability to adapt to environmental influences over a lifetime. (Source: Roberts and Hartsfield, 2004. Reproduced with permission of Elsevier.)

of fibrocartilage that can be eroded internally and replaced with bone (Schacter et al., 1969; Okeson, 2003). Thereafter, the mechanism of the adaptation of the fossa and condyle are different. Since the articulating surfaces of the long bones are covered with hyaline cartilage, which has no proliferative zone, there is limited capacity for growth, adaptation, or healing. On the other hand, animal and clinical studies have demonstrated that the normal TMJ has a remarkable ability to heal and adapt over a lifetime (Roberts, 1997, 2000a; Voudouris et al., 2003a, 2003b; Roberts and Hartsfield, 2004). For a review of the genetic influences on TMJ development and growth in murine models, and TMJ disorders clinically, the reader is referred to Hinton et al. (2015), and Sangani et al. (2015), respectively.

Tooth movement and bone modeling

The rate-limiting factor in orthodontics is the efficiency with which bone is removed in the path of tooth movement. Figure 6.27 is a histological section of frontal resorption along the PDL/bone margin with a remodeling event in the path of movement. The rate of tooth movement is related to the efficiency of the bone modeling and remodeling responses in the alveolar process. Coordinated PDL and periosteal bone modeling allows a tooth to maintain its periodontal support while changing its position relative to the apical base. Anabolic modeling along the periosteal surface in the direction of tooth movement is the critical process for maintaining alveolar bone support during tooth movement.

Subperiosteal hypertrophy is triggered by an elevated compressive strain at the bone surface. The anabolic response originates in the perivascular soft tissue of the widened PDL. Bone surface resorption during sustained tooth movement could be an atrophic response to suboptimal loading, or a fatigue failure reaction to excessive tensile strain (Figure 6.19). The initial PDL osteoclastic response to tooth movement appears to be related to hypertrophic and fatigue failure mechanisms (Figure 6.28) (Katona et al., 1995; Roberts, 1999; Roberts, 2000b). Orthodontic force is a static load superimposed on function (Roberts, 1984). Once the PDL is maximally compressed, heavy functional loads are transferred directly to a relatively small area of the lamina dura. It is hypothesized that the dynamic (repetitive) loading of mastication results in accelerated fatigue damage in bone adjacent to the necrotic PDL. Subsequently, undermining resorption removes the resisting bone, allowing the tooth to move (Figure 6.29).

The PDL has unique biomechanical properties that allow it to generate a bone modeling response to even light postural loads (Yoshida et al., 2001; Poppe et al., 2002). However, the bone modeling of the alveolar process, during sustained tooth movement (Figure 6.30), appears to be the same atrophic and hypertrophic mechanisms that are operative for functional adaptation throughout the skeleton (Figure 6.31). Both bone modeling and remodeling are involved in the orthodontic response as previously discussed. Figure 6.32 demonstrates anabolic and catabolic modeling in the alveolar process in the direction of tooth movement. As the alveolar process is thinned by bone resorption on the PDL surface, the labial plate of bone is exposed to excessive functional strain.

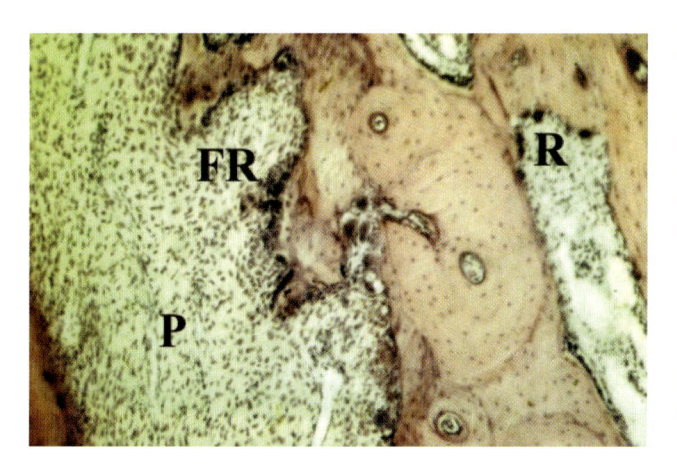

Figure 6.27 Premolar movement to the right in a monkey illustrates frontal bone resorption (FR) along the PDL (P) bone surface. The catabolic phase of remodeling (R) is noted in adjacent bone in the direction of tooth movement. (Source: Roberts et al., 2006. Reproduced with permission of Elsevier.)

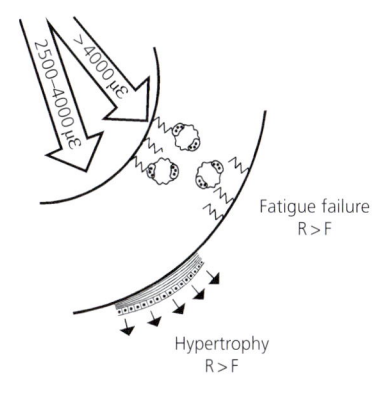

Figure 6.28 Initiation of tooth movement is a set of bone modeling reactions involving hypertrophy (resorption < formation) and fatigue failure (resorption > formation). R, resorption; F, formation. (Source: Roberts and Hartsfield, 2004. Reproduced with permission of Elsevier.)

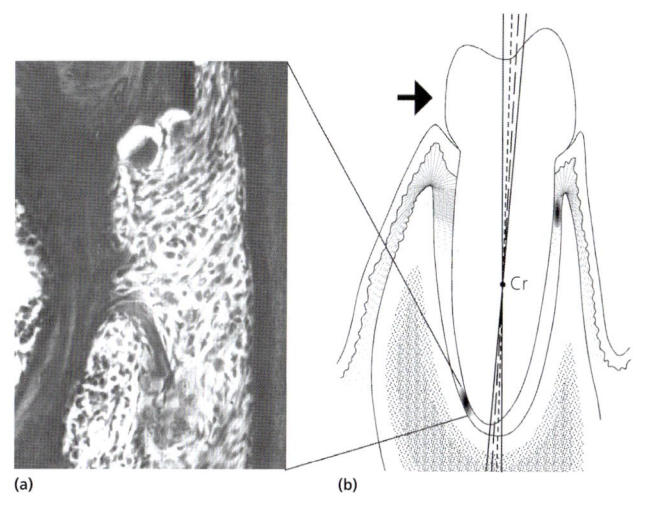

Figure 6.29 (a) The histological picture of undermining remodeling is related to (b) the zone of maximal PDL compression as a mandibular premolar is tipped labially. The tooth is rotating around the center of rotation (Cr). (Source: a, Roberts et al., 2004. Reproduced with permission of Elsevier. b, Roberts and Hartsfield, 2004. Reproduced with permission of Elsevier.)

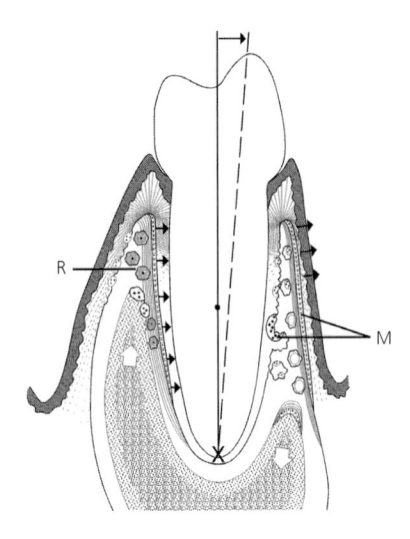

Figure 6.30 In the direction of tooth movement, catabolic and anabolic modeling (M) reposition the alveolar process relative to the apical base of bone. Remodeling (R) restructures primary bone into secondary osteons. (Source: Roberts and Hartsfield, 2004. Reproduced with permission of Elsevier.)

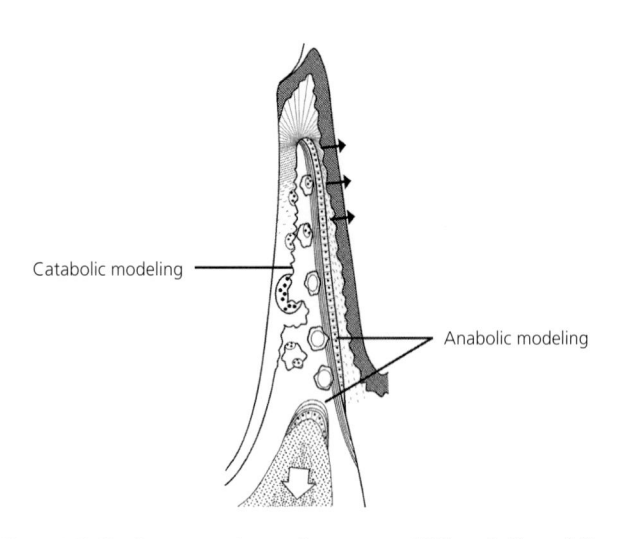

Figure 6.32 During progressive tooth movement, PDL catabolic modeling is driven primarily by inflammatory cytokines. Anabolic modeling on the endosteal and periosteal surfaces is driven by elevated strain as the alveolar process thins. (Source: Roberts and Hartsfield, 2004. Reproduced with permission of Elsevier.)

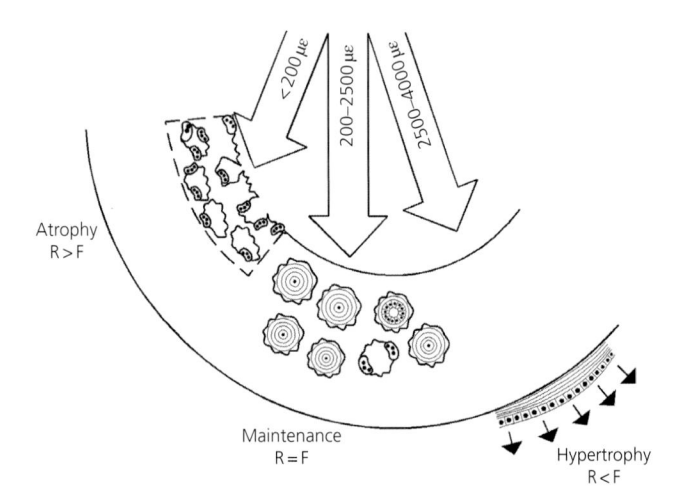

Figure 6.31 Subperiosteal formation in the direction of tooth movement is a hypertrophic reaction in response to increased functional flexure of the thinned alveolar process. Subperiosteal resorption of the trailing alveolar process is an example of disuse atrophy. (Source: Roberts and Hartsfield, 2004. Reproduced with permission of Elsevier.)

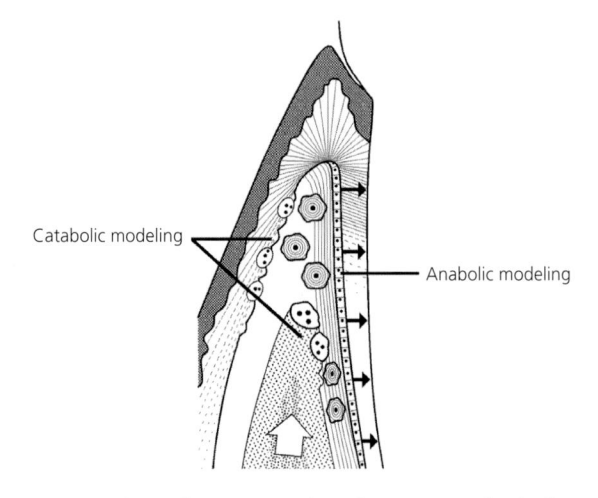

Figure 6.33 As the tooth moves away from the supporting alveolar bone, catabolic and anabolic modeling repositions the alveolar crest to maintain optimal periodontal support for the tooth. (Source: Roberts and Hartsfield, 2004. Reproduced with permission of Elsevier.)

A hypertrophic reaction on the periosteal surface adds bone to restore the strain levels to the optimal (physiologic maintenance) range. Figure 6.33 shows the complimentary reaction in the alveolar process that trails the moving tooth. As the alveolar process is thickened by bone apposition on the PDL surface, the periosteal surface is exposed to inadequate functional strain. Catabolic modeling is triggered by the atrophic mechanism. The alveolar process is thinned until the surface strain on the resorbing surface returns to the optimal physiologic range.

In summary, the coordinated modeling and remodeling responses of supporting bone during tooth movement are controlled independently from the PDL response (Figures 6.28 and 6.31). Both within the PDL and along periosteal surfaces, the osteogenic reaction is via the hypertrophic mechanism. However, the osteoclastic response at the PDL/bone interface, at least at the initiation of tooth movement, appears to be a fatigue failure response. Catabolic modeling at the periosteal surface is related to disuse atrophy (Figures 6.30 and 6.33) (Roberts et al., 2004).

Dental facial orthopedics and bone modeling

The TMJ is an area of high modeling and remodeling activity in response to growth, function, and therapeutic loads. Sequential bone labeling studies in rabbits demonstrated a high rate of remodeling of cortical and trabecular bone in the condyles of growing and adult animals (Roberts, 2005). Studies on fixed functional appliances in rats (Oudet et al., 1984; Petrovic et al., 1991) and monkeys (Elgoyhen et al., 1972; McNamara, 1973; McNamara and Carlson, 1979) revealed enhanced condylar growth of the mandible and/or resulted in a repositioning of the temporal fossa (Voudouris et al., 2003a, 2003b). There is some evidence that static therapeutic loads influence the modeling and remodeling of craniofacial structures (Turley et al., 1988), but few studies have directly addressed the problem. Headgear delivers orthopedic forces that strain the zygomatic process and temporomandibular eminence (Oberheim and Mao, 2002) and the Herbst appliance is known to orthopedically advance the mandible and retract the maxilla (Pancherz et al., 1998), at least in the short term. Modeling changes of facial bones are routinely documented on clinical radiographs; however, evaluation of remodeling activity requires bone scans and/or histology. Neither of the latter methods is routinely applied in clinical orthodontics. Consequently, little is known about therapeutically induced bone remodeling of the craniofacial complex in humans.

Calcium metabolism and tooth movement

Renal deficiency is associated with elevated PTH levels that enhance bone remodeling of the alveolar process. Although there was no difference in bone densitometry of the alveolar processes of renal deficient rats, the rate of tooth movement was enhanced. These data indicate that an underlying elevation in remodeling activity of alveolar bone assists the tooth-movement response (Shirazi et al., 2001). The active metabolite of vitamin D, which enhances the osteoclastic (remodeling) response in alveolar bone, is associated with increased rates of tooth movement (Takano-Yamamoto et al., 1992). It has been hypothesized that enhanced bone remodeling is the mechanism for the increased rates of tooth movements associated with magnetic forces (Steger and Blechman, 1995). From a variety of experiments, it is clear that teeth move more rapidly in bone with elevated rates of remodeling (Roberts et al., 1981). Metabolically weakened bone of rats with renal deficiency, as well as calcium or vitamin D deficiency, continues to respond to the mechanical demands of orthodontic force (Kiliaridis et al., 1996; Shirazi et al., 2001). From an orthodontic perspective, both biomechanics and calcium metabolism have powerful interactive influences on alveolar bone. For instance, the rate of tooth movement is substantially elevated in metabolically compromised rats with elevated PTH levels (Midgett et al., 1981, Kiliaridis et al., 1996, Shirazi et al., 2001). Another endocrine condition that enhances skeletal turnover and increases the rate of tooth movement is elevated estrogen level in pregnancy (Hellsing and Hammarstrom, 1991; Roberts et al., 2006).

Conclusion

Understanding bone/skeletal growth and metabolism is important to orthodontists. This applies whether they treat growing patients, older patients, medically compromised patients, or, as most do, some combination of the three. Applying the basics of bone biology to the specific situation of each patient advances the care of the patient. Future investigation of the interaction between environmental (including treatment) factors and each patient's unique genetic factors on bone biology through large-scale genome-wide association studies, familial genetic linkage studies, and genomic deep sequencing will refine the application of treatment on a personal basis (Hartsfield Jr et al., 2017).

Acknowledgement

This chapter is essentially a compilation of material previously published by Eugene Roberts, along with James Hartsfield and others, in two issues of Seminars in Orthodontics (Roberts and Hartsfield, 2004; Roberts et al., 2006). For the previous edition they, along with Dr. Song Chen, developed an outline of material to be compiled from their previous publications to facilitate editing and the addition of supporting material as indicated. The authors thank Dr. P. Lionel Sadowsky, editor of Seminars in Orthodontics at the time of the first edition, and his publisher, Elsevier, for their permission to reprint their previously published material. For this edition, Dr. Priyanka Gudsoorkar and Dr. Lorri Ann Morford were brought in to replace Dr. Chen for updating the chapter.

References

Al-Qawasmi, R. A., Hartsfield, J. K., Everett, E. T. et al. (2003) Genetic predisposition to external apical root resorption. American Journal of Orthodontics and Dentofacial Orthopedics 123, 242–252.

Arnold, J. S. (1951) A method for embedding undecalcified bone for histologic sectioning, and its application to radioautography. Science 114, 178–180.

Arun, R. M., Lakkakula, B. V. and Chitharanjan, A. B. (2016) Role of myosin 1H gene polymorphisms in mandibular retrognathism. American Journal of Orthodontics and Dentofacial Orthopedics 149, 699–704.

Ashmore, C. R. and Summers, P. J. (1981) Stretch-induced growth in chicken wing muscles: myofibrillar proliferation. American Journal of Physiology 241, C93–97.

Bagge, M. (2000) A model of bone adaptation as an optimization process. Journal of Biomechanics 33, 1349–1357.

Bakker, A. D., Soejima, K., Klein-Nulend, J. and Burger, E. H. (2001) The production of nitric oxide and prostaglandin E(2) by primary bone cells is shear stress dependent. Journal of Biomechanics 34, 671–677.

Barnett, J. G., Holly, R. G. and Ashmore, C. R. (1980) Stretch-induced growth in chicken wing muscles: biochemical and morphological characterization. American Journal of Physiology 239, C39–46.

Baumrind, S., Bravo, L. A., Ben-Bassat, Y. et al. (1997) Lower molar and incisor displacement associated with mandibular remodeling. The Angle Orthodontist 67, 93–102.

Beck, B. R., Qin, Y. X., Mcleod, K. J. and Otter, M. W. (2002) On the relationship between streaming potential and strain in an in vivo bone preparation. Calcified Tissue International 71, 335–343.

Becker, A. R., Handick, K. E., Roberts, W. E. and Garetto, L. P. (1997) Osteoporosis risk factors in female dental patients. A preliminary report. Journal (Indiana Dental Association) 76, 15–19; quiz 20.

Bentolila, V., Boyce, T. M., Fyhrie, D. P. et al. (1998) Intracortical remodeling in adult rat long bones after fatigue loading. Bone 23, 275–281.

Bidez, M. W. and Misch, C. E. (1992) Issues in bone mechanics related to oral implants. Implant Dentistry 1, 289–294.

Bloore, J. A., Furstman, L. and Bernick, S. (1969) Postnatal development of the cat palate. American Journal of Orthodontics 56, 505–515.

Bouvier, M. and Hylander, W. L. (1981) Effect of bone strain on cortical bone structure in macaques (Macaca mulatta). Journal of Morphology 167, 1–12.

Boyce, B. F., Aufdemorte, T. B., Garrett, I. R. et al. (1989) Effects of interleukin-1 on bone turnover in normal mice. Endocrinology 125, 1142–1150.

Boyce, B. F. and Xing, L. (2008) Functions of RANKL/RANK/OPG in bone modeling and remodeling. Archives of Biochemistry and Biochemistry 473, 139–146.

Boyde, A., Wolfe, L. A., Jones, S. J. et al. (1992) Microscopy of bone cells, bone tissue, and bone healing around implants. Implant Dentistry 1, 117–125.

Boyle, W. J., Simonet, W. S. and Lacey, D. L. (2003) Osteoclast differentiation and activation. Nature 423, 337–342.

Braschi, B., Denny, P., Gray, K. et al. (2018) Genenames. org: the HGNC and VGNC resources in (2019) Nucleic Acids Research 47, D786–D792.

Brockstedt, H., Bollerslev, J., Melsen, F. and Mosekilde, L. (1996) Cortical bone remodeling in autosomal dominant osteopetrosis: a study of two different phenotypes. Bone 18, 67–72.

Bronner-Fraser, M. (1993) Mechanisms of neural crest cell migration. Bioessays 15, 221–230.

Burr, D. B. (1993) Remodeling and the repair of fatigue damage. Calcified Tissue International 53 (Suppl. 1), S75–80; discussion S80–81.

Burr, D. B. (2002) Targeted and nontargeted remodeling. Bone 30, 2–4.

Burr, D. B., Schaffler, M. B., Yang, K. H. et al. (1989) The effects of altered strain environments on bone tissue kinetics. Bone 10, 215–221.

Chai, Y., Jiang, X., Ito, Y. et al. (2000) Fate of the mammalian cranial neural crest during tooth and mandibular morphogenesis. Development 127, 1671–1679.

Chai, Y., Zhao, J., Mogharei, A. et al. (1999) Inhibition of transforming growth factor-β type II receptor signaling accelerates tooth formation in mouse first branchial arch explants. Mechanisms of Development 86, 63–74.

Chang, H. N., Garetto, L. P., Katona, T. R. et al. (1996) Angiogenic induction and cell migration in an orthopaedically expanded maxillary suture in the rat. *Archives of Oral Biology* **41**, 985–994.

Chang, H. N., Garetto, L. P., Potter, R. H. et al. (1997) Angiogenesis and osteogenesis in an orthopedically expanded suture. *American Journal of Orthodontics and Dentofacial Orthopedics* **111**, 382–390.

Chang, J. H., Chen, P.-J., Arul, M. R. et al. (2019) Injectable RANKL sustained release formulations to accelerate orthodontic tooth movement. *European Journal of Orthodontics* **42**, 317–325.

Chen, J. C. and Carter, D. R. (2005) Important concepts of mechanical regulation of bone formation and growth. *Current Opinion in Orthopaedics* **16**, 338–345.

Chen, T.-H., Weber, F. E., Malina-Altzinger, J. and Ghayor, C. (2019) Epigenetic drugs as new therapy for tumor necrosis factor-α-compromised bone healing. *Bone* **127**, 49–58.

Claes, P., Roosenboom, J., White, J. D. et al. (2018) Genome-wide mapping of global-to-local genetic effects on human facial shape. *Nature Genetics* **50**, 414–423.

Cobourne, M. T. (2000) Construction for the modern head: current concepts in craniofacial development. *Journal of Orthodontics* **27**, 307–314.

Cruz, C. V., Mattos, C. T., Maia, J. C. et al. (2017) Genetic polymorphisms underlying the skeletal Class III phenotype. *American Journal of Orthodontics and Dentofacial Orthopedics* **151**, 700–707.

Cunha, A., Nelson-Filho, P., Marañón-Vásquez, G. A. et al. (2019) Genetic variants in ACTN3 and MYO1H are associated with sagittal and vertical craniofacial skeletal patterns. *Archives of Oral Biology* **97**, 85–90.

da Fontoura, C. G., Miller, S., Wehby, G. et al. (2015) Candidate gene analyses of skeletal variation in malocclusion. *Journal of Dental Research* **94**, 913–920.

Deguchi, T., Takano-Yamamoto, T., Kanomi, R. et al. (2003) The use of small titanium screws for orthodontic anchorage. *Journal of Dental Research* **82**, 377–381.

Desh, H., Gray, S. L., Horton, M. J. et al. (2014) Molecular motor MYO1C, acetyltransferase KAT6B and osteogenetic transcription factor RUNX2 expression in human masseter muscle contributes to development of malocclusion. *Archives of Oral Biology* **59**, 601–607.

Duncan, R. L. and Turner, C. H. (1995) Mechanotransduction and the functional response of bone to mechanical strain. *Calcified Tissue International* **57**, 344–358.

Elgoyhen, J. C., Moyers, R. E., Mcnamara, J. A., Jr. and Riolo, M. L. (1972) Craniofacial adaptation of protrusive function in young rhesus monkeys. *American Journal of Orthodontics* **62**, 469–480.

Enlow, D. H. (1962) A study of the post-natal growth and remodeling of bone. *American Journal of Anatomy* **110**, 79–101.

Enlow, D. H. and Bang, S. (1965) Growth and remodeling of the human maxilla. *American Journal of Orthodontics* **51**, 446–464.

Epker, B. N. (1967) Bone remodeling and balance and the development of osteoporosis. *Annual meeting – American Institute of Oral Biology* 3–15.

Eriksen, E. F., Langdahl, B., Vesterby, A. et al. (1999) Hormone replacement therapy prevents osteoclastic hyperactivity: A histomorphometric study in early postmenopausal women. *Journal of Bone and Mineral Research* **14**, 1217–1221.

Eriksen, E. F., Mosekilde, L. and Melsen, F. (1985) Trabecular bone remodeling and bone balance in hyperthyroidism. *Bone* **6**, 421–428.

Eriksen, E. F., Mosekilde, L. and Melsen, F. (1986) Trabecular bone remodeling and balance in primary hyperparathyroidism. *Bone* **7**, 213–221.

Everts, V., Delaisse, J. M., Korper, W. et al. (2002) The bone lining cell: its role in cleaning Howship's lacunae and initiating bone formation. *Journal of Bone and Mineral Research* **17**, 77–90.

Frost, H. M. (1969) Tetracycline-based histological analysis of bone remodeling. *Calcified Tissue International* **3**, 211–237.

Frost, H. M. (1983) The regional accelerating phenomenon: a review. *Henry Ford Hospital Medical Journal* **31**, 3–9.

Frost, H. M. (1987) Bone "mass" and the "mechanostat": a proposal. *The Anatomical Record* **219**, 1–9.

Frost, H. M. (1990) Skeletal structural adaptations to mechanical usage (SATMU): 1. Redefining Wolff's law: the bone modeling problem. *The Anatomical Record* **226**, 403–413.

Frost, H. M. (1991) Some ABC's of skeletal pathophysiology. 6. The growth/modeling/remodeling distinction. *Calcified Tissue International* **49**, 301–302.

Frost, H. M. (1994) Wolff's Law and bone's structural adaptations to mechanical usage: an overview for clinicians. *The Angle Orthodontist* **64**, 175–188.

Frost, H. M. (1998) Osteoporoses: a rationale for further definitions? *Calcified Tissue International* **62**, 89–94.

Frost, H. M., Villanueva, A. R., Roth, H. and Stanisavljevic, S. (1961) Tetracycline bone labeling. *The Journal of New Drugs* **1**, 206–216.

Fujiyoshi, Y., Yamashiro, T., Deguchi, T. et al. (2000) The difference in temporal distribution of c-Fos immunoreactive neurons between the medullary dorsal horn and the trigeminal subnucleus oralis in the rat following experimental tooth movement. *Neuroscience Letters* **283**, 205–208.

Furstman, L., Bernick, S. and Mahan, P. Z. (1971) The role of the nasal septum in the development of the secondary palate of the rat. *American Journal of Orthodontics* **60**, 244–256.

Gilbert, S. F.(2000) *Developmental Biology*. Sinauer Associates, Inc., Sunderland, MA.

Gilhuus-Moe, O. (1971) Fractures of the mandibular condyle in the growth period: histologic and autoradiographic observations in the contralateral, nontraumatized condyle. *Acta Odontologica Scandinavica* **29**, 53–63.

Goldberg, K. E. (1982) The skeleton: fantastic framework, in *The Human Body* (ed. J. Gersten). US News Books, Washington, DC.

Griffiths, D. L., Furstman, L. and Bernick, S. (1967) Postnatal development of the mouse palate. *American Journal of Orthodontics* **53**, 757–768.

Hamrick, M. W. (2003) Increased bone mineral density in the femora of GDF8 knock-out mice. *The Anatomical Record. Part A, Discoveries in Molecular, Cellular, and Evolutionary Biology* **272**, 388–391.

Hartsfield, J. K. (2007) Review of the etiologic heterogeneity of the oculo-auriculo-vertebral spectrum (hemifacial microsomia). *Orthodontics and Craniofacial Research* **10**, 121–128.

Hartsfield, J. K., Jr. (2009) Pathways in external apical root resorption associated with orthodontia. *Orthodontics and Craniofacial Research* **12**, 236–242.

Hartsfield, J.K. (2015) Personalized orthodontics: Limitations and possibilities in orthodontic practice, in *Biological Mechanisms of Tooth Movement* (eds. V. Krishnan and Z. Davidovitch). Wiley Blackwell, Chichester, pp. 164–172.

Hartsfield, J. K., Morford, L. A., Otero, L. M. and Fardo, D. W. (2013) Genetics and non-syndromic facial growth. *Journal of Pediatric Genetics* **2**, 009–020.

Hartsfield Jr, J. K., Jacob, G. J. and Morford, L. A. (2017) Heredity, genetics and orthodontics: How much has this research really helped? *Seminars in Orthodontics* **23**, 336–347.

Hasegawa, M., Kondo, M., Suzuki, I. et al. (2012) ERK is Involved in Tooth-pressure-induced Fos Expression in Vc Neurons. *Journal of Dental Research* **91**, 1141–1146.

Havers, C. (1691) *Osteologica Nova [Some new observations on bone]*. Berlin.

He, D., Kou, X., Luo, Q. et al. (2015) Enhanced M1/M2 macrophage ratio promotes orthodontic root resorption. *Journal of Dental Research* **94**, 129–139.

Hellsing, E. and Hammarstrom, L. (1991) The effects of pregnancy and fluoride on orthodontic tooth movements in rats. *European Journal of Orthodontics* **13**, 223–230.

High, W. B., Capen, C. C. and Black, H. E. (1981) Effects of thyroxine on cortical bone remodeling in adult dogs: a histomorphometric study. *American Journal of Pathology*, **102**, 438–446.

Hinton, R. J., Jing, J. and Feng, J. Q. (2015) Genetic influences on temporomandibular joint development and growth. *Current Topics in Developmental Biology* **115**, 85–109.

Hofbauer, L. C. and Schoppet, M. (2004) Clinical implications of the osteoprotegerin/RANKL/RANK system for bone and vascular diseases. *Journal of the American Medical Association* **292**, 490–495.

Holick, M. F. (1998) Perspective on the impact of weightlessness on calcium and bone metabolism. *Bone* **22**, 105S–111S.

Huang, H., Williams, R. C. and Kyrkanides, S. (2014) Accelerated orthodontic tooth movement: Molecular mechanisms. *American Journal of Orthodontics and Dentofacial Orthopedics* **146**, 620–632.

Hughes, L. V., Furstman, L. and Bernick, S. (1967) Prenatal development of the rat palate. *Journal of Dental Research* **46**, 373–379.

Huh, A., Horton, M. J., Cuenco, K. T. et al. (2013) Epigenetic influence of KAT6B and HDAC4 in the development of skeletal malocclusion. *American Journal of Orthodontics and Dentofacial Orthopedics* **144**, 568–576.

Hunt, P., Clarke, J. D., Buxton, P. et al. (1998) Segmentation, crest prespecification and the control of facial form. *European Journal of Oral Sciences* **106**(Suppl. 1), 12–8.

Hunter, J. 1778. *The Natural History of the Human Teeth*, London.

Iglesias-Linares, A., Morford, L. A. and Hartsfield, J. K. (2016) Bone density and dental external apical root resorption. *Current Osteoporosis Reports* **14**, 292–309.

Isaacson, R. J., Worms, F. W. and Speidel, T. M. (1976) Measurement of tooth movement. *American Journal of Orthodontics* **70**, 290–303.

Ishii-Suzuki, M., Suda, N., Yamazaki, K. et al. (1999) Differential responses to parathyroid hormone-related protein (PTHrP) deficiency in the various craniofacial cartilages. *Anatomical Record* **255**, 452–457.

Ito, G., Mitani, S. and Kim, J. H. (1988) Effect of soft diets on craniofacial growth in mice. *Anatomischer Anzeiger* **165**, 151–66.

Iwasaki, L. R., Gibson, C. S., Crouch, L. D. et al. (2006) Speed of tooth movement is related to stress and IL-1 gene polymorphisms. *American Journal of Orthodontics and Dentofacial Orthopedics* **130**, 698 e1–9.

Jee, W. S. (2005) The past, present, and future of bone morphometry: its contribution to an improved understanding of bone biology. *Journal of Bone and Mineral Metabolism* **23**(Suppl.), 1–10.

Jee, W. S., Blackwood, E. L., Dockum, N. L. et al. (1966) Bio-assay of responses of growing bones to cortisol. *Clinical Orthopaedics and Related Research*, **49**, 39–63.

Jee, W. S., Mori, S., Li, X. J. and Chan, S. (1990) Prostaglandin E2 enhances cortical bone mass and activates intracortical bone remodeling in intact and ovariectomized female rats. *Bone* **11**, 253–266.

Jerome, C. P., Burr, D. B., Van Bibber, T. *et al.* (2001) Treatment with human parathyroid hormone (1–34) for 18 months increases cancellous bone volume and improves trabecular architecture in ovariectomized cynomolgus monkeys (Macaca fascicularis). *Bone* **28**, 150–159.

Jilka, R. L., Noble, B. and Weinstein, R. S. (2013) Osteocyte apoptosis. *Bone* **54**, 264–271.

Kanzaki, H., Chiba, M., Takahashi, I. *et al.* (2004) Local OPG gene transfer to periodontal tissue inhibits orthodontic tooth movement. *Journal of Dental Research* **83**, 920–925.

Karsenty, G. (2003) The complexities of skeletal biology. *Nature* **423**, 316–318.

Katona, T. R., Paydar, N. H., Akay, H. U. and Roberts, W. E. (1995) Stress analysis of bone modeling response to rat molar orthodontics. *Journal of Biomechanics* **28**, 27–38.

Khosla, S. (2001) Minireview: the OPG/RANKL/RANK system. *Endocrinology* **142**, 5050–5055.

Kiliaridis, S., Engstrom, C., Lindskog-Stokland, B. and Katsaros, C. (1996) Craniofacial bone remodeling in growing rats fed a low-calcium and vitamin-D-deficient diet and the influence of masticatory muscle function. *Acta Odontologica Scandinavica* **54**, 320–326.

Kluemper, G. T., Morford, L. A. and Hartsfield, J. K., JR. (2019) The quest and reality of personalized treatment for the skeletal class III patient, in *Effective, Efficient and Personalized Orthodontics: Patient-Centered Approaches and Innovations* (eds. H. Kim-Berman, L. FranchI and A. Ruellas). The University of Michigan Craniofacial Growth Series, Ann Arbor, MI.

Kornak, U. and Mundlos, S. (2003) Genetic disorders of the skeleton: a developmental approach. *American Journal of Human Genetics* **73**, 447–474.

Krishnan, V. and Davidovitch, Z. E. (2006) Cellular, molecular, and tissue-level reactions to orthodontic force. *American Journal of Orthodontics and Dentofacial Orthopedics* **129**, 469. e1–469. e32.

Kronenberg, H. M. (2003) Developmental regulation of the growth plate. *Nature* **423**, 332–336.

Lattanzi, W., Barba, M., Di Pietro, L. and Boyadjiev, S. A. (2017) Genetic advances in craniosynostosis. *American Journal of Medical Genetics Part A* **173**, 1406–1429.

Le Douarin, N. M., Dupin, E. and Ziller, C. (1994) Genetic and epigenetic control in neural crest development. *Current Opinion in Genetics and Development* **4**, 685–695.

Li, C., Chung, C. J., Hwang, C.-J. and Lee, K.-J. (2019) Local injection of RANKL facilitates tooth movement and alveolar bone remodelling. *Oral Diseases* **25**, 550–560.

Li, J., Mashiba, T. and Burr, D. B. (2001) Bisphosphonate treatment suppresses not only stochastic remodeling but also the targeted repair of microdamage. *Calcified Tissue International* **69**, 281–286.

Lund, K. (1974) Mandibular growth and remodelling processes after condylar fracture. A longitudinal roentgencephalometric study. *Acta Odontologica Scandinavica. Supplementum*, **32**, 3–117.

MacGinitie, L. A., Seiz, K. G., Otter, M. W. and Cochran, G. V. (1994) Streaming potential measurements at low ionic concentrations reflect bone microstructure. *Journal of Biomechanics* **27**, 969–978.

Manocha, S., Farokhnia, N., Khosropanah, S. *et al.* (2019) Systematic review of hormonal and genetic factors involved in the nonsyndromic disorders of the lower jaw. *Developmental Dynamics* **248**, 162–172.

Manolagas, S. C., Kousteni, S. and Jilka, R. L. (2002) Sex steroids and bone. *Recent Progress in Hormone Research* **57**, 385–409.

Marcucio, R., Hallgrimsson, B. and Young, N. M. (2015) Facial morphogenesis: physical and molecular interactions between the brain and the face. *Current Topics in Developmental Biology* **115**, 299–320.

Martin, R. B. (2002) Is all cortical bone remodeling initiated by microdamage? *Bone* **30**, 8–13.

Mavropoulos, A., Bresin, A. and Kiliaridis, S. (2004) Morphometric analysis of the mandible in growing rats with different masticatory functional demands: adaptation to an upper posterior bite block. *European Journal of Oral Sciences* **112**, 259–266.

McNamara, J. A., Jr. (1973) Neuromuscular and skeletal adaptations to altered function in the orofacial region. *American Journal of Orthodontics* **64**, 578–606.

McNamara, J. A., Jr. and Carlson, D. S. (1979) Quantitative analysis of temporomandibular joint adaptations to protrusive function. *American Journal of Orthodontics* **76**, 593–611.

Meyers, G. A., Day, D., Goldberg, R. *et al.* (1996) FGFR2 exon IIIa and IIIc mutations in Crouzon, Jackson-Weiss, and Pfeiffer syndromes: evidence for missense changes, insertions, and a deletion due to alternative RNA splicing. *American Journal of Human Genetics* **58**, 491.

Midgett, R. J., Shaye, R. and Fruge, J. F., Jr. (1981) The effect of altered bone metabolism on orthodontic tooth movement. *American Journal of Orthodontics* **80**, 256–262.

Miller, S. C. and Marks, S. C., Jr. (1993) Local stimulation of new bone formation by prostaglandin E1: quantitative histomorphometry and comparison of delivery by minipumps and controlled-release pellets. *Bone* **14**, 143–151.

Minaire, P. (1989) Immobilization osteoporosis: a review. *Clinical Rheumatology* **8**(Suppl. 2), 95–103.

Mori, S. and Burr, D. B. (1993) Increased intracortical remodeling following fatigue damage. *Bone* **14**, 103–109.

Mosley, J. R. and Lanyon, L. E. (1998) Strain rate as a controlling influence on adaptive modeling in response to dynamic loading of the ulna in growing male rats. *Bone* **23**, 313–318.

Mulvihill, J. J. (1995) Craniofacial syndromes: no such thing as a single gene disease. *Nature Genetics* **9**, 101.

Mundlos, S., Otto, F., Mundlos, C. *et al.* (1997) Mutations involving the transcription factor CBFA1 cause cleidocranial dysplasia. *Cell* **89**, 773–779.

Nevill, A. M., Holder, R. L. and Stewart, A. D. (2003) Modeling elite male athletes' peripheral bone mass, assessed using regional dual x-ray absorptiometry. *Bone* **32**, 62–68.

Noble, B. S., Peet, N., Stevens, H. Y. *et al.* (2003) Mechanical loading: biphasic osteocyte survival and targeting of osteoclasts for bone destruction in rat cortical bone. *American Journal of Physiology. Cell Physiology* **284**, C934–943.

Noden, D. M. (1983) The role of the neural crest in patterning of avian cranial skeletal, connective, and muscle tissues. *Developmental Biology* **96**, 144–165.

Nomura, S. and Takano-Yamamoto, T. (2000) Molecular events caused by mechanical stress in bone. *Matrix Biology* **19**, 91–96.

Novak, M. L. and Koh, T. J. (2013) Phenotypic transitions of macrophages orchestrate tissue repair. *American Journal of Pathology* **183**, 1352–1363.

Oberheim, M. C. and Mao, J. J. (2002) Bone strain patterns of the zygomatic complex in response to simulated orthopedic forces. *Journal of Dental Research* **81**, 608–612.

Okeson, J. (2003) *Management of Temporomandibular Disorders and Occlusion*. Mosby, St Louis.

Oldridge, M., Zackai, E. H., McDonald-McGinn, D. M. *et al.* (1999) De novo alu-element insertions in FGFR2 identify a distinct pathological basis for Apert syndrome. *American Journal of Human Genetics* **64**, 446–461.

Oudet, C., Petrovic, A. and Stutzmann, J. (1984) Time-dependent effects of a 'functional'-type orthopedic appliance on the rat mandible growth. *Chronobiology International* **1**, 51–57.

Owan, I., Burr, D. B., Turner, C. H. *et al.* (1997) Mechanotransduction in bone: osteoblasts are more responsive to fluid forces than mechanical strain. *American Journal of Physiology* **273**, C810–815.

Pancherz, H., Ruf, S. and Kohlhas, P. (1998) "Effective condylar growth" and chin position changes in Herbst treatment: a cephalometric roentgenographic long-term study. *American Journal of Orthodontics and Dentofacial Orthopedics* **114**, 437–446.

Parfitt, A. M. (1976) The actions of parathyroid hormone on bone: relation to bone remodeling and turnover, calcium homeostasis, and metabolic bone disease. Part I of IV parts: mechanisms of calcium transfer between blood and bone and their cellular basis: morphological and kinetic approaches to bone turnover. *Metabolism* **25**, 809–844.

Parfitt, A. M. (2002) Targeted and nontargeted bone remodeling: relationship to basic multicellular unit origination and progression. *Bone* **30**, 5–7.

Parfitt, A. M. (2003) Renal bone disease: a new conceptual framework for the interpretation of bone histomorphometry. *Current Opinion in Nephrology and Hypertension* **12**, 387–403.

Parfitt, A. M., Drezner, M. K., Glorieux, F. H. *et al.* (1987) Bone histomorphometry: standardization of nomenclature, symbols, and units. Report of the ASBMR Histomorphometry Nomenclature Committee. *Journal of Bone and Mineral Research* **2**, 595–610.

Pavalko, F. M., Norvell, S. M., Burr, D. B. *et al.* (2003) A model for mechanotransduction in bone cells: the load-bearing mechanosomes. *Journal of Cellular Biochemistry* **88**, 104–112.

Petrovic, A., Stutzmann, J., Lavergne, J. and Shaye, R. (1991) Is it possible to modulate the growth of the human mandible with a functional appliance? *International Journal of Orthodontics* **29**, 3–8.

Pfeilschifter, J., Chenu, C., Bird, A. *et al.* (1989) Interleukin-1 and tumor necrosis factor stimulate the formation of human osteoclastlike cells in vitro. *Journal of Bone and Mineral Research* **4**, 113–118.

Pirttiniemi, P., Peltomäki, T., Müller, L. and Luder, H. U. (2009) Abnormal mandibular growth and the condylar cartilage. *European Journal of Orthodontics* **31**, 1–11.

Poppe, M., Bourauel, C. and Jager, A. (2002) Determination of the elasticity parameters of the human periodontal ligament and the location of the center of resistance of single-rooted teeth *a study of autopsy specimens and their conversion into finite element models. Journal of Orofacial Orthopedics* **63**, 358–370.

Proffit, W. R., Vig, K. W. and Turvey, T. A. (1980) Early fracture of the mandibular condyles: frequently an unsuspected cause of growth disturbances. *American Journal of Orthodontics* **78**, 1–24.

Provot, S. and Schipani, E. (2005) Molecular mechanisms of endochondral bone development. *Biochemical and Biophysical Research Communications* **328**, 658–665.

Qin, L., Raggatt, L. J. and Partridge, N. C. (2004) Parathyroid hormone: a double-edged sword for bone metabolism. *Trends in Endocrinology and Metabolism* **15**, 60–65.

Qin, Y. X., Kaplan, T., Saldanha, A. and Rubin, C. (2003) Fluid pressure gradients, arising from oscillations in intramedullary pressure, is correlated with the formation of bone and inhibition of intracortical porosity. *Journal of Biomechanics* **36**, 1427–1437.

Qin, Y. X., Rubin, C. T. and Mcleod, K. J. (1998) Nonlinear dependence of loading intensity and cycle number in the maintenance of bone mass and morphology. *Journal of Orthopaedic Research* **16**, 482–489.

Rabie, A. B. M., She, T. T. and Harley, V. R. (2003) Forward mandibular positioning up-regulates SOX9 and Type II collagen expression in the glenoid fossa. *Journal of Dental Research*, **82**, 725–730.

Raoul, G., Rowlerson, A., Sciote, J. et al. (2011) Masseter myosin heavy chain composition varies with mandibular asymmetry. *Journal of Craniofacial Surgery* **22**, 1093–1098.

Recker, R. R. (1983) *Bone Histomorphometry: Techniques and Interpretation*. CRC Press, Boca Raton, FL.

Renaud, S., Auffray, J.-C. and De La Porte, S. (2010) Epigenetic effects on the mouse mandible: common features and discrepancies in remodeling due to muscular dystrophy and response to food consistency. *BMC Evolutionary Biology* **10**, 28.

Roberts, W. E. (1984) Rigid endosseous anchorage and tricalcium phosphate (TCP)-coated implants. *CDA Journal California Dental Association* **12**, 158–161.

Roberts, W. E. (1988) Bone tissue interface. *International Journal of Oral Implantology: Implantologist* **5**, 71-74.

Roberts, W. E. (1994) Bone physiology, metabolism and biomechanics in orthodontic practice, in *Orthodontics: Current Principles and Techniques* (eds. T. M. Graber and R. L. Vanarsdall). Mosby, St Louis.

Roberts, W. E. (1997) Adjunctive orthodontic therapy in adults over 50 years of age. Clinical management of compensated, partially edentulous malocclusion. *Journal (Indiana Dental Association)* **76**, 33–34, 36–38, 40–41.

Roberts, W. E. (1999) Bone dynamics of osseointegration, ankylosis, and tooth movement. *Journal (Indiana Dental Association)* **78**, 24–32.

Roberts, W. E. (2000a) Bone physiology of tooth movement, ankylosis, and osseointegration. *Seminars in Orthodontics* **6**, 173–182.

Roberts, W. E. (2000b) Bone physiology, metabolism, and biomechanics in orthodontic practice, in *Orthodontics: Current Principles and Techniques* (eds. T. M. Graber and R. L. Vanarsdall). Mosby, St Louis.

Roberts, W. E. (2005) Bone physiology, metabolism, and biomechanics in orthodontic practice, in *Orthodontics: Current Principles and Techniques* (eds. T. M. Graber, R. L. Vanarsdall and K. W. L. Vig). Mosby, St Louis.

Roberts, W. E., Garetto, L. P., Arbuckle, G. R. et al. (1991) What are the risk factors of osteoporosis? Assessing bone health. *Journal of the American Dental Association* **122**, 59–61.

Roberts, W. E., Goodwin, W. C., Jr. and Heiner, S. R. (1981) Cellular response to orthodontic force. *Dental Clinics of North America*, **25**, 3–17.

Roberts, W. E. and Hartsfield, J. K. (1997) Multidisciplinary management of congenital and acquired compensated malocclusions: diagnosis, etiology and treatment planning. *Journal of the Dental Association* **76**, 42–43, 45–48, 50–51; quiz 52.

Roberts, W. E. and Hartsfield, J. K., JR. (2004) Bone development and function: genetic and environmental mechanisms. *Seminars in Orthodontics* **10**, 100–122.

Roberts, W. E., Huja, S. and Roberts, J. A. (2004) Bone modeling: biomechanics, molecular mechanisms and clinical perspectives. *Seminars in Orthodontics* **10**, 123–161.

Roberts, W. E. and Morey, E. R. (1985) Proliferation and differentiation sequence of osteoblast histogenesis under physiological conditions in rat periodontal ligament. *American Journal of Anatomy* **174**, 105–118.

Roberts, W. E., Mozsary, P. G. and Klingler, E. (1982) Nuclear size as a cell-kinetic marker for osteoblast differentiation. *American Journal of Anatomy* **165**, 373–384.

Roberts, W. E., Roberts, J. A., Epker, B. N. et al. (2006) Remodeling of mineralized tissues, part I: The Frost Legacy. *Seminars in Orthodontics* **12**, 216–237.

Roberts, W. E., Simmons, K. E., Garetto, L. P. and Decastro, R. A. (1992) Bone physiology and metabolism in dental implantology: risk factors for osteoporosis and other metabolic bone diseases. *Implant Dentistry* **1**, 11–21.

Roberts, W. E. and Stocum, D. L. (2018) Part II: Temporomandibular joint (TMJ) – regeneration, degeneration, and adaptation. *Current Osteoporosis Reports* **16**, 369–379.

Roberts, W. E., Turley, P. K., Brezniak, N. and Fielder, P. J. (1987a) Implants: Bone physiology and metabolism. *CDA Journal California Dental Association* **15**, 54–61.

Roberts, W. E., Viecilli, R. F., Chang, C. et al. (2015) Biology of biomechanics: Finite element analysis of a statically determinate system to rotate the occlusal plane for correction of a skeletal Class III open-bite malocclusion. *American Journal of Orthodontics and Dentofacial Orthopedics* **148**, 943–955.

Roberts, W. E., Wood, H. B., Chambers, D. W. and Burk, D. T. (1987b) Vascularly oriented differentiation gradient of osteoblast precursor cells in rat periodontal ligament: implications for osteoblast histogenesis and periodontal bone loss. *Journal of Periodontal Research* **22**, 461–467.

Robey, P. G., Fedarko, N. S., Hefferan, T. E. et al. (1993) Structure and molecular regulation of bone matrix proteins. *Journal of Bone and Mineral Research* **8**(Suppl. 2), S483–487.

Rowlerson, A., Raoul, G., Daniel, Y. et al. (2005) Fiber-type differences in masseter muscle associated with different facial morphologies. *American Journal of Orthodontics and Dentofacial Orthopedics* **127**, 37–46.

Rubin, J., Styner, M. and Uzer, G. (2018) Physical signals may affect mesenchymal stem cell differentiation via epigenetic controls. *Exercise and Sport Sciences Reviews* **46**, 42–47.

Sabatini, M., Boyce, B., Aufdemorte, T. et al. (1988) Infusions of recombinant human interleukins 1 alpha and 1 beta cause hypercalcemia in normal mice. *Proceedings of The National Academy of Sciences of the United States of America* **85**, 5235–5239.

Sangani, D., Suzuki, A., Vonville, H. et al. (2015) Gene mutations associated with temporomandibular joint disorders: a systematic review. *OAlib*, **2**.

Santagati, F. and Rijli, F. M. (2003) Cranial neural crest and the building of the vertebrate head. *Nature Reviews* **4**, 806–818.

Schacter, R. I., Furstman, L. and Bernick, S. (1969) Postnatal development of the mandible of the cat. *American Journal of Orthodontics* **56**, 354–364.

Sciote, J. J., Horton, M. J., Rowlerson, A. M. et al. (2012) Human masseter muscle fiber type properties, skeletal malocclusions, and muscle growth factor expression. *Journal of Oral and Maxillofacial Surgery* **70**, 440–448.

Sciote, J. J., Raoul, G., Ferri, J. et al. (2013) Masseter function and skeletal malocclusion. *Revue de Stomatologie de Chirugie Maxillofaciale et de Chirugie Orale* **114**, 79–85.

Seeman, E. and Delmas, P. D. (2001) Reconstructing the skeleton with intermittent parathyroid hormone. *Trends in Endocrinology and Metabolism* **12**, 281–283.

Shaw, N. E. and Lacey, E. (1975) The influence of corticosteroids on the normal and papain-treated epiphysial growth plate in the rabbit. *Journal of Bone and Joint Surgery* **57**, 228–233.

Shirazi, M., Khosrowshahi, M. and Dehpour, A. R. (2001) The effect of chronic renal insufficiency on orthodontic tooth movement in rats. *The Angle Orthodontist* **71**, 494–498.

Sperber, G. H., Sperber, S. M. and Guttmann, G. D. (2010) *Craniofacial Embryogenetics And Development*, PMPH-USA.

Steger, E. R. and Blechman, A. M. (1995) Case reports: molar distalization with static repelling magnets. Part II. *American Journal of Orthodontics and Dentofacial Orthopedics* **108**, 547–555.

Stocum, D. L. and Roberts, W. E. (2018) Part I: development and physiology of the temporomandibular joint. *Current Osteoporosis Reports* **16**, 360–368.

Storey, E. (1972) Growth and remodeling of bone and bones. *American Journal of Orthodontics* **62**, 142–165.

Takano-Yamamoto, T., Kawakami, M., Kobayashi, Y. et al. (1992) The effect of local application of 1,25-dihydroxycholecalciferol on osteoclast numbers in orthodontically treated rats. *Journal of Dental Research* **71**, 53–59.

Terai, K., Takano-Yamamoto, T., Ohba, Y. et al. (1999) Role of osteopontin in bone remodeling caused by mechanical stress. *Journal of Bone and Mineral Research* **14**, 839–849.

Turley, P. K., Kean, C., Schur, J. et al. (1988) Orthodontic force application to titanium endosseous implants. *The Angle Orthodontist* **58**, 151–162.

Vajo, Z., Francomano, C. A. and Wilkin, D. J. (2000) The molecular and genetic basis of fibroblast growth factor receptor 3 disorders: the achondroplasia family of skeletal dysplasias, Muenke craniosynostosis, and Crouzon syndrome with acanthosis nigricans. *Endocrine Reviews* **21**, 23–39.

Van't Hof, R. J., Macphee, J., Libouban, H. et al. (2004) Regulation of bone mass and bone turnover by neuronal nitric oxide synthase. *Endocrinology* **145**, 5068–5074.

Vasconcelos, B. C. D. E., Gonçalves, F., Andrade, A. et al. (2012) Assimetria mandibular: revisão de literatura e relato de caso. *Brazilian Journal of Otorhinolaryngology* **78**, 137.

Verborgt, O., Gibson, G. J. and Schaffler, M. B.(2000) Loss of osteocyte integrity in association with microdamage and bone remodeling after fatigue in vivo. *Journal of Bone and Mineral Research* **15**, 60–67.

Verna, C., Dalstra, M., Lee, T. C. et al. (2004) Microcracks in the alveolar bone following orthodontic tooth movement: a morphological and morphometric study. *European Journal of Orthodontics* **26**, 459–467.

Verna, C. and Melsen, B. (2003) Tissue reaction to orthodontic tooth movement in different bone turnover conditions. *Orthodontics and Craniofacial Research* **6**, 155–163.

Viecilli, R., Kar-Kuri, M., Varriale, J. et al. (2013) Effects of initial stresses and time on orthodontic external root resorption. *Journal of Dental Research* **92**, 346–351.

Voudouris, J. C., Woodside, D. G., Altuna, G. et al. (2003a) Condyle-fossa modifications and muscle interactions during Herbst treatment, Part 2. Results and conclusions. *American Journal of Orthodontics and Dentofacial Orthopedics* **124**, 13–29.

Voudouris, J. C., Woodside, D. G., Altuna, G. et al. (2003b) Condyle-fossa modifications and muscle interactions during herbst treatment, part 1. New technological methods. *American Journal of Orthodontics and Dentofacial Orthopedics* **123**, 604–613.

Wan, Q. and Li, Z.-B. (2010) Intra-articular injection of parathyroid hormone in the temporomandibular joint as a novel therapy for mandibular asymmetry. *Medical Hypotheses* **74**, 685–687.

Weinmann, J. P. and Sicher, H. (1955) *Bone and Bones: Fundamentals of Bone Biology*, 2nd edn. Henry Kimpton, London.

Weinstein, S. (1967) Minimal forces in tooth movement. *American Journal of Orthodontics* **53**, 881–903.

Widmer, C. G., English, A. W., Carrasco, D. I. and Malick, C. L. (2002) Modeling rabbit temporomandibular joint torques during a power stroke. *The Angle Orthodontist* **72**, 331–337.

Wilcox, W. R., Tavormina, P. L., Krakow, D. et al. (1998) Molecular, radiologic, and histopathologic correlations in thanatophoric dysplasia. *American Journal of Medical Genetics* **78**, 274–281.

Wong, S. K., Mohamad, N.-V., Ibrahim, N. I. et al. (2019) The molecular mechanism of vitamin E as a bone-protecting agent: a review on current evidence. *International Journal of Molecular Sciences* **20**, 1453.

Yamashiro, T., Aberg, T., Levanon, D. et al. (2002) Expression of Runx1, -2 and -3 during tooth, palate and craniofacial bone development. *Gene Expression Patterns* **2**, 109–112.

Yamashiro, T., Fujiyama, K., Fujiyoshi, Y. et al. (2000a) Inferior alveolar nerve transection inhibits increase in osteoclast appearance during experimental tooth movement. *Bone* **26**, 663–669.

Yamashiro, T., Fukunaga, T., Kabuto, H. et al. (2001a) Activation of the bulbospinal serotonergic system during experimental tooth movement in the rat. *Journal of Dental Research* **80**, 1854–1857.

Yamashiro, T., Fukunaga, T., Kobashi, N. et al. (2001b) Mechanical stimulation induces CTGF expression in rat osteocytes. *Journal of Dental Research* **80**, 461–465.

Yamashiro, T., Fukunaga, T., Yamashita, K. et al. (2001c) Gene and protein expression of brain-derived neurotrophic factor and TrkB in bone and cartilage. *Bone* **28**, 404–409.

Yamashiro, T., Kabuto, H., Fukunaga, T. et al. (2000b) Medullary monoamine levels during experimental tooth movement. *Brain Research* **878**, 199–203.

Yamashiro, T., Nakagawa, K., Satoh, K. et al. (1997) c-fos expression in the trigeminal sensory complex and pontine parabrachial areas following experimental tooth movement. *Neuroreport* **8**, 2351–2353.

Yamashiro, T., Satoh, K., Nakagawa, K. et al. (1998) Expression of Fos in the rat forebrain following experimental tooth movement. *Journal of Dental Research* **77**, 1920–1925.

Yang, Y.-Q., Tan, Y.-Y., Wong, R. et al. (2012) The role of vascular endothelial growth factor in ossification. *International Journal Of Oral Science* **4**, 64.

Yao, W., Jee, W. S., Zhou, H. et al. (1999) Anabolic effect of prostaglandin E2 on cortical bone of aged male rats comes mainly from modeling-dependent bone gain. *Bone* **25**, 697–702.

Yoshida, N., Koga, Y., Peng, C. L. et al. (2001) In vivo measurement of the elastic modulus of the human periodontal ligament. *Medical Engineering and Phys*, **23**, 567–572.

You, J., Yellowley, C. E., Donahue, H. J. et al. (2000) Substrate deformation levels associated with routine physical activity are less stimulatory to bone cells relative to loading-induced oscillatory fluid flow. *Journal of Biomechanical Engineering*, **122**, 387–393.

Zebrick, B., Teeramongkolgul, T., Nicot, R. et al. (2014) ACTN3 R577X genotypes associate with Class II and deepbite malocclusions. *American Journal of Orthodontics and Dentofacial Orthopedics* **146**, 603–611.

Zelzer, E. and Olsen, B. R. (2003) The genetic basis for skeletal diseases. *Nature* **423**, 343–348.

Zhao, Y. and Westphal, H. (2002) Homeobox genes and human genetic disorders. *Current Molecular Medicine* **2**, 13–23.

CHAPTER 7
Mechanical Load, Sex Hormones, and Bone Modeling

Sara H. Windahl and Ulf H. Lerner

> **Summary**
>
> Mechanical loading as a result of load-bearing physical activity is an important regulator of both bone mass and bone microarchitecture. Sex hormone receptor signaling involves several separate signaling cascades in a tissue-specific manner, affecting osteoclastic resorption, osteoblastic bone formation, bone modeling and remodeling, and is also an important determinant of bone mass. Interestingly, estrogen receptors play an important role in load-induced modeling of bone, an effect surprisingly found to be independent of estrogen. Modeling of jaw bones in response to orthodontic tooth movement is dependent on several factors where reshaping of bone by osteoclast and osteoblast activities are of major importance. Although not much studied, loading, sex hormones, and their receptors are likely to affect orthodontic tooth movement. This chapter gives an overview of bone cell differentiation and function and describes the role of sex hormone receptors in mechanical loading, and their possible role in orthodontic tooth movement.

Introduction

Skeletal tissue is made up of two structurally different types of bone: cortical (compact) bone, forming an outer shell in all flat and long bones, and cancellous (trabecular) bone arranged in spicules in the inner marrow cavity of some bones. Both types are formed by osteoblasts, but why some osteoblasts make cortical and others cancellous bone is unknown, as are the mechanisms involved. Cortical bone makes up 80% of bone mass and cancellous bone the remaining part. However, both types of bone are important for bone strength. Although characterized as compact bone, cortical bone contains many Haversian canals along the long axis, and Volkman's canal in the transverse axis, harboring blood vessels and nerves. In addition, many lacunae exist containing osteocytes, which are connected to each other by cellular extensions in small canals (canaliculi). Cortical bone is therefore far from being made exclusively of mineralized extracellular matrix.

The skeleton has many functions (Figure 7.1), the most well known being part of the musculoskeletal system. The skeleton is also important for the protection of vital organs like the brain, spinal cord, and the chest. It harbors the hematopoietic bone marrow, and research during the 2000s has shown that cells present in the bone marrow communicate with the bone cells and vice versa in the so called osteoimmune interplay (Tsukasaki and Takayanagi, 2019).

Furthermore, bone takes part in the regulation of calcium and phosphate metabolism, together with the kidneys and the gastrointestinal tract. The activities of bone cells are controlled by a variety of peptide and steroid hormones. This list includes, among others, parathyroid hormone, calcitonin, $1,25(OH)_2$-vitamin D3, vitamin A (retinoids), thyroid hormones, glucocorticoids, and sex steroids (estrogens and androgens).

Three cells are mainly regarded as bone cells – osteoblasts, osteocytes, and osteoclasts – although mesenchymal stromal cells in bone marrow are also important for bone. Osteoblasts and osteocytes are mesenchymally derived cells, while osteoclasts are of hematopoietic origin (see further later). Osteoclasts are bone-resorbing cells, whereas osteoblasts are cells that produce bone and have important roles as regulators of osteoclast differentiation. Osteocytes are embedded in bone tissue and exhibit many extensions, which can recognize mechanical loading and transmit signals to osteoblasts and osteoclasts on the bone surface, regulating both their differentiation and activity. These three cells extensively communicate with each other through several paracrine signaling molecules in a complex network of interactions. Bone cells sense increases in strain generated when the bone is loaded. This leads to site-specific increases in bone formation, thereby resulting in a bone mass and architecture that matches the load. This relationship between load/strain and

---

Biological Mechanisms of Tooth Movement, Third Edition. Edited by Vinod Krishnan, Anne Marie Kuijpers-Jagtman and Ze'ev Davidovitch.
© 2021 John Wiley & Sons Ltd. Published 2021 by John Wiley & Sons Ltd.

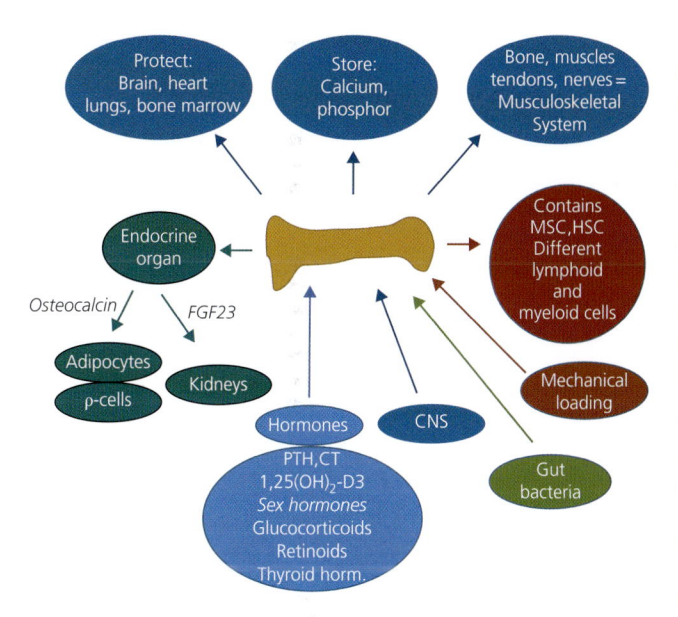

Figure 7.1 Bone interacts with many organs – the functions played by skeletal tissue. MSC, Mesenchymal stem cells; HSC, haemopoietic stem cells; FGF23, fibroblast growth factor 23, CNS, central nervous system; PTH, parathyroid hormone; 1,25(OH)$_2$-D3, 1,25, dihydroxycholecalciferol:

bone mass/structure was first reported by Wolff (Wolff, 1870) and was later termed "the mechanostat" (Frost, 1996, 1987).

Interestingly, bone cells are also controlled by signaling molecules in the peripheral and central nervous system such as catecholamines and serotonin (Karsenty and Yadav, 2011), and by bacteria in the gastrointestinal tract (Sjogren et al., 2012; Ohlsson and Sjogren 2018). One mechanism by which gut microbiota can affect the skeleton is through regulation of sex steroids. Thus, germ-free mice are resistant to bone loss induced by sex steroid withdrawal (Li et al., 2016). Gut microbiota also influence androgen metabolism in the intestine resulting in extremely high levels of free dihydrotestosterone, the most potent androgen, in colon (Colldén et al., 2019). In addition to the endocrine and paracrine regulation, mechanical loading is important for bone cell activities and bone mass (Price et al., 2011; Klein-Nulend et al., 2012). Thus, the cells in bone integrate a wide variety of signaling molecules which act in concert to regulate physiological and pathophysiological bone metabolism.

In recent years it has become evident that bone might be an endocrine organ in itself (Karsenty and Oury, 2012). Deletion of the osteocalcin gene in mice, thought to play an important role for mineralization of extracellular matrix proteins, does not result in any major defects in the skeleton, but the mice become fat and hyperglycemic (Lee et al., 2007). Thus, it seems that osteocalcin is a hormone with effects on adipocytes and β-cells in the pancreas, rather than being important for bone formation. Moreover, fibroblast growth factor-23 (FGF-23), which takes part in phosphate metabolism in the kidneys, is expressed by osteocytes and, therefore, is another example of a hormone produced by bone cells (Hu et al., 2013). In addition, it was recently shown that osteocytes also regulate cells in fat and thymus, as mice without osteocytes display lymphopenia and a complete loss of white adipose tissue (Sato et al., 2013). A new loading-dependent mechanism regulating body weight mediated through osteocytes, the "gravitostat", has recently been discovered (Jansson et al., 2018). Thus, bone cells regulate not only bone, but also other tissues such as adipose tissue in many ways, but this is beyond the scope of this chapter.

As we grow, bone mass increases and reaches its peak (peak bone mass) after final height is achieved. Individuals with high peak bone mass are less likely to get osteoporosis and fractures later in life. The adult skeleton is not static tissue but is rebuilt continuously by two different processes called modeling and remodeling (Martin and Seeman, 2008). Modeling of bone is a process that changes the size and shape of bone either by bone resorption without subsequent bone formation or by bone formation without prior bone resorption. Remodeling of bone is the process by which old bone is replaced by new bone. It starts by formation of osteoclasts, which resorb the old, damaged bone, and is followed by osteoblasts filling in the resorption lacuna with new bone. This process does not change the size or shape of the bones. When the amount of new bone formed is equal to that which is being resorbed, bone remodeling is in balance and bone mass is preserved. Remodeling takes place on surfaces of cancellous and cortical bones, as well as within cortical bone in the Haversian canals. It is more frequent in cancellous bone, which is the reason why metabolic bone diseases like osteoporosis mainly affect bones containing cancellous bone, like the vertebrae, distal radius, and proximal femur. It is not known in detail how osteoclasts can recognize damaged bone, but remodeling is believed to be initiated by osteocytes sensing microcracks in the mineralized bone extracellular matrix, resulting in osteocyte apoptosis, which triggers osteoclast formation and resorption of the microdamaged bone (Martin and Seeman, 2008).

Recent observations indicate that remodeling takes place under a canopy of inactive osteoblasts on the bone surface called bone lining cells (Martin et al., 2009). When the osteoclasts finish resorbing bone, osteoblasts are recruited to form new bone and, therefore, remodeling of bone has long been regarded as a coupled process. The coupling factors are not known although several locally produced signaling molecules, produced by the osteoclasts or released from bone matrix during the resorption, have been suggested to play a role (Sims and Martin, 2020). Remodeling takes place in a defined unit and engages both bone-forming and resorbing cells. The unit is called a bone multicellular unit (BMU). It is estimated that $1-2 \times 10^6$ of such BMUs are present throughout the entire skeleton under normal conditions and that 10% of the adult skeleton is remodeled each year. In estrogen deficiency, the number of BMUs is dramatically enhanced, which, together with reduced capacity of osteoblasts to refill the numerous resorption lacunae, is the reason why bone is lost in postmenopausal osteoporosis.

The effect of orthodontic treatment on the jawbone is often called remodeling. It has similarities to inflammation-induced bone remodeling. It is, however, probably improper to characterize these processes as remodeling (see above for definition), and the responses in bone surrounding tooth roots targeted for orthodontic loading should rather be called modeling to reshape the bone.

Osteoblast/osteocyte differentiation and function

Osteoblast differentiation

Osteoblasts are derived from mesenchymal stem cells, which are similar to pluripotent stromal cells in bone marrow, giving rise to osteoblasts, osteocytes, chondrocytes, adipocytes, fibroblasts, tenocytes, muscle cells, and endothelial cells (Knothe Tate et al., 2008). Stromal cells in bone marrow are the most closely related progenitors and are likely to be the cells from which endosteal osteoblasts on cancellous and endocortical bone are derived. Whether periosteal osteoblasts are also derived from these cells is more uncertain.

Differentiated osteoblasts are the cells that form new bone, and at the same time are crucial for differentiation of bone-resorbing osteoclasts (reviewed in Lerner, 2000). It is thus an intricate balance in the regulation of osteoblasts as anabolic cells versus their role as procatabolic cells. Parathyroid hormone was the first hormone shown to stimulate osteoclast formation, and patients with hyperparathyroidism suffer from hypercalcemia and secondary osteoporosis. However, if patients with osteoporosis are treated with intermittent administration of the same hormone, bone mass will increase due to enhanced bone formation. This is because the receptors for parathyroid hormone are present on osteoblasts, and that robust stimulation causes the osteoblasts to increase osteoclast formation, whereas mild activation enhances their bone-forming activity. The intracellular mechanisms responsible for these two different events are not fully understood. These circumstances have a large impact on the strategies to find specific anabolic parathyroid hormone-mimicking drugs causing enhanced bone mass.

Regulation of osteoblast differentiation is controlled by expression of transcription factors which are intracellular proteins binding to promoter regions of genes. Many of the transcription factors involved in osteoblast differentiation are also involved in differentiation of other cells. Two of these have been shown to be crucial for osteoblasts. Runt-related transcription factor-2 (*Runx2*), also called core binding factor α1 (*cbfa1*), and osterix, are necessary for osteoblast differentiation. This was demonstrated by the observations that mice that are deficient of both alleles in either *Runx2* or *Osterix* die, because they cannot form any bone tissue although they make a normal cartilaginous skeleton during embryonic life (Ducy *et al.*, 1997). These molecules are not expressed in early osteoblast progenitors but need to be expressed in the more differentiated osteoblasts. Mice lacking one of the two alleles for *Runx2* have a phenotype similar to patients with *Dysostosis cleidocranialis* and it was later shown that these patients have mutations in the *RUNX2* gene (Zhou *et al.*, 1999).

Osteoblasts as bone-forming cells

Osteoblasts make bone in a two-step process, which starts with formation of the extracellular matrix. The next step is the deposition of mineral crystals in this matrix. Not all parts of the matrix are mineralized and a zone most close to the osteoblasts remains unmineralized and is called the osteoid. The main protein in the matrix is type I collagen, which consists of a triple helix formed by two α1 subunits and one α2 subunit. Many collagen type I molecules form the collagen fiber, which is the dominating constituent of bone extracellular matrix. During bone resorption, collagen degradation products such as carboxy-terminal collagen crosslinks (CTX) are released and can be measured in serum as parameters reflecting the degree of bone resorption. Osteoblasts also make other proteins, which are deposited in the matrix. Several of them are proteins produced also by other cells, but osteocalcin and bone sialoprotein are believed to be specific for bone and thus anticipated to be involved in mineralization. It was, therefore, expected that mice lacking osteocalcin would exhibit defects in their skeleton. As mentioned above, the skeleton was rather normal, but the mice showed a phenotype similar to patients with the metabolic syndrome, indicating that osteocalcin might be a hormone (Lee *et al.*, 2007). There are also other hormone-like proteins in the matrix, which are rather abundant in bone, such as transforming growth factor-β (TGF-β), insulin-like growth factors (IGFs) and bone morphogenetic proteins (BMPs). It is assumed that these proteins are released intact during the resorption process and function as autocrine factors stimulating osteoblasts during remodeling.

How osteoblasts form hydroxyapatite crystals, and how the crystals are deposited in the matrix, remains elusive. The enzyme alkaline phosphatase is likely to play a role because active osteoblasts express large amounts of this enzyme and mice with deletion of the gene encoding this enzyme have disturbances in their mineralization (Wennberg *et al.*, 2000). Analysis of serum levels of alkaline phosphatase serves as an indicator of bone formation in patients with skeletal disorders.

Besides the findings that intermittent parathyroid hormone, and proteins in the TGF-β superfamily like TGF-β1, BMPs, activins, inhibins, and myostatin, can regulate osteoblast activities, knowledge of how bone formation is regulated is sparse. However, in recent years much attention has been paid to the role of the Wnt/Frizzled signaling system (Baron and Kneissel, 2013; Lerner and Ohlsson, 2015, and references therein). The Wnt/Frizzled signaling system is made up of the cell membrane co-receptor lipoprotein receptor-related protein (Lrp5), which dimerizes with the signaling subunit Frizzled in the presence of the ligand Wnt (Figure 7.2(a)). This system was first found to be important for bone when it was discovered that patients in some families with high bone mass had a gain-of-function mutation in the *LRP5* gene. In addition, patients with osteoporosis pseudoglioma syndrome, exhibiting low bone mass, have a loss-of-function mutation in the same gene. In humans, 10 Frizzleds and 19 different Wnts have been found and it is not known which of those components are crucial for bone formation. Several different inhibitors exist, one being sclerostin which binds to Lrp5 and inhibits the association to Frizzled (Figure 7.2(b)). Patients with van Buchem's disease or with sclerostosis have extremely high bone mass, which is explained by loss-of-function mutations in the gene *SOST* encoding sclerostin. Interestingly, and important from a bone biology point of view, *SOST* seems to be specifically expressed by osteocytes and is found to be involved in the mechanisms by which load stimulates bone formation (Figure 7.2(c), see further later). Antibodies neutralizing sclerostin have been developed and found to decrease bone loss due to estrogen deficiency. Two phase III studies using the humanized antibody romosozumab have been performed (Cosman *et al.* 2016; Saag *et al.* 2017). These studies showed that 12-month treatment decreased new vertebral fractures in postmenopausal women by 48% and 75%, respectively, with no or less effect on non-vertebral fractures. Although the treatment increased the numbers of serious cardiovascular adverse effects in one of the studies (Cosman *et al.* 2016), the drug is now approved in USA and EU.

Osteoblasts as regulators of osteoclast formation

It was unexpectedly found (McSheehy and Chambers, 1986) that the receptors for well-known stimulators of bone resorption like parathyroid hormone and 1,25(OH)$_2$-vitamin D3 were not present in osteoclasts or their progenitors, but in osteoblasts (reviewed in Lerner, 2000). Since then it has been found that receptors for most hormones and cytokines stimulating osteoclast formation are expressed by osteoblasts, as initially hypothesized by Rodan and Martin (1982). More recent work has revealed that osteoclasts are in their turn capable of affecting osteoblastogenesis through secretion of several different signaling molecules (Henriksen *et al.*, 2014). Differentiation of osteoclast progenitors depends on expression of receptor activator of nuclear factor κB ligand (RANKL) by

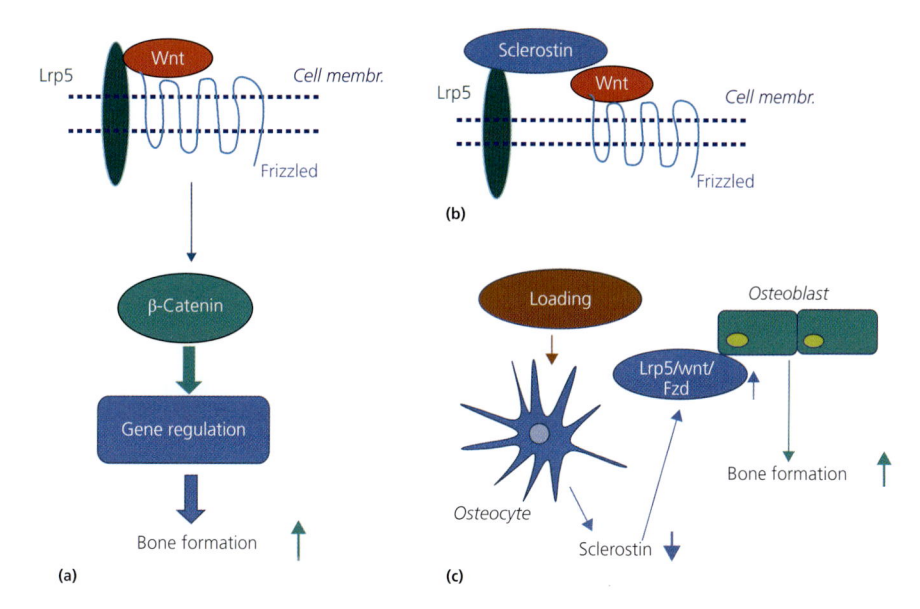

Figure 7.2 The canonical Wnt signaling pathway is involved in bone formation. (a) In the presence of the ligand Wnt, the co-receptor Lrp5 and the signaling receptor Frizzled form a complex in osteoblasts leading to activation of the transcription factor β-catenin, which is important for bone formation. (b) This receptor can be inactivated by several extracellular molecules, one being sclerostin, which binds to Lrp5 and inhibits Lrp5 binding to Frizzled and, thereby, bone formation is decreased. (c) Sclerostin is specifically expressed in osteocytes and its expression is downregulated by loading, which may be a mechanism by which loading enhances bone formation.

osteoblasts, which binds to the cognate receptor RANK on osteoclast progenitors. RANK signaling is the most crucial event for the progenitors to differentiate along the osteoclastic lineage (see further later). RANKL is expressed on the surface of osteoblasts, and osteoclastogenesis, therefore, requires cell-to-cell contact between osteoblasts and osteoclast progenitors. The activation of RANK is depressed by osteoprotegerin (OPG), which binds to RANKL and inhibits its binding to RANK. Therefore, the relative expression of RANKL/OPG is rate limiting in osteoclastogenesis. These observations demonstrate that osteoblasts are not only bone-forming cells, but also crucial for osteoclast formation. Antibodies neutralizing RANKL are currently used for treatment of patients with excessive osteoclast formation.

Osteocytes

Osteocytes are nonproliferative and terminally differentiated cells of the osteoblast lineage present in lacunae within cortical and cancellous bone. These cells have characteristic, nerve-like cell extensions through which they communicate with each other, and with similar extensions from osteoblasts on bone surfaces. They also communicate with osteoclasts by secretion of molecules (reviewed in Bonewald, 2017). Osteocytes reside near each other and are the most common bone cells, making up more than 95% of the bone cell number (Noble, 2008; extensively reviewed in Dallas et al., 2013). Thus, extracellular matrix in bone exhibits an extensive network of osteocytic/osteoblastic/osteoclastic communication, through which osteocytes are believed to orchestrate osteoblast and osteoclast activity.

Osteocytes as bone-remodeling cells

Osteocytes, like their predecessors osteoblasts, are able to form bone in their peri-lacunar matrix as visualized by fluorescent labeling using markers of mineralization like tetracycline. Little is known about the regulation of the bone-forming capacity of osteocytes, but recent studies have shown that it is dependent on matrix metalloproteinase-13 (MMP-13) and the parathyroid hormone type-1 receptor (O'Brien et al., 2008; Tang et al., 2012).

In the event of a microcrack appearing, the osteocytes enter apoptosis, releasing apoptotic bodies that initiate osteoclast recruitment and bone resorption (Noble et al., 2003; Kogianni et al., 2008). Recently, it has been found that osteocytes, or late osteoblasts soon to become osteocytes, not only express the main regulator of osteoclastogenesis, RANKL, but are the main RANKL-expressing cells in bone (see later). Osteocytes also express osteoclast proteins, for example RANK, cathepsin K, and MMPs, and it is suggested that the osteocytes themselves can resorb bone to adjust their canaliculi (see Noble, 2008; Bonewald, 2011 and references therein). The resorptive activity of osteocytes is enhanced during lactation when the calcium demand is high (Qing et al., 2012). Both bone mass and bone resorption-associated genes, such as *Acp5* (encoding the enzyme tartrate resistant acid phosphatase, TRAP) and *Ctsk* (encoding the collagen degrading enzyme cathepsin K), return to normal after weaning. These observations have led to revitalization of the idea of osteocytic osteolysis (Bonewald, 2011).

Osteocytes regulate phosphate and mineralization homeostasis through expression of X-linked phosphate-regulating neutral endopeptidase (Phex/Pex), dentin matrix protein 1 (DMP-1), matrix extracellular phosphoglycoprotein (MEPE), and FGF-23 (Bonewald, 2007; Rowe, 2012). The exact function of the metalloproteinase Phex is not clear, but it seems to be involved in both phosphate homeostasis and mineralization because deletion, or loss of function, of Phex leads to X-linked hypophosphatemic rickets (HYP/XLH). Interestingly, deletion of DMP-1 in mice also leads to hypophosphatemic rickets. FGF23 is released into the circulation by the osteocytes, leading to enhanced phosphate excretion by the kidney, and thereby reduced circulating phosphate. It has therefore been proposed that osteocytes can function as endocrine cells. Thus, the osteocytes seem to be able not only to recruit osteoclasts, or adjust their own lacunar and canalicular compartment, but they might also take an active part in mineral metabolism. Considering the large bone surface facing osteocytes, compared with the bone surface facing osteoblasts and osteoclasts, and their role in FGF23-signaling, the role of osteocytes have previously most likely been underestimated in bone metabolism as well as in phosphate and calcium homeostasis.

Osteocytes as mechano-sensory cells

The osteocyte network is important for sensing mechanical load on bone. Mice lacking osteocytes are insensitive to unloading (Tatsumi et al., 2007). The exact mechanism through which the osteocytes sense load is not fully established, but ciliae on the osteocytes respond to mechanical stimuli, and so-called mechano-sensory membrane channels, for example connexin 43, also respond to strain/loading. Moreover, osteocytes respond to mechanical load through membrane-bound receptors, for example the insulin-like growth factor receptors (IGF-1R, see Noble, 2008 and below).

Osteoclast differentiation and function

Osteoclasts are the main cells in nature able to resorb bone. The reason is that bone must be demineralized before the matrix is accessible for matrix degrading enzymes, and it is the capacity to produce acid in a closed milieu (the resorption lacuna) that provides the osteoclasts with the unique ability to resorb bone. Therefore, physiological and pathological remodeling and modeling of bone requires osteoclasts. Thus, loss of bone in periodontal disease does not take place unless osteoclasts are formed locally in the periodontium. Similarly, modeling of bone during orthodontic tooth movement (OTM) requires local formation of osteoclasts.

Osteoclast differentiation

Osteoclasts are giant, multinucleated cells, which are formed by fusion of mononucleated osteoclast progenitors derived from hematopoietic tissues. The progenitors belong to the myeloid lineage, and the progenitor cells giving rise to osteoclasts, macrophages, and dendritic cells in the immune system are very closely related. All these cells require stimulation by macrophage colony-stimulating factor (M-CSF), a cytokine expressed by osteoblasts, and by many other cell types. M-CSF is needed for the proliferation and survival of the progenitor cells. As mentioned previously, RANKL is the cytokine which specifically drives the progenitors along the osteoclastic lineage (Figure 7.3(a)). It is expressed by stromal cells in bone marrow and osteoblasts at the bone surfaces. The expression of RANKL can also be induced in fibroblasts from synovial tissues and from periodontal ligament, whereas gingival fibroblasts seem not to express RANKL. During physiological bone remodeling, RANKL is predominantly expressed by osteocytes/late osteoblasts (Nakashima et al., 2011; Xiong et al., 2011).

Effects of RANKL are counterbalanced by OPG acting extracellularly by binding to RANKL (Nakashima et al., 2012). Thus, OPG

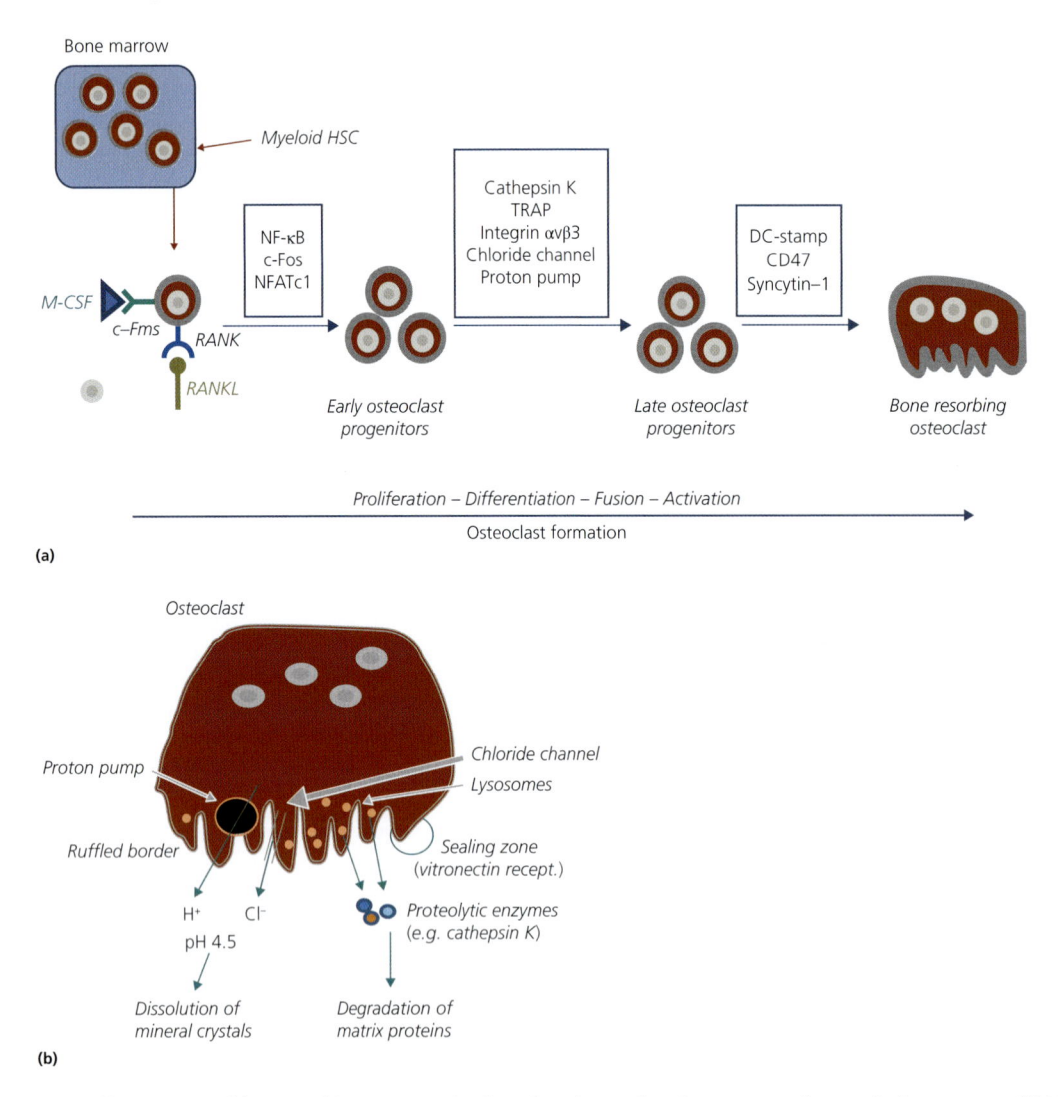

Figure 7.3 Osteoclast differentiation and function. (a) Formation of multinucleated osteoclasts from mononuclear myeloid progenitors. (b) Mature osteoclasts are attached to bone through αvβ3-expressing vitronectin receptors and in the sealing zone. Osteoclasts form the ruffled border in which proton pump subunits and a chloride channel pump are present. These pumps are important for hydroxyapatite crystal dissolution. Lysosomes releasing proteolytic enzymes involved in bone matrix degradation are also abundant in the ruffled border.

is a soluble decoy receptor in the TNF receptor superfamily. Osteoprotegerin is expressed by osteoblasts and stromal cells in bone marrow and most hormones and cytokines stimulating osteoclastogenesis not only increase RANKL but also decrease OPG and, thereby, increase the RANKL/OPG ratio. Because of the crucial role of RANKL/RANK/OPG in osteoclast formation, antibodies have been developed neutralizing RANKL. Treatment of patients with osteoporosis by injections of humanized anti-RANKL antibodies twice per year results in increased bone mass and reduced number of fractures (Sinningen et al., 2012). RANKL is a member of the TNF superfamily and RANK, as well as OPG, are members of the TNF receptor superfamily.

For differentiation of osteoclast progenitors to mature osteoclasts, not only is activation of the receptors for RANKL and M-CSF important, but also activation of co-stimulatory immunoglobulin-like receptors present on the surface of the progenitor cells. These receptors are heterodimeric complexes made up by the ligand-binding domain OSCAR and the signal-transducing component FcRγ and by the ligand-binding domain TREM-2 and its signaling partner DAP12. Compound gene deletion, but not single deletion, of FcRγ and DAP12 results in lack of osteoclasts and a high bone mass phenotype, demonstrating a redundancy of the osteoclastogenic importance. For an extensive review of osteoclast differentiation see Guerrini and Takayangi (2014).

It is most likely that local RANKL expression is the reason for osteoclast formation during tooth movement. Thus, compressive force to co-cultures of human periodontal ligament cells and peripheral blood monocytes results in increased osteoclast formation and enhanced RANKL mRNA and protein expression, effects decreased by inhibition of prostaglandin production (Kanzaki et al., 2002). The pressure/compression areas of OTM in humans is associated with increased RANKL and decreased OPG in the gingival crevicular fluid 24 hours after initiation of force (Nishijima et al., 2006). The fact that tooth movement and osteoclast formation in the periodontium are enhanced in mice deficient of OPG (Oshiro et al., 2002) argues for the role of RANKL in orthodontically induced osteoclastogenesis. Furthermore, local injection of a plasmid expressing OPG decreases OTM and osteoclast formation in rats (Kanzaki et al., 2004). Interestingly, a similar treatment has also been found to inhibit relapse of OTM (Zhao et al., 2012). Indirect evidence for the view that RANKL/RANK/OPG signaling is important for orthodontically induced osteoclastogenesis is also provided by the observations that increased RANKL mRNA in periodontal ligament, and enhanced RANKL protein in periodontal fibroblasts, have been reported in rats during OTM (Garlet et al., 2007; Brooks et al., 2009). Further evidence is the report that local gene transfer of RANKL enhances osteoclast formation and OTM (Kanzaki et al., 2006). The crucial role of RANKL produced by periodontal ligament cells for OTM has recently been shown using tamoxifen-induced genetic deletion of the gene encoding RANKL (*Tnfsf11*) in mice in which the Cre recombinase was driven by the osteoblast-specific promoter for the *Col1a1* gene (Yang et al., 2018). The tooth movement caused by an orthodontic force in these mice was completely inhibited. However, the mechanism(s) by which RANKL is induced by orthodontic treatment is unknown. One possibility might be formation of microcracks and osteocytic RANKL expression caused by the load, similar to the events causing physiological remodeling of bone. Another possibility may be local inflammation and production of prostaglandins induced by cytokines in periodontal ligament cells (reviewed in Lerner, 2012), maybe in concert with bradykinin and thrombin (Marklund et al., 1994; Ransjo et al., 1998), subsequently stimulating RANKL expression. Other regulatory mechanisms shown recently to regulate RANKL during OTM are GDF15 (growth differentiation factor 15) produced by periodontal ligament cells (Li et al., 2020) and micro RNA-21 (Wu et al., 2020).

Osteoclast function

Osteoclasts attach to bone surfaces by binding of vitronectin receptors (αvβ3 integrin), expressed on the osteoclast cell membrane, to RGD sequences in bone matrix proteins such as osteopontin or bone sialoprotein (Figure 7.3(b), Vaananen and Laitala-Leinonen, 2008). This attachment forms a sealing zone surrounding the active resorption area exhibiting a characteristic ruffled border. In this ruffled border, osteoclasts express a proton pump, which together with a chloride channel, facilitates release of hydrochloric acid into the Howship´s resorption lacunae. Mineral crystals are thereby dissolved, and bone matrix proteins will become accessible for proteolytic enzymes, which are also released into the lacuna. It is not known exactly which enzymes are involved, but cathepsin K is known to play a crucial role.

Osteoclast-dependent factors important for osteoblast stimulation during bone remodeling

Physiological bone remodeling is a process important for the maintenance of a healthy skeleton in adults. It is a process in which damaged bone is substituted by new bone without any change in bone mass or shape. It takes place at the surfaces of trabecular and endocortical bone and in the Haversian canals present in cortical bone. The remodeling process is initiated by formation of osteoclasts in the area with damaged bone followed by resorption of the old bone. The resorption lacunae are subsequently filled in by bone-forming osteoblasts which during healthy conditions form equal amounts of bone to that being removed by resorption in order to keep bone mass constant. These areas are called BMUs and can be found at $1-2 \times 10^6$ different places in the skeleton which are geographically and chronologically separated. The resorption phase takes 3–4 weeks, whereas the formation phase lasts for 3–4 months. It has been estimated that it takes 2–5 years until a new BMU is formed at a place where a BMU has been completed, and that 10% of the skeleton is renewed each year. These circumstances suggest that the cellular activities in BMUs are controlled by local, rather than systemic, factors.

The recruitment and activation of osteoblasts in BMUs are due to factors released during resorption, either from the osteoclasts or from the bone matrix. Osteoclast-derived factors include osteoblast-stimulating factors such as Wnt10b, BMP6, cardiotrophin-1 and sphingosine-1-phosphate, as well as microvesicles containing microRNA. Bone matrix-derived factors include BMP2, TGF-β and IGF-1. Also, factors bound to osteoclast cell membranes such as semaphorin4D and ephrinB2 have been implicated as coupling factors. For an excellent review of bone remodeling and coupling factors, see Sims and Martin (2020).

Sex hormones and their receptors

The sex hormones (estrogens and androgens) derive from cholesterol (Figure 7.4) and are mainly produced in the gonads (ovaries and testes, respectively) and in humans (but not rodents) also in the adrenal cortex (for example dehydroepiandrosterone/DHEA, DHEA-S, and androstenedione). Estrogens can also be synthesized from adrenal androgen precursors in other tissues such as fat, brain,

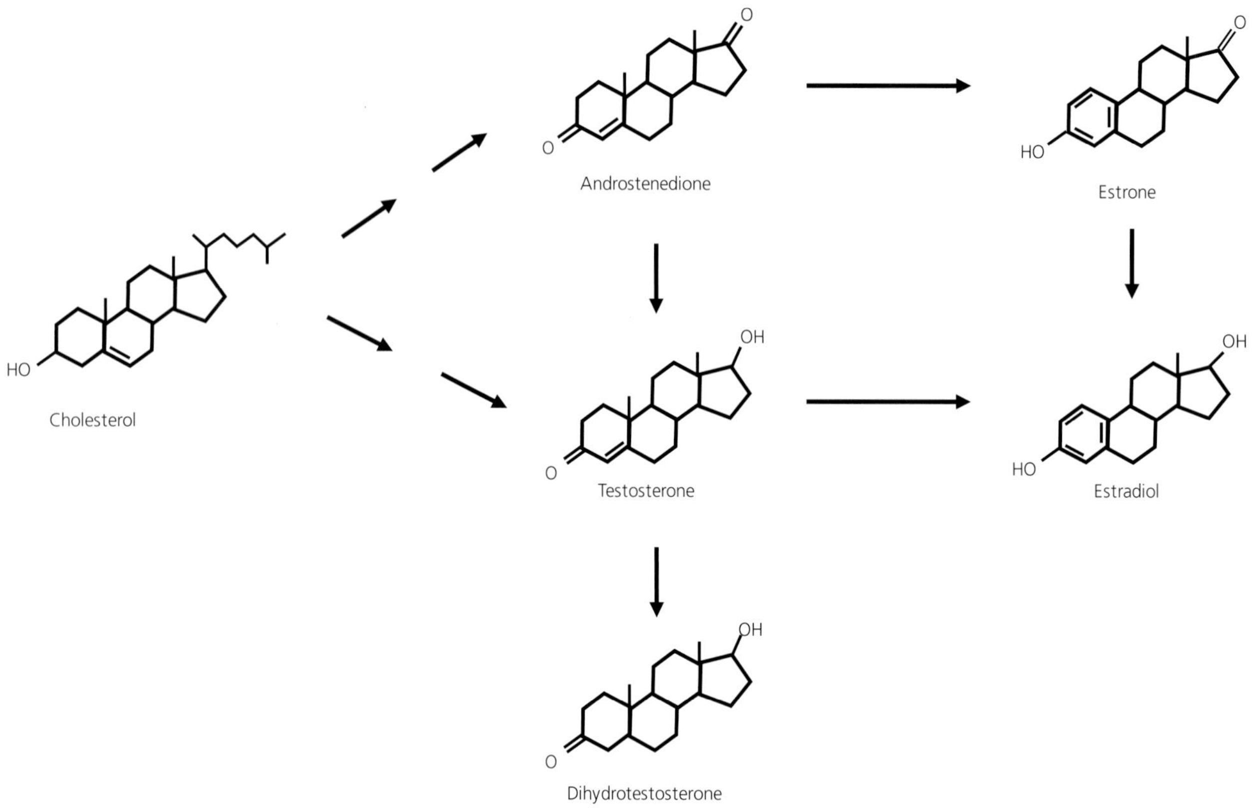

Figure 7.4 Sex steroid synthesis. Cholesterol is, through several steps, converted to androstenedione and testosterone. Androstenedione is a weak androgen and precursor of both the androgen testosterone and the estrogen estrone. The most potent androgen, dihydrotestosterone (DHT), is converted from testosterone, while the most potent estrogen, 17β-estradiol, is converted from both estrone and testosterone.

and bone (Barakat et al., 2016). The production and secretion of the sex hormones are under the control of follicle-stimulating hormone (FSH) and luteinizing hormone (LH) from the brain.

The biological effects of sex hormones are mediated by receptors belonging to the nuclear receptor superfamily of transcription factors. The androgen receptor (AR) is encoded by the androgen receptor gene (*Ar*), and the estrogen receptors (ERs) α and β (ERα and ERβ), are encoded by the *Esr1* and the *Esr2* genes, respectively. The sex-hormone receptors are also expressed as several splice variants, adding complexity to the picture. In male bone, the sex hormones exert their functions through the AR and ERα, while in female bone, estrogen also exerts its function via ERβ to modulate the effects of ERα (Börjesson et al., 2013; Laurent et al., 2014; Almeida et al., 2017). The molecular mechanisms of sex hormone receptors and their involvement in the osteogenic bone response to loading are described in more detail later.

Genomic signaling through sex-hormone receptors in bone

The sex-hormone receptors contain stretches of amino acids called nuclear localization signals, which cooperate in the transfer of the steroid receptors to the nucleus, where they are mainly located in most cells. While in the nucleus, the receptors can be activated by their hormones and by hormone-independent phosphorylation (Figure 7.5). Upon activation in the nucleus, the sex-hormone receptors bind directly to DNA through response elements present in promoter regions of different genes (androgen response element, ARE or estrogen response element, ERE). Interestingly, the sex-hormone receptors can also regulate genes that contain response elements for other transcription factor proteins, e.g., AP-1, SP-1 and NF-κB. By binding to these transcription factors, the sex hormone receptors can recruit co-factors and thereby regulate transcription from the response element of those transcription factors. Due to the DNA binding capacity of the sex hormone receptors and their nuclear localization, most studies so far have focused on the direct transcriptional (genomic) effects of these receptors.

When the sex hormones bind to their receptors, conformational changes within the receptors are induced that enables binding of specific coregulatory factors, such as SRC 1-3 and NCoR. Upon DNA binding, the sex hormone receptors regulate transcription via direct contact with the general transcription machinery and/or indirectly by binding coregulatory factors bridging to the general transcription machinery (Figure 7.5). Depending on the coregulators bound, transcription is either enhanced or inhibited.

Non-genomic signaling by sex-hormone receptors

In addition to the well-known transcriptional regulatory activity of the sex hormone receptors, data describing the so-called non-genomic effects of sex-hormone receptors have accumulated. The sex-hormone receptors are phosphoproteins. Thus, growth factors such as epidermal growth factor and IGF-1, cAMP and protein kinase A (PKA) activators have been shown to be involved in the activation of the sex-hormone receptors by phosphorylating the receptors in the absence of hormones (Figure 7.5). Although controversial, evidence is accumulating that the sex-hormone

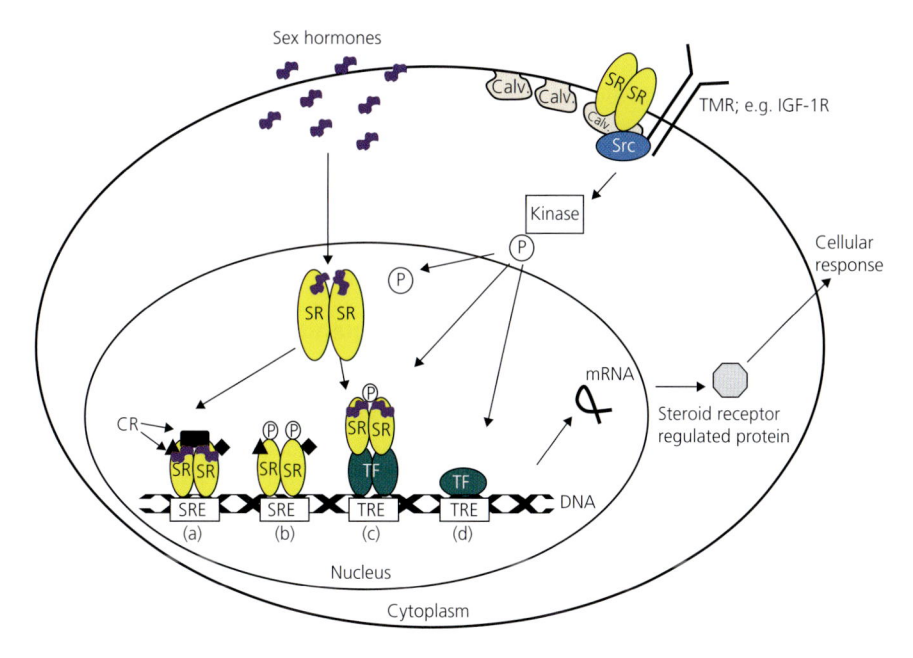

Figure 7.5 Sex-hormone signaling pathways. The sex-hormone receptors (SR) can be activated by either (A) hormone binding or by (B) phosphorylation (P). Upon activation, the SRs regulate gene transcription by binding to their different response element (SRE) and to several coregulators (CR). This SR-coregulator complex targets the transcriptional initiation machinery and, thereby, regulates transcription of mRNA and subsequent translation of steroid receptor regulated proteins and finally a cellular response. (C) The SRs can also bind to transcription factors (TF), and, thereby, regulate gene transcription from their response elements (TRE). Although still controversial, the steroid receptors also seem to be located at the cell membrane together with calveolae (Calv.) and from there they interact physically with transmembrane receptors (TMR), e.g., growth factor receptors such as insulin like growth factor 1 receptor (IGF-1R). The SRs are thus also involved in signaling cascades such as phosphorylation cascades through kinases acting upon the SR themselves and/or (D) other transcription factors. Thus, the SRs can regulate gene transcription by at least four different pathways (A–D).

receptors not only reside in the nucleus but also in the cytoplasm and at the cell membrane within calveoli that are suggested to serve as mechanotransduction sites within the plasma membrane (Chambliss et al., 2002; Liedert et al., 2006; Bennett et al., 2010). In the presence of estrogen, ERα is de-palmitoylated and thus dissociates from calveolin-1. ERα can then bind to and facilitate signaling from Src and phosphatidylinositide-3-kinase (PI3K). This way, a membrane-bound sex-hormone receptor can physically interact with both the tyrosine kinase Src and IGF-1R to enhance downstream signaling through mitogen activation protein kinase (MAPK), specifically the extracellular signal-regulated kinase ERK1/2. This results in a further stimulation of the steroid receptors themselves, or other transcription factors, by phosphorylation (Figure 7.5). Consistent with this notion, membrane-bound ERs have been shown to mediate ERK activation in osteoblasts and osteocytes in response to strain *in vitro*.

Osteoblasts and osteocytes respond to load-induced modeling

The adult skeleton is continuously rebuilt through modeling to withstand the habitual load that is placed onto it. It is the growth rate, rather than gender, that affects the size of the load-related changes in bone formation in the growing skeleton. When bone is loaded, the first initial phase (within days) involves osteoblast recruitment from nondividing preosteoblasts and/or bone-lining cells (Turner et al., 1998; Zannit and Silva, 2019). Within a week, new osteoblasts formed from proliferation and differentiation of osteoprogenitor cells are also observed (Matthews et al., 2020). Thus, a strong increase in bone formation rate can be seen during the first weeks following loading, which then gradually decreases and becomes normalized in fewer than 6 weeks (Schriefer et al., 2005).

Extensive studies have been performed to delineate the different pathways underlying the bone anabolic effects of loading on a molecular level, revealing the involvement of a wide range of signaling pathways. The response in bone to load can be divided into time-dependent patterns of gene expression; early upregulated genes (within hours, for example AP-1, and cytokines), genes upregulated during matrix formation (within days, for example growth factors, calcium- and Wnt-signaling and matrix proteins) and genes downregulated during matrix formation (for example inhibitors of the Wnt-pathway) (Mantila Roosa et al., 2011).

Load-induced proliferation of bone cells is dependent on ERα and possibly inhibited by ERβ acting independently of estrogen through nongenomic signaling and/or signaling through binding to other transcription factors, such as AP-1. Here we will concentrate on the pathways that are modeled by the sex-hormone receptors in response to load, mainly using data from studies of ERα as a model system involved in the osteogenic response to loading.

Wnt/β-catenin pathway

Loading leads to increased expression of genes coding for proteins involved in the Wnt-pathway, e.g., β-catenin, and to decreased expression of genes coding for proteins inhibiting the Wnt-pathway, e.g., sclerostin and, thus, to enhanced expression of genes associated with bone formation (Figure 7.6(a)). One example of a gene regulated by load through the Wnt-pathway is the extracellular bone matrix protein osteopontin (OPN). The OPN promoter, which contains response elements for the transcription factors

LEF/TCF, is activated by strain through the Wnt-pathway, and is dependent on ERs via hitherto unknown mechanism/s.

ERα is involved in the expression and activity of several stages of the Wnt-pathway in response to load resulting in enhanced osteoblast proliferation and activity (Figure 7.6(a)). First, loading results in upregulation of Frizzled 2 (*Fzd2*), a process involving ERα. Second, strain induces translocation of β-catenin to the nucleus, which also is an effect mediated by ERα. Third, ERα and β-catenin reciprocally enhance the activity of promoters containing their respective DNA-binding sites (Figure 7.6(a)).

ERβ is involved in strain-mediated downregulation of the Wnt inhibitor sclerostin via a kinase-dependent pathway, and thereby further enhances the activity of the Wnt-pathway. In contrast, AR seems to inhibit the strain-mediated downregulation of sclerostin, which in part can explain the finding that the cortical osteogenic effects of loading are enhanced in the absence of the AR.

IGF-1 pathway

Growth hormone and IGF-1 are important determinants of bone formation and resorption, bone mass, and bone size (reviewed in Kopchick et al., 2014). The osteogenic effects of loading are dependent on local osteoblast- and osteocyte-derived IGF-1, but independent on serum IGF-1.

Strain mediates activation of the IGF-I receptor (IGF-IR) through an ERα-dependent pathway. This leads to activation and nuclear translocation of β-catenin and activation of promoters such as the OPN promoter and enhanced bone formation (Figure 7.6(b)). The mechanism for this is unclear, but it is possible that mechanical strain "primes" ERα via hitherto unidentified mechanisms to interact with and activate the IGF-IR by enhancing the phosphorylation of IGF-1R. This activation then results in initiation of a phosphorylation cascade including a PI3K/Akt-dependent activation of β-catenin and altered gene regulation, which in turn results in increased bone formation (Sunters et al., 2010; Windahl et al., 2013b).

Mechanical loading also inhibits apoptosis through an IGF-I/Akt-dependent pathway (Figure 7.6(b)). Since ERα is known to interact physically with IGF-1, as well as to regulate Akt (Simoncini et al., 2002; Yu et al., 2013), it is possible that ERα can regulate load-induced inhibition of apoptosis of osteoblasts and osteocytes via this pathway. It is not known if AR can affect the bone anabolic effects of loading through the IGF-1-pathway.

Nitric oxide signaling

In response to fluid shear stress, membrane-bound endothelial cell nitric oxide synthase (ecNOS) produces nitric oxide (NO), which has a positive effect on bone mass by acting on osteocytes, osteoblasts, and osteoclasts. Osteoblast proliferation is decreased, while osteoblast differentiation is increased by NO, thereby resulting in enhanced bone formation (Figure 7.6(c)). In situations of low strain, osteocyte apoptosis is increased due to low levels of NO (Burger et al., 2003; Ford et al., 2014). This results in enhanced osteoclast recruitment and resorption.

In contrast, during high strain, osteocyte apoptosis is inhibited by a high NO concentration (Liedert et al., 2006). The high NO concentration also promotes osteoclast retraction and detachment, thereby inhibiting bone resorption. The capability of NO to decrease RANKL and increase OPG expression (Fan et al., 2004) could, at least in part, explain the decrease in osteoclast activity and increase in bone formations seen in response to NO stimulation. The mechanisms underlying the NO-induced osteoclast retraction and detachments need to be investigated further.

The rapid increase in NO production by osteoblasts and osteocytes by load/strain is dependent on ERα, but not AR (Figure 7.6(c); Jessop et al., 2004; Callewaert et al., 2010). Thus, ERs exert anabolic effects on bone by increasing NO production. However, strain-mediated release of NO can be inhibited by AR-dependent testosterone treatment *in vitro*. It is still unclear if AR by itself can inhibit the osteogenic effects of loading by inhibiting NO release.

Prostaglandin pathway

Cyclooxygenase-2 (Cox-2) is a membrane-bound enzyme that catalyzes the conversion of arachidonic acid to prostaglandins (e.g., PGE_2) and is enhanced in response to inflammation and loading. Mechanical stimulation of osteoblast cells leads to activation of Cox-2/PGE_2-signaling *in vivo* and *in vitro*, resulting in a bone anabolic effect (Figure 7.6(d)).

Strain-mediated upregulation of *Cox-2* mRNA is not dependent on AR, nor is it affected by testosterone (Callewaert et al., 2010). In contrast, ERα has the possibility to regulate Cox-2 mediated synthesis of PGE_2 at different levels (Figure 7.6(d)). First, Cox-2, like ERα, interacts with calveolin-1 at the cell membrane, facilitating the possibility for a direct interaction of ERα with *Cox-2*. Second, the *Cox-2* promoter itself contains AP-1 and NF-κB-sites that can be regulated by the ERs, thereby providing another possibility for ERs to regulate Cox-2 dependent activation of bone formation (Kang et al., 2007; Liedert et al., 2010).

In conclusion, when bone is loaded, osteoblasts are recruited from nondividing preosteoblasts and/or bone-lining cells. This is followed by proliferation and differentiation of preosteoblasts and a subsequent increase in bone formation. The response in bone to load can be divided into time-dependent patterns of gene expression; early upregulated genes, genes upregulated during matrix formation, and genes downregulated during matrix formation. The sex-hormone receptors are involved in the cellular response to load/strain through a complex mesh of signaling pathways including among others, the *Wnt* and IGF-1 pathways. These signals result in enhanced differentiation and activation, and reduced apoptosis, of osteoblasts and osteocytes, leading to increased bone formation and bone strength.

Loading-induced anabolic response and vitamin A

The biologically active form of vitamin A is all-*trans*-retinoic acid (ATRA), which is formed in the body by conversion of retinyl esters and carotenoids provided by food intake. ATRA is bound to nuclear receptors in target cells called retinoic acid receptors (RARs) which form heterodimers with closely related retinoic X receptors (RXRs). The complex acts as ligand-dependent transcription factor regulating transcription of a wide variety of genes. Hypervitaminosis A is most well known as a risk factor for secondary osteoporosis due to stimulation of cortical bone resorption (Conaway et al. 2013; Henning et al. 2015). We have recently shown that vitamin A in clinically relevant doses causes decreased cortical bone mass not only by increased bone resorption but also by decreased bone formation (Lionikaite et al., 2018). Surprisingly, such doses of vitamin A were found to abolish new bone formation induced by loading through a mechanism which could be attributed to both decreased osteoblast numbers and activity (Lionikaite et al., 2019). These observations suggest the possibility that vitamin A may influence the rate of OTM.

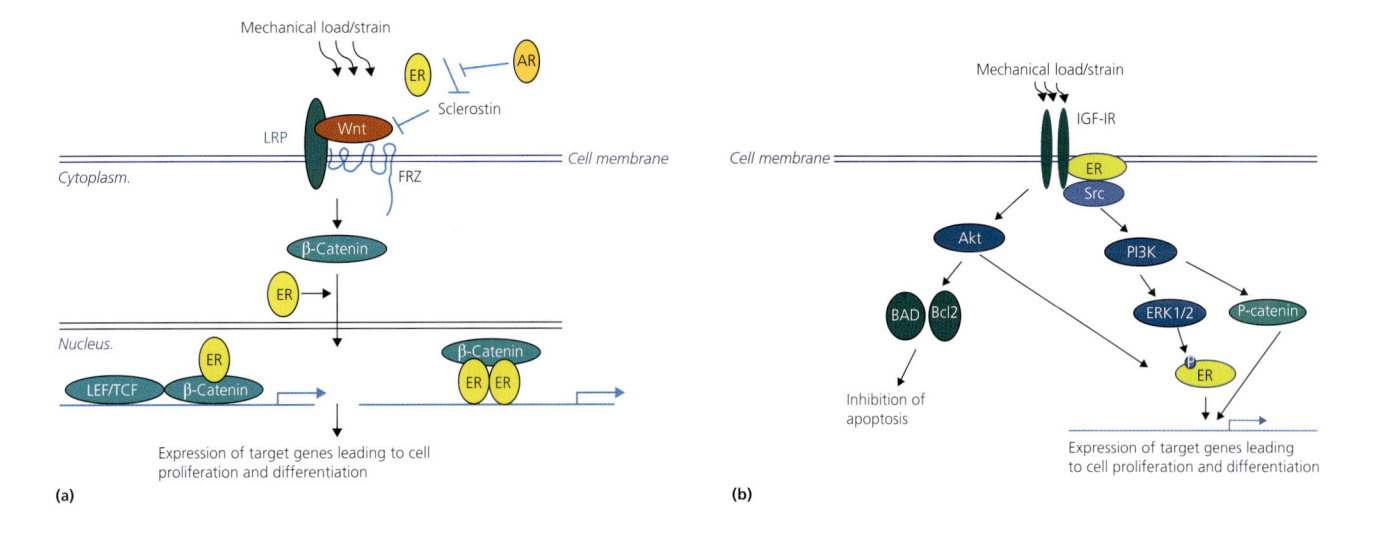

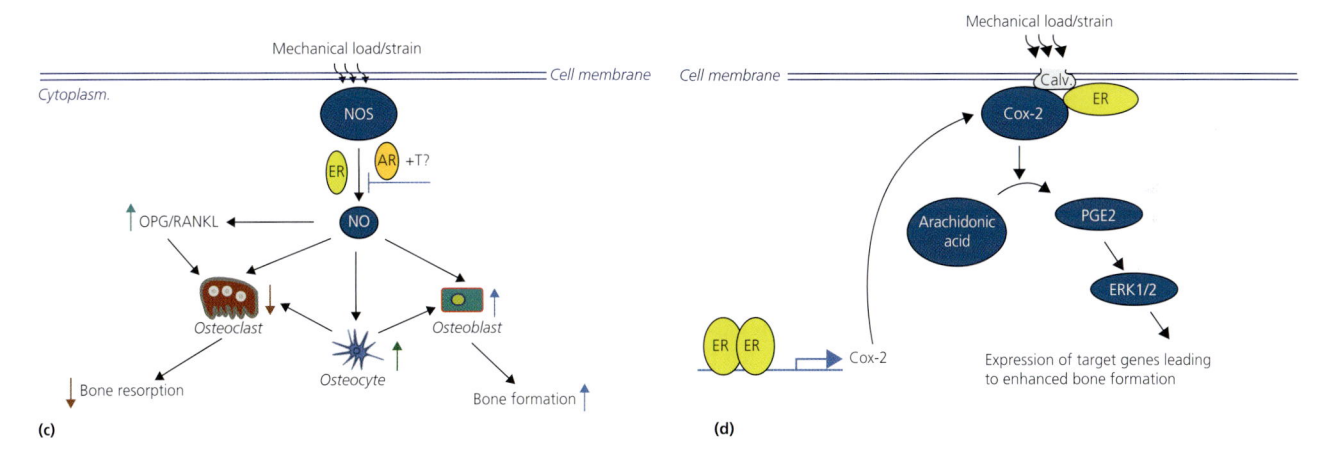

Figure 7.6 Pathways involved in sex hormone receptor mediated bone anabolic response to strain. (a) Mechanical load/strain activates the canonical Wnt-signaling pathway and an ERα-dependent translocation of β-catenin to the nucleus. (b) Mechanical load/strain also enhances osteoblast proliferation and differentiation by activating the IGF-1 receptor through unknown mechanism/s. (c) Mechanical load/strain leads to activation of nitric oxide synthase (NOS), and consequently to an increase in nitric oxide (NO). High concentrations of NO inhibit osteocyte apoptosis, enabling osteocytes to regulate both osteoclast and osteoblast activity. (d) Mechanical load/strain leads, in an ER-dependent manner, to an activation of COX-2 resulting in increased synthesis of prostaglandins, e.g., PGE_2, and subsequent activation of an ERK-1/2 mediated phosphorylation cascade and enhanced gene regulation and bone formation. IGF-1R, insulin-like growth factor 1 receptor; LRP, lipoprotein receptor-related protein; FRZ, frizzled; ER, estrogen receptor; LEF, lymphoid enhancer-binding factor; TCF, transcription factor.

Osteoclast response to load-induced modeling

The involvement of osteoclasts in load-induced bone modeling is currently not sufficiently investigated, but seems to involve both direct effects on preosteoclasts, and indirect effects via osteocytes stimulating preosteoclast recruitment from the bone marrow and their differentiation into mature bone-resorbing osteoclasts. As described in the section on NO-signaling above, osteocytes are suggested to regulate osteoclast differentiation and activity in response to altered strain on the skeleton, and, thereby, mediate an indirect effect of loading/unloading on osteoclasts. In response to mechanical loading *in vitro*, osteocytes not only upregulate NO, but they also upregulate the expression of MEPE. This upregulation results in enhanced OPG expression and inhibition of osteoclastogenesis in response to loading (Figure 7.7; Kulkarni et al., 2010). Consequently, unloading *in vivo* leads to enhanced osteoclast formation due to increased RANKL expression, indicating that osteocytes/osteoblasts enhance osteoclast formation in response to unloading (Lloyd et al., 2013). These data fit well with the net anabolic results seen in long bones in response to loading and unloading.

During OTM, there is pressure on the periodontal ligament, while the adjacent bone surface is being bent by the orthodontic force (becoming convex), which is a signal for bone resorption leading to an increased osteoclast number and activity on the "pressure side." Although stretching *in vitro* of mouse preosteoclasts show that low magnitude strain results in decreased RANK expression and osteoclast cell differentiation; high magnitude strain increases RANK and MMP-9 expression as well as osteoclast cell differentiation (Figure 7.7). Fluid pressure *in vivo* in rats enhances osteoclast recruitment and activation, a process involving enhanced expression of the inflammatory-related genes prostaglandin E synthase (Pges), inducible nitric oxide synthase (iNOS), interleukin 6 (IL-6) and chemokine (C-C motif) ligand (CCL2) in bone (Nilsson

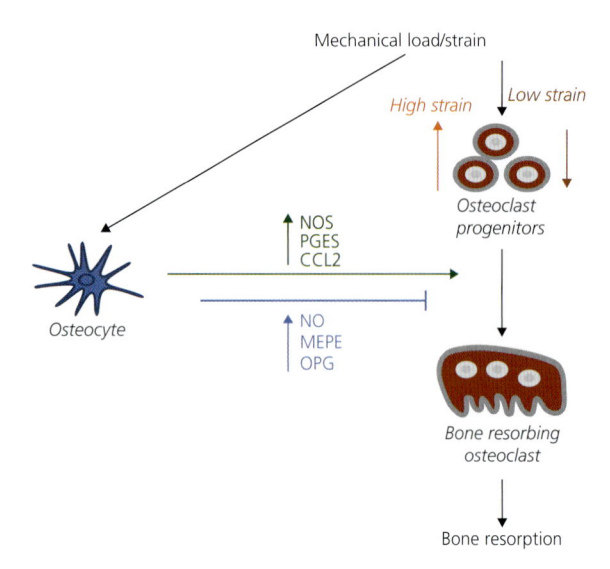

Figure 7.7 Impact of strain on osteoclast formation and activity. Loaded/strained osteocytes increase the expression of nitric oxide (NO), matrix extracellular phosphoglycoprotein (MEPE), and osteoprotegrin (OPG), and, thereby, decrease osteoclast differentiation. NOS, Nitric oxide synthase; PGE, prostaglandin E; CCL2, Chemokine (C-C motif) ligand 2; MEPE, Matrix extracellular phosphoglycoprotein; OPG, Osteoprotegerin.

et al., 2012). Interestingly, CCL2, which is involved in migration of inflammatory cells, is also upregulated during OTM (Garlet et al., 2008).

Thus, depending on the magnitude, strain can either result in enhanced or decreased osteoclast formation and/or activity. It is the balance of osteoblast and osteoclast formation and activity that determine whether the alteration in strain shall lead to a net bone loss (unloading) or bone gain (loading of long bones). It remains to be determined whether sex hormones and their receptors affect osteoclasts directly and/or indirectly in response to loading *in vivo* and *in vitro*.

Role of sex hormones for the osteogenic effect of loading

Male sex hormones and loading

The AR is expressed in human and rodent chondrocytes, osteoblasts and osteocytes, and in murine osteoclasts, but possibly not in human osteoclasts. The expression of AR mRNA is similar in bone from men and women, and AR is therefore likely to play an important role in both genders. Interestingly, the expression of AR varies between different sites in the skeleton. Osteoblast cells derived from mandibular bone and from cortical long bones express higher AR mRNA and more AR binding sites than osteoblasts in cancellous bone either in the long bones or in iliac crest. Thus, a site-specific response to androgens is to be expected. In line with the higher AR expression, mandibular osteoblasts exhibit a higher mitogenic response to dihydrotestosterone (DHT)-treatment than osteoblasts from the iliac crest. Whether this leads to a different response to mechanical load in different skeletal sites is unknown. Both androgens and estrogens (e.g., 17β-estradiol) enhance AR expression. This could be one possible explanation for the additive effects of estrogens and androgens on bone mass.

Mutations or deletion of the AR gene, as can be seen in XY-women with androgen insensitivity syndrome, result in reduced bone mineral density compared with control women and men. In contrast, these patients have normal pubertal growth spurts and a normal closure of their growth-plates. Interestingly, women with XY-karyotype and androgen insensitivity or lack of androgens, have larger maxillary arch dimensions than both male and female controls, and larger mandibular arch dimensions than their female controls. Thus, dysfunctional AR-signaling in human bone affects peak bone mass as well as maxillary and mandibular arch dimensions, but not longitudinal growth. It should be considered, though, that these patients with deficient AR-signaling are often surgically castrated during childhood and are not always sufficiently treated or do not comply with their treatment, phenomena that could affect the bone phenotype. Treatment of mice with testosterone shortly after birth does not affect femur or mandibular length or condylar height (Marquez Hernandez et al., 2011). The phenotype of the facial bones of AR deficient mice has not been reported, indicating that AR in mice has no drastic impact on facial bones.

AR deficient mice have decreased cancellous bone mineral density and cortical bone size of long bones due to increased bone turnover and decreased periosteal expansion (Kawano et al., 2003; Venken et al., 2006; Ophoff et al., 2009). ARs react to loading in a strain-dependent manner. Low intense loading of the skeleton, such as running, increases cancellous bone mineral density and trabecular number in AR deficient mice (Ophoff et al., 2009). However, possibly due to the low strain, running could not increase cortical dimensions in the femur of these AR-deficient mice. Thus, ARs are not needed for a trabecular anabolic effect in response to low strain load. In contrast, the normal increase in cortical periosteal bone formation rate (BFR) seen in response to high strain axial mechanical loading in wild-type mice was enhanced in AR-deficient male mice, indicating that ARs play an inhibitory role in the cortical anabolic effects of high strain load (Callewaert et al., 2010). This inhibitory role of ARs on cortical bone formation involves stimulation of *Sost/Sclerostin* expression leading to inhibition of the Wnt-pathway and bone formation. Testosterone and AR also inhibit NO release induced by pulsatile fluid flow (Figure 7.6(c)).

Although osteocytes are believed to be the load-sensitive bone cells, male mice depleted of ARs specifically in osteocytes respond normally to dynamic axial loading of the tibia (Sinnesael et al., 2012), indicating that it is ARs present in cells other than osteocytes that are involved in AR regulation of the bone anabolic effects of loading. The involvement of ARs in the osteogenic response to loading in females has not been reported, and information regarding the loading response in mice with ARs specifically depleted in bone cells other than osteocytes; for example, chondrocytes, osteoblasts, and osteoclasts, would be valuable.

Female sex hormones and loading

Both subtypes of the ERs are expressed in cells of the epiphyseal growth plates at the ends of long bones (proliferative, prehypertophic, and hypertrophic chondrocytes) and condylar cartilage cells of humans and rodents. The ERs are also expressed in osteoblasts and osteocytes of human and rodent bone tissue, as well as in human and avian osteoclasts and human giant cell tumors of bone. Interestingly, the ERs, like ARs, seem to be concentrated in different areas of the human bone. ERα is largely expressed in osteoblasts and osteocytes of the periosteal region of cortical bone, whereas ERβ is highly expressed in osteoblasts and osteocytes of cancellous bone. Thus, a site-specific response to ERα and ERβ activation would be expected.

The expression of ERs in bone indicates that estrogen can exert direct effects on bone cells. Indeed, several genes are direct targets of estrogen in bone cells (Krum, 2011). TGF-β and alkaline phosphatase (ALP) are early estrogen-responsive target genes involved in bone formation, which are upregulated in osteoblasts within 3–4 hours after estrogen administration. Late-responsive genes, involved in the anabolic effects of ER in osteoblasts during remodeling, are detected after 24 hours and include, for instance, OPG and BMP-2. ERs inhibit osteoclast formation and activity, and early estrogen target genes found in osteoclasts are FBJ murine osteosarcoma viral oncogene homolog (c-fos) and jun proto-oncogene (c-jun) and cathepsin K, which are all downregulated by estrogen.

The expression level of ERs during aging is not clear. Some studies report that ERα and/or ERβ expression is decreased in male and female fracture callus, female bone biopsies, and rat osteocytes, during ageing and decreased estrogen production. In contrast, ER expression levels were increased in osteoblast-like cells from female donors during ageing, although the ER-activity measured by collagen synthesis and the activity from a synthetic ERE-containing promoter was decreased. However, loading still leads to increased cancellous bone mineral density in the distal radius of elderly women, albeit to a lower extent than in young women.

The absence of a functional ERα in humans has been reported for one man and one woman (Smith et al., 1994, 2008; Quaynor et al., 2013). ER deficiency in the man lead to severe osteoporosis, an extended growth period long into adulthood (up to age 35), and low bone age (when 28 years old, he had a bone-age of 15). At the age of 18, the woman with a dysfunctional ERα had a lower than expected bone mass for her age and increased bone turnover. She had not reached peak bone mass; her epiphyses were open, and she was still growing. The phenotype of the facial bones of this man and woman without a functional ERα has not been reported, indicating that depletion of functional ERα in humans has no drastic impact on facial bones.

The bones of ERα and ERβ-depleted mice are normal before puberty. However, adult male mice depleted of ERα have osteopenia as the man with ERα deficiency, and female mice depleted of ERα display increased longitudinal growth as both the man and woman with ERα deficiency (Vidal et al., 2000; Sims et al., 2002; Börjesson et al., 2012). In contrast, male mice depleted of ERβ have normal bones, while young adult female ERβ-depleted mice display a transient increase in femur length, and mainly a cortical bone phenotype with increased cortical bone mineral density, area, and periosteal circumference. Interestingly, ageing ERβ-depleted female mice are partially protected from age-related cancellous bone loss (Windahl et al., 2001; Ke et al., 2002), indicating that ERβ plays an inhibitory role in the ageing skeleton, possibly by counteracting the stimulatory action of ERα. In contrast to ERβ-depleted mice, treatment with an ERβ-antagonist decreased femur and mandibular length in mice of both genders shortly after birth (Marquez Hernandez et al., 2011). In addition, ERβ plays an inhibitory role in condylar growth in female mice by inhibiting fibrocartilage turnover (Kamiya et al., 2013).

In order to analyze bone formation during a specific time interval, it is common to use fluorescent labels such as calcein (green) and alizarin (red) that bind to newly formed bone surfaces. By injecting the labels at two time-points within a specific time interval, green and red lines will be found in bone sections. In some areas both labels will be seen with a distance in between, in other areas only one of the labels is observed. Where two lines are found, the distance in between can be measured and the mineral apposition rate (MAR) can be calculated. The BFR is estimated by multiplying the MAR with the extent of bone surface that is labeled. This technique is widely used to assess actual BFR *in vivo* (see next paragraph for further discussion).

Estrogen treatment suppresses strain-induced periosteal bone formation in male rats (Saxon and Turner, 2006), whereas ERα depletion has been reported to both stimulate (Saxon et al., 2012) or have no effect (Callewaert et al., 2010) on loading-induced cortical bone formation in male mice. Thus, the involvement of estrogens and their receptors in the osteogenic response to load in male rodents is presently unclear. In female mice, ERα is essential for the cortical, but not cancellous, osteogenic effects of loading in a ligand-independent manner (Hagino et al., 1993; Lee et al., 2003; Pajamaki et al., 2008; Windahl et al., 2013b), as demonstrated in Figure 7.8 using dynamic labeling with calcein and alizarin. Interestingly, this effect seems to involve AP-1 rather than ERE-dependent promoters (Jessop et al., 2004; Windahl et al., 2013a), the Wnt-signaling pathway, and enhanced NO-release, as described above. The involvement of ERβ in the osteogenic effects of loading is more complex and may be dependent on the magnitude of the load applied (Saxon et al., 2012). At low magnitude, but not intermediate strain, ERβ may mediate the cortical osteogenic effects of loading. In contrast, ERβ seem to counteract the osteogenic effect of loading in cortical bone at high-magnitude strain.

As described above, osteocytes are believed to mediate the bone response to mechanical loading. Interestingly, female mice with ERα depleted specifically in osteocytes or late osteoblasts display a normal osteogenic response to loading, indicating that it is not osteocytic ERα, or ERα in late osteoblasts, which modifies the osteogenic response to loading in mice. However, the osteogenic response to loading is abrogated in mice where ERα is depleted from osteoblast progenitor cells, indicating that ERα in early osteoblast progenitor cells are essential for the osteogenic response to loading in female mice (Figure 7.9).

In conclusion, in female mice, ERα expressed in osteoblast progenitor cells is involved in mediating the anabolic response to loading in cortical, but not in cancellous bone. The relative importance of AR for the anabolic effects of loading in females remains to be elucidated. In male mice, nonosteocytic AR, and possibly also nonosteocytic ERα and ERβ, all counteract the osteogenic effects of loading in cortical, but not in cancellous bone. It remains to be further investigated which cell type harbors the sex-hormone receptors that are involved in the osteogenic effects of loading, and which splice variants of the steroid receptors that are involved. A more detailed knowledge of the underlying mechanisms of how the steroid receptors affect the osteogenic effects of loading is warranted. The notion that sex-hormone receptor expression, at least ERα expression, decreases during ageing may in part explain the decrease in the anabolic response to loading during aging. The relative importance of the steroid receptors for the response to loading in the ageing human bone remains to be investigated.

Sex hormones and OTM

Sex hormones regulate bone remodeling by promoting bone formation through enhanced osteoblast differentiation and activity and

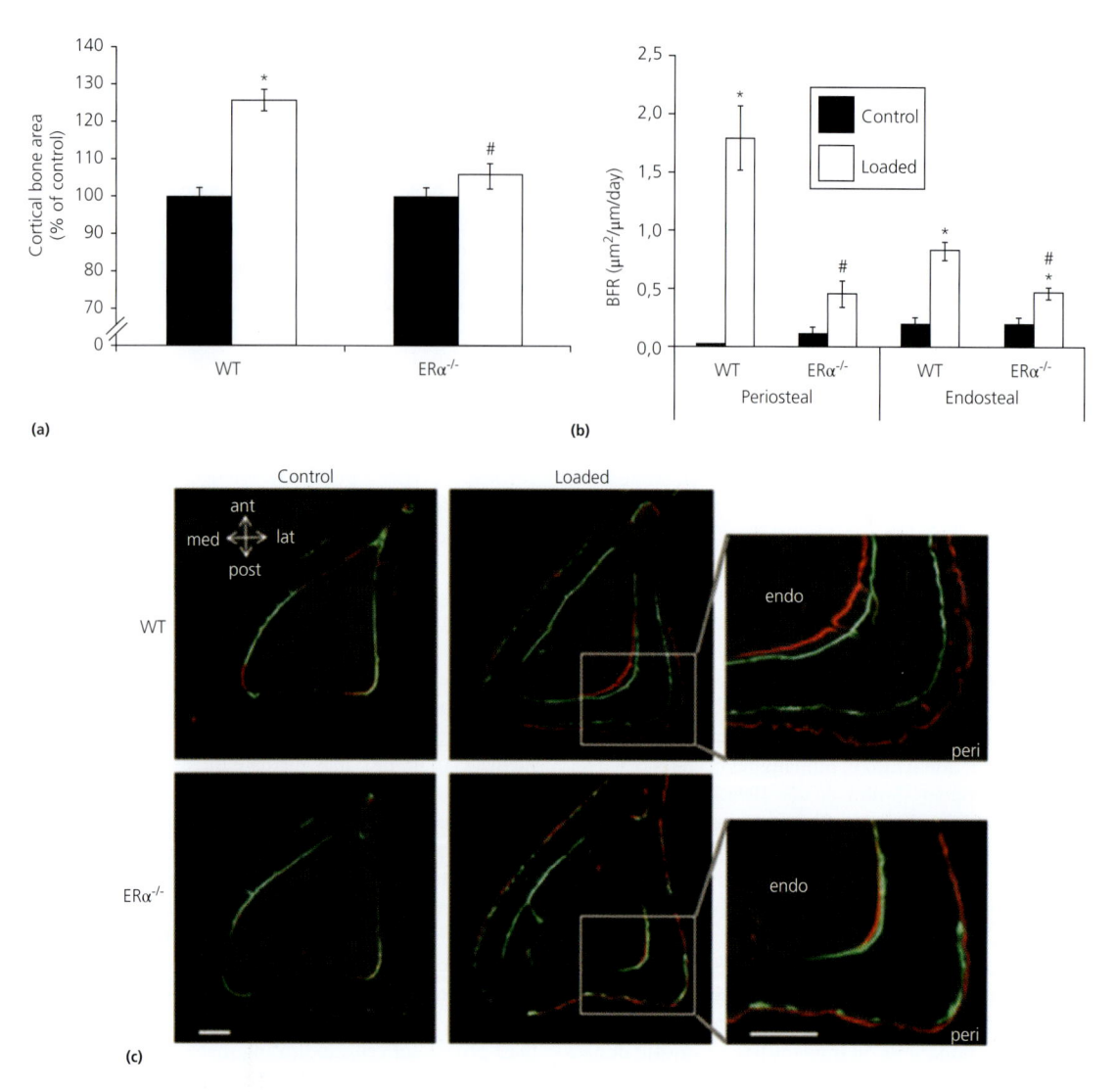

Figure 7.8 Bone formation as visualized and measured with dual fluorescent labeling. ERα is required for the cortical osteogenic response to mechanical loading in female mice tibial bone. Calcein (green) and alizarin (red) are both fluorescent labels that are incorporated in newly formed bone. By injecting the labels with a specific time interval, the bone formed between the time-points will appear between the labels. Thus, by measuring the length and the distance between the two lines, the bone formation rate (BFR) and mineral apposition rate (MAR) can be calculated. (a) µCT analyses of cortical cross-sectional bone area of the mid-diaphyseal region of the non-loaded (control) and loaded (loaded) tibia in wild-type (WT) and estrogen receptor-α inactivated (ERα$^{-/-}$) mice. (b, c) Dynamic histomorphometric analyses of the cortical periosteal and endosteal surfaces. In (b) bone formation rate (BFR) data are presented as mean ± SEM. *$P<0.05$ versus control; #$P<0.05$ the effect of loading in ERα$^{-/-}$ versus the effect of loading in WT mice, Student's t-test. (c) Representative sections show that the loading-induced bone formation was severely reduced at the periosteal and slightly reduced at the endosteal surface in ERα$^{-/-}$ compared with WT mice (calcein/green and alizarin/red). The white bars represent 200 mm. endo, endosteal side; peri, periosteal side of the cortical bone. (Source: Windahl et al., 2013b. Reproduced with permission of American Society for Bone and Mineral Research.)

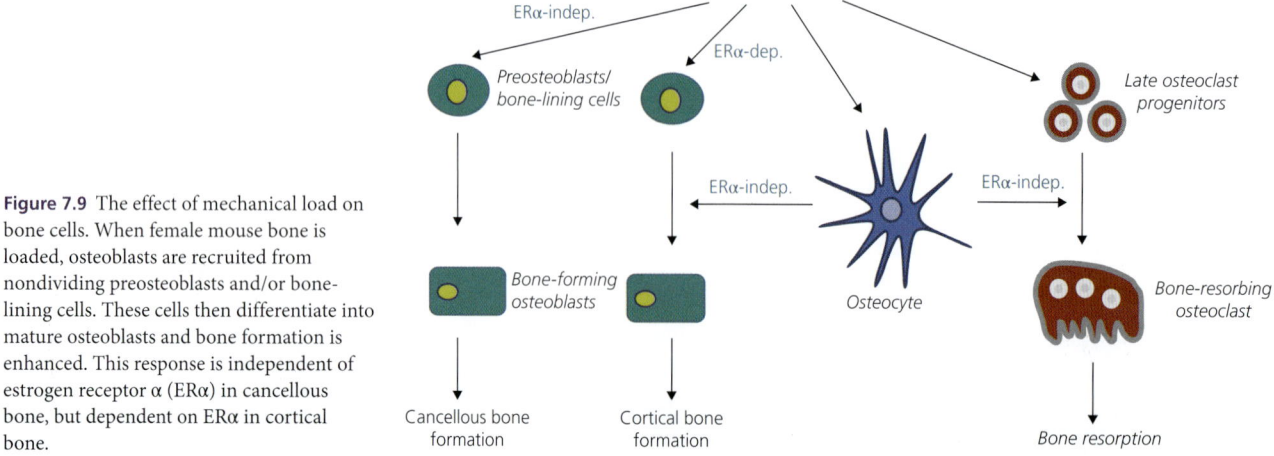

Figure 7.9 The effect of mechanical load on bone cells. When female mouse bone is loaded, osteoblasts are recruited from nondividing preosteoblasts and/or bone-lining cells. These cells then differentiate into mature osteoblasts and bone formation is enhanced. This response is independent of estrogen receptor α (ERα) in cancellous bone, but dependent on ERα in cortical bone.

Table 7.1 The sex hormones have different effects on the osteogenic response to mechanical loading.

Knockout	Depletion	Response to dynamic axial mechanical loading vs. WT		References
Males				
AR°	Global AR	PsBFR increase	↑	Callewaert et al., 2010
		SOST inhibition	↑	
Ot-AR°	Osteocytic AR	Normal		Sinnesael et al., 2012
ERα°	Global ERα	Cortical area increase	↑	Callewaert et al., 2010; Saxon et al., 2012;
		PsBFR increase	↔	
ERβ°	Global ERβ	Cortical area increase	↑ ↔	Lee et al., 2004; Saxon et al., 2007, 2012
		BFR increase	↑ ↔	
Females				
AR°	Global AR	Not reported		
ERα°	Global ERα	Cortical area increase	↓	Lee et al. 2003, 2004; Callewaert et al., 2010; Saxon et al., 2012; Windahl et al., 2013b
		PsBFR increase	↓	
ERα AF-1°	Global ERα AF-1	Cortical area increase	↓	Windahl et al., 2013b
		PsBFR increase	↓	
ERα AF-2°	Global ERα AF-2	Normal		Windahl et al., 2013b
Ot-ERα°	Osteocytic ERα	Normal		Windahl et al., 2013a
ERβ°	Global ERβ	Cortical area increase	↑ ↓	Lee et al., 2004; Saxon et al., 2007, 2012
		BFR increase	↑ ↓	

AR° = androgen receptor deficient mice, Ot-AR° = mice deficient of androgen receptors specifically in osteocytes, ERα° = estrogen receptor α deficient mice, ERβ° = estrogen receptor β deficient mice, ERα AF-1° = mice expressing ERα lacking the activation function 1 domain, ERα AF-2° = mice expressing ERα lacking the activation function 2 domain, PsBFR = periosteal bone formation rate, ↑ = the osteogenic response to loading in the knockout mouse model is increased compared to wild-type mice, ↓ = the osteogenic response to loading in the knockout mouse model is decreased compared to wild-type mice, ↔ = the osteogenic response to loading in the knockout mouse model is normal.

decreased osteoblast apoptosis (Table 7.1). In addition, estrogens decrease bone resorption by decreasing osteoclast differentiation and activity and increasing osteoclast apoptosis during normal bone maintenance. The effects of androgens on osteoclasts are contradictory where both repression of osteoclast formation and enhancement of bone resorption has been reported (Laurent et al., 2014).

There is rising interest in the effects of sex steroids on OTM. Hsieh et al. suggested already in 1995 that loss of estrogen through ovariectomy in rats could affect bone turnover after tooth extraction (Hsieh et al., 1995). Later studies using the ovariectomized rat model showed that loss of estrogen enhanced experimental tooth movement and orthodontically induced root resorption (Yamashiro and Takano-Yamamoto, 2001; Arslan et al., 2007; Sirisoontorn et al., 2011).

Bone histomorphometric analysis shows that hormone depletion due to ovariectomy or orchidectomy leads to decreased mandibular alveolar bone thickness in rats (Armada et al., 2006). However, the periodontal ligament thickness was unaffected by hormone depletion in these rats. In experimental rat models of OTM, ovariectomy elevated both osteoclast density and number at both the pressure and tension sites, indicating enhanced bone resorption and enhanced OTM in the absence of estrogen (Yamashiro and Takano-Yamamoto, 2001; Arslan et al., 2007, Seifi et al., 2015). Interestingly, this could be predicted by a computed model of OTM (Van Schepdael et al., 2013). The increase in osteoclasts in ovariectomized mice subjected to orthodontic treatment was accompanied by an increase in osteoblast density at the bone resorbing pressure site, while it was unchanged in response to ovariectomy at the bone forming tension site (Yamashiro and Takano-Yamamoto, 2001; Van Schepdael et al., 2013). In contrast, Arslan et al. (2007), using a similar experimental design, report that osteoblast numbers are decreased at both sites. The increase in OTM in rats induced by decreased estrogen levels could be partially inhibited by cotreatment with bisphosphonates such as risedronate (Wu et al., 2019).

Using pregnant rats in an experimental model of tooth movement, the authors showed that increased estrogen levels during pregnancy lead to an expected significant decrease in osteoclast numbers at the movement (pressure) side. However, no change in OTM was seen compared with control mice (Ghajar et al., 2013). However, OTM was significantly decreased following oral contraceptive treatment in rats (Olyaee et al., 2013). In line with these studies, cycling estrogen levels during the estrus cycle affects tooth movement in rats and cats (Haruyama et al., 2002; Celebi et al., 2012). The rate of OTM was decreased when estrogen levels peaked, whereas the opposite was seen when estrogen levels were low. The inflammatory mediators, PGE_2 and IL-1β, reached their lowest levels when estrogen levels peaked. Furthermore, it has been proposed that orthodontic force after ovulation could promote tooth movement and shorten the time for orthodontic treatment in women (Xu *et al.*, 2010). Estrogen may inhibit OTM through ERα-mediated mechanisms in both male and female mice, as octeoclast numbers are increased and osteoblast numbers are decreased during OTM in ERα deficient mice (Macari *et al.*, 2016). The authors further showed that deletion of ERα is associated with an increase in inflammatory cytokines like IL-33, TNF-α and IL-1β which are known to stimulate osteoclasts. These observations indicate that the response to OTM is reduced by estrogen through ERα-mediated mechanisms which may either be due to effects on osteoclast activating inflammatory mediators and/or direct effects on osteoclasts. The effects of androgens on OTM are more controversial, where studies in rats show that androgen treatment (Karakida *et al.*, 2017) and androgen depletion through castration (Seifi *et al.*, 2015) both enhance OTM. Further studies are needed to confirm the effects of androgens on OTM and delineate the underlying mechanisms.

Using a mouse model of osteocyte ablation, it was shown that osteoclast number and activity was reduced in osteocyte deficient mice, resulting in a reduction in OTM (Matsumoto *et al.*, 2013). Thus, osteocytes are involved in regulating osteoclast activity in OTM in mice, possibly through expression of RANKL by osteocytes similar to observations in physiological bone remodeling.

In conclusion, estrogen, both endogenously produced and pharmacologically administered, most likely inhibits OTM and alveolar bone resorption. The role of androgen regulation of OTM is not sufficiently investigated. Since androgens are involved in the regulation of osteoclast activity, the development of jaw bones, and bone formation, it is possible that androgens may also affect OTM. Further studies are needed to extend our knowledge of the underlying mechanisms of estrogen inhibition, and androgen effects, of OTM, including genomic and nongenomic effects of the sex steroid receptors, and to confirm that the effects of sex steroids on OTM shown in preclinical studies are reproducible in humans.

Acknowledgements

Studies performed in the authors' laboratories were supported by grants from the Swedish Research Council, Swedish Dental Society, the Royal 80 Year Fund of King Gustav V, the Swedish Rheumatism Association, the Lundberg foundation, the Medical Faculty at Umeå University, Combine, the Marie Curie Initial Training Network (FP7-People-2013-ITN, Grant 607446, Euroclast), the Swedish state under the agreement between the Swedish government and the county council (the ALF agreement) grants from the Sahlgrenska University Hospital and the County Council of Västerbotten.

References

Almeida, M., Laurent, M.R., Dubois, V. et al (2017) Estrogens and androgens in skeletal physiology and pathophysiology. *Physiological Review* **97**, 135–187.

Armada, L., Nogueira, C. R., Neves, U. L. *et al.* (2006) Mandible analysis in sex steroid-deficient rats. *Oral Diseases* **12**, 181–186.

Arslan, S. G., Arslan, H., Ketani, A. and Hamamci, O. (2007) Effects of estrogen deficiency on tooth movement after force application: an experimental study in ovariectomized rats. *Acta Odontologica Scandinavica* **65**, 319–323.

Barakat, R., Oakley, O., Kom, H. *et al.* (2016) Extra-gonadal sites of estrogen biosynthesis and function. *BMB Reports* **49**, 488–496.

Baron, R. and Kneissel, M. (2013) WNT signaling in bone homeostasis and disease: from human mutations to treatments. *Nature Medicine* **19**, 179–192.

Bennett, N. C., Gardiner, R. A., Hooper, J. D. *et al.* (2010) Molecular cell biology of androgen receptor signalling. *International Journal of Biochemical and Cellular Biology* **42**, 813–827.

Bonewald, L. F. (2007) Osteocytes as dynamic multifunctional cells. *Annals of the New York Academy of Science* **1116**, 281–290.

Bonewald, L. F. (2011) The amazing osteocyte. *Journal of Bone and Mineral Research* **26**, 229–238.

Bonewald, L.F. (2017) The role of the osteocyte in bone and nonbone disease. *Endocrinology and Metabolism Clinics North America* **46**, 1–18.

Börjesson, A. E., Windahl, S. H., Karimian, E. *et al.* (2012) The role of estrogen receptor-alpha and its activation function-1 for growth plate closure in female mice. *American Journal of Physiology, Endocrinology and Metabolism* **302**, E1381–1389.

Börjesson, A.E., Lagerquist, M.K., Windahl, S.H., *et al.* (2013) The role of estrogen receptor α in the regulation of bone and growth plate cartilage. *Cellular and Molecular Life Sciences* **70**, 4023–4037.

Brooks, P. J., Nilforoushan, D., Manolson, M. F. *et al.* (2009) Molecular markers of early orthodontic tooth movement. *The Angle Orthodontist* **79**, 1108–1113.

Burger, E. H., Klein-Nulend, J. and Smit, T. H. (2003) Strain-derived canalicular fluid flow regulates osteoclast activity in a remodelling osteon – a proposal. *Journal of Biomechanics* **36**, 1453–1459.

Callewaert, F., Bakker, A., Schrooten, J. *et al.* (2010) Androgen receptor disruption increases the osteogenic response to mechanical loading in male mice. *Journal of Bone and Mineral Research* **25**, 124–131.

Celebi, A. A., Demirer, S., Catalbas, B. and Arikan, S. (2012) Effect of ovarian activity on orthodontic tooth movement and gingival crevicular fluid levels of interleukin-1beta and prostaglandin E(2) in cats. *The Angle Orthodontist* **83**, 70–75.

Chambliss, K. L., Yuhanna, I. S., Anderson, R. G. *et al.* (2002) ERbeta has nongenomic action in caveolae. *Molecular Endocrinology* **16**, 938–946.

Colldén, H., Landin, A., Wallenius, V. *et al.* (2019) The gut microbiota is major regulator of androgen metabolism in intestinal contents. *American Journal of Endocrinology and Metabolism* **317**, E1182–E1192.

Conaway, H.H., Henning, P. and Lerner, U.H. (2013) Vitamin A metabolism, action and role in skeletal homeostasis. *Endocrine Reviews* **34**, 766–797.

Cosman, F., Crittenden, D.B. Adachi, J.D. *et al.* (2016) Romosozumab treatment in postmenopausal women with osteoporosis. *New England Journal of Medicine* **375**, 1532–1543.

Dallas, S. L., Prideaux, M. and Bonewald, L. F. (2013) The osteocyte: An endocrine cell and more. *Endocrine Reviews* **34**, 658–690.

Ducy, P., Zhang, R., Geoffroy, V. *et al.* (1997) Osf2/Cbfa1: a transcriptional activator of osteoblast differentiation. *Cell* **89**, 747–754.

Fan, X., Roy, E., Zhu, L. *et al.* (2004) Nitric oxide regulates receptor activator of nuclear factor-kappaB ligand and osteoprotegerin expression in bone marrow stromal cells. *Endocrinology* **145**, 751–759.

Ford, H., Suri, S., Nilforoushan, D. *et al.* (2014). Nitric oxide in human gingival crevicular fluid after orthodontic force application. *Archives of Oral Biolog* **59**(11), 1211–1216.

Frost, H.M. (1987) The mechanostat: a proposed pathogenic mechanism of osteoporoses and the bone mass effects of mechanical and nonmechanical agents. *Bone and Mineral* **2**(**2**), 73–-85.

Frost, H.M. (1996) Perspectives: a proposed general model of the "mechanostat" (suggestions from a new skeletal-biologic paradigm). *Anatomical Record* **244**(2), 139–147.

Garlet, T. P., Coelho, U., Repeke, C. E. *et al.* (2008) Differential expression of osteoblast and osteoclast chemoattractants in compression and tension sides during orthodontic movement. *Cytokine* **42**, 330–335.

Garlet, T. P., Coelho, U., Silva, J. S. and Garlet, G. P. (2007) Cytokine expression pattern in compression and tension sides of the periodontal ligament during orthodontic tooth movement in humans. *European Journal of Oral Science* **115**, 355–362.

Ghajar, K., Olyaee, P., Mirzakouchaki, B. *et al.* (2013) The effect of pregnancy on orthodontic tooth movement in rats. *Medicina Oral Patologia Oral y Cirugia Bucal* **18**, e351–355.

Guerrini, M.M. and Takayanagi, H. (2014) The immune system, bone and RANKL. *Archives of Biochemistry and Biophysics* **561**, 118–123.

Hagino, H., Raab, D. M., Kimmel, D. B. *et al.* (1993) Effect of ovariectomy on bone response to in vivo external loading. *Journal of Bone and Mineral Research* **8**, 347–357.

Haruyama, N., Igarashi, K., Saeki, S. *et al.* (2002) Estrous-cycle-dependent variation in orthodontic tooth movement. *Journal of Dental Research* **81**, 406–410.

Henriksen, K., Karsdal, M. A. and John Martin, T. (2014) Osteoclast-derived coupling factors in bone remodeling. *Calcified Tissue International* **94**(1), 88–97.

Henning, P., Conaway, H. H. and Lerner, U. H. (2015). Retinoid receptors in bone and their role in bone remodeling. *Frontiers in Endocrinology* **6**, 31.

Hsieh, Y. D., Devlin, H. and McCord, F. (1995) The effect of ovariectomy on the healing tooth socket of the rat. *Archives of Oral Biology* **40**, 529–531.

Hu, M. C., Shiizaki, K., Kuro-O, M. and Moe, O. W. (2013) Fibroblast growth factor 23 and Klotho: physiology and pathophysiology of an endocrine network of mineral metabolism. *Annual Review of Physiology* **75**, 503–533.

Jansson, J.O., Palsdottir, V., Hägg, D.A. *et al.* (2018) Body weight homeostat that regulates fat mass independently of leptin in rats and mice. *Proceedings of the National Academy of Science USA* **115**, 427–435.

Jessop, H. L., Suswillo, R. F., Rawlinson, S. C. *et al.* (2004) Osteoblast-like cells from estrogen receptor alpha knockout mice have deficient responses to mechanical strain. *Journal of Bone and Mineral Research* **19**, 938–946.

Kamiya, Y., Chen, J., Xu, M. et al. (2013) Increased mandibular condylar growth in mice with estrogen receptor beta deficiency. *Journal of Bone and Mineral Research* **28**, 1127–1134.

Kang, Y. J., Mbonye, U. R., Delong, C. J. et al. (2007) Regulation of intracellular cyclooxygenase levels by gene transcription and protein degradation. *Progress in Lipid Research* **46**, 108–125.

Kanzaki, H., Chiba, M., Arai, K. et al. (2006) Local RANKL gene transfer to the periodontal tissue accelerates orthodontic tooth movement. *Gene Therapy* **13**, 678–685.

Kanzaki, H., Chiba, M., Shimizu, Y. and Mitani, H. (2002) Periodontal ligament cells under mechanical stress induce osteoclastogenesis by receptor activator of nuclear factor kappaB ligand up-regulation via prostaglandin E2 synthesis. *Journal of Bone and Mineral Research* **17**, 210–220.

Kanzaki, H., Chiba, M., Takahashi, I. et al. (2004) Local OPG gene transfer to periodontal tissue inhibits orthodontic tooth movement. *Journal of Dental Research* **83**, 920–925.

Karakida, L.M., de Arujo, C. M., Johann, A.C.B.R., et al.et al.et al. (2017) Interaction of anabolic androgenic steroids and induced tooth movement in rats. *Brazilian Dental Journal* **28**, 504–510.

Karsenty, G. and Oury, F. (2012) Biology without walls: the novel endocrinology of bone. *Annual Review of Physiology* **74**, 87–105.

Karsenty, G. and Yadav, V. K. (2011) Regulation of bone mass by serotonin: molecular biology and therapeutic implications. *Annual Review of Medicine* **62**, 323–331.

Kawano, H., Sato, T., Yamada, T. et al. (2003) Suppressive function of androgen receptor in bone resorption. *Proceedings of the National Academy of Sciences of the United States of America* **100**, 9416–9421.

Ke, H. Z., Brown, T. A., Qi, H. et al. (2002) The role of estrogen receptor-beta, in the early age-related bone gain and later age-related bone loss in female mice. *Journal of Musculoskeletal and Neuronal Interaction* **2**, 479–488.

Klein-Nulend, J., Bacabac, R. G. and Bakker, A. D. (2012) Mechanical loading and how it affects bone cells: the role of the osteocyte cytoskeleton in maintaining our skeleton. *European Cells and Materials Journal* **24**, 278–291.

Knothe Tate, M. L., Falls, T. D., McBride, S. H. et al. (2008) Mechanical modulation of osteochondroprogenitor cell fate. *International Journal of Biochemistry and Cell Biology* **40**, 2720–2738.

Kogianni, G., Mann, V. and Noble, B. S. (2008) Apoptotic bodies convey activity capable of initiating osteoclastogenesis and localized bone destruction. *Journal of Bone and Mineral Research* **23**, 915–927.

Kopchick, J. J., List, E. O., Kelder, B. et al. (2014) Evaluation of growth hormone (GH) action in mice: Discovery of GH receptor antagonists and clinical indications. *Mollecular and Cellular Endocrinology* **386**(1–2), 34–45.

Krum, S. A. (2011) Direct transcriptional targets of sex steroid hormones in bone. *Journal of Cell Biochemistry* **112**, 401–408.

Kulkarni, R. N., Bakker, A. D., Everts, V. and Klein-Nulend, J. (2010) Inhibition of osteoclastogenesis by mechanically loaded osteocytes: involvement of MEPE. *Calcified Tissue International* **87**, 461–468.

Laurent, M., Antonio, L., Sinnesael, M., et al (2014) Androgens and estrogens in skeletal sexual dimorphism. *Asian Journal of Andrology* **16**, 213–222

Lee, K., Jessop, H., Suswillo, R. et al. (2003) Endocrinology: bone adaptation requires oestrogen receptor-alpha. *Nature* **424**, 389.

Lee, K., Jessop, H., Suswillo, R. et al. (2004) The adaptive response of bone to mechanical loading in female transgenic mice is deficient in the absence of oestrogen receptor-alpha and -beta. *Journal of Endocrinology* **182**, 193–201.

Lee, N. K., Sowa, H., Hinoi, E. et al. (2007) Endocrine regulation of energy metabolism by the skeleton. *Cell* **130**, 456–469.

Lerner, U. H. (2000) Osteoclast formation and resorption. *Matrix Biology* **19**, 107–120.

Lerner, U. H. (2012) Osteoblasts, osteoclasts, and osteocytes: unveiling their intimate-associated responses to applied orthodontic forces. *Seminars in Orthodontics* **18**, 237–248.

Lerner, U.H. and Ohlsson, C. (2015) The WNT system: background and its role in bone. *Journal of Internal Medicine* **277**, 630–649.

Li, J.Y., Chassaing, B., Tyagi, A.M. et al. (2016) Sex steroid deficiency-associated bone loss is microbiota dependent and prevented by probiotics. *Journal of Clinical Investigation* **126**, 2049–2063.

Li, S., Li, Q., Zhu, Y. et al. (2020) GDF15 induced by compressive force contributes to osteoclast differentiation in human periodontal ligament cells. *Experimental Cell Research* **387**, 111745.

Liedert, A., Kaspar, D., Blakytny, R. et al. (2006) Signal transduction pathways involved in mechanotransduction in bone cells. *Biochemical and Biophysical Research Communications* **349**, 1–5.

Liedert, A., Wagner, L., Seefried, L. et al. (2010) Estrogen receptor and Wnt signaling interact to regulate early gene expression in response to mechanical strain in osteoblastic cells. *Biochemical and Biophysical Research Communications* **394**, 755–759.

Lionikaite, V., Gustafsson, K.L., Westerlund, A. et al. (2018) Clinically relevant doses of vitamin A decrease cortical bone mass in mice. *Journal of Endocrinology* **239**, 389–402.

Lionikaite, V., Henning, P., Drevinge, C. et al. (2019) Vitamin A decreases the anabolic bone response to mechanical loading by suppressing bone formation. *The Faseb Journal* **33**, 5237–5247.

Lloyd, S. A., Loiselle, A. E., Zhang, Y. and Donahue, H. J. (2013) Connexin 43 deficiency desensitizes bone to the effects of mechanical unloading through modulation of both arms of bone remodeling. *Bone* **57**, 76–83.

Macari, S., Sharma, L.A., Wyatt, A. et al. (2016) Osteoprotective effects of estrogen in the maxillary bone depend on ERα. *Journal of Dental Research* **95**, 689–696

Mantila Roosa, S. M., Liu, Y. and Turner, C. H. (2011) Gene expression patterns in bone following mechanical loading. *Journal of Bone and Mineral Research* **26**, 100–112.

Marklund, M., Lerner, U. H., Persson, M. and Ransjo, M. (1994) Bradykinin and thrombin stimulate release of arachidonic acid and formation of prostanoids in human periodontal ligament cells. *European Journal of Orthodontics* **16**, 213–221.

Marquez Hernandez, R. A., Ohtani, J., Fujita, T. et al. (2011) Sex hormones receptors play a crucial role in the control of femoral and mandibular growth in newborn mice. *European Journal of Orthodontics* **33**, 564–569.

Martin, T., Gooi, J. H. and Sims, N. A. (2009) Molecular mechanisms in coupling of bone formation to resorption. *Critical Reviews in Eukaryotic Gene Expression* **19**, 73–88.

Martin, T. J. and Seeman, E. (2008) Bone remodelling: its local regulation and the emergence of bone fragility. *Best Practice and Research: Clinical Endocrinology and Metabolism* **22**, 701–722.

Matsumoto, T., Iimura, T., Ogura, K. et al. (2013) The role of osteocytes in bone resorption during orthodontic tooth movement. *Journal of Dental Research* **92**, 340–345.

Matthews, B. G., Wee, N.K., Widjaja, V. N. et al. (2020) αSMA osteoprogenitor cells contribute to the increase in osteoblast numbers in response to mechanical loading. *Calcified Tissue International* **106**, 208–217.

McSheehy, P. M. and Chambers, T. J. (1986) Osteoblastic cells mediate osteoclastic responsiveness to parathyroid hormone. *Endocrinology* **118**, 824–828.

Nakashima, T., Hayashi, M., Fukunaga, T. et al. (2011) Evidence for osteocyte regulation of bone homeostasis through RANKL expression. *Nature Medicine* **17**, 1231–1234.

Nakashima, T., Hayashi, M. and Takayanagi, H. (2012) New insights into osteoclastogenic signaling mechanisms. *Trends in Endocrinology and Metabolism* **23**, 582–590.

Nilsson, A., Norgard, M., Andersson, G. and Fahlgren, A. (2012) Fluid pressure induces osteoclast differentiation comparably to titanium particles but through a molecular pathway only partly involving TNFalpha. *Journal of Cellular Biochemistry* **113**, 1224–1234.

Nishijima, Y., Yamaguchi, M., Kojima, T. et al. (2006) Levels of RANKL and OPG in gingival crevicular fluid during orthodontic tooth movement and effect of compression force on releases from periodontal ligament cells in vitro. *Orthodontics and Craniofacial Research* **9**, 63–70.

Noble, B. S. (2008) The osteocyte lineage. *Archives of Biochemistry and Biophysics* **473**, 106–111.

Noble, B. S., Peet, N., Stevens, H. Y. et al. (2003) Mechanical loading: biphasic osteocyte survival and targeting of osteoclasts for bone destruction in rat cortical bone. *American Journal of Physiology – Cell Physiology* **284**, C934–943.

O'Brien, C. A., Plotkin, L. I., Galli, C. et al. (2008) Control of bone mass and remodeling by PTH receptor signaling in osteocytes. *PLoS One* **3**, e2942.

Ohlsson, C. and Sjogren, K. (2018) Osteomicrobiology: A new cross-disciplinary research field. *Calcified Tissue International* **102**, 426–432.

Olyaee, P., Mirzakouchaki, B., Ghajar, K. et al. (2013) The effect of oral contraceptives on orthodontic tooth movement in rat. *Medicina Oral Patologia Oral y Cirugia Bucal* **18**, e146–150.

Ophoff, J., Callewaert, F., Venken, K. et al. (2009) Physical activity in the androgen receptor knockout mouse: evidence for reversal of androgen deficiency on cancellous bone. *Biochemical and Biophysical Research Communications* **378**, 139–144.

Oshiro, T., Shiotani, A., Shibasaki, Y. and Sasaki, T. (2002) Osteoclast induction in periodontal tissue during experimental movement of incisors in osteoprotegerin-deficient mice. *Anatomical Record* **266**, 218–225.

Pajamaki, I., Sievanen, H., Kannus, P. et al. (2008) Skeletal effects of estrogen and mechanical loading are structurally distinct. *Bone* **43**, 748–757.

Price, J. S., Sugiyama, T., Galea, G. L. et al. (2011) Role of endocrine and paracrine factors in the adaptation of bone to mechanical loading. *Current Osteoporosis Reports* **9**, 76–82.

Qing, H., Ardeshirpour, L., Pajevic et al. (2012) Demonstration of osteocytic perilacunar/canalicular remodeling in mice during lactation. *Journal of Bone and Mineral Research* **27**, 1018–1029.

Quaynor, S. D., Stradtman, E. W., Jr., Kim, H. G. et al. (2013) Delayed puberty and estrogen resistance in a woman with estrogen receptor alpha variant. *New England Journal of Medicine* **369**, 164–171.

Ransjo, M., Marklund, M., Persson, M. and Lerner, U. H. (1998) Synergistic interactions of bradykinin, thrombin, interleukin 1 and tumor necrosis factor on prostanoid biosynthesis in human periodontal-ligament cells. *Archives of Oral Biology* **43**, 253–260.

Rodan, G.A. and Martin, T.J. (1982) Role of osteoblasts in hormonal control of bone resorption – a hypothesis. *Calcified Tissue International* **34**, 311.

Rowe, P. S. (2012) Regulation of bone-renal mineral and energy metabolism: the PHEX, FGF23, DMP1, MEPE ASARM pathway. *Critical Reviews in Eukaryotic Gene Expression* **22**, 61–86.

Saag, K.G., Petersen, J., Brandi, M.L. *et al.* (2017) Romsozumab or alendronate for fracture prevention in women with osteoporosis. *New England Journal of Medicine* **377**, 1417–1427.

Sato, M., Asada, N., Kawano, Y. *et al.* (2013) Osteocytes regulate primary lymphoid organs and fat metabolism. *Cell Metabolism* **18**, 749–758.

Saxon, L. K., Galea, G., Meakin, L. *et al.* (2012) Estrogen receptors alpha and beta have different gender-dependent effects on the adaptive responses to load bearing in cancellous and cortical bone. *Endocrinology* **153**, 2254–2266.

Saxon, L. K., Robling, A. G., Castillo, A. B. *et al.* (2007) The skeletal responsiveness to mechanical loading is enhanced in mice with a null mutation in estrogen receptor-beta. *American Journal of Physiology: Endocrinology and Metabolism* **293**, E484–491.

Saxon, L. K. and Turner, C. H. (2006) Low-dose estrogen treatment suppresses periosteal bone formation in response to mechanical loading. *Bone* **39**, 1261–1267.

Schriefer, J. L., Warden, S. J., Saxon, L. K. *et al.* (2005) Cellular accommodation and the response of bone to mechanical loading. *Journal of Biomechanics* **38**, 1838–1845.

Seifi, M., Ezzati, B., Saedi, S., et al.et al.et al.et al. (2015) The effect of ovariectomy and orchiectomy on orthodontic tooth movement and root resorption in Wistar rats. *Journal of Dentistry (Shiraz University of Medical Sciences)* **16**, 302–309.

Simoncini, T., Genazzani, A. R. and Liao, J. K. (2002) Nongenomic mechanisms of endothelial nitric oxide synthase activation by the selective estrogen receptor modulator raloxifene. *Circulation* **105**, 1368–1373.

Sims, N.A. and Martin, T.J. (2020) Osteoclasts provide coupling signals to osteoblast lineage cells through multiple mechanisms. *Annual Review of Physiology* **82**, 507–529.

Sims, N. A., Dupont, S., Krust, A. *et al.* (2002) Deletion of estrogen receptors reveals a regulatory role for estrogen receptors-beta in bone remodeling in females but not in males. *Bone* **30**, 18–25.

Sinnesael, M., Claessens, F., Laurent, M. and Vanderschueren, D. (2012) Androgen receptor (AR) in osteocytes is important for the maintenance of male skeletal integrity: evidence from targeted AR disruption in mouse osteocytes. *Journal of Bone and Mineral Research* **27**, 2535–2543.

Sinningen, K., Tsourdi, E., Rauner, M. *et al.* (2012) Skeletal and extraskeletal actions of denosumab. *Endocrine* **42**, 52–62.

Sirisoontorn, I., Hotokezaka, H., Hashimoto, M. *et al.* (2011) Tooth movement and root resorption; the effect of ovariectomy on orthodontic force application in rats. *The Angle Orthodontist* **81**, 570–577.

Sjogren, K., Engdahl, C., Henning, P. *et al.* (2012) The gut microbiota regulates bone mass in mice. *Journal of Bone and Mineral Research* **27**, 1357–1367.

Smith, E. P., Boyd, J., Frank, G. R. *et al.* (1994) Estrogen resistance caused by a mutation in the estrogen-receptor gene in a man. *New England Journal of Medicine* **331**, 1056–1061.

Smith, E. P., Specker, B., Bachrach, B. E. *et al.* (2008) Impact on bone of an estrogen receptor-alpha gene loss of function mutation. *Journal of Clinical Endocrinology and Metabolism* **93**, 3088–3096.

Sunters, A., Armstrong, V. J., Zaman, G. *et al.* (2010) Mechano-transduction in osteoblastic cells involves strain-regulated estrogen receptor alpha-mediated control of insulin-like growth factor (IGF) I receptor sensitivity to Ambient IGF, leading to phosphatidylinositol 3-kinase/AKT-dependent Wnt/LRP5 receptor-independent activation of beta-catenin signaling. *Journal of Biological Chemistry* **285**, 8743–8758.

Tang, S. Y., Herber, R. P., Ho, S. P. and Alliston, T. (2012) Matrix metalloproteinase-13 is required for osteocytic perilacunar remodeling and maintains bone fracture resistance. *Journal of Bone and Mineral Research* **27**, 1936–1950.

Tatsumi, S., Ishii, K., Amizuka, N. *et al.* (2007) Targeted ablation of osteocytes induces osteoporosis with defective mechanotransduction. *Cell Metabolism* **5**, 464–475.

Tsukasaki, M. and Takayanagi, H. (2019) Osteoimmunology: evolving concepts in bone-immune interactions in health and disease. *Nature Review Immunology* **19**, 626–642.

Turner, C. H., Owan, I., Alvey, T. *et al.* (1998) Recruitment and proliferative responses of osteoblasts after mechanical loading in vivo determined using sustained-release bromodeoxyuridine. *Bone* **22**, 463–469.

Vaananen, H. K. and Laitala-Leinonen, T. (2008) Osteoclast lineage and function. *Archives of Biochemistry and Biophysics* **473**, 132–138.

Van Schepdael, A., Vander Sloten, J. and Geris, L. (2013) Mechanobiological modeling can explain orthodontic tooth movement: three case studies. *Journal of Biomechanics* **46**, 470–477.

Venken, K., De Gendt, K., Boonen, S. *et al.* (2006) Relative impact of androgen and estrogen receptor activation in the effects of androgens on trabecular and cortical bone in growing male mice: a study in the androgen receptor knockout mouse model. *Journal of Bone and Mineral Research* **21**, 576–585.

Vidal, O., Lindberg, M. K., Hollberg, K. *et al.* (2000) Estrogen receptor specificity in the regulation of skeletal growth and maturation in male mice. *Proceedings of the National Academy of Science of the United States of America* **97**, 5474–5479.

Wennberg, C., Hessle, L., Lundberg, P. *et al.* (2000) Functional characterization of osteoblasts and osteoclasts from alkaline phosphatase knockout mice. *Journal of Bone and Mineral Research* **15**, 1879–1888.

Windahl, S. H., Borjesson, A. E., Farman, H. H. *et al.* (2013a) Estrogen receptor-alpha in osteocytes is important for trabecular bone formation in male mice. *Proceedings of the National Academy of Science of the United States of America* **110**, 2294–2299.

Windahl, S. H., Hollberg, K., Vidal, O. *et al.* (2001) Female estrogen receptor beta-/ mice are partially protected against age-related trabecular bone loss. *Journal of Bone and Mineral Research* **16**, 1388–1398.

Windahl, S. H., Saxon, L., Borjesson, A. E. *et al.* (2013b) Estrogen receptor-alpha is required for the osteogenic response to mechanical loading in a ligand-independent manner involving its activation function 1 but not 2. *Journal of Bone and Mineral Research* **28**, 291–301.

Wolff, J. (1870) Ueber die innere Architectur der Knochen und ihre Bedeutung für die Frage vom Knochenwachsthum. *Virchows Archiv für Pathologische Anatomie und Physiologie* **50**, 389–450. Available in English (2010) *Clinical Orthopaedics and Related Research* **468**, 1056–1065.

Wu, D., Meng, B., Cheng, Y. *et al.* (2019) The effect of risedronate on orthodontic tooth movement in ovariectomized rats. *Archives of Oral Biology* **105**, 59–64

Wu, L., Su, Y., Lin, F. *et al.* (2020) MicroRNA-21 promotes orthodontic tooth movement by modulating the RANKL/OPG balance in T cells. *Oral Diseases* **26**, 370–380.

Xiong, J., Onal, M., Jilka, R. L. *et al.* (2011) Matrix-embedded cells control osteoclast formation. *Nature Medicine* **17**, 1235–1241.

Xu, X., Zhao, Q., Yang, S. *et al.* (2010) A new approach to accelerate orthodontic tooth movement in women: Orthodontic force application after ovulation. *Medical Hypotheses* **75**, 405–407.

Yamashiro, T. and Takano-Yamamoto, T. (2001) Influences of ovariectomy on experimental tooth movement in the rat. *Journal of Dental Research* **80**, 1858–1861.

Yang, C.Y., Jeon, H.H., Alshabab, A. *et al.* (2018) RANKL deletion in periodontal ligament and bone lining cells blocks orthodontic tooth movement. *International Journal of Oral Science* **10**(1), 3.

Yu, Z., Gao, W., Jiang, E. *et al.* (2013) Interaction between IGF-IR and ER Induced by E2 and IGF-I. *PLoS One*, **8**, e62642.

Zannit, M., Silva, M.J. (2019) Proliferation and activation of osterix-lineage cells contribute to loading-induced periosteal bone formation in mice. *JBMR Plus* **3**, e10227

Zhao, N., Lin, J., Kanzaki, H. *et al.* (2012) Local osteoprotegerin gene transfer inhibits relapse of orthodontic tooth movement. *American Journal of Orthodontics and Dentofacial Orthopedics* **141**, 30–40.

Zhou, G., Chen, Y., Zhou, L. *et al.* (1999) CBFA1 mutation analysis and functional correlation with phenotypic variability in cleidocranial dysplasia. *Human Molecular Genetics* **8**, 2311–2316.

CHAPTER 8
Biological Reactions to Temporary Anchorage Devices

Gang Wu, Jiangyue Wang, Ding Bai, Jing Guo, Haikun Hu, and Vincent Everts

> **Summary**
>
> Mini implant-based temporary anchorage devices (TADs), such as miniscrews and miniplates, are widely used in orthodontics for the correction of various orofacial deformities and malocclusions. The success rate is 84.6% for miniscrews and 92.7% for miniplates. In this chapter, we review the current knowledge of the biological reactions to TADs and the factors that affect a successful application of TADs.

Introduction

Force is an essential element to achieve (orthodontic) tooth movement. An appropriate anchorage is of paramount importance to exert a force that is proper in both strength and three-dimensional direction. An ideal anchorage should meet the following requirements: it can (i) provide sufficient anchorage in the proper direction; (ii) maximally avoid any undesired tooth movement; (iii) obtain good patient compliance; (iv) be easily used in the clinic; and (v) function without side effects. Continuous efforts have been made to search for appropriate anchorage devices. The pioneering work by Brånemark, who discovered osseointegration of titanium implants in 1953, provided a novel and promising anchorage possibility for orthodontic treatments. Based on the concept of dental implants, skeletal anchorage was incorporated into orthodontic treatment (Creekmore and Eklund, 1983). The quest for absolute anchorage began with conventional dental implants (Higuchi and Slack, 1991), retromolar implants (Roberts et al., 1990), and palatal implants (Wehrbein et al., 1996). However, the limitation in space, cost of the implants, and difficulties with connecting to the orthodontic appliances encouraged the rapid development of smaller devices that could be placed in various locations in the dental arch; these were miniscrews and miniplates. Miniscrews (Kanomi, 1997) and miniplates (Jenner and Fitzpatrick, 1985) that are specifically designed for orthodontic treatment satisfy most of the requirements for an ideal anchorage and are being progressively adopted into clinical practice.

These miniscrews and miniplates are implanted temporarily for orthodontic treatment and are removed afterwards. Consequently, they are termed as temporary anchorage devices (TADs). Miniscrews are advantageous over miniplates because of their small size, good compliance, broader applicability, and ease of surgical implantation and removal. Consequently, miniscrews are more widely used than miniplates in orthodontics. On the other hand, miniplates have a stronger anchorage, a relatively high success rate, are safe for host teeth, and replacement is not required during treatment.

Paradigms have started to shift in the orthodontic world since the introduction of mini-implants in the anchorage armamentarium (Leung et al., 2008). For example, miniscrews have allowed the management of larger discrepancies than those treatable by conventional biomechanics because force can be applied directly from the bone-borne anchor unit. Therefore, miniscrews not only help orthodontists in anchorage-demanding cases, but they also enable clinicians to have good control over tooth movement in three dimensions (Leung et al., 2008). Miniscrew-based TADs have been extensively used for the correction of various orofacial deformities and malocclusions, such as retraction of anterior teeth, protraction of molars or the whole dentition, molar distalization, intrusion or extrusion of individual teeth, and correction of crossbite (Figure 8.1).

Biological Mechanisms of Tooth Movement, Third Edition. Edited by Vinod Krishnan, Anne Marie Kuijpers-Jagtman and Ze'ev Davidovitch.
© 2021 John Wiley & Sons Ltd. Published 2021 by John Wiley & Sons Ltd.

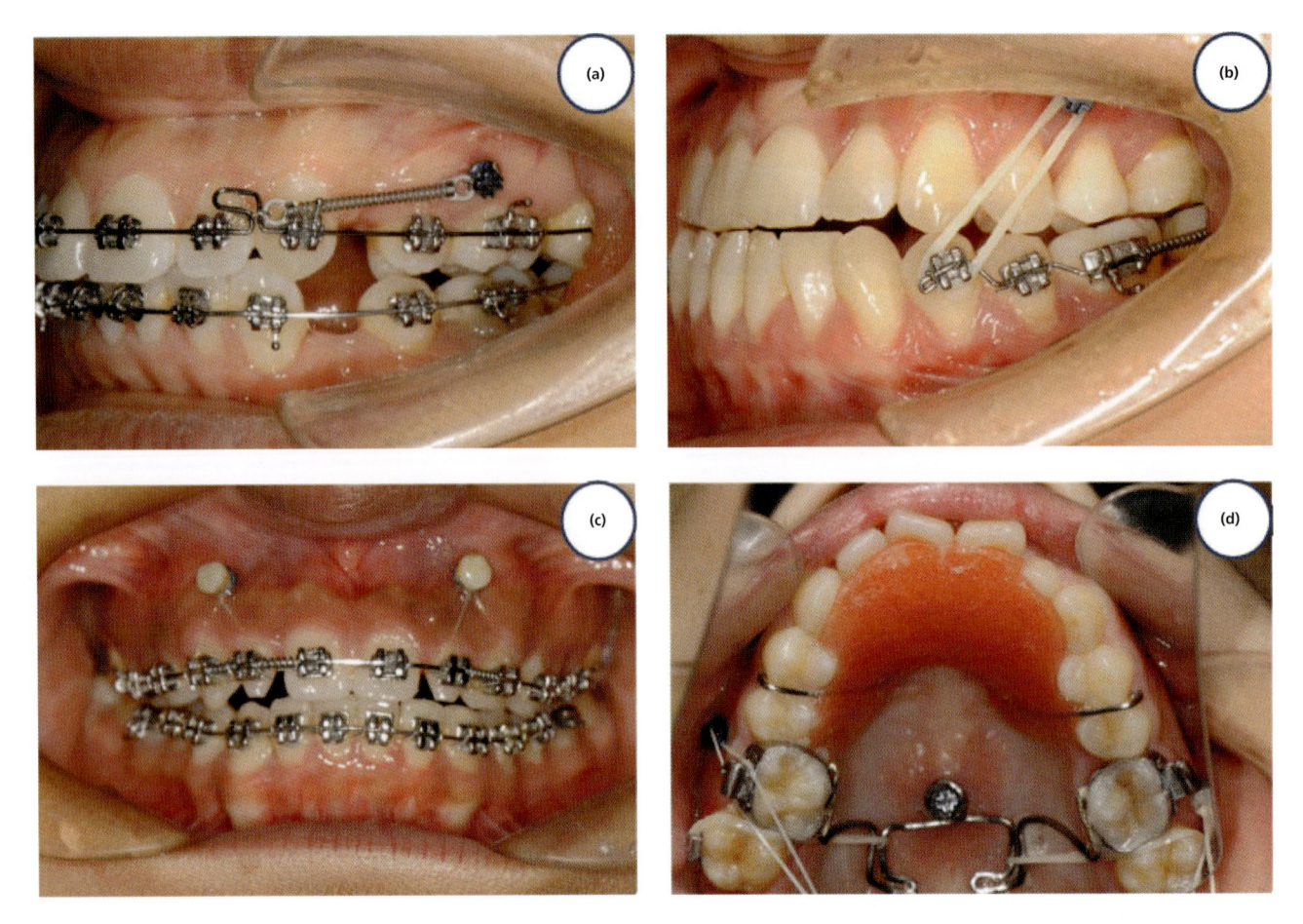

Figure 8.1 Temporary anchorage devices are applied for the correction of various orofacial deformities and malocclusions, such as (a) the retraction of anterior teeth, (b) the protraction of molars, (c) intrusion of individual teeth, and (d) correction of crossbite.

Clinical factors in the success of TADs

Miniscrew-based TADs are used during orthodontic treatment to obtain an absolute anchorage and to ensure that teeth move predictably and with minimal reciprocal movement (Liou et al., 2004). Although TADs have been widely used in various conditions in orthodontic treatment (Iwasa et al., 2017; Marusamy et al., 2018), a certain failure rate has been reported. By analysis of 46 studies, which included 3466 miniscrews, Alharbi et al. (2018) calculated a 13.5% pooled failure rate (95% CI 11.5–15.9, $P = 0.001$, $I^2 = 57.1\%$).

Many clinical studies have been performed to investigate risk factors for miniscrew failure (Suzuki et al., 2013; Migliorati et al., 2016; Elshebiny et al., 2018). Hitherto, the failure of TADs has been found to be associated with the following clinical factors: (i) age of the patient, (ii) loading time points, (iii) implantation site and local inflammation, (iv) implantation torque, (v) mobility, and (vi) miniscrew diameter.

Age of the patient

In a meta-analysis including 41 studies and 3250 orthodontic miniscrews, Alharbi et al. (2018) found that the failure rate of patients under 18 years old was 8.6%, while in patients 18 years old and older, the failure rate was 11.2%, suggesting that age of the patient is one of the factors affecting the success of miniscrews. However, in a similar meta-analysis, Papageorgiou et al. (2012) excluded age from factors associating with the success of miniscrews with a failure rate of 12.6% in patients under 20 years old and a failure rate of 15.5% in patients 20 years old and older. The different results between the two studies may be related to the variation of the included studies. Chen et al. (2007) proposed a reason why younger patients have a greater failure rate. They suggested that as patients became older, bone density increased and cortical bone thickened, which contributes to a more stable skeletal anchorage system.

Loading time point

It is known that a miniscrew does not maintain its primary stability and capability of sustaining clinical strength through osteointegration. Therefore, some studies suggested that immediate loading is possible and does not lead to loosening. In a clinical evaluation on immediate loading of orthodontic miniscrews as anchorage control in en masse retraction, Chopra and Chakranarayan (2015) had an overall 83% success rate, similar to the 84–85% success rate reported by Miyawaki et al. (2003). The only complication observed was peri-implant inflammation. Papageorgiou et al. (2012) came to the same conclusion in their review. By measuring the miniscrews' torque during insertion, 1 week after insertion and at the end of treatment, Migliorati et al. (2016) found that the immediate loading group had a significant lower torque decrease compared with the group loaded after one week, which suggested a stronger bone-to-implant contact in the immediate loading group. However, Büchter et al. (2005) suggested that once the load-related biomechanics exceeded an upper limit, immediate loading may lead to loss of stability. According to Miyawaki et al. (2003) less-than-2 N applied force was recommended.

Implantation site

TADs should be inserted into a region with high bone density and thin epithelial tissue. The chosen location should be the optimal one in terms of both the patient's safety and biomechanical tooth movement. Bone density and soft-tissue health are the key determinants that affect the success of TADs (Miyawaki et al., 2003).

Misch et al. (1999) classified bone density in the oral and maxillofacial region into four groups – D1, D2, D3, and D4 – by measuring the number of Hounsfield units (HU) using computed tomographic scanning (Figure 8.2). A D1 region contains more than 1250 HU and is a region with the densest cortical bone. D1 regions can be found in the anterior mandible, buccal shelf, and midpalatal region. A D2 region contains 850–1250 HU and is porous cortical bone with coarse trabeculae. D2 regions can be found in the anterior maxilla, the midpalatal region and the posterior mandible. A D3 region contains 350–850 HU and is thin and porous cortical bone with fine trabeculae. D3 regions can be found in the posterior maxilla and mandible. A D4 region contains 150–350 HU and is fine trabecular bone. D4 regions can be found in the tuberosity region. Regions of D1 to D3 bone are adequate for TAD implantation. TADs placed in D1 bone may require a drilled purchase point to perforate the thick outer cortical plate. D1 and D2 bone are suitable for TADs placement with lower stress at the screw-bone interface (Sevimay et al., 2005). D4 bone is not recommended for TADs placement owing to the high failure rate associated with it (35–50%) (Jaffin and Berman, 1991; Hutton et al., 1995).

The bone density, the quality, and quantity of cortical bone is crucial in sustaining primary stability, which represents the mechanical locking between the miniscrew and the bone. The bone hardness, the mean buccal bone thickness, and cortical bone mineral density all show significant relevance to the mean failure rate of miniscrews (Iijima et al., 2012). Hence the differences in properties between maxilla and mandible suggest that the failure rate also varies with the jaw of insertion. In a subgroup meta-analysis on prognostic factors, Hong et al. (2016) found that a miniscrew inserted in the maxilla had a higher success rate than one inserted in the mandible (Hong et al., 2016), a finding similar to a previous study (Dalessandri et al., 2013). Although the mandible has a greater bone density, the higher failure rate can be attributed to the following factors: (i) a higher density requires greater torque during insertion, which may lead to unwanted results; (ii) overheat during insertion; (iii) less cortical bone around the miniscrew in the mandible; (iv) the shape of the vestibule is narrower than the maxilla, which adds to the difficulty in maintaining oral hygiene (Papageorgiou et al., 2012); and (v) the mandible has a more loose attached gingiva which adds to the risk of inflammation.

Although Antoszewska et al. (2009) and Lin et al. (2013) have reported a higher success rate for miniscrews inserted in the left side, the difference did not reach statistical significance. Possible explanations are that most dentists are right-handed which makes inserting miniscrews in the left part of the jaw easier, and most of the patients are also right-handed suggesting a better oral hygiene maintenance on the left side.

One of the most common insertion sites of miniscrews is the interradicular site. Thus, root proximity must be taken into consideration. Watanabe et al. (2013) reported that root proximity is a major factor for miniscrew failure, especially in the mandible. Deguchi et al. (2006) found that the greatest distance between teeth was found between the maxillary second premolar and the mesial root of the maxillary first molar. This appears in agreement with the conclusion of Kuroda et al. (2007b) that the maxilla premolar area is the optimal site for miniscrew insertion with a success rate of 95%. Clinically, it is suggested that a three-dimensional (3D) cone beam computed tomography (CBCT) evaluation should be performed before insertion in case of unwanted root proximity (Watanabe et al., 2013).

In a meta-analysis including 63 studies, Mohammed et al. (2018) evaluated the insertion site at the palate, the buccal maxilla, and the mandible and found that the sites with the highest success rate were: the midpalatal area, the site between the maxillary second premolar and maxillary first molar, and the site between the mandibular canine and mandibular premolar. By measuring the cortical bone thickness, buccal shelf bone width, and insertion depth, Elshebiny et al. (2018) suggested that the most favorable insertion site in a patient's mandible was buccal to the second molar.

Insertion torque

The force delivered when inserting the miniscrew is called insertion torque. It is determined both by host factors (Seifi and Matini, 2016), such as bone density, cortical bone thickness, and by material factors (Inoue et al., 2014), such as length, type, and diameter of the miniscrew. Measuring the insertion torque has proven to be a reliable way to predict the primary stability of the miniscrews (Migliorati et al., 2016). Either an excessive or a low torque will decrease the stability of the miniscrew and increase the failure rate. Watanabe et al. (2017) reported a higher insertion torque (10.7±1.9 N·cm) in the failure group than that (8.5±2.1 N·cm) in the success group and suggested that an excessive insertion torque may cause damage to the cortical bone. Similarly, McManus et al. (2011) found that when the maximum insertion torque was less than 5 N·cm, there was a statistically significant lower resistance to miniscrew movement and increasing deflection. However, considering the host factors which may vary between individuals and are hard to control, Inoue et al. (2014) came upon with a new concept – torque ratio which equaled maximum insertion torque (MIT) divided by maximum removal torque (MRT). They found that the torque ratio was significantly lower in the failure group when MIT and MRT were not related to the success of miniscrews.

Implant diameter and length

Due to their small diameter, miniscrews bear several advantages, such as maximum comfort and minimal chance of damage to

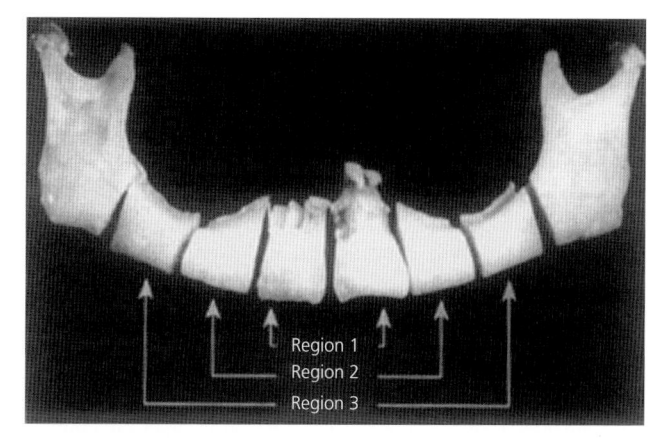

Figure 8.2 Mandible sectioned into three regions bilaterally. Region 1 includes the incisors and canines, region 2 includes the premolars, and region 3 includes the molars. (Source: Misch et al., 1999. Reproduced with permission of Elsevier.)

adjacent teeth. Many researchers have tried to identify the optimal diameter and length of miniscrews.

In a meta-analysis, Alharbi et al. (2018) grouped miniscrews into <8mm and >8mm length groups and found that the shorter group had a slightly higher failure rate. In a retrospective study, Topouzelis and Tsaousoglou (2012) found that 8mm miniscrews had an almost six times higher success probability than 10mm miniscrews. This could be due to a higher risk of damaging teeth roots or peripheral structures, such as the maxillary sinus. By measuring the success rate among 105 patients, Suzuki et al. (2013) suggested that the optimal miniscrew length for the maxilla was 5mm, while in the mandible the length should not be less than 6mm. They also suggested that miniscrews of at least 3.8mm in length should be placed in mandibles.

Alharbi et al. (2018) found that when the diameter of miniscrews was less than 1.3mm, it had a higher success rate than miniscrews with 1.4–1.6mm diameter. This is consistent with the conclusion of Topouzelis and Tsaousoglou (2012) who found that compared with the 1.4mm miniscrew, the 1.2mm miniscrew had a 5.6 times higher probability of success. With the increase in diameter, there is higher risk of root proximity or root contact. Chen et al. (2009) found the miniscrew with a diameter larger than 1.6mm was not superior. Other studies reported that miniscrews with diameters of 1.2, 1.3, and 1.5mm had similar or higher success rates in comparison with the 1.6mm miniscrew (Miyawaki et al., 2003; Kuroda et al., 2007a; Park et al., 2006). Miyawaki et al. (2003) also reported no success with 1.0mm diameter miniscrews. Papageorgiou et al. (2012), on the other hand, suggested no significant relation between the length and diameter of miniscrews and the success rate.

Mobility

Mobility is a significant risk factor for orthodontic miniscrew failure as shown in the meta-analysis by Papageorgiou et al. (2012). Therefore, it has been used as one of the criteria when defining miniscrew success (Moon et al., 2008; Son et al., 2014; Iwai et al., 2015). In most cases, a successful miniscrew implant is defined as having no mobility or withstanding orthodontic force application during treatment (Papageorgiou et al., 2012). The presence of any inflammation, infection, or mobility may lead to premature loss of miniscrews (Alharbi et al., 2018). However, mobility does not necessarily mean the failure of TADs. Park et al. (2006) found that mobility was a risk factor but 34 of 45 minimally mobile screw implants were successful. Screw implants with minimal mobility could still be used as anchorage under comparatively low force. When an excessive load is applied, partly osseointegrated screw implants can become severely mobile and eventually fail. Dental implants are usually loaded in all directions, but orthodontic screw implants are usually loaded with unidirectional lateral forces, which may allow minimal mobility in orthodontic screw implants.

Mechanical analysis using finite element models

In addition to clinical investigations, finite element analysis is also extensively used to analyze the factors related to the mechanical stress surrounding TADs. Finite element methods (FEMs) provide an approximate solution for the response of 3D structures to the applied external loads under certain given conditions. FEMs appear to be suitable for simulating complex mechanical stress situations in the maxillofacial region (Basciftci et al., 2008).

The first step of FEMs is to subdivide the complex geometry into a suitable set of smaller elements of finite dimensions, all of which, when combined, form the mesh model of the investigated structures. Each element can be a specific geometric shape (i.e., triangle, square, or tetrahedron) with a specific internal strain function. By using these functions and the actual geometry of the element, the equilibrium equations can be determined between the external forces acting on the element and the displacements occurring on its nodes (Jasmine et al., 2012).

With FEMs, the stability of TADs is found to be associated with several factors: (i) cortical bone thickness; (ii) insertion angulation; (iii) thread location and mechanical anisotropy; and (iv) exposed length.

Cortical bone thickness

Cortical bone thickness is an important factor influencing the success of TADs in the clinic (Papageorgiou et al., 2012; Watanabe et al., 2013). Researchers also adopted FEMs to identify the exact influence of cortical bone thickness on the mechanical stress surrounding TADs.

Motoyoshi et al. (2007) used FEMs to investigate the influence of cortical bone thickness from 0.5 to 1.5mm, at 0.25mm intervals on the stress surrounding TADs. They constructed cortical bone models with and without cancellous bone to examine the biomechanical influence on cortical bone after bone resorption. When cortical bone thickness was less than 1mm, the cancellous bone models exhibited von Mises stresses exceeding 6 MPa, and the cortical bone models without cancellous bone showed von Mises stresses exceeding 28 MPa. This study verified that a clinical cortical bone thickness threshold of 1mm improves the success rate of miniscrews.

By constructing a 3D model with a bone block integrated with a miniscrew, Liu et al. (2012) studied the effect cortical bone thickness had on stress distribution and displacement of the miniscrew. They found that the peak von Mises stress on the cortex increased as the cortex thickness decreased from 3.0 to 0.5 mm under the same loading conditions and, if the cortex thickness was reduced from 1.2 to 0.5 mm, there was a significant 20–25% increase in the peak von Mises stress. When it came to displacement, the result was similar. If the cortex thickness and the Young's modulus of cancellous bone were reduced simultaneously to 0.5 mm and one eighth of normal, the maximum displacement of the miniscrew increased by 27%. However, the density of the cancellous bone had a minor effect on the cortex bone stress. Liu et al. (2012) offered two reasonable explanations: with a higher Young's modulus, cortical bone sustains higher loads than cancellous bone, and the bending mode has more effect at the base support region.

In combination with cortical bone thickness, the distance of TADs to the adjacent teeth was also found to influence significantly the mechanical stress surrounding TADs. The interradicular site has become the most common miniscrew insertion place, but this comes with an increasing risk of root proximity. Motoyoshi et al. (2009b) established four different FEMs and found that the maximum stress on the bone increased when the miniscrew was close to the root. When the miniscrew touched the root, stress increased to 140 MPa or more, and bone resorption could be predicted. Stress was higher for a cortical bone thickness of 2mm than for 1mm or 3mm (Figure 8.3(b)). Cortical bone of 2mm thick had a higher risk for resorption (Motoyoshi et al., 2009b). By using computed tomography (CT) imaging, Albogha and Takahashi (2018) reconstructed

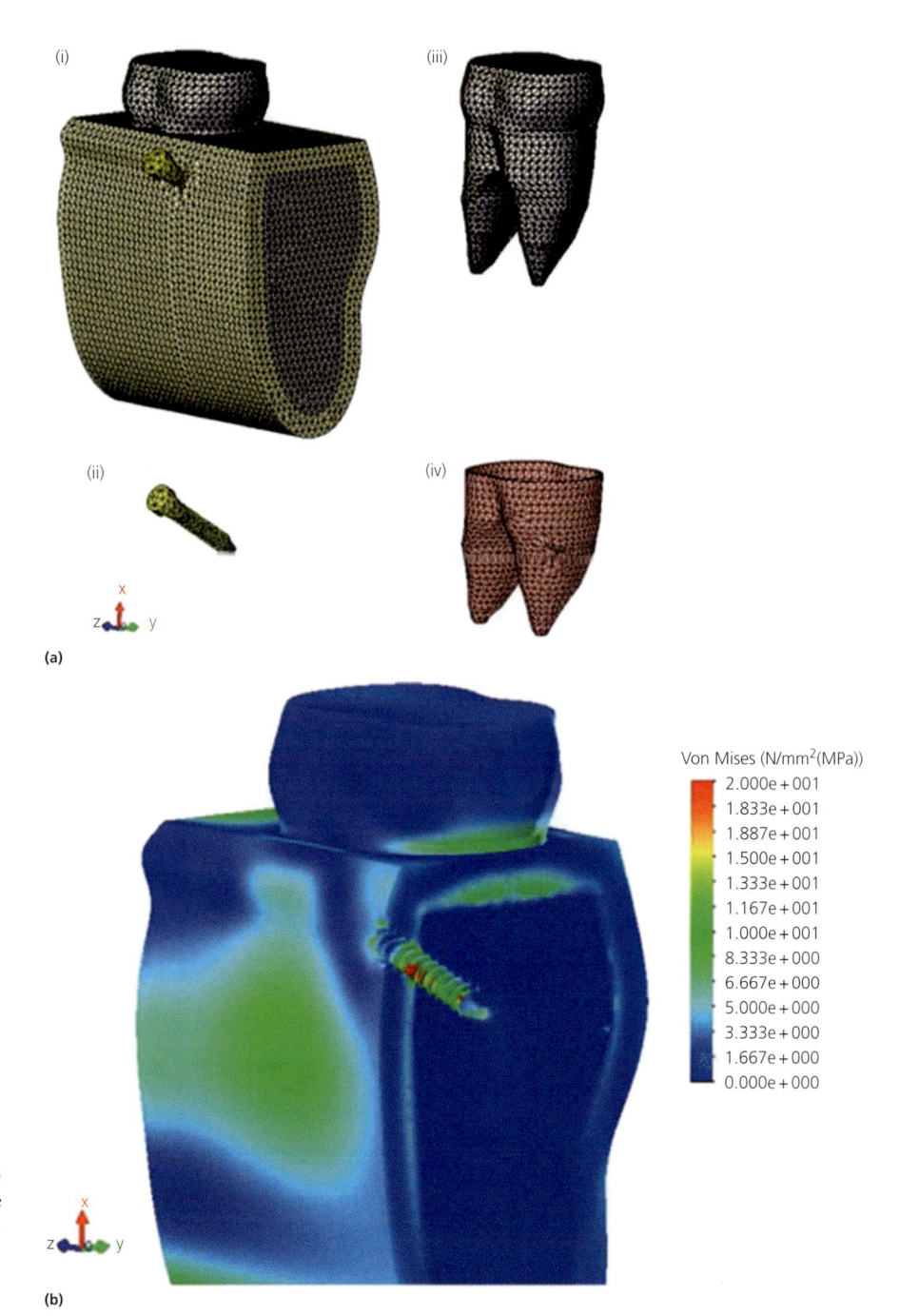

Figure 8.3 (a) (i) Finite element model consisting of (ii) miniscrew, (iii) tooth, (iv) periodontal membrane and bone elements. (b) von Mises stress distribution in the bone elements of the FEM for model (iii) with the screw thread of the miniscrew embedded in the periodontal membrane. (Source: Motoyoshi et al., 2007. Reproduced with permission of Elsevier.)

patient-specific finite element models and studied the compressive stress of PDL with different adjacent distance. They found that the compressive stress remained low when retracting the canine with a 2 N force, if the miniscrew implant stayed more than 0.5 mm away from the PDL. Thus, they recommended a minimum distance of 0.5 mm from the PDL and a minimum distance of 1.0 mm from the root (Albogha and Takahashi, 2018).

Insertion angulations

The proper angle of insertion is important for cortical anchorage, patient safety, and biomechanical control. However, the proper clinical insertion angle has been a controversial field. Some suggested inserting miniscrews at angles of 30° to 40° in the maxilla and 10° to 20° in the mandible in order to avoid root damage (Kyung et al., 2003), while others reported that placing miniscrews 90° to the bone surface reduced the stress concentration, and that placing miniscrews at angles less than 90° did not offer advantages in terms of anchorage resistance force (Woodall et al., 2011). Because it is difficult to measure the exact stress around the miniscrew *in vivo*, finite element analysis has been introduced to offer an insight into the proper insertion angle.

Jasmine et al. (2012) performed finite element analysis through established FEMs of a maxilla and a mandible with types of D3 and D2 bone quality, and of miniscrews with a diameter of 1.3 mm and lengths of 8 and 7 mm. They found that the maximum von Mises stresses in the miniscrews and the cortical bone decreased as the

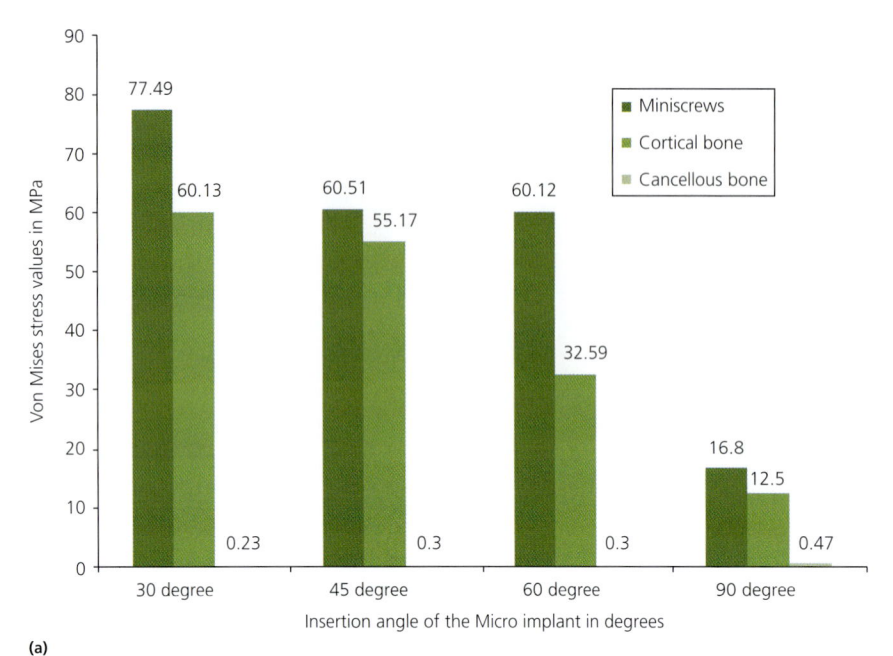

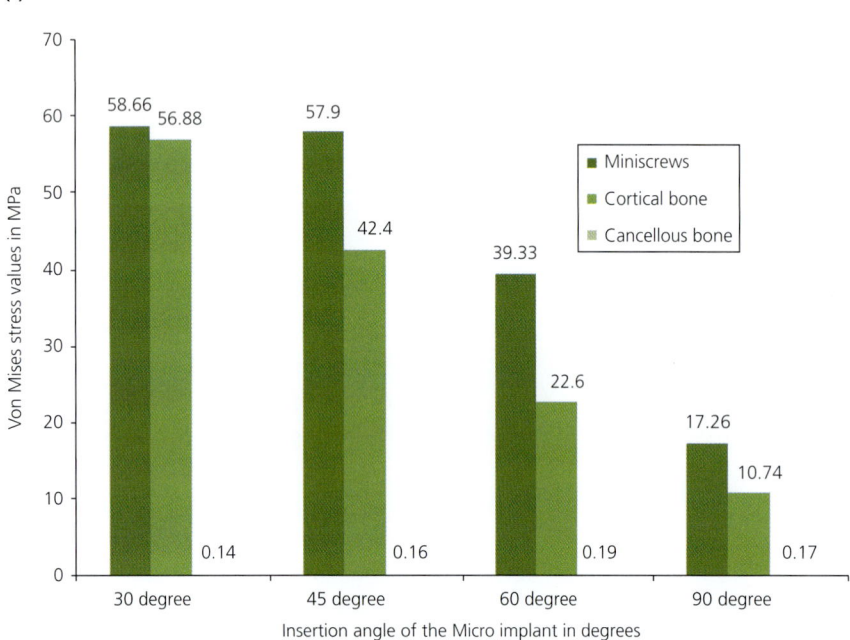

Figure 8.4 Maximum von Mises stress values (in MPa) induced at various insertion angulations of miniscrews in a finite element model. (a) Maxilla and (b) mandible. (Source: Jasmine et al., 2012. Reproduced with permission of Elsevier.)

insertion angle increased (Figure 8.4) The maximum von Mises stress was higher in type D3 bone quality than type D2 bone quality. They concluded that placement of miniscrews at a 90° angulation in the bone reduced the stress concentration, thereby increasing the likelihood of implant stabilization. Perillo et al. (2015) also found that cortical and trabecular bone stress was least when miniscrews were 90° to the alveolar process when investigating the stress distribution of 30°, 60°, 90°, 12°, and 150° insertion degrees. However, Kuroda et al. (2017) suggested that when analyzing the principal stress distribution in surrounding bone, the compressive and tensile stresses increased with the angle of insertion up to 30°. For larger insertion angles, the increase almost vanished. Thus, they concluded that with care during placement and removal, the obliquely inserted miniscrew could generally provide sufficient anchorage for 2 N loading.

Thread location, properties, and mechanical anisotropy

The stability of a miniscrew can be significantly influenced by its thread shape (Chun et al., 2002) and pitch (Motoyoshi et al., 2005). For most miniscrews, the thread coils to the right, so that the screw is geometrically asymmetric. The location of the thread ridge of the screw in the bone is determined haphazardly in the clinic. To identify the influence of thread location on stress distribution in the bone around orthodontic mini-implants, Motoyoshi et al. (2009a) used FEMs for conventional and cervical threadless miniscrews with cortical bone 1 or 3 mm thick (Figure 8.5). They found a high compressive stress of −55 MPa in the model of the conventional screw with 1 mm thick cortical bone when the traction was fixed in the direction of the tip of the thread ridge at the bone surface.

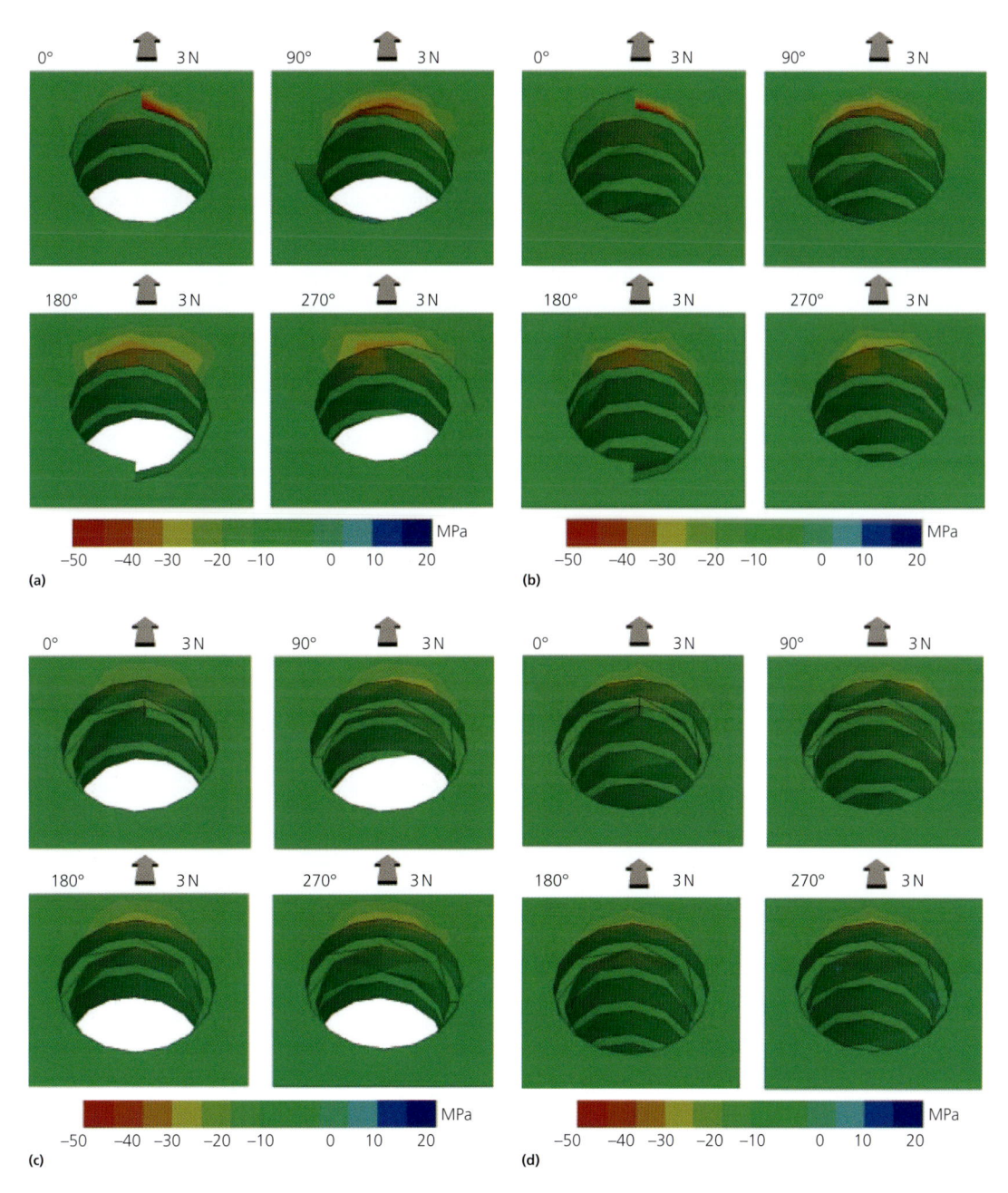

Figure 8.5 (a) Stress distributions for a conventional screw with 1 mm thick cortical bone. The arrows indicate the direction of traction. When the traction was at 0°, stress was concentrated (red area) at the sharp bone edge located in that direction. (b) Stress distributions for a conventional screw with 3 mm thick cortical bone. (c) Stress distributions for a cervical threadless screw with 1 mm thick cortical bone. (d) Stress distributions for a cervical threadless screw with 3 mm thick cortical bone. (Source: Based on Motoyoshi *et al.*, 2007. Reproduced with permission of Elsevier.)

Although a thicker cortical bone is believed to favor the stability of miniscrews, the peak compressive stress was reduced by only a few MPa in the model and still exceeded −50 MPa with thicker cortical bone (3 mm). This means that thicker cortical bone does not always enhance the stability of a miniscrew. Consequently, mechanical anisotropy contributed to miniscrew failure. The location of the thread ridge cannot be aligned with the bone margin when placing a miniscrew in the implant hole. To reduce the negative influence of mechanical anisotropy, the authors designed a new type of miniscrew – a cervical threadless miniscrew. The miniscrew has a flat surface at the part in contact with the bone margin. The peak compressive stress was also observed at the superior margin of the bone surface of a cervical threadless miniscrew, but the value was reduced to between −22 and −26 MPa. The mechanical anisotropy decreased in the cervical threadless model, while cortical bone thickness had no effect. The screw-thread increases the contact area between the miniscrew and bone, facilitating rigid support. It was concluded that the screw-thread in the superior part of the cortical bone might reduce the stability of the miniscrew. The cervical threadless miniscrew is equivalent to inserting a conventional screw deep beyond the thread part, and it is expected to improve the clinical success rate of the miniscrew (Motoyoshi *et al.*, 2009a).

Thread properties, such as thread height, taper shape, and taper length also play a role in affecting the stability of miniscrews. By using a 3D finite element model, Shen *et al.* (2015) studied the optimal range of the thread height and pitch using bivariate analysis. They found that thread height played a significant role in reducing maxillary stress and enhancing miniscrew stability and a pitch around 1.2 mm was the best for orthodontic miniscrews in the maxillary posterior region. Chang *et al.* (2012) found that the maximum values of stress concentration on the threads decreased as the taper degrees increased. The values of relative displacement also decreased as the taper degrees increased. The possible explanation for that was as the core diameter increased in the tapered portion, the thread profile changed from a sharp triangular shape to a more trapezoidal shape. The trapezoidal threads engaged more bone than did the triangular threads, and the increased core diameter in the tapered portion also helped to decrease the chance for breakage or bending failure in this high-stress area.

Exposed length

Studies that evaluated the miniscrew-length effect had inconsistent or inconclusive results (Stahl *et al.*, 2009), but Liu *et al.* (2012) pointed out that the exposed screw length (screw length above the cortex or total screw length minus the implanted depth) was the dominant factor in a 3D finite element analysis. Therefore, both screw length and implanted depth of the miniscrew should be considered. A longer miniscrew might not be able to provide extra stability if it cannot be implanted deeply enough to reduce the lever arm.

A study performed by Lin *et al.* (2013) indicated that the exposed length of a miniscrew could significantly influence the stress distribution surrounding miniscrews. The authors constructed 27 FEMs simulating the biomechanical response of the alveolar bone adjacent to the miniscrews. Factorial analysis was performed to investigate the comparative influence of each factor. The simulation results showed that the exposed length of the miniscrews had a statistically significant influence on bone stress, with a contribution of 82.35%. Increased exposure length resulted in higher bone stress adjacent to the miniscrews. Whereas all investigated factors had a statistically significant influence on cancellous bone stress, the stress values associated with cancellous bone were much less than those with cortical bone. The authors concluded that an increased exposed length resulted in higher bone stresses adjacent to the miniscrew. The percentage of contribution of the insertion angle of the miniscrew (6%) was also statistically significant but much less than that of the exposed length (82%).

Histological reactions

Although extensive studies have been performed to investigate the clinical factors for, and mechanical reactions to TADs, the tissue reactions to TADs still remain to be elucidated. TADs were developed based on the principle of dental implants. The tissue reactions to TADs should also contain two phases: the primary stability (mechanical) that is derived from a mechanical engraving of the titanium screw implant in the bone tissue; and the secondary stability (biological) that results from the ongoing process of osseointegration. For the endosseous implants, when the healing process is completed, the primary stability is fully replaced by the secondary stability, and the transition from primary to secondary stability roughly starts at the 5th week after insertion and lasts till the 8th week (Raghavendra *et al.*, 2005). However, for the TAD used in the field of orthodontics, the full establishment of secondary stability may add some disadvantages. In contrast to the endosseous implant, TADs need to be removed after fulfilling their function as skeletal anchorage, which suggests that full osseointegration makes removal of TADs difficult (Vande Vannet *et al.*, 2007). Criteria for the success of orthodontic mini-implants are: absence of inflammation, absence of clinically detectable mobility, and capability of sustaining the anchorage function throughout the course of orthodontic treatment (Wiechmann *et al.*, 2007). It is reported that the osseointegration of titanium miniscrews is less than half that of conventional dental implants (Costa *et al.*, 1998).

Osseointegration process

To understand the tissue reactions to TADs under loading, knowledge about the osseointegration process is needed. In 1952, Brånemark accidently found that a titanium chamber placed in rabbit bone was completely integrated by surrounding bone. He named the phenomenon as "osseointegration". Osseointegration is defined as direct bone deposition on an implant surface. It generally follows three stages: (i) incorporation by woven bone, (ii) adaptation of bone mass to load and (iii) adaptation of bone structure to load (bone remodeling) (Schenk and Buser, 1998). Vande Vannet *et al.* (2007) conducted a study to examine the osseointegration extent by inserting four bracket screw bone anchors in the alveolar process of the lower jaw in each of five male Beagle dogs. After 6 months, histological evaluation of the eight remaining screws was performed to evaluate the extent of osseointegration. All eight screws showed partial osseointegration with a mean of 74% osseointegration. They concluded that a small size titanium screw could stand orthodontic loading for 12–24 months with only partial osteointegration (Vande Vannet *et al.*, 2007). Histology suggested that woven bone or fibrous tissue contact at the miniscrew–bone surface is not a sign of successful integration of the miniscrew but rather indicative of an overload situation and suggestive of impending failure (Huja, 2015). Under normal conditions, with functional loading, the bony structures will be adapted to the load by replacing pre-existing, necrotic, and/or initially formed woven bone and establishing mature lamellar bone. This leads to functional adaptation of the bony structures with changes in dimension as well as structural orientation of bony trabeculae to the load. The adaption process continues with time and changes of loading.

Immediate loading of orthodontic miniscrews

Although immediate loading of orthodontic miniscrews can be clinically successful, there are still few histological data available. Luzi *et al.* (2009) investigated the tissue reactions to immediate loading in an animal model. Fifty orthodontic titanium miniscrews were inserted in four adult male monkeys at four time intervals. Forty-two devices were loaded with 0.5 N super-elastic coil springs immediately after insertion while eight were left unloaded and served as the controls. In this study, a wide variation between animals was found for bone-miniscrew contact areas, mineralized surface area, and number of resorptive surfaces (Figure 8.6). There was a decrease of bone–miniscrew contact between one week and one month followed by a significantly progressive increase. Miniscrews that showed as little as 3% bone–miniscrew contact successfully resisted loading. Mineralized surface increased significantly between one week and one month, followed by a progressive decrease. Resorptive surfaces were found to decrease between one week and one month, followed by a progressive increase. The authors concluded that immediate loading with light forces did not negatively affect the bone healing pattern. Trabecular bone volume density did not show any particular trend while bone-miniscrew contact was a time-dependent factor.

Nakagaki *et al.* (2014) used μCT and histology of bone surrounding miniscrews to investigate the bone response to immediate loading. Ten miniscrews were placed in the mandibles of three Beagle dogs. Five pairs of miniscrews were immediately loaded with 150 g of continuous force using nickel–titanium coil springs for 8 weeks. The compression region in cortical bone showed a significantly higher bone mineral density value than the tension region. Scanning electron microscopy of the retrieved miniscrews showed, besides a small amount of titanium, vanadium, calcium, phosphorus, and a large amount of carbon on the surface. There were no significant differences in the bone-to-implant contact of the tension side compared with the compression side. On the compression side there was a significant higher bone mineralization of cortical bone compared with the tension side. The authors concluded that immediate loading of miniscrews may help to activate bone remodeling and increase the mineral content at the loaded region.

Time point of loading

The osseointegration process is significantly influenced by the timing, magnitude, and duration of the load. Oltramari-Navarro *et al.* (2013) conducted a histomorphometric study on miniscrew stability to evaluate healing time before loading. Miniscrews were inserted in six minipigs with four different loading regimes: unloaded, immediate loading, after 15 days, and after 30 days. Tissue blocks were harvested after 120 days and used for histomorphometric analysis. Although the immediate loading group had a 50% survival rate compared with other groups and the overall survival rate, there was no significant difference among the groups. There was also no significant difference in the direct bone-to-miniscrew contact and the area of bone observed between the thread of the screws. Microscopic findings showed that after 120 days, bone remodelling was in progress, with woven bone mineralization between the screw and lamellar bone. The authors indicated that immediate low intensity loading or early orthodontic static loads did not affect miniscrew stability. This is in line with other studies reporting that loading *per se* does not cause the loss of stability until an overload limit is reached (Büchter *et al.*, 2005).

The diameter ratio of pilot hole to miniscrew

Uemura *et al.* (2012) evaluated the relationship between miniscrew mobility during the healing phase and the prognosis for miniscrew stability. They used drills with diameters of 0.8, 0.9, 1.0, and 1.1 mm to make pilot holes in tibiae of 40 male Wistar rats (aged 20 weeks). The inserted miniscrews (diameter 1.4 mm; spearhead 1.2 mm; halfway between maximum and minimum 1.3 mm; length 4.0 mm) were subjected to an experimental traction force for 3 weeks, and the bone–miniscrew contact (BIC) was analyzed histologically. Twenty rats were used to evaluate the bone–miniscrew contact and the other 20 were used to measure the stability of the miniscrews using the Periotest before and after traction. The authors found that the BIC ratios of the 0.9 and 1.0 mm groups were significantly greater than those of the other groups. The Periotest values measured 3 weeks after implant insertion were significantly lower than those measured at insertion, except for the 1.1 mm group. The authors concluded that a pilot hole of 69–77% miniscrew diameter was optimal for the stability of the miniscrews. A significant decrease in the mobility of the miniscrews 3 weeks postinsertion implies a good prognosis for the subsequent miniscrew stability.

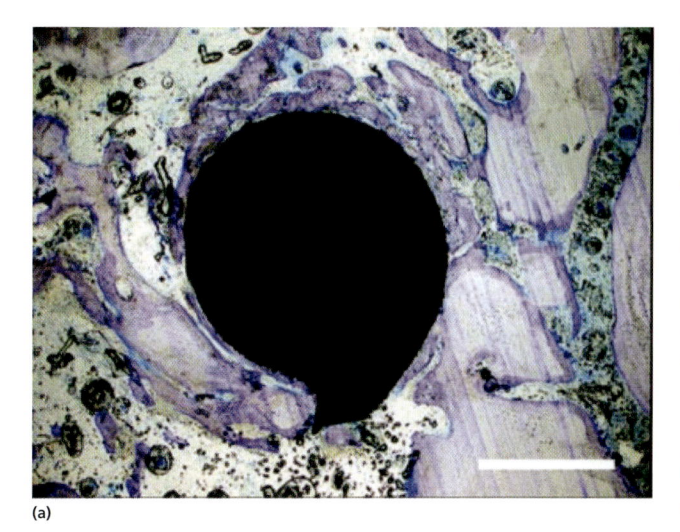

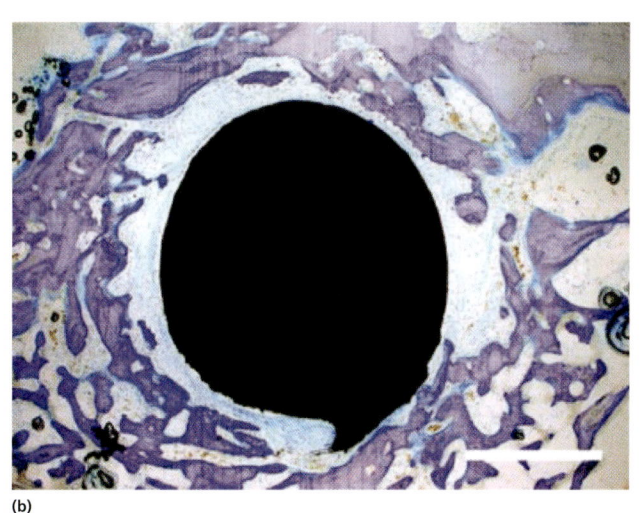

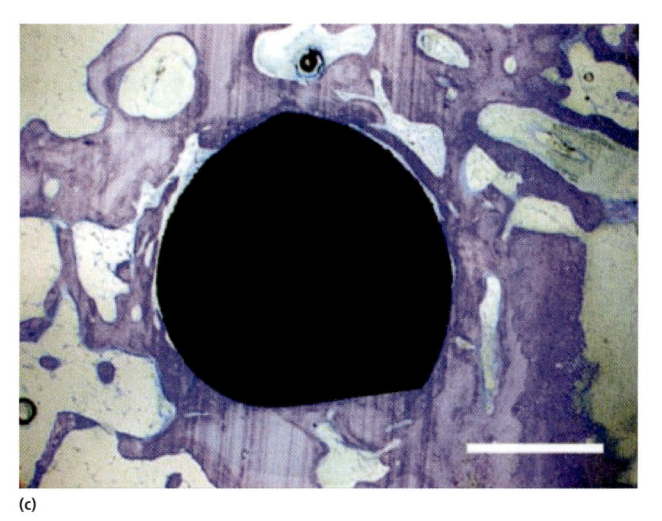

Figure 8.6 Histological section taken to assess bone-to-miniscrew contact (BIC): (a) and (b) are taken from different animals (*Macaca fascicularis* monkeys) at the 1 month observation, while (b) and (c) are taken from the same animal at the 1 and 3 months observations, respectively. Note the interanimal variability at the same time interval and the time-dependent increase in BIC in the same animal. Bar, 1 mm. (Source: Luzi *et al.*, 2009. Reproduced with permission of Oxford University Press.)

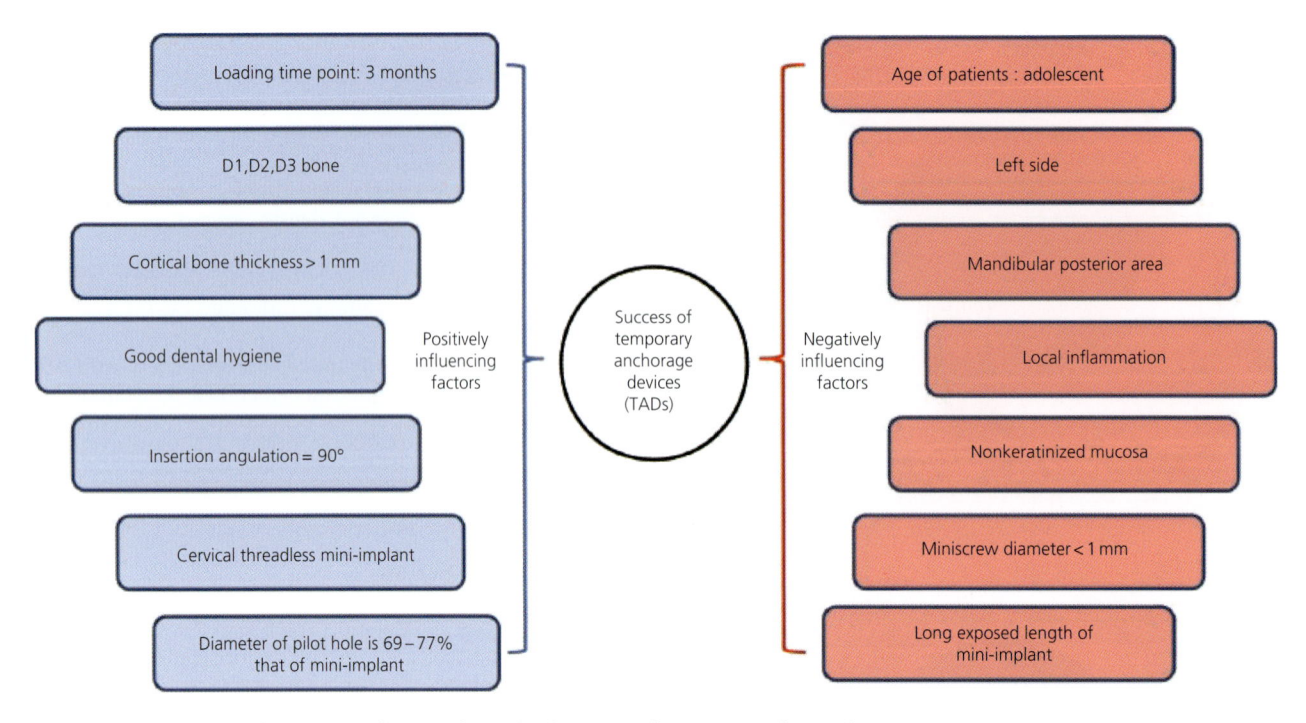

Figure 8.7 The positively and negatively influencing factors for the success of temporary anchorage devices.

Inflammatory reactions

Despite continuous efforts, no TAD-system has provided a 100% success rate (Antoszewska et al., 2010). Peri-implantitis is one of the main causes for the failure of dental implants. In clinical investigations, the failure of TADs was partially attributed to a local infection and inflammation (Antoszewska et al., 2009). Therefore, the assessment of factors involved in inflammation has become crucial to increase TAD stability in orthodontics. Unfortunately, hitherto, the inflammatory response surrounding TADs was seldom studied.

One way to monitor the inflammation level around the orthodontic TADs is to measure the biomarkers including IL-1, IL-2, IL-6, IL-8 and RANKL/OPG in the peri-miniscrew implant crevicular fluid (PMICF), which is an inflammatory exudate secreted in the crevice between miniscrew and peri-miniscrew tissue (Kaur et al., 2017). Sari and Ucar (2007) studied the level of IL-1β in PMICF surrounding 20 miniscrews used as direct anchorage and found no significant difference in IL-1β at different time points between the miniscrew and the control groups. However, when using miniscrews as indirect anchorage, Monga et al. (2014) reported that the level of IL-1β was significantly higher 1 hour after miniscrew placement and 1 day after loading compared with the baseline. Hamamci et al. (2012) examined the level of IL-2, IL-6, and IL-8 in the PMICF when using miniscrews as direct anchorage to retracting anterior teeth. The levels of IL-2 and IL-8 were higher in the implant group than in the control group at 24 hours after loading; IL-6 levels remained unchanged at all observation time points. These observations suggest that the force applied to miniscrews during orthodontic loading may lead to cytokine secretion, which may result in screw loosening.

TADs show good cytocompatibility to human osteogenic sarcoma cells, permanent keratinocytes (HaCat), and primary gingival fibroblasts in a neutral condition. However, in an acidic condition TADs appear to have a cytotoxic effect (Galeotti et al., 2013). This finding suggested that TADs might harm surrounding tissue in an inflammatory site with acidified microenvironments.

Conclusions

TADs are widely used in orthodontics for the correction of various orofacial deformities and malocclusions. The success rate is 87% for miniscrews (Alharbi et al., 2018) and 97% for miniplates (Findik et al., 2017). Clinical and mechanical studies indicate that the success of TADs can be significantly influenced by the following factors: age of the patients, loading time points, implant site and presence of local inflammation, implantation torque, mobility, design of implants, insertion angulation, and exposed length (Figure 8.7). Very few data are available on the histological and inflammatory reactions to TADs. Further studies are urgently needed to identify the biological mechanisms for the failure and success of TADs.

References

Albogha, M. H. and Takahashi, I. (2018) Effect of loaded orthodontic miniscrew implant on compressive stresses in adjacent periodontal ligament. *The Angle Orthodontist* **89**, 235–241. doi:10.2319/122017-873.1.

Alharbi, F., Almuzian, M. and Bearn, D. (2018) Miniscrews failure rate in orthodontics: systematic review and meta-analysis. *European Journal of Orthodontics* **40**, 519–530. doi:10.1093/ejo/cjx093.

Antoszewska, J., Papadopoulos, M. A., Park, H. S. and Ludwig, B. (2009) Five-year experience with orthodontic miniscrew implants: a retrospective investigation of factors influencing success rates. *American Journal of Orthodontics and Dentofacial Orthopedics* **136**, 158.e151–110; discussion 158–159. doi:10.1016/j.ajodo.2009.03.031.

Antoszewska, J., Raftowicz-Wojcik, K., Kawala, B. and Matthews-Brzozowska, T. (2010) Biological factors involved in implant-anchored orthodontics and in prosthetic-implant therapy: a literature review. *Archivum Immunologiae et Therapie Experimentalis (Warsz)* **58**, 379–383. doi:10.1007/s00005-010-0088-8.

Büchter, A., Wiechmann, D., Koerdt, S. et al. (2005) Load-related implant reaction of mini-implants used for orthodontic anchorage. *Clinical Oral Implants Research* **16**, 473–479. doi:10.1111/j.1600-0501.2005.01149.x.

Basciftci, F. A., Korkmaz, H. H., Üşümez, S. and Eraslan, O. (2008) Biomechanical evaluation of chincup treatment with various force vectors. *American Journal of Orthodontics and Dentofacial Orthopedics* **134**, 773–781. doi:https://doi.org/10.1016/j.ajodo.2006.10.035.

Chang, J. Z.-C., Chen, Y.-J., Tung, Y.-Y. et al. (2012) Effects of thread depth, taper shape, and taper length on the mechanical properties of mini-implants. *American Journal* of Orthodontics and Dentofacial Orthopedics **141**, 279–288. doi:https://doi.org/10.1016/j.ajodo.2011.09.008.

Chen, Y.-J., Chang, H.-H., Huang, C.-Y. et al. (2007) A retrospective analysis of the failure rate of three different orthodontic skeletal anchorage systems. *Clinical Oral Implants Research* **18**, 768–775. doi:10.1111/j.1600-0501.2007.01405.x.

Chen, Y., Kyung, H. M., Zhao, W. T. and Yu, W. J. (2009) Critical factors for the success of orthodontic mini-implants: A systematic review. *American Journal of Orthodontics and Dentofacial Orthopedics* **135**, 284–291. doi:https://doi.org/10.1016/j.ajodo.2007.08.017.

Chopra, S. S. and Chakranarayan, A. (2015) Clinical evaluation of immediate loading of titanium orthodontic implants. *Medical Journal, Armed Forces India* **71**, 165–170. doi:10.1016/j.mjafi.2012.06.020.

Chun, H.-J., Cheong, S.-Y., Han, J.-H. et al. (2002) Evaluation of design parameters of osseointegrated dental implants using finite element analysis. *Journal of Oral Rehabilitation* **29**, 565–574. doi:10.1046/j.1365-2842.2002.00891.x.

Costa, A., Raffainl, M. and Melsen, B. (1998) Miniscrews as orthodontic anchorage: a preliminary report. *International Journal of Adult Orthodontics and Orthognathic Surgery* **13**, 201–209.

Creekmore, T. D. and Eklund, M. K. (1983) The possibility of skeletal anchorage. *Journal of Clinical Orthodontics* **17**, 266–269.

Dalessandri, D., Salgarello, S., Dalessandri, M. et al. (2013) Determinants for success rates of temporary anchorage devices in orthodontics: a meta-analysis (n > 50). *European Journal of Orthodontics* **36**, 303–313. doi:10.1093/ejo/cjt049.

Deguchi, T., Nasu, M., Murakami, K. et al. (2006) Quantitative evaluation of cortical bone thickness with computed tomographic scanning for orthodontic implants. *American Journal of Orthodontics and Dentofacial Orthopedics* **129**, 721.e727–721.e712. doi:https://doi.org/10.1016/j.ajodo.2006.02.026.

Elshebiny, T., Palomo, J. M. and Baumgaertel, S. (2018) Anatomic assessment of the mandibular buccal shelf for miniscrew insertion in white patients. *American Journal of Orthodontics and Dentofacial Orthopedics* **153**, 505–511. doi:https://doi.org/10.1016/j.ajodo.2017.08.014.

Findik, Y., Baykul, T., Esenlik, E. and Turkkahraman, M. H. (2017) Surgical difficulties, success, and complication rates of orthodontic miniplate anchorage systems: Experience with 382 miniplates. *Nigerian Journal of Clinical Practice* **20**, 512–516. doi:10.4103/1119-3077.187320.

Galeotti, A., Uomo, R., Spagnuolo, G. et al. (2013) Effect of pH on in vitro biocompatibility of orthodontic miniscrew implants. *Progress in Orthodontics* **14**, 15. doi:10.1186/2196-1042-14-15.

Hamamci, N., Acun Kaya, F., Uysal, E. and Yokus, B. (2012) Identification of interleukin 2, 6, and 8 levels around miniscrews during orthodontic tooth movement. *European Journal of Orthodontics* **34**, 357–361. doi:10.1093/ejo/cjr019.

Higuchi, K. W. and Slack, J. M. (1991) The use of titanium fixtures for intraoral anchorage to facilitate orthodontic tooth movement. *International Journal of Oral and Maxillofacial Implants* **6**, 338–344.

Hong, S.-B., Kusnoto, B., Kim, E.-J. et al. (2016) Prognostic factors associated with the success rates of posterior orthodontic miniscrew implants: A subgroup meta-analysis. *Korean Journal of Orthodontics* **46**, 111–126. doi:10.4041/kjod.2016.46.2.111.

Huja, S. S. (2015) Bone anchors – can you hitch up your wagon? *Orthodontics and Craniofacial Research* **18**, 109–116. doi:10.1111/ocr.12082.

Hutton, J. E., Heath, M. R., Chai, J. Y. et al. (1995) Factors related to success and failure rates at 3-year follow-up in a multicenter study of overdentures supported by Branemark implants. *International Journal of Oral and Maxillofacial Implants* **10**, 33–42.

Iijima, M., Takano, M., Yasuda, Y. et al. (2012) Effect of the quantity and quality of cortical bone on the failure force of a miniscrew implant. *European Journal of Orthodontics* **35**, 583–589. doi:10.1093/ejo/cjs066.

Inoue, M., Kuroda, S., Yasue, A. et al. (2014) Torque ratio as a predictable factor on primary stability of orthodontic miniscrew implants. *Implant Dentistry* **23**, 576–581. doi:10.1097/id.0000000000000138.

Iwai, H., Motoyoshi, M., Uchida, Y. et al. (2015) Effects of tooth root contact on the stability of orthodontic anchor screws in the maxilla: Comparison between self-drilling and self-tapping methods. *American Journal of Orthodontics and Dentofacial Orthopedics* **147**, 483–491. doi:https://doi.org/10.1016/j.ajodo.2014.12.017.

Iwasa, A., Horiuchi, S., Kinouchi, N. et al. (2017) Skeletal anchorage for intrusion of bimaxillary molars in a patient with skeletal open bite and temporomandibular disorders. *Journal of Orthodontic Science* **6**, 152–158. doi:10.4103/jos.JOS_63_17.

Jaffin, R. A. and Berman, C. L. (1991) The excessive loss of Branemark fixtures in type IV bone: a 5-year analysis. *Journal of Periodontology* **62**, 2–4. doi:10.1902/jop.1991.62.1.2.

Jasmine, M. I. F., Yezdani, A. A., Tajir, F. and Venu, R. M. (2012) Analysis of stress in bone and microimplants during en-masse retraction of maxillary and mandibular anterior teeth with different insertion angulations: A 3-dimensional finite element analysis study. *American Journal of Orthodontics and Dentofacial Orthopedics* **141**, 71–80. doi:https://doi.org/10.1016/j.ajodo.2011.06.031.

Jenner, J. D. and Fitzpatrick, B. N. (1985) Skeletal anchorage utilising bone plates. *Australian Orthodontic Journal* **9**, 231–233.

Kanomi, R. (1997) Mini-implant for orthodontic anchorage. *Journal of Clinical Orthodontics* **31**, 763–767.

Kaur, A., Kharbanda, O. P., Kapoor, P. and Kalyanasundaram, D. (2017) A review of biomarkers in peri-miniscrew implant crevicular fluid (PMICF). *Progress in Orthodontics* **18**, 42. doi:10.1186/s40510-017-0195-8.

Kuroda, S., Inoue, M., Kyung, H. M. et al. (2017) Stress distribution in obliquely inserted orthodontic miniscrews evaluated by three-dimensional finite-element analysis. *International Journal of Oral and Maxillofacial Implants* **32**, 344–349. doi:10.11607/jomi.5061.

Kuroda, S., Sugawara, Y., Deguchi, T. et al. (2007a) Clinical use of miniscrew implants as orthodontic anchorage: Success rates and postoperative discomfort. *American Journal of Orthodontics and Dentofacial Orthopedics* **131**, 9–15. doi:https://doi.org/10.1016/j.ajodo.2005.02.032.

Kuroda, S., Yamada, K., Deguchi, T. et al. (2007b) Root proximity is a major factor for screw failure in orthodontic anchorage. *American Journal of Orthodontics and Dentofacial Orthopedics* **131**, S68–S73. doi:https://doi.org/10.1016/j.ajodo.2006.06.017.

Kyung, H. M., Park, H. S., Bae, S. M. et al. (2003) Development of orthodontic micro-implants for intraoral anchorage. *Journal of Clinical Orthodontics* **37**, 321–328; quiz 314.

Leung, M. T., Lee, T. C., Rabie, A. B. and Wong, R. W. (2008) Use of miniscrews and miniplates in orthodontics. *Journal of Oral and Maxillofacial Surgery* **66**, 1461–1466. doi:10.1016/j.joms.2007.12.029.

Lin, T.-S., Tsai, F.-D., Chen, C.-Y. and Lin, L.-W. (2013) Factorial analysis of variables affecting bone stress adjacent to the orthodontic anchorage mini-implant with finite element analysis. *American Journal of Orthodontics and Dentofacial Orthopedics* **143**, 182–189. doi:https://doi.org/10.1016/j.ajodo.2012.09.012.

Liou, E. J. W., Pai, B. C. J. and Lin, J. C. Y. (2004) Do miniscrews remain stationary under orthodontic forces? *American Journal of Orthodontics and Dentofacial Orthopedics* **126**, 42–47. doi:https://doi.org/10.1016/j.ajodo.2003.06.018.

Liu, T.-C., Chang, C.-H., Wong, T.-Y. and Liu, J.-K. (2012) Finite element analysis of miniscrew implants used for orthodontic anchorage. *American Journal of Orthodontics and Dentofacial Orthopedics* **141**, 468–476. doi:https://doi.org/10.1016/j.ajodo.2011.11.012.

Luzi, C., Verna, C. and Melsen, B. (2009) Immediate loading of orthodontic mini-implants: a histomorphometric evaluation of tissue reaction. *European Journal of Orthodontics* **31**, 21–29. doi:10.1093/ejo/cjn087.

Marusamy, K. O., Ramasamy, S. and Wali, O. (2018) Molar protraction using miniscrews (temporary anchorage device) with simultaneous correction of lateral crossbite: an orthodontic case report. *Journal of International Society of Preventive and Community Dentistry* **8**, 271–276. doi:10.4103/jispcd.JISPCD_447_17.

McManus, M. M., Qian, F., Grosland, N. M. et al. (2011) Effect of miniscrew placement torque on resistance to miniscrew movement under load. *American Journal of Orthodontics and Dentofacial Orthopedics* **140**, e93–e98. doi:https://doi.org/10.1016/j.ajodo.2011.04.017.

Migliorati, M., Drago, S., Gallo, F. et al. (2016) Immediate versus delayed loading: comparison of primary stability loss after miniscrew placement in orthodontic patients – a single-centre blinded randomized clinical trial. *European Journal of Orthodontics* **38**, 652–659. doi:10.1093/ejo/cjv095.

Misch, C. E., Qu, Z. and Bidez, M.W. (1999) Mechanical properties of trabecular bone in the human mandible: implications for dental implant treatment planning and surgical placement. *Journal of Oral and Maxillofacial Surgery* **57**, 700–708.

Miyawaki, S., Koyama, I., Inoue, M. et al. (2003) Factors associated with the stability of titanium screws placed in the posterior region for orthodontic anchorage. *American Journal of Orthodontics and Dentofacial Orthopedics* **124**, 373–378. doi:https://doi.org/10.1016/S0889-5406(03)00565-1.

Mohammed, H., Wafaie, K., Rizk, M. Z. et al. (2018) Role of anatomical sites and correlated risk factors on the survival of orthodontic miniscrew implants: a systematic review and meta-analysis. *Progress in Orthodontics* **19**, 36–36. doi:10.1186/s40510-018-0225-1.

Monga, N., Chaurasia, S., Kharbanda, O. P. et al. (2014) A study of interleukin 1β levels in peri-miniscrew crevicular fluid (PMCF). *Progress in Orthodontics* **15**, 30–30. doi:10.1186/s40510-014-0030-4.

Moon, C.-H., Lee, D.-G., Lee, H.-S. et al. (2008) Factors associated with the success rate of orthodontic miniscrews placed in the upper and lower posterior buccal region. *The Angle Orthodontist* **78**, 101–106. doi:10.2319/121706-515.1.

Motoyoshi, M., Yoshida, T., Ono, A. and Shimizu, N. (2007) Effect of cortical bone thickness and implant placement torque on stability of orthodontic mini-implants. *International Journal of Oral and Maxillofacial Implants* **22**, 779–784.

Motoyoshi, M., Inaba, M., Ueno, S. and Shimizu, N. (2009a) Mechanical anisotropy of orthodontic mini-implants. *International Journal of Oral and Maxillofacial Surgery* **38**, 972–977. doi:https://doi.org/10.1016/j.ijom.2009.05.009.

Motoyoshi, M., Ueno, S., Okazaki, K. and Shimizu, N. (2009b) Bone stress for a mini-implant close to the roots of adjacent teeth - 3D finite element analysis. *International Journal of Oral and Maxillofacial Surgery* **38**, 363–368. doi:https://doi.org/10.1016/j.ijom.2009.02.011.

Motoyoshi, M., Yano, S., Tsuruoka, T. and Shimizu, N. (2005) Biomechanical effect of abutment on stability of orthodontic mini-implant. A finite element analysis. *Clinical Oral Implants Research* **16**, 480–485. doi:10.1111/j.1600-0501.2005.01130.x.

Nakagaki, S., Iijima, M., Handa, K. et al. (2014) Micro-CT and histologic analyses of bone surrounding immediately loaded miniscrew implants: comparing compression and tension loading. *Dental Materials Journal* **33**, 196–202.

Oltramari-Navarro, P. V. P., Navarro, R. L., Henriques, J. F. C. et al. (2013) The impact of healing time before loading on orthodontic mini-implant stability: A histomorphometric study in minipigs. *Archives of Oral Biology* **58**, 806–812. doi:https://doi.org/10.1016/j.archoralbio.2012.12.010.

Papageorgiou, S. N., Zogakis, I. P. and Papadopoulos, M. A. (2012) Failure rates and associated risk factors of orthodontic miniscrew implants: A meta-analysis. *American Journal of Orthodontics and Dentofacial Orthopedics* **142**, 577–595.e577. doi:https://doi.org/10.1016/j.ajodo.2012.05.016.

Park, H.-S., Jeong, S.-H. and Kwon, O.-W. (2006) Factors affecting the clinical success of screw implants used as orthodontic anchorage. *American Journal of Orthodontics and Dentofacial Orthopedics* **130**, 18–25. doi:https://doi.org/10.1016/j.ajodo.2004.11.032.

Perillo, L., Jamilian, A., Shafieyoon, A. et al. (2015) Finite element analysis of miniscrew placement in mandibular alveolar bone with varied angulations. *European Journal of Orthodontics* **37**, 56–59. Doi:10.1093/ejo/cju006.

Raghavendra, S., Wood, M. C. and Taylor, T. D. (2005) Early wound healing around endosseous implants: a review of the literature. *International Journal of Oral and Maxillofacial Implants* **20**, 425–431.

Roberts, W. E., Marshall, K. J. and Mozsary, P. G. (1990) Rigid endosseous implant utilized as anchorage to protract molars and close an atrophic extraction site. *The Angle Orthodontics* **60**, 135–152. doi:10.1043/0003-3219(1990)060<0135:Reiuaa>2.0.Co;2.

Sari, E. and Ucar, C. (2007) Interleukin 1beta levels around microscrew implants during orthodontic tooth movement. *The Angle Orthodontist* **77**, 1073–1078. doi:10.2319/100506-405.1.

Schenk, R. K. and Buser, D. (1998) Osseointegration: a reality. *Periodontology 2000* **17**, 22–35. doi:10.1111/j.1600-0757.1998.tb00120.x.

Seifi, M. and Matini, N.-S. (2016) Evaluation of primary stability of innovated orthodontic miniscrew system (STS): An ex-vivo study. *Journal of Clinical and Experimental Dentistry* **8**, e255–e259. doi:10.4317/jced.52676.

Sevimay, M., Turhan, F., Kilicarslan, M. A. and Eskitascioglu, G. (2005) Three-dimensional finite element analysis of the effect of different bone quality on stress distribution in an implant-supported crown. *Journal of Prosthetic Dentistry* **93**, 227–234. doi:10.1016/j.prosdent.2004.12.019.

Shen, S., Sun, Y., Zhang, C., Yang, Y. et al. (2015) Bivariate optimization of orthodontic mini-implant thread height and pitch. *International Journal of Computer Assisted Radiology and Surgery* **10**, 109–116. doi:10.1007/s11548-014-1107-8.

Son, S., Motoyoshi, M., Uchida, Y. and Shimizu, N. (2014) Comparative study of the primary stability of self-drilling and self-tapping orthodontic miniscrews. *American Journal of Orthodontics and Dentofacial Orthopedics* **145**, 480–485. doi:https://doi.org/10.1016/j.ajodo.2013.12.020.

Stahl, E., Keilig, L., Abdelgader, I. et al. (2009) Numerical analyses of biomechanical behavior of various orthodontic anchorage implants. *Journal of Orofacial Orthopedics / Fortschritte der Kieferorthopädie* **70**, 115–127. doi:10.1007/s00056-009-0817-y.

Suzuki, M., Deguchi, T., Watanabe, H. et al. (2013) Evaluation of optimal length and insertion torque for miniscrews. *American Journal of Orthodontics and Dentofacial Orthopedics* **144**, 251–259. doi:https://doi.org/10.1016/j.ajodo.2013.03.021.

Topouzelis, N. and Tsaousoglou, P. (2012) Clinical factors correlated with the success rate of miniscrews in orthodontic treatment. *International Journal of Oral Science* **4**, 38–44. doi:10.1038/ijos.2012.1.

Uemura, M., Motoyoshi, M., Yano, S. et al. (2012) Orthodontic mini-implant stability and the ratio of pilot hole implant diameter. *European Journal of Orthodontics* **34**, 52–56. doi:10.1093/ejo/cjq157.

Vande Vannet, B., Sabzevar, M. M., Wehrbein, H. and Asscherickx, K. (2007) Osseointegration of miniscrews: a histomorphometric evaluation. *European Journal of Orthodontics* **29**, 437–442. doi:10.1093/ejo/cjm078.

Watanabe, H., Deguchi, T., Hasegawa, M. et al. (2013) Orthodontic miniscrew failure rate and root proximity, insertion angle, bone contact length, and bone density. *Orthodontics and Craniofacial Research* **16**, 44–55. doi:10.1111/ocr.12003.

Watanabe, T., Miyazawa, K., Fujiwara, T. et al. (2017) Insertion torque and Periotest values are important factors predicting outcome after orthodontic miniscrew placement. *American Journal of Orthodontics and Dentofacial Orthopedics* **152**, 483–488. doi:10.1016/j.ajodo.2017.01.026.

Wehrbein, H., Merz, B. R., Diedrich, P. and Glatzmaier, J. (1996) The use of palatal implants for orthodontic anchorage. Design and clinical application of the orthosystem. *Clinical and Oral Implants Research* **7**, 410–416.

Wiechmann, D., Meyer, U. and Buchter, A. (2007) Success rate of mini- and microimplants used for orthodontic anchorage: a prospective clinical study. *Clinical and Oral Implants Research* **18**, 263–267. doi:10.1111/j.1600-0501.2006.01325.x.

Woodall, N., Tadepalli, S. C., Qian, F. et al. (2011) Effect of miniscrew angulation on anchorage resistance. *American Journal of Orthodontics and Dentofacial Orthopedics* **139**, e147–e152. doi:https://doi.org/10.1016/j.ajodo.2010.08.017.

CHAPTER 9
Tissue Reaction to Orthodontic Force Systems. Are we in Control?

Birte Melsen, Michel Dalstra, and Paolo M. Cattaneo

Summary

The purpose of this chapter is to assess how an updated analysis of the biomechanical assumptions for segmented appliances as formulated by Burstone (1962) would influence clinical behavior. The focus is mainly on renewed discussion of the pressure–tension theory, the influence of the material properties, the influence of the morphology of the alveolar wall, the influence of the force level, and the influence of the interaction with occlusion. Theoretically, the idea of applying a force system in a well-determined relationship to the center of resistance makes sense, but clinically the observed displacement may not be what is expected based on the calculations, and the observed displacements will indicate which modifications are needed. The reported analysis of factors influencing the type of tooth movement when applying a force, which from a mathematical point of view should deliver a specific displacement, indicate the necessity of carefully analysing the observed movement and adapting the force system accordingly.

Introduction

During orthodontic treatment, forces are applied to teeth and consequently the teeth are being displaced in a manner determined by the line of action of the force applied. As the shortest distance between two points is a straight line, this could according to Burstone (1962) be formulated in orthodontic terms as: for a well-defined tooth movement, there is only one correct line of action of the force. This force, however, can be generated by many different appliances. Already the description of the change in tooth position can pose a problem. When a tooth is being translated, all parts of the tooth have the same amount of movement in the same direction, and when submitted to a couple, all parts are rotated around the centre of resistance (CR), the position of which may be in different localizations in different planes of space (Figure 9.1). Apart from the situations where a tooth is purely translated or rotated, all other displacements are combinations of translations and rotations. These movements are expressed by the distance between the CR and the CRot (centre of rotation). When analysing tooth movement, Viecilli calculated the localization of the CR in various teeth in three-dimensions (3D) mostly focusing on the tooth morphology only mentioning the influence of the surrounding periodontium (Viecilli et al., 2008; Viecilli, 2015). Indeed, when localizing the CR in the three planes of space in addition to the morphology of the various teeth, tooth position and quality and level of the surrounding bone play a decisive role.

The existence of a CR and its importance for the prediction of tooth displacement when submitted to an orthodontic force was introduced by Burstone in the 1960s and 1970s (Burstone, 1962; Burstone et al., 1978). For an ideal ellipsoid-shaped root, the CR can be mathematically calculated, and it is located on the longitudinal axis of the tooth at one-third of the root's length seen in a sagittal view. However, holographic analysis (Burstone and Pryputniewicz, 1980) demonstrated that for an actual single-rooted tooth, this location was closer to 40% of its root's length.

The line of action of an orthodontic force with respect to the CR is controlling the displacement of the tooth and thereby the load transfer from tooth to the periodontium. The perpendicular distance from the CR to the line-of-action of the applied force can be expressed as the moment-to-force ratio (M/F) of a force applied at the bracket. In relation to an incisor with the longitudinal axis vertical, a M/F of respectively 0, –5, –10 and –12 mm at the bracket is associated with an M/F of 10, 5, 0 and –2 mm at the CR, consequently resulting in an uncontrolled tipping, a controlled tipping, a pure translation, and a root movement, respectively

---

Biological Mechanisms of Tooth Movement, Third Edition. Edited by Vinod Krishnan, Anne Marie Kuijpers-Jagtman and Ze'ev Davidovitch.
© 2021 John Wiley & Sons Ltd. Published 2021 by John Wiley & Sons Ltd.

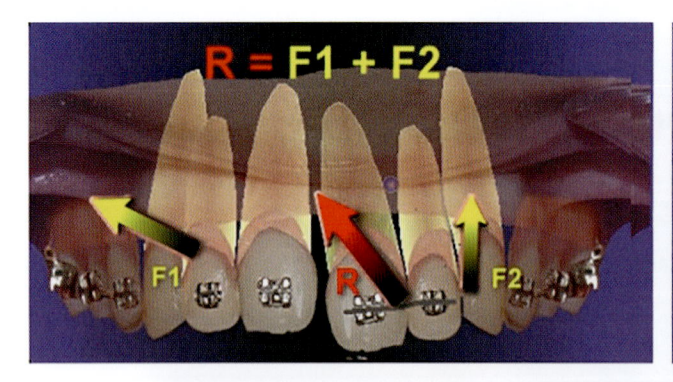

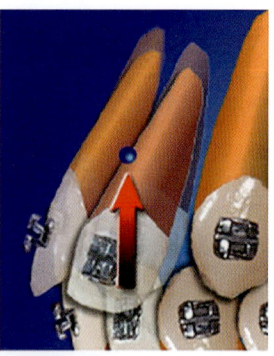

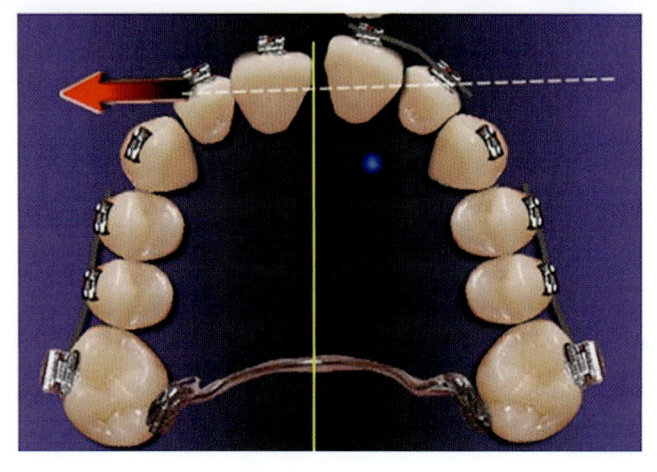

Figure 9.1 Localization of the CR in 3D. Line of action of a force applied for the intrusion and intrusion of two maxillary incisors. It can be seen that the CR cannot be defined as the same point in all three planes of space. (Source: Fiorelli, G. and Melsen, B., 2013. *Biomechanics in Orthodontics. A Multimedia Textbook*. Libro Orthodonzia, Arezzo, Italy. With permission.)

(Burstone, 1962). These theories are based on four assumptions, which since the introduction of the rationale of segmented arch (Burstone, 1966) have received little attention:

1. The force added to a tooth is via the periodontal ligament (PDL) transferred to the alveolar wall, the area of which is assumed to be mirroring the root surface;
2. The PDL behaves linearly and generates equal (yet oppositely directed) reaction forces to both the tension and compression side of the alveolus;
3. The root is uniformly supported on all sides by alveolar bone, and therefore the CR is located on the central axis of the root;
4. The magnitude of the external force has no influence on the load transfer, as it appears both above and below the division line of the M/F, and is thus cancelled out and of no further consequence.

However, none of these assumptions have, since the introduction of this treatment approach, been supported by research.

An additional problem receiving little attention is the tissue reaction to the application of an orthodontic force system. According to the classic "pressure–tension" hypothesis, the pressure generated when displacing a tooth within the PDL is directly related to resorption, either directly or indirectly in relation to a hyalinization. However, bone biologists generally demonstrated that loading of bone with pressure is related to increase in bone density, e.g., in case of bruxism and weightlifting. When a long bone is bent, apposition is occurring on the compressed concave side and resorption on the stretched convex side. In spite of several attempts to solve this controversy with studies of the reaction to deformation (Verna and Melsen, 2012), this theory is still being referred to in recent orthodontic literature (Proffit, 2019). Histological studies disclose that reactions of the PDL and the alveolar bone occur simultaneously, but what is the mechanism of this relationship?

The perception of the reaction to force application has been based on different interpretations of clinical observations or mathematical considerations (Reitan, 1951; Baumrind, 1969; Heller and Nanda, 1979; Melsen, 2001). Since 1987, Finite Element Analysis (FEA) has been the method of preference to study the effect of a force system, applied at the bracket level, on the alveolar support tissues (Tanne et al., 1987). The clinical consequences of an FEA are, however, completely dependent on the realism of the input, i.e., the size of the elements in relation to the question asked and the validity of the material properties assigned to the included structures (Cattaneo et al., 2005). As an FEA is only illustrating one particular case, the results are also dependent on how well the model represents the region for which the question is asked.

This chapter will focus on factors influencing both the tissue reaction and the clinical result of application of various force systems to the tooth.

The following factors influencing the results of a force application will be discussed:

1. Renewed discussion of the pressure–tension theory;
2. The influence of the material properties;
3. The influence of the morphology of the alveolar wall;
4. The influence of the force level;
5. The influence of the interaction with occlusion.

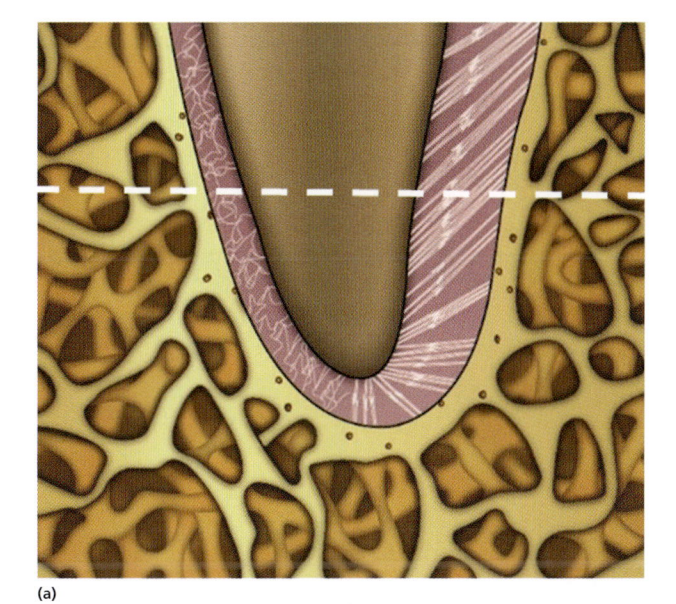

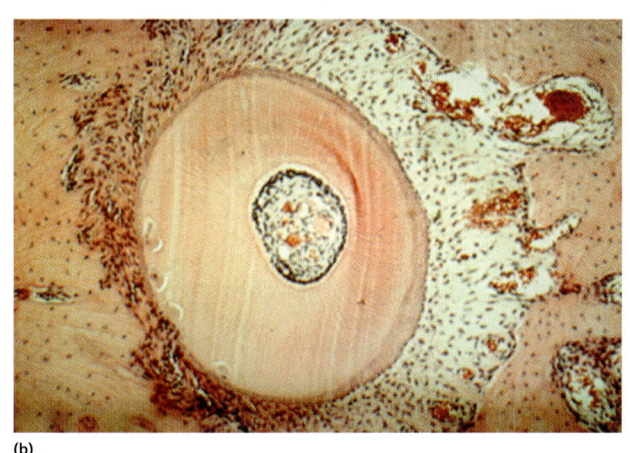

Figure 9.2 (a) Sagittal view of a tooth being displaced within the PDL resulting in a curling of the fibers on the "pressure side". (b) Horizontal section of a tooth being displaced within the periodontal ligament. The displacement results in a narrowing of the PDL in the direction of the force. This leads to a curling of the fibers crossing the PDL which means that the osteocytes will not receive any stimulus when chewing forces are applied to the tooth. Therefore, the result will be a removal of bone that is not loaded as indicated in Figure 9.1. (Source: Dr. Birte Melsen.)

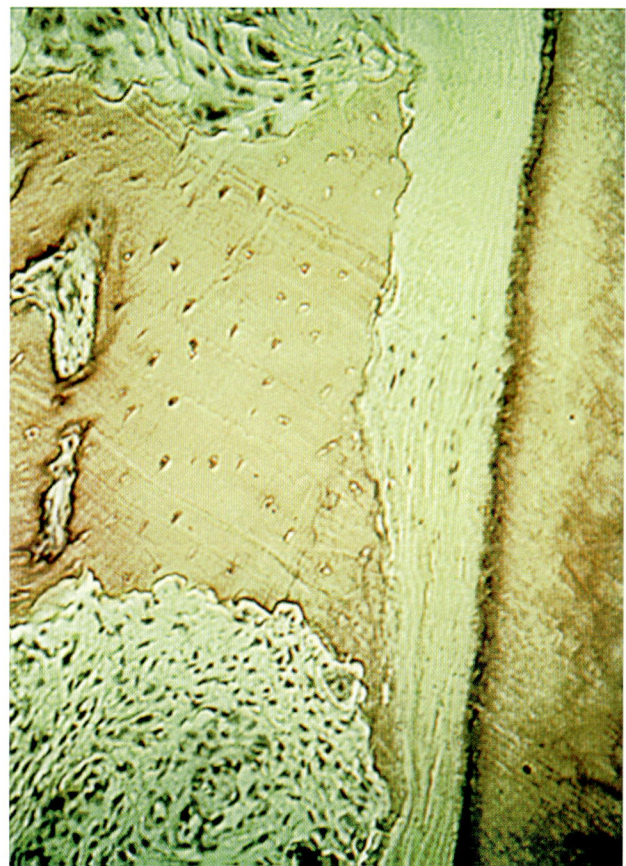

Figure 9.3 Hyalinization and the so-called indirect resorption. There are no lining cells and the osteocytes lacunae in the bone below the hyalinization are empty. An apoptosis has taken place when the ischemia lead to death of the lining cells. The indirect resorption can therefore be perceived as a repair removing necrotic tissue. (Source: Dr. Birte Melsen.)

Pressure–tension theory: Still valid?

In 1999, and also in 2001, Melsen and collaborators focused on the controversy between orthodontists and orthopedists on the perceived biological response of bone to pressure (Melsen, 1999; Melsen., 2001) (Figure 9.2). The displacement of the tooth within the PDL is the first reaction to a force application and is universally agreed upon. A remodeling of the connection of the fibers extending from the cementum and from the alveolar wall takes place, allowing the tooth to be replaced with respect to the alveolar wall. Simultaneously, the alveolar wall is rebuilt as a result of a reaction monitored by the osteocytes. According to Frost (1994), the strain determines whether an anabolic or a catabolic process is taking place, i.e., whether the density of the bone is increasing or decreasing. On the periosteal and the endosteal surface, resorption or apposition will take place. The lining cells are important, however, and when they disappear because of ischemia as a result of high pressure, the underlying cells become apoptotic as a sign of the local necrosis (Hauge *et al.*, 2009) (Figure 9.3). The indirect resorption should, therefore, according to bone biologists, reflect removal of necrotic tissue as part of a repair. This explanation can be accepted by bone biologists and form the frame for interdisciplinary research.

The influence of the material properties

The *in vivo* displacement of a tooth following an application of a force was described by Burstone and Pryputniewics (1980), based on holographic analysis of a standard-sized central incisor. In an attempt at a deeper understanding, the tissue reaction was analyzed using FE models, where tooth displacement within the PDL space was assessed. The PDL is a closed system, anticipating a linear reaction, which is stated in most published FEA studies of orthodontic load transfer. This does not, however, describe the real situation. The PDL displays a behavior that is compatible with the composition and organization of the PDL: a poro-elastic material constituted by a fluid or semifluid matrix material in which the fibers are embedded. The interaction between the solid and the fluid component gives the material its time-dependent behavior (van Driel *et al.*, 2000) and the fluid phase can be pressed from the PDL into the surrounding alveolar bone, which is characterized by a high porosity (Dalstra et al., 2006, 2015). As a consequence, the PDL can be expected to be anisotropic, nonlinear, and visco-elastic, thus setting special conditions for FEA. Recently, a group of Indian researchers confirmed the validity of modeling the material property as being nonlinear (Hemanth et al., 2015). The comparison of linear and nonlinear material properties for the PDL was assessed by Cattaneo et al. (2008) in an FEA study (Figure 9.4). The morphology of the teeth and supporting tissues used in the FE models were based on µCT-scanned jaw sections, obtained at autopsy, thus providing detailed descriptions of both the external and the internal morphology of the alveolar bone (Figure 9.5).

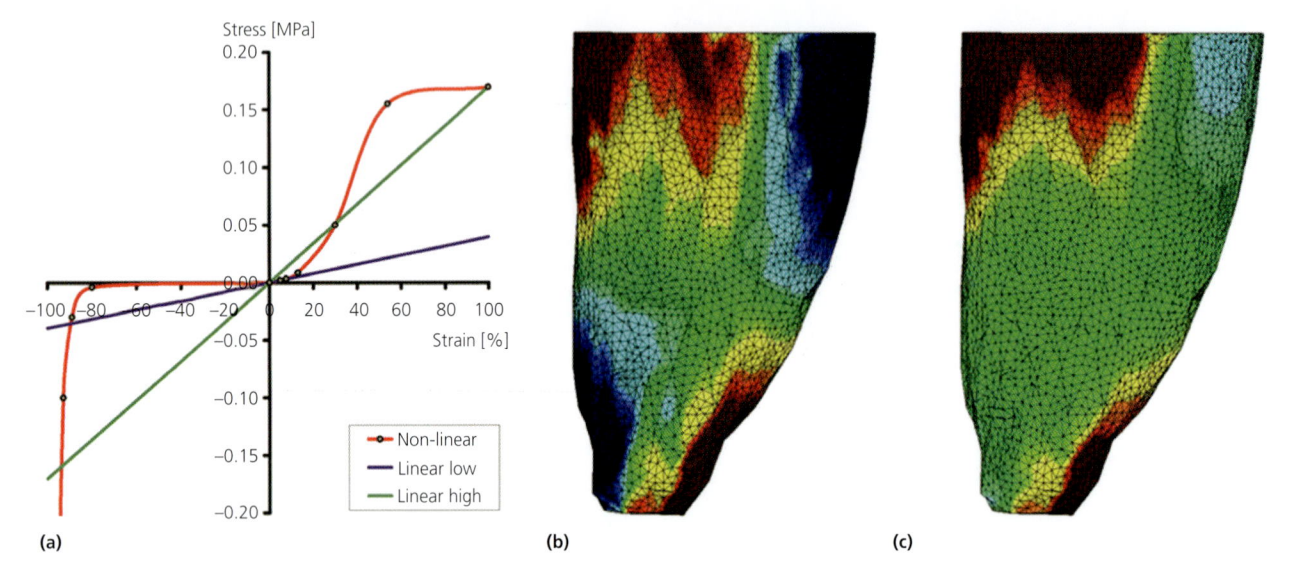

Figure 9.4 Three constitutive models for the PDL are depicted (a), showing the different behavior in a stress–strain plot: physiologic nonlinear behavior (red + dots); linear behavior with a low Young's modulus (purple); and linear behavior with a high Young's modulus (green). The stresses in the PDL of an incisor are shown for an uncontrolled tipping (F = 100 cN, direction ligual–buccal), assuming linear (b) and nonlinear material properties (c). Note the antisymmetry of tensile (red) and compressive stresses (blue) in the linear PDL, and the absence of compressive stresses in the nonlinear PDL. (Source: Based on Cattaneo et al., 2008.)

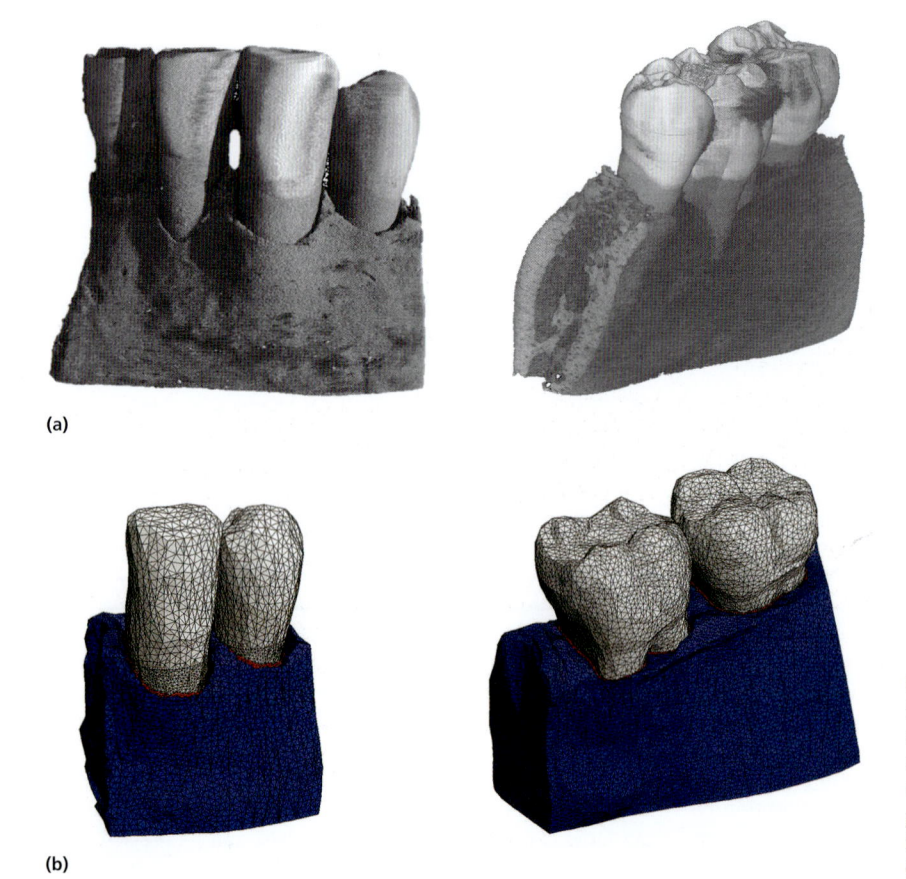

Figure 9.5 (a) Rendering of the 3D µ-CT dataset (voxel dimension: 37 micron) of two bone segments obtained at autopsy. (b) The corresponding FE models (where only portions of the original samples were used) comprising the lower premolar and canine (left) and the mandibular first and second molar (right). (Source: Based on Cattaneo et al., 2009.)

Moreover, a nonlinear stress–strain formulation of the PDL, based on experimental results (Vollmer et al., 1999; Poppe et al., 2002; Nishihira et al., 2003) was used. In contrast to the holographic studies, where the focus was on a model of a central incisor, the aim of the FE studies was to see whether different types of teeth (i.e., incisors, canines, premolars, and molars) complied with the classic "Burstone model."

These detailed FE models demonstrated that the transfer mechanism of forces and moment applied at the bracket to the alveolar supporting structures cannot be explained using the simplistic formulation of the compression and tension zones. By modeling the thin cortical shell of the alveolar edges it is evident that the load transfer mechanisms result in stress distributions that are exactly opposite to those that might be expected based on the "pressure–tension" theory (Reitan, 1951). Defining of the PDL as linear will generate the "traditional" compression and tension zones in case of uncontrolled tipping and translation, once again marking the influence of correct modeling of the alveolar support structures in FE models.

One main consequence of the abovementioned FE studies is that direct bone resorption in the alveolar bone along the direction of movement may be the consequence of a hypophysiological loading, which is in agreement with the suggestion by Binderman et al. (2002) in a study on alveolar bone modeling in orthodontics triggered by a "strain relaxation." On the other hand, in areas where the PDL is undergoing large compressive deformation, ischemia occurs, and the lining cells disappear. The existence of lining cells is crucial for the viability of the osteocytes and, in the classic images of Reitan illustrating undermining resorption, it is obvious that the osteocytic lacunae in the alveolar wall facing the hyalinization are empty, indicating that the bone is necrotized and that the indirect resorption should be perceived as a removal of dead bone – a repair process (Figure 9.3). Hyalinization will occur as result of local ischemia of the PDL (Thilander et al., 2005). Hyalinization is known to be an almost unavoidable phenomenon associated with orthodontic movement, and this was already shown in the innovative research on tooth movement performed by Sandstedt at the beginning of last century (Persson, 2005).

The influence of the morphology of the alveolar wall

As stated above, the CR of a tooth is where all reaction forces generated by the alveolar support tissues are thought to be concentrated. Assuming a regularly shaped and uniformly supported root, the CR can be located exactly on the longitudinal axis of the tooth. If the root is a perfect ellipsoid, then the CR would be located at 33% of its length; in the case of a perfect cylinder (this would be less anatomical, but purely from a mathematical point of view), it would be located at 50% of its length. But are these assumptions valid for the anatomical shape of a root? Burstone and Pryputniewicz (1980) already showed that the actual location of the CR for single-rooted teeth was close to 40% of the root length – so, the real anatomical shape of a single-rooted tooth is a mix somewhere between an ideal ellipsoid and a cylinder in the cervico-apical aspect. Yet what about the actual location of the CR in the mesio-distal and bucco-lingual aspects? The CR can only be located on the central axis of the tooth, when the root is uniformly supported radially. However, looking at μCT-scanned jaw sections obtained at autopsy, it is evident that the bony support of the roots is not uniform around all sides of the root or along its length (Figures 9.6 and 9.7). Cervically, the root is surrounded by cortical bone as it penetrates the cortex of the jaw. Apically, the root is only supported by a very thin layer of lamina dura, not much thicker than the PDL, which in itself is supported mostly by low density trabecular bone. In the mesio-distal aspect, the roots are contained by cortical bone in the cervical area, while apically there is only trabecular bone surrounding the lamina dura. In the bucco-lingual

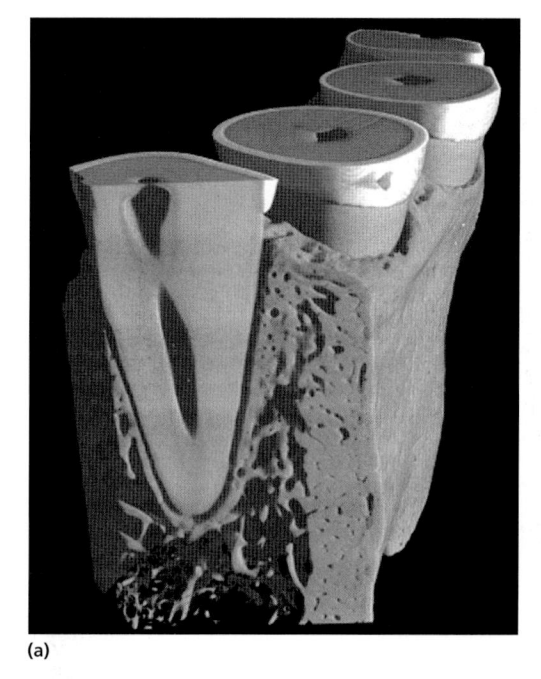

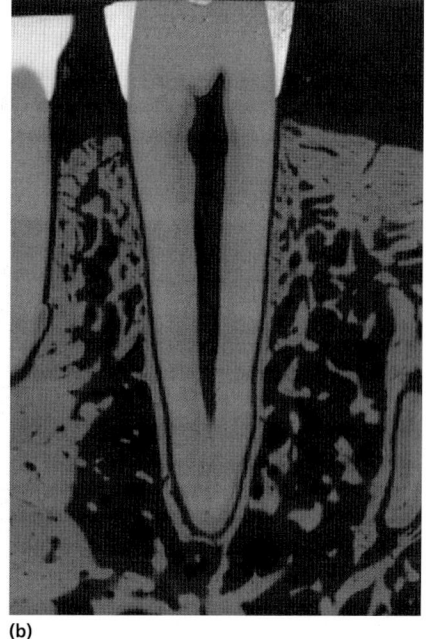

Figure 9.6 3D reconstruction of a μ-CT scanned jaw segment of a 19-year-old male donor with a cut view of the canine (a). The mesio-distal cut view through the first premolar shows the reduced bony support at the apical root (b). (Source: Based on Cattaneo et al., 2009.)

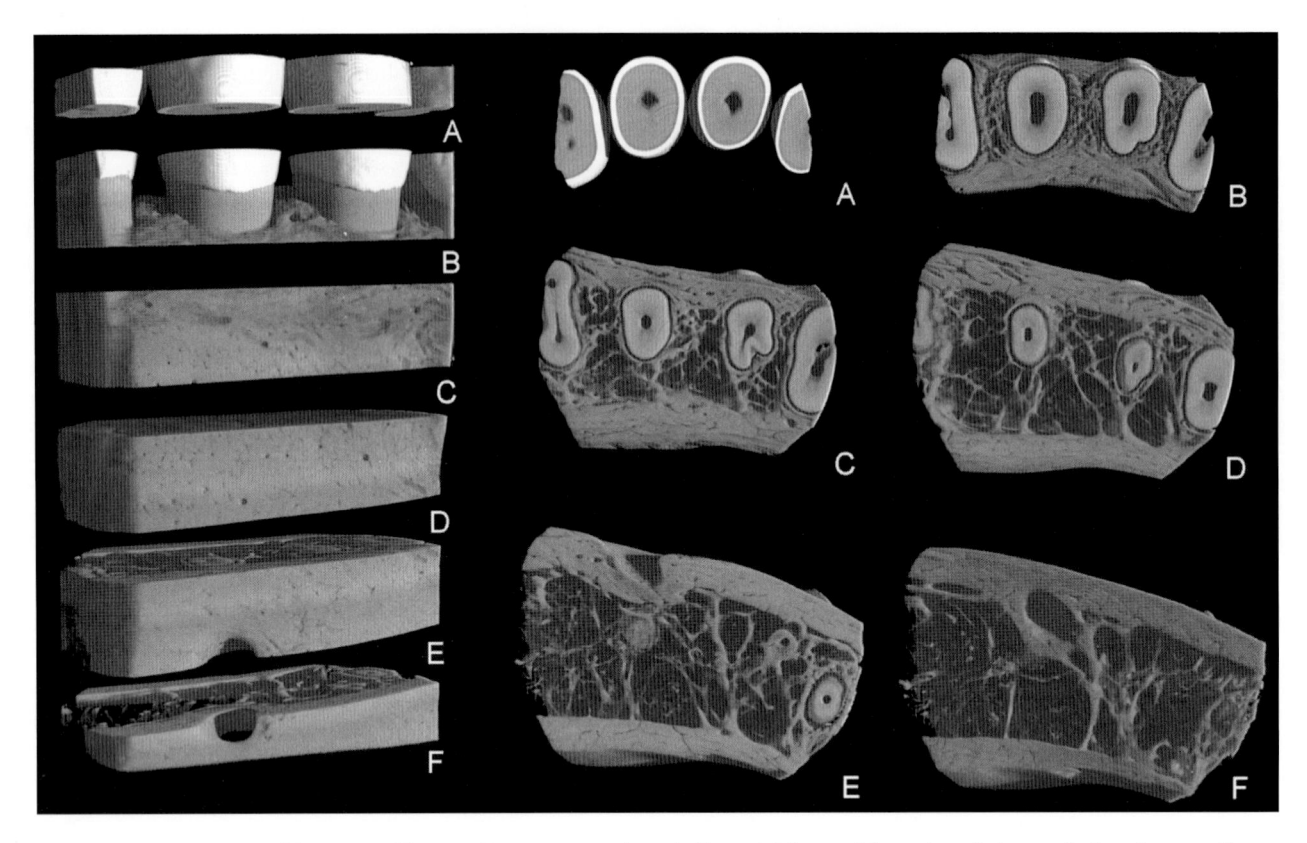

Figure 9.7 3D reconstruction of the same μ-CT scanned jaw segment as shown in Figure 9.6. Sequential cuts through the sample show the nonuniform bony support of the roots. (Source: Dr. Michel Dalstra.)

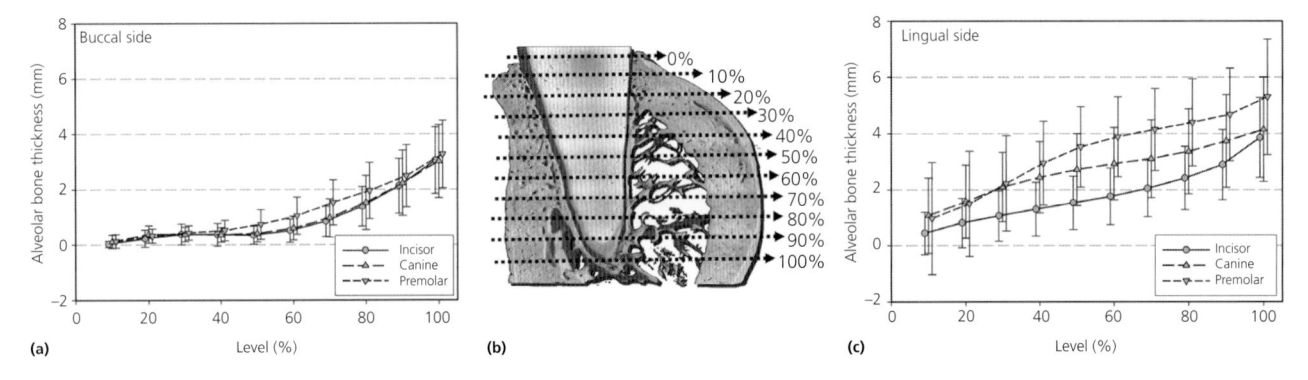

Figure 9.8 Measurements of the thickness of the alveolar bone for incisors, canines, and premolars on the buccal and lingual side. Note that for the first 50% of the root length, the bone thickness on the buccal side is less than 1 mm. (Source: Dr. Michel Dalstra.)

aspect, the lamina dura is much more integrated with the cortex of the jaw, but this is not symmetrical on the buccal and lingual side (Figure 9.8). On the buccal side, the lamina dura is integrated for one-third to half of its length with the cortex, whereas on the lingual side this only occurs cervically. All these deviations from a uniform distribution of the alveolar support tissues will have their own contribution to the exact location of the CR and it is therefore to be expected that this location is not conveniently placed on the central axis of the tooth.

Another aspect of the shape of the alveolar wall has not so much to do with the CR, but rather with the loading of the alveolar wall itself. When considering the stresses on the alveolar wall exerted by an orthodontically moving tooth, usually a smooth surface of the alveolus is assumed. However, μCT-scans of samples of dental roots with the surrounding tissues show that this is not the case. The bony surface features a far from smooth surface with thin bony spicules sticking out into the PDL space (Figures 9.9 and 9.10). It has been shown that these spicules contain osteocyte lacunae (Dalstra et al., 2015) and as such will register even minor local deformation. While the level of forces applied normally ranges between 50 and 300 cN, Weinstein demonstrated that only a few cNs were necessary to displace a tooth, when other forces such as occlusal forces and pressure from the internal and external muscle matrix were excluded (Weinstein, 1967). An explanation

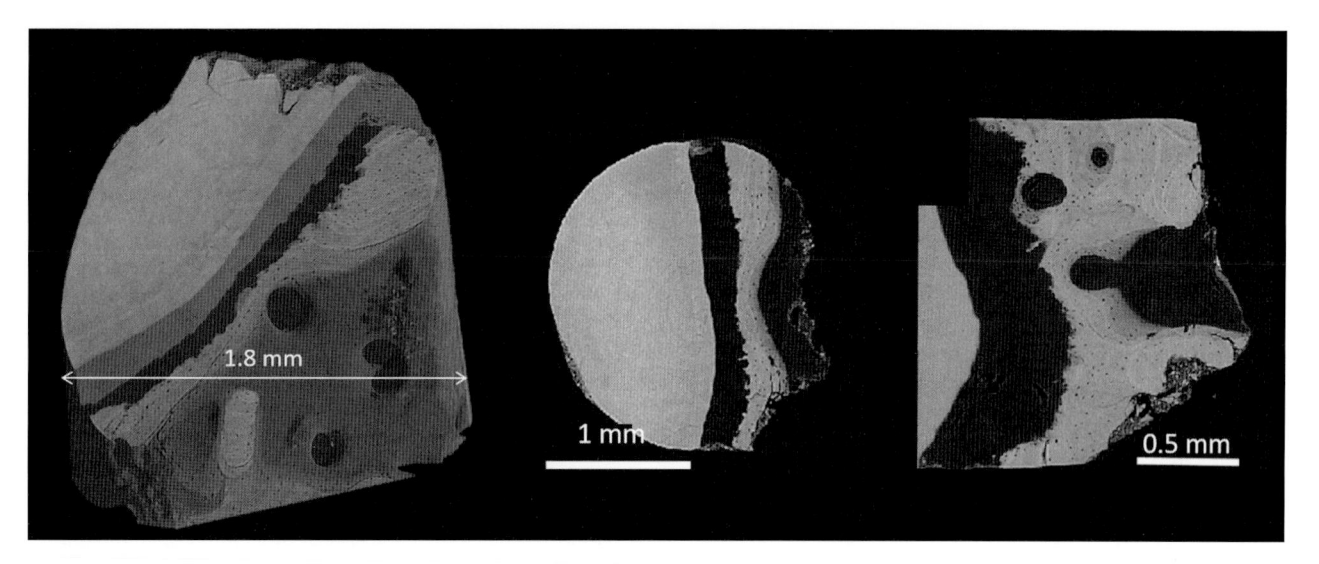

Figure 9.9 3D reconstruction of a detail of the root-PDL-bone complex. Note the smooth surface of the root versus the rough inner surface of the alveolus. (Source: Dr. Michel Dalstra.)

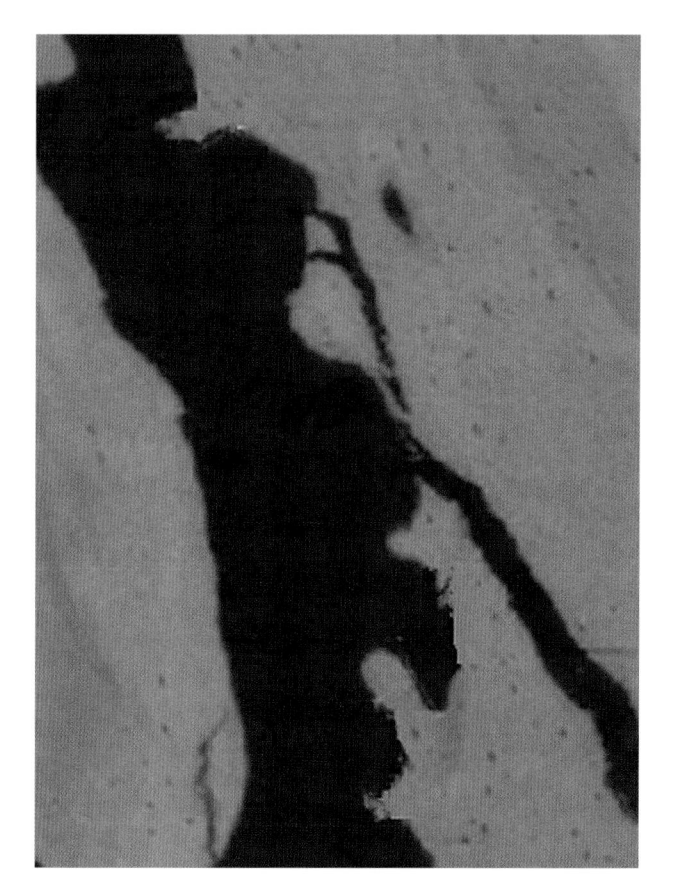

Figure 9.10 Detailed 3D reconstruction of the root-PDL-alveolus complex. Note the bony spicules going into the PDL space and the osteocyte lacunae evenly distributed through the alveolar bone. (Source: Dr. Michel Dalstra.)

may be that the forces are first perceived by the spicules, where a local hyalinization and necrosis will take place with even very low forces. This indicates clinically that the initial force can never be too low. Orthodontic loading generally involves low forces compared with physiological loading. These spicules could act as a kind of "load magnifier" as the load becomes locally concentrated there.

The nonuniformity and the amount of bony support will also play a role, when its integrity is affected by trauma or surgical intervention. Verna *et al.* (2018) have assumed that corticotomies will therefore alter the modus and amount of orthodontic tooth movement. A M/F, normally associated with pure translation can, in the case of corticotomy of the alveolar bone, lead to a tipping.

The influence of force level

An FEA with the purpose of analysing how changes in the force level would influence the type of tooth movement was performed to understand the clinical implications (Cattaneo *et al.*, 2008). It is well known that the decay rate of a force and the decay of the moment associated with this force are not linearly related, thus the actual force system applied at the brackets is changing during the deactivation phase (Burstone, 1982).

In a series of experiments, where the material property of the PDL was assumed to be nonlinear and nonsymmetric, it was found that the M/F, at which pure translation would occur, varied with different tooth morphology. Secondly, it was found that the magnitude of the force in fact did have an influence on the location of the CRot. Interestingly, this behavior was already noted in 1969 by Christiansen and Burstone in their clinical experiments even with forces below 50 cN, yet they wrongly attributed this phenomenon to inaccuracies in the measuring technique and instrumentation (Christiansen and Burstone, 1969). In our in-silico simulation for large forces (>150 cN), the deviation of the actual location of the CRot and the location according to the classic theory do not differ much. However, for smaller forces (up to 50 cN) this deviation could amount to 6–8 mm (Figure 9.11). The explanation for this is that a nonlinear PDL cannot resist tension and compression equally. Thus, the fibers loaded in tension contribute more to the localization of the CRot than the fibers loaded in compression (Figure 9.12). Furthermore, the flat toe region of the nonlinear stress–strain curve of the PDL determines how

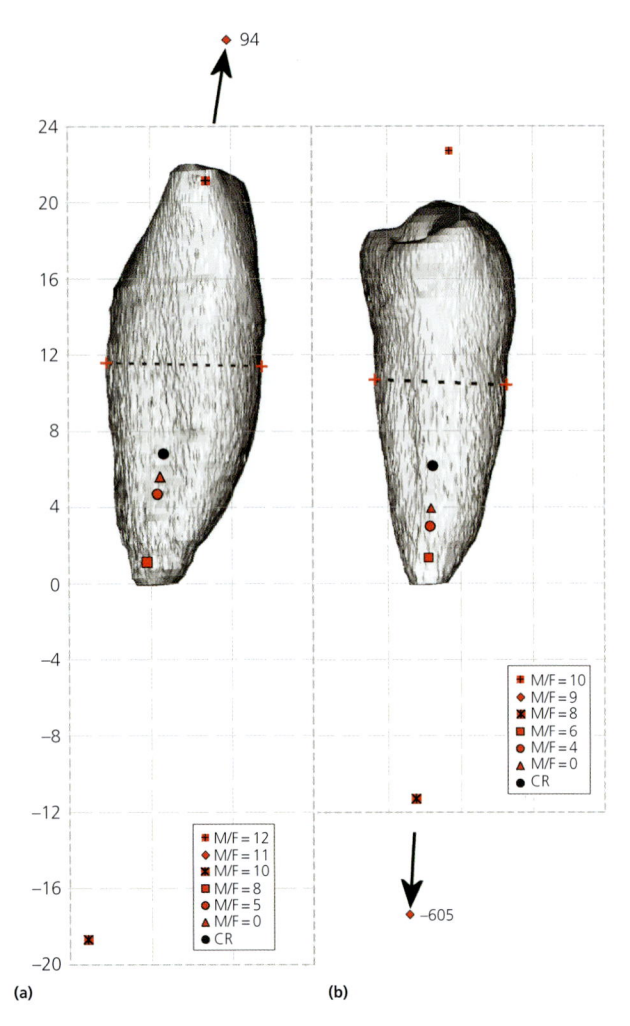

Figure 9.11 Changes of the position of the CRot when the applied force at the bracket of the canine is fixed at 100 cN, while the M/F ratio varies from 0 to 12 (a): location of the CRot when the force on the premolar is kept constant at 100 cN and the M/F ratio is changed from 0 to 10 (b).

many of its fibers deliver a contribution to the localization of the CRot for a given external load, and to what extent. This explains the dependency of the position of the CRot on the magnitude of the external force.

From a clinical point of view, the findings underline the importance of monitoring the force system during treatment when comparing the outcome with the anticipated tooth movement. When there is a discrepancy between the predicted and the actual tooth movement, the clinician should adjust the force system to achieve the desired tooth movement.

The influence of the interaction with occlusion

It is known that continuous or static forces do not influence the remodeling process, while this is influenced by dynamic loading. This is consistent with the fact that in nature no purely static loadings exist (Hert et al., 1971; Lanyon and Rubin, 1984). Therefore, the reasons why bone modeling occurs when an orthodontic continuous force is applied cannot be found. Consequently, in a series of analyses, occlusal vertical forces ranging from 0 to 20,000 cN were superimposed to an orthodontic force of 100 cN, using a M/F of 0 (Cattaneo et al., 2009). By simulating a vertical occlusive force, the stress and strain distribution in the PDL resembled the distribution seen with the pure orthodontic loading up to when the occlusive force reached a magnitude of about 500 cN. Beyond this level, the stress and strain distribution in both the PDL and the surrounding structures became completely different, and the behavior of the tooth changed from uncontrolled tipping (due to the pure orthodontic force) to an intrusive movement (due to the occlusive loading) (Figure 9.13).

As a consequence, the continuous orthodontic forces are perceived by the periodontium as noncontinuous forces, due to their interaction with the intermittent occlusal forces, which, given their magnitude, completely conceal the effect of orthodontics forces.

Conclusions

The results of studies of the morphology of the periodontium by μ-CT have demonstrated that predicting a tooth displacement by an initial estimation of the localization of the CR for the tooth or a block of teeth may not lead to the expected result. A number of factors influence the stress–strain distribution and the reaction of the alveolus to orthodontic forces applied to a tooth.

The irregularity of the alveolar wall will, with even the lowest possible forces, initially lead to a local pressure zone characterized by necrosis of the lining cells and a local necrosis of the underlying bony spicules.

The difference in bone density and quality of the alveolar bone, cervically characterized by dominance of cortical bone and apically by trabecular bone, indicates that the periodontal bone may react differently to an appliance delivering a force with the line of action passing close to the crown, and an identical force with the line of action localized apically to the CRot. This further leads to a demonstration of how the applied force is influenced by the localization of the CRot.

FEM analyses have demonstrated that both the proper description of the anatomical geometry and material properties will result in distributions of the stresses and strains in the alveolar support tissues, which reject the "pressure–tension" theory.

Finally, it had been demonstrated that the occlusal forces interact with the applied force system and thereby the predicted displacement.

Clinically, the idea of applying a force system in a well-determined relationship to the CR makes sense, but the observed displacement may not be the calculated and the observed displacements will indicate which modifications are needed. The reported analysis of factors influencing the type of tooth movement when applying a force that, from a mathematical point of view, should deliver a specific displacement, indicates the necessity of carefully analyzing the observed movement and adapting the force system accordingly. It is thus not possible even with detailed calculations to predict the exact result of an orthodontic force system. In addition, this paper has completely ignored the influence of growth, which in children is responsible for the largest impact on the treatment result.

Where are we now? How should we continue?

The finite element method in orthodontics was introduced by Tanne in 1987 and was soon considered "state of the art." It was anticipated that more important information could be obtained with the increased validity of the input data reflecting the material and morphology (Tanne et al., 1987). However, the input data only represents

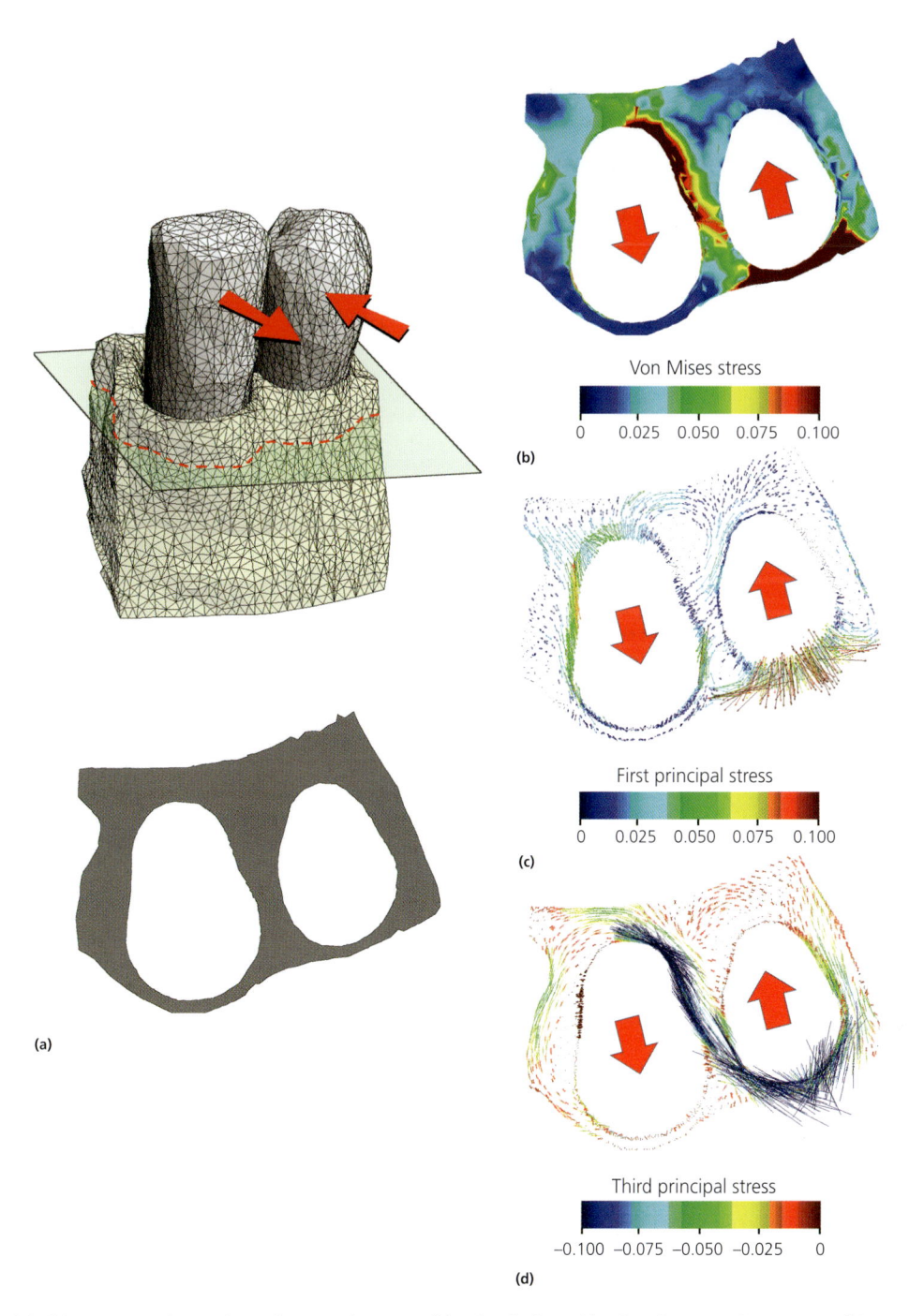

Figure 9.12 FE model of the canine and premolar and a coronal section of the alveolar bone (a), when the material properties of the PDL is considered nonlinear and not symmetric; the corresponding Von Mises' stress (b), first principal stress (c), and third principal stress (d) in the coronal section of the alveolar bone are depicted, when a tipping movement is simulated (red arrows).

a static situation for one individual, and neither function nor individual variation in bone turnover is taken into consideration.

Perhaps we have to realize that we are treating individual patients and to try to fit all patients into the same "Procrustes" appliance is not possible. Pilon *et al.* (1996), in an animal experiment, demonstrated that the rate of tooth movement was more related to the individual dog than to the level of force. Through finite element modeling we have improved our theoretical knowledge on tissue reaction of one individual at one time point, but we are treating individuals that are functioning. Using the information gained from an FE-model can be the basis for the first appliance, but the reaction observed will dictate the monitoring of the appliance. The segmented appliance, separating the active and the passive units, is still preferential to a straight wire approach, where the "Procrustes" idea dominates.

The standard treatments carried out on growing individuals are frequently successful, sometimes in spite of treatment, because growth of the craniofacial skeleton is responsible for most of the changes as stated by Tweed in 1968 (Melsen, 2017).

When planning a treatment, it is important to differentiate between the recommended approach based on randomized con-

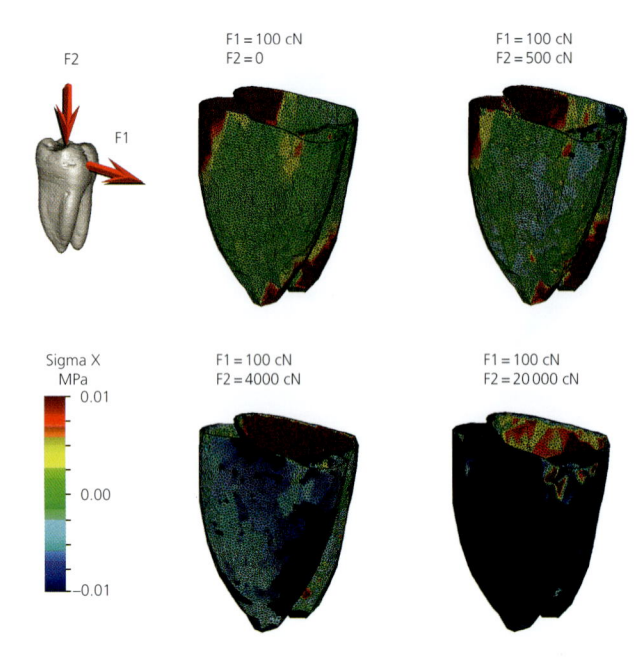

Figure 9.13 Stress in the bone–PDL interface along the buccal–lingual direction around the root of the first molar. The negative values represent compression while the positive values represent tension. In this simulation, the orthodontic force was kept constant (F1 = 100 cN and M/F = 0), while the occlusal force acting along the vertical direction (F2) was increased up to 20 000 N: it can be noticed that the stress distribution substantially changes when the occlusal force is bigger than 500 cN. (Source: Based on Frost, 1994).

trolled trials and meta-analyses, and the force system necessary to solve a particular treatment requiring a well-defined tooth movement. As orthodontists we have been enthusiastic about "methods" and predictions, but we must realize that Nature, through individual patients' growth, function, and metabolism, cannot be overruled.

References

Baumrind, S. (1969) A reconsideration of the propriety of the "pressure-tension" hypothesis. *American Journal of Orthodontic and Dentofacial Orthopedics* **55**, 12–22.

Binderman, I., Bahar, H. and Yaffe, A. (2002) Strain relaxation of fibroblasts in the marginal periodontium is the common trigger for alveolar bone resorption: a novel hypothesis. *Journal of Periodontology* **73**, 1210–1215.

Burstone, C.J. (1962) The biomechanics of tooth movement, in *Vistas in Orthodontics* (eds B.S. Kraus and A. Ripamonti). Lea and Febiger, Philadelphia, pp. 197–213.

Burstone, C.J. (1966) The mechanics of the segmented arch techniques. *The Angle Orthodontist* **36**, 99–120.

Burstone, C.J. (1982) The segmented arch approach to space closure. *American Journal of Orthodontics* **82**, 361–378.

Burstone, C.J. and Pryputniewicz, R.J. (1980) Holographic determination of centers of rotation produced by orthodontic forces. *American Journal of Orthodontic and Dentofacial Orthopedics* **77**, 396–409.

Burstone, C.J., Pryputniewicz, R.J. and Bowley, W.W. (1978) Holographic measurement of tooth mobility in three dimensions. *Journal of Periodontal Research* **13**, 283–294.

Cattaneo, P.M., Dalstra, M. and Melsen, B. (2005) The finite element method: a tool to study orthodontic tooth movement. *Journal of Dental Research* **84**, 428–433.

Cattaneo, P.M., Dalstra, M. and Melsen, B. (2008) Moment-to-force ratio, center of rotation, and force level: a finite element study predicting their interdependency for simulated orthodontic loading regimens. *American Journal of Orthodontic and Dentofacial Orthopedics* **133**, 681–689.

Cattaneo, P.M., Dalstra, M. and Melsen, B. (2009) Strains in periodontal ligament and alveolar bone associated with orthodontic tooth movement analyzed by finite element. *Orthodontic and Craniofacial Research* **12**, 120–128.

Christiansen, R.L. and Burstone, C.J. (1969) Centers of rotation within the periodontal space. *American Journal of Orthodontic and Dentofacial Orthopedics* **55**, 353–369.

Dalstra, M., Cattaneo, P.M. and Beckmann, F. (2006) Synchrotron radiation-based microtomography of alveolar support tissues. *Orthodontics and Craniofacial Research* **9**, 199–205.

Dalstra, M., Cattaneo, P.M., Laursen, M.G. et al. (2015) Multi-level synchrotron radiation-based microtomography of the dental alveolus and its consequences for orthodontics. *Journal of Biomechanics* **48**, 801–806.

Frost, H.M. (1994) Wolff's Law and bone's structural adaptations to mechanical usage: an overview for clinicians. *The Angle Orthodontics* **64**, 175–188.

Hauge, E.M., Qvesel, D., Eriksen, E.F. et al. (2009) Cancellous bone remodeling occurs in specialized compartments lined by cells expressing osteoblastic markers. *Journal of Bone and Mineral Research* **16**, 1575–1582.

Heller, I.J. and Nanda, R. (1979) Effect of metabolic alteration of periodontal fibers on orthodontic tooth movement. *An experimental study. American Journal of Orthodontic and Dentofacial Orthopedics* **75**, 239–258.

Hert, J., Lisková, M. and Landa, J. (1971) Reaction of bone to mechanical stimuli. 1. Continuous and intermittent loading of tibia in rabbit. *Folia Morphologica (Praha)* **19**, 290–300.

Hemanth, M., Deoli, S., Raghuveer, H.P. et al. (2015) Stress induced in periodontal ligament under orthodontic loading (Part II): A comparison of linear versus non-linear FEM study. *Journal of International Oral Health* **7**, 114–118.

Lanyon, L.E. and Rubin, C.T. (1984) Static vs dynamic loads as an influence on bone remodelling. *Journal of Biomechanics* **17**, 897–905.

Melsen, B. (1999). Biological reaction of alveolar bone to orthodontic tooth movement. *The Angle Orthodontist* **69**(2), 151–158.

Melsen, B. (2001) Tissue reaction to orthodontic tooth movement – a new paradigm. *European Journal of Orthodontics* **23**, 671–681.

Melsen, B. (2017) JPO Interviews Dr. *Charles H. Tweed. Journal of Clinical Orthodontics* **51**, 516–519.

Nishihira, M., Yamamoto, K., Sato, Y. et al. (2003) Mechanics of periodontal ligament, in *Dental Biomechanics* (ed. A.N. Natali). CRC Press, Boca Raton.

Persson, M. (2005) A 100th anniversary: Sandstedt's experiments on tissue changes during tooth movement. *Journal of Orthodontics* **32**, 27–28.

Pilon, J.J., Kuijpers-Jagtman, A.M. and Maltha, J.C. (1996) Magnitude of orthodontic forces and rate of bodily tooth movement. An experimental study. *American Journal of Orthodontic and Dentofacial Orthopedics* **110**, 16–23.

Poppe, M., Bourauel, C. and Jager, A. (2002) Determination of the elasticity parameters of the human periodontal ligament and the location of the center of resistance of single-rooted teeth. *A study of autopsy specimens and their conversion into finite element models. Journal of Orofacial Orthopedics* **63**, 358–370.

Proffit, W.R. (2019) The biologic basis of orthodontic therapy, in *Contemporary Orthodontics*, 6th edn (eds. W.R. Proffit, H.W. Jr. Fields, B.E. Larson and D.M. Sarver), Elsevier, Amsterdam, pp. 248–275.

Reitan, K. (1951) The initial tissue reaction incident to orthodontic tooth movement as related to the influence of function. *Acta Odontologica Scandinavica* (Suppl 6)

Tanne, K., Sakuda, M. and Burstone, C.J. (1987) Three-dimensional finite element analysis for stress in the periodontal tissue by orthodontic forces. *American Journal of Orthodontic and Dentofacial Orthopedics* **92**, 499–505.

Thilander, B., Rygh, P. and Reitan, K. (2005) Tissue reactions in orthodontics, in *Orthodontics – Current Principles and Techniques* (eds. L.W. Graber, R.L. Vanarsdall and K.W.L. Vig), Elsevier, St Louis, MO, pp. 145–219.

van Driel, W.D., van Leeuwen, E.J., Von den Hoff, J.W. et al. (2000) Time-dependent mechanical behaviour of the periodontal ligament. *Proceedings of the Institution of Mechanical Engineers [H]* **214**, 497–504.

Verna, C., Cattaneo, P.M. and Dalstra, M. (2018) Corticotomy affects both the modus and magnitude of orthodontic tooth movement. *European Journal of Orthodontics* **40**, 107–112.

Verna, C. and Melsen, B. (2012) What can orthodontists learn from orthopaedists engaged in basic research?, in *Integrated Clinical Orthodontics* (eds. V. Krishnan and Z. Davidovitch). Wiley-Blackwell, Chichester, pp. 168–181.

Viecilli, R.F. (2015) 3D concepts in tooth movement, in *The Biomechanical Foundation of Clinical Orthodontics* (eds C.J. Burstone and K. Choy). Quintessence, Batavia, IL, pp. 193–198.

Viecilli, R.F., Katona, T.R., Chen, J. et al. (2008) Three-dimensional mechanical environment of orthodontic tooth movement and root resorption. *American Journal of Orthodontic and Dentofacial Orthopedics* **133**, 791–726.

Vollmer, D., Bourauel, C., Maier. K. and Jäger A. (1999) *Determination of the centre of resistance in an upper human canine and idealized tooth model. European Journal of Orthodontics* **21**, 633–648.

Weinstein, S. (1967) Minimal forces in tooth movement. *American Journal of Orthodontics* **53**, 881–903.

PART 3

Inflammation and Orthodontics

CHAPTER 10
The Influence of Orthodontic Treatment on Oral Microbiology

Alessandra Lucchese and Lars Bondemark

> **Summary**
>
> The positioning of biomaterials in the oral cavity, such as prostheses or orthodontic appliances, can induce alterations to the oral microbiota. Orthodontic appliances have been associated with increased cariogenic risk and exacerbation of pre-existing periodontal pathologies. This is because different types of brackets, such as conventional, self-ligating, and lingual brackets, or different bracket materials, such as metallic, ceramic, and plastic, or also removable orthodontic appliances, can often cause colonization of bacteria followed by enamel demineralization and gingival inflammation. Hence, insertion of orthodontic appliances may result in an increase in retentive sites at which the bacterial plaque and potentially pathogenic species, such as periodontal or cariogenic bacteria or fungi, are able to proliferate more easily, damaging oral health and potentially general health.
>
> Another significant variable for microbial alterations is the duration the device is used inside the oral cavity; for this reason, it is evident that removable appliances have a significantly lower impact on oral microorganisms than fixed orthodontic appliances. Although changes taking place in the microbial system involve all types of orthodontic appliances, changes occur more rapidly during fixed orthodontic treatment; such alterations can be recorded only a few months after the start of treatment and can lead to deterioration in periodontal health. Furthermore, being able to remove the orthodontic appliance in order to clean both the appliance and the teeth seems to be more important for maintaining oral health than the duration of treatment.
>
> Considering the variations in the microbiota which occur with the introduction of biomaterials in the oral cavity, in particular orthodontic appliances, it is appropriate for patients to undergo personalized hygiene protocols so that the oral bacterial load is controlled and the risk of developing carious and periodontal disease is reduced.

Introduction

The oral microbiome was recognized for the first time by the Dutchman Antoni van Leeuwenhoek, using a microscope of his own construction. In 1670 he reported to the British Royal Society that various forms of microbes were present in the plaque found on the surface of the teeth. This observation came at a time when bacteriology had not yet been established, and van Leeuwenhoek was fascinated by the kinetics of the microbiome. His report described individual differences in the oral microbiome, and although he did not directly refer to it, he realized that individual differences in the microbiome could affect the health of the oral cavity. Subsequently, 200 years later, we developed a systematic theory on the correlation between the microbiome and oral cavity pathologies.

Later, at the end of the nineteenth century, the American dentist W.D. Miller studied the association between oral microbes and oral cavity diseases in a small laboratory in Berlin. Miller was motivated by R. Koch, who at about the same time had reported cutting-edge results in studies on the association between microbes and infectious diseases (Miller, 1890). In his book, *The Micro-organisms of the Human Mouth*, Miller proposed the "chemicoparasitic theory," which stated that the main cause of dental caries was the acid metabolism from sugar in foods by oral microbes. However, his research failed to identify cariogenic bacteria and focused on acids as bacterial metabolites rather than on the bacteria that produced these metabolites. In addition, until the mid-twentieth century, Miller's theory was thought to have misled his research successors who classified the *Lactobacillus* species as cariogenic bacteria and according to Koch's hypothesis.

Humans, like all complex multicellular eukaryotes, are not autonomous organisms but biological units that include numerous symbiotic microorganisms with their genomes (Kilian et al., 2016). Thus, the microorganisms present in our body constitute a fundamental functional organ for our health and physiology. Together with our symbiotic microbes, we form a "super-organism," or "holobiont." The microbial component of the human "holobiont" is fundamental and is at least equivalent to the number of our cells

---

Biological Mechanisms of Tooth Movement, Third Edition. Edited by Vinod Krishnan, Anne Marie Kuijpers-Jagtman and Ze'ev Davidovitch.
© 2021 John Wiley & Sons Ltd. Published 2021 by John Wiley & Sons Ltd.

(Kilian et al., 2016; Sender et al., 2016). The community of microbial residents who colonize us is defined as our "microbiota," which indicates the ecological community of commensal, symbiotic, and pathogenic microorganisms that literally share space in our body. None of them is considered decisive for the state of health of the host (Kilian et al., 2016). The emergence of new genomic technologies, including the "new generation sequencing" (NGS) and bioinformatics tools, have provided powerful agents to understand the contribution of the human microbiota to health status.

To date we have learned that we are not randomly colonized, but that our microorganisms have co-evolved with us over millions of years. Consequently, the relationship that is created between the microbiota and the host is dynamic and is influenced by many aspects of our modern lifestyle such as diet, tobacco consumption, and stress. These parameters can alter our microbiota and its properties, and thereby induce a state in which this finely tuned ecosystem is no longer in balance (Kilian et al., 2016). To address this divergence and maintain a harmonious state in order to protect health and prevent disease, we must not only focus on the host and its residents as separate units, but instead consider the "holobiont" as a single unit. The oral cavity is one of the most colonized parts of our body, and different distinct habitats within the mouth support heterogeneous microbial communities which constitute an important link between oral and general health (Kilian et al., 2016).

An alteration of the bacterial flora is called "dysbiosis," which can make the organism more vulnerable to pathogens and contribute to the development of diseases (O'Hara and Shanahan, 2006). Recent studies suggest a causal relationship between microbiota alterations and various pathologies such as obesity (Turnbaugh and Gordon, 2009), diabetes (Zhang et al., 2013), irritable bowel syndrome, inflammatory bowel disease (Li et al., 2012), colorectal cancer (Ahn et al., 2013), and autism (Adams et al., 2011).

The oral cavity contains about 700 different species, most of which are not cultivable *in vitro* (Keijser et al., 2008). This great diversity is guaranteed above all by the impressive variety of environmental conditions which we can find in the different sites of the mouth: mucous surfaces (back of the tongue, cheeks, lips) and hard surfaces (the teeth with all their surfaces). The oral mucosa is composed of lining mucosa (oral floor, cheeks, and soft palate), masticatory mucosa (gums and hard palate), and specialized mucosa (back of the tongue). Although the entire oral mucosa is covered by a layer of squamous epithelium, each structure is different. The covering mucosa is coated by a nonkeratinized epithelium, while the masticatory mucosa is covered by a keratinized epithelium, and finally the specialized mucosal surface comprises different types of papillae and has a complex structure (Ritz, 1967). In principle, the surfaces which are the most difficult to colonize for bacteria are the hard ones because the mucous membranes tend to peel and therefore do not guarantee bacteria a stable adhesion. The only exception is the tongue, which despite being a mucous surface due to the papillae, is very easily colonized.

From an ecological point of view, the oral cavity is an "open microbial growth system" in which nutrients and microorganisms are constantly introduced and removed (Antonelli et al., 2012). In this ecosystem a dynamic equilibrium is created so that the composition of the oral flora itself will vary based on a series of exogenous factors such as prosthetic or orthodontic materials, and endogenous factors which include:

- Temperature: in the oral cavity it is about 35–36°C which is ideal for the growth of many microorganisms, but in the case of periodontal pathology with inflammation it can reach 39°C at the level of the pockets.
- Redox potential: most species in the oral cavity are facultative, microaerophilic, and obligate anaerobias; the latter manage to survive only due to the fact that the aerobic species present consume oxygen and allow them to survive.
- pH: the optimal pH of the oral cavity for the growth of most species is neutral (pH 7) and is maintained above all by the buffering power of saliva. On the other hand, the cariogenic and parodontopathogenic species tend to prefer an acidic (pH <7) and basic pH (>7), and therefore do not proliferate in an environment with a neutral pH.
- Nutrients: exogenous nutrients (diet) and, particularly, endogenous nutrients (saliva, crevicular fluid) are essential for the survival and differentiation of oral flora in various individuals.
- Habitat: in the course of life the oral cavity undergoes a series of modifications, causing changes in the oral flora; the newborn is initially colonized only on the mucous surfaces, but when the deciduous as well as permanent teeth erupt a whole series of species appear which then adhere to the tooth surfaces.

Contrary to what one might think, during pregnancy the fetus is not sterile. In more than 70% of pregnant women, the intrauterine environment is colonized by *Fusobacterium nucleatum*. During birth the first colonization with microorganisms occurs. During a natural birth the fetus will come into contact with the resident flora of the vagina and rectum, while during a cesarean section the newborn child has contact with the maternal skin flora.

Nutrition, respiration, and above all maternal contact during the first 3 days after birth favor the colonization of the child by *viridans Staphylococci* and *Streptococci*.

In the newborn, the absence of teeth means that only the soft tissues are colonized; *Streptococcus salivarius* makes up 98% of the microorganisms. Over time, the microbiota of the child is increasingly different from that of the mother. After 5 months the anaerobic bacteria appear: *Firmicutes*, *Proteobacteria*, *Actinobacteria*, *Bacteroides*, *Fusobacteria*, and *Spirochaetes*, and among these the prevailing genera are *Streptococcus*, *Haemophilus*, *Neisseria*, and *Veillonella*.

As previously mentioned, the oral flora depends on the substrate on which the bacteria can adhere, so once dental eruption begins, there is a net change in the oral microbiota. This change occurs because the surface of the teeth is not subject to desquamation, as is the case for oral soft tissues. This change in habitat will influence bacterial adhesion.

The most numerous species at this point are *Streptococcus mutans* and *S. sanguis*, accompanied to a lesser extent by anaerobic species, which find a favorable habitat in the area of the gingival collar. With the onset of permanent dentition, *Veillonellaceae* and *Prevotella* increase in number, to the detriment of the *Coriobacteriaceae* which decrease. Moreover, puberty involves significant hormonal changes that also affect the oral cavity, when *Spirochaetes* and Gram anaerobes increase.

From birth until adulthood there will be many changes in the oral cavity flora, i.e., allogenic (due to chemical–physical factors of the ecosystem) and autogenic (from interaction between the various microorganisms). In fact, with increasing age, bacterial load tends to increase, but the diversity of the various species decreases (Antonelli et al., 2012).

Microbiology of periodontal disease

Studies during "the golden age" of microbiology (1880–1930) suggested four essential microorganisms as the main etiological agents of periodontitis: *Amoeba*, *Spirochete*, *Fusobacteria*, and *Streptococci*.

After this period, there was no interest in finding a specific etiological agent that could cause periodontitis until the 1960s (Socransky and Haffajee, 2000). Research is continuing today, and over the past 25 years more than 200 studies using culture techniques or molecular methods such as DNA probes and PCR (Loesche and Grossman, 2001) have evaluated periodontal-associated bacteria and bacterias associated with periodontitis. However, there are inherent difficulties in identifying periodontal pathogens, especially because periodontitis occurs in sites with a pre-existing overall normal flora, making the discrimination of opportunistic pathogens from species compatible with the health of the host a real challenge. In particular, it is believed that pathogens may be present, in smaller percentages, in a state of health (carrier state) (Haffajee and Socransky, 1994). It should also be considered that many of the periodontal bacteria are difficult or impossible to cultivate in vitro, and moreover, periodontal infections seem to be of a mixed nature involving more than one bacterial species.

For this and for other reasons, Koch's hypotheses have been replaced by a series of criteria for defining periodontal pathogens. These criteria include: (i) association, meaning the species is found more frequently and in higher numbers in cases of disease compared with a healthy periodontal state, (ii) elimination, i.e., elimination of the bacterial species is associated with regression of the disease, (iii) presence of an immune response by the host against the determined bacterial species, (iv) presence of virulence factors, and (v) the possibility of inducing the disease in animals (Haffajee and Socransky, 1994). In light of these criteria, some microorganisms have been identified as etiological agents of periodontitis (Haffajee and Socransky, 1994), such as the species belonging to the so-called red complex, and to a lesser extent, the orange complex, which are strongly associated with the clinical signs of periodontitis. The bacteria in other complexes do not show an association with periodontitis, and therefore seem to be compatible with a healthy periodontal state (Socransky et al., 1998). It is also worth mentioning that periodontal pathogens have also been detected in the supragingival plaque associated with periodontitis (Ximenez-Fyvie et al., 2000).

Recently, some attention has also been paid to the bacteria that until now could not be cultured. Studies which use 16 S rRNA genetic analysis suggest that some still noncultivable species may also be involved in the etiology of periodontal disease (Dewhirst et al., 2000; Sakamoto et al., 2002).

Some studies have recently evaluated the role of other microorganisms in the etiology of periodontitis. A growing number of studies support the belief that viruses such as cytomegalovirus can contribute to the severity of periodontal disease, probably by changing the host's immune control on bacteria present in the plaque (Slots, 2004). Moreover, the Archaea, in particular Methanobrevibacter oralis-like phylotype was indicated as a possible etiological factor for periodontitis (Lepp et al., 2004).

Strong evidence supports the involvement of Porphyromonas gingivalis and Bacteroides forsythus (current name: Tannerella forsythia) as the etiological agents of adult periodontitis (now classified as chronic periodontitis) and of Actinobacillus actinomycetemcomitans known as Aggregatibacter actinomycetemcomitans in juvenile periodontitis (now classified as aggressive periodontitis). Furthermore, there is also moderate evidence regarding the involvement of other species such as Treponema denticola, Fusobacterium nucleatum, Prevotella intermedia, P. nigrescens, Peptostreptococcus micros, Eubacterium nodatum and Campylobacter rectus (Genco et al., 1996). It is known that established and presumed periodontal pathogens, as well as other periodontal bacteria, exist within real "bacterial complexes" in the subgingival plaque.

Microbiology of dental caries

In 1890, Miller established the role of microorganisms in enamel demineralization. Miller was able to demonstrate the ability of bacteria present in saliva to produce acid from fermentable carbohydrates in an amount sufficient to decalcify dental enamel (Kleinberg, 2002). However, he failed to identify a specific bacterium, thus providing the basis for the "nonspecific plaque hypothesis" (NSPH) at the origin of the etiology of dental caries (Loesche, 1967). After Miller's discoveries, there has been extensive investigations into the causative agents of the carious process during the twentieth century. A systematic review of literature from 1966 to 2000 identified 2730 publications that investigated the role of bacteria in dental caries in animals and humans (Tanzer et al., 2001).

It is well known that four main groups of bacteria are associated with dental caries: S. mutans, Lactobacillus spp. (L. acidophilus, L. casei, L. paracasei, L. rhamnosus, and L. fermentum), Actinomyces, and Streptococcus non-mutans. In the first half of the twentieth century, Lactobacilli were widely considered the main suspects in the etiology of caries (the Lactobacilli era), mainly because they were frequently isolated in the presence of deep carious lesions (Hamilton, 2000) and that these bacteria are highly acidogenic and acidic (Van Houte, 1994). Lactobacilli, however, have a low affinity for teeth and they prefer to colonize the back of the tongue and be transported by saliva (Tanzer et al., 2001) and are therefore not essential for the development of carious lesions. However, Lactobacilli are frequently detected in advanced caries lesions and are also considered to be important for the progression of consolidated lesions (Loesche, 1986; Van Houte, 1994). Lactobacilli isolated from human dental caries include: L. acidophilus, L. casei, L. paracasei, L. rhamnosus and L. fermentum (Martin et al., 2002). Moreover, a recent study has also identified other Lactobacilli species in advanced lesions such as: L. gasseri, L. ultunensis, L. crispatus, L. gallinarum, and L. delbrueckii as well as new filotypes, suggesting that Lactobacilli in advanced caries are more diverse than previously assumed (Byun et al., 2004).

In 1924, Clark isolated S. mutans from carious lesions, but it was not until the 1960s, when S. mutans was used to demonstrate the infectious nature and transmission of dental caries in experimental animal models (Keyes, 1960), that S. mutans became the primary fulcrum in the microbiology of caries. Hundreds of cross-sectional, longitudinal, case-controlled, and experimental clinical studies have been conducted and have provided strong evidence for the central role of S. mutans in the initiation of carious lesions (Tanzer et al., 2001). Recognizing the remarkable serological and genetic heterogeneity of human and animal S. mutans strains, these have been grouped into eight species, collectively referred to as Streptococci (MS) mutans. The prevalent species in humans are S. mutans (serotype c, e, f) and S. sobrinus (serotype d, g) with the occasional isolation of S. rattus (serotype b) and S. cricetus (serotype a). S. mutans serotype c represents 70–100% of human MS isolates (Loesche, 1986).

In addition, the biological and virulence properties of S. mutans have been the subject of many studies (Loesche, 1986; Van Houte, 1994). The virulence factors of S. mutans are mainly adhesion, acidogenicity, and acid tolerance. S. mutans adheres to the surfaces of the teeth by saccharose-dependent and saccharose-independent mechanisms.

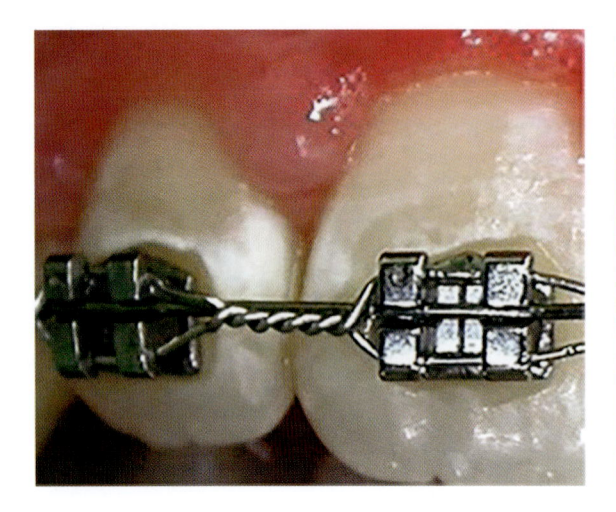

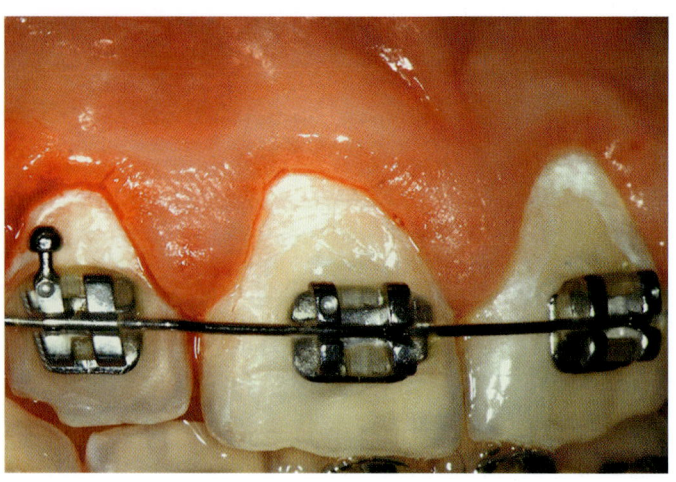

Figure 10.1 White spot lesions. Initial decalcification of the enamel with chalky colour during orthodontic treatment with fixed appliances. (Source: Dr. Alessandra Lucchese.)

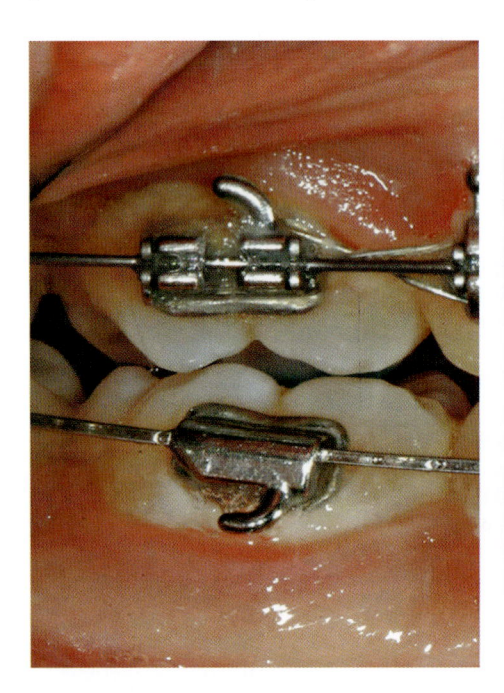

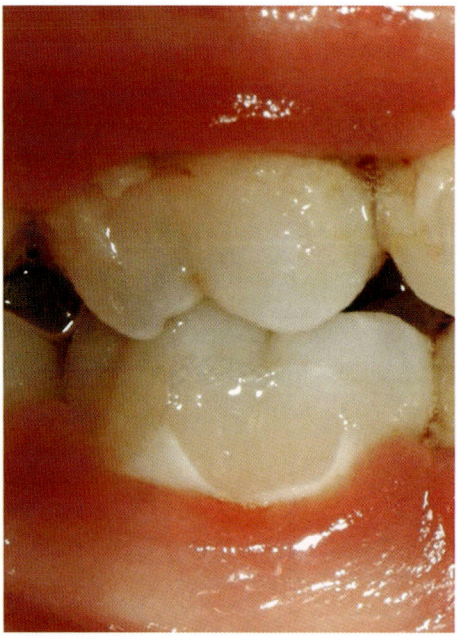

Figure 10.2 In the most serious cases, white spot lesions can turn brown in color. White spot and brown spot lesions on the gingival margins of upper and lower molars, during and after orthodontic treatment. (Source: Dr. Alessandra Lucchese.)

Despite the strong association between *MS* and caries, some cases of carious lesions with no or low incidence of *MS* have been reported. These results indicate that there are other species which should be taken into consideration as potential etiological agents (Hamilton, 2000). Indeed, analyzing the association between *non-mutans Streptococci* (*non-MS*) and carious lesions in humans it has been demonstrated that these *non-MS* are able to generate acid at reduced pH, and thereby are able to create pH lower than 4.4 (Van Houte *et al.*, 1991; Sansone *et al.*, 1993; Van Houte *et al.*, 1996). Information on the individual species of these *non-MS* living at "low pH" is not known, but *S. mitis* can be considered an important member among these species (Hamilton, 2000).

Regarding root caries, a consist association has been found with *Actinomyces* and *A. naeslundii* genospecies 1 and 2 (formerly *A. viscosus*) (Bowden *et al.*, 1999). However, evidence exists to suggest a polymicrobial etiology in carious lesions at root level. Recent studies have shown a large number of microorganisms are involved such as *Prevotella*, *Capnocytophaga*, *Eubacterium*, *Corynebacterium*, and *Clostridium* (Hamilton, 2000). This diversity has also been observed using molecular methods in caries at the coronal level (Chhour *et al.*, 2005). In addition to the onset of caries, the alteration of the microbial flora can lead to the beginning of white spot lesions (WSLs) with the increase in acidity in the oral cavity. WSLs indicate areas of initial decalcification of dental enamel and are named for their chalky color in the initial stages (Figure 10.1). In the most serious cases WSLs can turn brown in color and have an irregular surface (Figure 10.2). WSLs in the esthetic zone can cause ugly discolorations of the teeth which dissatisfy patients (Ogaard, 1989).

Changes in the oral microbiome with removable orthodontic appliances

Changes in the oral microbiota during treatment with removable orthodontic devices involve various bacterial species. The placement of removable orthodontic appliances creates a favorable environment for the accumulation of bacterial plaque and food residues which over time can cause cavities or exacerbate any pre-existing periodontal disease (Zachrisson, 1974; Bjerklin et al., 1983; Jabur, 2008).

The surface characteristics of an orthodontic device influence the type of bacterial adhesion, i.e., surface roughness and free energy. Removable orthodontic devices can be made of various materials including resins and silicones (including the new biomedical silicones), which are highly biocompatible materials with smooth surfaces without microporosity and that are not resilient to bacteria. Any type of removable orthodontic device positioned in the oral cavity causes an increase in the accumulation of bacterial plaque and therefore an alteration of the oral microbiota. Moreover, orthodontic treatment with removable devices induces an alteration of physiological pH values; during therapy pH is more acidic, but tends to return to physiological values within 6 months from the end of orthodontic treatment (D'Ercole et al., 2014; Lucchese et al., 2020). Nevertheless, there are fewer changes than with fixed orthodontic appliances. Unfortunately, however, in the majority of studies published to date, the specifications on the type of removable appliance are lacking. As a result, it is not possible to state which material guarantees better control of the bacterial load, although devices made of new biomedical materials may provide a better control of bacterial proliferation due to their intrinsic characteristics, but further investigations are needed (Figure 10.3).

Periodontal bacteria

Among the various removable orthodontic appliances, clear aligners are increasingly common in adult orthodontics and also in the treatment of younger subjects. The efficiency and effectiveness of these devices is correlated with their wearing time and use is recommended for about 22 hours a day (Rossini et al., 2015), which induces changes in oral flora. It was observed that oral flora remained healthy for up to 6 months from the beginning of removable appliance treatment and that there were no significant differences with respect to fixed orthodontic treatment if good levels of oral hygiene were maintained (Petti et al., 1997).

Cariogenic bacteria

In studies conducted on removable appliances, all with a 6-year follow-up (Batoni et al., 2001; Topaloglu-Ak et al., 2011; Kundu et al., 2016), it was concluded that the removable orthodontic appliances represent a promoter factor for the colonization of S. mutans. The samples taken from unstimulated saliva (Topaloglu-Ak et al., 2011; Kundu et al., 2016) and gingival crevicular fluid (Batoni et al., 2001) were all analyzed in bacterial culture. Kundu et al. (2016) observed a statistically significant increase ($P< 0.001$) of S. mutans from baseline to 6 months of treatment. Furthermore, the bacterial count of S. mutans was significantly higher than those of Lactobacillus spp. and Candida albicans at various time intervals (Kundu et al., 2016). Moreover, a constant increase in Lactobacillus and an increase in S. mutans after 15 days has been shown followed by a progressive decrease after 30 and 60 days (Topaloglu-Ak et al., 2011). Likewise, the number of S. mutans colonies showed a continuous increase ($P< 0.05$) from the start and to one month of treatment (Batoni et al., 2001).

Regarding the presence of Lactobacillus spp. the quantitative and qualitative bacterial charge of Lactobacillus spp. increased with the use of removable devices both in children and adolescents (Topaloglu-Ak et al., 2011; Kundu et al., 2016; Lucchese et al., 2018).

Fungi

Candida is one of the most analyzed fungi in microbiological investigations of orthodontic appliances and many studies have highlighted an increase of Candida during therapy with removable appliances (Addy et al., 1982; Arendorf and Addy, 1985; Khanpayeh et al., 2014; Kundu et al., 2016; Lucchese et al., 2018).

According to Jabur (2008), removable orthodontic appliances induce an increase in Candida level up to 13.3% after an average of 5 weeks and 20% after a 4-month period. In contrast, in the investigations of Addy et al. (1982) and Khanpayeh et al. (2014), the increase in Candida was slight after a period of 3 weeks (Addy et al., 1982) and 6 months (Khanpayeh et al., 2014) in children and adolescents.

The study by Arendorf and Addy (1985) analyzed 33 patients, from 8 to 27 years of age, while wearing an acrylic removable maxillary orthodontic appliance. Six intraoral mucosal sites (anterior palate, posterior palate, anterior tongue, posterior tongue, left cheek, and right cheek) were sampled for Candida spp. using square foam pads. The samples were collected immediately prior to appliance positioning (T0), 5 months after the insertion of the appliance (T1), and 5 months after the removal of the appliance (T2). The prevalence of Candida was 57.6% in all subjects, but the interesting aspect was that 39.4% of the subjects in the sample were already carriers of Candida before orthodontic treatment. Therefore, only 18.2% of the subjects became new carriers of this fungus 5 months after treatment. Furthermore, a significant overall increase in

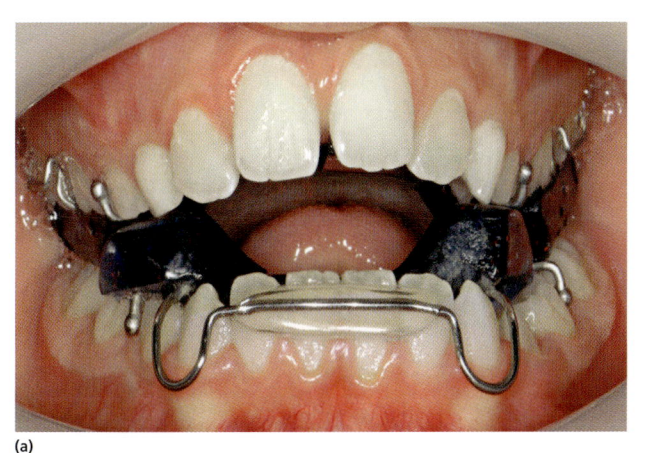

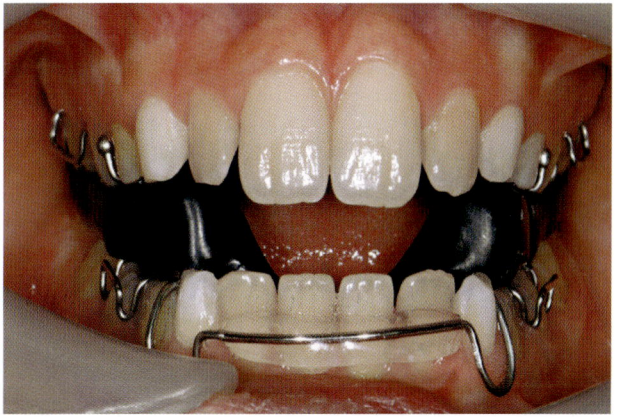

Figure 10.3 Absence of gingivitis, white spot lesions, and caries in the upper and lower jaw. (a) Before orthopaedic treatment and (b) at the end of the orthopaedic treatment with a removable appliance in a patient with skeletal Class II malocclusion. (Source: Dr. Alessandra Lucchese.)

Candida using the device (*P* < 0.001) was found and especially in the posterior and anterior palatal sites. However, this increase was then followed by a significant reduction after removal of the device (*P* < 0.001). Consequently, after 5 months of treatment, 42.4% reported *Candida* colonies, which implies that removable orthodontic appliances have led to an increase in *Candida* colonies by only 3% (Arendorf and Addy, 1985).

The average number (*P* = 0.001) of *Candida* colonies isolated from saliva 6 months after start of treatment was: *Candida albicans*, 25%; *Candida tropicalis*, 3%; *Candida parapsylosis*, 2%; *Candida krusei*, 1%; and *Candida kefyr*, 0%. (Khanpayeh *et al.*, 2014). *Candida* species were identified by performing the germ tube test, hyphae/pseudo hyphae and chlamydoconidia growth on corn meal agar, as well as using the identification system API 20C test on 40 patients (mean age: 11.7 years) (Khanpayeh *et al.*, 2014).

Perkowski *et al.* (2019) analyzed 25 patients, aged 6–13 years old. Swabs were taken from 10 sites of the periodontium, dental plaques, and from dental pockets to isolate and identify oral microbiota. They found that the use of removable appliances can increase *Candida albicans* but often this increase is not significant compared with patients who have not used orthodontic appliances (Perkowski *et al.*, 2019).

Changes in the oral microbiome with fixed orthodontic appliances

The introduction of a biomaterial within the oral cavity creates an additional retentive surface on which the bacterial species are able to reproduce and where there is a greater difficulty in maintaining oral hygiene. As revealed by the literature review of Øilo and Bakken (2015), the presence of biomaterials in the oral cavity leads to an increase in the quantity of plaque and alterations in the oral microbiota (Claro-Pereira *et al.*, 2011; Sampaio-Maia *et al.*, 2012). Hence, on the basis of these evaluations it seems reasonable to state that the degree of bacterial colonization correlated to orthodontic appliances is influenced by the surface energy and by the roughness of the surfaces of the equipment itself. Moreover, the structure and dimensions of the appliance can be a key factor in the ability to perform procedures for maintaining oral hygiene effectively. Another significant variable for microbial alterations is the duration that the device is used inside the oral cavity. For this reason, it is evident that fixed orthodontic appliances (24 hours/day) have a significantly greater impact on oral microorganisms compared with removable orthodontic appliances (Lucchese *et al.*, 2018).

Even though changes in the microbial system involve all types of orthodontic appliance, changes are more rapid, both from a qualitative and quantitative point of view, in fixed compared with removable orthodontic treatment. Such alterations may already be recorded after 1 month of treatment and can lead to a decrease in periodontal, and more generally, oral health of patients (Boyd *et al.*, 1989; Lucchese *et al.*, 2018). However, as stated by Lucchese *et al.* (2018), the role of subgingival bacteria in periodontal changes must be evaluated together with the action of enzymes that are activated in response to the stimuli of orthodontic forces.

Periodontal bacteria

Numerous studies in the literature have evaluated the modifications of the periodontal microbiota following fixed orthodontic therapy (Sinclair *et al.*, 1987; Paolantonio *et al.*, 1999; Perinetti *et al.*, 2004; Leung *et al.*, 2006; Ristic *et al.*, 2007, 2008; Alves de Souza *et al.*, 2008; Thornberg *et al.*, 2009; Van Gastel *et al.*, 2011; Kim *et al.*, 2012; Torlakovic *et al.*, 2013; Ghijselings *et al.*, 2014) and many of these have shown that the use of these devices is able to determine an increase of microbiota with regard to the percentage of Gram-negative species and *Aggregatibacter actinomicetemcomitans* (Sinclair *et al.*, 1987; Paolantonio *et al.*, 1999; Perinetti *et al.*, 2004; Leung *et al.*, 2006; Ristic *et al.*, 2007, 2008; Alves de Souza *et al.*, 2008; Thornberg *et al.*, 2009; Van Gastel *et al.*, 2011; Kim *et al.*, 2012; Ghijselings *et al.*, 2014).

However, the changes that occur in the oral flora do not seem to be permanent, in fact the prevalence of periodontal bacteria, including *Treponema denticola*, decreases significantly (*P* = 0.039) 10 days after removal of the appliance, showing that local factors associated with use of a fixed orthodontic appliance affect changes in the subgingival plaque and lead to increased inflammation and bleeding, which decrease when the orthodontic device is removed (Yáñez-Vico *et al.*, 2015) (Figure 10.4).

However, after the removal of the orthodontic appliance the periodontal changes induced by the latter return to normal only partially and not completely even 3 months after appliance removal (Pan *et al.*, 2017). In addition, there appears to be a greater subgingival prevalence of *A. actinomycetemcomitans* and *Tannerella forsythia* in orthodontic patients up to 6 months after removal of the device compared with untreated patients. Therefore, the presence of fixed orthodontic appliances seems to be associated with a qualitative and quantitative change in the subgingival microbiota which returns to a certain extent, but not entirely to normality in the first months after removal of the appliance. Likewise, there is limited evidence on the timing and extent of these changes (Papageorgiou *et al.*, 2018).

It also appears that the type of ligation used in the fixed appliances may also be associated with changes in the oral microbiota. Thus, a study has evaluated the influence of the type of ligatures used, i.e., comparing elastic and metal modules, and revealed a significant increase in the Gram-negative species with the use of elastic ligatures (Alves de Souza *et al.*, 2008).

Cariogenic bacteria

Most of the studies available in the literature analyzing the Gram-positive species associated with caries show the presence of *S. mutans* and *Lactobacillus* spp., highlighting in almost all cases an increase of these species due to the use of conventional orthodontic bonded brackets (Mattingly *et al.*, 1983; Sinclair *et al.*, 1987;

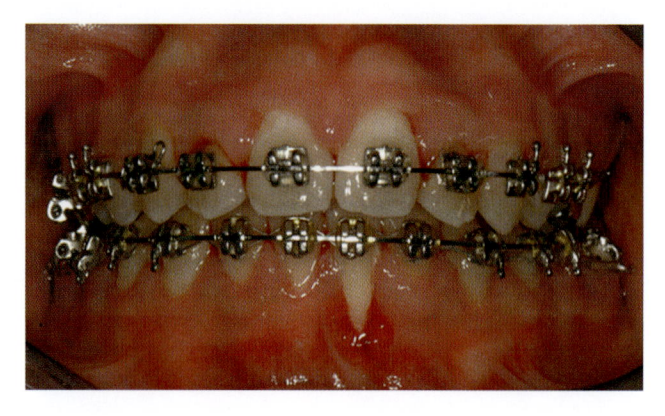

Figure 10.4 Gingivitis, gingival enlargement, and inflammation associated with the placement of fixed orthodontic appliances. (Source: Dr. Alessandra Lucchese.)

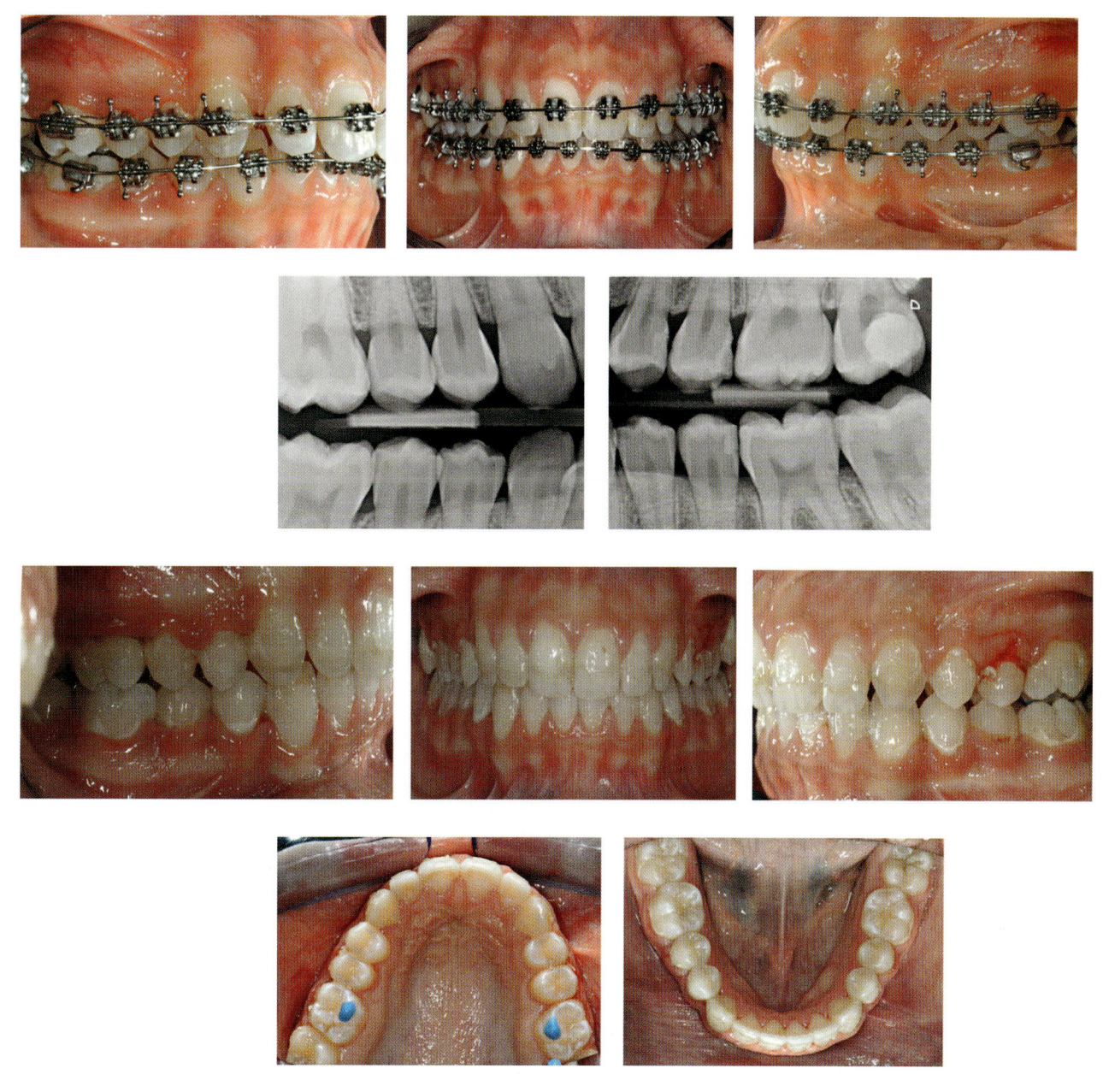

Figure 10.5 Inadequate oral hygiene during orthodontic treatment with fixed appliances. Presence of generalized gingivitis. Development of white spot lesions and caries on the molars, typically at the gingival margin, and in the interproximal and tooth cervical level. The orthodontic treatment had to be ended earlier than planned because of poor oral hygiene. (Source: Dr. Alessandra Lucchese.)

Forsberg et al., 1991; Liu et al., 2004; Ai et al., 2005; Kupietzky et al., 2005; Turkkahraman et al., 2005; Leung et al., 2006; Miura et al., 2007; Lara-Carrillo et al., 2010a, 2010b; Peros et al., 2011; Van Gastel et al., 2011; Wichelhaus et al., 2011; Torlakovic et al., 2013; Ghijselings et al., 2014; Maret et al., 2014; Sudarević et al., 2014; Arab et al., 2016; Shukla et al., 2016, 2017).

The incidence of *S. mutans* in patients with a fixed orthodontic appliance tends to increase significantly in the long treatment period when also white spot lesions can occur (Figure 10.5). However, it seems that the incidence of *Lactobacillus* in the oral microenvironment may increase, albeit not significantly, with fixed orthodontic treatment (Jing et al., 2019).

Fungi

Some studies have evaluated the incidence of *Candida* spp. and all have revealed that *Candida* colonization increases significantly (Arslan et al., 2008; Hägg et al., 2004; Arab et al., 2016; Hernández-Solís et al., 2016; Zheng et al., 2016; Shukla et al., 2017). The percentage of patients with candidiasis and the total number of colony forming units (CFU) increased significantly after 2 months of fixed orthodontic treatment (Zheng et al., 2016). Often, despite clinical advice and oral hygiene instruction, patients were still unable to completely eliminate the possible harmful effects caused by plaque accumulation and the onset and increase of *Candida spp.* (Arslan et al., 2008).

Effects of different orthodontic bracket types on oral microbiome

Conventional brackets

As mentioned previously, conventional brackets cause a significant increase in the BOP (bleeding on probing) and PI (plaque index) (Paoloantonio et al., 1999; Perinetti et al., 2004; Ristic et al., 2007). However, Sinclair et al. (1987), Lara-Carrillo et al. (2010a), and Torlakovic et al. (2013) showed that clinical and microbiological evaluations carried out at different times from the beginning of orthodontic treatment (at 1, 3, 5, 6, and 12 months) did not show significant changes that indicates an increase of the PI. In addition, from the bacterial analyzes conducted on this type of brackets, an increase of the percentage of Gram-negative species and *Aggregatibacter actinomicetemcomitans* in relation to the days elapsed since the beginning of treatment was found (Paolantonio et al., 1999; Perinetti et al., 2004; Leung et al., 2006; Alves de Souza et al., 2008; Ristic et al., 2007, 2008; Thornberg et al., 2009; Van Gastel et al., 2011; Kim et al., 2012; Ghijselings et al., 2014). These assessments are also confirmed for *S. Mutans* and *Lactobacillus* spp., which, in most cases, are subject to an increase with the use of conventional brackets (Mattingly et al., 1983; Sinclair et al., 1987; Forsberg et al., 1991; Liu et al., 2004; Turkkahraman et al., 2005; Kupietzky et al., 2005; Leung et al., 2006; Miura et al., 2007; Lara-Carrillo et al., 2010a, 2010b; Peros et al., 2011; Van Gastel et al., 2011; Wichelhaus et al., 2011; Torlakovic et al., 2013; Ghijselings et al., 2014; Sudarević et al., 2014; Maret et al., 2014; Arab et al., 2016; Shukla et al., 2016, 2017).

Self-ligating brackets

As far as periodontal indexes are concerned, the study by Al-Anezi (2014) showed that at 3 months the use of elastic chain ligatures with self-ligating brackets did not cause a significant worsening of the PI or BOP compared with the use of self-ligating brackets without chain ligatures. Other studies that compared self-ligating brackets with conventional brackets showed a deterioration of the PI and BOP with the use of both conventional brackets and self-ligating ones (Baka et al., 2013; Pejda et al., 2013; Nalçacı et al., 2014; Uzuner et al., 2014).

As for the worsening of clinical parameters with the use of self-ligating brackets compared with the use of conventional brackets, the results are contradictory. In fact, the studies of Baka et al. (2013) and of Pejda et al. (2013), underlined that there are no differences between these two groups while Nalçacı et al. (2014) showed a worsening of the BOP with the use of conventional brackets while Uzuner et al. (2014) presented a worsening of clinical parameters using self-ligating brackets.

Furthermore, Baka et al. (2013) showed an increase in Gram-postive bacteria, in particular *S. mutans and Lactobacillus* spp., at 3 months with the use of self-ligating brackets compared with controls without bonded brackets. On the other hand, other studies that have compared self-ligating with conventional brackets have not revealed any significant differences with regard to Gram-positive bacteria (Pandis et al., 2010; Baka et al., 2013; Pejda et al., 2013; Nalçacı et al., 2014; Uzuner et al., 2014) except the study by Pellegrini et al. (2009), who showed less *Streptococci* when using self-ligating brackets.

Lingual brackets

The use of lingual brackets causes a worsening of the PI and BOP (Demling et al., 2009; Demling et al., 2010; Lombardo et al., 2013; Yener et al., 2020). Both lingual and conventional brackets increase the plaque index and bleeding on probing without any statistically difference between them (Lombardo et al., 2013) (Figure 10.6). Also, an increase of *S. mutans* with lingual brackets could be associated with a greater occurrence of caries (Sfondrini et al., 2012). The lingual positioning of the brackets can increase the amount of *A. actinomycetemcomitans* after 4 weeks due to more difficult oral hygiene (Demling et al., 2010).

Conventional metallic versus aesthetic brackets (composite or ceramic)

Orthodontic brackets can be manufactured of stainless steel, titanium, gold, plastic, composite, and ceramic.

A study that compared composite and conventional metallic brackets did not show any statistically significant differences at 12 weeks for the bacterial species *S. mutans* and *S. sobrinus* (Jurela et al., 2013). Considering the periodontopathogenic bacteria it seems that on metallic brackets there is a greater quantity of *Treponema denticola, A. actinomycetemcomitans, Fusobacterium nucleatum* ss *vincentii, Streptococcus anginosus,* and *Eubacterium nodatum,* while on ceramic brackets an increase of *Eikenella corrodens, Campylobacter showae* and *Selomonas* was observed (Anhoury

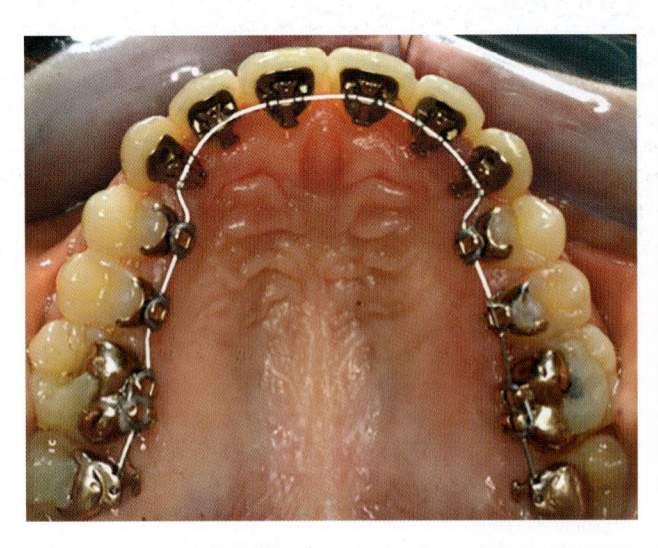

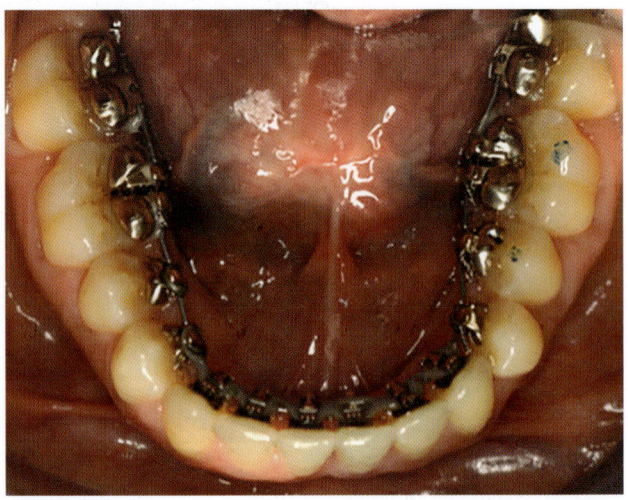

Figure 10.6 Patient with a fixed lingual orthodontic appliance, with widespread gingivitis. (Source: Dr. Alessandra Lucchese.)

et al., 2002). However, other studies affirm that ceramic brackets show, in the long term, a lower accumulation of biofilm than the metallic ones (Lindel et al., 2011). This emphasizes the need for further studies.

Comparing the effects of stainless steel, gold, ceramic, and plastic brackets on the *in vivo* presence of *S. mutans* and *S. sobrinus* and their correlation with the visible plaque index (VPI) and the gingival bleeding index (GBI), at 1 month from the beginning of the orthodontic treatment, it emerged that there were fewer *S. mutans* and *S. sobrinus* on the surface of the gold and stainless steel brackets compared with the plastic and ceramic ones, and a statistically significant difference was observed in the prevalence of *S. mutans* and *S. sobrinus* between metallic and aesthetic brackets. There were no statistically significant differences in the prevalence of *S. mutans* and *S. sobrinus* when the gold and stainless steel brackets were compared, and the comparison between plastic and ceramic brackets revealed similar results. Furthermore, a significant correlation between the *in vivo* prevalence of *S. mutans* and *S. sobrinus* and the indexes of oral hygiene ($P < 0.05$) was found, suggesting that oral hygiene indices could be a good indicator of prevalence of *S. mutans* and *S. sobrinus* (Pramod et al., 2011).

Recent studies have analyzed the *in vivo* adhesion of *S. mutans* (*MS*) to self-ligating ceramic brackets (Clarity-SL [CSL], 3M Unitek, Monrovia, California, USA; Clippy-C [CC], Tomy, Tokyo, Japan) and the relationships between bacterial adhesion and oral hygiene indexes. The main limitation of such investigations, however, is the fact that this type of bracket presents a complex configuration that can significantly influence bacterial adhesion. These analyzes have shown that oral bacteria, including *MS*, can adhere to self-ligating ceramic brackets. In particular, CSL has shown greater adhesion both in total bacteria and in *S. mutans*, which may be due to its bulky size and complex configuration. However, the indexes of oral hygiene were not significantly correlated with the total bacterial adhesion, and of the *MS*, to the brackets (Jung et al., 2015).

In conclusion, it can be stated that conventional brackets are still a good choice with respect to the development of oral biofilm, although there is a lack of high quality scientific evidence and the literature shows contradictory results. Above all, there are not enough studies that affirm a better bacterial control regarding self-ligating, aesthetic, and lingual brackets.

Changes in the oral microbiome with orthodontic retainers

Removable orthodontic retainers
Cariogenic bacteria

Retention is considered an integral part of orthodontic therapy and during this phase stability and occlusal balance should coexist. Numerous removable retention devices are available on the market and among the main ones are the thermo-molded retainers and the Hawley plate. Studies have shown how the use of removable retention devices can influence the quality of the patient's oral hygiene and in the oral cavity promote bacterial differentiation which may lead to carious lesions, white spot lesions, and gingivitis (Klukowska et al., 2011; Lucchese and Gherlone, 2013). The thermo-molded retention appliance covers the palatal, lingual and vestibular surfaces of the teeth and this could influence the microbial flora during the retention period as they hinder the salivary flow on the dental and mucous tissues. Addy et al. (1982) have shown that plaque indices in the palatal region are higher in the group wearing removable retention than in a control group without a retention device. It was also presented that the plaque indices in the vestibular portion were higher than in the control group (Addy et al., 1982).

The bacteria most involved in the colonization of removable retention appliances are *S. mutans* and *Lactobacilli*. *S. mutans* plays a major role in the early development of the cariogenic process. On the other hand, the *Lactobacilli* are found in the progression of this process over time (Lif Holgerson et al., 2015). Even though a statistically significant increase in *S. mutans* and *Lactobacilli* in plaque samples has been found, no statistically significant change of the same bacteria was found in saliva. This is in agreement with other studies which do not show significant changes and this could be explained by an insufficient flow of saliva on dental and gingival tissues (Lara-Carrillo et al., 2010b).

In a study by Türköz et al. (2012), 40 subjects between the ages of 14 and 20 were evaluated and a correlation was found between the use of thermo-molded retainers and colonization by *S. mutans* and *Lactobacilli*. No statistically significant difference in the presence of these bacteria was detected between the maxilla and the mandible.

It is important to know that the bacterial adhesion on the thermo-molded retainers is influenced by two surface characteristics: surface roughness and free energy. A rough surface creates an environment conducive to bacterial colonization and a material with a high surface free energy attracts many bacteria (Lessa et al., 2007). In addition, it should also be remembered that thermo-molded retainers do not have a completely smooth surface, but a surface with microabrasions and surface irregularities that could contribute to bacterial adhesion (Low et al., 2011).

In order to evaluate which retention device has less influence on oral microbiology, studies were carried out to compare fixed and removable retention appliances. It can be concluded that after debonding, patients with either fixed orthodontic retainers (bonding of 0.0215 inch five stranded wire) or removable retention devices (thermo-molded retainers or Hawley's plate), generally showed an increase in the levels of *S. mutans* and *Lactobacillus casei*. However, bacteria levels tend to decrease after 13 weeks, underlining the fact that if correct oral hygiene is performed the condition of the oral cavity after orthodontic treatment tends to return quickly to normal.

Studies that examined *S. mutans* in saliva before, during, and after orthodontic treatment with a fixed multibrackets appliance showed that the salivary levels of *S. mutans* statistically significantly increased during orthodontic treatment. After treatment and during the retention (fixed and/or removable retainers) phase *S. mutans* decreased and subsequently reached the same levels as in the phase prior to orthodontic treatment (Rosenbloom and Tinanoff, 1991). Similarly, a statistically significant decrease in total salivary bacterial levels was found 5 weeks after debonding due to greater ease in home oral hygiene (Jung et al., 2014). However, a statistically significant increase in total bacteria was found for *S. mutans* and *S. sobrinus*, 5 and 13 weeks after debonding (Jung et al., 2014). Contrary to the results of Jung et al. (2014), the *S. mutans* levels in another study (Eroglu et al., 2019) were found to decrease from 5 weeks to 13 weeks after debonding for the Hawley retainer and a significant decrease in the *S. mutans* count occurred for thermo-molded retainers at 13 weeks after debonding in patients with conventional brackets (Eroglu et al., 2019).

Despite contradictory findings regarding the 5-week analyzes from debonding, it seems that all studies agree that with time after debonding the levels of *S. mutans* tend to decrease with all types of retention devices (fixed and/or removable retainers), and it emerges that the use of thermo-molded retainers, compared with other types of retention devices, enables better control of the bacterial load following debonding (Rosenbloom and Tinanoff, 1991; Jung et al., 2014; Eroglu et al., 2019).

In recent years more and more attention has been paid to biomaterials and treatments aimed at reducing the bacterial load in patients subjected to both orthodontic treatment and retention. In a study by Farhadian et al. (2016), it was evaluated if silver nanoparticles incorporated in the acrylic base of the Hawley plate could affect the CFU of *S. mutans*. It was shown that the use of silver nanoparticles modifies the bacterial count of *S. mutants* along the palatal surfaces of the teeth and the silver nanoparticles incorporated in the acrylic base of the retainers (concentration of 500 ppm and a size of 40 nm) showed a strong antimicrobial effect against *S. mutans* (Farhadian et al., 2016).

Periodontal bacteria
No statistically significant differences in PI, BOP depth values ($P > 0.05$) were found between a Hawley plate group and a group with thermo-molded retention (Eroglu et al., 2019). Furthermore, after debonding, the oral hygiene or the PI as well as the gingival index were compared between patients with thermo-molded retainers in the upper arch and a Hawley plate in the lower arch. It was observed that all periodontal parameters decreased immediately after debonding and oral hygiene improved markedly (Kim et al., 2016). Also, Heier et al. (1997) have evaluated the periodontal indices at T0 (shortly before debonding) and at 1, 3, and 6 months after debonding and reported an increase in gingival health.

Since analyzes regarding the presence of periodontopathogenic bacteria during and after using removable orthodontic retainers are lacking, further studies are needed to elucidate this issue.

Fungi
There are few studies that relate to removable retention appliances and fungal species. One study has shown that opportunistic, non-oral pathogenic microorganisms, such as *Staphylococcus* spp. and *Candida* spp., may be present in patients using a retention appliance (Al Groosh et al., 2011). However, it seems that the type of retention device has no effect on the colonization of *Candida*, at least in regards to the palatal mucosa (Yitschaky et al., 2016).

Fixed orthodontic retainers
Cariogenic bacteria
One of the main indications for the use of fixed retention is the prevention of recurrences in the places where rotations and crowding of the maxillary and mandibular six front teeth have been corrected. Forde et al. (2018) evaluated the plaque and gingival index as well as the presence of calculus on upper and lower retainers after 12 months. They reported that compared with thermo-molded retainers, fixed retainers were associated with a greater accumulation of plaque and gingival inflammation. Many studies have revealed that *S. mutans* subsequently decreases 13 weeks after debonding, but no statistically significant difference was found in salivary count of *S. mutans* and *Lactobacillus casei* between fixed and removable retainers (Rosenbloom and Tinanoff, 1991; Jung et al., 2014; Eroglu et al., 2019).

In vitro studies have shown that the design and shape of the fixed retention device influences the number of microorganisms present in the biofilm of the device itself (Jongsma et al., 2013). Thus, it has been demonstrated that the biofilm present on the interwoven fixed retention devices is less susceptible to oral antimicrobials than the biofilm present on single-wire containment devices (Figure 10.7).

The biofilm that adheres to the fixed retention device has a higher percentage of *Lactobacilli* and *S. sobrinus* than the biofilm that adheres to dental enamel surfaces (Jongsma et al., 2013). Moreover, it seems that the bacteria are generally located in the cracks of the multistranded wires while in the single-strand-wires retention devices bacteria are located at the level of surface irregularities (Jongsma et al., 2013). It has also been found that use of toothpaste containing triclosan and mouthwash with essential oils in patients with fixed retainers result in a lower presence of *Lactobacilli*, *S. sobrinus* and *S. mutans* (Jongsma et al., 2013). Finally, the use of retention wires covered with silver ions may also reduce the bacterial load and the risk of caries in patients with fixed retainers. Consequently, wires covered with silver ions showed a greater antibacterial activity compared with wires without silver ions ($P < 0.05$) (Morita et al., 2014).

Periodontal bacteria
Studies have shown that following debonding and insertion of fixed retainers, the plaque and gingival index as well as BOP improve (Eroglu et al., 2019; Heier et al., 1997). Furthermore, no statistically significant difference for recessions and BOP was found between single and multistranded fixed retainers (Corbett et al., 2015). Periodontal indices of individuals wearing or not wearing a bonded retention device showed no statistically significant difference (Kaji et al., 2013). These results were found in patients with good oral hygiene which indicates that oral hygiene is essential with fixed retention (Kaji et al., 2013).

Importance of oral hygiene

Carious and periodontal diseases are related to the presence of dental plaque and for this reason good oral hygiene procedures are essential in patients undergoing orthodontic treatment (Bondemark, 1998; Eckley at al., 2012). In fact, patients undergoing fixed orthodontic therapy have an increase in bacterial species, plaque accumulation, depth of probing, and microbial activity that may be associated with periodontal destruction (Lucchese et al., 2018). However, 30 days after the removal of the orthodontic fixed appliance the plaque index, probing depth, and microbial activity return almost to the basal level (Eckley et al., 2012).

Removable orthodontic appliances can be completely cleaned and thereby provide conditions for better oral hygiene without the presence of further retentive surfaces (Rossini et al., 2015). Thus, removable appliances like clear aligners do not induce deterioration of oral health nor significant biodiversity changes in oral bacterial communities as long as the correct oral hygiene procedures are followed (Zhao et al., 2019). Accordingly, it seems more important to be able to remove the orthodontic appliances and clean both the device and the teeth to maintain a correct bacterial load; the wearing time of the orthodontic device seems less important, which in the case of aligners can reach 22 hours (Rossini et al., 2015).

In any case, it has to be remembered that various investigations in children and adolescents have confirmed that oral hygiene is essential during orthodontic treatment with fixed and removable orthodontic appliances (Lundström et al., 1980; Paolantonio et al.,1997; Koopman et al., 2015; Gizani et al., 2016), and furthermore, if an adequate protocol of oral hygiene is followed with periodic reminders, good gingival health prevails after the placement of orthodontic appliances (Gkantidis et al., 2010). Moreover, numerous studies have reported the importance of good oral health on periodontal tissues during treatment with fixed orthodontic

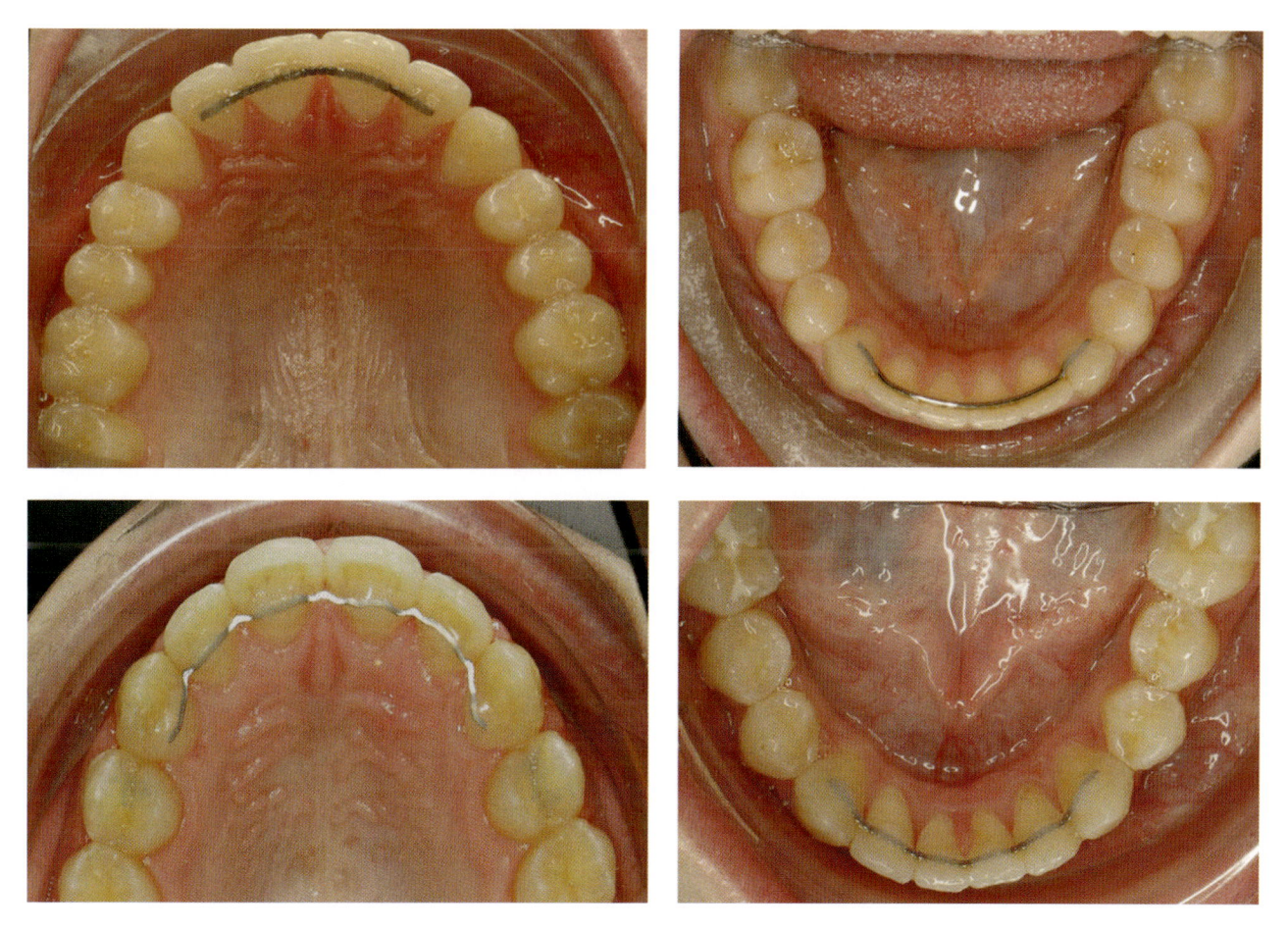

Figure 10.7 Different types of fixed orthodontics retainers: the morphology of the fixed orthodontic retainer influences the number of microorganisms present in the biofilm of the device itself. (Source: Dr. Alessandra Lucchese.)

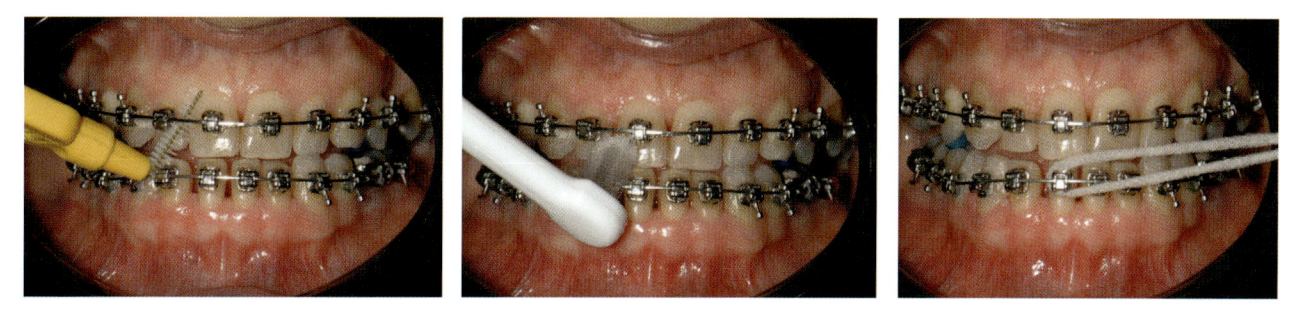

Figure 10.8 Procedures for good oral hygiene with fixed appliances. (Source: Dr. Alessandra Lucchese.)

multibrackets in order to avoid the proliferation of pathogenic species (Kloehn and Pfeiffer, 1974; Diamanti-Kipioti et al., 1987; Petti et al. 1997; Kouraki et al., 2005; Sonesson et al. 2014) (Figure 10.8). In addition, from a recent study by Klaus et al. (2016), which aimed to study the prevalence of *Candida* species, *S. mutans*, and *Lactobacilli* in patients with multibracket appliances, it was found that the use of multibracket appliances resulted in a high presence of oral *Candida* species. It was also revealed that in patients with white spot lesion formation during treatment, a higher count of *Candida* and *Lactobacilli* was evident compared with patients with good oral hygiene (Klaus et al., 2016).

In order to perform appropriate oral hygiene procedures, there are numerous products available to the orthodontic patient, but the literature in relation to this topic is very heterogeneous. For example, the use of fluoride mouthwash in subjects aged between 10 and 17 years resulted in only slight alterations in the composition of the oral microbiome (Koopman et al., 2015). On the other hand, Silin et al. (2017) have stated that although fixed orthodontic appliances result in a deterioration of the patient's oral hygiene, increase the viscosity of the saliva, and reduce its mineralization capacity, the use of Parodontax sodium bicarbonate toothpaste may normalize the oral microbiota and reduce the salivary viscosity with an increase in its mineralization capacity. In addition, daily intake of lozenges (DSM 17938 and ATCC PTA 5289; Biogaia AB, Lund, Sweden) containing the probiotic bacterium *Lactobacillus reuteri* during orthodontic treatment did not influence the development of white spot lesions during orthodontic treatment with fixed appliance as long as proper oral hygiene was maintained. Consequently, good oral hygiene and motivation in orthodontic patients seems to be fundamental. The individual susceptibility of the host linked to their genetic predisposition to caries and periodontal disease and the host's genetic microbial heritage should be also be considered (Shungin et al., 2019).

Finally, it is important to note that children and adolescents undergoing orthodontic treatment are more aware of the importance of good oral hygiene compared with children who have not experienced any kind of orthodontic therapy. This depends on the repeated oral hygiene information that is provided by the orthodontic staff during the orthodontic patient's regular visits to the orthodontic clinic (Davies et al., 1991; Paolantonio et al., 1997; Sari and Birinci, 2007).

Impacted teeth, mini-implants, orthognathic surgery and changes in oral microbiota

Impacted teeth

The maxillary canine is the second most frequently impacted tooth, occurring in 1–2% of the population (Jacobs, 1996). A palatally impacted maxillary canine occurs three times more often than those buccally impacted and rarely erupts spontaneously (Jacoby, 1983). The mandibular canine accounts for about 0.4% of impacted teeth (Thilander and Myrberg, 1973). Women are three times more likely to have impacted maxillary canines than men (Johnston, 1969).

Periodontal complications associated with orthodontic eruption of impacted teeth arise from inadequate oral hygiene. Surgical uncovering of impacted teeth exposes deeper areas of the periodontium to the destructive effects of poor plaque control. In addition to established plaque patterns, new and extensive plaque accumulation patterns result from the resin-bonded brackets (Figure 10.9). Gwinnett and Ceen (1979) demonstrated that plaque accumulates on brackets and resins even when the patient's oral hygiene is good. They also showed that the surface area of resin, the size of the particles, and the type of bracket were important factors in plaque accumulation. Removing excess bonding material from around an attachment, especially in the gingival area, is recommended (Gwinnett and Ceen, 1979). Most patients develop generalized gingivitis shortly after appliance placement. Orthodontic appliances complicate plaque control by interfering with brushing, mastication, and salivary flow. Additionally, the mere presence of orthodontic attachments or cement irritates soft tissues (Alexander, 1991; Atack et al., 1996). Orthodontic tooth movement in the presence of gingival inflammation and inadequate plaque control is not recommended and can result in loss of bone support or apical migration of gingival attachment (Hansson and Linder-Aronson, 1972; Wise, 1981; Alexander, 1991 Vanarsdall, 1991; Ong et al., 1998). Lindhe and Svanberg (1974) reported that the breakdown of the periodontium can be rapid and irreversible. Impacted teeth frequently are moved in a partially erupted state over long distances for relatively long periods, and damage to the periodontium can occur at any time (Figure 10.10).

The periodontal architecture, created by exposing the impacted canines, is more or less comparable with those seen in localized moderate-to-severe periodontal disease. Therefore, the patient's supragingival plaque control should be supplemented with frequent professional cleaning since, generally, canine surgical sites experience profound periodontal destruction.

In conclusion, no single local factor is responsible for periodontal destruction; rather, it is the interaction of local factors resulting in the rapid and profound destruction of the periodontium. The relationship between the impacted canine crown and the adjacent teeth or the surgery uncovering the impacted teeth can create a more vulnerable periodontal architecture. The interaction of inadequate plaque control, the presence of periopathogens, and a vulnerable periodontium during the orthodontic eruption of the maxillary canine are thought to cause the periodontal destruction. Thus, the orthodontist should take active measures to avoid periodontal destruction. If radiographs cannot separate the impacted tooth from the root of an adjacent tooth, a 3-dimensional image should be obtained. The surgical procedure should be designed to minimize the destruction or vulnerability of the periodontium of impacted or adjacent teeth. Supplementary plaque control measures (frequent professional cleaning, antimicrobial rinses or irrigation, electric toothbrush) should be used. Furthermore, an increase in putative periopathogens should be expected after placing an orthodontic attachment. If monitoring reveals pathologic levels of periopathogens, site-specific antibiotic use may be indicated.

Mini-implants

Mini-implants are routinely used to anchor retraction of the anterior segment, mesiodistal movement of the posterior teeth, asymmetrical tooth movement, intrusive mechanics, and orthopaedic corrections. Some authors, in retrospective studies, have identified co-factors that could increase the rate of success or failure of mini-implants (Park et al., 2005; Prabhu and Cousley, 2006). Among the contributing factors for mini-implant failure is the colonization of the surfaces by pathogenic bacteria.

Apel et al. (2009) conducted an analysis of the microflora collected around the head of orthodontic mini-implants with and without mobility and did not observe a cause–effect relationship between the observed bacteria and clinical failure of the implants. In fact, the bacterial analysis did not reveal any major difference in the total amount or species composition between control and failed mini-implants. However, *Actinomyces viscosus* was found in four (100%) and *Campylobacter gracilis* in three (75%) stable controls, whereas both species were rarely found (12.5%) in connection with failed implants (Apel et al., 2009).

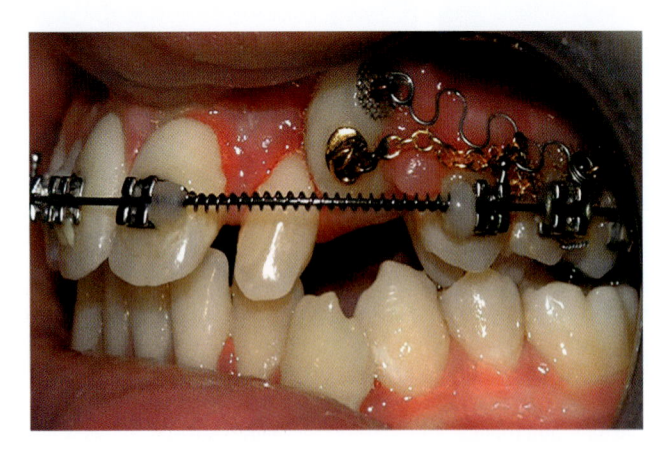

Figure 10.9 Poor oral hygiene. Gingivitis with hyperplasia between canine (23) and premolar (24) in a patient subjected to canine disimpaction, with the Nicodemo spring system and fixed multibracketed therapy. (Source: Dr. Alessandra Lucchese.)

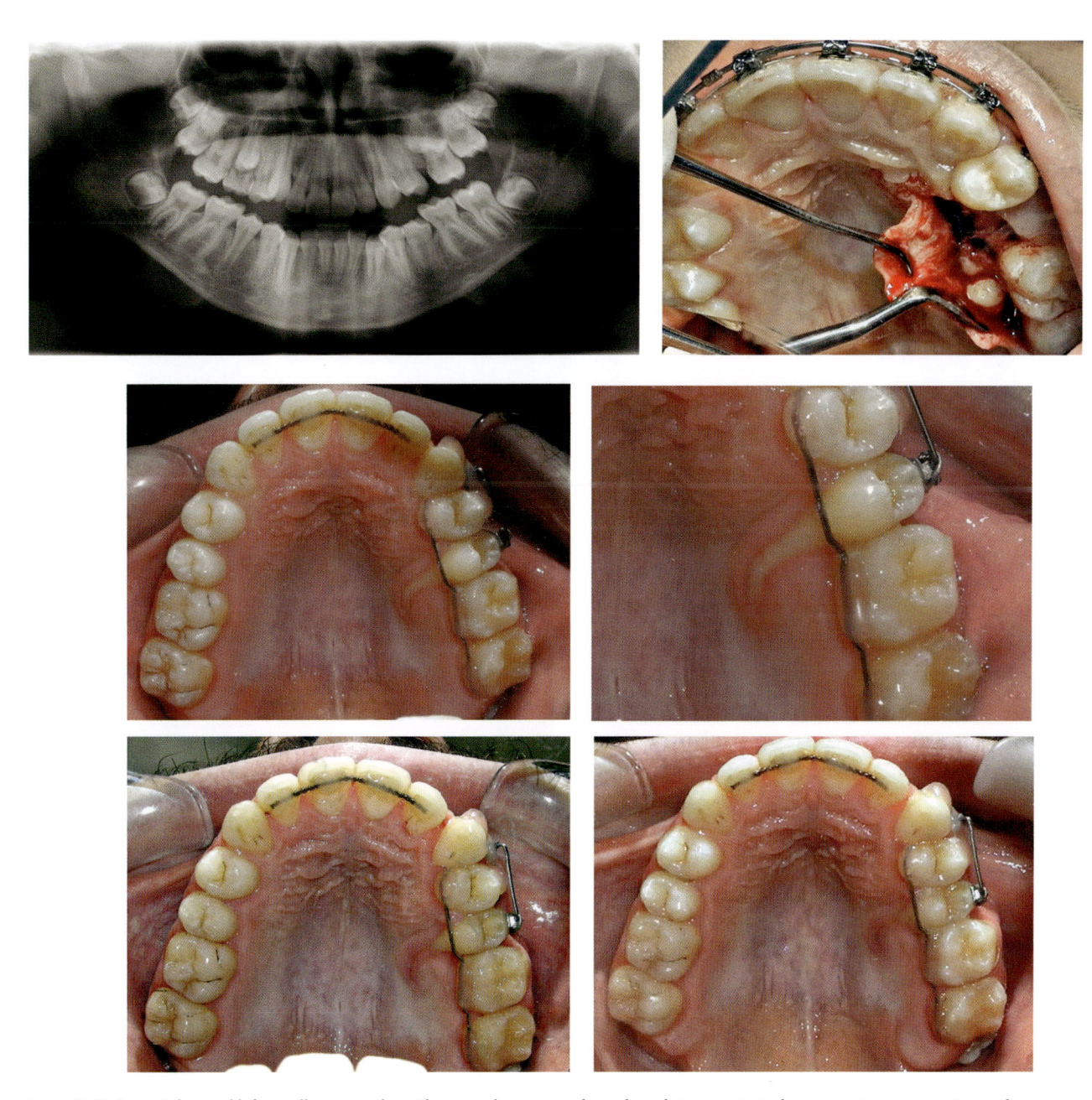

Figure 10.10 Impacted second left maxillary premolar with a curved root, moved over long distances; gingival recession; torque correction with a titanium–molybdenum alloy (TMA) wire cantilever in the management of gingival recession. (Source: Dr. Alessandra Lucchese.)

Apel *et al.* (2009) described that species of oral origin associated with peri-implantitis, including *P. gingivalis,* were absent in healthy implants. *Streptococcus* spp. (*S. gordonii*, as well as *S. mitis*) were found in all successful devices. These findings corroborate with the results of Freitas *et al.* (2012). Several studies using microbial culture techniques, polymerase chain reaction (PCR), and microarray (Apel *et al.*, 2009; Freitas *et al.*, 2012; Tortamano *et al.*, 2012) have identified periodontopathogenic microorganisms in the peri-implant sulci or surfaces of mini-implants.

Andrucioli *et al.,* (2018) have evaluated the contamination of mini-implant surfaces using checkerboard DNA-DNA hybridization. In this analysis, 40 microbial species including the *Actinomyces* group, purple, yellow, green, orange, red complexes, and other species were evaluated. All 40 microbial species of the *Actinomyces* group were observed in both groups (successful and failed mini-implants), although no significant difference ($P = 0.2824$) was found between successful and failed mini-implants considering the frequency of the microbial complexes (Andrucioli *et al.*, 2018). In addition, Tortamano *et al.* (2012) found that the presence of *A. actinomycetemcomitans*, *P. gingivalis*, and *P. intermedia* were not the primary causal factors for the mobility of mini-implants. Instead, bacterial infection responsible for peri-implantitis begins in soft tissues due to poor oral hygiene and slowly extends over the implants, causing mobility and consequently clinical failure (Lindhe and Meyle, 2008).

Since progression of peri-implantitis as well as chronic periodontitis is usually slow and often takes several years, peri-implant inflammation may not be so important from a practical point of

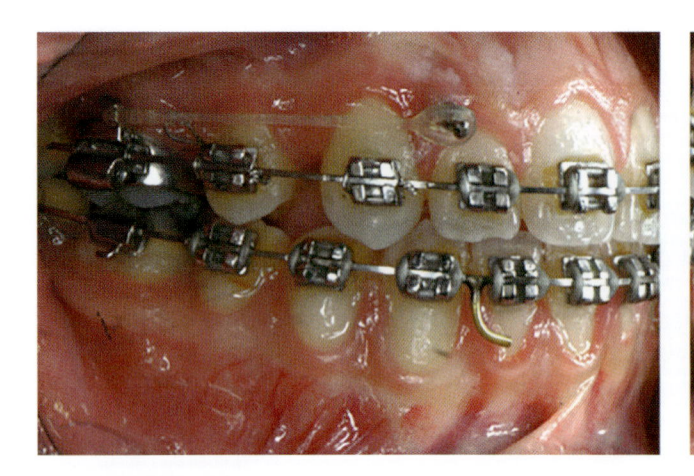

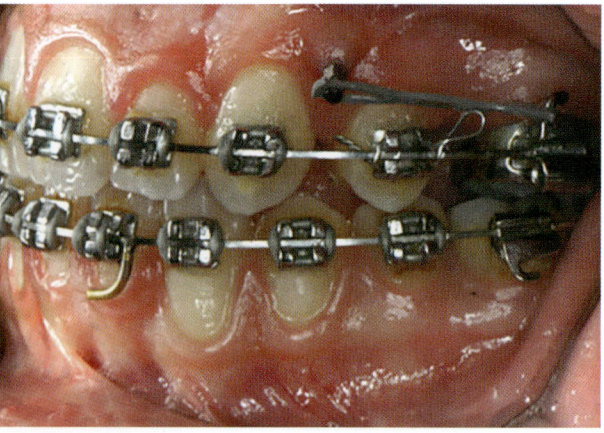

Figure 10.11 Mini-implant used to anchor retraction of the anterior segment. Absence of inflammation and gingivitis around the orthodontic mini-implant. Early failures seem to be more a result of mini-implant mobility than bacterial colonization. (Source: Dr. Alessandra Lucchese.)

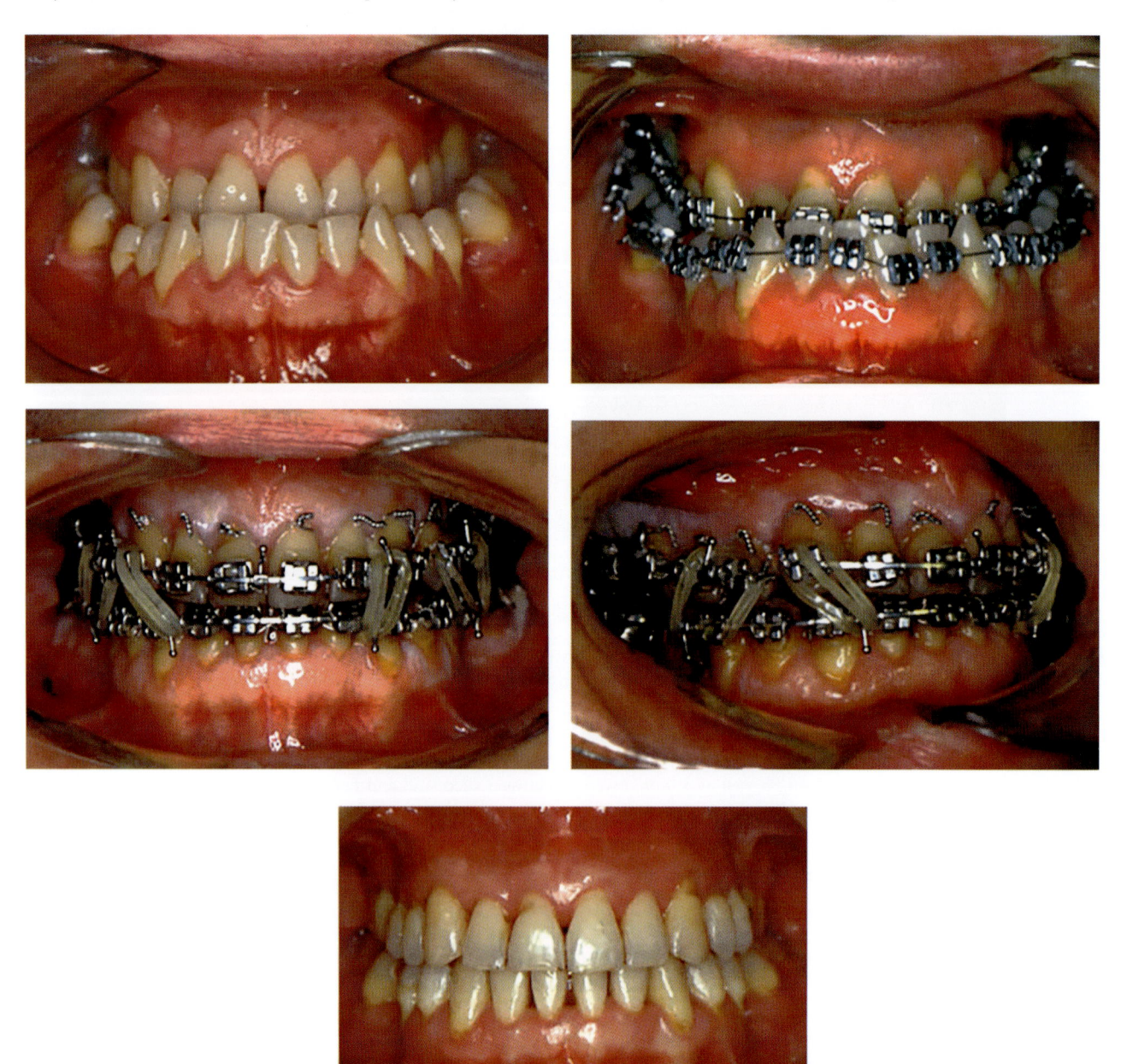

Figure 10.12 Orthognathic surgery may cause statistically significant changes of periodontal parameters. (Source: Dr. Alessandra Lucchese.)

view in determining the clinical short-term function and effectiveness of a temporary anchorage device. Even if the lack of primary stability of mini-implant or temporary anchorage devices can be responsible for early failures, this seems to be more associated with technical, mechanical, or bone quality reasons rather than bacterial colonization (Lindhe and Meyle, 2008) (Figure 10.11).

Orthognathic surgery

Weinspach et al. (2012) evaluated the influence of orthognathic surgery on the development of periodontal and microbiological changes. Plaque index and concentrations of 11 periodonto-pathogenic bacteria were recorded 1 day prior to surgery, 1 week, and 6 weeks postsurgery. In addition, a complete periodontal examination including pocket probing depth, gingival recession, clinical attachment level, BOP, and width of keratinized gingiva was performed prior and after surgery. A significant increase in plaque index during the first week followed by a significant decrease was found. Apart from *Eikenella corrodens* ($P = 0.036$), no significant microbiological changes were recorded. The pocket probing depth significantly increased on oral sites ($P = 0.045$) and gingival recessions especially on buccal sites ($P = 0.001$) (Weinspach et al., 2012) (Figure 10.12). Consequently, orthognathic surgery may cause statistically significant changes of periodontal parameters, but these changes do not necessarily impair the aesthetic appearance of the gingival margin (Weinspach et al., 2012).

Conclusions

The presence of orthodontic appliances including for example metallic brackets or self-ligating brackets and removable appliances represents a risk for an increase in quantity of plaque due to the difficulty that the patient may have in the management of daily hygiene on the surfaces of these devices. The accumulation of plaque during orthodontic treatment appears to be the main cause of gingivitis, halitosis, and demineralization of dental enamel. Since 1983, much research has been performed considering the interaction between orthodontic appliances and oral cavity bacteria (Mattingly et al., 1983). However, the heterogeneity of orthodontic appliances as well as of different bacteria and fungi studied, and also because of the technological evolution of the methods used for microbiological analysis, have led to different and sometimes conflicting results over time.

The research literature confirms that orthodontic appliances influence the oral microbiota regardless of the type of device, but removable appliances have less impact on the oral flora than fixed orthodontic appliances. Since the oral microbiota will change, and plaque accumulation will increase during orthodontic treatment, it is strongly recommended from the beginning of treatment to use adequate protocols of professional oral hygiene and oral home care for all orthodontic patients.

References

Adams, J. B., Johansen, L. J., Powell, L. D. et al. (2011) Gastrointestinal flora and gastrointestinal status in children with autism – comparisons to typical children and correlation with autism severity. *BMC Gastroenterology* **11**, 22.

Addy, M., Shaw, W. C., Hansford, P. and Hopkins, M. (1982) The effect of orthodontic appliances on the distribution of Candida and plaque in adolescents. *British Journal of Orthodontics* **9**(3), 158–163.

Ahn, J., Sinha, R., Pei, Z. et al. (2013) Human gut microbiome and risk of colorectal cancer. *Journal of the National Cancer Institute* **105**(24), 1907–1911.

Ai, H., Lu, H. F., Liang, H. Y. et al. (2005) Influences of bracket bonding on mutans streptococcus in plaque detected by real time fluorescence-quantitative polymerase chain reaction. *Chinese Medical Journal (Engl)* **118**, 2005–2010.

Al Groosh, D., Roudsari, G. B., Moles, D. R. et al. (2011) The prevalence of opportunistic pathogens associated with intraoral implants. *Letters in Applied Microbiology* **52**(5), 501–505.

Al-Anezi, S. A. (2014) Dental plaque associated with self-ligating brackets during the initial phase of orthodontic treatment: A 3-month preliminary study. *Journal of Orthodontic Science* **3**, 7–11.

Alexander, S. A. (1991) Effects of orthodontic attachments on the gingival health of permanent second molars. *American Journal of Orthodontics and Dentofacial Orthopedics* **100**, 337–340.

Alves de Souza, R., Borges de Araújo Magnanib, M. B., Nouerc, D. F. et al. (2008) Periodontal and microbiologic evaluation of 2 methods of archwire ligation: Ligature wires and elastomeric rings. *American Journal of Orthodontics and Dentofacial Orthopedics* **134**(4), 506–512.

Andrucioli, M. C. D., Matsumoto, M. C. N., Saraiva, M. C. P. et al. (2018) Successful and failed mini-implants: microbiological evaluation and quantification of bacterial endotoxin. *Journal of Applied Oral Science* **26**, 20170631.

Anhoury, P., Nathanson, D., Huges, C. V. et al. (2002) Microbial profile on metallic and ceramic bracket materials. *The Angle Orthodontist* **73**, 338–343.

Antonelli, G., Clementi, M., Pozzi, G. and Rossolini, G. M. (2012) *Principi di microbiologia medica: II edizione*. Milano: Casa Editrice Ambrosiana ISBN 978-88-08-18073-5.

Apel, S., Apel, C., Morea, C. et al. (2009) Microflora associated with successful and failed orthodontic mini-implants. *Clinical Oral Implants Research* **20**, 1186–1190.

Arab, S., Nouhzadeh Malekshah, S., Abouei Mehrizi, E. et al. (2016) Effect of fixed orthodontic treatment on salivary flow, pH and microbial count. *Journal of Dentistry (Tehran)* **13**(1), 18–22.

Arendorf, T. and Addy, M. (1985) Candidal carriage and plaque distribution before, during and after removable orthodontic appliance therapy. *Journal of Clinical Periodontology* **12**(5), 360–368.

Arslan, S. G., Akpolat, N., Kama, J. D. et al. (2008) One-year follow-up of the effect of fixed orthodontic treatment on colonization by oral Candida. *Journal of Oral Pathology and Medicine* **37**(1), 26–29.

Atack, N. E., Sandy, J. R. and Addy, M. (1996) Periodontal and microbiological changes associated with the placement of orthodontic appliances. A review. *Journal of Periodontology* **67**, 78–85.

Baka, Z. M., Basciftci, F. A. and Arslan, U. (2013) Effects of 2 bracket and ligation types on plaque retention: A quantitative microbiologic analysis with real-time polymerase chain reaction. *American Journal of Orthodontics and Dentofacial Orthopedics* **144**, 260–267.

Batoni, G., Pardini, M., Giannotti, A. et al. (2001) Effect of removable orthodontic appliances on oral colonisation by mutans streptococci in children. *European Journal of Oral Sciences* **109**(6), 388–392.

Bjerklin, K., Garskog, B. and Ronnerman, A. (1983) Proximal caries increment in connection with orthodontic treatment with removable appliances. *British Journal of Orthodontics* **10**, 21–24.

Bondemark, L. (1998) Interdental bone changes after orthodontic treatment: a 5-year longitudinal study. *American Journal of Orthodontics and Dentofacial Orthopedics* **114**(1), 25–31.

Bowden, G. H., Nolette, N., Ryding, H. and Cleghorn, B. M. (1999) The diversity and distribution of the predominant ribotypes of Actinomyces naeslundii genospecies 1 and 2 in samples from enamel and from healthy and carious root surfaces of teeth. *Journal of Dental Research* **78**(12), 1800–1809.

Boyd, R. L., Leggott, P. J., Quinn, R. S. et al. (1989) Periodontal implications of orthodontic treatment in adults with reduced or normal periodontal tissues versus those of adolescents. *American Journal of Orthodontics and Dentofacial Orthopedics* **96**, 191–198.

Byun, R., Nadkarni, M. A., Chhour, K. L. et al. (2004) Quantitative analysis of diverse Lactobacillus species present in advanced dental caries. *Journal of Clinical Microbiology* **42**(7), 3128–3136.

Chhour, K. L., Nadkarni, M. A., Byun, R. et al. (2005) Molecular analysis of microbial diversity in advanced caries. *Journal of Clinical Microbiology* **43**(2), 843–849.

Claro-Pereira, D., Sampaio-Maia, B., Ferreira, C. et al. (2011) In situ evaluation of a new silorane-based composite resin's bioadhesion properties. *Dental Materials* **27**, 1238–1245.

Corbett, A. I., Leggitt, V. L., Angelov, N. et al. (2015) Periodontal health of anterior teeth with two types of fixed retainers. *The Angle Orthodontist* **85**(4), 699–705.

Davies, T. M., Shaw, W. C., Worthington, H. V. et al. (1991) The effect of orthodontic treatment on plaque and gingivitis. *American Journal of Orthodontics and Dentofacial Orthopedics* **99**(2), 155–161.

Demling, A., Demling, C., Schwestka-Polly, R. et al. (2009) Influence of lingual orthodontic therapy on microbial parameters and periodontal status in adults. *European Journal of Orthodontics* **31**(6), 638–642.

Demling, A., Demling, C., Schwestka-Polly, R. et al. (2010) Short-term influence of lingual orthodontic therapy on microbial parameters and periodontal status. A preliminary study. *The Angle Orthodontics* **80**, 480–484.

D'Ercole, S., Martinelli, D. and Tripodi, D. (2014) Influence of sport mouthguards on the ecological factors of the children oral cavity. *BMC Oral Health* **14**, 97.

Dewhirst, F. E., Tamer, M. A., Ericson, R. E. et al. (2000) The diversity of periodontal spirochetes by 16S rRNA analysis. *Oral Microbiology and Immunology* **15**(3), 196–202.

Diamanti-Kipioti, A., Gusberti, F. A. and Lang, N. P. (1987) Clinical and microbiological effects of fixed orthodontic appliances. *Journal of Clinical Periodontology* **14**(6), 326–333.

Eckley, B., Thomas, J., Crout, R. and Ngan, P. (2012) Periodontal and microbiological status of patients undergoing orthodontic therapy. *Hong Kong Dental Journal* **9**, 11–20.

Eroglu, A. K., Baka, Z. M. and Arslan, U. (2019) Comparative evaluation of salivary microbial levels and periodontal status of patients wearing fixed and removable orthodontic retainers. *American Journal of Orthodontics and Dentofacial Orthopedics* **156**(2), 186–192.

Farhadian, N., Usefi Mashoof, R., Khanizadeh, S. et al. (2016) Streptococcus mutans counts in patients wearing removable retainers with silver nanoparticles vs those wearing conventional retainers: A randomized clinical trial. *American Journal of Orthodontics and Dentofacial Orthopedics* **149**(2), 155–160.

Forde, K., Storey, M., Littlewood, S. J. et al. (2018) Bonded versus vacuum-formed retainers: A randomized controlled trial. Part 1: Stability, retainer survival, and patient satisfaction outcomes after 12 months. *European Journal of Orthodontics* **40**(4), 387–398.

Forsberg, C. M., Brattström, V., Malmberg, E. and Nord, C. E. (1991) Ligature wires and elastomeric rings: two methods of ligation, and their association with microbial colonization of Streptococcus mutans and lactobacilli. *European Journal of Orthodontics* **13**(5), 416–420.

Freitas, A. O., Alviano, C. S., Alviano, D. S. et al. (2012) Microbial colonization in orthodontic mini-implants. *Brazilian Dental Journal* **23**(4), 422–427.

Genco, R., Kornman, K., Williams, R. et al. (1996) Consensus report. Periodontal diseases: pathogenesis and microbial factors. *Annals of Periodontology* **1**(1), 926–932.

Ghijselings, E., Coucke, W., Verdonck, A. et al. (2014) Long-term changes in microbiology and clinical periodontal variables after completion of fixed orthodontic appliances. *Orthodontics and Craniofacial Research* **17**(1), 49–59.

Gizani, S., Petsi, G., Twetman, S. et al. (2016) Effect of the probiotic bacterium Lactobacillus reuteri on white spot lesion development in orthodontic patients. *European Journal of Orthodontics* **38**(1), 85–89.

Gkantidis, N., Christou, P. and Topouzelis, N. (2010) The orthodontic-periodontic interrelationship in integrated treatment challenges: a systematic review. *Journal of Oral Rehabilitation* **37**(5), 377–390.

Gwinnett, A. J. and Ceen, R. F. (1979) Plaque distribution on bonded brackets: a scanning microscope study. *American Journal of Orthodontics* **75**, 667–677.

Haffajee, A. D. and Socransky, S. S. (1994) Microbial etiological agents of destructive periodontal diseases. *Periodontology 2000* **5**, 78–111.

Hägg, U., Kaveewatcharanont, P., Samaranayake, Y. H. and Samaranayake, L. P. (2004) The effect of fixed orthodontic appliances on the oral carriage of Candida species and Enterobacteriaceae. *European Journal of Orthodontics* **26**(6), 623–629.

Hamilton, I. R. (2000) Ecological basis for dental caries, in *Oral Bacterial Ecology: The Molecular Basis* (eds. R.P. Ellen and H.K. Kuramitsu). Horizon Scientific Press Wymondham, pp. 219–274.

Hansson, C. and Linder-Aronson, S. (1972) Gingival status after orthodontic treatment of impacted upper canines. *Transactions European Orthodontic Society* 48th Congress; Oslo, Norway, pp. 433–41.

Heier, E. E., De Smit, A. A., Wijgaerts, I. A. and Adriaens, P. A. (1997) Periodontal implications of bonded versus removable retainers. *American Journal of Orthodontics and Dentofacial Orthopedics* **112**(6), 607–616.

Hernández-Solís, S. E., Rueda-Gordillo, F., Flota-Alcocer, A. D. et al. (2016) Influence of orthodontic appliances on the occurrence of Candida spp. in the oral cavity. *Revista Chilena de Infectologia* **33**(3), 293–297.

Jabur, S. F. (2008) Influence of removable orthodontic appliance on oral microbiological status. *Journal of the Faculty of Medicine Baghdad* **50**(2), 199–202.

Jacobs, S. G. (1996) The impacted maxillary canine. Further observations on aetiology, radiographic localization, prevention/interception of impaction, and when to suspect impaction. *Australian Dental Journal* **4**, 310–316.

Jacoby, H. (1983) The etiology of maxillary canine impactions. *American Journal of Orthodontics* **84**, 125–132.

Jing, D., Hao, J., Shen, Y. et al. (2019) Effect of fixed orthodontic treatment on oral microbiota and salivary proteins. *Experimental and Therapeutic Medicine* **17**(5), 4237–4243.

Johnston, W. D. (1969) Treatment of palatally impacted canine teeth. *American Journal of Orthodontics* **56**, 589–596.

Jongsma, M. A., Pelser, F. D., van der Mei, H. C. et al. (2013) Biofilm formation on stainless steel and gold wires for bonded retainers in vitro and in vivo and their susceptibility to oral antimicrobials. *Clinical Oral Investigation* **17**(4), 1209–1218.

Jung, W. S., Kim, H., Park, S. Y. et al. (2014) Quantitative analysis of changes in salivary mutans streptococci after orthodontic treatment. *American Journal of Orthodontics and Dentofacial Orthopedics* **145**(5), 603–609.

Jung, W. S., Yang, I. H., Lim, W. H. et al. (2015) Adhesion of mutans streptococci to self-ligating ceramic brackets: in vivo quantitative analysis with real-time polymerase chain reaction. *European Journal of Orthodontics* **37**(6), 565–569.

Jurela, A., Repic, D., Pejda, S. et al. (2013) The effect of two different bracket types on the salivary levels of S mutans and S sobrinus in the early phase of orthodontic treatment. *The Angle Orthodontist* **83**(1), 140–145.

Kaji, A., Sekino, S., Ito, H. and Numabe, Y. (2013) Influence of a mandibular fixed orthodontic retainer on periodontal health. *Australian Orthodontic Journal* **29**(1), 76–85.

Keijser, B. J., Zaura, E., Huse, S. M. et al. (2008) Pyrosequencing analysis of the oral microflora of healthy adults. *Journal of Dental Research* **87**, 1016–1020.

Keyes, P. H. (1960) The infectious and transmissible nature of experimental dental caries. Findings and implications. *Archives of Oral Biology* **1**, 304–320.

Khanpayeh, E., Jafari, A. A. and Tabatabaei, Z. (2014) Comparison of salivary Candida profile in patients with fixed and removable orthodontic appliances therapy. *Iranian Journal of Microbiology* **6**(4), 263–268.

Kilian, M., Chapple, I. L. C., Hannig, M. et al. (2016) The oral microbiome – an update for oral healthcare professionals. *British Dental Journal* **221**, 657–666.

Kim, K., Jung, W. S., Cho, S. and Ahn, S. J. (2016) Changes in salivary periodontal pathogens after orthodontic treatment: An in vivo prospective study. *The Angle Orthodontist* **86**(6), 998–1003.

Kim, S. H., Choi, D. S., Jang, I. et al. (2012) Microbiologic changes in subgingival plaque before and during the early period of orthodontic treatment. *The Angle Orthodontist* **82**(2), 254–260.

Klaus, K., Eichenauer, J., Sprenger, R. and Ruf, S. (2016) Oral microbiota carriage in patients with multibracket appliance in relation to the quality of oral hygiene. *Head and Face Medicine* **12**(1), 28.

Kleinberg, I. (2002) A mixed-bacteria ecological approach to understanding the role of the oral bacteria in dental caries causation: an alternative to Streptococcus mutans and the specific plaque hypothesis. *Critical Reviews in Oral Biology and Medicine* **13**(2), 108–25.

Kloehn, J. S. and Pfeifer, J. S. (1974) The effect of orthodontic treatment on the periodontium. *The Angle Orthodontist* **44**(2), 127–134.

Klukowska, M., Bader, A., Erbe, C. et al. (2011) Plaque levels of patients with fixed orthodontic appliances measured by digital plaque image analysis. *American Journal of Orthodontics and Dentofacial Orthopedics* **139**(5), 463–470.

Koopman, J. E., van der Kaaij, N. C., Buijs, M. J. et al. (2015) The effect of fixed orthodontic appliances and fluoride mouthwash on the oral microbiome of adolescents - a randomized controlled clinical trial. *PLOS One* **10**(9), 137318.

Kouraki, E., Bissada, N. F., Palomo, J. M. and Ficara, A. J. (2005) Gingival enlargement and resolution during and after orthodontic treatment. *New York State Dental Journal* **71**(4), 34–37.

Kundu, R., Tripathi, A., Jaiswal, J. et al. (2016) Effect of fixed space maintainers and removable appliances on oral microflora in children: An in vivo study. *Journal of Indian Society of Pedodontics and Preventive Dentistry* **34**(1), 3–9.

Kupietzky, A., Majumdar, A. K., Shey, Z. et al. (2005) Colony forming unit levels of salivary Lactobacilli and Streptococcus mutans in orthodontic patients. *Journal of Clinical Pediatric Dentistry* **30**(1), 51–53.

Lara-Carrillo, E., Montiel-Bastida, N. M., Sánchez-Pérez, L. and Alanís-Tavira, J. (2010a) Changes in the oral environment during four stages of orthodontic treatment. *Korean Journal of Orthodontics* **40**(2), 95–105.

Lara-Carrillo, E., Montiel-Bastida, N. M., Sánchez-Pérez, L. and Alanís-Tavira, J. (2010b) Effect of orthodontic treatment on saliva, plaque and the levels of Streptococcus mutans and Lactobacillus. *Medicina Oral Patologia Oral y Cirugia Bucal* **15**(6), 924–929.

Lepp, P. W., Brinig, M. M., Ouverney, C. C. et al. (2004) Methanogenic Archaea and human periodontal disease. *Proceedings of the National Academy of Sciences of the United States of America* **101**(16), 6176–6181.

Lessa, F. C., Enoki, C., Ito, I. Y. et al. (2007) In-vivo evaluation of the bacterial contamination and disinfection of acrylic baseplates of removable orthodontic appliances. *American Journal of Orthodontics and Dentofacial Orthopedics* **131**(6), 70511–70517.

Leung, N. M., Chen, R. and Rudney, J. D. (2006) Oral bacteria in plaque and invading buccal cells of young orthodontic patients. *American Journal of Orthodontics and Dentofacial Orthopedics* **130**(6), 69811–69818.

Li, Q., Wang, C., Tang, C. et al. (2012) Molecular-phylogenetic characterization of the microbiota in ulcerated and non-ulcerated regions in the patients with Crohn's disease. *PLOS One* **7**(4), e3493.

Lif Holgerson, P., Öhman, C., Rönnlund, A. and Johansson, I. (2015) Maturation of oral microbiota in children with or without dental caries. *PLOS One* **10**(5), e0128534.

Lindel, I. D., Elter, C., Heuer, W. et al. (2011) Comparative analysis of long-term biofilm formation on metal and ceramic brackets. *The Angle Orthodontist* **81**(5), 907–914.

Lindhe, J. and Meyle, J. (2008) Peri-implant diseases: consensus report of the sixth European workshop on Periodontology. *Journal of Clinical Periodontology* **35**, 282–285.

Lindhe, J. and Svanberg, G. (1974) Influence of trauma from occlusion on progression of experimental periodontitis in the beagle dog. *Journal of Clinical Periodontology* **1**, 3–14.

Liu, J., Bian, Z., Fan, M. et al. (2004) Typing of mutans streptococci by arbitrarily primed PCR in patients undergoing orthodontic treatment. *Caries Research* **38**(6), 523–529.

Loesche, W. J. (1967) Chemotherapy of dental plaque infections. *Oral Sciences Reviews* **9**, 65–107.

Loesche, W. J. (1986) Role of Streptococcus mutans in human dental decay. *Microbiological Reviews* **50**(4), 353–380.

Loesche, W. J. and Grossman, N. S. (2001) Periodontal disease as a specific, albeit chronic, infection: diagnosis and treatment. *Clinical Microbiology Reviews* **14**(4), 727–752.

Lombardo, L., Ortan, Y. Ö., Gorgun, Ö. et al. (2013) Changes in the oral environment after placement of lingual and labial orthodontic appliances. *Progress in Orthodontics* **14**, 28.

Low, B., Lee, W., Seneviratne, C.J. et al. (2011) Ultrastructure and morphology of biofilms on thermoplastic orthodontic appliances in 'fast' and 'slow' plaque formers. *European Journal of Orthodontics* **33**(5), 577–583.

Lucchese, A., Bondemark, L., Marcolina, M. and Manuelli, M. (2018) Changes in oral microbiota due to orthodontic appliances: a systematic review. *Journal of Oral Microbiology* **10**(1), 1476645.

Lucchese, A. and Gherlone, E. (2013) Prevalence of white-spot lesions before and during orthodontic treatment with fixed appliances. *European Journal of Orthodontics* **35**(5), 664–668.

Lucchese, A., Manuelli, M. et al. (2021) The effect of removable orthodontic appliances on oral microbiota: systematic review. *Materials Journal (in press)*.

Lundström, F., Hamp, S. E. and Nyman, S. (1980) Systematic plaque control in children undergoing long-term orthodontic treatment. *European Journal of Orthodontics* **2**(1), 27–39.

Maret, D., Marchal-Sixou, C., Vergnes, J. N. et al. (2014) Effect of fixed orthodontic appliances on salivary microbial parameters at 6 months: a controlled observational study. *Journal of Applied Oral Science* **22**(1), 38–43.

Martin, F. E., Nadkarni, M. A., Jacques, N. A. and Hunter, N. (2002) Quantitative microbiological study of human carious dentine by culture and real-time PCR: association of anaerobes with histopathological changes in chronic pulpitis. *Journal of Clinical Microbiology* **40**(5), 1698–1704.

Mattingly, J. A., Sauer, G. J., Yancey, J. M. and Arnold, R. R. (1983) Enhancement of Streptococcus mutans colonization by direct bonded orthodontic appliances. *Journal of Dental Research* **62**(12), 1209–1211.

Miller, W. D. (1890) *The Micro-Organisms of the Human Mouth: The Local and General Diseases Which Are Caused By Them.* University of Glasgow. S.S. White Dental Manufacturing Co., Library Philadelphia, PA.

Miura, K. K., Ito, I. Y., Enoki, C. et al. (2007) Anticariogenic effect of fluoride-releasing elastomers in orthodontic patients. *Brazilian Oral Research* **21**(3), 228–233.

Morita, Y., Imai, S., Hanyuda, A. et al. (2014) Effect of silver ion coating of fixed orthodontic retainers on the growth of oral pathogenic bacteria. *Dental Materials Journal* **33**(2), 268–274.

Nalçacı, R., Özat, Y., Çokakoğlu, S. et al. (2014) Effect of bracket type on halitosis, periodontal status, and microbial colonization. *The Angle Orthodontist* **84**, 479–485.

O'Hara, A. M. and Shanahan, F. (2006) The gut flora as a forgotten organ. *EMBO Reports* **7**, 688–693.

Ogaard, B. (1989) Prevalence of white spot lesions in 19-year-olds: A study on untreated and orthodontically treated persons 5 years after treatment. *American Journal of Orthodontics and Dentofacial Orthopedics* **96**, 423–427.

Øilo, M. and Bakken, V. (2015) Biofilm and Dental Biomaterials. *Materials* **8**, 2887–2900.

Ong, M. A., Wang, H. L. and Smith, F. N. (1998) Interrelationship between periodontics and adult orthodontics. *Journal of Clinical Periodontology* **25**, 271–277.

Pan, S., Liu, Y., Zhang, L. et al. (2017) Profiling of subgingival plaque biofilm microbiota in adolescents after completion of orthodontic therapy. *PLOS One* **12**(2), 171550.

Pandis, N., Papaioannou, W., Kontou, E. et al. (2010) Salivary Streptococcus mutans levels in patients with conventional and self-ligating brackets. *European Journal of Orthodontics* **32**(1), 94–99.

Paolantonio, M., Festa, F., di Placido, G. et al. (1999) Site-specific subgingival colonization by Actinobacillus actinomycetemcomitans in orthodontic patients. *American Journal of Orthodontics and Dentofacial Orthopedics* **115**(4), 423–428.

Paolantonio, M., Pedrazzoli, V., di Murro, C. et al. (1997) Clinical significance of Actinobacillus actinomycetemcomitans in young individuals during orthodontic treatment. A 3-year longitudinal study. *Journal of Clinical Periodontology* **24**, 610–617.

Papageorgiou, S. N., Xavier, G. M., Cobourne, M. T. and Eliades, T. (2018) Effect of orthodontic treatment on the subgingival microbiota: A systematic review and meta-analysis. *Orthodontics and Craniofacial Research* **21**(4), 175–185.

Park, H. S., Lee, S.K. and Kwon, K. (2005) Group distal movement of teeth using mini-screw implant anchorage. *The Angle Orthodontist* **75**, 602–609.

Pejda, S., Varga, M. L., Milosevic, S. A. et al. (2013) Clinical and microbiological parameters in patients with self-ligating and conventional brackets during early phase of orthodontic treatment. *The Angle Orthodontist* **83**, 133–139.

Pellegrini, P., Sauerwein, R., Finlayson, T. et al. (2009) Plaque retention by self-ligating vs elastomeric orthodontic brackets: quantitative comparison of oral bacteria and detection with adenosine triphosphate-driven bioluminescence. *American Journal of Orthodontics and Dentofacial Orthopedics* **135**, 426–429.

Perinetti, G., Paolantonio, M., Serra, E. et al. (2004) Longitudinal monitoring of subgingival colonization by Actinobacillus actinomycetemcomitans, and crevicular alkaline phosphatase and aspartate aminotransferase activities around orthodontically treated teeth. *Journal of Clinical Periodontology* **31**(1), 60–67.

Perkowski, K., Baltaza, W., Conn, D. B. et al. (2019) Examination of oral biofilm microbiota in patients using fixed orthodontic appliances in order to prevent risk factors for health complications. *Annals of Agricultural and Environmental Medicine* **26**(2), 231–235.

Peros, K., Mestrovic, S., Anic-Milosevic, S. and Slaj, M. (2011) Salivary microbial and nonmicrobial parameters in children with fixed orthodontic appliances. *The Angle Orthodontist* **81**(5), 901–906.

Petti, S., Barbato, E. and Simonetti D'Arca, A. (1997) Effect of orthodontic therapy with fixed and removable appliances on oral microbiota: a six-month longitudinal study. *New Microbiologica* **20**(1), 55–62.

Prabhu, J. and Cousley R. R. J. (2006) Current products and practice: bone anchorage devices in orthodontics. *Journal of Orthodontics* **33**, 288–307.

Pramod, S., Kailasam, V., Padmanabhan, S. and Chitharanjan, A. B. (2011) Presence of cariogenic streptococci on various bracket materials detected by polymerase chain reaction. *Australian Orthodontic Journal* **27**(1), 46–51.

Ristic, M., Vlahovic Svabic, M., Sasic, M. and Zelic, O. (2007) Clinical and microbiological effects of fixed orthodontic appliances on periodontal tissues in adolescents. *Orthodontics and Craniofacial Research* **10**, 187–195.

Ristic, M., Vlahovic Svabic, M., Sasic, M. and Zelic, O. (2008) Effects of fixed orthodontic appliances on subgingival microflora. *International Journal of Dental Hygiene* **6**, 129–136.

Ritz, H. L. (1967) Microbial population shifts in developing human dental plaque. *Archives of Oral Biology* **12**(12), 1561–1568.

Rosenbloom, R. G. and Tinanoff, N. (1991) Salivary Streptococcus mutans levels in patients before, during, and after orthodontic treatment. *American Journal of Orthodontics and Dentofacial Orthopedics* **100**(1), 35–37.

Rossini, G., Parrini, S., Castroflorio, T. et al. (2015) Periodontal health during clear aligners treatment: a systematic review. *European Journal of Orthodontics* **37**(5), 539–543.

Sakamoto, M., Huang, Y., Umeda, M. et al. (2002) Detection of novel oral phylotypes associated with periodontitis. *FEMS Microbiology Letters* **217**(1), 65–69.

Sampaio-Maia, B., Figueiral, M. H., Sousa-Rodrigues, P. et al. (2012) The effect of denture adhesives on Candida albicans growth in vitro. *Gerodontology* **29**, 348–356.

Sansone, C., Van Houte, J., Joshipura, K. et al. (1993) The association of mutans streptococci and non-mutans streptococci capable of acidogenesis at a low pH with dental caries on enamel and root surfaces. *Journal of Dental Research* **72**(2), 508–516.

Sari, E. and Birinci, I. (2007) Microbiological evaluation of 0,2% chlorhexidine gluconate mouth rinse in orthodontic patients. *The Angle Orthodontist* **77**, 881–884.

Sender, R., Fuchs, S. and Milo, R. (2016) Are we really vastly outnumbered? Revisiting the ratio of bacterial to host cells in humans. *Cell* **164**, 337–340.

Sfondrini, M. F., Debiaggi, M., Zara, F. et al. (2012) Influence of lingual bracket position on microbial and periodontal parameters in vivo. *Journal of Applied Oral Science* **20**(3), 357–361.

Shukla, C., Maurya, R., Singh, V. and Tijare, M. (2017) Evaluation of role of fixed orthodontics in changing oral ecological flora of opportunistic microbes in children and adolescent. *Journal of Indian Society of Pedodontics and Preventive Dentistry* **35**(1), 34–40.

Shukla, C., Maurya, R.K., Singh, V. and Tijare, M. (2016) Evaluation of changes in Streptococcus mutans colonies in microflora of the Indian population with fixed orthodontics appliances. *Dental Research Journal (Isfahan)* **13**(4), 309–314.

Shungin, D., Haworth, S., Divaris, K. et al. (2019) Genome-wide analysis of dental caries and periodontitis combining clinical and self-reported data. *Nature Communications* **10**(1), 2773.

Silin, A. V., Satygo, E. A. and Reutskaya, K. V. (2017) Effectiveness of Paradontax toothpaste in patients undergoing orthodontic treatment. *Stomatologiia (Mosk)* **96**(4), 20–22.

Sinclair, P. M., Berry, C. W., Bennett, C. L. and Israelson, H. (1987) Changes in gingiva and gingival flora with bonding and banding. *The Angle Orthodontist* **57**(4), 271–278.

Slots, J. (2004) Update on human cytomegalovirus in destructive periodontal disease. *Oral Microbiology and Immunology* **19**(4), 217–223.

Socransky, S. S. and Haffajee, A. D. (1994) Evidence of bacterial etiology: a historical perspective. *Periodontology 2000* **5**, 7–25.

Socransky, S. S., Haffajee, A. D., Cugini, M. A. *et al.* (1998) Microbial complexes in subgingival plaque. *Journal of Clinical Periodontology* **25**(2), 134–144.

Sonesson, M., Twetman, S. and Bondemark, L. (2014) Effectiveness of high-fluoride toothpaste on enamel demineralization during orthodontic treatment-a multicenter randomized controlled trial. *European Journal of Orthodontics* **36**(6), 678–682.

Sudarević, K., Jurela, A., Repić, D. *et al.* (2014) Oral health changes during early phase of orthodontic treatment. *Acta Clinica Croatica* **53**, 399–404.

Tanzer, J. M., Livingston, J. and Thompson, A. M. (2001) The microbiology of primary dental caries in humans. *Journal of Dental Education* **65**(10), 1028–1037.

Thilander, B. and Myrberg, N. (1973) The prevalence of malocclusion in Swedish schoolchildren. *Scandinavian Journal of Dental Research* **81**, 12–20.

Thornberg, M. J., Riolo, C. S., Bayirli, B. *et al.* (2009) Periodontal pathogen levels in adolescents before, during, and after fixed orthodontic appliance therapy. *American Journal of Orthodontics and Dentofacial Orthopedics* **135**(1), 95–98.

Topaloglu-Ak, A., Ertugrul, F., Eden, E. *et al.* (2011) Effect of orthodontic appliances on oral microbiota – 6 month follow-up. *Journal of Clinical Pediatric Dentistry* **35**(4), 433–436.

Torlakovic, L., Paster, B. J., Øgaard, B. and Olsen, I. (2013) Changes in the supragingival microbiota surrounding brackets of upper central incisors during orthodontic treatment. *Acta Odontologica Scandinavica* **71**(6), 1547–1554.

Tortamano, A., Dominguez, G. C., Haddad, A. C. *et al.* (2012) Periodontopathogens around the surface of mini-implants removed from orthodontic patients. *The Angle Orthodontist* **82**(4), 591–595.

Turkkahraman, H., Sayın, M. O., Bozkurt, F. Y. *et al.* (2005) Archwire ligation techniques, microbial colonization, and periodontal status in orthodontically treated patients. *The Angle Orthodontist* **75**, 231–236.

Türköz, C., Canigür Bavbek, N., Kale Varlik, S. and Akça, G. (2012) Influence of thermoplastic retainers on Streptococcus mutans and Lactobacillus adhesion. *American Journal of Orthodontics and Dentofacial Orthopedics* **141**(5), 598–603.

Turnbaugh, P. J. and Gordon, J. I. (2009) The core gut microbiome, energy balance and obesity. *Journal of Physiology* **1**;587(Pt 17), 4153–4158.

Uzuner, F. D., Kaygisiz, E. and Cankaya, Z. T. (2014) Effect of the bracket types on microbial colonization and periodontal status. *The Angle Orthodontist* **84**, 1062–1067.

Vanarsdall, R. L. (1991) Complications of orthodontic treatment. *Current Opinion in Dentistry* **1**, 622–633.

Van Gastel, J., Teughels, W., Quirynen, M. *et al.* (2011) Longitudinal changes in gingival crevicular fluid after placement of fixed orthodontic appliances. *American Journal of Orthodontics and Dentofacial Orthopedics* **139**(6), 735–744.

Van Houte, J. (1994) Role of micro-organisms in caries etiology. *Journal of Dental Research* **73**(3), 672–681.

Van Houte, J., Lopman, J. and Kent, R. (1996) The final pH of bacteria comprising the predominant flora on sound and carious human root and enamel surface. *Journal of Dental Research* **75**(4), 1008–1014.

Van Houte, J., Sansone, C., Joshipura, K. and Kent, R. (1991) Mutans streptococci and non-mutans streptococci acidogenic at low pH, and in vitro acidogenic potential of dental plaque in two different areas of the human dentition. *Journal of Dental Research* **70**(12), 1503–1507.

Weinspach, K., Demling, A., Günay, H. *et al.* (2012) Short-term periodontal and microbiological changes following orthognathic surgery. *Journal of Cranio-Maxillofacial Surgery* **40**(5), 467–472.

Wichelhaus, A., Brauchli, L., Song, Q. *et al.* (2011) Prevalence of Helicobacter pylori in the adolescent oral cavity: dependence on orthodontic therapy, oral flora and hygiene. *Journal of Orofacial Orthopedics* **72**(3), 187–195.

Wise, R. J. (1981) Periodontal diagnosis and management of the impacted maxillary canine. *International Journal of Periodontics and Restorative Dentistry* **1**, 56–73.

Ximenez-Fyvie, L. A., Haffajee, A. D. and Socransky, S. S. (2000) Microbial composition of supra- and subgingival plaque in subjects with adult periodontitis. *Journal of Clinical Periodontology* **27**(10), 722–732.

Yáñez-Vico, R. M., Iglesias-Linares, A., Ballesta-Mudarra, S. *et al.* (2015) Short-term effect of removal of fixed orthodontic appliances on gingival health and subgingival microbiota: a prospective cohort study. *Acta Odontologica Scandinavica* **73**(7), 496–502.

Yener, S.,B. Özsoy, Ö.P. (2020) Quantitative Analysis of Biofilm Formation On Labial and Lingual Bracket Surfaces. *Angle Orthod* **90**(1), 100–108.

Yitschaky, O., Katorza, A., Zini, A. *et al.* (2016) Acrylic orthodontic retainer is not a risk factor for focal Candida colonization in young healthy patients: a pilot study. *Oral Surgery Oral Medicine Oral Pathology and Oral Radiology* **121**(1), 39–42.

Zachrisson, B. U. (1974) Oral hygiene for orthodontic patients: Current concepts and practical advice. *American Journal of Orthodontics* **66**(5), 487–497.

Zhang, X., Shen, D., Fang, Z. *et al.* (2013) Human gut microbiota changes reveal the progression of glucose intolerance. *PLOS One* **8** (8).

Zhao, R., Huang, R., Long, H. *et al.* (2019) The dynamics of the oral microbiome and oral health among patients receiving clear aligner orthodontic treatment. *Oral Diseases* 26(2):473–483.

Zheng, Y., Li, Z. and He, X. (2016) Influence of fixed orthodontic appliances on the change in oral Candida strains among adolescents. *Journal of Dental Sciences* **11**(1), 17–12.

CHAPTER 11
Markers of Paradental Tissue Remodeling in the Gingival Crevicular Fluid and Saliva of Orthodontic Patients

Taylor E. Glovsky and Laura R. Iwasaki

Summary

Oral fluid markers of the mechanisms associated with paradental tissue changes that account for tooth movement could help identify, assess, and improve tooth movement. Identified markers fit three main categories: metabolic products of paradental remodeling, inflammatory mediators, and patient-response modifiers, and enzymes and enzyme-inhibitors that are patient-derived. To develop useful clinical tools, these markers must be quantified and linked to clinically meaningful phenomena, such as the type and speed of orthodontic tooth movement, retention of tooth positions, resorption of tooth roots, and pain experience or developmental stage of the patient. Currently, progress in this area has been limited because of the paucity of studies that have measured both the applied variables and outcomes of orthodontic stimuli. This chapter will present an overview of the study of markers in oral fluids during orthodontic tooth movement to date and prospects for the future.

Why study oral fluids?

Both saliva and gingival crevicular fluid (GCF) are inexpensive potential sources of personalized oral and general health information that are easily and noninvasively collectable. Over the past 15 years, major advancements have occurred in salivary testing for oral and systemic health and disease (Schipper et al., 2007; Genco, 2012; Al Kawas et al., 2012; Dawes and Wong, 2019), known as salivary diagnostics or "salivaomics" (Wong, 2012). Salivaomics involves the development and validation of saliva-based technologies aimed at early detection of diseases, such as cancer and periodontal disease, and at screening for conditions such as drug use. The components of saliva have a number of different sources: multiple salivary glands, GCF, nasopharyngeal discharge, food debris, and microorganisms (Genco, 2012) and are influenced by time of day, mechanical and chemical stimuli, medications, flow rate, plus sample storage and handling methods (de Jong et al., 2011; Giannobile, 2012; Lamy and Mau, 2012). Advances in the salivary research field have accelerated recently because of novel approaches that can characterize potential biomarkers of the genome, epigenome, microbiome, transcriptome, proteome, and metabolome within an individual sample (Dawes and Wong, 2019). However, saliva has unique and complex properties from biochemical, physicochemical, and rheological aspects that vary depending on where and how it is collected and stored (Schipper et al., 2007; Al Kawas et al., 2012). Standardized protocols for collection, handling, and analyses of saliva have yet to be established (Vitorino et al., 2012; Justino et al., 2017). Even when collection and handling variables are controlled, intra- and interindividual variabilities in measurable components are high (Quintana et al., 2009; Thomas et al., 2009).

Orthodontic forces cause local inflammation and increase capillary permeability in paradental tissues, and hence, because GCF is closer to the sites of these activities and likely less diluted, it has more diagnostic potential than saliva for markers of these activities (Rody et al., 2011). GCF was acknowledged more than 100 years ago (Black, 1899) but research to investigate its origins, dynamic nature, and composition began about 50 years later. Descriptive and mathematical models of GCF, supported by subsequent experimental findings, indicate that the initial fluid accumulated in a healthy gingival crevice is a transudate of interstitial fluid whereas in inflamed or stimulated conditions GCF is an exudate that reflects serum concentrations of metabolites (Griffiths, 2003). GCF is also isolated and different from saliva (Goodson, 2003); for example, it is free of salivary amylase when sampled carefully (Burke et al., 2002).

Initial GCF studies were aimed at improving clinical judgment, prevention, and treatment of periodontitis. However, improved knowledge of humoral immune responses, genomics, proteomics, and metabolomics has broadened the prospective applications of GCF and saliva analyses. If an individual's immune and inflammatory

---

Biological Mechanisms of Tooth Movement, Third Edition. Edited by Vinod Krishnan, Anne Marie Kuijpers-Jagtman and Ze'ev Davidovitch.
© 2021 John Wiley & Sons Ltd. Published 2021 by John Wiley & Sons Ltd.

responses to stimuli can be measured through analyses of these oral fluids, these results could constitute an assessment of the relative risk of the individual not only for periodontitis, but also for other systemic conditions (Genco, 2012; Giannobile, 2012). Consequently, considerable on-going efforts aim to improve technologies for analyzing oral fluids and to establish which components (DNA, proteins, mRNAs, micro-RNAs, extracellular vesicles, metabolites, and microbes) are keys to condition-specific diagnostic tests.

What is known about markers in oral fluids during orthodontic tooth movement?

Studies with respect to orthodontic therapy have followed the periodontal research and technology of the day based on expectations that mechanical stimuli applied to move teeth affect oral fluid amounts and constituents. GCF studies associated with orthodontic tooth movement (OTM) have so far predominated compared with saliva studies. Furthermore, although GCF and saliva are expected to have similar constituents, concentrations are higher in GCF. For example, measurement of myeloperoxidase as an indicator of anti-inflammatory defenses in both GCF and whole saliva sampled at the same time during orthodontic treatment showed concentrations 10–100-fold higher in GCF compared with saliva (Marcaccini et al., 2010; Navarro-Palacios et al., 2014).

Saliva studies

In general, relatively short term studies (≤6 months), compared to the duration of orthodontic treatment have shown that salivary flow rates significantly increased during the period 1–3 months after delivery of fixed appliances relative to baseline before fixed orthodontic appliances (Chang et al., 1999; Peros et al., 2011) and control levels (Li et al., 2009). However, 1.5–2 months after the completion of treatment, rates returned closer to baseline and control levels. Similarly, cariogenic bacterial counts in whole saliva samples increased significantly 3 months after placement of fixed appliances compared with baseline levels, but thereafter decreased closer to baseline levels (Chang et al., 1999; Peros et al., 2011).

Only a few proof-of-concept studies so far have demonstrated that some markers are measurable in whole saliva and vary across groups with and without orthodontic appliances and periodontal disease (Zhang et al., 2012) and with orthodontic appliances with or without root resorption (Kaczor-Urbanowicz et al., 2017) or over time (Ellias et al., 2012; Florez-Moreno et al., 2012, 2013; Corega et al., 2014) with fixed orthodontic appliances alone and with corticotomies (Wu et al., 2018). One study showed differences in salivary leptin levels between obese and normal weight subjects with the aim of associating these results with differences in rate of space closure after extraction of maxillary first premolars (Jayachandran et al., 2017). The authors reported significantly slower space closure in obese compared with normal weight subjects. However, these results could have been affected by factors such as the subjects' age range of 14–30 years. This age range likely represented individuals who were and were not actively growing and who would be expected to show significant differences in rates of tooth movement (Iwasaki and Nickel, 2018).

Previous studies have demonstrated associations between specific host genotypes and a number of phenomena of orthodontic importance; for example, susceptibility to root resorption (Al-Qawasmi et al., 2003; Sharab et al., 2015), speed of tooth movement (Iwasaki et al., 2009), and primary failure of eruption (Grippaudo et al., 2018). Historically, whole blood and buccal swabs have been used for assesment of root resorption susceptibility analysis, but more recently DNA has been successfully extracted for genotyping from properly handled saliva samples of sufficient volume (Pulford et al., 2013) and using array-based (such as Infinium HumanMethylation450 BeadChip array) analyses (Bruinsma et al., 2018). Although whole blood yields the best quality DNA, saliva has the advantage of being relatively noninvasively collected and storable long-term at room temperature with appropriate preservatives (Nunes et al., 2012). Hence, saliva samples are likely to be commonly used in future for genetic analysis of the host and the host's microbiome (Tapia et al., 2019).

GCF studies

Early studies lead to the conclusion that in children with good oral hygiene, GCF volumes were not significantly different between teeth with or without orthodontic forces (Tersin, 1978). A recent survey confirmed further that GCF volumes were not indicative of tissue remodeling associated with OTM (Perinetti et al., 2013). Measurement of GCF constituents in relation to orthodontics began to be reported in the late 1980s. A literature search using the keywords "GCF" and "orthodontic" reveals that the number of papers published between 1985 and 2000 was 15, between 2001 and 2010 was 55, and so far from 2011-to date more than 104 (PubMed, 2019). This trend followed the growing wealth of information from in vitro and animal studies about the links between physical, cellular, and molecular events that result in paradental tissue remodeling and tooth movement. To date, more than 10 reviews (Waddington and Embery, 2001; Kavadia-Tsatala et al., 2002; Yamaguchi and Kasai, 2005; Ren and Vissink, 2008; d'Apuzzo et al., 2013; Perinetti et al., 2013; Kapoor et al., 2014; Alhadlaq, 2015; Kumar et al., 2015; de Aguiar et al., 2017; Vansant et al., 2018; Kapoor et al., 2019) and more than 100 studies concerning the effect of mechanical stimuli, applied to move teeth, on GCF measured in vivo in humans have been published in the English peer-reviewed literature. Most of these studies identified specific GCF markers associated with orthodontic forces. These markers can be broadly categorized into three groups (Table 11.1): metabolic products of paradental remodeling, inflammatory mediators and patient-response modifiers, and enzymes and enzyme-inhibitors that are patient-derived.

Evidence that a given marker was measurable in GCF as a result of a mechanical stimulus was the first step for in vivo human studies. Generally, research designs have evolved to those comparing GCF markers in experimental and control sites in the same subjects (split-mouth design), where the control tooth (teeth) is (are) the contralateral or antagonist tooth (or both) and where data are collected at multiple time-points. Short-term studies, up to 10 days long with GCF sampling at least once before the mechanical stimulus and at 2–7 time-points after the application of the stimulus, have generally shown that peak levels of substances occur, on average, at 1–2 days after the application of the stimulus and then appear to return to baseline after about 1 week (see * in Table 11.1) (Uematsu et al., 1996a, 1996b; Hoshino-Itoh et al., 2005; Giannopoulou et al., 2006; Karacay et al., 2007; Kawasaki et al., 2006). A 2013 investigation showed similar results for inflammatory markers measured in GCF of maxillary canines retracted 6 months after maxillary first premolars extractions (Alikhani et al., 2013). In addition, on the contralateral side, small bony perforations were made just prior to the canine retraction and GCF from these teeth demonstrated significantly even higher levels of these inflammatory markers compared with the other side, indicating that GCF constituents reflect the degree of inflammatory stimuli. Some of the early longer-term studies compared levels of markers in GCF

Table 11.1 Example GCF markers that have been correlated to orthodontic mechanical stimuli.

Metabolic products of paradental remodeling:
- chondroitin sulphate (CS), deoxy-pyridinoline, hyaluronic acid (HA), insulin-like growth factor-I (IGF-I), IGF binding protein-3 (IGFBP-3), n-telopeptide of type I collagen (NTx), osteocalcin, osteopontin (OPN), pyridinoline (Pyr)

Inflammatory mediators and patient-response modifiers:
- Beta$_2$-microglobulin (β_2-MG), *epidermal growth factor (EGF), granulocyte-macrophage colony-stimulating factor (GM-CSF), *interleukin-1alpha (IL-1α), *IL-1β, IL-1 receptor antagonist (IL-1RA), IL-2, IL-4, IL-5, *IL-6, *IL-8, IL-10, leptin, *macrophage inflammatory protein-1α (MIP-1α or CCL3), *monocyte chemotactic protein (MCP-1 or CCL2), osteoprotegerin (OPG), pentraxin-3 (PTX-3), *plasminogen activator inhibitor (PAI)-2, *prostaglandin E$_2$ (PGE$_2$), receptor activator of nuclear factor kappa-B (RANK), *RANK ligand (RANKL), *regulated on activation normal T cell expressed and secreted (RANTES or CCL5), *substance P, *transforming growth factor-β_1 (TGF-β_1), *tumor necrosis factor-α (TNF-α), *tissue plasminogen factor (t-PA)

Patient-derived enzymes and enzyme-inhibitors:
- acid phosphatase (ACP), alkaline phosphatase (ALP), aspartate aminotransferase (AST), β-Glucuronidase (β-G), *cathepsin B, collagenase, cystatins, interferon-gamma (IFN-γ), lactate dehydrogenase (LDH), matrix metalloproteinase (MMP)-1, MMP-2, MMP-3, MMP-7, MMP-8, MMP-9, MMP-12, MMP-13, myeloperoxidase, tissue inhibitor of metalloproteinase (TIMP)-1, TIMP-2

*Markers that have demonstrated peak levels 1–2 days after stimulus application and then return to baseline after about 1 week.

before, during, and after orthodontic treatment (Pender et al., 1994; Griffiths et al., 1998) but failed to show differences between untreated teeth and teeth in treatment and retention. Other longer-term studies, intended to investigate the relative levels of markers in GCF during orthodontic treatment, followed teeth in different subjects at different stages of treatment (Ren et al., 2002) or with different orthodontic appliances (Insoft et al., 1996) and the same teeth at multiple time-points for up to 201 days after stimulus application.

The major problems with these short-term and longer-term studies were that the investigators did not quantify the associated changes in the force magnitude and the amount of tooth movement. That is, the mechanical stimulus was estimated or only measured at initial delivery, and/or changes in tooth position over time-points in the study were unknown (although some studies reported the average tooth movement). In other studies where tooth movement was measured serially, anchorage was not controlled so the amounts of tooth movement were not solely attributable to the experimental teeth. Therefore, in these cases, the changes in the amounts of GCF markers with the applied stimulus or the amount and type of tooth movement that resulted cannot be reliably correlated. Furthermore, most of the orthodontic treatment regimens applied involved the tipping of teeth where, although it was not measured in these studies, the crown and root of the tooth likely did not move by the same amount in the same direction.

A more controlled mechanical system by which to study the nature and speed of tooth movement is one that yields bodily movement, that is, translation of the tooth crown and root in the same direction by the same amount. In this situation, the stress and strain distributions along the length of the periodontal ligament are more determinant in that the sign of the principal stress (or strain) is homogeneously negative on the leading side of the tooth and homogeneously positive on the trailing side. Few studies to date have used orthodontic appliances designed for tooth translation (Karacay et al., 2007; Lee et al., 2004; Iwasaki et al., 2017). Even fewer studies have measured three-dimensional tooth movement.

An additional problem common to over 90% of the previous longer-term studies is the collection of longitudinal data, while the analysis of these data is performed in a cross-sectional manner by averaging results for each time-point based on pooled sites measured in different subjects. Studies of controlled tooth movement have shown that teeth moved by the same applied stress can move more than 21-fold faster in some subjects than in others and at least five-fold faster within groups of similar growth status (Iwasaki and Nickel, 2018). Furthermore, individuals who were actively growing compared with those who were not showed average speeds of tooth movement that were 1.5-fold faster (Iwasaki and Nickel, 2018). There is further evidence that the results from subjects in different stages of development should not be pooled: this includes the findings that higher GCF volumes (Ren et al., 2002) and ratios of RANKL/OPG in GCF (Kawasaki et al., 2006; Rody et al., 2014b) while lower levels of PGE$_2$ (Chibebe et al., 2010) were measured in adolescents compared with adults. A possible circadian pattern to the amount of GCF measurable was previously reported (Bissada et al., 1967) but has not been supported by subsequent studies (Suppipat et al., 1977; Deinzer et al., 2000; Gunday et al., 2014). In addition, the possible influence of sex hormones has been suggested (Cimasoni, 1983). Following the secretion of total protein, IL-1β, and IL-1RA in GCF longitudinally, however, has shown that for both females and males (Figure 11.1) there is generally a fluctuation with a variable periodicity.

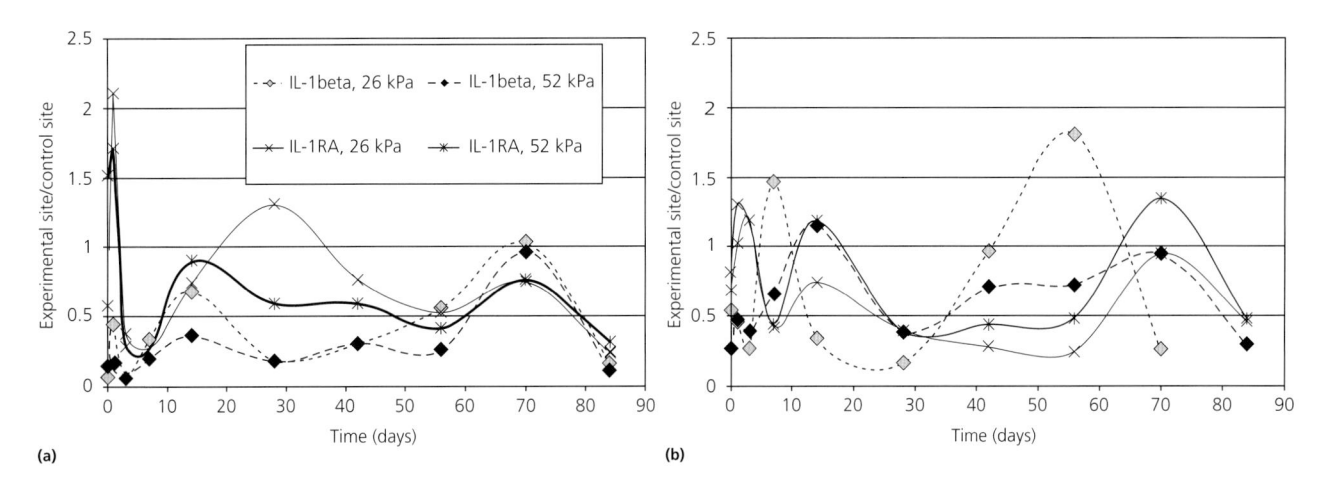

Figure 11.1 Cytokines in GCF from experimental site/control site versus time (days) for (a) a female subject and (b) a male subject for maxillary canines moved by 26 or 52 kPa.

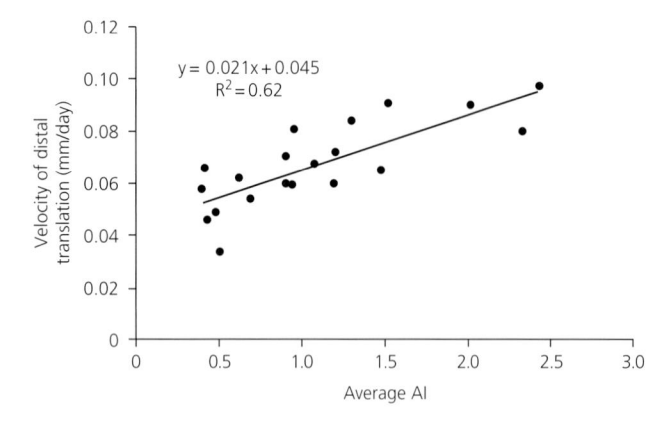

Figure 11.2 Velocity of distal translation (speed of tooth movement in mm/day) versus average activity index (AI) for 20 maxillary canines. (Source: Iwasaki et al., 2006. Reproduced with permission of Elsevier.)

A number of substances are known to function synergistically (e.g., IL-1β and TNF-α), modify (e.g., IL-1β induces or modulates IL-1RA, IL-6, IL-8 and PGE_2), or inhibit one another (e.g., MMPs and TIMPs). Although relative ratios of substances in GCF that could reflect homeostatic balance or the lack thereof have been considered infrequently, higher RANKL/OPG in adolescent than adult subjects was associated with faster tooth movement (Kawasaki et al., 2006) and increased MMP-9/TIMP-1 was found at compression sites after force-application (Grant et al., 2013). Furthermore, a series of studies showed IL-1β/IL-1RA in GCF at experimental versus control sites (activity index, AI) accounted for up to 82% of the variability in the speed of maxillary canine translation (Iwasaki et al., 2001, 2005, 2006, 2009; Iwasaki and Nickel, 2018) (Figure 11.2).

GCF analysis has also tested indirectly the effectiveness of preventive products that could combat the effects of plaque accumulation during orthodontic treatment (Skold-Larsson et al., 2003; Paschos et al., 2008). It has also been used to test if states of root resorption are detectable. GCF from teeth with marked compared with mild root resorption, and mild compared with no root resorption showed higher amounts of extracellular matrix proteins associated with dentin mineralization (Mah and Prasad, 2004; Balducci et al., 2007). Although dentin was not expected to be remodeled like paradental structures, measurable amounts of extracellular matrix proteins were found in GCF from teeth with no clinically detectable root resorption after 12 weeks of orthodontic treatment compared with baseline (Mah and Prasad, 2004; Balducci et al., 2007; Kereshanan et al., 2008). In addition, GCF RANKL/OPG was significantly increased in cases where apical root resorption was >2 mm compared with controls (George and Evans, 2009) and granulocyte-macrophage colony-stimulating factor was significantly decreased in teeth with high compared with low amounts of root resorption induced by tooth tipping (Ahuja et al., 2017). Liquid chromatography–mass spectrometry has been applied to compare protein profiles of GCF from second primary molars with evidence of root resorption and first permanent molars without evidence of root resorption in 11 subjects (Rody et al., 2016). This approach showed thousands of nonredundant proteins are identifiable from both sites and that protein profiles are highly variable between individuals. Nevertheless, pooled results indicated smaller numbers of candidate proteins for future investigation; 37 that were upregulated and 55 that were downregulated, in GCF from teeth with actively resorbing roots compared with teeth with intact roots.

Although the research to date implies that markers are important for assessing the effects of orthodontic therapy, improved diagnostic trials are needed before oral fluid markers can be useful as predictive or analytical clinical tools. The following sections will outline the variables that need to be addressed in future diagnostic trials by presenting an overview of the knowledge gained from and the limitations of the previous research with respect to these variables.

What is needed for improved diagnostic trials of markers in oral fluids during orthodontic treatment?

Diagnostic trials are studies conducted to find better tests or procedures for detecting and identifying particular conditions. To design a good diagnostic trial, therefore, the tests or procedures must comprise variables that are controlled and measured at an appropriate frequency over a sufficient duration. In addition, the particular condition of interest must be clearly defined and also measured. Finally, attention must be paid to recruitment of sufficient numbers of suitably characterized subjects and the application of appropriate statistical methods. The split-mouth design (Hujoel, 1998; Pandis et al., 2013; Zhu et al., 2017) holds promise for diagnostic trials of GCF markers during OTM, especially if standardized guidelines are followed (Lesaffre et al., 2007). Future diagnostic trials of oral fluid markers during OTM should also consider the current Consolidated Standards of Reporting Trials (CONSORT) (Boutron et al., 2017). Because of the current advantages of GCF over saliva for the study of the local effects of orthodontic mechanical stimuli, the following sections will focus on GCF.

Variables associated with the collection and analysis of GCF

GCF collection during orthodontic therapy

Inflammation, as well as chemical or mechanical/traumatic stimulations, will cause increased fluid accumulation in the gingival crevice (Egelberg, 1966a, b; Goodson, 2003). A GCF sample reflects the resting volume and the influx of fluid during the time that it was collected (rate of GCF flow × time of sample collection). Both resting volume and rate of GCF flow are characteristics of a given sampling location and the health of the associated tissues. In healthy populations, GCF resting volume and rate of flow can be stable over time. For example, average measures of resting volume and rate of GCF flow for 102 healthy 18-year-old male subjects were: 0.100 μL and 6.0 μL/h, respectively, for the maxillary left first permanent molar, and 0.050 μL and 3.0 μL/h, respectively, for the mandibular right canine and were similar a year later (Griffiths et al., 1992). The degree of inflammation, however, has a positive effect on resting volume, rate of GCF flow, and time-to-fill a healthy crevice or periodontal pocket (Goodson, 2003). Many studies have demonstrated positive correlations between the amount of GCF collected and clinical indices of inflammation (Cimasoni, 1983; Pender et al., 1994). In addition, other factors such as stage of development and smoking appear to be important. That is, significantly larger volumes of GCF were collected from adolescent subjects compared with adult subjects from sites with and without mechanical orthodontic stimuli (Ren et al., 2002; Kawasaki et al., 2006). In smokers, significantly smaller volumes of GCF have been measured compared with nonsmokers (Hedin et al., 1981).

Studies involving multiple sampling from the same sites have shown that the protein concentration of the initial sample was relatively low and resembled that of interstitial fluid (i.e., transudate-like) (Curtis *et al.*, 1988). The protein concentration in subsequent samples from healthy sites with no sign of inflammation remained about the same, but from inflamed sites the protein concentration was significantly higher and resembled that of serum (i.e., exudate-like).

Constituents of GCF are a reflection of systemic as well as local conditions (Ebersole, 2003). Multiple genes and interactions with other genes and environmental factors over time ultimately affect how the individual responds to pathogens or other stimuli, including response to treatment. Genetic effects have been investigated in individuals with similar states of periodontal disease and health, where differences in IL-1 levels in GCF were related to IL-1 gene cluster polymorphisms in some studies (Engebretson *et al.* 1999; Lopez *et al.* 2005). However, given the heterogeneity of periodontal diseases, the ethnic and regional variations in genotype and allele frequencies, and epigenetic variations (inherited changes in gene function that are influenced by the environment), most studies in this arena have so far been under-powered and tested single rather than multiple genes (Laine *et al.*, 2012). Nevertheless, there is some evidence that when mechanical stimuli, stage of development, and oral health are controlled, IL-1 gene cluster polymorphisms are related to the speed of tooth movement, as well as the amounts of IL-1β and IL-1RA in GCF during tooth movement (Iwasaki *et al.*, 2009) (Figure 11.3). Furthermore, average AIs in GCF during tooth movement and stimulated whole blood showed significant correlations (Iwasaki *et al.*, 2005).

These results demonstrate the importance of the following for studies of GCF during orthodontic therapy:
- Measures to maintain, monitor, and confirm health of paradental tissues.
- Careful selection of site, duration, number, and interval of GCF collections.
- Careful and consistent preparation of collection sites, sample handling, and storage.
- Consideration of health status, stage of development, and genetic background of the subjects.

Methods of collection

There is consensus regarding the preparation of a gingival crevice for collection of fluid. The preparatory steps may or may not begin with a wash of the area with water, followed by isolation of the tooth with cotton rolls, removal of supragingival plaque by gentle wiping, and finally careful drying with a stream of air. The major sources of contamination are saliva, plaque, and blood. Careful isolation has been shown to be sufficient to prevent contamination by saliva and plaque (Griffiths *et al.*, 1997). It is also important to note the timing of GCF collection relative to other clinical procedures. If completed prior to GCF sampling, procedures such as probing can result in blood contamination of the GCF sample (Wassall and Preshaw, 2016).

A variety of methods and products have been reported for GCF collection; for example: microcapillary tubules, custom intraoral appliance with peristaltic pump, absorbent string, strips of polyvinylidene difluoride membrane, gingival washing techniques, and immunomagnetic beads (Oppenheim, 1970; Rossomando *et al.*, 1990; Nakashima *et al.*, 1994; de Aguiar *et al.*, 2017). However, by far the most prevalent collection method for GCF is via paper strips (Figure 11.4). The intracrevicular approach has two commonly used standardized methods: one where the end of the paper

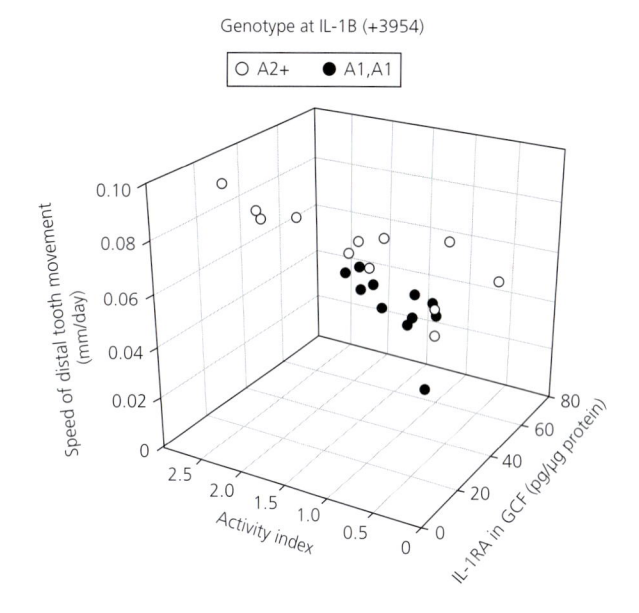

Figure 11.3 Graph showing effects of IL-1B genotype (○ ≥1 copy of allele 2, A2+; ● homozygous for allele 1, A1A1), activity index (AI), and IL1-RA in GCF at experimental sites on speed of distal movement of maxillary canines. (Source: Reprinted from Iwasaki *et al.*, 2009. Reproduced with permission of John Wiley & Sons.)

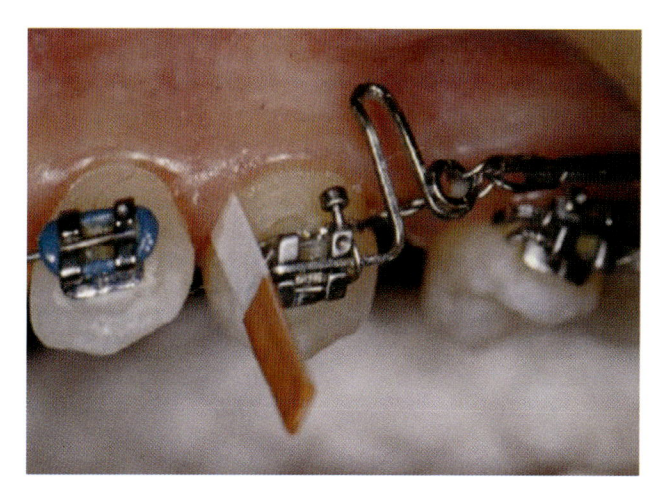

Figure 11.4 Buccal view of isolated site showing GCF collection via paper strip. (Source: Photograph by J. Haack.)

strip is inserted in the crevice until minimum resistance is felt, and the other where the strip is placed at the entrance of the crevice (Loe and Holm-Pedersen, 1965) or at a set distance, e.g., 1 mm, into the crevice (Offenbacher *et al.*, 1981). The former method tends to increase the amount of fluid collected, in theory because the delivery of the paper strip to the bottom of the crevice causes local mechanical irritation or trauma and results in increased local vascular permeability. In conditions of healthy paradental structures, however, with minimal periodontal pocket depths, the two methods probably give similar results (Griffiths, 2003).

The amount of time the paper strip is held in the gingival sulcus is a matter for debate (Wassall and Preshaw, 2016). The most common method is to hold the paper strip in place for a predetermined amount of time, typically 30 seconds, but some researchers opt to hold the paper in place until it is 'visibly wet.' The latter method has the potential to cause complications due to variable levels of inflammation and thus flow of GCF at collection sites. This can result in the paper strip becoming oversaturated quickly or relatively long wait-times for the paper to become visibly wet. For these reasons, a standardized protocol of inserting each paper strip into the gingival sulcus for 30 seconds has been widely adopted.

To calculate the volume of fluid collected on a paper strip, a calibrated scale or machine such as a "Periotron" (Golub and Kleinberg, 1976), which measures and converts the electrical capacitance of the strips, may be used. It is critical that this measurement occurs as quickly as possible after collection and that the paper strips are stored in sealed containers before analysis because evaporation can affect the volumetric quantification. Samples are routinely stored dry or in a buffer solution at a recommended temperature of -80°C in order to avoid proteolysis. Most paper strips have a maximum capacity of 1.2 μL (up to 2 μL strips are available for larger volumes), so if the amount of fluid is an important measure, care must be taken that the duration of collection is not so long as to exceed the maximum capacity of the strip (Goodson, 2003; Wassall and Preshaw, 2016).

Quantification of GCF constituents

Expression of the amount of a given constituent as a concentration relative to the amount of GCF collected has limitations when comparing results from different samples because of the small volumes expected in healthy conditions and the many variables that affect the GCF volume collected. Other approaches are to express the amount of the analyte relative to total protein in the sample, or as a total amount per sample using standardized collection methods, or to compare two or more analytes as a ratio within a sample.

Prior to analytical techniques, sampled GCF must be eluted from the paper strip. Although dependent on the analyte being studied, elution is commonly completed through a combination of low and high shaking, vortexing, or centrifugation at observed temperatures. Preliminary studies to test elution methods for optimum recovery of the analytes of interest are essential because these methods will be analyte- and laboratory-dependent (Wassall and Preshaw, 2016). This is especially critical for GCF analytes that are present in amounts near the minimum detection levels of the assay.

The accuracy in quantifying and the sensitivity of the assay methods have improved since research on the GCF constituents first began. Enzyme-linked immunosorbent assays (ELISAs) are commonly used and highly specific for a particular analyte but have the disadvantages of measuring only one analyte at a time and being relatively costly. Measuring GCF analytes from healthy tissues can be challenging in other ways because when the sample volume is small, the amount of the analyte of interest will also be small and may be below the detection limit of the assay. More recently, multiplexed assays using fluorescent microspheres (Capelli et al., 2011; Grant et al., 2013), microarrays (Rody et al., 2016), and mass spectroscopy (Rody et al., 2012, 2014a) for measurements of multiple biomarkers from the same sample have been applied. Raman spectroscopy has also been applied to analyze the biochemical composition of GCF and how this changes during OTM (Jung et al., 2014; d'Apuzzo et al., 2017). Raman spectroscopy uses radiated energy to determine the vibrational modes of molecules and thus can identify changes in the protein content and conformation in biological samples. Raman microspectroscopy, in particular, shows promise because it requires little to no sample preparation (Jung et al., 2014; d'Apuzzo et al., 2017). Further developments in these and other technologies are likely to address some of the past problems and limitations associated with assaying techniques.

How the analytes measurable in GCF are organized or "packaged" may also be an important factor to consider in the future. Recent research on the regulation of intercellular functions shows that extracellular vesicles, including exosomes and microvesicles with important analytes within or attached, play key roles in tissue responses to stimuli, and therefore could be important GCF biomarkers linked to OTM or root resorption (Holliday et al., 2019).

Outcomes associated with orthodontic treatment

A major challenge in the design of good diagnostic studies is that the dependent variable for orthodontic treatment outcome must be defined and quantified, and the variables affecting it must be controlled. This has not been addressed suitably in most previous studies, where in many cases the mechanical stimulus has been simply "orthodontic treatment" and where the tooth movement (or other effect) has not even been measured.

Possible candidates for dependent variables of interest for orthodontic treatment are the type and nature of tooth movement, the speed of tooth movement, the retention of tooth positions, the amount of root resorption, and the pain experience and the developmental stage of the patient. Standard protocols to control and quantify these dependent variables have not been definitively established to date. There is growing evidence that environmental and genetic factors affect a tooth's response to a known mechanical stimulus, which implies that pooling data from different individuals without attention to these environmental and genetic factors is unlikely to yield informative results.

The future

"Markers" that are physical or biological characteristics of specific underlying conditions in living humans can be valuable if they can be used to identify susceptibility to disease, risk of treatment, stage of a disease state, or progress of physiological responses. Blood pressure, sugar, and cholesterol levels are examples of well-known physical and biological markers. The new improved technologies and the findings that result from current research efforts on "salivaomics" (Wong, 2012) could help to overcome some of the problems associated with oral fluid analysis as a diagnostic test for tooth movement and stabilization, root resorption, and other outcomes of orthodontic treatment. Once research has established what to measure and what measures are meaningful, this knowledge needs to be translated to the point of care, where orthodontists can assess important markers in-office on a patient-by-patient basis. Most key molecules have a promoting and repressing function, which implies that a single analyte measurement, without study of its effects on other analytes, will not be meaningful in most cases. In addition, multiple samples from each patient will likely need to be collected longitudinally. New technologies and findings will hopefully provide easy, non-painful, and inexpensive sampling methods along with accurate, portable, and easy-to-use evaluative equipment.

Conclusions

Unlike complex chronic disease conditions, OTM has stimuli that can be quantified and controlled to study the cascade of associated events and the outcomes. The stimuli and outcomes simply need to be measured. If this can be done, not only might the analyses of oral fluids during tooth movement in the future be useful to assess and predict individual responses in terms of orthodontic results, but these analyses also might provide adjunctive information about other individual-specific paradental tissue characteristics and potential for systemic disease or anomalous developmental conditions.

References

Ahuja, R., Almuzian, M., Khan, A. et al. (2017) A preliminary investigation of short-term cytokine expression in gingival crevicular fluid secondary to high-level orthodontic forces and the associated root resorption: case series analytical study. *Progress in Orthodontics* **18**, 23.

Al-Qawasmi, R. A., Hartsfield, J. K., Jr., Everett, E. T. et al. (2003) Genetic predisposition to external apical root resorption. *American Journal of Orthodontics and Dentofacial Orthopedics* **123**, 242–252.

Al Kawas, S., Rahim, Z. H. and Ferguson, D. B. (2012) Potential uses of human salivary protein and peptide analysis in the diagnosis of disease. *Archives of Oral Biology* **57**, 1–9.

Alhadlaq, A. M. 2015. Biomarkers of orthodontic tooth movement in gingival crevicular fluid: a systematic review. *Journal of Contemporary Dental Practice* **16**, 578–587.

Alikhani, M., Raptis, M., Zoldan, B. et al. (2013) Effect of micro-osteoperforations on the rate of tooth movement. *American Journal of Orthodontics and Dentofacial Orthopedics* **144**, 639–648.

Balducci, L., Ramachandran, A., Hao, J. et al. (2007) Biological markers for evaluation of root resorption. *Archives of Oral Biology* **52**, 203–208.

Bissada, N. F., Schaffer, E. M. and Haus, E. (1967) Circadian periodicity of human crevicular fluid flow. *Journal of Periodontology* **38**, 36–40.

Black, G. V. (1899) The fibers and glands of the peridental membrane. *Dental Cosmos* **41**.

Boutron, I., Altman, D. G., Moher, D. et al. (2017) CONSORT statement for randomized trials of nonpharmacologic treatments: A 2017 update and a CONSORT Extension for Nonpharmacologic Trial Abstracts. *Annals of Internal Medicine* **167**, 40–47.

Bruinsma, F. J., Joo, J. E., Wong, E. M. et al. (2018) The utility of DNA extracted from saliva for genome-wide molecular research platforms. *BMC Research Notes* **11**, 8.

Burke, J. C., Evans, C. A., Crosby, T. R. and Mednieks, M. I. (2002). Expression of secretory proteins in oral fluid after orthodontic tooth movement. *American Journal of Orthodontics and Dentofacial Orthopedics* **121**, 310–315.

Capelli, J., Jr., Kantarci, A., Haffajee, A. et al. (2011) Matrix metalloproteinases and chemokines in the gingival crevicular fluid during orthodontic tooth movement. *European Journal of Orthodontics* **33**, 705–711.

Chang, H. S., Walsh, L. J. and Freer, T. J. (1999) The effect of orthodontic treatment on salivary flow, pH, buffer capacity, and levels of mutans streptococci and lactobacilli. *Australian Orthodontic Journal* **15**, 229–234.

Chibebe, P. C., Starobinas, N. and Pallos, D. (2010) Juveniles versus adults: differences in PGE2 levels in the gingival crevicular fluid during orthodontic tooth movement. *Brazilian Oral Research* **24**, 108–113.

Cimasoni, G. (1983) Crevicular fluid updated. *Monographs in Oral Science* **12**, III–VII, 1–152.

Corega, C., Vaida, L., Festila, D.G. et al. (2014) Salivary levels of IGA in healthy subjects undergoing active orthodontic treatment. *Minerva Stomatologica,* January 2014.

Curtis, M. A., Griffiths, G. S., Price, S. J. et al. (1988) The total protein concentration of gingival crevicular fluid. Variation with sampling time and gingival inflammation. *Journal of Clinical Periodontology* **15**, 628–632.

D'Apuzzo, F., Cappabianca, S., Ciavarella, D. et al. (2013) Biomarkers of periodontal tissue remodeling during orthodontic tooth movement in mice and men: overview and clinical relevance. *Scientific World Journal*, 2013, 105873.

D'Apuzzo, F., Perillo, L., Delfino, I. et al. (2017) Monitoring early phases of orthodontic treatment by means of Raman spectroscopies. *Journal of Biomedical Optics* **22**, 1–10.

Dawes, C. and Wong, D. T. W. (2019) Role of saliva and salivary diagnostics in the advancement of oral health. *Journal of Dental Research* **98**, 133–141.

De Aguiar, M. C., Perinetti, G. and Capelli, J., Jr. (2017) The gingival crevicular fluid as a source of biomarkers to enhance efficiency of orthodontic and functional treatment of growing patients. *Biomedical Research International* 2017, 3257235.

De Jong, E. P., Van Riper, S. K., Koopmeiners, J. S. et al. (2011) Sample collection and handling considerations for peptidomic studies in whole saliva; implications for biomarker discovery. *Clinica Chimica Acta* **412**, 2284–2288.

Deinzer, R., Mossanen, B. S. and Herforth, A. (2000) Methodological considerations in the assessment of gingival crevicular fluid volume. *Journal of Clinical Periodontology* **27**, 481–488.

Ebersole, J. L. (2003) Humoral immune responses in gingival crevice fluid: local and systemic implications. *Periodontology 2000* **31**, 135–166.

Egelberg, J. (1966a) Permeability of the dento-gingival blood vessels. 1. Application of the vascular labelling method and gingival fluid measurements. *Journal of Periodontal Research* **1**, 180–191.

Egelberg, J. (1966b) Permeability of the dento-gingival blood vessels. II. Clinically healthy gingivae. *Journal of Periodontal Research* **1**, 276–286.

Ellias, M. F., Ariffin, S. H. Z., Karsani, S.A. et al. (2012) Proteomic analysis of saliva identifies potential biomarkers for orthodontic tooth movement. *Scientific World Journal* 2012, 647240.

Engebretson, S. P., Lamster, I. B., Herrera-Abreu, M. et al. (1999) The influence of interleukin gene polymorphism on expression of interleukin-1beta and tumor necrosis factor-alpha in periodontal tissue and gingival crevicular fluid. *Journal of Periodontology* **70**, 567–573.

Florez-Moreno, G. A., Isaza-Guzman, D. M., Isaza-Guzman, D. M. (2013a) Time-rlated changes in salivary levels of the osterotropic factors sRANKL and OPG through orthodontic tooth movement. *American Journal of Orthodontics and Dentofacial Orthopedics* **143**, 92–100.

Florez-Moreno, G. A., Marin-Restrepo, L. M., Isaza-Guzman, D. M., Isaza-Guzman, D. M. (2013b) Screening for salivary levels of deoxypyridinoline and bone-specific alkaline phosphatase during orthodontic tooth movement: a pilot study. *European Journal of Orthodontics* **35**, 361–368.

Genco, R. J. (2012) Salivary diagnostic tests. *Journal of the American Dental Association* **143**, 3S–5S.

George, A. and Evans, C. A. (2009) Detection of root resorption using dentin and bone markers. *Orthodontic and Craniofacial Research* **12**, 229–235.

Giannobile, W. V. (2012) Salivary diagnostics for periodontal diseases. *Journal of the American Dental Association* **143**, 6S–11S.

Giannopoulou, C., Dudic, A. and Kiliaridis, S. (2006) Pain discomfort and crevicular fluid changes induced by orthodontic elastic separators in children. *Journal of Pain* **7**, 367–376.

Golub, L. M. and Kleinberg, I. (1976) Gingival crevicular fluid: a new diagnostic aid in managing the periodontal patient. *Oral Science Review* 49–61.

Goodson, J. M. (2003) Gingival crevice fluid flow. *Periodontology 2000* **31**, 43–54.

Grant, M., Wilson, J., Rock, P. and Chapple, I. (2013) Induction of cytokines, MMP9, TIMPs, RANKL and OPG during orthodontic tooth movement. *European Journal of Orthodontics* **35**, 644–651.

Griffiths, G. S. (2003) Formation, collection and significance of gingival crevice fluid. *Periodontology 2000* **31**, 32–42.

Griffiths, G. S., Moulson, A. M., Petrie, A. and James, I. T. (1998) Evaluation of osteocalcin and pyridinium crosslinks of bone collagen as markers of bone turnover in gingival crevicular fluid during different stages of orthodontic treatment. *Journal of Clinical Periodontology* **25**, 492–498.

Griffiths, G. S., Sterne, J. A., Wilton, J. M. et al. (1992) Associations between volume and flow rate of gingival crevicular fluid and clinical assessments of gingival inflammation in a population of British male adolescents. *Journal of Clinical Periodontology* **19**, 464–470.

Griffiths, G. S., Wilton, J. M. and Curtis, M. A. (1997) Permeability of the gingival tissues to IgM during an experimental gingivitis study in man. *Archives of Oral Biology* **42**, 129–136.

Grippaudo, C., Cafiero, C., D'apolito, I. et al. (2018) Primary failure of eruption: Clinical and genetic findings in the mixed dentition. *The Angle Orthodontist* **88**, 275–282.

Gunday, S., Topcu, A. O., Ercan, E. and Yamalik, N. (2014) Analysis of daytime variations in gingival crevicular fluid: a circadian periodicity? *Journal of Periodontology* **85**, e47–56.

Hedin, C. A., Ronquist, G. and Forsberg, O. (1981) Cyclic nucleotide content in gingival tissue of smokers and non-smokers. *Journal of Periodontal Research* **16**, 337–343.

Holliday, L. S., Truzman, E., Zuo, J. et al. (2019) Extracellular vesicle identification in tooth movement models. *Orthodontic and Craniofacial Research* **22**(Suppl. 1), 101–106.

Hoshino-Itoh, J., Kurokawa, A., Yamaguchi, M. and Kasai, K. (2005) Levels of t-PA and PAI-2 in gingival crevicular fluid during orthodontic tooth movement in adults. *Australian Orthodontic Journal* **21**, 31–37.

Hujoel, P. P. (1998) Design and analysis issues in split mouth clinical trials. *Community Dentistry and Oral Epidemiology* **26**, 85–86.

Insoft, M., King, G. J. and Keeling, S. D. (1996) The measurement of acid and alkaline phosphatase in gingival crevicular fluid during orthodontic tooth movement. *American Journal of Orthodontics and Dentofacial Orthopedics* **109**, 287–296.

Iwasaki, L. R., Chandler, J. R., Marx, D. B. et al. (2009) IL-1 gene polymorphisms, secretion in gingival crevicular fluid, and speed of human orthodontic tooth movement. *Orthodontic and Craniofacial Research* **12**, 129–140.

Iwasaki, L. R., Crouch, L. D., Tutor, A. et al. (2005) Tooth movement and cytokines in gingival crevicular fluid and whole blood in growing and adult subjects. *American Journal of Orthodontics and Dentofacial Orthopedics* **128**, 483–491.

Iwasaki, L. R., Gibson, C. S., Crouch, L. D. et al. (2006) Speed of tooth movement is related to stress and IL-1 gene polymorphisms. *American Journal of Orthodontics and Dentofacial Orthopedics* **130**, 698 e1–9.

Iwasaki, L. R., Haack, J. E., Nickel, J. C. et al. (2001) Human interleukin-1 beta and interleukin-1 receptor antagonist secretion and velocity of tooth movement. *Archives of Oral Biology* **46**, 185–189.

Iwasaki, L. R., Liu, Y., Liu, H. and Nickel, J. C. (2017) Speed of human tooth movement in growers and non-growers: Selection of applied stress matters. *Orthodontic and Craniofacial Research* **20** Suppl 1, 63–67.

Iwasaki, L. R. and Nickel, J. C. (2018) Mechanics and gingival crevicular fluid biomarkers associated with speed of human tooth movement, in *Effective, Efficient and Personalized Orthodontics: Patient-centered Approaches and Innovations* (eds H. Kim-Berman, L. Franchi and A. Ruellas). The University of Michigan, Ann Arbor.

Jayachandran, T., Srinivasan, B. and Padmanabhan, S. (2017) Salivary leptin levels in normal weight and overweight individuals and their correlation with orthodontic tooth movement. *The Angle Orthodontist* **87**, 739–744.

Jung, G. B., Kim, K. A., Han, I. et al. (2014) Biochemical characterization of human gingival crevicular fluid during orthodontic tooth movement using Raman spectroscopy. *Biomedical Optics Express* **5**, 3508–3520.

Justino, A. B., Teixeira, R. R., Peixoto, L. G. et al. (2017) Effect of saliva collection methods and oral hygiene on salivary biomarkers. *Scandinavian Journal of Clinical and Laboratory Investigation* **77**, 415–422.

Kaczor-Urbanowicz, K. E., Deutsch, O., Zaks, B. et al. (2017) Identification of salivary protein biomarkers for orthodontically induced inflammatory root resorption. *Proteomics – Clinical Applications* **11**.

Kapoor, P., Kharbanda, O. P., Monga, N. et al. (2014) Effect of orthodontic forces on cytokine and receptor levels in gingival crevicular fluid: a systematic review. *Progress in Orthodontics* **15**, 65.

Kapoor, P., Monga, N., Kharbanda, O. P. et al. (2019) Effect of orthodontic forces on levels of enzymes in gingival crevicular fluid (GCF): A systematic review. *Dental Press Journal of Orthodontics* **24**, 40 e1–40 e22.

Karacay, S., Saygun, I., Bengi, A. O. and Serdar, M. (2007) Tumor necrosis factor-alpha levels during two different canine distalization techniques. *The Angle Orthodontist* **77**, 142–147.

Kavadia-Tsatala, S., Kaklamanos, E. G. and Tsalikis, L. (2002) Effects of orthodontic treatment on gingival crevicular fluid flow rate and composition: clinical implications and applications. *International Journal of Adult Orthodontic and Orthognathic Surgery* **17**, 191–205.

Kawasaki, K., Takahashi, T., Yamaguchi, M. and Kasai, K. (2006) Effects of aging on RANKL and OPG levels in gingival crevicular fluid during orthodontic tooth movement. *Orthodontic and Craniofacial Research* **9**, 137–142.

Kereshanan, S., Stephenson, P. and Waddington, R. (2008) Identification of dentine sialoprotein in gingival crevicular fluid during physiological root resorption and orthodontic tooth movement. *European Journal of Orthodontics* **30**, 307–214.

Kumar, A. A., Saravanan, K., Kohila, K. and Kumar, S. S. (2015) Biomarkers in orthodontic tooth movement. *Journal of Pharmacology and Bioallied Sciences* **7**, S325–330.

Laine, M. L., Crielaard, W. and Loos, B. G. (2012) Genetic susceptibility to periodontitis. *Periodontology 2000* **58**, 37–68.

Lamy, E. and Mau, M. (2012) Saliva proteomics as an emerging, non-invasive tool to study livestock physiology, nutrition and diseases. *Journal of Proteomics* **75**, 4251–4258.

Lee, K. J., Park, Y. C., Yu, H. S. et al. (2004) Effects of continuous and interrupted orthodontic force on interleukin-1beta and prostaglandin E2 production in gingival crevicular fluid. *American Journal of Orthodontics and Dentofacial Orthopedics* **125**, 168–177.

Lesaffre, E., Garcia Zattera, M. J., Redmond, C. et al. (2007) Reported methodological quality of split-mouth studies. *Journal of Clinical Periodontology* **34**, 756–761.

Li, Y., Hu, B., Liu, Y. et al. (2009) The effects of fixed orthodontic appliances on saliva flow rate and saliva electrolyte concentrations. *Journal of Oral Rehabilitation* **36**, 781–785.

Loe, H. and Holm-Pedersen, P. (1965) Absence and presence of fluid from normal and inflamed gingivae. *Periodontics* **3**, 171–177.

Lopez, N. J., Jara, L. and Valenzuela, C. Y. (2005) Association of interleukin-1 polymorphisms with periodontal disease. *Journal of Periodontology* **76**, 234–243.

Mah, J. and Prasad, N. (2004) Dentine phosphoproteins in gingival crevicular fluid during root resorption. *European Journal of Orthodontics* **26**, 25–30.

Marcaccini, A. M., Amato, P. A., Leao, F. V. et al. (2010) Myeloperoxidase activity is increased in gingival crevicular fluid and whole saliva after fixed orthodontic appliance activation. *American Journal of Orthodontics and Dentofacial Orthopedics* **138**, 613–636.

Nakashima, K., Demeurisse, C. and Cimasoni, G. (1994) The recovery efficiency of various materials for sampling enzymes and polymorphonuclear leukocytes from gingival crevices. *Journal of Clinical Periodontology* **21**, 479–483.

Navarro-Palacios, A., Garcia-Lopez, E., Meza-Rios, A. et al. (2014) Myeloperoxidase enzymatic activity is increased in patients with different levels of dental crowding after initial orthodontic activation. *American Journal of Orthodontics and Dentofacial Orthopedics* **146**, 92–97.

Nunes, A. P., Oliveira, I. O., Santos, B. R. et al. (2012) Quality of DNA extracted from saliva samples collected with the Oragene DNA self-collection kit. *BMC Medical Research Methodology* **12**, 65.

Offenbacher, S., Farr, D. H. and Goodson, J. M. (1981) Measurement of prostaglandin E in crevicular fluid. *Journal of Clinical Periodontology* **8**, 359–367.

Oppenheim, F. G. (1970) Preliminary observations on the presence and origin of serum albumin in human saliva. *Helvetica Odontologica Acta* **14**, 10–17.

Pachos, E., Limbach, m., Teichmann, M. et al. (2008) Orthdontic attachments and chlorhexidine-containing varnish effects on gingival health. *The The Angle Orthodontist* **78**, 98–916.

Pandis, N., Walsh, T., Polychronopoulou, A. et al. (2013) Split-mouth designs in orthodontics: an overview with applications to orthodontic clinical trials. *European Journal of Orthodontics* **35**(6), 783–789.

Pender, N., Samuels, R. H. and Last, K. S. (1994) The monitoring of orthodontic tooth movement over a 2-year period by analysis of gingival crevicular fluid. *European Journal of Orthodontics* **16**, 511–520.

Perinetti, G., Primozic, J., Castaldo, A. et al. (2013) Is gingival crevicular fluid volume sensitive to orthodontic tooth movement? A systematic review of split-mouth longitudinal studies. *Orthodontic and Craniofacial Research* **16**, 1–19.

Peros, K., Mestrovic, S., Anic-Milosevic, S. and Slaj, M. (2011) Salivary microbial and nonmicrobial parameters in children with fixed orthodontic appliances. *The Angle Orthodontist* **81**, 901–906.

PubMed (2019) [online] available at: https://www.ncbi.nlm.nih.gov/pubmed/?term=GCF+AND+orthodontic [Accessed July 23, 2019].

Pulford, D. J., Mosteller, M., Briley, J. D. et al. (2013) Saliva sampling in global clinical studies: the impact of low sampling volume on performance of DNA in downstream genotyping experiments. *BMC Medical Genomics* **6**, 20.

Quintana, M., Palicki, O., Lucchi, G. et al. (2009) Inter-individual variability of protein patterns in saliva of healthy adults. *Journal of Proteomics* **72**, 822–830.

Ren, Y., Maltha, J. C., Van't Hof, M. A. et al. (2002) Cytokine levels in crevicular fluid are less responsive to orthodontic force in adults than in juveniles. *Journal of Clinical Periodontology* **29**, 757–762.

Ren, Y. and Vissink, A. (2008) Cytokines in crevicular fluid and orthodontic tooth movement. *European Journal of Oral Sciences* **116**, 89–97.

Rody, W. J., Jr., Akhlaghi, H., Akyalcin, S. et al. (2011) Impact of orthodontic retainers on periodontal health status assessed by biomarkers in gingival crevicular fluid. *The Angle Orthodontist* **81**, 1083–1089.

Rody, W. J., Jr., Holliday, L. S., Mchugh, K. P. et al. (2014a) Mass spectrometry analysis of gingival crevicular fluid in the presence of external root resorption. *American Journal of Orthodontics and Dentofacial Orthopedics* **145**, 787–798.

Rody, W. J., Jr., Iwasaki, L. R. and Krokhin, O. (2012) Oral fluid-based diagnostics and applications in orthodontics, in *Taking Advantage of Emerging Technologies in Clinical Practice* (ed. J. A. McNamara Jr.). The University of Michigan, Ann Arbor.

Rody, W. J., Jr., Wijegunasinghe, M., Holliday, L. S. et al. (2016) Immunoassay analysis of proteins in gingival crevicular fluid samples from resorbing teeth. *The Angle Orthodontist* **86**, 187–192.

Rody, W. J., Jr., Wijegunasinghe, M., Wiltshire, W. A. and Dufault, B. (2014b) Differences in the gingival crevicular fluid composition between adults and adolescents undergoing orthodontic treatment. *The Angle Orthodontist* **84**, 120–126.

Rossomando, E. F., Kennedy, J. E. and Hadjimichael, J. (1990) Tumour necrosis factor alpha in gingival crevicular fluid as a possible indicator of periodontal disease in humans. *Archives of Oral Biology* **35**, 431–434.

Schipper, R. G., Silletti, E. and Vingerhoeds, M. H. (2007) Saliva as research material: biochemical, physicochemical and practical aspects. *Archives of Oral Biology* **52**, 1114–1135.

Sharab, L. Y., Morford, L. A., Dempsey, J. et al. (2015) Genetic and treatment-related risk factors associated with external apical root resorption (EARR) concurrent with orthodontia. *Orthodontic and Craniofacial Research* **18**(Suppl. 1), 71–82.

Skold-Larsson, K., Yucel-Linberg, T., Twetman, S. and Modeer, T. (2003) Effect of a triclosan-containing dental gel on the levels of prostaglandin I2 and interleukin-1beta in gingival crevicular fluid from adolescents with fixed orthodontic appliances. *Acta Ondontologica Scandinavica* **61**, 193–196.

Suppipat, N., Johansen, J. R. and Gjermo, P. (1977) Influence of "time of day", pocket depth and scaling on gingival fluid flow. *Journal of Clinical Periodontology* **4**, 48–55.

Tapia, C. V., Batarce, C., Amaro, J. et al. (2019) Microbiological characterisation of the colonisation by Candida sp in patients with orthodontic fixed appliances and evaluation of host responses in saliva. *Mycoses* **62**, 247–251.

Tersin, J. (1978) Studies of gingival conditions in relation to orthodontic treatment. IV. The effect of oral hygiene measures on gingival exudation during the course of orthodontic treatment. *Swedish Dental Journal* **2**, 131–136.

Thomas, M. V., Branscum, A., Miller, C. S. et al. (2009) Within-subject variability in repeated measures of salivary analytes in healthy adults. *Journal of Periodontology* **80**, 1146–1153.

Uematsu, S., Mogi, M. and Deguchi, T. (1996a) Increase of transforming growth factor-beta 1 in gingival crevicular fluid during human orthodontic tooth movement. *Archives of Oral Biology* **41**, 1091–1095.

Uematsu, S., Mogi, M. and Deguchi, T. (1996b) Interleukin (IL)-1 beta, IL-6, tumor necrosis factor-alpha, epidermal growth factor, and beta 2-microglobulin levels are elevated in gingival crevicular fluid during human orthodontic tooth movement. *Journal of Dental Research* **75**, 562–567.

Vansant, L., Cadenas De Llano-Perula, M., Verdonck, A. and Willems, G. (2018) Expression of biological mediators during orthodontic tooth movement: A systematic review. *Archives of Oral Biology* **95**, 170–186.

Vitorino, R., Guedes, S., Manadas, B. et al. (2012) Toward a standardized saliva proteome analysis methodology. *Journal of Proteomics* **75**, 5140–5165.

Waddington, R. J. and Embery, G. (2001) Proteoglycans and orthodontic tooth movement. *Journal of Orthodontics* **28**, 281–290.

Wassall, R. R. and Preshaw, P. M. (2016) Clinical and technical considerations in the analysis of gingival crevicular fluid. *Periodontology 2000* **70**, 65–79.

Wong, D. T. (2012) Salivaomics. *Journal of the American Dental Association* **143**, 19S–24S.

Wu, J. Q., Jiang, J. H., Xu, L. et al. (2018) magnetic bead-based salivary peptidome profiling for accelerated osteogenic orthodontic treatments. *Chinese Journal of Dental Research* **21**, 41–49.

Yamaguchi, M. and Kasai, K. (2005) Inflammation in periodontal tissues in response to mechanical forces. *Archivum Immunologiae et Therapiae Experimentalis (Warsz)* **53**, 388–398.

Zhang, J., Zhou, S., Li, R. et al. (2012) Magnetic bead-based salivary peptidome profiling for periodontal-orthodontic treatment. *Proteome Science* **10**, 63.

Zhu, H., Zhang, S. and Ahn, C. (2017) Sample size considerations for split-mouth design. *Statistical Methods in Medical Research* **26**, 2543–2551.

PART 4

Personalized Diagnosis and Treatment

CHAPTER 12
Genetic Influences on Orthodontic Tooth Movement

Margarita Zeichner-David

> **Summary**
>
> The application of orthodontic forces to move teeth generates numerous reactions from the tooth itself as well as from the surrounding tissues, including changes in the expression of hundreds of genes in cells contained in the periodontal tissues. Orthodontic tooth movement is achieved by a delicate balance between alveolar bone resorption and deposition of new bone mediated by physical, cellular, biochemical, and molecular events taking place in the periodontal tissues surrounding the roots. The expression of genes such as neurotransmitters, signaling molecules, extracellular matrix components, cytokines, chemokines, growth factors, transcription factors, proteases, mineralization-associated proteins, and many other molecules which control periodontal ligament and bone remodeling to achieve tooth movement have been reported. Understanding these changes, as well as the sequence of events responsible for the expression of these genes during orthodontic tooth movement, is crucial to fully comprehend this process, to develop new therapeutics, to optimize the treatment outcomes, and to prevent undesirable side-effects. In this chapter, we will focus on the changes in gene expression currently known to have an influence on orthodontic tooth movement. It is our goal that by the end of this chapter, the reader will have a better appreciation of the molecular events associated with the application of forces to move teeth and of how important these genetic influences are on a successful outcome of orthodontic tooth movement.

Introduction

There is one major principle behind every single biological process: every action has a reaction. This is the basic principle behind the ability to induce orthodontic tooth movement (OTM) as well. The application of orthodontic forces to teeth generates numerous reactions from the tooth itself and the surrounding tissues, including changes in the expression of hundreds of genes in cells contained in the periodontal tissues resulting in the remodeling of the periodontium. Although all cells in the body contain the same genes, it is the timely, sequential, and specific expression of these genes that determines the identity, shape, and function of a cell. Understanding the changes in gene expression, as well as the sequence of events responsible for the expression of these genes during OTM, is crucial to comprehend this process fully, to develop new therapeutics, to optimize the treatment outcomes, and to prevent undesirable side-effects.

This chapter will focus on the changes in gene expression currently known to have an influence on OTM. As the reader will realize, this is an overly complex event involving the expression of numerous genes in different tissues, and with a great deal of redundancy. To facilitate the comprehension of these events, this chapter is organized by the tissue involved. It is, however, particularly important to keep in mind that these events sometimes take place sequentially and sometimes they take place simultaneously in all the tissues. Furthermore, what happens in one tissue not only influences the surrounding tissues but also can have a systemic effect in the whole body. For example, animal studies have shown that diabetes prolongs the degradation of periodontal ligament (PDL) and alveolar bone and the recovery from the damage caused by orthodontic movement will be slower (Li et al., 2010) or the application of orthodontic forces in teeth can cause release of the hormone relaxin from ovaries (Yang et al., 2011).

One could ask why a practicing orthodontist needs to know about the changes in gene expression and molecular events that take place while applying orthodontic forces to move teeth in patients. As the reader will see in the pages that follow, there are molecules whose expression (presence) or inhibition (absence) can increase, decrease, or inhibit the speed at which a tooth can be moved. There are reactions from the tooth itself and surrounding tissues that will determine if and how long the treated teeth will survive. There are genetic disorders, traits, and polymorphisms (slight differences in DNA sequence amongst the same gene in different individuals; groups or populations) that will determine which patients will be easier to treat, which patients will require more work, and which patients should probably not be treated at all. The numerous studies emerging, which correlate application of orthodontic forces with mechanosensing and biochemical/molecular cell responses, and our ability to follow this process by using gingival crevicular fluid (GCF) or salivary biomarkers is changing the face of orthodontics. The future of therapeutic interventions in orthodontics will be based on the application of personalized biomedicine based on principles of evidence-based dentistry (King, 2009; Jheon et al., 2017).

As acknowledged by Meikle (2006), "After 100 years of research in OTM, there is a good understanding of the sequence of events at both tissue and cellular levels and now it is time to focus the research at the molecular level." Molecular biology has made it possible to understand the interactions and reactions between the various cells that constitute the different tissues of any system. Therefore, to fully understand the genetic influences on tooth movement associated with orthodontic forces, we need to understand the molecular mechanisms behind the process of bone remodeling (reviewed in Proff and Romer, 2009). We need to understand the molecular interactions between the periodontal tissues: bone (osteoblasts, osteocytes, osteoclasts, and their precursors), PDL (fibroblasts and stem cells), cementum (cementoblasts and cementoclasts), pulp (fibroblasts, stem cells, odontoblasts, odontoclasts), gingiva (epithelial and mesenchymal cells), blood vessels (hematopoietic and endothelial cells), and the neural fibers (dendritic and neural cells) and their interactions with the surrounding extracellular matrix (ECM). The ECM is a multicomponent tissue that enables internal and external mechanical strains to effect changes in organ structure and function, through mechanotransduction (Krishnan and Davidovitch, 2009).

This chapter will review some of the major changes in gene expression that are associated with the application of orthodontic forces to induce tooth movement. In no way does the author claim that this chapter is an exhaustive compilation of all genes affected by these processes. Furthermore, there are numerous new studies being carried out and new methodologies being applied to this field so that a considerable volume of new information is likely to be published at the same time as this book. For example, new data has emerged from using saliva (Ellias et al., 2012; Zhang et al., 2012a; Allen et al., 2019) and GCF (Atsawasuwan et al., 2018; Wu et al., 2020) to detect biomarkers for tooth movement. The molecular mapping of the process of tooth movement has also resulted in new therapeutic conditions that can accelerate tooth movement like the regulation of RANKL (Iglesias-Linares et al., 2011; Küchler et al., 2019) There are numerous excellent articles and reviews that describe in detail the mechanistic, physical, biological, cellular, and molecular events associated with the application of orthodontic forces to achieve tooth movement. The following articles were used profusely to guide this chapter and are highly recommended to readers that desire more in depth detail about specific topics: Davidovitch et al. (1988); Davidovitch (1991); Zernik and Minken (1992); Isaacson et al. (1993); Redlich et al. (1999); Kerrigan et al. (2000); Hall et al. (2001); Karanth and Shetty (2001); Melsen (2001); Shimono et al. (2003); Ren et al. (2004); Mussig et al. (2005); Yamaguchi and Kasai (2005); Krishnan and Davidovitch (2006a, 2006b); Masella and Meister (2006); Meikle (2006, 2007); Krishnan (2007); Pizzo et al. (2007); Henneman et al. (2008); Krishnan and Davidovitch (2009); Von Böhl and Kuijpers-Jagtman (2009); Zainal Ariffin et al. (2011); Gritsch et al. (2012); d'Apuzzo et al. (2013); Patil et al. (2013); Vansant et al. (2018); Theodorou et al. (2019).

Tissue reactions to application of mechanical forces

Reaction of the periodontal ligament

Histological and immunohistochemical studies have clearly demonstrated that orthodontic forces stimulate remodeling of the PDL. Widening of the PDL in tension sites and an increase in the number of connective tissue cells has been established. The reactions to the applied mechanical loads involve interactions between extracellular and intracellular structural elements: the ECM surrounding the cells and the cell cytoskeleton through cell surface proteins. After a few hours of application of the orthodontic force, osteoclasts appear in the PDL along the alveolar bone surface (King et al., 1997; Rody et al., 2001), suggesting that the PDL might be both the means of force transfer and the way by which alveolar bone remodels in response to applied forces (Beertsen et al., 1997).

In order to achieve remodeling, the collagen fibers and other macromolecules need to be removed, and this removal is achieved by the action of several enzymes that have been identified in the remodeling ECM, for example serine proteases, aspartate proteases, and cysteine proteases, matrix metalloproteinases (MMPs), such as collagenases, gelatinases, stromelysin, and membrane-type MMPs, along with their inhibitor, TIMP (tissue inhibitor of MMPs), indicating that these enzymes play a major role in ECM remodeling (Bolcato-Bellemin et al., 2000; Kerrigan et al., 2000; Waddington and Embery, 2001; Apajalahti et al., 2003; Holliday et al., 2003; Takahashi et al., 2003). Specifically, it has been shown that expression of MMP-8 and MMP-13 mRNA transiently increased in both the compression and tension sides during active tooth movement *in vivo* (Takahashi et al., 2003, 2006). MMP-8 has also been associated with the physiological PDL remodeling that takes place during tooth eruption. However, MMP-13 appears to be associated with a small population of osteoblasts and osteocytes in alveolar bone, suggesting a more defined role in bone remodeling (Tsubota et al., 2002; Reyna et al., 2006). The expression of MMP-2, MMP-9, and TIMPs 1–3 is increased transiently during OTM at both the tension and compression sides. It appears, however, that the expression of these genes is regulated differentially in the periodontal tissue of the tension side and compression side. This altered pattern of gene expression has been associated with determination of the rate and extent of remodeling of the collagenous ECM in periodontal tissues during OTM (Takahashi et al., 2006). Although changes in gene expression for these molecules are strongly suggestive of a role in OTM, the actual proof of their function comes from studies where the particular molecule is rendered nonfunctional.

In order to complete the remodeling, molecules that have been degraded need to be replenished. It has been shown that responses to mechanical forces include stimulation of cell division and cell secretion, which leads to increased collagen synthesis and stimulation of alkaline phosphatase (ALP) activity (Bumann et al., 1997). *In vitro* studies with isolated PDL cells have also shown that there is a significant time-dependent up-regulation of the tropoelastin gene after external pressure simulating orthodontic force fibroblasts (Redlich et al., 2004). The density of cells expressing a positive signal for type I collagen mRNA after tooth movement appeared to be much greater on the tension side than on the pressure side (Yoshimatsu et al., 2008; Olson et al., 2012). On both sides, the distribution of collagen-positive cells was uniform along the principal fibers of the ligament. This characteristic distribution appeared a few hours after the initiation of tooth movement and persisted for a couple of weeks during the treatment (Nakagawa et al., 1994).

Expression of type XII collagen was also noted but took place after the expression of type I and was more obvious in the tension side. The activation of types I and XII collagen expression in the remodeling occurred in a pattern similar to that found during the development of the PDL, suggesting that type XII collagen expression may be closely associated with the functional regeneration of the PDL (Karimbux and Nishimura, 1995). The effects of OTM on the synthesis of other collagen types (III, V, and VI) have also been analyzed in the human PDL subjected to OTM. Synthesis of all collagens was seen in both compression and tension sides. However, whereas collagen synthesis in the tension zone of the treated teeth did not change significantly when compared with the control teeth, significantly higher rates of selected types of collagen were found in the corresponding compression zones (Bumann et al., 1997). This finding was unexpected because it had been believed that there is a prevalence of proliferative processes in the tension zones, as opposed to degradation in the compression zones. This data suggests that, in addition to bone resorption, there is active tissue remodeling in zones of compression following the disappearance of the hyalinized areas (Bumann et al., 1997).

Recently, Sulakshana et al. (2019), while evaluating the expression pattern of type I collagen, lysyl oxidase, and tropoelastin, observed a time dependent variation in mRNA expression with orthodontic force application. They reported expression peaks of type I collagen and lysyl oxidase mRNA at 14 days, while a decreased expression pattern for tropoelastin mRNA was observed. After subjecting human PDL fibroblasts and human osteoblasts to 5 and 10% compressive force in a Flexcell system, Nettelhoff et al. (2016) concluded that 10% force application reduced the viability of the cells but was capable of inducing apoptosis. They identified differential gene expression with varied force levels; increased ALP gene expression, osteopontin (OPN) upregulation and the highest RANKL/OPG ratio was observed after 5% compressive force in human PDL fibroblasts, and RANKL/OPG ratio expression increased after 10% compressive force in human osteoblasts. Human PDL fibroblasts showed an upregulation of MMP-8-synthesis and an increased MMP-8/TIMP-1 ratio.

In addition to the expression of the molecules described before, several *in vivo* and *in vitro* studies have indicated that PDL cells exposed to orthodontic forces can undergo self-destruction by the process of apoptosis in both compression and tension sites (Hatai et al., 2001; Rana et al., 2001; Mabuchi et al., 2002). Several molecules in the apoptotic signal pathway have been identified: amongst them members of the tumor necrosis factor ligand family (TNFSF8), tumor necrosis factor receptor family (FAS, TNFRSF10B, TNFRSF11B, TNFRSF25, and CD27), the Bcl-2 family (BAG3, BAK1, BCL2L11, and BCLAF1), the caspase family (CASP5 and CASP7), the inhibitor of apoptosis proteins family (BIRC3, BIRC6 and NAIP), the caspase recruitment domain family (RIPK2 and PYCARD) and the death domain family (DAPK1), as well as an oncogene (*BRAF*) (Xu et al., 2011). Another protein associated with the self-destruction by necrosis that has been detected in the PDL of tissues undergoing application of orthodontic forces is HMGB1 (high mobility group box protein 1), which is a nuclear protein that binds DNA and regulates gene expression. It also serves as a multifunctional cytokine that mediates proinflammatory responses, but at the same time promotes wound healing. Outside the cell, HMGB1 can serve as an alarmin (signal tissue and cell damage) to activate the innate immune system and mediate a wide range of physiological and pathological responses (Wolf et al., 2013, 2014). A time and force-dependent regulation and role of HMGB1 expression during OTM leading to decrease in areas of active periodontal remodeling and increase in extracellular sites were identified through a Sprague–Dawley rat study by Zou et al. (2019). Previously, it was also shown that administration of $1\alpha,25(OH)_2D_3$ (calcitriol) greatly reduced the expression of HMGB1, thereby a time-dependent reduction in expression of the early inflammatory cytokines, IL-6 and TNF-α. (Cui et al., 2016).

As we can see, PDL cells respond to the application of orthodontic forces by inducing the expression of many different genes associated with the process of remodeling. Furthermore, the PDL also contains stem cells that have the potential to differentiate into the different components of the periodontium, and it has been shown that the application of mechanical forces can induce the differentiation of these cells into an osteogenic pathway and form osteoblasts (Ku et al., 2009; Zhang et al., 2012b; Jacobs et al., 2013). The molecules involved in PDL remodeling are illustrated in Figure 12.1 and Table 12.1.

How do changes in the PDL affect tissues?

As we previously described, application of orthodontic forces elicits a physical, cellular, and molecular response from the PDL. This is further elucidated in Chapters 3, 4, and 5 of this book. These changes affect all tissues that constitute the periodontium including blood vessels. Through a rat experiment, Sprogar et al. (2010) demonstrated that the endothelial cells lining the luminal surface of the blood vessels secrete endothelins, a family of three closely related

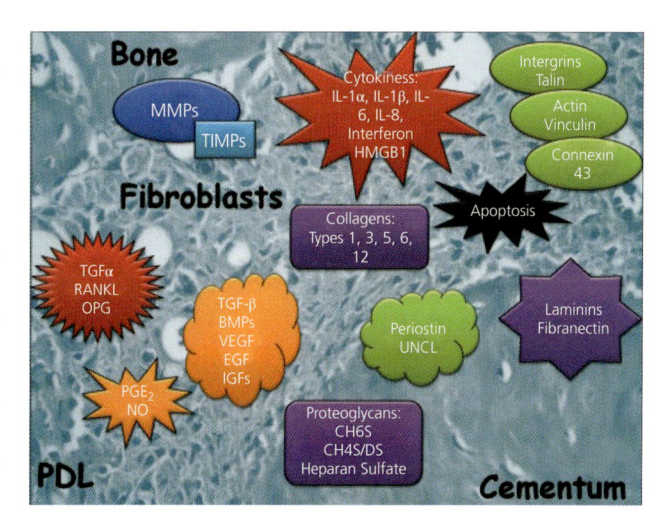

Figure 12.1 Gene expression in the PDL following orthodontic force application. BMPs, bone morphogenetic proteins; CH6S, chondroitin 6-sulfate; CH4S, chondroitin 4-sulfate; DS, dermatan sulfate; EGF, epithelial growth factor; HMGB1, high mobility group box protein 1; IGF, insulin-like growth factor; IL-1α, interleukin-1α; IL-1β, interleukin-1β; IL-6, interleukin-6; IL-8, interleukin-8; MMPs, matrix metalloproteases; NO, nitrous oxidase; OPG, osteoprotegerin; PDL, periodontal ligament; PGE_2, prostaglandin E_2; RANKL, receptor activator of nuclear factor kappa B ligand; TGF-β, transforming growth factor-beta; TIMPs, tissue inhibitor of metalloproteases; TNF-α, tumor necrosis factor-alpha; VEGF, vascular endothelial growth factor; UNCL, uncoordinated-like.

Table 12.1 Molecules associated with OTM.

Gene	Cell expression	Function	Effect on tooth movement	Effect on root resorption
Neural tissues				
Calcitonin gene-related peptide (CGRP)	Neurons, pulp, PDL and marginal gingivae	Neurotransmitter, vasodilator, increases osteoblast differentiation, inhibits osteoclast formation	Bone remodeling	
Vasoactive intestinal polypeptide (VIP)	PDL, pulp	Neurotransmitter, vasodilator, increases osteoblast differentiation	Bone remodeling	
Neuropeptide Y (NPY)	Neurons	Neurotransmitter, vasodilator, increases osteoblast differentiation	Bone remodeling	
Substance P	Pulp, PDL and marginal gingivae	Neurotransmitter, vasodilator, increases osteoblast differentiation	Bone remodeling	
Preproenkephalin	Neurons	Neurotransmitter, vasodilator, increases osteoblast differentiation	Bone remodeling	
Dynorphin	Neurons	Neurotransmitter, vasodilator, increases osteoblast differentiation	Bone remodeling	
Protein gene product (PGP)-5	Neurons	Neurotransmitter, vasodilator, increases osteoblast differentiation	Bone remodeling	
Proteases				
MMP-1, MMP-2, MMP-8, MMP-9, MMP-13	PDL, fibroblast cells, osteoblasts and cementoblasts	Removal of tissue, protein digestion	ECM and bone remodeling. Inhibition of MMPs results in no tooth movement	
Tissue inhibitor of MMP (TIMP 1–3)	ECM, fibroblast cells, osteoblasts, osteocytes	Inhibit action of MMPs	Regulate ECM and bone remodeling.	
Lysosomal cystein proteases: cathepsin B, cathepsin G, cathepsin L, cathepsin K	Odontoclasts and osteoclasts	Removal of proteins from bone	Bone resorption/bone remodeling	
ECM				
Collagen I, collagen III, collagen V, collagen VI, collagen XII	Fibroblasts, ECM, osteoblasts	ECM and bone formation, PDL fibers	ECM and bone remodeling	
Proteoglycans: chondroitin 6-sulphate (CH-6S), chondroitin 4-sulphate (CH-4S), dermatan sulphate, sulphated glycosaminoglycans, heparan sulphate	ECM, fibroblasts	Provide support for the PDL fibers and cells	Markers for ECM remodeling	
Laminin	ECM, fibroblasts	Cell attachment and differentiation	ECM remodeling	
Fibronectin	ECM, fibroblasts	Cell shape and migration	ECM and bone remodeling	
Elastin	ECM, fibroblasts	Provide ECM elasticity	ECM remodeling	
Connexin 43	Fibroblasts, osteoblasts, osteocytes	Cell–cell communication	ECM and bone remodeling	
Integrins	Fibroblasts, osteoblasts, osteocytes	Cell–ECM communication, bind to fibronectin	ECM and bone remodeling	
Periostin	PDL fibroblasts, osteoblasts	ECM and bone remodeling	Inhibition of periostin results in PDL deficiency	
Uncoordinated-like (UNCL)	PDL fibroblasts, Cementoblasts	Signaling, mechanotransduction	ECM mechanotransduction	
Cytokines chemokines				
Interleukin-1a (IL-1α)	Odontoclasts, fibroblasts, macrophages, pulp	Proliferation and differentiation, osteoclast function	ECM remodeling, bone resorption	
Interleukin-1b (IL-1β)	PDL, alveolar bone	Stimulates osteoclasts. Promotes bone resorption /inhibits bone formation	ECM remodeling, bone resorption. Inhibitors reduce rate of tooth movement	Polymorphisms have been associated with root resorption
Interleukin-2 (IL-2)	PDL, fibroblasts	Stimulates osteoclasts. Promotes bone resorption/inhibits bone formation	ECM remodeling, bone resorption	
Interleukin-3 (IL-3)	Pulp	Stimulates osteoclasts. Promotes bone resorption/inhibits bone formation	ECM remodeling, bone resorption	
Interleukin-4 (IL-4)	Fibroblasts	Increases osteoprotegerin (OPG) and inhibits osteoclasts	Inhibits bone resorption	
Interleukin-6 (IL-6)	Pulp, fibroblasts	Stimulates osteoclasts. Promotes bone resorption/inhibits bone formation	ECM remodeling, bone resorption	
Interleukin-8 (IL-8)	PDL tension site	Stimulates osteoclasts. Promotes bone resorption/inhibits bone formation	ECM remodeling, bone resorption. Inhibitors reduce rate of tooth movement	
Interleukin-13 (IL-13)	Fibroblasts, osteoblasts	Increases OPG and inhibits osteoclasts	Inhibits bone resorption	
Tumor necrosis factor ligand family (TNF)	PDL, pulp	Stimulates osteoclasts. Promotes bone resorption/inhibits bone formation	ECM remodeling, bone resorption. Inhibitors reduce rate of tooth movement	
Tumor necrosis factor receptor family (FAS, TNFRSF 10B, TNFRSF11B, TNFRSF26 and CD27)	PDL	Stimulates osteoclasts. Promotes bone resorption/inhibits bone formation	ECM remodeling, bone resorption. Inhibitors reduce rate of tooth movement	
Interferon gamma	Fibroblasts	Stimulates osteoclasts. Promotes bone resorptio /inhibits bone formation	ECM remodeling, bone resorption	
Osteoclast differentiation factor (ODF)	Osteoblasts	Stimulates osteoclasts. Promotes bone resorption /inhibits bone formation	Bone resorption	
OPG	Osteoblasts	Inhibits osteoclast differentiation. Inhibition severely increased of bone resorption	Inhibits bone resorption	
Receptor activator of nuclear factor kappa B ligand (RANKL)	Osteoblast, osteoclasts, fibroblasts, pulp	Promotes osteoclast formation	Stimulates bone resorption	
Monocyte chemotactic protein -1 (MCP-1)	Fibroblasts	Promotes osteoclast formation	Stimulates bone resorption	

Molecule	Source/Location	Function	Notes
Regulated on activation normal T expressed and secreted (RANTES/CCL5)	Fibroblasts	Promotes osteoclast formation	Stimulates bone resorption
Macrophage inflammatory protein -2 (MIP/CXCL2)	Fibroblasts	Promotes osteoclast formation	Stimulates bone resorption
High mobility group box protein 1 (HMGB1)	PDL	Promotes proinflammatory responses. Also wound healing	PDL remodeling
Growth factors			
Connective tissue growth factor (CTGF)	ECM, osteoblasts and osteocytes	Proliferation and differentiation of osteoblast/bone formation	Stimulates bone formation
Transforming growth factor-beta-1 (TGF-β1)	PDL, osteoblasts, pulp	Induce osteoclast apoptosis	Stimulates bone formation
Epithelial growth factor (EGF)	Fibroblasts, pulp	Remodeling	ECM and bone remodeling
Vascular endothelial growth factor (VEGF)	Pulp, osteoblasts	Neovascularization, osteoclast recruitment	Stimulates bone resorption, accelerates movement
Bone morphogenetic proteins (BMPs)	Fibroblasts, osteoblasts	Osteoblast formation	Stimulates bone formation
Macrophage colony stimulating factor (M-CSF)	Fibroblasts	Osteoclast differentiation	Stimulates bone resorption
Fibroblast growth factor (FGF)	Osteoblasts, pulp	Osteoblast differentiation	Stimulates bone formation
Insulin-like growth factor (IGF)	Fibroblasts, osteoblasts, osteocytes	Stimulates osteoblast and osteoclasts function/bone remodeling	Bone remodeling
Platelet-derived growth factor (PDGF)	Pulp, fibroblasts	Osteoblast proliferation mediates through PGE	Stimulates bone formation
Transcription factors			
NF-kappaB (RANK)	Osteoclasts	Receptor, osteoclast differentiation	Stimulates bone resorption. Its gene (TNFRSF11A) has been linked to external apical root resorption (EARR)
Runx/Cbfa1	Osteoblasts	Osteoblast differentiation	Stimulates bone formation, inhibition results in no bone mineralization
Osterix	Osteoblasts	Osteoblast differentiation	Stimulates bone formation
Mineralization			
Osteonectin	Fibroblasts, osteoblasts, pulp		
Osteopontin (OPN)	PDL, osteocytes, osteoblasts, pulp	Chemoattractant for osteoclasts/remodeling	Bone remodeling. Inhibition does not remodel bone in response to stress
Osteocalcin (OCN)	Pulp, osteoblasts	Bone formation	Bone remodeling, accelerates tooth movement
Bone sialoprotein (BSP)	Osteoblasts	Bone formation	Bone remodeling
Alkaline phosphatase (ALP)	Osteoblasts	Bone formation	Bone remodeling
Hormones/vitamins			
Estrogen	Ovaries	Multiple functions, suppresses bone resorption/reduces osteoclast number	Bone formation
Testosterone	Testis, ovaries	Multiple functions, promotes bone formation	Bone formation
Leptin	Adipose tissue, bone marrow and other tissues	Multiple functions, increases angiogenesis, suppresses osteoblast function/reduces bone formation	Bone remodeling
Vitamin D_3	Skin exposed to UV	Calcium homeostasis/induces both differentiation of osteoclasts and osteoblasts	Bone remodeling. Enhances tooth movement
Parathyroid hormone (PTH)	Parathyroid glands	Regulates calcium and phosphate homeostasis, stimulates vitamin D production, stimulates osteoblasts to produce RANKL, inhibits osteoclast apoptosis	Bone remodeling
Calcitonin	Thyroid gland	Regulates calcium and phosphate homeostasis, decreases osteoclast activity	Bone remodeling
Endothelins (ET-1, ET-2, and ET-3)	Blood vessels	Diverse physiological actions; bone resorption	Bone remodeling
Signaling molecules			
cAMP pathway	Multiple tissues, fibroblasts, osteoblasts, pulp	Mechanotransduction, inflammation	ECM and bone remodeling
NO-NOS pathway	Multiple tissues, fibroblasts, osteoblasts, pulp	Neurotransmission, vasodilatation, inflammation	ECM and bone remodeling. Inhibition accelerates tooth movement
Phosphoinositide (PI) (pathway)	Multiple tissues, fibroblasts, osteoblasts, pulp	Mechanotransduction, inflammation	ECM and bone remodeling
Cyclooxygenase-2 (COX-2)	Multiple tissues, fibroblasts, osteoblasts, pulp	Mechanotransduction, inflammation	ECM and bone remodeling. Inhibition slows tooth movement
PGE_1, PGE_2	Multiple tissues, fibroblasts, osteoblasts, pulp	Stimulates bone resorption	Accelerates tooth movement
Apoptosis pathway (Bcl-2 family, caspase family, caspase recruitment domain family, death domain family)	PDL	Self-destruction proteins	PDL remodeling

peptide hormones: ET-1, ET-2, and ET-3. With diverse physiological actions in response to mechanical force application, ET-1 and ET-3 were equally important during the initial and lag phase, but ET-1 was mainly found in the late phase. ET-2 seems to be of minor importance during OTM. The ET-1 gene expression level was probably increased because ET-1 is released due to intravascular shear stress and hypoxia, which are both present after orthodontic force application. TBC3214, an ET1 antagonist, significantly decreased osteoclast volume and significantly increased alveolar bone volume and therefore probably decreased bone resorption in the late stage of OTM. This suggests that ET-1 increases osteoclastic bone resorption during tooth movement in rats.

Amongst other molecules whose expression in the PDL has been reported to be affected by the application of orthodontic forces are periostin and uncoordinated-like (UNCL). Periostin is an ECM protein preferentially expressed in the periosteum and in the PDL. It appears to be involved in cell adhesion (Horiuchi et al., 1999), and might play a role in bone metabolism and remodeling. In control specimens, expression of periostin mRNA was uniformly observed in the PDL surrounding the mesial and distal roots of the upper molars and was weak in the PDL of the root furcation area. The divergent expression of periostin mRNA in the PDL began to be observed at 3 hours and continued up to 96 hours after the onset of tooth movement. The maximum changes, which showed stronger staining in the pressure sites than in the tension sites, were observed at 24 hours. These results suggest that periostin is one of the local contributing factors in bone and periodontal tissue remodeling following mechanical stress during experimental tooth movement (Wilde et al., 2003; Cobo et al., 2016). UNCL is found to be preferentially expressed in PDL fibroblasts. After application of orthodontic forces, strong UNCL expression was observed in PDL fibroblasts and in the differentiating cementoblasts at the site of tension, suggesting a role associated with the mechanotransduction of PDL fibroblasts (Kim et al., 2007).

Jiang and Tang (2018) could observe continuous and time-dependent upregulation in mRNA expression levels of ALP, OPN, Col I, osteocalcin, and bone sialoprotein (BSP) in human PDL fibroblasts subjected to mechanical stress. Following addition of specific inhibitors of extracellular signal-regulated kinase (ERK)1/2 and p38 mitogen-activated protein kinase (MAPK), they reported a reduction in all the genes listed above indicating the important roles these kinases play in PDL remodeling associated with orthodontic force application. Küchler et al. (2020) could identify genetic polymorphisms in genes associated with OTM, such as TT genotype in *RANKL* polymorphism rs9594738 and GG genotype in *COX2* polymorphism rs5275 leading to upregulation of RANK and downregulation of COX-2 respectively in human PDL fibroblasts, resulting in either increase or decrease in the rate of tooth movement. Rankovic et al. (2020) applied static compressive forces on human PDL-derived fibroblasts and observed high molecular activity over a period of 6 days resulting in significant upregulation of cFOS, IL-6, and TNFα expression and downregulation of P2RX7. For a summary of the genetic expression in PDL tissues see Table 12.1.

Reaction of neural tissues

Tooth movement-associated tissue remodeling has been shown to be associated with an inflammatory process, which more often than not results in painful sensations, particularly after activation of the orthodontic appliance. Normal PDL and alveolar bone innervation are essential for periodontal remodeling because healthy innervations promote maximum blood flow during OTM.

OTM affects the number, functional properties, and distribution of both mechanosensitive and nociceptive periodontal nerve fibers. The mechanoreceptors are silent in physiological conditions, but contain various neuropeptides, such as substance P, vasoactive intestinal polypeptide (VIP), and calcitonin gene-related peptide (CGRP) (Jacobsen and Heyerans, 1997). These neuropeptides are stored in peripheral and central nerve terminals and are released when these terminals are strained. Increased immunoreactivity of substance P has been demonstrated in the PDL in the early phases of tooth movement. This neuropeptide has been shown to cause vasodilatation and increased vascular permeability, contributing to the increased local blood flow that accompanies inflammation (Davidovitch, 1995). Incubation of substance P with human PDL fibroblasts *in vitro* significantly increased the concentration of cAMP in the cells and the release of PGE_2 in the medium (Davidovitch et al., 1988). Studies in rats localized CGRP in the PDL and the dental pulp during tooth movement, particularly in the tension sites (Kvinnsland and Kvinnsland, 1990; Norevall et al., 1995). CGRP and substance P act as neurotransmitters, as well as vasodilators, inducers of increased vascular flow and permeability, and stimulators of plasma extravasations and leukocyte migration into tissues. Receptors for CGRP are found on osteoblasts, monocytes, lymphocytes, and mast cells. CGRP induces bone formation through osteoblast proliferation and osteoclast inhibition (Anderson and Seybold, 2004), as is illustrated in Figure 12.2. Strong reactivity to VIP in the compressed PDL and in the pulp of moving teeth in cats has been reported (Saito et al., 1990). In other studies, CGRP and protein gene product (PGP) 9.5 were found to be expressed more at the apical PDL and distributed towards the alveolar bone, and frequently found in bone resorption lacunae. Nerve sprouting was also present both in the root and coronal pulp, and an increased nerve and blood vessel density generally appeared together.

Levels of pre-proenkephalin mRNA expression in trigeminal subnucleus complex increased as a result of tooth-movement stimuli, suggesting that enkephalinergic inhibitory systems could be activated during tooth movement (Balam et al., 2005). It has also been reported that experimental tooth movement induced the expression of dynorphin in the superficial layers of the

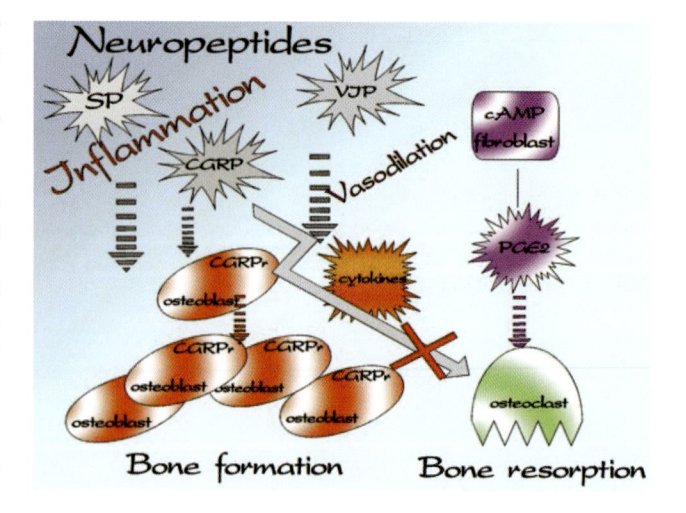

Figure 12.2 Reaction of neural tissues to the applied orthodontic forces. cAMP, cyclic adenosine monophosphate; CGRP, calcitonin gene-related peptide; CGRPr, calcitonin gene-related peptide receptor; PGE_2, prostaglandin E_2; SP, substance P; VIP, vasoactive intestinal peptide.

subnucleus caudalis, which might play an important part in modulation of the discomfort and pain evoked by tooth movement (Kato et al., 1995). A report on administration of MK-801 (a noncompetitive antagonist of N-methyl-D-aspartate receptors) before tooth movement in rats showed that a blockade of N-methyl-D-aspartate receptors resulted in the suppression of the trigeminal sensory nuclear complex. These effects were found to increase the neuronal activity in the descending antinociceptive system, including nuclear raphe magnus, ventrolateral PAG, dorsal raphe nucleus, and Edinger–Westphal nucleus. These results suggest a pharmacological way to decrease pain perception during OTM (Hattori et al., 2004).

The abundant presence of PGP 9.5, a neural-specific marker and neuronal growth factor (NGF), mediating inflammatory pain during orthodontic treatment in PDL fibroblasts was demonstrated by Kyrkanides et al. (2016). NGF binds with high affinity to its cell membrane tyrosine kinase A receptor (TrkA) and NGF-TrkA complex gets transported to the primary sensory neuron body and upregulates the expression of substance P and CGRP (Kyrkanides et al., 2016). An et al. (2019), through an experiment on Sprague–Dawley rats injecting substance P systemically, found an increase in levels of TRAP-positive osteoclasts on day 3 and further increase on days 7 and 14 leading to increased alveolar bone remodeling. They could also observe an increase in serum concentrations of IFN-γ and TNF-α in peripheral blood on days 7 and 14. A summary of the genetic expression in neural tissues is presented in Figure 12.2. and Table 12.1.

Reaction of the alveolar bone

In order to achieve tooth movement, remodeling of the alveolar bone surrounding the dental roots is required. Bone remodeling involves a complex network of cells (osteoblasts, osteoclasts, and osteocytes), cell interactions and cell–matrix interactions, all of which are regulated by hormones, growth factors, and cytokines (some of which are the result of the strained PDL). The appearance of osteoclasts is the first step in this process, and bone resorption is a much faster process than bone apposition; it can take 3 months to replace bone resorbed in only 2–3 weeks (Roberts et al., 2004).

Gene expression and osteoclasts

Osteoclasts are specialized multinucleated giant cells not seen normally in the PDL, but when orthodontic forces are applied, they can be observed shortly thereafter. It is widely accepted that osteoclasts are derived from stem cells in hematopoietic organs, and granulocyte–macrophage colony-forming units are the earliest identifiable precursors of osteoclasts (Mundy and Roodman, 1987). In bone remodeling during experimental tooth movement, osteoclast induction first occurred in vascular canals of the alveolar bone crest in the pressure side, and then in the PDL in the pressure side. Osteoclasts and preosteoclastic cells can be identified by immunohistochemistry for H(+)-ATPase (Yokoya et al., 1997).

There are many genes involved in osteoclast proliferation, differentiation, and regulation. Amongst the key players for these functions are genes like osteoprotegerin (*OPG*), cathepsin K (*CTSK*), and chloride channel 7 (*ClCN7*), which are rate-limiting agents for osteoclast differentiation and function (Harada and Rodan, 2003). *OPG* blocks the transcription factor receptor activator of NF-kB (RANK) and RANK ligand (RANKL) binding, while *CTSK* destroys bone matrix proteins whereas *ClCN7* maintains osteoclast neutrality by shuffling chloride ions through the cell membrane. RANK and RANKL are also key proteins regulating osteoclast function. Synthesis of these proteins takes place in osteoblasts and their expression is dependent on the magnitude of the force being applied; *OPG* synthesis increased with the force while RANKL mRNA expression decreased in an *in vitro* system. Furthermore, the induction of *OPG* mRNA expression by stretching was inhibited by indomethacin or genistein, and the stretch-induced reduction of RANKL mRNA was inhibited by PD098059 (Tang et al., 2006). Synthesis of RANKL by osteoblasts and its role in promoting osteoclast differentiation supports the hypothesis that osteoblasts control osteoclast differentiation. Recently the responsiveness of transcription factor TEA domain family member 1 (TEAD1) to mechanical force was investigated and it was reported that knockdown of TEAD1 in human PDL fibroblasts downregulated expression of *OPG* and promotes osteoclast differentiation (Li et al., 2019). The role played by growth differentiation factor 15 (*GDF15*, a novel compressive force responsive gene) in osteoclastogenesis associated with orthodontic force application was elicited by Li et al. (2020b). They suggested that *GDF15* will promote the expression of several proinflammatory cytokines and RANKL/OPG ratio in PDLCs, while its knockdown impaired the process of osteoclastogenesis.

Another important player in the osteoclast life is macrophage colony-stimulating factor (M-CSF), which is necessary for osteoclast recruitment and survival (Sanuki et al., 2010). Many interleukins also play a key role in osteoclast function associated with mechanical forces; expression levels of IL-17s and their receptors increased depending on the compressive force. The addition of IL-17A increased the expression of IL-17-receptors as well as RANKL, and M-CSF, whereas it decreased *OPG* expression (Zhang et al., 2010). Vascular endothelial growth factor (VEGF) is another important factor as it can induce neovascularization as well as osteoclast recruitment, and it has been shown that osteoclasts express VEGF receptor 1 (VEGFR-1) (Niida et al., 1999). Expression of VEGF plays a role in the early remodeling of periodontal tissues during OTM (Yue et al., 2018). Application of mechanical forces to induce tooth movement increases the expression of VEGF in osteoblasts on the alveolar bone surface in PDL tension sites. Furthermore, the number of osteoclasts can be enhanced by the injection of recombinant human VEGF, which significantly increases the rate of tooth movement. These results suggested that tooth movement is accelerated by endogenous VEGF (Kohno et al., 2003). Treatment with anti-VEGF polyclonal antibody markedly reduced the osteoclast number and inhibited the amount of tooth movement and relapse of moved teeth (Kohno et al., 2005).

The end of bone resorption and the start of bone formation occur through a coupling mechanism that ensures that an equivalent amount of bone is laid down after the previous resorption phase. Whether activation of osteoblasts begins simultaneously with osteoclast recruitment or at a later stage during lacunae development is still controversial. It has been proposed that growth factors such as TGF-β, IGF-I, and IGF-II, and proteases such as plasminogen activators, play a major role in this coupling mechanism (Hill, 1998). Zhang et al. (2020) identified the role played by long noncoding RNAs (lncRNAs), the newly identified class of functional RNAs regulating gene expression and translation regulation, in OTM. Their study revealed that lncRNA Nron (long noncoding RNA repressor of the nuclear factor of activated T cells) is highly expressed in osteoclast precursors and which when overexpressed resulted in reduction in tooth movement through reduced osteoclastogenesis. The expression of molecules associated with osteoclast function and formation is depicted in Figure 12.3.

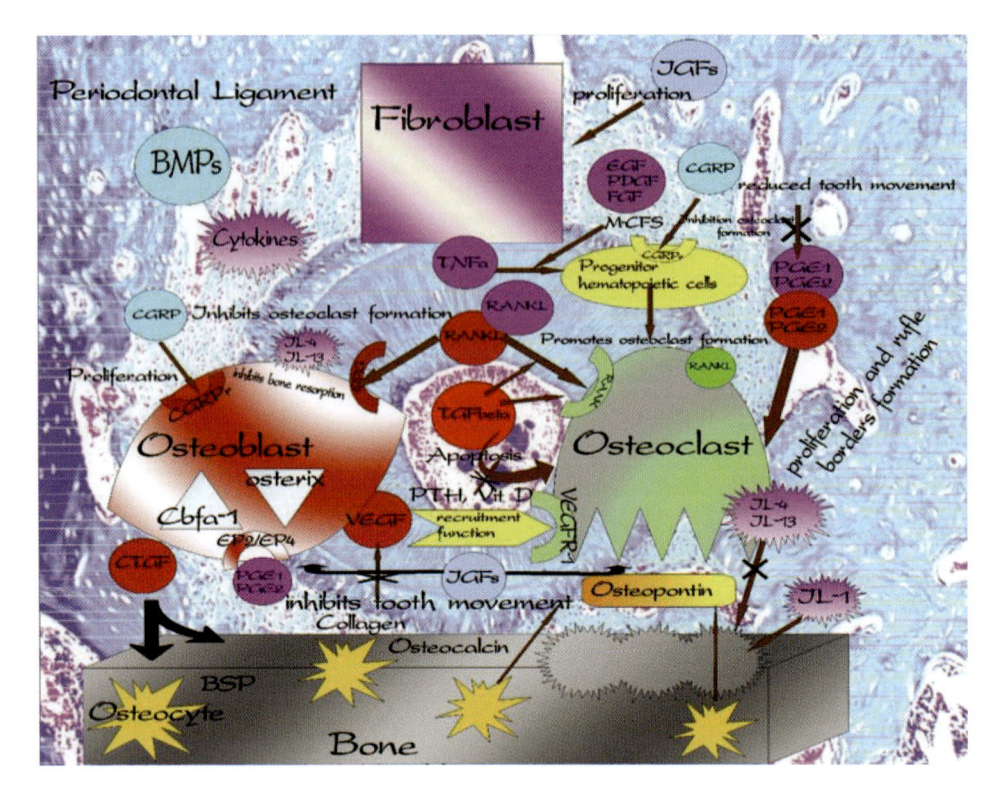

Figure 12.3 Remodeling of the PDL and alveolar bone following orthodontic force application. BMPs, bone morphogenetic proteins; BSP, bone sialoprotein; Cbfa-1, core binding factor alpha-1; CGRP, calcitonin gene-related peptide; CGRPr, calcitonin gene-related peptide receptor; CTGF, connective tissue growth factor; EGF, epithelial growth factor; EP2, prostaglandin EP2 receptor; EP4, prostaglandin EP4 receptor; FGF, fibroblast growth factor; IGFs, insulin-like growth factors; IL-1, interleukin-1; IL-4, interleukin-4; IL-13, interleukin-13; M-CSF, macrophage colony-stimulating factor; OPG, osteoprotegerin; PDGF, platelet-derived growth factor; PGE_2, prostaglandin E_2; PGE_1, prostaglandin E_1; PTH, parathyroid hormone; RANK, receptor activator of nuclear factor kappa B; RANKL, receptor activator of nuclear factor kappa B ligand; TGF-β, transforming growth factor-beta; TNFα, tumor necrosis factor-alpha; VEGF, vascular endothelial growth factor; VEGF R1, vascular endothelial growth factor receptor 1; Vit D, vitamin D.

Gene expression and osteoblasts/osteocytes

Bone formation results from differentiation of osteoblast precursor cells from primitive mesenchymal cells, maturation of osteoblasts, and formation of a mineralized ECM. Osteoblast differentiation and proliferation are separate processes, controlled by different genes. Although many genes control the complex process of osteogenesis, the transcription factor core-binding factor 1 (*Cbfa1*, also known as *Runx2* or *OSF2*) is the earliest expressed, and it is considered the most specific marker for bone formation (Karsenty, 2003). The initial event in bone formation is chemoattraction of osteoblasts or their precursors to the site of bone formation. During OTM, bone formation starts with stem-cell migration from blood-vessel walls, or mesenchymal stem cells (MSC) and preosteoblast formation. Osteoblasts that become surrounded by calcified matrix and remain in the bone are known as osteocytes. Osteocytes connect with each other by narrow processes located in canaliculi throughout the bone matrix. The osteocytes are important mechanosensors and transducers of applied mechanical strain, transforming strain into chemical signaling towards the effector cells, i.e., osteoblasts and osteoclasts (Tresguerres et al., 2020).

Transcription factors such as *Cbfa1/Runx2* and *osterix* are key factors for bone formation. *Cbfa1/Runx2* is essential for osteoblast differentiation and bone formation. *Runx2* null mice completely lack mineralized tissue and die soon after birth, while *Runx2* heterozygous knock-out mice stay alive but show morphological defects in the skeletal system as observed in cleidocranial dysplasia in humans. Mechanical stress-induced tooth movement was similar between *Runx2* heterozygotes and normal animals in terms of movement distance. However, while rotational movement between the first and third weeks was increased in wild-type mice, it was not altered in heterozygous animals (Chung et al., 2004).

After application of a mechanical force, increases in TGF-β1 and OPG mRNA were observed in the stretched cells on the tension side of the distal bone surface, simultaneously with the loss of osteoclasts. Both of these factors are known to have a negative effect on osteoclast recruitment and survival. Some of these stretched cells were identified as cuboidal osteoblasts showing intense signals for both factors, suggesting that there might be a sequential link in tensional force applied on the bone lining cells, upregulation of TGF-β1/OPG, and disappearance of osteoclasts (Kobayashi et al., 2000). Connective tissue growth factor (CTGF) has been shown to be expressed in osteoblasts, fibroblasts, and chondrocytes. During experimental tooth movement, CTGF mRNA expression increased in osteoblasts and in osteocytes, suggesting that CTGF might regulate osteocytes function during the mechanical stimulation of bone (Yamashiro et al., 2001). Osteoblasts contain a rich array of functional cell surface receptors open to protein binding. Bone morphogenetic proteins (BMPs) bind to such receptors, triggering a signaling pathway that promotes osteoprogenitor cell differentiation and upregulation of osteoblast function (Massague et al., 2000; Miyazono, 2000). BMPs can induce *Cbfa1/Runx2* expression and, in turn, BMP expression and signaling might be controlled by other signaling molecules and Hedgehog genes (Miyazono, 2000). An increased phospho-Ser9-GSK-3β expression and β-catenin signaling pathway activity was observed through a rat study by Mao et al. (2018). They also observed increased bone parameters (bone mineral density, bone volume to tissue volume, and trabecular thickness), as well as ALP- and osterix-positive cells at tension sites during tooth movement while downregulating GSK-3β activity. Yoneda et al. (2019) studied mechano-sensory behavior of osteoblastic MC3T3-E1 cells and observed high mRNA expression of *Piezo1* and *Trpv4* and increased Ca^{2+} response (one of the earliest events in osteoblasts to induce a mechanical stimulus) with Yoda1, a PIEZO1 agonist. Osteoblast receptor–ligand binding not only changes cell form and function, and initiates signaling, but also serves as a potential point for therapeutic modifications. Drugs that enhance or block activity of osteoblast receptors can modulate bone remodeling and tooth movement.

The effect of orthodontic mechanical loading on the expression of bone proteins like ALP, collagens type I and osteocalcin has been determined. ALP mRNA levels were increased shortly after application of the forces and remained elevated for several days. In contrast, collagen I mRNA levels were not changed at that time but were greatly increased after a few days of force application (Pavlin et al., 2000). As expected, expression of collagen type I was higher at the tension side as was the expression of BSP, both of which were negligible in the compression site (Domon et al., 2001). The levels of osteocalcin increased considerably after 2–48 hours of treatment. Symmank et al. (2019), through their study in male Wistar rats, provided evidence for a potential role of *GDF15* in translating mechanical stimuli into cellular changes in immature osteoblasts and resulting in an increased transcription of osteogenic marker genes like *RUNX2*, osteocalcin and ALP. Taken together, these studies suggest that mechanical stress induces deposition of bone matrix primarily by stimulating gene expression and differentiation of osteoblasts (Pavlin et al., 2001). The effect of local administration of osteocalcin on tooth movement was examined in rats and it was determined that tooth movement was significantly higher in the injected rats than in the controls, particularly in the early stages of the experimental period. The accelerated movement was accompanied by a larger number of osteoclasts accumulated on the mesial alveolar bone surface, suggesting that osteocalcin accelerates OTM due to enhancement of osteoclastogenesis on the pressure side (Hashimoto et al., 2001).

Other genes that are expressed during mechanically induced bone remodeling are nitric oxide synthetase (NOS), prostaglandin G/H synthetase, glutamate/aspartate transporter, parathyroid hormone (PTH), IGFs and estrogen receptor-β (Roberts et al., 2004). The low-density lipoprotein receptor-related protein 5 (*LRP5*) gene was found to control bone formation through modifying osteoblast proliferation and increasing bone mass. *LRP5* mutation in both alleles causes loss of osteoblast function and an osteoporosis–pseudoglioma syndrome, characterized by a very low bone mass. Single-gene mutations in *LRP5* might cause a gain in function, resulting in osteoblast hyperactivity and increased bone mass. *LRP5* might mediate other molecular genetic processes, including cancer (Harada and Rodan, 2003). Using osteoblastic cell lines, it has been shown that mechanical stress also induces the production of inflammatory cytokines and their receptors in these cells. The expression of IL-1β, IL-1 receptor, IL-6, IL-6 receptor, IL-8 receptor, IL-11 and tumor necrosis factor-alpha (TNF-α) increased depending on the strength and duration of the compressive force, whereas the expression of IL-8, IL-11 receptor and TNF-α receptor did not change with the application of compressive force (Koyama et al., 2008). The expression of genes associated with orthodontic forces in osteoblasts and osteocytes is illustrated in Figure 12.3 and Table 12.1.

Bone remodeling

Bone remodeling in response to orthodontic forces requires the synchronized action of osteoblasts, osteoclasts, osteocytes, and PDL cells. Cell-to-cell communication via gap junctions has been implicated as an important factor in the transduction mechanism between force, as applied to bone during OTM, and bone remodeling. The presence of Connexin 43, a protein forming gap junctions connecting cells, was found to increase in the PDL after exposure to mechanical forces suggesting that this protein plays a role in the coordination of events during experimentally induced alveolar bone remodeling (Su et al., 1997). Increased expression in osteoblasts and osteocytes, at both formation and resorption sites has also been documented (Gluhak-Heinrich et al., 2006).

Changes in expression for OPN mRNA during experimental tooth movement were detected in the osteocytes on the pressure side at early stages, and gradually spread to those on the tension side, and also to the osteoblasts and bone-lining cells in the alveolar bone. Following the increased expression of OPN, a 17-fold greater number of osteoclasts and numerous resorption pits were observed on the pressure side of the alveolar bone, suggesting that OPN is an important factor in bone remodeling caused by mechanical forces (Terai et al., 1999). Furthermore, bone remodeling in response to mechanical stress was suppressed in OPN knockout mice. These results indicate the critical role of OPN in the process of bone remodeling and suggest the presence of an *in vivo* mechanical stress response element in the 5.5-kb upstream region of the *OPN* gene (Fujihara et al., 2006).

Ongoing research activities elucidate the role of many more genetic pathways in the complex bone remodeling process associated with mechanical force application. The role played by the *Cas* (Crk-Associated Substrate) protein family in mechanically induced bone remodeling through its association with NF-κB, altering the mechanosensing by osteocytes, was demonstrated by Miyazaki et al. (2019). The influence of micro RNA -21 (MiR 21) in bone remodeling through the RANKL/OPG mechanism, wherein increased secretion of RANKL from activated T-cells and downregulation of OPG inducing more osteoclasts, is demonstrated through two separate studies on mid-palatal suture remodeling (Li et al., 2020a) and OTM (Wu et al., 2020). Further, the expression of Gli1+ cells in PDL, which will proliferate and differentiate into osteoblastic cells under tensile force were demonstrated by Liu et al. (2020). They demonstrated the force responsive nature of Gli1+ cells and its role in bone remodeling through conditional ablation of the *Yap* gene, which is a classical mechanotransduction factor which will get elevated upon force application.

Role of growth factors in bone remodeling

Bone is a rich depository of growth factors, and many of them are responsive to the application of mechanical forces (Pinkerton et al., 2008). Amongst the most abundant growth factors associated with cell growth, differentiation, apoptosis, bone formation, and remodeling are the members of the transforming growth factor family: TGF-β1, activins, inhibins, and BMPs (Katagiri and Takahashi, 2002). Davidovitch (1995) demonstrated an increase in the presence of TGF-β in cat PDL cells and alveolar bone osteoblasts during OTM, while control PDL and alveolar bone showed no staining for TGF-β. This factor has been shown to enhance osteoblast protein synthesis, including collagen (ten Dijke et al., 1990), and also enhance osteoclast differentiation from hematopoietic cells stimulated with RANKL and M-CSF (Quinn et al., 2001). Orthodontic forces result in an increase in epidermal growth factor (EGF) concentrations in paradental cells in cats, suggesting that it participates in tissue remodeling associated with tooth movement (Guajardo et al., 2000). Another growth factor important in bone formation is fibroblast growth factor (FGF). It has been shown that bone marrow cells treated with FGF increase DNA synthesis, ALP activity, and formation of bone-like nodules (Noff et al., 1989). Osteoblasts can synthesize FGF and secrete it into the surrounding ECM, where it might act as an autocrine or paracrine signal (Globus et al., 1989). It has been suggested that FGFs are sequestered in the cells responsible for their synthesis and are released only when there is a disruption of the plasma membrane. Plasma membrane disruption in PDL tension sites after orthodontic force application has been demonstrated, and it was suggested that this process could support uptake and release of large signaling molecules (Orellana et al., 2002).

Insulin-like growth factor (IGF) I and II represent a family of endocrine-, paracrine-, and autocrine-acting polypeptide growth factors controlling pre- and postnatal development and growth processes. In general, IGF-I and II are involved in various cellular processes, including differentiation, proliferation, morphogenesis, growth, control of metabolic functions, and carcinogenesis. In bone cells, the action of IGF-I is regulated by various systemic and local factors, including growth hormone, PTH, vitamin D_3, corticosteroids, TGF-α, IL-1, and PDGF. When added to PDL cells in culture, IGF-I causes an increase in DNA synthesis (Blom et al., 1992), and when injected into newborn lambs it stimulates osteoblastic function, mediated through rapid and sustained release of osteocalcin (Coxam et al., 1992). To investigate their roles in tooth movement, root resorption, and repair, the presence of components of the IGF system was determined by immunohistochemistry on sections from rat maxillae where the first molar had been moved mesially by means of an orthodontic appliance. Increased immunostaining for nearly all components in pressure sides and resorption lacunae suggests an active involvement in the resorption processes (Götz et al., 2006).

Platelets are a major source of growth factors such as PDGF, and when mechanical damage to the periodontal vasculature is created by orthodontic force, platelets migrate from the blood vessels to the extravascular space. When PDGF binds to the PDGF receptor, it releases arachidonic acid, which, via cyclooxygenase (COX) and lipooxygenase activity, leads to formation of prostaglandins and leukotrienes. It has been proposed that this pathway is important for mitogenesis in bone cells (Davidai et al., 1992; Sandy, 1998). CTGF is also associated with the ECM during anabolic bone remodeling (Safadi et al., 2003). This signal molecule enhances vascular invasion, stimulates proliferation of osteoblast precursors, and promotes mineralization of new bone by osteoblasts. In alveolar bone, CTGF is localized in osteoblasts and osteocytes near the PDL. After 12 hours of experimental tooth movement, CTGF is expressed in osteoblasts and extends to osteocytes deep in the bone on both sides of the moving root (Yamashiro et al., 2001).

Colony-stimulating factors (CSF) include those related to granulocytes (G-CSF), to macrophages (M-CSF), or to both cell types (GM-CSF), and might have particular implications in bone remodeling through osteoclast formation and thereby during tooth movement. These molecules interact to regulate the production, maturation, and function of granulocytes and monocyte-macrophages. Fibroblasts and endothelial cells synthesize M-CSF (Davidovitch, 1995). It was shown that osteoclasts can form as a result of culturing bone-marrow cells with M-CSF for 10 days. It has also been demonstrated that stimulation of fibroblasts with EGF, PDGF, FGF, and IL-1 induces M-CSF expression by these cells. In terms of potency, M-CSF is the most potent in stimulating bone-marrow cells to produce osteoclasts, followed by GM-CSF, IL-3, and G-CSF (Kahn and Simmons, 1975; Falkenberg et al., 1990; Takashi et al., 1991).

As can be seen from the description presented above, tooth movement is the result of the effect of mechanotransduction on the expression of numerous genes which regulate the remodeling of the periodontal tissues. This process is quite complex, with numerous molecules acting on several tissues resulting in their inhibition or stimulation. An attempt to simplify and summarize the molecules involved and their actions is illustrated in Figure 12.3. A compilation of molecules and their functions is described in Table 12.1.

Reaction of the pulp tissues

As expected, OTM evokes a pronounced biological reaction in the dental pulp as well. The pulpal response to orthodontic force involves cell damage, inflammation, and wound healing, processes that could adversely affect the dental pulp. It is important to understand how the pulp tissues are affected, since these responses can have a serious impact on the long-term vitality of teeth subjected to orthodontic movement (Von Böhl et al., 2012). Derringer et al. (1996) demonstrated an increase in the number of microvessels after the application of mechanical forces suggesting an increase in angiogenic growth factors in the dental pulp. Vasodilatation in the pulp of an orthodontically stressed tooth has also been observed (Wong et al., 1999), which might be the result of the increase in nitric oxide synthase (NOS) associated with orthodontic forces (Leone et al., 2002; Di Nardo Di Maio et al., 2004). The expression of angiogenic growth factors like VEGF, fibroblast growth factor-2 (FGF-2), platelet-derived growth factor (PDGF), and transforming growth factor-beta (TGF-β) in pulp tissues following the application of orthodontic forces were identified by Derringer and Linden (2004). The progression of the inflammatory process in human pulp fibroblasts apparently depends on stimulation by neuropeptides and production of inflammatory cytokines, such as IL-1, IL-3, IL-6, and TNF-α. Yu et al. (2016) demonstrated inflammation and elevated IL-17A secretion in the dental pulp leading to self-renewal and differentiation of dental pulp stem cells during OTM. Han et al. (2020) demonstrated upregulation of c-Fos and MMP-9 expression in the dental pulp of tooth subjected to extreme intrusive forces and Charoenpong et al. (2019) concluded that mechanical stress induced expression of s100 proteins (especially S100A7) by human dental pulp cells promoting root resorption by inducing osteoclast differentiation and activity. Perinetti et al. (2004) demonstrated that an enzyme, aspartate aminotransferase (which is released extracellularly upon cell death), is significantly elevated after orthodontic force application. More recent studies showed that insertion of elastic bands between molars resulted in proliferation and vasodilatation of capillaries followed by apoptosis in the pulp. Interestingly, expression of HSP70, OPN and osteocalcin mRNAs in the experimental groups was higher than that in the control group, suggesting that OTM causes degenerative changes and apoptosis in pulp cells, while pulp homeostasis is maintained at the genetic level (Shigehara et al., 2006). As previously stated, expression of substance P was increased in the pulp after application of orthodontic forces. PGE_2, COX-2 and RANKL increased in the presence of substance P (Kojima et al., 2006).

It has been shown that the application of orthodontic forces increases the levels of EGF in paradental cells in human subjects (Sismanidou et al., 1996), in human GCF (Uematsu et al., 1996) and in the cat canine PDL (Guajardo et al., 2000). EGF is a mitogen for fibroblasts and endothelial cells *in vitro*, promoting angiogenesis *in vivo*, and it has been isolated in low concentrations from human dentine (Roberts-Clark and Smith, 2000). Previous studies have found angiogenic changes in the human dental pulp in response to orthodontic force, and it was concluded that the EGF released following orthodontic force application plays a part in the angiogenic response of the pulp (Derringer et al., 1996; Derringer and Linden, 2003, 2004, 2007). The molecules expressed in the pulp are depicted in Figure 12.4 and Table 12.1.

In summary, application of orthodontic forces not only affects the periodontal tissues but also may have a significant effect on the vitality of the pulpal tissue. Changes in gene expression associated with inflammation, programmed cell death, and/or tertiary dentin formation (Reyna et al., 2006) have been reported. These data indicate that during OTM there is a fine balance between maintaining a healthy pulp or ending up with a tooth that might need a root canal in the long term. However, it is important to note that a systematic review performed to investigate the relationship between orthodontic force level and pulp reaction in humans concluded that there is limited scientific support for the notion that orthodontic forces have an effect on the blood supply of the pulp regardless of the force level used (Von Böhl et al., 2012). They also found limited scientific support for the role of VEGF, FGF-2, PDGF, TGF-β, and EGF in the angiogenic response of the pulp, but they did find strong scientific support for changes in pulpal enzyme activity; reduction of ALP activity and increase of AST activity because of force application. In conclusion, although many studies have demonstrated that orthodontic force application may lead to pathologic changes in the dental pulp tissue, this systematic review showed that our knowledge concerning dental pulp reactions and orthodontic force application is still limited (Von Böhl et al., 2012). It is important to keep in mind that this systematic review was restricted to humans and human studies in this area are very limited.

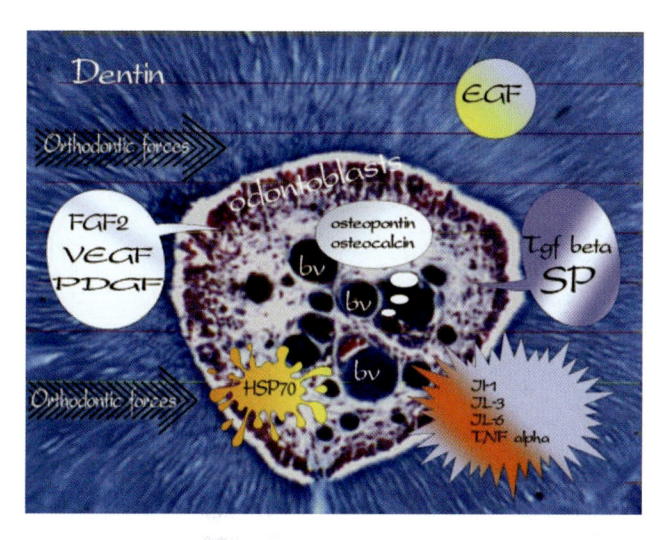

Figure 12.4 Reaction of the dental pulp to applied orthodontic forces. bv, blood vessels; EGF, epithelial growth factor; FGF-2, fibroblast growth factor-2; HSP70, heat shock protein 70; IL-1, interleukin-1; IL-3, interleukin-3; IL-6, interleukin-6; PDGF, platelet-derived growth factor; SP, substance P; TGF-β, transforming growth factor-beta; TNF-α, tumor necrosis factor-alpha; VEGF, vascular endothelial growth factor.

Genetic influences and translational applications

Information related to the genetic, cellular, biochemical, and molecular events associated with OTM have not only advanced our basic need to know the mechanisms involved in this process, but they are now being used as "proof of principle" in translational studies. These studies are slowly finding their way to the practice of orthodontics by managing and controlling the process and complications that might arise during treatment. Stimulation of the expression of proinflammatory cytokines by osteoperforation near the moving teeth increases the rate of tooth movement (Teixeira et al., 2010; Chandran et al., 2018; Feizbakhsh et al., 2018) while local administration of soluble receptors for IL-1 or TNF-α or the use of neutralizing antibodies to VEGF to block the function of these proteins retards OTM (Jäger et al., 2005; Kohno et al., 2005).

Numerous studies are being performed to determine the genetic, biologic, and mechanical factors that affect speed of human tooth movement. Relaxin, a member of the insulin/relaxin family of structurally related hormones is one of those factors. Relaxin is related to many physiological processes, such as collagen turnover, angiogenesis, and antifibrosis in both males and females. It has been reported that relaxin decreased the release and expression of Col-I and increased the expression of MMP-1 in human PDL cells *in vitro*. In an experimental model for tooth movement in dogs, relaxin stimulated the velocity of tooth movement *in vivo* (Takano et al., 2009). Therefore, this hormone is thus considered to possibly influence OTM through alterations of the PDL (Stewart et al., 2005). However, a randomized, placebo-controlled clinical trial in humans did not show any effect of relaxin on rate of tooth movement for 8 weeks or on short-term relapse (McGorray et al., 2012). Based on the results that are currently available Swidi et al. (2018) concluded that relaxin treatment is a dead-end for further exploration of orthodontic applications.

Some studies found that three factors significantly affected speed of movement: (i) an increased activity index (AI = experimental [IL-1β /IL-1RA]/control [IL-1β /IL-1RA]), (ii) decreased presence of IL-1RA in GCF, and (iii) having the allele 2 at IL-1β (+3954), were associated with faster tooth movement (Iwasaki et al., 2006, 2009). As is quite evident from the previous sections and chapters, the main influences on the process of bone resorption, and therefore tooth movement, are the interplay between RANK/RANKL and its antagonist OPG, so numerous studies have focused on the modulation of these molecules to accelerate or slow down tooth movement using different types of molecules. A schematic representation of a summary of these events is presented in Figure 12.5 and a detailed description of all these molecules and their effect on orthodontic treatment can be found in Chapter 15.

Complications of OTM and its genetic implications

As with every therapeutic procedure, OTM can be complicated by several different factors. Knowledge derived from understanding the molecular aspects of the process can also provide solutions for some of these problems. A few examples are provided below.

Eruption failure/primary failure of eruption

Primary failure of eruption (PFE) is characterized by nonsyndromic eruption failure of permanent teeth in the absence of mechanical obstruction. The hallmark features of this condition are infraocclusion of affected teeth, increasing significant posterior

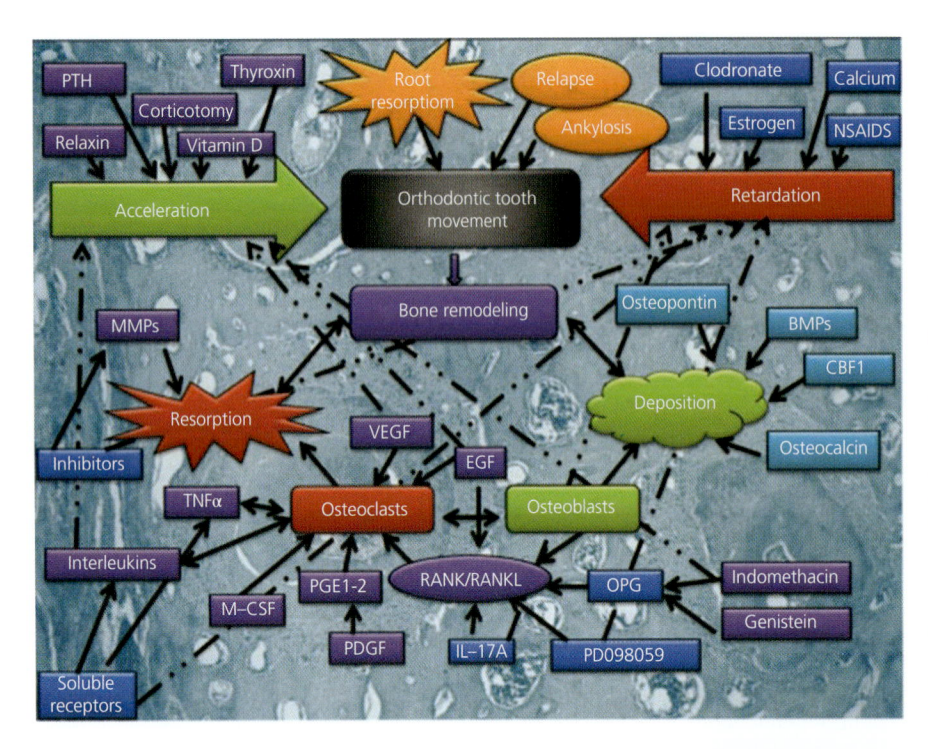

Figure 12.5 Summary of the events that can accelerate or slow down OTM. PTH, parathormone; NSAIDs, nonsteroidal anti-inflammatory drugs; MMPs, matrix metalloproteinases; BMPs, bone morphogenetic proteins; CBF1, core binding factor 1; HSP70, heat shock protein 70; IL-17A, interleukin-17A; PDGF, platelet-derived growth factor; TNF-α, tumor necrosis factor-alpha; VEGF, vascular endothelial growth factor; EGF, epidermal growth factor; M-CSF, macrophage colony stimulating factor; PGE_{1-2}, prostaglandin E1-2; RANK/RANKL, receptor activator for nuclear factor kappa and ligand.

open-bite malocclusion accompanying normal vertical facial growth, and inability to move affected teeth orthodontically. Many studies have noted the heritable basis of this dental phenotype and recently mutations in parathyroid hormone receptor 1 (PTH1R) have been identified in several familial cases of PFE. This knowledge can provide a novel diagnostic tool as well as the means to overcome this problem in the clinical management of orthodontic patients with failure of tooth eruption (Frazier-Bowers et al., 2010). A detailed description on PFE and its genetic implications are provided in Chapter 13.

Tooth relapse

The relapse of teeth that have moved during orthodontic treatment is a major clinical issue that undermines the outcomes of a successful treatment. It is believed that this relapse is a physiologic response of the supporting tissues and can be attributed to occlusal instability and increased mechanical tension exerted by the transseptal fibers of the PDL (reviewed in detail in Chapter 19). These fibers are the major component of the PDL, travel from the cementum to adjacent cementum and from the cementum to the gingival papillae, and consist of collagen and oxytalan fibers (Pareker et al., 1972; Yoshida et al., 1999). Based on this knowledge, different biomedical agents are being tested to determine their effect on avoiding this problem like RANKL inhibitors OPG and denosumab, bisphosphonates, bone morphogenic proteins (BMPs), Simvastatin, and strontium. Local OPG gene transfer to periodontal tissues can inhibit relapse after OTM, through the inhibition of osteoclastogenesis (Zhao et al., 2012a). So far, the RANKL inhibitor agent denosumab seems to be the most promising agent for preventing relapse. However, further studies are needed before a clinical application is on the horizon (Swidi et al., 2018).

Root resorption

The association of root resorption as an unwelcome effect of OTM has been postulated since 1914 (Ottolengui, 1914; Reitan, 1972) (Figure 12.6). There are several factors, for example corticosteroids,

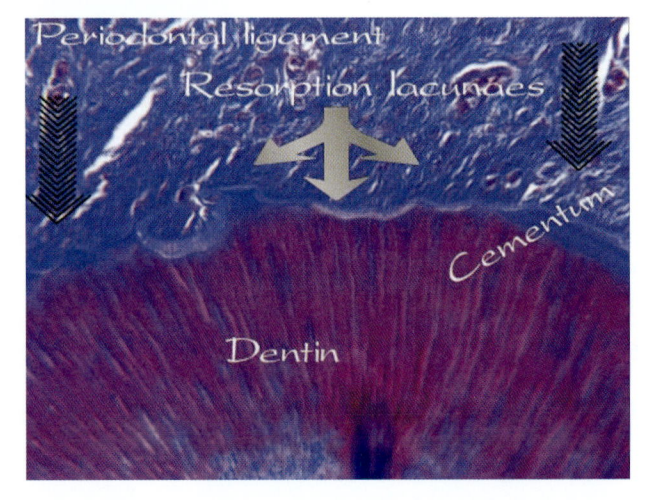

Figure 12.6 The resorptive lacunae destroying the cementum and dentin layers of roots. This is the initial process of root resorption associated with the application of an orthodontic force.

alcohol use, asthma, and allergies, that have been proposed to predispose individuals for root resorption (Krishnan, 2005; Armstrong et al., 2006). It is easy to believe that the magnitude of an orthodontic force is an important factor for root resorption, but this assumption has not been confirmed in recent systematic reviews (Theodorou et al., 2019; Currell et al., 2020; Sondeijker et al., 2020).

Many studies have attempted to identify the gene(s) responsible for root resorption with the hope that one day there could be a way to monitor patients while undergoing orthodontic treatment and provide early detection of root resorption while it is reversible. Some of the genes expressed during OTM have been associated with root resorption. For example, increased amounts of IL-1α and β have been found in cells in resorption lacunae in cat canines (Davidovitch et al., 1988). Rossi et al. (1996) attempted to correlate the high levels of TNF-α and IL-1β produced by monocytes with patients presenting with severe root shortening. No differences, however, were found between the patients and the controls.

Considering the role of PGE_2 in bone remodeling, it was considered a candidate for root resorption. Studies by Sinha (1996), however, found that local injections of PGE_2 near maxillary rat molars did not induce root resorption. Furthermore, no differences were found among different concentrations and different periods of time (Boekenoogen, 1996). Other studies have suggested that BSP, OPN, and the cell adhesion molecules such as αvβ3 integrins could be related to external root resorption. Shigeyama et al. (1996) reported increased concentrations of OPN and its associated integrin (αvβ3) at resorption sites, and the presence of BSP on the mineralized areas of the roots in cats, but no direct relation to root resorption has been demonstrated. Cysteine proteinases, for example cathepsins B and G, have been found in odontoclasts during physiological root resorption, and were assumed to be involved in the formation of the resorption lacunae by degradation of collagen and other noncollagenous proteins (Sasaki and Ueno-Matsuda, 1992). Although high collagenolytic activity has been detected in resorbing tissues of deciduous teeth, the cellular origin of collagenolytic enzymes in root-resorbing tissue caused by tooth movement has not been identified.

Domon et al. (1999) subjected rats to experimental tooth movement to induce root resorption, and then performed in situ hybridization with digoxigenin-labeled RNA probes to detect mRNAs that encode matrix metalloproteinase-1 (MMP-1) and cathepsin K in root-resorbing tissue. MMP-1 mRNA was detected in fibroblastic cells, cementoblasts, and osteoblasts, but not in either odontoclasts or osteoclasts, suggesting that these enzymes are not directly involved in root resorption. In contrast, cathepsin K mRNA was expressed only in odontoclasts and osteoclasts, suggesting a possible involvement. However, cathepsin K appears to operate at later stages of the process and it is not the initial "trigger" for root resorption.

Recently, hundreds of genes expressed as a consequence of OTM and/or root resorption in the rat were identified using cDNA microarrays, including a higher level of expression of MMP-13 both at the mRNA and protein levels in the roots showing resorption (Reyna et al., 2006). However, a direct correlation of these genes to root resorption has not yet been demonstrated. The functional coordination of the OPG/RANKL/RANK system contributes not only to alveolar remodeling, but it has been suggested that it also relates to physiological root resorption as well as orthodontic-induced root resorption. It has been postulated that determination of OPG and RANKL concentrations in serum and/or GCF might be useful for predicting the rate of bone remodeling, the net effect between bone remodeling and root resorption, and the degree of root resorption (Tyrovola et al., 2008). This is particularly difficult since it has not been actually demonstrated that this coordination is different in root resorption compared with tooth movement.

It has been proposed that external apical root resorption (EARR) is likely to be influenced by a combination of environmental and host factors in a multifactor cascade, and that there may be a familial (genetic) factor in susceptibility (Harris et al., 1997; Hartsfield et al., 2004). In an attempt to separate the contribution made by genetic factors from those due to environmental factors, 16 monozygotic and 10 dizygotic twins were studied. The genetic contribution to EARR was assessed using concordance and heritability estimates. External apical root resorption was not dependent on the pretreatment root length. Qualitative and quantitative estimates of concordance indicate a genetic component to root resorption

(Ngan et al., 2004). The effect of the genotype on susceptibility or resistance to develop root resorption as a consequence of OTM was studied in mice from different inbred strains. The results showed that some inbred mouse strains (DBA/2 J, BALB/cJ, and 129P3/J) are highly susceptible to root resorption, while other strains (A/J, C57BL/6 J, and SJL/J) are much more resistant. The variation in the severity of root resorption associated with orthodontic force among different inbred strains of mice, when all other variables were controlled, points strongly towards a genetic influence on susceptibility or resistance to root resorption associated with orthodontic force (Al-Qawasmi et al., 2006; Abass et al., 2008).

Evidence of linkage disequilibrium of an IL-1β polymorphism with the clinical manifestation of EARR has been reported. Individuals homozygous for the IL-1β (+3953) allele 1 have a 5.6-fold increased risk of EARR as compared with individuals who are not homozygous for the IL-1β (+3953) allele 1. The IL-1β gene diallelic variation at +3953 is associated with variable IL-1β protein production, and individuals homozygous for IL-1β (+3953) allele 1 have reduced production of secreted IL-1β as compared with individuals homozygous for IL-1β (+3953) allele 2, and even individuals heterozygous for IL-1β (+3953) alleles 1 and 2 (Al-Qawasmi et al., 2004). These results were confirmed in a Brazilian population and significant statistical differences among the frequencies of the alleles and genotypes of the IL-1β gene polymorphism between the affected and unaffected groups were found, supporting the notion that allele 1 predisposed the subjects to EARR (Bastos-Lages et al., 2009; Iglesias-Linares et al., 2012).

Interestingly, Rossi et al. (1996) examined IL-1β and TNF-α production in monocytes from a group of orthodontic patients with severe root shortening and found no significant differences in mean levels between resorption and nonresorption groups. This supports the likelihood that EARR is genetically heterogeneous. Expanding on the possible mechanism of the association of the IL-1β allele 1 and EARR, a relatively decreased IL-1β production in the case of allele 1 may result in relatively less catabolic bone modeling (resorption) at the cortical bone interface with the PDL (Al-Qawasmi et al., 2004). Stress analysis of orthodontically stimulated rat molars suggests that the initiation of mechanically induced bone resorption is due to fatigue failure within the bone itself (Katona et al., 1995; Roberts, 1999). This hypothesis would suggest that a deficiency of IL-1β inhibits the resorptive response to orthodontic loads. A slower rate of bone resorption may result in a prolonged stress that is concentrated in the root of the tooth, which in turn could trigger a cascade of fatigue-related events leading to root resorption. This scenario contradicts the hypothesis that increased severity of root resorption after orthodontic treatment is related to an increase in alveolar bone resorption (Engstrom et al., 1988). On the contrary, root resorption may be related to reduced rates of bone resorption at the PDL interface of the root and the alveolar socket. Interestingly studies by Iwasaki et al. (2006, 2009) have found that the ratio of IL-1β/IL-1RA in GCF, and the presence of IL-1 gene cluster polymorphisms, are associated with faster tooth movement. Additional support for the role of IL-1β in root resorption comes from mice lacking the P2X7 receptor which is crucial in bone biology. P2X7 is an adenosine triphosphate (ATP)-gated ionotropic channel and a key mediator of inflammation and bone adaptation responses. After mechanical trauma, damaged cells release ATP that leads to the activation of P2X7 in macrophages and other cell types, which in turn release IL-1 cytokines; therefore, the P2X7 receptor plays a significant role in mechanotransduction. It is hypothesized that variability in the expression of the P2X7 receptor is an important factor in the individual variation to applied orthodontic loads when the mechanical environment is controlled. In the areas of higher stress, the lack of P2X7 receptor (and consequently IL-1β) caused about a 20% increase in EARR in these roots (Viecilli et al., 2009). However, a recent systematic review by Nowrin et al. (2018) could not find any association of the IL-1β (+3954) polymorphism and the risk of EARR and pointed to the need for more research to elucidate it.

Using a candidate gene approach, a possible linkage between orthodontic treatment-related EARR and the TNSALP, TNF-α, and TNFRSF11A gene loci was analyzed. No evidence of linkage was found between EARR and the TNF-α and TNSALP genes. There was, however, linkage to the TNFRSF11A locus, or another tightly linked gene associated with EARR. It should be noted that the TNFRSF11A gene codes for the protein RANK (Al-Qawasmi et al., 2003a, 2003b). Through a recent review, Iglesias-Linares and Hartsfield (2017) stated that many highly complex autocrine and paracrine chemical signaling pathways mediate the three key cellular aspects of cell fusion/activation, clastic cell adhesion, and mineralized tissue reparative capabilities as far as root resorption and repair process is concerned. The molecular pathway leading to root resorption cannot be attributed to a single regulating factor but several of the molecular pathways and factors interact in a crosstalk and influence effector cells for resorption at the level of fusion, activation, and cell adhesion.

Several ways to slow down or treat orthodontic root resorption have been described previously, including the administration of drugs, hormones, growth factors, and low-intensity pulsed ultrasound. Some of these results are promising, demonstrating also an ability to reduce the extent of root resorption (Loberg and Engstrom, 1994; Igarashi et al., 1996; El-Bialy et al., 2004; Jerome et al., 2005; Villa et al., 2005; Krishnan and Davidovitch, 2006b; Sanuki et al., 2010). The use of local OPG gene transfection was tested in rats and suggested that the presence of OPG enhanced the repair of EARR (Zhao et al., 2012b). A systematic review to evaluate the effectiveness of interventions in the management of EARR in humans was conducted by Ahangari et al. (2010). The authors concluded that there is a lack of any high-level evidence on this topic and they suggested that clinicians decide on the most appropriate means of managing this condition according to their clinical experience with regard to patient-related factors. Similar conclusions were obtained by Weltman et al. (2010) and Sondeijker et al. (2020), thus indicating the need for increased research in this area.

Conclusions

As we can see from the information presented in this and other chapters, application of molecular biology to understand the process of tooth movement has begun to unveil the identity of genes that control the cellular and ECM components associated with OTM. The application of new methodologies to this field has resulted in an accelerated rate of information arising in the last few years that no doubt will continue to increase in the future. This information, which now appears quite complex and irrelevant, allows us to start discerning the molecular pathways that control mechanotransduction, PDL and bone remodeling, tooth vitality, and even pain associated with tooth movement. As we can see from the information presented, manipulation of the presence or absence of some molecules, or interference with their function, will result in slow down or acceleration of tooth movement. Furthermore, the general systemic status of an individual will also have a great influence on how that patient will react to the application of the orthodontic forces.

It is clear that the RANKL–RANK–OPG pathway is very important for OTM. It is clear from the discussion that the complex controls osteoclast activity, which in turn controls bone remodeling and therefore tooth movement. It is also becoming apparent that this system will have a major role in the genetic component associated with root resorption. It is not far-fetched to think that in the near future there will be a genetic test that will determine root-resorption-associated polymorphisms in patients prior to orthodontic treatment. This in turn will determine the course and length of the appropriate treatment or might preclude some individuals from getting any treatment at all. We have just begun to scratch the surface. As research continues, new molecules and pathways will be identified and their role in OTM determined. This information will eventually lead to the development of new diagnostic, preventive and therapeutic means that will facilitate the work of orthodontists by optimizing the treatment course, benefiting the patient and increasing the successful outcomes of the treatment.

References

Abass, S. K., Hartsfield, J. K. Jr, Al-Qawasmi, R. A. et al. (2008) Inheritance of susceptibility to root resorption associated with orthodontic force in mice. *American Journal of Orthodontics and Dentofacial Orthopedics* **134**, 742–750.

Ahangari, Z., Nasser, M., Mahdian, M. et al. (2010) Interventions for the management of external root resorption. *Cochrane Database Systematic Reviews* 10.1002/14651858.

Allen, R. K., Edelmann, A. R., Abdulmajeed, A. and Bencharit, S. (2019) Salivary protein biomarkers associated with orthodontic tooth movement: a systematic review. *Orthodontics and Craniofacial Research* **22**, 14–20.

Al-Qawasmi, R. A., Hartsfield, J. K. Jr, Everett, E. T. et al. (2003a) Genetic predisposition to external apical root resorption in orthodontic patients: linkage of chromosome-18 marker. *Journal of Dental Research* **82**, 356–360.

Al-Qawasmi, R. A., Hartsfield, J. K. Jr, Everett, E. T. et al. (2003b) Genetic predisposition to external apical root resorption. *American Journal of Orthodontics and Dentofacial Orthopedics* **123**, 242–252.

Al-Qawasmi, R. A., Hartsfield, J. K. Jr., Everett, E. T. et al. (2004) Root resorption associated with orthodontic force in IL-1Beta knockout mouse. *Journal of Musculoskeletal Neuronal Interactions* **4**, 383–385.

Al-Qawasmi, R. A., Hartsfield, J. K. Jr., Everett, E. T. et al. (2006) Root resorption associated with orthodontic force in inbred mice: genetic contributions. *European Journal of Orthodontics* **28**, 13–29.

An, S., Zhang, Y., Chen, Q. et al. (2019) Effect of systemic delivery of Substance P on experimental tooth movement in rats. *American Journal of Orthodontics and Dentofacial Orthopedics* **155**(5), 642–649.

Anderson, L. E. and Seybold, V. S. (2004) Calcitonin gene-related peptide regulates gene transcription in primary afferent neurons. *Journal of Neurochemistry* **91**, 1417–1429.

Apajalahti, S., Sorsa, T., Railavo, S. and Ingman, T. (2003) The *in vivo* levels of matrix metalloproteinase-1 and -8 in gingival crevicular fluid during initial orthodontic tooth movement. *Journal of Dental Research* **82**, 1018–1022.

Armstrong, D., Kharbanda, O. P., Petocz, P. and Darendeliler, M. A. (2006) Root resorption after orthodontic treatment. *Australian Orthodontic Journal* **22**, 153–160.

Atsawasuwan, P., Lazari, P., Chen, Y. et al. (2018) Secretory microRNA-29 expression in gingival crevicular fluid during orthodontic tooth movement. *PloS one* **13**(3), e0194238.

Balam, T. A., Yamashiro, T., Zheng, L. et al. (2005) Experimental tooth movement upregulates preproenkephalin mRNA in the rat trigeminal nucleus caudalis and oralis. *Brain Research* **1036**, 196–201.

Bastos-Lages, E. M., Drummond, A. F., Pretti, H. et al. (2009) Association of functional gene polymorphism IL-1beta in patients with external apical root resorption. *American Journal of Orthodontics and Dentofacial Orthopedics* **136**(4), 542–546.

Beertsen, W., McColloch, C. A. and Sodek, J. (1997) The periodontal ligament: a unique multifunctional connective tissue. *Periodontology 2000* (13), 20–40.

Blom, S., Holmstrup, P. and Dabelsteen, E. (1992) The effect of insulin like growth factor 1 and human growth hormone on periodontal ligament fibroblast morphology, growth pattern, DNA synthesis and receptor binding. *Journal of Periodontology* **63**, 960–968.

Boekenoogen, D. (1996) The effects of exogenous prostaglandin E2 on root resorption in rats. *American Journal of Orthodontics and Dentofacial Orthopedics* **109**, 277–286.

Bolcato-Bellemin, A. L., Elkaim, R., Abehsera, A. et al. (2000) Expression of mRNAs encoding for alpha and beta integrin subunits, MMPs, and TIMPs in stretched human periodontal ligament and gingival fibroblasts. *Journal of Dental Research* **79**, 1712–1716.

Bumann, A., Carvalho, R. S., Schwarzer, C. L. and Yen, E. H. (1997) Collagen synthesis from human PDL cells following orthodontic tooth movement. *European Journal of Orthodontics* **9**, 29–37.

Chandran, M., Muddaiah, S., Nair, S. et al. (2018) Clinical and molecular-level comparison between conventional and corticotomy-assisted canine retraction techniques. *Journal of the World Federation of Orthodontists* **7**(4), 128–133

Charoenpong, H., Osathanon, T., Pavasant, P. et al. (2019) Mechanical stress induced S100A7 expression in human dental pulp cells to augment osteoclast differentiation. *Oral Diseases* **25**(3), 812–821.

Chung, C. R., Tsuji, K., Nifuji, A. et al. (2004) Micro-CT evaluation of tooth, calvaria and mechanical stress-induced tooth movement in adult Runx2/Cbfa1 heterozygous knock-out mice. *Journal of Medical and Dental Sciences* **51**, 105–113.

Cobo, T., Viloria, C. G., Solares, L. et al. (2016) Role of periostin in adhesion and migration of bone remodeling cells. *PLoS One* **11**(1), e0147837.

Coxam, V., Davicco, M. J., Pastoureau, P. et al. (1992) Insulin-like growth factor II increases plasma osteocalcin concentration in newborn lambs. *Bone Mineralization* **17**, 177–186.

Cui, J., Li, J., Wang, W. et al. (2016) The effect of calcitriol on high mobility group box 1 expression in periodontal ligament cells during orthodontic tooth movement in rats. *Journal of Molecular Histology* **47**(2), 221–228.

Currell, S. D., Liaw, A., Blackmore Grant, P. D. et al. (2019) Orthodontic mechanotherapies and their influence on external root resorption: a systematic review. *American Journal of Orthodontics and Dentofacial Orthopedics* **155**(3), 313–329.

d'Apuzzo, F., Cappabianca, S., Ciavarella, D. et al. (2013) Biomarkers of periodontal tissue remodeling during orthodontic tooth movement in mice and men: overview and clinical relevance. *Scientific World Journal* 2013, 105873.

Davidai, G., Lee, A., Schvartz, I. and Hazum, E. (1992) PDGF induces tyrosine phosphorylation in osteoblast like cells – relevance to mitogenesis. *American Journal of Physiology* **263**, 205–209.

Davidovitch, Z. (1991) Tooth movement. *Critical Reviews in Oral Biology and Medicine* **2**, 411–450.

Davidovitch, Z. (1995) Cell biology associated with orthodontic tooth movement, in *The Periodontal Ligament in Health and Disease* (eds. B. B. Berkovitz, B. J. Moxham and H. N. Newman). Mosby, St Louis, MO, pp. 47–75.

Davidovitch, Z., Nicolay, O. F., Ngan, P. W. and Shanfeld, J. L. (1988) Neurotransmitters, cytokines, and the control of alveolar bone remodeling in orthodontics. *Dental Clinics of North America* **32**, 411–435.

Derringer, K. A., Jaggers, D. C. and Linden, R. W. (1996) Angiogenesis in human dental pulp following orthodontic tooth movement. *Journal of Dental Research* **75**, 1761–1766.

Derringer, K. A. and Linden, R. W. (2003) Angiogenic growth factors released in human dental pulp following orthodontic force. *Archives of Oral Biology* **48**, 285–291.

Derringer, K. A. and Linden, R. W. (2004) Vascular endothelial growth factor, fibroblast growth factor 2, platelet derived growth factor and transforming growth factor beta released in human dental pulp following orthodontic force. *Archives of Oral Biology* **49**, 631–641.

Derringer, K. A. and Linden, R. W. (2007) Epidermal growth factor released in human dental pulp following orthodontic force. *European Journal of Orthodontics* **29**, 67–71.

Di Nardo Di Maio, F., Lohinai, Z., D'Arcangelo, C. et al. (2004) Nitric oxide synthase in healthy and inflamed human dental pulp. *Journal of Dental Research* **83**, 312–316.

Domon, S., Shimokawa, H., Matsumoto, Y. et al. (1999) In situ hybridization for matrix metalloproteinase-1 and cathepsin K in rat root-resorbing tissue induced by tooth movement. *Archives of Oral Biology* **44**, 907–915.

Domon, S., Shimokawa, H., Yamaguchi, S. and Soma, K. (2001) Temporal and spatial mRNA expression of bone sialoprotein and type I collagen during rodent tooth movement. *European Journal of Orthodontics* **23**, 339–348.

El-Bialy, T., El-Shamy, I. and Graber, T. M. (2004) Repair of orthodontically induced root resorption by ultrasound in humans. *American Journal of Orthodontics and Dentofacial Orthopedics* **126**, 186–193.

Ellias, M. F., Zainal Ariffin, S. H., Karsani, S. A. et al. (2012) Proteomic analysis of saliva identifies potential biomarkers for orthodontic tooth movement. *Scientific World Journal* **2012**, 647240.

Engstrom, C., Granstrom, G. and Thilander, B. (1988) Effect of orthodontic force on periodontal tissue metabolism: a histologic and biochemical study in normal and hypocalcemic young rats. *American Journal of Orthodontics and Dentofacial Orthopedics* **93**, 486–495.

Falkenberg, J. H. F., Harrington, M. A., Walsh, W. K. et al. (1990) Gene expression and release of macrophage colony stimulating factor in quiescent and proliferating fibroblasts: effects of serum, fibroblast growth promoting factors and IL-1. *Journal of Immunology* **144**, 4657–4662.

Feizbakhsh, M., Zandian, D., Heidarpour, M. et al. (2018) The use of micro-osteoperforation concept for accelerating differential tooth movement. *Journal of the World Federation of Orthodontists* **7**(2), 56–60.

Frazier-Bowers, S. A., Simmons, D., Wright, J. T. et al. (2010) Primary failure of eruption and PTH1R: the importance of a genetic diagnosis for orthodontic treatment planning. *American Journal of Orthodontics and Dentofacial Orthopedics* **137**, 160.

Fujihara, S., Yokozeki, M., Oba, Y. et al. (2006) Function and regulation of osteopontin in response to mechanical stress. *Journal of Bone and Mineral Research* **21**, 956–964.

Globus, K. B., Plouet, J. and Gospodarowicz, D. (1989) Cultured bovine bone cells synthesize basic fibroblast growth factor and store it in extracellular matrix. *Endocrinology* **12**, 1539–1547.

Gluhak-Heinrich, J., Gu, S., Pavlin, D. and Jiang, J. X. (2006) Mechanical loading stimulates expression of connexin 43 in alveolar bone cells in the tooth movement model. *Cell Communication and Adhesion* **13**, 115–125.

Götz, W., Kunert, D., Zhang, D. et al. (2006) Insulin-like growth factor system components in the periodontium during tooth root resorption and early repair processes in the rat. *European Journal of Oral Sciences* **114**, 318–327.

Gritsch, K., Laroche, N., Morgon, L. et al. (2012) A systematic review of methods for tissue analysis in animal studies on orthodontic mini-implants. *Orthodontics and Craniofacial Research* **15**, 135–147.

Guajardo, G., Okamoto, Y., Gogen, H. et al. (2000) Immunohistochemical localization of epidermal growth factor in cat paradental tissues during tooth movement. *Amercian Journal of Orthodontics and Dentofacial Orthopedics* **118**, 210–219.

Hall, M., Masella, R. and Meister, M. (2001) PDL neuron-associated neurotransmitters in orthodontic tooth movement: identification and proposed mechanism of action. *Todays FDA* **13**, 24–25.

Han, G., Liu, W., Jiang, H. et al. (2020) Extreme intrusive force affects the expression of c-Fos and matrix metallopeptidase 9 in human dental pulp tissues. *Medicine*, **99**(9), e19394.

Harada, S. and Rodan, G. A. (2003) Control of osteoblast function and regulation of bone mass. *Nature* **423**, 349–355.

Harris, E. F., Kineret, S. E. and Tolley, E. A. (1997) A heritable component for external apical root resorption in patients treated orthodontically. *American Journal of Orthodontics and Dentofacial Orthopedics* **111**, 301–309.

Hartsfield, J. K. Jr, Everett, E. T. and Al-Qawasmi, R. A. (2004) Genetic factors in external apical root resorption and orthodontic treatment. *Critical Reviews in Oral Biology and Medicine* **15**, 115–122.

Hashimoto, F., Kobayashi, Y., Mataki, S. et al. (2001) Administration of osteocalcin accelerates orthodontic tooth movement induced by a closed coil spring in rats. *European Journal of Orthodontics* **23**, 535–545.

Hatai, T., Yokozeki, M., Funato, N. et al. (2001) Apoptosis of periodontal ligament cells induced by mechanical stress during tooth movement. *Oral Diseases* **7**, 287–290.

Hattori, Y., Watanabe, M., Iwabe, T. et al. (2004) Administration of MK-801 decreases c-Fos expression in the trigeminal sensory nuclear complex but increases it in the midbrain during experimental movement of rat molars. *Brain Research* **1021**, 183–191.

Henneman, S., Von den Hoff, J. W. and Maltha, J. C. (2008) Mechanobiology of tooth movement. *European Journal of Orthodontics* **30**, 299–306.

Hill, P. A. (1998) Bone remodeling. *British Journal of Orthodontics* **25**, 101–107.

Holliday, L.S., Vakani, A., Archer, L. and Dolce, C. (2003) Effects of matrix metalloproteinase inhibitors on bone resorption and orthodontic tooth movement. *Journal of Dental Research* **82**, 687–691.

Horiuchi, K., Amizuka, N., Takeshita, S. et al. (1999) Identification and characterization of a novel protein, periostin, with restricted expression to periosteum and periodontal ligament and increased expression by transforming growth factor beta. *Journal of Bone and Mineral Research* **14**, 1239–1249.

Igarashi, K., Adachi, H., Mitani, H. and Shinoda, H. (1996) Inhibitory effect of topical administration of a bisphosphonate (risedronate) on root resorption incident to orthodontic tooth movement in rats. *Journal of Dental Research* **75**, 1644–1649.

Iglesias-Linares, A., Moreno-Fernandez, A. M., Yañez-Vico, R. et al. (2011) The use of gene therapy vs. corticotomy surgery in accelerating orthodontic tooth movement. *Orthodontics Craniofacial Research* **14**, 138–148.

Iglesias-Linares, A, Yañez-Vico, R. M., Ortiz-Ariza, E. et al. (2012) Post orthodontic external root resorption in root-filled teeth is influenced by interleukin-1β polymorphism. *Journal of Endodontics* **38**, 283–287.

Iglesias-Linares, A. and Hartsfield Jr, J. K. (2017) Cellular and molecular pathways leading to external root resorption. *Journal of Dental Research* **96**(2), 145–152.

Isaacson, R. J., Lindauer, S. J. and Davidovitch, M. (1993) On tooth movement. *The Angle Orthodontist* **63**, 305–309.

Iwasaki, L. R., Chandler, J. R., Marx, D. B. et al. (2009) IL-1 gene polymorphisms, secretion in gingival crevicular fluid, and speed of human orthodontic tooth movement. *Orthodontics Craniofacial Research* **12**, 129–140.

Iwasaki, L. R., Gibson, C. S., Crouch, L. D. et al. (2006) Speed of tooth movement is related to stress and IL-1 gene polymorphisms. *American Journal of Orthodontics and Dentofacial Orthopedics* **130**, 698.e1–9.

Jacobs, C., Grimm, S., Ziebart, T. et al. (2013) Osteogenic differentiation of periodontal fibroblasts is dependent on the strength of mechanical strain. *Archives of Oral Biology* **58**, 896–904.

Jacobsen, E. B. and Heyerans, K. J. (1997) Pulpal interstitial tissue fluid pressure and blood flow after denervation and electrical tooth stimulation in the ferret. *Archives of Oral Biology*, **42**, 407–15.

Jäger, A., Zhang, D., Kawarizadeh, A. et al. (2005) Soluble cytokine receptor treatment in experimental orthodontic tooth movement in the rat. *European Journal of Orthodontics* **27**, 1–11.

Jerome, J., Brunson, T., Takeoka, G. et al. (2005) Celebrex offers a small protection from root resorption associated with orthodontic tooth movement. *California Dental Association Journal* **33**, 951–959.

Jheon, A. H., Oberoi, S., Solem, R. C. and Kapila, S. (2017) Moving towards precision orthodontics: An evolving paradigm shift in the planning and delivery of customized orthodontic therapy. *Orthodontics and Craniofacial Research* **20**, 106–113.

Jiang, L. and Tang, Z. (2018) Expression and regulation of the ERK1/2 and p38 MAPK signaling pathways in periodontal tissue remodeling of orthodontic tooth movement. *Molecular Medicine Reports*, **17**(1), 1499–1506.

Kahn, A. J. and Simmons, D. J. (1975) Investigations of cell lineage in bone using a chimera of chick and quail embryonic tissue. *Nature* **258**, 325–327.

Karanth, H. S. and Shetty, K. S. (2001) Orthodontic tooth movement and bioelectricity. *Indian Journal of Dental Research* **12**, 212–221.

Karimbux, N. Y. and Nishimura, I. (1995) Temporal and spatial expressions of type XII collagen in the remodeling periodontal ligament during experimental tooth movement. *Journal of Dental Research* **74**, 313–318.

Karsenty, G. (2003) The complexities of skeletal biology. *Nature* **423**, 316–318.

Katagiri, T. and Takahashi, N. (2002) Regulatory mechanisms of osteoblast and osteoclast differentiation. *Oral Diseases* **8**, 147–159.

Kato, J., Wakisaka, S., Tabata, M. J. et al. (1995) Appearance of dynorphin in the spinal trigeminal nucleus complex following experimental tooth movement in the rat. *Archives of Oral Biology* **40**, 79–81.

Katona, T. R., Paydar, N. H., Akay, H. U. and Roberts, W. E. (1995) Stress analysis of bone modeling response to rat molar orthodontics. *Journal of Biomechanics* **28**, 27–38.

Kerrigan, J. J., Mansell, J. P. and Sandy, J. R. (2000) Matrix turnover. *Journal of Orthodontics* **27**, 227–233.

Kim, H. J., Choi, Y. S., Jeong, M. J. et al. (2007) Expression of UNCL during development of periodontal tissue and response of periodontal ligament fibroblasts to mechanical stress *in vivo* and in vitro. *Cell and Tissue Research* **327**, 25–31.

King, G. (2009) Biomedicine in orthodontics: from tooth movement to facial growth. *Orthodontics and Craniofacial Research* **12**, 53–58.

King, G. J., Latta, L., Ruttenberg, A. O. and Keeling, S. D. (1997) Alveolar bone turnover and tooth movement in male rats after removal of orthodontic appliances. *American Journal of Orthodontics and Dentofacial Orthopedics* **111**, 266–275.

Kobayashi, Y., Hashimoto, F., Miyamoto, H. et al. (2000) Force-induced osteoclast apoptosis *in vivo* is accompanied by elevation in transforming growth factor beta and osteoprotegerin expression. *Journal of Bone and Mineral Research* **15**, 1924–1934.

Kohno, S., Kaku, M., Kawata, T. et al. (2005) Neutralizing effects of an antivascular endothelial growth factor antibody on tooth movement. *The Angle Orthodontist* **75**, 797–804.

Kohno, S., Kaku, M., Tsutsui, K. et al. (2003) Expression of vascular endothelial growth factor and the effects on bone remodeling during experimental tooth movement. *Journal of Dental Research* **82**, 177–182.

Kojima, T., Yamaguchi, M. and Kasai, K. (2006) Substance P stimulates release of RANKL via COX-2 expression in human dental pulp cells. *Inflammation Research* **55**, 78–84.

Koyama, Y., Mitsui, N., Suzuki, N. et al. (2008) Effect of compressive force on the expression of inflammatory cytokines and their receptors in osteoblastic Saos-2 cells. *Archives of Oral Biology* **53**, 488–496.

Krishnan, V. (2005) Critical issues concerning root resorption: a contemporary review. *World Journal of Orthodontics* **6**, 30–40.

Krishnan, V. (2007) Orthodontic pain: from causes to management – a review. *European Journal of Orthodontics* **29**, 170–179.

Krishnan, V. and Davidovitch, Z. (2006a) Cellular, molecular, and tissue-level reactions to orthodontic force. *American Journal of Orthodontics and Dentofacial Orthopedics* **129**, 469.e1–32.

Krishnan, V. and Davidovitch, Z. (2006b) The effect of drugs on orthodontic tooth movement. *Orthodontics and Craniofacial Research* **9**, 163–171.

Krishnan, V. and Davidovitch, Z. (2009) On a path to unfolding the biological mechanisms of orthodontic tooth movement. *Journal of Dental Research* **88**, 597–608.

Ku, S. J., Chang, Y. I., Chae, C. H. et al. (2009) Static tensional forces increase osteogenic gene expression in three-dimensional periodontal ligament cell culture. *BMB Reports* **42**, 427–432.

Küchler, E. C., Schröder, A., Corso, P. et al. (2020) Genetic polymorphisms influence gene expression of human periodontal ligament fibroblasts in the early phases of orthodontic tooth movement. *Odontology* **108**, 493–502.

Kvinnsland, I. and Kvinnsland, S. (1990) Changes in CGRP-immunoreactive nerve fibres during experimental tooth movement in rats. *European Journal of Orthodontics* **12**, 320–329.

Kyrkanides, S., Huang, H. and Faber, R. D. (2016) Neurologic regulation and orthodontic tooth movement. *Frontiers in Oral Biology* **18**, 64–74.

Leone, A., Patel, M., Uzzo, M. L. et al. (2002) Expression and modification of NO synthase in human dental pulps during orthodontic treatment. *Bulletin du Groupement International pour la Recherche Scientifique en Stomatologieet Odontologie* **44**, 57–60.

Li, Q., Han, G., Liu, D., & Zhou, Y. (2019) Force-induced decline of TEA domain family member 1 contributes to osteoclastogenesis via regulation of osteoprotegerin. *Archives of Oral Biology* **100**, 23–32.

Li, M., Zhang, Z., Gu, X. et al. (2020a) MicroRNA-21 affects mechanical force-induced midpalatal suture remodelling. *Cell Proliferation* **53**(1), e12697.

Li, S., Li, Q., Zhu, Y. and Hu, W. (2020b) GDF15 induced by compressive force contributes to osteoclast differentiation in human periodontal ligament cells. *Experimental Cell Research* **387**(1), 111745.

Li, X., Zhang, L., Wang, N. et al. (2010) Periodontal ligament remodeling and alveolar bone resorption during orthodontic tooth movement in rats with diabetes. *Diabetes Technology and Therapeutics* **12**, 65–73.

Liu, A. Q., Zhang, L. S., Chen, J. et al. (2020) Mechanosensing by Gli1$^+$ cells contributes to the orthodontic force-induced bone remodelling. *Cell Proliferation* **53**(5), e12810.

Loberg, E. L. and Engstrom, C. (1994) Thyroid administration to reduce root resorption. *The Angle Orthodontist* **64**, 395–399.

Mabuchi, R., Matsuzaka, K. and Shimono, M. (2002) Cell proliferation and cell death in periodontal ligaments during orthodontic tooth movement. *Journal of Periodontal Research* **37**, 118–124.

Mao, Y., Wang, L., Zhu, Y. et al. (2018) Tension force-induced bone formation in orthodontic tooth movement via modulation of the GSK-3β/β-catenin signaling pathway. *Journal of Molecular Histology* **49**(1), 75–84.

Masella, R. S. and Meister, M. (2006) Current concepts in the biology of orthodontic tooth movement. *American Journal of Orthodontics and Dentofacial Orthopedics* **129**, 458–468.

Massague, J., Blain, S. W. and Lo, R. S. (2000) TGF beta signaling in growth control, cancer, and heritable disorders. *Cell* **103**, 295–309.

McGorray, S. P., Dolce, C., Kramer, S. et al. (2012) A randomized, placebo-controlled clinical trial on the effects of recombinant human relaxin on tooth movement and short-term stability. *American Journal of Orthodontics and Dentofacial Orthopedics* **141**(2), 196–203.

Meikle, M. C. (2006) The tissue, cellular, and molecular regulation of orthodontic tooth movement: 100 years after Carl Sandstedt. *European Journal of Orthodontics* **28**, 221–240.

Meikle, M. C. (2007) Remodeling the dentofacial skeleton: the biological basis of orthodontics and dentofacial orthopedics. *Journal of Dental Research* **86**, 12–24.

Melsen, B. (2001) Tissue reaction to orthodontic tooth movement – a new paradigm. *European Journal of Orthodontics* **23**, 671–681.

Miyazaki, T., Zhao, Z., Ichihara, Y. et al. (2019) Mechanical regulation of bone homeostasis through p130Cas-mediated alleviation of NF-κB activity. *Science Advances* **5**(9), eaau7802.

Miyazono, K. (2000) TGF-beta signaling by Smad proteins. *Cytokine and Growth Factor Reviews* **11**, 15–22.

Mundy, G. R. and Roodman, G. D. (1987) Osteoclast ontogeny and function, in *Bone and Mineral Research* (ed. W. A. Peck). Elsevier, Amsterdam, pp. 209–279.

Mussig, E., Tomakidi, P. and Steinberg, T. (2005) Molecules contributing to the maintenance of periodontal tissues. Their possible association with orthodontic tooth movement. *Journal of Orofacial Orthopedics* **66**, 422–433.

Nakagawa, M., Kukita, T., Nakasima, A. and Kurisu, K. (1994) Expression of the type I collagen gene in rat periodontal ligament during tooth movement as revealed by in situ hybridization. *Archives of Oral Biology* **39**, 289–294.

Nettelhoff, L., Grimm, S., Jacobs, C. et al. (2016) Influence of mechanical compression on human periodontal ligament fibroblasts and osteoblasts. *Clinical Oral Investigations* **20**(3), 621–629.

Ngan, D. C., Kharbanda, O. P., Byloff, F. K. and Darendeliler, M. A. (2004) The genetic contribution to orthodontic root resorption: a retrospective twin study. *Australian Orthodontic Journal* **20**, 1–9.

Niida, S., Kaku, M., Amano, H. *et al.* (1999) Vascular endothelial growth factor can substitute for macrophage colony-stimulating factor in the support of osteoclastic bone resorption. *Journal of Experimental Medicine* **190**, 293–298.

Noff, D., Pitaru, S. and Savion, N. (1989) Basic fibroblast growth factor enhances the capacity of bone marrow cells to form bone-like nodules in vitro. *FEBS Letters* **250**, 619–621.

Norevall, L. I., Forsgren, S. and Matsson, L. (1995) Expression of neuropeptides (CGRP, substance P) during and after orthodontic tooth movement in the rat. *European Journal of Orthodontics* **17**, 311–325.

Nowrin, S. A., Jaafar, S., Ab Rahman, N. *et al.* (2018) Association between genetic polymorphisms and external apical root resorption: a systematic review and meta-analysis. *The Korean Journal of Orthodontics* **48**(6), 395–404.

Olson, C., Uribe, F., Kalajzic, Z. *et al.* (2012) Orthodontic tooth movement causes decreased promoter expression of collagen type 1, bone sialoprotein and alpha-smooth muscle actin in the periodontal ligament. *Orthodontics and Craniofacial Research* **15**, 52–61.

Orellana, M. F., Smith, A. K., Waller, J. L. *et al.* (2002) Plasma membrane disruption in orthodontic tooth movement in rats. *Journal of Dental Research* **81**, 43–47.

Ottolengui, R. (1914) The physiological and pathological resorption of tooth roots. *Item of Interest* **36**, 332–362.

Pareker, G.R. (1972) Transseptal fibers and relapse following bodily retraction of teeth: a histologic study. *American Journal of Orthodontics* **61**, 331–344.

Patil, A. K., Shetty, A. S., Setty, S. and Thakur, S. (2013) Understanding the advances in biology of orthodontic tooth movement for improved ortho-perio interdisciplinary approach. *Journal of Indian Society of Periodontology* **17**, 309–318.

Pavlin, D., Dove, S. B., Zadro, R. and Gluhak-Heinrich, J. (2000) Mechanical loading stimulates differentiation of periodontal osteoblasts in a mouse osteoinduction model: effect on type I collagen and alkaline phosphatase genes. *Calcified Tissue International* **67**, 163–172.

Pavlin, D., Zadro, R. and Gluhak-Heinrich, J. (2001) Temporal pattern of stimulation of osteoblast-associated genes during mechanically-induced osteogenesis *in vivo*: early responses of osteocalcin and type I collagen. *Connective Tissue Research* **42**, 135–148.

Perinetti, G., Varvara, G., Festa, F. and Esposito, P. (2004) Aspartate aminotransferase activity in pulp of orthodontically treated teeth. *American Journal of Orthodontics and Dentofacial Orthopedics* **125**, 88–92.

Pinkerton, M. N., Wescott, D. C., Gaffey, B. J. *et al.* (2008) Cultured human periodontal ligament cells constitutively express multiple osteotropic cytokines and growth factors, several of which are responsive to mechanical deformation. *Journal of Periodontal Research* **43**, 343–351.

Pizzo, G, Licata, M. E., Guiglia, R. and Giuliana, G. (2007) Root resorption and orthodontic treatment. Review of the literature. *Minerva Stomatology* **56**, 31–44.

Proff, P. and Romer, P. (2009) The molecular mechanism behind bone remodeling – a review. *Clinical Oral Investigations* **13**(4), 355–362.

Quinn, J. M., Itoh, K., Udagawa, N. *et al.* (2001) Transforming growth factor β effects on osteoclast differentiation via direct and indirect actions. *Journal of Bone and Mineral Research* **16**, 1787–1794.

Rana M. W., Pothisiri, V., Killiany, D. M. and Xu, X. M. (2001) Detection of apoptosis during orthodontic tooth movement in rats. *American Journal of Orthodontics and Dentofacial Orthopedics* **119**, 516–521.

Rankovic, M. J., Docheva, D., Wichelhaus, A. and Baumert, U. (2020) Effect of static compressive force on in vitro cultured PDL fibroblasts: monitoring of viability and gene expression over 6 days. *Clinical Oral Investigations* **24**, 2497–2511.

Redlich, M., Asher Roos, H., Reichenberg, E. *et al.* (2004) Expression of tropoelastin in human periodontal ligament fibroblasts after simulation of orthodontic force. *Archives of Oral Biology* **49**, 119–124.

Redlich, M., Shoshan, S. and Palmon, A. (1999) Gingival response to orthodontic force. *American Journal of Orthodontics and Dentofacial Orthopedics* **116**, 152–158.

Reitan, K. (1972) Mechanism of apical root resorption. *Transactions of the European Orthodontics Society* 363–379.

Ren, Y., Maltha, J. C. and Kuijpers-Jagtman, A. M. (2004) The rat as a model for orthodontic tooth movement – a critical review and a proposed solution. *European Journal of Orthodontics* **26**, 483–490.

Reyna, J., Moon, H. B., Maung, V. *et al.* (2006) Gene expression induced by orthodontic tooth movement and/or root resorption, in *Biological Mechanisms of Tooth Eruption, Resorption and Movement* (eds. Z. Davidovitch, J. Mah and S. Suthanarak). Harvard Society for the Advancement of Orthodontics, Boston, MA, pp. 45–75.

Roberts, W. E. (1999) Bone dynamics of osseointegration, ankylosis, and tooth movement. *Journal of Indiana Dental Association* **78**, 24–32.

Roberts, W. E., Huja, S. and Roberts, J. A. (2004) Bone modeling – biomechanics, molecular mechanisms and clinical perspectives. *Seminars in Orthodontics* **10**, 123–161.

Roberts-Clark, D. J. and Smith, A. J. (2000) Angiogenic growth factors in human dentine matrix. *Archives of Oral Biology* **45**, 1013–1016.

Rody, W. J., King, J. and Gu, G. (2001) Osteoclast recruitment to sites of compression in orthodontic tooth movement. *American Journal of Orthodontics and Dentofacial Orthopedics* **120**, 477–489.

Rossi, M., Whitcomb, S. and Lindemann, R. (1996) Interleukin-1 beta and tumor necrosis factor-alpha production by human monocytes cultured with L-thyroxine and thyrocalcitonin: relation to severe root shortening. *American Journal of Orthodontics and Dentofacial Orthopedics* **110**, 399–404.

Safadi, F. F., Xu, J., Smock, S. L. *et al.* (2003) Expression of connective tissue growth factor in bone – its role in osteoblast proliferation and differentiation in vitro and bone formation *in vivo*. *Journal of Cell Physiology* **196**, 51–62.

Saito, S., Ngan, P., Saito, M. *et al.* (1990) Effect of cytokines of prostaglandin E and cAMP in human periodontal ligament fibroblasts in vivo. *Archives of Oral Biology* **35**, 387–395.

Sandy, J. R. (1998) Signal transduction. *British Journal of Orthodontics* **25**, 269–274.

Sanuki, R., Shionome, C., Kuwabara, A. *et al.* (2010) Compressive force induces osteoclast differentiation via prostaglandin E(2) production in MC3T3-E1 cells. *Connective Tissue Research* **51**, 150–158.

Sasaki, T. and Ueno-Matsuda, E. (1992) Immunocytochemical localization of cathepsins B and G in odontoclasts of human deciduous teeth. *Journal of Dental Research* **71**, 1881–1884.

Shigehara, S., Matsuzaka, K. and Inoue, T. (2006) Morphohistological change and expression of HSP70, osteopontin and osteocalcin mRNAs in rat dental pulp cells with orthodontic tooth movement. *Bulletin of Tokyo Dental College* **47**, 117–124.

Shigeyama, Y., Grove, T. K., Strayhorn, C. and Somerman, M. J. (1996) Expression of adhesion molecules during tooth resorption in feline teeth: a model system for aggressive osteoclastic activity. *Journal of Dental Research* **75**, 1650–1657.

Shimono, M., Ishikawa, T., Ishikawa, H. *et al.* (2003) Regulatory mechanisms of periodontal regeneration. *Microscopy Research and Techniques* **60**, 491–502.

Sinha, P. (1996) The relationship between orthodontic tooth movement and root resorption in PGE2 and non-PGE2 treated sides in a rat model, in *Biological Mechanisms of Tooth Movement and Craniofacial Adaptation* (ed. Z. Davidovitch). Harvard Society for the Advancement of Orthodontics, Boston, MA, pp. 337–348.

Sismanidou, C., Hilliges, M. and Lindskog, S. (1996) Healing of the root surface-associated periodontium: an immunohistochemical study of orthodontic root resorption in man. *European Journal of Orthodontics* **18**, 435–444.

Sondeijker, C., Lamberts, A. A., Beckmann, S. H. *et al.* (2020) Development of a clinical practice guideline for orthodontically induced external apical root resorption. *European Journal of Orthodontics* **42**(2), 115–124.

Sprogar, S., Meh, A., Vaupotic, T. *et al.* (2010) Expression levels of endothelin-1, endothelin-2, and endothelin-3 vary during the initial, lag, and late phase of orthodontic tooth movement in rats. *European Journal of Orthodontics*, **32**(3), 324–328.

Stewart, D. R., Sherick, P., Kramer, S., and Breining, P. (2005) Use of relaxin in orthodontics. *Annals of New York Academy of Science* **1041**, 379–387.

Su, M., Borke, J. L., Donahue, H. J. *et al.* (1997) Expression of connexin 43 in rat mandibular bone and periodontal ligament (PDL) cells during experimental tooth movement. *Journal of Dental Research* **76**(7), 1357–1366.

Sulakshana, K., Vijayaraghavan, N. and Krishnan, V. (2019) Time–dependent variation in expression patterns of Lysyl Oxidase, Type I Collagen and tropoelastin mRNA in response to orthodontic force application. *Archives of Oral Biology* **102**, 218–224.

Symmank, J., Zimmermann, S., Goldschmitt, J. *et al.* (2019) Mechanically induced GDF15 secretion by periodontal ligament fibroblasts regulates osteogenic transcription. *Scientific Reports* **9**(1), 1–8.

Swidi, A. J., Taylor, R. W., Tadlock, L. P. and Buschang, P. H. (2018) Recent advances in orthodontic retention methods: a review article. *Journal of the World Federation of Orthodontics* **7**, 6–12.

Takahashi, I., Nishimura, M., Onodera, K. *et al.* (2003) Expression of MMP-8 and MMP-13 genes in the periodontal ligament during tooth movement in rats. *Journal of Dental Research* **82**, 646–651.

Takahashi, I., Onodera, K., Nishimura, M. *et al.* (2006) Expression of genes for gelatinases and tissue inhibitors of metalloproteinases in periodontal tissues during orthodontic tooth movement. *Journal of Molecular Histology* **37**, 333–342.

Takano, M., Yamaguchi, M., Nakajima, R. *et al.* (2009) Effects of relaxin on collagen type I released by stretched human periodontal ligament cells. *Orthodontics and Craniofacial Research* **12**, 282–288.

Takashi, N., Udagawa, N., Akatsu, T. *et al.* (1991) Role of colony stimulating factors in osteoclast development. *Journal of Bone and Mineral Research* **6**, 977–985.

Tang, L., Lin, Z. and Li, Y. M. (2006) Effects of different magnitudes of mechanical strain on Osteoblasts in vitro. *Biochemical and Biophysical Research Communications* **344**, 122–128.

Teixeira, C. C., Khoo, E., Tran, J. et al. (2010) Cytokine expression and accelerated tooth movement. *Journal of Dental Research* **89**, 1135–1141.

ten Dijke, P., Iwata, K. K., Goddard, C. et al. (1990) Recombinant transforming growth factor type ß3: biological activities and receptor binding properties in isolated bone cells. *Molecular and Cellular Biology* **10**, 4473–4479.

Terai, K., Takano-Yamamoto, T., Ohba, Y. et al. (1999) Role of osteopontin in bone remodeling caused by mechanical stress. *Journal of Bone and Mineral Research* **14**, 839–849.

Theodorou, C. I., Kuijpers-Jagtman, A. M., Bronkhorst, E. M. and Wagener, F. (2019) Optimal force magnitude for bodily orthodontic tooth movement with fixed appliances: a systematic review. *American Journal of Orthodontics and Dentofacial Orthopedics* **156**(5), 582–592.

Tresguerres, F. G. F., Torres, J., López-Quiles, J. et al. (2020) The osteocyte: a multifunctional cell within the bone. *Annals of Anatomy* **227**, 151422.

Tsubota, M., Sasano, Y., Takahashi, I. et al. (2002) Expression of MMP-8 and MMP-13 mRNAs in rat periodontium during tooth eruption. *Journal of Dental Research* **81**, 673–678.

Tyrovola, J. B., Spyropoulos, M. N., Makou, M. and Perrea, D. (2008) Root resorption and the OPG/RANKL/RANK system: a mini review. *Journal of Oral Sciences* **50**, 367–376.

Uematsu, S., Mogi, M. and Deguchi, T. (1996) Interleukin (IL)-1beta, IL-6, tumor necrosis factor-alpha, epidermal growth factor and beta2 microglobulin are elevated in gingival crevicular fluid during human orthodontic tooth movement. *Journal of Dental Research* **75**, 562–567.

Vansant, L., Cadenas De Llano-Pérula, M., Verdonck, A. and Willems, G. (2018) Expression of biological mediators during orthodontic tooth movement: a systematic review. *Archives of Oral Biology* **95**, 170–186.

Viecilli, R. F., Katona, T. R., Chen, J. et al. (2009) Orthodontic mechanotransduction and the role of the P2X7 receptor. *American Journal of Orthodontics and Dentofacial Orthopedics* **135**, 694.

Villa, P. A., Oberti, G., Moncada, C. A. et al. (2005) Pulp–dentine complex changes and root resorption during intrusive orthodontic tooth movement in patients prescribed nabumetone. *Journal of Endodontics* **31**, 61–66.

Von Böhl, M., Ren, Y., Kuijpers-Jagtman, A. M. et al. (2016) Age-related changes of dental pulp tissue after experimental tooth movement in rats. *PeerJ* **4**, e1625.

Von Böhl, M. and Kuijpers-Jagtman, A. M. (2009) Hyalinization during orthodontic tooth movement: a systematic review on tissue reactions. *European Journal of Orthodontics* **31**, 30–36.

Von Böhl, M., Ren, Y., Fudalej, P. S. and Kuijpers-Jagtman, A. M. (2012) Pulpal reactions to orthodontic force application in humans: a systematic review. *Journal of Endodontics* **38**, 1463–1469.

Waddington, R. J. and Embery, G. (2001) Proteoglycans and orthodontic tooth movement. *Journal of Orthodontics* **28**, 281–290.

Weltman, B., Vig, K. W., Fields, H. W. et al. (2010) Root resorption associated with orthodontic tooth movement: a systematic review. *American Journal of Orthodontics and Dentofacial Orthopedics* **137**, 462–476.

Wilde, J., Yokozeki, M., Terai, K. et al. (2003) The divergent expression of periostin mRNA in the periodontal ligament during experimental tooth movement. *Cell and Tissue Research* **312**, 345–351.

Wolf, M., Lossdörfer, S., Küpper, K. and Jäger, A. (2014) Regulation of high mobility group box protein 1 expression following mechanical loading by orthodontic forces in vitro and in vivo. *European Journal of Orthodontics* **36**(6), 624–631.

Wolf, M., Lossdörfer, S., Abuduwali, N. and Jäger, A. (2013) Potential role of high mobility group box protein 1 and intermittent PTH (1-34) in periodontal tissue repair following orthodontic tooth movement in rats. *Clinical Oral Investigations* **17**, 989–997.

Wong, V. S., Freer, T. J., Joseph, B. K. and Daley, T. J. (1999) Tooth movement and vascularity of the dental pulp: a pilot study. *Australian Orthodontic Journal* **15**, 246–250.

Wu, L., Su, Y., Lin, F. et al. (2020) MicroRNA-21 promotes orthodontic tooth movement by modulating the RANKL/OPG balance in T cells. *Oral Diseases* **26**(2), 370–380.

Xu, C., Hao, Y., Wei, B. et al. (2011) Apoptotic gene expression by human periodontal ligament cells following cyclic stretch. *Journal of Periodontal Research* **46**, 742–748.

Yamaguchi, M. and Kasai, K. (2005) Inflammation in periodontal tissues in response to mechanical forces. *Archivum Immunologiae et Therapiae Experimentalis (Warsz)* **53**, 388–398.

Yamashiro, T., Fukunaga, T., Kobashi, N. et al. (2001) Mechanical stimulation induces CTGF expression in rat osteocytes. *Journal of Dental Research* **80**, 461–465.

Yang, S. Y., Ko, H. M., Kang, J. H. et al. (2011) Relaxin is upregulated in the rat ovary by orthodontic tooth movement. *European Journal of Oral Sciences* **119**(2), 115–120.

Yokoya, K., Sasaki, T. and Shibasaki, Y. (1997) Distributional changes of osteoclasts and pre-osteoclastic cells in periodontal tissues during experimental tooth movement as revealed by quantitative immunohistochemistry of H(+)-ATPase. *Journal of Dental Research* **76**, 580–587.

Yoneda, M., Suzuki, H., Hatano, N. et al. (2019) PIEZO1 and TRPV4, which are distinct mechano-sensors in the osteoblastic MC3T3-E1 cells, modify cell-proliferation. *International Journal of Molecular Sciences* **20**(19), 4960.

Yoshida, Y., Sasaki, T., Yokoya, K. et al. (1999) Cellular roles in relapse processes of experimentally moved rat molars. *Journal of Electron Microscopy* **48**, 147–157.

Yoshimatsu, M., Uehara, M. and Yoshida, N. (2008) Expression of heat shock protein 47 in the periodontal ligament during orthodontic tooth movement. *Archives of Oral Biology* **53**, 890–895.

Yu, W., Zhang, Y., Jiang, C. et al. (2016) Orthodontic treatment mediates dental pulp microenvironment via IL17A. *Archives of Oral Biology* **66**, 22–29.

Yue, Y., Chen, Z., Xie, B. and Yao, H. L. (2018) Expression of vascular endothelial growth factor in periodontal tissues during orthodontic tooth movement and its role in bone remodelling. *Shanghai Journal of Stomatology* **27**(1), 18–21.

Zainal Ariffin, S. H., Yamamoto, Z., ZainolAbidin, I. Z. et al. (2011) Cellular and molecular changes in orthodontic tooth movement. *Scientific World Journal* **11**, 1788–1803.

Zernik, J. H. and Minken, C. (1992) Genetic control of bone remodeling. *Journal of the California Dental Association* **20**, 14–19.

Zhang, F., Wang, C. L., Koyama, Y. et al. (2010) Compressive force stimulates the gene expression of IL-17 s and their receptors in MC3T3-E1 cells. *Connective Tissue Research* **51**, 359–369.

Zhang, J., Zhou, S., Zheng, H. et al. (2012a) Magnetic bead-based salivary peptidome profiling analysis during orthodontic treatment durations. *Biochemical and Biophysics Research Communications* **421**, 844–849.

Zhang, P., Wu, Y., Jiang, Z. et al. (2012b) Osteogenic response of mesenchymal stem cells to continuous mechanical strain is dependent on ERK1/2-Runx2 signaling. *International Journal of Molecular Medicine* **29**, 1083–1089.

Zhang, R., Li, J., Li, G. et al. (2020) LncRNA Nron regulates osteoclastogenesis during orthodontic bone resorption. *International Journal of Oral Science* **12**, 14.

Zhao, N., Lin, J., Kanzaki, H. et al. (2012a) Local osteoprotegerin gene transfer inhibits relapse of orthodontic tooth movement. *American Journal of Orthodontics and Dentofacial Orthopedics* **141**, 30–40.

Zhao, N., Liu, Y., Kanzaki, H. et al. (2012b) Effects of local osteoprotegerin gene transfection on orthodontic root resorption during retention: an *in vivo* micro-C analysis. *Orthodontics and Craniofacial Research* **15**, 10–20.

Zou, Y., Xu, L. and Lin, H. (2019) Stress overload-induced periodontal remodelling coupled with changes in high mobility group protein B1 during tooth movement: an in-vivo study. *European Journal of Oral Sciences* **127**(5), 396–407.

CHAPTER 13
Precision Orthodontics: Limitations and Possibilities in Practice

James K. Hartsfield, Jr., Priyanka Gudsoorkar, and Lorri A. Morford

---

Summary

Personalized medicine, now more frequently referred to as precision medicine, is the application of a specific type of treatment to an individual because that person belongs to a subpopulation of patients who are expected to develop disease and/or respond to treatment differently than the rest of the overall patient population. This use of specialized care is typically based on a unique set of clinical observations and/or the results from specific medical assessments (including but not limited to genetic, immunologic, and/or metabolic tests). For orthodontics, the application of precision medicine may be warranted when a patients' phenotype is driven or influenced by a specific etiology, when a variable response to treatment is observed, and/or when variation in stability following orthodontic treatment with or without surgical correction is noted. However, it remains to be seen how much precision medicine will impact orthodontics on the level of daily practice and into the future. What would precision orthodontics be based upon? How would the studies be undertaken and validated in practice? How will this be funded? Understanding the influence of and the interaction between genetic and environmental factors (e.g., orthodontic treatment) that can act on the treatment response of patients and the stability of that response is fundamental to the evidence-based practice of orthodontics (i.e., we must understand the impact of nature plus nurture together).

Introduction

Definition

"Personalized medicine" refers to the adaptation of medical care to the individual characteristics of each patient. Although the use of the word "personalized" is sometimes taken to mean treatment implemented to address the unique needs of a single patient, the terminology "personalized medicine" was intended to describe the process of classifying individuals into subpopulations that differ in their susceptibility to a disease and/or their response to a specific treatment (also termed population stratification) so that a subpopulation of patients could benefit from targeted treatment. In order to avoid this type of confusion, the terminology "precision medicine" is now often preferred over "personalized medicine".

The label "precision medicine" may also reflect the goal of integrating genomic data towards a more molecularly based taxonomy of disease and its treatment, such as is seen with the field of pharmacogenetics (National Research Council, 2011). Preventive or therapeutic interventions can then be concentrated on those who will benefit most, sparing expense and side effects for those who will not (Behrens, 2008). Others have noted that the treatment outcomes of an individual patient, including his or her response(s) to drug therapy, are not and are unlikely to ever be determined exclusively by genomic variation, even as analyzed by entire genome sequencing (Roden and Tyndale, 2013). Although the focus can be on genomic variation, precision healthcare includes a variety of "-omics," e.g., epigenomics, transcriptomics, proteomics, metabolomics, lipidomics, ionomics, as well as social determinants of health, etc. facilitated by advancing technology, increasingly large-scale databases, and bioinformatics (Figure 13.1) (National Research Council, 2011; Yan et al., 2015; Khoury et al., 2016; Allareddy et al., 2019; Meyer, 2020).

Evidence-based guidelines practice versus precision medicine practice

Evidence-based practice guidelines are founded on the clinical data available for a specific question. There are varying levels of evidence used to produce these important guidelines, with meta-analyses and randomized clinical trials at the top of the evidence pyramid (Paul and Leibovici, 2014). Although evidence-based guidelines are designed to promote optimized clinical care for the majority of patients, there are some individuals who will not respond to the

---

Biological Mechanisms of Tooth Movement, Third Edition. Edited by Vinod Krishnan, Anne Marie Kuijpers-Jagtman and Ze'ev Davidovitch.
© 2021 John Wiley & Sons Ltd. Published 2021 by John Wiley & Sons Ltd.

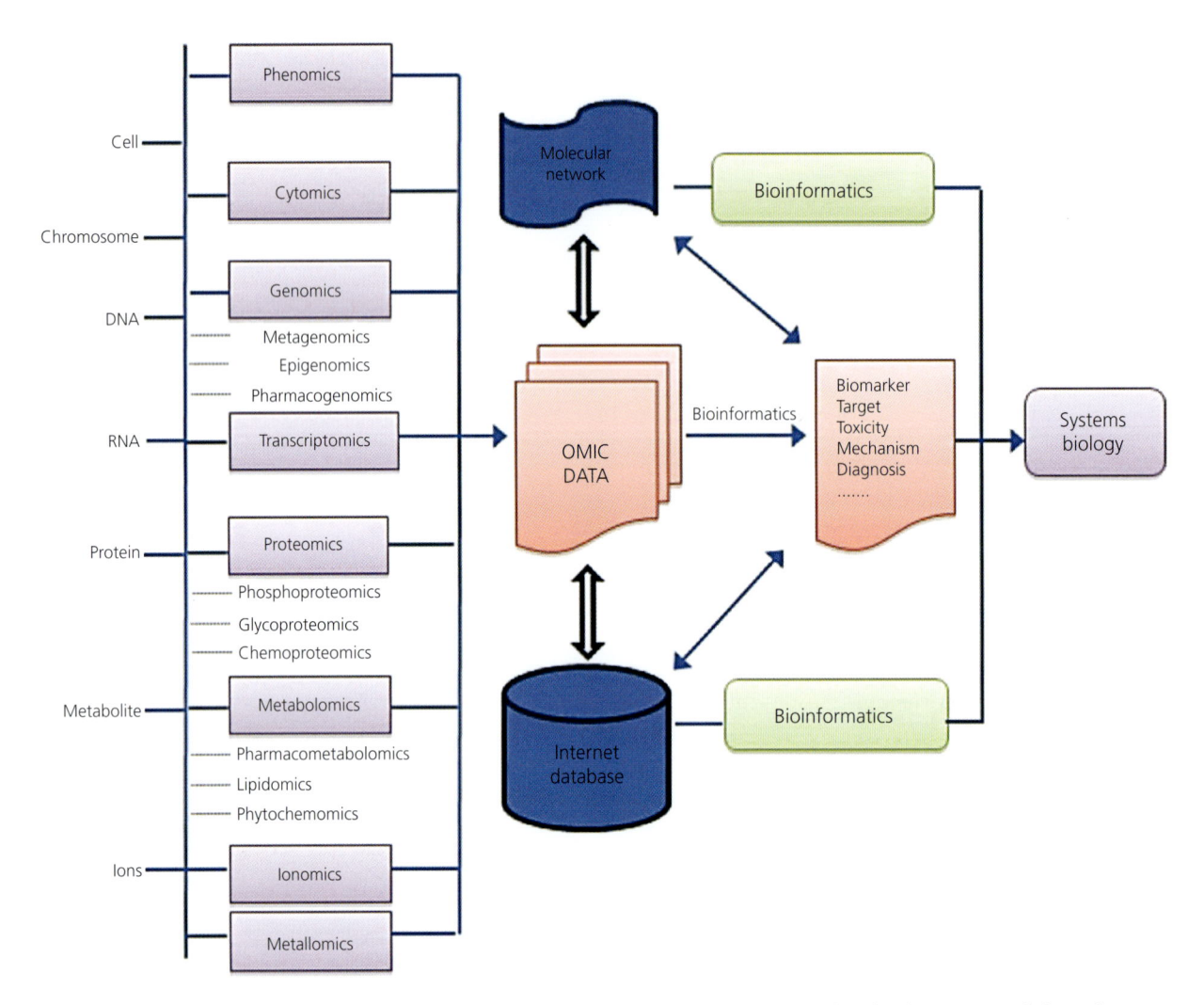

Figure 13.1 Various "omics" techniques and their roles in systems biology. (Source: Yan *et al.*, 2015. Reproduced with permission of Elsevier.)

same degree as those falling within the population norm (Berlin *et al.*, 2002; Schmid *et al.*, 2004), despite even the highest level of patient compliance during treatment. This heterogeneity in response to treatment may in part be due to genetic variation among the patients receiving treatment and/or could be due to other treatment-related factors. An analysis claiming that a single characteristic influences a treatment outcome (e.g., the association of a specific genetic marker allele with the occurrence of external apical root resorption concurrent with orthodontia) may be of limited clinical significance unless variables that may modify the importance of that single characteristic (e.g., length of treatment, type of tooth movement, tooth extraction versus non-extraction, etc.) are also considered (Van der Weele and Knol, 2011).

Precision medicine is an approach aimed at individualizing the diagnosis and treatment of disease using genetic, biomarker, phenotypic, and/or psychosocial characteristics. This approach allows practitioners and researchers to predict more accurately which treatment and prevention strategies for a specific disease will work best in which groups of people. It contrasts with a one-size-fits-all approach. However, high-quality evidence is lacking for effectiveness in many applications as will be discussed later regarding gene testing. Although the paradigms of evidence-based medicine and precision medicine both have strengths and weaknesses (Beckmann and Lew, 2016), the ever-growing amount of high-resolution data generated by transformative tools like high-resolution molecular omics, imaging, clinical measures, and analysis of large data sets ("big data") can and will lead to a profound shift in healthcare (Collins, 2015).

Progression in DNA analysis technology and its impact on clinical research and practice

The Human Genome Project

The landmark sequencing of the human genome (The Human Genome Project) was only one step toward developing a "map" or understanding of not only how our genomes are similar, but also how variation occurs and influences phenotypic differences among us (International Human Genome Sequencing Consortium, 2001; Venter *et al.*, 2001). A phenotype is an individual's observable traits, such as height, eye color, blood, or malocclusion in three planes of space (Hartsfield and Bixler, 2010; https://www.genome.gov/genetics-glossary/). Our genome varies from one individual to the next most often in terms of single base changes within the DNA code called single nucleotide polymorphisms (SNPs, pronounced "snips"). The main research use of a human SNP map has been to determine the contributions of genes to diseases (or nondisease) phenotypes that have a complex, multifactorial basis (Chakravarti, 2001).

Following the sequencing of the human genome, generation of a haplotype "map" of the human genome was undertaken. It consists of a high-density summary of the SNPs that define ancestral haplotypes (blocks of tightly correlated genetic variants that are in linkage disequilibrium for different ethnic backgrounds) in each region of the human genome. Using this genome-wide linkage disequilibrium map, microarray chips (i.e., panels containing many of the most highly informative SNPs) and analysis software have enabled comprehensive and efficient testing of the association of genes with pathology and other types of traits (International HapMap Consortium, 2005). In order to investigate and test this growing body of data, the Precision Medicine Initiative was introduced by the Obama administration in 2015 to promote the prevention and treatment of disease taking into account the variability in the patient's genome, environment, and lifestyle (Collins and Varmus, 2015).

Genome-wide association studies (GWAS)

A genetic association study is a method to determine whether a specific polymorphic variant (e.g., a SNP) is more frequently inherited by a group of subjects with a specific pathology or "trait of interest" when compared with a control group. This approach had been initially used to look for an association of polymorphic variants within or neighboring a candidate gene for association to a specific trait or phenotype based on previous knowledge regarding the function of the candidate gene and/or its possible role in the development of the trait of interest. The downside to this approach is that it lacks the capability of new gene discovery in connection with a trait or phenotype, particularly when a gene plays a cumulative or modifying role on the expression of the trait and/or phenotype.

The development of haplotype maps, microarray chips, and the software to analyze the large amount of data produced by such studies eventually led to the inception of the genome-wide association study (GWAS). This type of study allows for the simultaneous testing of over a million SNP markers on all chromosomes for an association to a trait via a hypothesis-free or "agnostic" approach, which could yield new gene associations not previously suspected. Additional confidence that the identified associations are strong and relevant in a population are gained by replicating studies using large sample sizes (International HapMap Consortium, 2005). As a result, thousands of DNA variants have been identified that are associated with diseases and traits through candidate gene and GWAS studies (Hindorff et al., 2009). Statistical association with a disease or trait, however, does not mean that the genetic variation is predictive of the disease or trait, particularly when a complex (multiple genetic and environmental factors) etiology is involved.

Next-generation sequencing

Next-generation technology has transformed the scale of sequencing. Compared with the methods used for the Human Genome Project, modern sequencers are 50,000-fold faster, and therefore proportionately cheaper. In addition to sequencing DNA, next-generation sequencing (NGS) has the advantage of detecting gene fusions and translocations in conjunction with RNA sequencing. Also known as massively parallel or deep sequencing, NGS has revolutionized genomic research and its application in clinical care (Shendure et al., 2017). In contrast to Sanger Sequencing, where only short DNA reads of 100 to 300 DNA bases (including variants) at a single gene loci could accurately be resolved, the fundamental advance that enabled the substantial throughput gains from next-generation sequencers was the ability to simultaneously generate millions of short anchored sequencing reads commonly of 150 base pairs (bp), in massive parallel fashion across the entire genome in a short amount of time.

Although generating high coverage across the entire genome (referred to as whole genome sequencing, or WGS) is decreasing in price, a common alternative is to use hybridization capture to enrich a DNA sample only for sequences in the exons of coding genes that make up approximately 1–2% of the whole genome (known as the 'exome'), resulting in whole exome sequencing (WES) (Bamshad et al., 2011). Determination of the genes responsible for still unknown Mendelian (Single-Gene) and Complex diseases and traits presents an immediate opportunity to use this technology to move from approaches using only partial information (genetic linkage and/or GWAS) to complete analysis of the relationship between genomic variation and phenotype (Kilpinen and Barrett, 2013). The use of WGS and WES is rapidly overtaking SNP chip or single-gene tests (Drmanac, 2011; Zettler et al., 2014).

Human phenotype ontology

Analysis of even the most complete genotype data depends on an accurate and consistent description and classification of the phenotype. The Human Phenotype Ontology project (https://hpo.jax.org/app/) provides a structured and controlled vocabulary for the phenotypic features encountered in human hereditary and other disease (Robinson et al., 2008). This standardization allows for description of patients (including those with an undiagnosed condition) in shared databases without exposing identifiable personal health information and facilitates computational analysis of the human phenome and its relation to the genome and other datasets. The precise and comprehensive analysis of phenotypic abnormalities in which the individual components of the phenotype are observed and described have been termed "deep phenotyping" (Köhler et al., 2019). The analysis of the relationship of genomic variation with phenotypic variation is enhanced with the standardized description of the patients' features, including digital imaging for facial phenotype analysis (Robinson, 2012).

Application in medical practice

Technology has outpaced its application to most aspects of practice in that WGS data is not used in most routine healthcare today (McGuire and Burke, 2008). Yet, there are many examples of personalized medicine in current practice, notably in cancer treatment with a steady growth in the availability of targeted therapeutics since the approval of trastuzumab for human epidermal growth factor receptor 2 (HER2) receptor-positive breast cancer (Ginsburg, 2013). The classification(s) of many types of cancer today are determined in part by their molecular drivers and expected responses to targeted therapies (Roden and Tyndale, 2013). Other examples of the clinically useful application of pharmacogenetics include a targeted dosing algorithm for warfarin based on cytochrome P450 *CYP2C9* genotype, and the reduction in the incidence of adverse events by checking for susceptible genotypes for drugs like abacavir, carbamazepine, and clozapine (Fernald et al., 2011).

In 2011, there were more than 1,000 genomic tests available in clinical practice for an estimated 2,500 conditions with approximately 30% specific to oncology (Gwinn et al., 2011). In 2013 the number was more than 2,000 tests (Green et al., 2013). Along with the accelerating pace of discovery and the relatively unregulated availability of genome-based tests for cancer prevention and care (Ramsey et al., 2011) little research has looked at the clinical utility of these applications. Although quality, safety, and efficacy standards must be met before a medication can be prescribed to patients, the value of a laboratory test does not have to be proven prior to its implementation (Bates, 2014). Not surprisingly, health insurers have struggled to determine which emerging genomic applications merit coverage, especially because, to date, there is insufficient evidence of clinical utility for most of these applications, leading to skepticism by some providers and their customers of the added value of genomics to improve patient care (Scheuner et al., 2008; Simonds et al., 2013).

Although there are over 2,000 genetic tests available, the American College of Medical Genetics and Genomics (ACMG) Working Group on reporting incidental findings in clinical exome and genome sequencing determined a "minimum list" of DNA variants in 57 genes for 37 conditions for which incidental findings in a clinical setting should be reported if the data are readable (Green et al., 2013). The ACMG Secondary Findings Maintenance Working Group later updated the minimum list by adding four genes and removing one gene from the 2013 list (Kalia et al., 2017). In effect, the ACMG working groups decided that out of all the genetic tests available, only a small number were of sufficient validity and clinically actionable (actually would result in a change in the care of the patient) to recommend that if they were discovered on WGS or WES, that they be reported to the patient and their healthcare provider for their discussion and possible implementation.

Genome interpretive services are emerging to assist clinicians in understanding the meaning and actionability of genome information in much the same way as radiologists perform interpretation for imaging (Ginsburg, 2013). The role of the clinical geneticist certified by the American Board of Medical Genetics, or the genetic counselor certified by the American Board of Genetic Counseling, should expand to help both practitioners and their patients understand the genetic data that has been collected for their care (Katsanis and Katsanis, 2013; Dorschner et al., 2014; Swanson et al., 2014). In the future, there will likely be a need for some individuals with dental medicine or dental hygiene degrees to undergo further education in basic and clinical genetics in general, and in craniofacial genetics in particular. These individuals could both educate dental students, residents, and practitioners, and act as practice consultants in the application of genome information in patient care.

Efficacy of risk prediction of Mendelian (single-gene) versus complex traits

Genetic diseases or traits that are strongly associated with a single gene (whether dominant or recessive in their inheritance) are referred to as Mendelian, after Gregor Mendel. The simplest description of a single gene trait inherited as an autosomal dominant is that anyone who inherits the causative variation in the gene of interest that results in the condition, will typically present with some form of the condition. Variable expression as to the severity of the condition may still occur, however, even among the affected members of the same family and/or with traits having an autosomal dominant pattern of inheritance.

There can even be examples where the condition "skips a generation," and for whatever reason, perhaps due to a unique interaction of other genes, is not evident in an individual who has the single-gene genotype that would have been expected to result in the disease or trait. This phenomenon is referred to as non- or incomplete penetrance of the genotype expressing itself in the phenotype. Variable expressivity and incomplete penetrance occur in many conditions that may have a dominant inheritance, including hypodontia, Crouzon syndrome, and Class III malocclusion (Everett et al., 1999; Cruz et al., 2008; Hartsfield and Bixler, 2010; Hartsfield, 2011). This variable expressivity and even nonpenetrance of diseases and traits that have a "strong" genetic basis can make predicting the occurrence and/or the severity of the being affected imprecise. This of course also has clinical ramifications in the use of genotypic data to predict phenotype.

There is even less accuracy expected when trying to predict a disease or trait that has a complex inheritance or etiology. A complex trait infers it is the result of many factors, both genetic and potentially environmental, which interact. With several if not many genes involved, the finding that any number of genes are statistically associated with a trait or increased risk of developing that trait does not mean that consideration of an associated gene will be predictive *a priori*. For example, a significant association between genetic variation within the *CYP19A1* gene (which encodes the testosterone-to-estrogen converting enzyme aromatase) and the average annualized sagittal growth of the mandible during puberty in Caucasian and Chinese males has been reported in the literature. This genetic variation, however, only explains a small part of the total variation observed in the sagittal jaw growth in males, and by itself does not give a useful clinical prediction of jaw growth (Hartsfield et al., 2010; He et al., 2012). Without an understanding of the potential interaction of multiple genes, and the environmental factors, even predictions based on polygenic factors may substantially lack power.

This is a concern even when large studies are undertaken for conditions such as type 2 diabetes, coronary artery disease, and prostate cancer, and necessitate robust modeling based on increasing sample sizes and inclusion of other data such as family history (Chatterjee et al., 2013). The study sizes examined for these conditions are typically exponentially many times the typical size of a study involving facial growth, dental development, or other orthodontic areas of interest. Hence, when we are looking at complex craniofacial and oral traits, we are highly unlikely to reach a level where useful clinical prediction is a reality until we have studies that are of sufficient size and construction to ask and answer the questions involving so many factors.

Precision oral healthcare

A combination of advancing materials, imaging, and other technologies along with genomics are evolving in dentistry. Some examples include: tissue reconstruction using stem cell biology, biomaterial science, and tissue engineering for patients with orofacial injuries (especially cancer patients) or developmental anomalies (Zhang et al., 2019). The multicenter study "Orofacial Pain: Prospective Evaluation and Risk Assessment" (OPPERA), investigated the risk factors for onset and persistence of temporomandibular muscle and joint disorders (TMD), including genomic variants (Maixner et al., 2011; Dworkin, 2013; Smith et al., 2019).

Perhaps the area in which precision medicine is currently applied most is in cancer treatment, particularly for the various genomic types of breast cancer (Heinemann et al., 2018; Sun et al., 2019). Although personalized treatment for oral pharyngeal cancer (primarily comprised of squamous cell carcinomas) is currently based on tumor stage and location, development of customized therapies based on the biology of the individual tumor, the use of immunotherapeutic agents and/or activation of the patient's immunity are ongoing (D'Silva, 2015; D'Silva and Gutkind, 2019).

The study or application of precision care is not just directed to the patient's genome. Oral diseases such as periodontitis and caries involve the oral microbiome in their pathogenicity. Modulating the pathogenesis of the oral microbiome may for example be used to decrease the prevalence and severity of caries (Baker *et al.*, 2019). In addition, "big-data" investigations into genomic variants associated with phenotypes including periodontitis and caries yield additional candidate loci to investigate for their role in the etiologic heterogeneity and possible population stratification (Allareddy *et al.*, 2019; Divaris, 2019; Shungin *et al.*, 2019).

From personalized to precision orthodontics

In recognition of the 100th year of the *American Journal of Orthodontics and Dentofacial Orthopedics*, Professor David Carlson reviewed evolving concepts of heredity and genetics in orthodontics. He noted that Hartsfield was perhaps first to use the term

"personalized orthodontics" for scientific purposes (Hartsfield, 2008; Carlson, 2015), reflecting the use of the term personalized medicine at the time. Hartsfield and Carlson concluded that patient outcomes in orthodontics may be affected by polymorphic genes, making it important to understand gene variants in quantitative terms. The key concept of investigating the effect of variants in developmental genes, and variants in genes and epigenetics that affect the response to treatment, is illustrated by Carlson in Figure 13.2 (Carlson, 2015).

Orthodontists do not, of course, treat all patients the same. They form a treatment plan based on the diagnosis of every patient based on several factors, usually maturity and physical features. Here, however, precision orthodontics refers specifically to considering genetic data as well. To achieve that goal, the need to incorporate modern and developing genomic methodologies into clinical research in orthodontics was stressed, including clinical trials using appropriately stratified samples based on the genomic profile (Figure 13.3) (Hartsfield, 2008; Carlson, 2015).

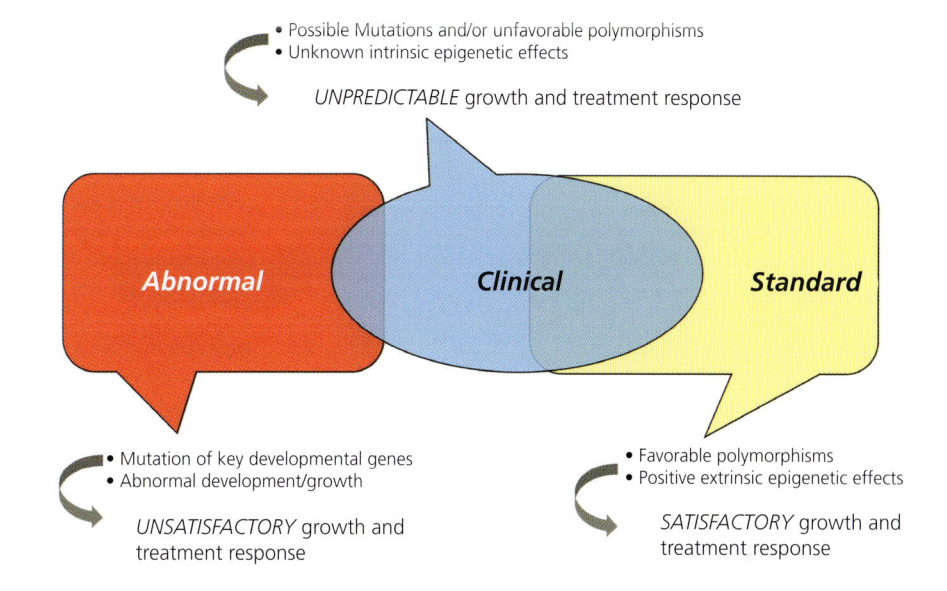

Figure 13.2 Heuristic model illustrating the basis and rationale for consideration of genomics in the treatment of malocclusion. (Source: Carlson, 2015. Reproduced with permission of Elsevier.)

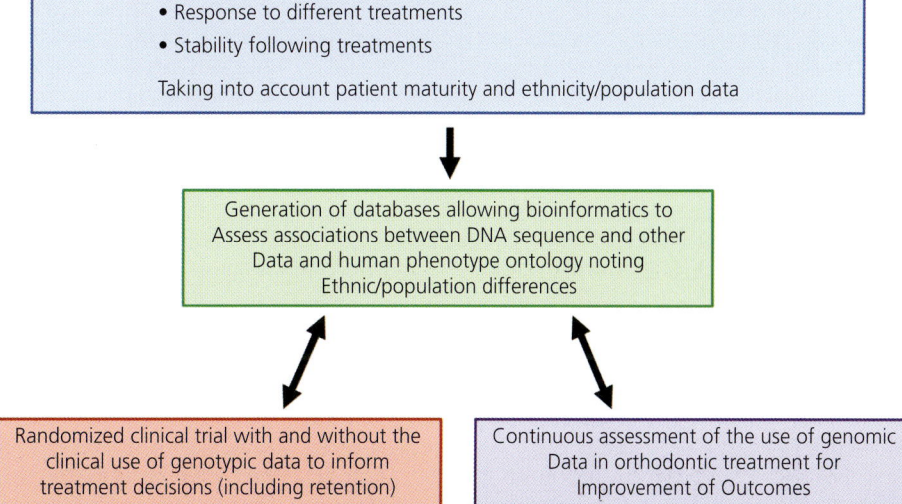

Figure 13.3 Development of precision orthodontics. *Human Phenotype Ontology Project (https://hpo.jax.org/app/). Genotyping would be performed on all patients, but only known in those randomly selected to have genomic data considered in the diagnosis and treatment planning of the patient. "Immediate" and longer term post-treatment assessments of all patients would be done with genomic data.

Class III malocclusion

We all realize there are patients with a Class III malocclusion who have distinctive jaw characteristics, (e.g., hypoplastic maxilla, hypertrophic mandible, or both), as well as variations in vertical and/or other facial dimensions. Analysis of the most common morphometric shapes among Class III patients have resulted in the delineation of different "subtypes" of Class III malocclusion, which appear to vary by ethnic background (Mackay et al., 1992; Singh et al., 1997; Singh et al., 1998; Bui et al., 2006; Staudt and Kiliaridis, 2009; Moreno Uribe et al., 2013; Li et al., 2016). In addition to better describing and understanding different Class III patients, this further classification has been proposed to define a characteristic morphology that is more likely to be correlated with a specific genetic variation.

Although it remains to be seen if these "subtypes" of Class III malocclusion correspond to one or more of the specific chromosomal locations or candidate genes associated with Class III so far or in the future (Hartsfield et al., 2012), this approach is a rational one to increase the likelihood of finding a genotype–phenotype correlation. If this is found, then the next step would be to determine which of the different treatment protocols would be more efficacious for certain subtypes than others. This type of analysis could of course be undertaken based solely on a morphometric classification, as we already do when we use different headgear vectors on Class II patients depending on their vertical dimension. However, the increased understanding of the biological factors involved may yield a better understanding of the treatment effect, and perhaps lead to new therapies.

Although many genetic markers on various chromosomes have been associated with Class III malocclusion through GWAS, the use of NGS in families has yielded a growing list of genetic variants associated with the malocclusion in those families, several of which are in key pathways of jaw development (Manocha et al., 2019). So far most families have had a different gene involved in the etiology of their malocclusion, emphasizing the genetic heterogeneity of Class III malocclusion, and the need for further investigation of the genetic variants associated with the malocclusion (Hartsfield Jr. et al., 2017; Kluemper et al., 2018; de Frutos-Valle et al., 2019; Genno et al., 2019; Kajii et al., 2019; Kantaputra et al., 2019; Rao et al., 2020). In addition, different variants in the same gene may be associated with Class III or Class II malocclusion (Jiang et al., 2019).

External apical root resorption concurrent with orthodontia

Another area of interest has been external apical root resorption (EARR) concurrent with orthodontia, starting with the first studies of specific genetic markers with its occurrence (Al-Qawasmi et al., 2003a, 2003b). Since then several groups have investigated some of the same and different genes and their variations (Bastos Lages et al., 2009; Gülden et al., 2009; Hartsfield, 2009; Tomoyasu et al., 2009; Fontana et al., 2012; Iglesias-Linares et al., 2012a, 2012b, 2014; Wu et al., 2012; Linhartova et al., 2013; Pereira et al., 2013; Sharab et al., 2015; Nowrin et al., 2018). The results have varied and, even when significant, indicate that the particular genetic marker being investigated has an effect size of 15% or less, showing that genetic variation plays a role in EARR, but no one factor is predictive. Larger studies in this area are needed particularly to look into the interaction of multiple gene products as well as other factors in EARR, such as length of treatment, premolar extractions, and distance of tooth movement.

Sagittal facial growth during puberty

Another aspect of clinical practice mentioned in the 2008 paper was the prediction of facial growth, particularly starting with a Class II malocclusion. We know from the Phase I treatment of Class II patients randomized clinical trial that, although there was a significant average difference among the control subjects, bionator subjects, and cervical headgear subjects at the end of Phase I, there was considerable variation in the growth of each group, with some controls growing more than individuals treated with either appliance (Tulloch et al., 1998). In addition, the average differences amongst the groups were not significant later after comprehensive treatment (Tulloch et al., 2004). This not only calls into question the efficacy of the treatment modalities long term, and but also suggests that individual growth potential is more significant than the treatment effects.

Investigations of the effect of one genetic factor on facial growth during puberty in orthodontic patients involved the cytochrome P450 *CYP19A1* gene. This gene codes for the enzyme aromatase, which converts testosterone and androstenedione to estradiol and estrone respectively (Guo et al., 2006). The rate of this conversion is critical for the testosterone/estrogen (T/E) ratio in the body. The T/E ratio is critical in the development of sex-indexed facial characteristics such as the growth of cheekbones, the mandible and chin, the prominence of eyebrow ridges and the lengthening of the lower face (Schaefer et al., 2005, 2006).

In one study, the difference in the average sagittal jaw growth between the two groups of Caucasian males with different alleles (different versions of the same gene) with the greatest differences in growth per year was just over 1.5 mm per year during treatment for the maxilla, and 2.5 mm per year for the mandible. There was no statistical difference for the particular *CYP19A1* genetic marker in females. This is particularly impressive since at the beginning of treatment there was no significant difference among the males based upon the *CYP19A1* genotype. The significant difference only expressed itself over the time of treatment during the cervical vertebral stage associated with increased growth velocity (Hartsfield et al., 2010).

Interestingly, the same result was found in a group of Chinese males and females, strongly suggesting that this variation in the *CYP19A1* gene may be a multiethnic marker for sagittal facial growth (He et al., 2012). Although the difference in average annual sagittal mandibular and maxillary growth based upon this *CYP19A1* genotype was significant in males during pubertal orthodontic treatment, this one factor accounts for only a relatively small part of the variation seen in the complex trait of sagittal jaw growth, and therefore by itself has little predictive power. Further investigation of this and other genetic factors, their interactions with each other and with environmental factors, will help to explain what has up to now been an unknown component of individual variations in facial growth.

Primary failure of eruption

A specific condition not mentioned in the 2008 paper highlights the recent investigations into primary failure of eruption (PFE). Although relatively rare, PFE does occur and can have a marked effect on orthodontic treatment, whereby teeth affected by PFE act as natural anchors when orthodontic forces are placed on them for their extrusion. In some families it has an autosomal dominant mode of inheritance, with variable expressivity. This means that family members who are affected are not necessarily affected in the same pattern or severity. Certainly, a family history of PFE, as with other conditions that can have a complex or single-gene mode of inheritance, are a strong indicator that the practitioner should be aware, particularly if the same lack of eruption is seen in the next family member. However, sometimes with the variation seen in the expression of PFE, or in cases in which there is no family history either perhaps by chance or a new mutation, then genetic analysis for the cause of PFE could be useful.

This was facilitated by the discovery of mutations in the parathyroid hormone 1 receptor (*PTH1R*) gene in patients with PFE (Decker *et al.*, 2008; Frazier-Bowers *et al.*, 2010; Stellzig-Eisenhauer *et al.*, 2010). This finding does not make the genetic testing necessarily fail proof for a diagnosis since as with most genetic conditions, more than one variation in the gene may be associated with the same or a similar condition. In addition, sometimes genetic variations outside of the part that codes for the protein vary, or may be influenced by outside factors, to change the transcription of the DNA sequence into its protein. Still, this is an interesting example of a specific single-gene condition that can have a marked effect on malocclusion and how it is treated, and that can be investigated by genetic analysis (Frazier-Bowers *et al.*, 2010).

These recent examples show how this is just the beginning of a potentially long process of understanding how variation in the gene(s) and therefore the product protein(s) interact with each other, and with environmental factors over time to lead to or influence the variation in growth or pathology of interest. This is particularly true when a gene that contributes some increased likelihood of growth variation or pathology is only one of several that may be involved. These are often referred to as susceptibility genes, as particular variations present in them may be associated with, but not guarantee, the likelihood that a variation in growth or pathology will be present or develop.

Support of next generation sequencing, other genetic studies, and the utility of their application in orthodontics

The introduction of innovative technologies has enabled researchers to utilize novel study designs to tackle previously unexplored research questions in human genomics. These new types of studies typically need large sample sizes to overcome the multiple testing challenges caused by the enormous number of interrogated genetic variants. As a consequence, large consortia-studies are at present the default in disease genetics research (Palotie *et al.*, 2013). These will also be required in orthodontics if any significant headway is to be made.

These large size studies will require the integration of genomic information with clinical and physical examination data. To that end, the NIH's Electronic Medical Records and Genomics (eMERGE) network seeks to develop and apply approaches to test whether electronic medical record systems can serve as resources for complex genomic analyses of disease and therapeutic outcomes (McCarty *et al.*, 2011). Unfortunately currently, there are no oral, dental, or craniofacial primary phenotypes under study within the eMERGE network, highlighting a significant future opportunity (Garcia *et al.*, 2013). Since most oral, dental, and craniofacial variations in growth and development, diseases, and disorders such as dental caries, periodontal diseases, oral and pharyngeal cancers, chronic orofacial pain, cleft lip/cleft palate, and malocclusion arise from a complex interaction of genetic, biological, behavioral, and environmental factors, the integration and analysis of substantial amounts of genetic and clinical data will be necessary (Hartsfield, 2011; Garcia *et al.*, 2013).

In a time of national budget constraints and a largely stagnant NIH budget for several years, the importance of studies to analyze the diagnosis for and outcome of orthodontic treatment is sometimes not appreciated by non-orthodontists. It will be imperative for the profession to support this type of research for it to proceed, to show its validity, and to attract NIH funding. Undoubtedly, significant challenges lie ahead, though none are insurmountable. Yet expectations must be realistic: the investigation and application of genomic information to healthcare will happen neither automatically nor overnight (Mirnezami *et al.*, 2012). Orthodontics in the era of big data analytics has gained popularity. Machine learning has become increasingly utilized in healthcare in recent years and has been successful in identifying disease subtypes as well as providing insights into rare diseases and associated outcomes, predictive modelling, and identification of targeted therapies (Handelman *et al.*, 2018). With increased awareness of the current and emerging technologies, facilitated translation of approaches toward precision orthodontics holds ever-increasing promise (Iwasaki *et al.*, 2015).

An important concept to investigate in the future is not only the contribution of genetic variation (and hence the protein variation in structure and or amount) to phenotype variability, but the genetic contribution to the patients response to treatment, and the genetic contribution to the stability of the treatment effect (retention). The genomic (proteomic) variation associated with clinical variation for etiology, treatment response, and retention may or may not be the same for these three areas of clinical interest (Figure 13.4).

A significant hurdle to overcome if personalized/precision orthodontics is to progress relates to the lack of large database information. As Allareddy *et al.* stated "There is a need for real-time, collaborative data pooling for the purpose of quality improvement in orthodontics" (Allareddy *et al.*, 2019). In addition to private practice surveys, and pooling clinical data from practices, clinics, and residency programs, research on facial morphology and genomics from non-orthodontic patient groups or databases will be useful to identify genomic variants that may be associated with facial morphological variation (Weinberg *et al.*, 2019), and to serve as a population sample for comparison with orthodontic patients.

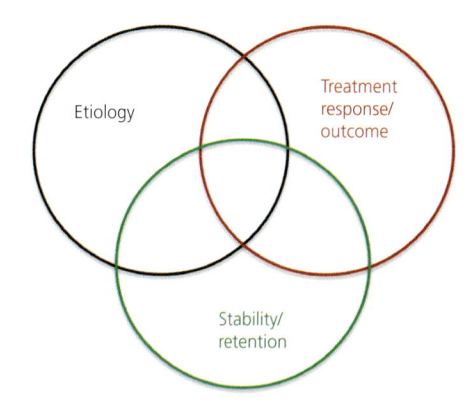

Figure 13.4 A Venn diagram illustrating the concept that the genomic/proteomic variation can be associated with clinical variation for etiology, treatment response, and retention. It is important to note that the genomic/proteomic variation that impacts one or two of these areas may or may not be the same for all three areas of clinical interest.

Education

As orthodontists, we are responsible for the correct interpretation of the pathology seen on a radiograph. Likewise, how do we interpret any future genetic testing and are we responsible for counselling the patient and family for possible diseases or conditions that may be associated with the analysis we asked for? Many genetic variations are associated with an increased or decreased likelihood of more than one condition developing in various parts or systems of the body.

For example, apolipoprotein E *(APOE)-ε4* has been associated with an increased risk of developing Alzheimer disease. It has also been found in some studies to be significantly associated with the presence of sleep apnea. In the future evaluation of a patient who has a Class II malocclusion, your recommendation on surgery may include consideration of whether the patient will likely develop sleep apnea if a mandibular advancement is not performed. Not everyone who has or develops sleep apnea is obese with a high BMI, so there are currently studies to investigate genetic factors in sleep apnea, especially in the patient who is not obese. What if one of the genetic markers for sleep apnea is identified as *APOE-ε4*, and the patient's report states that they are homozygous for *APOE-ε4*, a known risk factor for developing Alzheimer disease? Will you tell the patient, or refer them to their physician or clinical geneticist/genetic counselor, or ignore it since it is not in your area of practice (Roedig *et al.*, 2014)?

Practitioners in all fields, including dentists, need to learn more about genetics, genomics, and their interpretation and application to practice and other issues. As genetic testing becomes more common, it is unclear how well prepared healthcare providers, including dentists, will be to interpret them. Dental schools will need to incorporate genetics and genomics into their curricula, and dentists will need to keep up with rapidly changing technologies (Garcia *et al.*, 2013). There have been calls for teaching and learning objectives to be prepared, and text material to be published for genetics in dental school curricula, including pediatric dentistry, and graduate orthodontic programs (Collins and Tabak, 2004; Dudlicek *et al.*, 2004; Johnson *et al.*, 2008; Hartsfield and Bixler, 2010; Hartsfield, 2011).

Conclusion

Multiple factors and processes contribute to the response to orthodontic treatment. Some patients will exhibit unusual outcomes linked to or associated with polymorphic genes. Although it may be imprecise in informing patient care, taking a family history is still important because it reflects the presence, not only of single-gene disorders, but also of shared genes, shared environments, and complex gene–environment interactions, even if "genetic testing" is never contemplated (Khoury, 2003). Analysis of overall treatment response requires a systems analysis using informatics for integration of all relevant information. The influence of genetic factors on treatment outcome must be studied and understood in quantitative terms. Conclusions from retrospective studies must be evaluated by prospective testing to evaluate their value in practice. Genome-wide association, whole genome and exome sequencing studies are necessary to further the evidence base for the practice of orthodontics. Only then will we begin to truly understand how nature (genetic factors) and nurture (environment factors, including treatment) together affect the treatment of our patients.

References

Al-Qawasmi, R. A., Hartsfield, J. K., Jr., Everett, E. T. *et al.* (2003a) Genetic predisposition to external apical root resorption. *American Journal of Orthodontics and Dentofacial Orthopedics* **123**, 242–252.

Al-Qawasmi, R. A., Hartsfield, J. K., Jr., Everett, E. T. *et al.* (2003b) Genetic predisposition to external apical root resorption in orthodontic patients: linkage of chromosome-18 marker. *Journal of Dental Research* **82**, 356–360.

Allareddy, V., Rengasamy Venugopalan, S., Nalliah, R. P. *et al.* (2019) Orthodontics in the era of big data analytics. *Orthodontics and Craniofacial Research* **22**, 8–13.

Baker, J., He, X. and Shi, W. (2019) Precision reengineering of the oral microbiome for caries management. *Advances In Dental Research* **30**, 34–39.

Bamshad, M. J., Ng, S. B., Bigham, A. W. *et al.* (2011) Exome sequencing as a tool for Mendelian disease gene discovery. *Nature Reviews Genetics* **12**, 745–755.

Bastos Lages, E. M., Drummond, A. F., Pretti, H. *et al.* (2009) Association of functional gene polymorphism IL-1β in patients with external apical root resorption. *American Journal of Orthodontics and Dentofacial Orthopedics* **136**, 542–546.

Bates, S. E. (2014) It's all about the test: the complexity of companion diagnostic co-development in personalized medicine. *Clinical Cancer Research* **20**, 1418–1418.

Beckmann, J. S. and Lew, D. (2016) Reconciling evidence-based medicine and precision medicine in the era of big data: challenges and opportunities. *Genome Medicine* **8**, 134.

Behrens, M. K. (2008) *Priorities for Personalized Medicine* [Online]. President's Council of Advisors on Science and Technology. Available: https//bigdatawg.nist.gov/PCAST Personalized Medicine Priorities.pdf (accessed September 17, 2020).

Berlin, J. A., Santanna, J., Schmid, C. H. *et al.* (2002) Individual patient-versus group-level data meta-regressions for the investigation of treatment effect modifiers: ecological bias rears its ugly head. *Statistics in Medicine* **21**, 371–387.

Bui, C., King, T., Proffit, W. and Frazier-Bowers, S. (2006) Phenotypic characterization of Class III patients. *The Angle Orthodontist* **76**, 564–569.

Carlson, D. S. (2015) Evolving concepts of heredity and genetics in orthodontics. *American Journal of Orthodontics and Dentofacial Orthopedics* **148**, 922–938.

Chakravarti, A. (2001) Single nucleotide polymorphisms:. . . to a future of genetic medicine. *Nature* **409**, 822–823.

Chatterjee, N., Wheeler, B., Sampson, J. *et al.* (2013) Projecting the performance of risk prediction based on polygenic analyses of genome-wide association studies. *Nature Genetics* **45**, 400–405.

Collins, F. and Tabak, L. (2004) A call for increased education in genetics for dental health professionals. *Journal of Dental Education* **68**, 807–808.

Collins, F. S. (2015) Exceptional opportunities in medical science: a view from the National Institutes of Health. *JAMA* **313**, 131–132.

Collins, F. S. and Varmus, H. (2015) A new initiative on precision medicine. *New England Journal of Medicine* **372**, 793–795.

Cruz, R. M., Krieger, H., Ferreira, R. *et al.* (2008) Major gene and multifactorial inheritance of mandibular prognathism. *American Journal of Medical Genetics A* **146A**, 71–77.

D'Silva, N. and Gutkind, J. (2019) Oral cancer: integration of studies for diagnostic and therapeutic precision. *Advances in Dental Research* **30**, 45–49.

D'Silva, N. J. (2015) Biomarkers for individualized oral cancer therapy, in *Personalized Oral Health Care* (ed. P. J. Polverini). Springer, Berlin, pp. 43–60.

De Frutos-Valle, L., Martin, C., Alarcon, J. A. *et al.* (2019) Subclustering in skeletal class III phenotypes of different ethnic origins: a systematic review. *Journal of Evidence Based Dental Practice* **19**, 34–52.

Decker, E., Stellzig-Eisenhauer, A., Fiebig, B. S. *et al.* (2008) Loss-of-function mutations in familial, nonsyndromic primary failure of tooth eruption. *American Journal of Human Genetics* **83**, 781–786.

Divaris, K. (2019) Searching deep and wide: advances in the molecular understanding of dental caries and periodontal disease. *Advances in Dental Research* **30**, 40–44.

Dorschner, M. O., Amendola, L. M., Shirts, B. H. *et al.* (2014) Refining the structure and content of clinical genomic reports. *American Journal of Medical Genetics C: Seminars in Medical Genetics* **166**, 85–92.

Drmanac, R. (2011) The advent of personal genome sequencing. *Genetics in Medicine* **13**, 188–190.

Dudlicek, L. L., Gettig, E. A., Etzel, K. R. and Hart, T. C. (2004) Status of genetics education in US dental schools. *Journal of Dental Education* **68**, 809–818.

Dworkin, S. F. (2013) The OPPERA study: act two. *Journal of Pain* **14**, T1.

Everett, E. T., Britto, D. A., Ward, R. E. and Hartsfield, J. K., Jr. (1999) A novel FGFR2 gene mutation in Crouzon syndrome associated with apparent nonpenetrance. *Cleft Palate-Craniofacial Journal* **36**, 533–541.

Fernald, G. H., Capriotti, E., Daneshjou, R. *et al.* (2011) Bioinformatics challenges for personalized medicine. *Bioinformatics* **27**, 1741–1748.

Fontana, M. L. S., De Souza, C. M., Bernardino, J. F. *et al.* (2012) Association analysis of clinical aspects and vitamin D receptor gene polymorphism with external apical root resorption in orthodontic patients. *American Journal of Orthodontics and Dentofacial Orthopedics* **142**, 339–347.

Frazier-Bowers, S. A., Simmons, D., Wright, J. T. et al. (2010) Primary failure of eruption and PTH1R: the importance of a genetic diagnosis for orthodontic treatment planning. *American Journal of Orthodontics and Dentofacial Orthopedics* **137**, 160. e1–160. e7.

Garcia, I., Kuska, R. and Somerman, M. (2013) Expanding the foundation for personalized medicine implications and challenges for dentistry. *Journal of Dental Research* **92**, S3–S10.

Genno, P. G., Nemer, G. M., Eddine, S. B. Z. et al. (2019) Three novel genes tied to mandibular prognathism in eastern Mediterranean families. *American Journal of Orthodontics and Dentofacial Orthopedics* **156**, 104–112. e3.

Ginsburg, G. S. (2013) Realizing the opportunities of genomics in health care. *JAMA* **309**, 1463–1464.

Green, R. C., Berg, J. S., Grody, W. W. et al. (2013) ACMG recommendations for reporting of incidental findings in clinical exome and genome sequencing. *Genetics in Medicine* **15**, 565–574.

Gülden, N., Eggermann, T., Zerres, K. et al. (2009) Interleukin-1 polymorphisms in relation to external apical root resorption (EARR). *Journal of Orofacial Orthopedics* **70**, 20–38.

Guo, Y., Xiong, D. H., Yang, T. L. et al. (2006) Polymorphisms of estrogen-biosynthesis genes CYP17 and CYP19 may influence age at menarche: a genetic association study in Caucasian females. *Human Molecular Genetics* **15**, 2401–2408.

Gwinn, M., Grossniklaus, D. A., Yu, W. et al. (2011) Horizon scanning for new genomic tests. *Genetics in Medicine* **13**, 161–165.

Handelman, G. S., Kok, H. K., Chandra, R. V. et al. (2018) eDoctor: machine learning and the future of medicine. *Journal of Internal Medicine* **284**, 603–619.

Hartsfield, J. and James K. (2008) Personalized orthodontics, the future of genetics in practice. *Seminars in Orthodontics* **14**, 166–171.

Hartsfield, J., Morford, L. A. and Otero, L. M. (2012) Genetic factors affecting facial growth, in *Orthodontics – Basic Aspects and Clinical Considerations* (ed. F. Bourzgui). Intech, Rijeka.

Hartsfield, J. K., Jr. (2009) Pathways in external apical root resorption associated with orthodontia. *Orthod Craniofac Res* **12**, 236–242.

Hartsfield, J. K., Jr. (2011) Genetics and orthodontics, in *Orthodontics: Current Principles and Techniques*, 5th edn (eds. L. W. Graber, R. L Vanarsdall and K. W. LVig). Elsevier Mosby, St Louis.

Hartsfield, J. K., Jr. and Bixler, D. (2010) Clinical genetics for the dental practitioner, in *McDonald's and Avery's dentistry for the Child and Adolescent*, 9th edn. (eds. J. A. Dean, D. R. Avery and R. E McDonald) Mosby/Elsevier, St Louis.

Hartsfield, J. K., Jr., Zhou, J. and Chen, S. (2010) The importance of analyzing specific genetic factors in facial growth for diagnosis and treatment planning, in *Surgical Enhancement of Orthodontic Treatment* (eds. J.A. McNamara, Jr. and S.D. Kapila, S. D.). University of Michigan, Ann Arbor.

Hartsfield Jr, J. K., Jacob, G. J. and Morford, L. A. (2017) Heredity, genetics and orthodontics: how much has this research really helped? *Seminars in Orthodontics* **23**, 336–347.

He, S., Hartsfield Jr, J. K., Guo, Y. et al. (2012) Association between CYP19A1 genotype and pubertal sagittal jaw growth. *American Journal of Orthodontics and Dentofacial Orthopedics* **142**, 662–670.

Heinemann, F. S., Police, A., Lin, E. et al. (2018) Impact of genomics on personalization of breast cancer care, in *Genomics-Driven Healthcare* (ed. Y. Pathak). Springer, Berlin, pp. 331–372.

Hindorff, L. A., Sethupathy, P., Junkins, H. A. et al. (2009) Potential etiologic and functional implications of genome-wide association loci for human diseases and traits. *Proceedings of the National Academy of Sciences* **106**, 9362–9367. https://www.genome.gov/genetics-glossary/ (Accessed 2020).

Iglesias-Linares, A., Yanez-Vico, R. M., Moreno-Fernandez, A. M. et al. (2014) Osteopontin gene SNPs (rs9138, rs11730582) mediate susceptibility to external root resorption in orthodontic patients. *Oral Diseases* **20**, 307–312.

Iglesias-Linares, A., Yañez-Vico, R., Ballesta-Mudarra, S. et al. (2012a) Postorthodontic external root resorption is associated with IL1 receptor antagonist gene variations. *Oral Diseases* **18**, 198–205.

Iglesias-Linares, A., Yañez-Vico, R., Ballesta, S. et al. (2012b) Interleukin 1 gene cluster SNPs (rs1800587, rs1143634) influences post-orthodontic root resorption in endodontic and their contralateral vital control teeth differently. *International Endodontic Journal* **45**, 1018–1026.

Iglesias-Linares, A., Yañez-Vico, R. M., Moreno-Fernández, A. M. et al. (2014) Osteopontin gene SNPs (rs9138, rs11730582) mediate susceptibility to external root resorption in orthodontic patients. *Oral Diseases* **20**, 307–312.

International Hapmap Consortium (2005) A haplotype map of the human genome. *Nature* **437**, 1299–1320.

International Human Genome Sequencing Consortium (2001) Initial sequencing and analysis of the human genome. *Nature* **409**, 860–921.

Iwasaki, L. R., Covell, D. A., Jr., Frazier-Bowers, S. A. et al. (2015) Personalized and precision orthodontic therapy. *Orthodontics and Craniofacial Research* **18**(Suppl 1), 1–7.

Jiang, Q., Mei, L., Zou, Y. et al. (2019) Genetic polymorphisms in FGFR2 underlie skeletal malocclusion. *Journal of Dental Research* **98**, 1340–1347.

Johnson, L., Genco, R. J., Damsky, C. et al. (2008) Genetics and its implications for clinical dental practice and education: report of panel 3 of the Macy study. *Journal of Dental Education* **72**, 86–94.

Kajii, T. S., Oka, A., Saito, F. et al. (2019) Whole-exome sequencing in a Japanese pedigree implicates a rare non-synonymous single-nucleotide variant in BEST3 as a candidate for mandibular prognathism. *Bone* **122**, 193–198.

Kalia, S. S., Adelman, K., Bale, S. J. et al. (2017) Recommendations for reporting of secondary findings in clinical exome and genome sequencing, 2016 update (ACMG SF v2. 0): a policy statement of the American College of Medical Genetics and Genomics. *Genetics in Medicine* **19**, 249–255.

Kantaputra, P. N., Pruksametanan, A., Phondee, N. et al. (2019) ADAMTSL1 and mandibular prognathism. *Clinical Genetics* **95**, 507–515.

Katsanis, S. H. and Katsanis, N. (2013) Molecular genetic testing and the future of clinical genomics. *Nature Reviews Genetics* **14**, 415–426.

Khoury, M. J. (2003) Genetics and genomics in practice: the continuum from genetic disease to genetic information in health and disease. *Genetics in Medicine* **5**, 261–268.

Khoury, M. J., Iademarco, M. F. and Riley, W. T. (2016) Precision public health for the era of precision medicine. *American Journal of Preventive Medicine* **50**, 398–401.

Kilpinen, H. and Barrett, J. C. (2013) How next-generation sequencing is transforming complex disease genetics. *Trends in Genetics* **29**, 23–30.

Kluemper, G. T., Morford, L. A. and Hartsfield Jr., J. K. (2018) The quest and reality of personalized treatment for the skeletal class III patient, in *Forty-fifth Annual Moyers Symposium Effective, Efficient and Personalized Orthodontics: Patient-Centered Approaches and Innovations* (eds. H. Kim-Berman, L. Franchi and A. Ruellas). University of Michigan, pp. 125–149.

Köhler, S., Carmody, L., Vasilevsky, N. et al. (2019) Expansion of the human phenotype ontology (HPO) knowledge base and resources. *Nucleic Acids Research* **47**, D1018–D1027.

Li, C., Cai, Y., Chen, S. and Chen, F. (2016) Classification and characterization of class III malocclusion in Chinese individuals. *Head and Face Medicine* **12**, 31.

Linhartova, P., Cernochova, P. and Izakovicova Holla, L. (2013) IL1 gene polymorphisms in relation to external apical root resorption concurrent with orthodontia. *Oral Diseases* **19**, 262–270.

Mackay, F., Jones, J., Thompson, R. and Simpson, W. (1992) Craniofacial form in class III cases. *British Journal of Orthodontics* **19**, 15–20.

Maixner, W., Diatchenko, L., Dubner, R. et al. (2011) Orofacial pain prospective evaluation and risk assessment study–the OPPERA study. *Journal of Pain* **12**, T4–T11. e2.

Manocha, S., Farokhnia, N., Khosropanah, S. et al. (2019) Systematic review of hormonal and genetic factors involved in the nonsyndromic disorders of the lower jaw. *Developmental Dynamics* **248**, 162–172.

Mcguire, A. L. and Burke, W. (2008) An unwelcome side effect of direct-to-consumer personal genome testing: raiding the medical commons. *JAMA* **300**, 2669–2671.

Meyer, S. L. (2020) Toward precision public health. *Journal of Public Health Dentistry* **80**, S7–S13.

Mirnezami, R., Nicholson, J. and Darzi, A. (2012) Preparing for precision medicine. *New England Journal of Medicine* **366**, 489–491.

Moreno Uribe, L. M., Vela, K. C., Kummet, C. et al. (2013) Phenotypic diversity in white adults with moderate to severe Class III malocclusion. *American Journal of Orthodontic and Dentofacial Orthopedics* **144**, 32–42.

National Research Council (2011) *Toward Precision Medicine: Building a Knowledge Network for Biomedical Research and a New Taxonomy Of Disease*. National Academies Press.

Nowrin, S. A., Jaafar, S., Ab Rahman, N. et al. (2018). Association between genetic polymorphisms and external apical root resorption: a systematic review and meta-analysis. *Korean Journal of Orthodontics* **48**(6), 395–404.

Palotie, A., Widén, E. and Ripatti, S. (2013) From genetic discovery to future personalized health research. *New Biotechnology* **30**, 291–295.

Paul, M. and Leibovici, L. (2014) Systematic review or meta-analysis? Their place in the evidence hierarchy. *Clinical Microbiology and Infection* **20**, 97–100.

Pereira, S., Lavado, N., Nogueira, L. et al. (2013) Polymorphisms of genes encoding P2X7R, IL-1B, OPG and RANK in orthodontic-induced apical root resorption. *Oral Diseases* **20**, 659–667.

Ramsey, S. D., Veenstra, D., Tunis, S. R. et al. (2011) How comparative effectiveness research can help advance 'personalized medicine' in cancer treatment. *Health Affairs* **30**, 2259–2268.

Rao, C., Guan, B., Luo, D. et al. (2020) Identification of pathogenic variants of ERLEC1 in individuals with class III malocclusion by exome sequencing. *Human Mutation* **41**, 1435–1446.

Robinson, P. N. (2012) Deep phenotyping for precision medicine. *Human Mutation* **33**, 777–780.

Robinson, P. N., Köhler, S., Bauer, S. et al. (2008) The Human Phenotype Ontology: a tool for annotating and analyzing human hereditary disease. *American Journal of Human Genetics* **83**, 610–615.

Roden, D. and Tyndale, R. (2013) Genomic medicine, precision medicine, personalized medicine: what's in a name? *Clinical Pharmacology and Therapeutics* **94**, 169–172.

Roedig, J. J., Phillips, B. A., Morford, L. A. et al. (2014) Comparison of BMI, AHI, and apolipoprotein E ε4 (APOE-ε4) alleles among sleep apnea patients with different skeletal classifications. *Journal of Clinical Sleep Medicine* **10**, 397–402.

Schaefer, K., Fink, B., Grammer, K. et al. (2006) Female appearance: facial and bodily attractiveness as shape. *Psychological Science* **48**, 187–204.

Schaefer, K., Fink, B., Mitteroecker, P. et al. (2005) Visualizing facial shape regression upon 2nd to 4th digit ratio and testosterone. *Collegium Antropologicum* **29**, 415–419.

Scheuner, M. T., Sieverding, P. and Shekelle, P. G. (2008) Delivery of genomic medicine for common chronic adult diseases: a systematic review. *JAMA* **299**, 1320–1334.

Schmid, C. H., Stark, P. C., Berlin, J. A et al. (2004) Meta-regression detected associations between heterogeneous treatment effects and study-level, but not patient-level, factors. *Journal of Clinical Epidemiology* **57**, 683–697.

Sharab, L. Y., Morford, L. A., Dempsey, J. et al. (2015) Genetic and treatment-related risk factors associated with external apical root resorption (EARR) concurrent with orthodontia. *Orthodontics and Craniofacial Research* **18**, 71–82.

Shendure, J., Balasubramanian, S., Church, G. M. et al. (2017) DNA sequencing at 40: past, present and future. *Nature* **550**, 345–353.

Shungin, D., Haworth, S., Divaris, K. et al. (2019) Genome-wide analysis of dental caries and periodontitis combining clinical and self-reported data. *Nature Communications* **10**, 1–13.

Simonds, N. I., Khoury, M. J., Schully, S. D. et al. (2013) Comparative effectiveness research in cancer genomics and precision medicine: current landscape and future prospects. *Journal of the National Cancer Institute* **105**, 929–936.

Singh, G., McNamara Jr., J. and Lozanoff, S. (1998) Morphometry of the midfacial complex in subjects with class III malocclusions: Procrustes, Euclidean, and cephalometric analyses. *Clinical Anatomy* **11**, 162–170.

Singh, G. D., McNamara Jr., J. A. and Lozanoff, S. (1997) Morphometry of the cranial base in subjects with Class III malocclusion. *Journal of Dental Research* **76**, 694–703.

Smith, S. B., Parisien, M., Bair, E. et al. (2019) Genome-wide association reveals contribution of MRAS to painful temporomandibular disorder in males. *Pain* **160**, 579.

Staudt, C. B. and Kiliaridis, S. (2009) Different skeletal types underlying Class III malocclusion in a random population. *American Journal of Orthodontic and Dentofacial Orthopedics* **136**, 715–721.

Stellzig-Eisenhauer, A., Decker, E., Meyer-Marcotty, P. et al. (2010) Primary failure of eruption (PFE)–clinical and molecular genetics analysis. *Journal of Orofacial Orthopedics* **71**, 6–16.

Sun, L., Brentnall, A., Patel, S. et al. (2019) A cost-effectiveness analysis of multigene testing for all patients with breast cancer. *JAMA Oncology* **5**, 1718–1730.

Swanson, A., Ramos, E. and Snyder, H. (2014) Next generation sequencing is the impetus for the next generation of laboratory-based genetic counselors. *Journal of Genetic Counseling*, 1–8.

Tomoyasu, Y., Yamaguchi, T., Tajima, A. et al. (2009) External apical root resorption and the interleukin-1B gene polymorphism in the Japanese population. *Orthodontic Waves* **68**, 152–157.

Tulloch, J., Phillips, C. and Proffit, W. R. (1998) Benefit of early Class II treatment: progress report of a two-phase randomized clinical trial. *American Journal of Orthodontics and Dentofacial Orthopedics* **113**, 62–74.

Tulloch, J., Proffit, W. R. and Phillips, C. (2004) Outcomes in a 2-phase randomized clinical trial of early Class II treatment. *American Journal of Orthodontics and Dentofacial Orthopedics* **125**, 657–667.

Vanderweele, T. J. and Knol, M. J. (2011) Interpretation of subgroup analyses in randomized trials: heterogeneity versus secondary interventions. *Annals of Internal Medicine* **154**, 680–683.

Venter, J. C., Adams, M. D., Myers, E. W. et al. (2001) The sequence of the human genome. *Science* **291**, 1304–1351.

Weinberg, S. M., Roosenboom, J., Shaffer, J. R. et al. (2019) Hunting for genes that shape human faces: initial successes and challenges for the future. *Orthodontics and Craniofacial Research* **22**, 207–212.

Wu, F., Wang, L., Huang, Y. et al. (2012) Interleukin-1β+ 3954 polymorphisms and risk of external apical root resorption in orthodontic treatment: a meta-analysis. *Genetics and Molecular Research* **12**, 4678–4686.

Yan, S.-K., Liu, R.-H., Jin, H.-Z. et al. (2015) "Omics" in pharmaceutical research: overview, applications, challenges, and future perspectives. *Chinese Journal of Natural Medicines* **13**, 3–21.

Zettler, P. J., Sherkow, J. S. and Greely, H. T. (2014) 23andme, the food and drug administration, and the future of genetic testing. *JAMA Internal Medicine* **174**, 493–494.

Zhang, Q., Chen, C., Chang, M. et al. (2019) Oral rehabilitation of patients sustaining orofacial injuries: the UPenn initiative. *Advances in Dental Research* **30**, 50–56.

CHAPTER 14
The Effect of Drugs, Hormones, and Diet on Orthodontic Tooth Movement

Vinod Krishnan, James J. Zahrowski, and Ze'ev Davidovitch

> **Summary**
>
> The objective of this chapter is to review the published literature on the effects of various drugs and nutrition supplements consumed by patients for treatment of systemic diseases on the process of orthodontic tooth movement. The increase in the number of adults seeking orthodontic treatment has introduced more medical conditions and medication use, causing an additional set of factors in orthodontic tooth movement, with potential implications for mechanotherapy and retention protocols. Orthodontic tooth movement is first initiated by placing carefully directed forces upon teeth. These forces cause many biological processes and mediators to occur within the periodontal ligament causing inflammation and bone turnover. Medications, nutrition supplements, and molecules produced in various diseased tissues and organs can reach the mechanically stressed paradental tissues through the circulation and interact with local target cells. The combined effect of mechanical forces and one or more of these agents may be inhibitory, additive, or synergistic. All the medications reviewed have systemic therapeutic effects. However, the potential adverse effects on OTM are probably overshadowed by the medical benefit. These adverse effects may change the desired outcome of tooth position or health of surrounding tissues. Therefore, it is imperative that the orthodontist pays close attention to the medical and drug consumption history of each patient before and during orthodontic treatment. The medication benefits and risks for tissue systems must be explored to determine the best orthodontic mechanotherapy and health outcome for our patients.

Introduction

A US National Center for Health Statistics brief (Martin et al., NCHS Data Brief No. 334, May 2019) stated that "45.8% of the US population used prescription drugs in the past 30 days and the use of prescription drug use increased with age, from 18.0% of children under age 12 years to 85.0% of adults aged 60 and over. It was found to be highest among non-Hispanic white persons followed by non-Hispanic black persons, and lowest among non-Hispanic Asian and Hispanic persons." It continues: "the most commonly used types of drugs included bronchodilators for ages 0–11 years, central nervous system stimulants for ages 12–19, antidepressants for ages 20–59, and lipid-lowering drugs for ages 60 and over." Furthermore, the use and abuse of over-the-counter (OTC) medications has also increased significantly in recent years, making it difficult to elicit accurately the drug history in many patients. A Mayo Clinic study (Zhong et al., 2013) also commented on the high prevalence of prescription drug use. In their defined population, they stated that the percentage of 1,42,377 individuals taking prescription medications was 68% using one drug, 50% using two drugs, and 21% using five drugs. Their defined population included all ages with 22% below the age of 18 years old. Orthodontists should be aware of the disease processes of their patients as well as any effects medication may have on the orthodontic tooth movement (OTM) process. Clinicians must also be cognizant of methods to manage untoward effects of any medication in order to optimize the orthodontic treatment rendered to the patient.

In the USA, the Food and Drug Administration (FDA) approves all medications, whether they can be purchased with or without a prescription, to assure safety and effectiveness to treat the intended medical conditions. Medications, which are relatively safe and effective for nonserious medical conditions, are approved for OTC purchase and self-supervised use. Some OTC medications have many adverse effects yet have had a long history of public use and grandfathered into an OTC drug status, such as aspirin. Some medications start off as prescription medications and later change to the OTC category after a track record of effectiveness and safety has been established, such as ibuprofen.

Prescription drugs form the mainstay of the medical profession, in order to treat, control, or prevent diseases. Medications, approved for prescription use only, are intended to treat serious medical conditions

---

Biological Mechanisms of Tooth Movement, Third Edition. Edited by Vinod Krishnan, Anne Marie Kuijpers-Jagtman and Ze'ev Davidovitch.
© 2021 John Wiley & Sons Ltd. Published 2021 by John Wiley & Sons Ltd.

with more adverse drug effects and ensure supervised use. Every prescription drug must go through four phases of rigorous human testing before being released for public use. Large random controlled human trials, the highest level of evidence, are required to evaluate the drug's effectiveness (benefit) versus the drug's adverse effects (harm). During the clinical controlled trials, the observed adverse drug effects are quantified for incidence and severity by the investigators. All evidence for each drug is evaluated by a panel of independent experts to make sure the intended medical benefit outweighs the risk of harm. Although most adverse drug effects are noted during these large clinical trials, some adverse effects are rare or unexpected and not found until after the drug is approved for prescription use, such as bisphosphonate osteonecrosis.

Remodeling of paradental tissues in response to mechanical force application is a complicated process. The synthesis, release, as well as the role of various inflammatory mediators, neurotransmitters, growth factors, and other cytokines in response to applied mechanical forces were elucidated and have become targets of thorough reviews in the past (Roberts-Harry and Sandy, 2004; Krishnan and Davidovitch, 2006a; Meikle, 2006). These endogenous molecules have been found to play important roles in the initiation, maintenance, and cessation of tooth movement. However, some of these ligands can also cause unwanted side effects, such as pain and root resorption. Current orthodontic research is aiming at developing methods to increase the tissue concentrations of those molecules which promote tooth movement, while simultaneously decreasing the concentration of unwanted elements which can produce harmful side effects.

An extensive review performed by the authors of this chapter (Krishnan and Davidovitch, 2006b) and the systematic review by Bartzela et al. (2009), outlined the effects of various classes of drugs on OTM. Following these publications, an editorial by Turpin (2009) emphasized the importance of obtaining a detailed drug intake history from all prospective orthodontic patients, so that any untoward effects on the course of OTM are well managed. Apart from medications, patients also consume vitamins, minerals, and other compounds, as dietary supplements for the prevention or treatment of various diseases. Some medications or supplements may have effects on the short- and long-term outcomes of orthodontic treatment. Clinical FDA drug trials do not evaluate adverse drug effects upon tooth movement. Most of the reported drug effects upon tooth movement are derived from studies with lower levels of evidence, such as animal studies or human case reports. From this evidence, it can only be assumed that a certain drug will affect OTM as the incidence of a drug's effect upon tooth movement may not have been studied sufficiently in humans. The purpose of this chapter is to supply as much information regarding medication effects upon orthodontic therapy that is known at this time.

Prostaglandins and analogues

Tissue remodeling activities associated with inflammatory reactions form the biological foundation of OTM. Certain eicosanoids (prostaglandins [PGs] and leukotrienes), released from paradental cells in sites of compression and tension, have significant stimulatory effects on bone remodeling (Salvi and Lang, 2005). This finding led researchers to inject PGs locally, at the site of OTM, to enhance the bone remodeling process, and thereby accelerate the pace of tooth movement. Yamasaki et al. (1982) found an increased number of osteoclasts in rats' alveolar bone after local injection of PGE_1. A similar regimen in human subjects significantly increased the rate of canine and premolar movement (Yamasaki et al., 1984). Apparently, PGs act by increasing the number of osteoclasts, and promoting the formation of ruffled borders, thereby stimulating bone resorption. Among the PGs that had been found to affect bone metabolism (E_1, E_2, A_1, and F_2-α), PGE_2 stimulated osteoblastic cell differentiation and new bone formation which coupled with bone resorption in vitro (Gustafson et al., 1977). Gurton et al. (2004) evaluated the effect of prostacyclin and thromboxane A_2 on OTM and revealed an increase in the number of osteoclasts and the amount of alveolar bone resorption by these analogs.

In a human split mouth study in 15 patients having three PGE_1 injections on days 1, 6, and 17, it was found that canine retraction increased 1.7 times compared with the control tooth (Patil et al., 2005). Through the histological study on young adult rabbits, Cağlaroğlu and Erdem (2012) have demonstrated that the intraligamentous route of prostaglandin administration seems to be more effective in comparison to submucous and intravenous route to accelerate OTM (Figure 14.1).

The main side effect associated with local injection of PGs is hyperalgesia due to the release of noxious agents, such as histamine, bradykinin, serotonin, acetylcholine, and substance P, from nerve endings, both peripherally and centrally (Leiker et al., 1995). Although PGs enhance OTM, their side effects are very serious and preclude their clinical use. Combining local anesthetics with PGs, in order to reduce pain while injected locally, is in the preliminary phase of research.

Implication

PGs and analogs are presently being used in orthodontic research in order to evaluate the possibility of increasing the pace of OTM for clinical use. Although medically prescribed PG analogs have the potential to achieve this goal, they probably do not affect clinical orthodontic practice due to their short duration of medical use.

Nonsteroidal anti-inflammatory drugs

The most common group of medications used in orthodontics to control pain following mechanical force application to teeth are nonsteroidal anti-inflammatory drugs (NSAIDs). These drugs are classified as being nonopioid and analgesic acting peripherally. They inhibit cyclooxygenase (COX), which modulates the transformation of PGs from arachidonic acid in the cellular plasma membrane (Polat et al., 2005; Arias and Marquez-Orozco, 2006). These PGs increase the levels of matrix metalloproteinases (MMPs) 9 and 2, including collagenase, followed by a reduction in procollagen synthesis, which is considered essential for bone and periodontal ligament (PDL) remodeling. The consumption of NSAIDs result in inhibition of COX activity, leading to altered vascular and extracellular matrix remodeling, and causing a possible reduction in the pace of OTM (Kyrkanides et al., 2000).

The first reports on the use of analgesics in orthodontics were published by Simmons and Brandt (1992), and by Paganelli (1993). The former group used acetaminophen in their trial, while the latter researcher applied flurbiprofen. The first effort to compare various drugs for their effectiveness in managing orthodontic pain was performed by Ngan et al. (1994). These investigators concluded that ibuprofen is more effective than aspirin and placebo in controlling pain. Subsequently, numerous studies evaluated the pain-reducing effects of various NSAIDs, including nonselective COX-1/COX-2 inhibitors like ibuprofen, acetyl salicylic acid, indomethacin, and naproxen sodium, and also rofecoxib, a selective COX-2 inhibitor

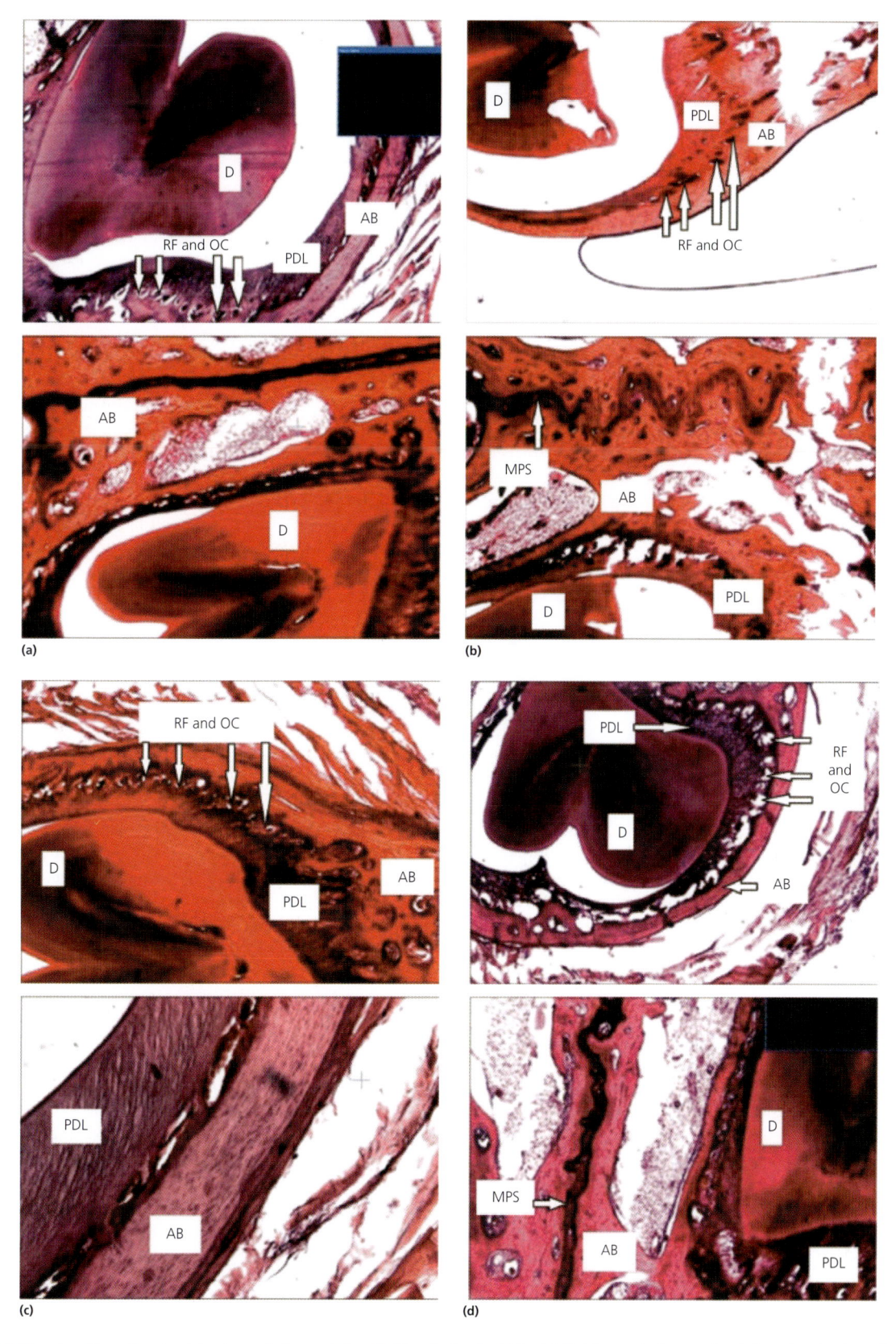

Figure 14.1 Hematoxylin and eosin-stained sample from adult male New Zealand rabbits. (a) Positive control group ($n = 10$), each animal was fitted with a spring exerting 20-g reciprocal force on the maxillary incisors, and PGE_2 was not administered. (b) Intravenous PGE_2 group, injected with 0.06 mL PGE_2 (10 µg/mL) in the bilateral auricular veins. (c) Submucosal PGE_2 group, injected to submucosa immediately distal to the maxillary incisors. (d) Intraligamentous PGE_2 group, injected to PDL surrounding the maxillary incisors. The pressure (top; rows 1 and 3) and tension (bottom; rows 2 and 4) sides are shown. Abbreviations: AB, alveolar bone; C, capillary; D, dentin; MPS, median palatine suture; OC, osteoclast; PDL, periodontal ligament; RF, resorption foci. (Source: Cağlaroğlu and Erdem, 2012.)

(Chumbley and Tuncay, 1986; Kehoe et al., 1996; Sari et al., 2004; de Carlos et al., 2007). These studies not only demonstrated that NSAIDs effectively reduce pain and discomfort caused by the periodic activation of orthodontic appliances but also may affect OTM by inhibiting or reducing the associated inflammatory and bone resorptive processes.

The development of a sterile inflammatory process following mechanical force application is of paramount importance in OTM. Consequentially, pain prevention with NSAIDs, which inhibits inflammation by altering the arachidonic acid pathway, has long been of concern. Knop et al. (2012) suggested that PG inhibition by NSAIDs triggers a cascade of events, leading to a reduction in the number of osteoclast-like cells, Howship lacunae, and blood vessels in the PDL throughout all treatment periods. Retamoso et al. (2011) demonstrated a lower rate of collagen maturation in the PDL with both NSAIDs and steroidal drugs, with steroidal drugs having a more pronounced effect. Shetty et al. (2013) found decreased PGE_2 levels in upper bicuspid extraction patients taking ibuprofen, but not for those patients taking acetaminophen. They implied a decreased OTM may occur from ibuprofen administration. Most of the reported studies have concentrated on PG inhibition, largely ignoring the fact that there are other mediators involved in OTM, such as leukotrienes, interleukins, cyclic AMP and cyclic GMP, and calcium. However, PGs may have an important role in the processes of mechanotransduction, inflammation, and pain sensation, but this involvement is short-lived, occurring in the presence of other mediators. Therefore, a long-term reduction of PGs after the administration of regular and repeated doses of NSAIDs would only reduce the efficiency of the inflammatory cells (Consolaro et al., 2010).

Research has evidenced reports on the use of NSAIDs for pain control during orthodontic treatment (Polat and Karaman, 2005; Arantes et al., 2009; Padisar et al., 2009; Kohli and Kohli, 2011). Padisar et al. (2009) compared the efficacy of four NSAIDs (ibuprofen 400 mg, naproxen 250 mg, mefenamic acid 250 mg, and aspirin 325 mg) in postoperative pain reduction and concluded that ibuprofen is the most effective in this regard. Arantes et al. (2009) evaluated the efficacy of tenoxicam (an oxicam derivative taken 20 mg orally for 3 days) and concluded that it does not interfere with OTM yet is effective in reducing acute postoperative pain. Administration of a single dose of these drugs preoperatively is considered to be effective in reducing orthodontic postoperative pain. The randomized controlled trial by Kohli and Kohli (2011) revealed that premedication with 20 mg of piroxicam, one hour before the separator placement, is more effective than 400 mg of ibuprofen in reducing pain after the procedure. A recent Cochrane review by Monk et al. (2017) concluded that there exists moderate-quality evidence that the use of analgesics reduces the pain associated with orthodontic treatment. It continues to say that "we remain uncertain whether the systemic NSAIDs are more effective than paracetamol, and whether topical NSAIDs are more effective than local anaesthetic, at reducing pain associated with orthodontic treatment. There is very low-quality evidence that the use of pre-emptive ibuprofen, taken one hour before orthodontic treatment, significantly reduces pain up to two hours after treatment."

All these reports suggest that NSAIDs are effective in reducing postoperative orthodontic pain without affecting OTM when a few doses are taken. Ibuprofen and most NSAIDs have a quick elimination and therefore a short anti-inflammatory action within the body (Brunton et al., 2011). The belief that PG inhibitors significantly reduce OTM may not be valid, as new pathways and molecules associated with tooth movement were discovered (Krishnan and Davidovitch, 2009). The drawbacks of all these studies is their limited number of subjects, evaluating analgesia with short-term studies, and not evaluating how long-term use affects OTM, such as in patients with arthritis or back pain. Correa et al. (2017) through their systematic review of six eligible studies out of 505 retrieved articles concluded that paracetamol is the only drug that does not interfere with orthodontic movement, while drugs such as aspirin, ibuprofen, sodium diclofenac, and selective COX-2 inhibitors caused a reduction in tooth movement when compared with the control group. Furthermore, Consolaro et al. (2010) reviewed the controversies regarding prescribing analgesics after orthodontic force application and pointed out the lack of consistent methodology in this research area, making comparisons among different studies difficult. Many of the parameters varied throughout studies and undermined the possibility of meaningful comparisons which included subject selection, amount and duration of mechanical force application, type of orthodontic appliances, the drug dosage, the duration of use, and route of administration.

Implication
Since NSAIDs have a short drug half-life, the anti-inflammatory action within the body is also of a short duration. Therefore, NSAIDs taken acutely (several days) to relieve orthodontic pain should not clinically affect OTM. However, NSAIDs taken chronically may slow OTM and the clinician should monitor the OTM rate. Should OTM be slowed to an unacceptable rate, a consultation with the patient's physician may reveal other acceptable temporary pain medications without anti-inflammatory properties, such as acetaminophen, until the major OTM is accomplished.

Antiresorptive agents
It is important for the orthodontist to know about antiresorptive medications as their modes of action directly interfere with bone resorption and formation, thereby inhibiting OTM and increasing tooth mobility (Zahrowski, 2007). Presently, the antiresorptive medications used are bisphosphonates (BP), denosumab (DN), estrogens, raloxifene, and calcitonin. BPs and DN are by far the most effective agents to decrease both bone resorption and bone formation.

BPs and DN have different pharmacological mechanisms of action but both severely decrease osteoclastic activity by 70–80% and decrease osteoblastic activity by 50–60% (Black et al., 2000; Cummings et al., 2009). The treatment doses are different for medical situations, such as bone cancer therapy compared with the most commonly used to treat osteoporosis. Uncommon medical uses for antiresorptive agents may also be osteogenesis imperfecta, Paget's bone disease, hypercalcemia, fibrous dysplasia, or Gaucher's disease.

Metastatic bone cancers, such as multiple myeloma and stage 4 breast or prostate cancers, change bone physiology by increasing osteoclastic activity, causing excessive bone resorption and severe pain. High doses of BPs, zoledronic acid, or pamidronate, given intravenously every 4 weeks, are used to treat bone cancer metastases by keeping the bone surface areas saturated with the drug which decreases bone resorption and pain, healing lytic bone lesions and possibly slowing cancer metastases (Zahrowski, 2007; Mhaskar et al., 2017). High doses of DN given subcutaneously every 4 weeks may also be used alternatively to treat bone cancer metastases (Stopeck et al., 2010; Fizazi et al., 2011; Henry et al., 2011).

In osteoporosis, internal cross links begin to break within the trabecular bone due to more resorption occurring within the trabecular bone than the outer cortical bone. The destabilized bone structure allows more fractures to occur in the hip and the lumbar vertebral regions (Rosen, 2005). Osteoporotic fractures, mostly in postmenopausal women, are a principal cause of disability and death, with approximately 1.5 million osteoporotic fractures occurring annually in the USA. Low doses of BPs, commonly oral alendronate, risedronate, or ibandronate, or annual intravenous zoledronic acid, are commonly prescribed for osteoporosis therapy with alendronate being the fifteenth most prescribed medication within the USA (Zahrowski, 2007). Low doses of DN given subcutaneously every 6 months have recently been used alternatively to treat osteoporosis (Cummings et al., 2009). Large random controlled clinical trials have found that BP or DN therapy can prevent 50–70% of vertebral and hip fractures (Black et al., 2000).

The common generic names for BPs are alendronate, risedronate, ibandronate, zoledronic acid, pamidronate, etidronate, tiludronate, and clodronate. The first five BPs are used commonly and are more potent by containing a nitrogen group (Hellstein et al., 2011). BPs have unique pharmacological characteristics, unlike those of any other drug group. Their backbone chemical structure, phosphorus-carbon-phosphorus, allows BPs to bind to free calcium or to the exposed hydroxyapatite in resorbing bone (Licata, 2005). The duration of action for BPs is complicated by the drug's elimination having possibly three elimination rates from the body. After the BP reaches the blood stream, approximately 50% of the drug binds to the bone surfaces and 50% is excreted through the kidneys within the first day (Licata, 2005). Small clinical trials have shown that after acute administration, the one-half of the BP remaining on the bone surface leaves the body via the kidneys in 3 months (Lin et al., 1999; Cremers et al., 2002). The remaining BP, approximately one fourth of the dose originally given, is integrated into the bone matrix by osteoblasts. The BP, which has integrated into bone, is released by osteoclasts when bone is being repaired throughout the body and during tooth movement through alveolar bone. The released BP is taken up by the osteoclast, inhibits the cell's function, and slows bone resorption. Once the BP is integrated into the bone, it is estimated to have a very long elimination half-life of 10 years (Lin et al., 1999; Cremers et al., 2002).

DN, a monoclonal antibody, is designed to mimic osteoprotegerin's action, which decreases mature osteoclast formation (http://pi.amgen.com/united_states/prolia/prolia_pi.pdf, accessed September 9, 2020). DN does not accumulate or integrate within the bone (unlike BP) and has a drug half-life of approximately 1 month (Cummings et al., 2009). The serum markers for osteoclastic and osteoblastic activity remain decreased for 6 months after DN administration and return to normal pretreatment levels within nine months after stopping (http://pi.amgen.com/united_states/prolia/prolia_pi.pdf). Therefore, the effect of DN to decrease OTM should subside 6 months after the last subcutaneous injection. Fernández-González et al. (2016) showed in rats that a local administration of zoledronic acid or a recombinant fusion protein osteoprotegerin inhibited tooth movement ~50%. However, recombinant osteoprotegerin was more effective in blocking the action of osteoclasts than zoledronic acid.

The American Association of Oral and Maxillofacial Surgeons (AAOMS) published a clinical definition of osteonecrosis of the jaw: an exposure of necrotic bone in the mandible or maxilla lasting more than 8 weeks in patients that have taken BP without a history of radiation treatment to the jaws (AAOMS, 2014). In 2011, the American Dental Association Council on Scientific Affairs called for the accepted name for this condition to be "anti-resorptive agent induced osteonecrosis of the jaw" (ARONJ), as osteonecrosis has been observed to result from DN, an antiresorptive agent which is not a BP (Hellstein et al., 2011). In 2014, the AAOMS renamed osteonecrosis of the jaw arising from medications to Medication-Related Osteonecrosis of the Jaw (MRONJ) (AAOMS, 2014). After BP or DN administration, osteonecrosis has been most commonly observed after tooth extractions (Urade et al., 2011; AAOMS, 2014). The frequency of osteonecrosis is dependent on dose and duration of use. During low dose BP use, a retrospective study suggests that frequency of osteonecrosis occurs 1 in 1000 patients (Lo et al., 2010). The effects of a low dose of DN have not been observed long enough to evaluate an osteonecrosis incidence but have been case reported (http://pi.amgen.com/united_states/prolia/prolia_pi.pdf). However, when high dose BP or DN is given to treat bone cancers, the osteonecrosis is more difficult to treat, and it occurs more frequently, in between 1 and 13 in 100 patients (Migliorati et al., 2010; Fizazi et al., 2011; Henry et al., 2011). Migliorati et al. (2013) demonstrated in a controlled human cohort that soft tissue healing after tooth extraction was impaired in patients exposed to BP and implying that BP also affects soft tissues surrounding bone. An interesting study showed prior to extraction of a maxillary molar in zoledronic acid-treated mice that a local injection of a non-nitrogen BP decreased the incidence and severity of osteonecrosis (Hokugo et al., 2019). It is believed that a non-nitrogen BP with less potency replaced zoledronic acid at the bone surface and allowed better bone healing. These authors suggested systemic administration of non-nitrogen BP not to be helpful, possibly due to its lower local levels thereby limiting the drug interchange. However, in humans, Yamaguchi et al. (2010) and Oizumi et al. (2016) suggested giving oral etidronate, a non-nitrogen BP, improved healing from osteonecrosis in patients having stage 2–3 osteonecrosis.

Orthodontic animal research has investigated effects of BP upon reducing the rate of OTM, decreasing root resorption, enhancing anchorage conservation, and reducing post-treatment relapse. Among the drugs investigated, risedronate appears to be the most effective in reducing OTM, followed by alendronate, and then clodronate (Iglesias-Linares et al., 2010). Kim et al. (1999) demonstrated that the enhancement of anchorage and reduction of OTM was due to the impairment of osteoclast structure, which included the disappearance of ruffled borders and clear zones, formation of irregular borders, and necrotic degeneration. Liu et al. (2004) demonstrated reduced root resorption, along with a reduction in OTM and the number of osteoclasts, with local injection of clodronate into the subperiosteal area adjacent to left maxillary molars in rats. Alatli et al. (1996) reported that a single BP injection in rats, before activation of an orthodontic device, generated the formation of atypical hyperplastic cementum, instead of the acellular cementum that protects against root resorption. This finding disagreed with their previous report, which revealed that these drugs produce cemental surface alterations by inhibiting acellular cementum formation and increasing the vulnerability of the dental root to the resorptive process (Alatli et al., 1996).

Zoledronic acid has been also used in orthodontic research to elucidate the effect of BP upon OTM and bone remodeling, since it is the most potent BP in injectable form. Sirisoontorn et al. (2012) demonstrated that zoledronic acid inhibited excessive OTM in ovariectomized rats and reduced the risk of severe orthodontically induced root resorption. Öztürk et al. (2011) demonstrated in rats that zoledronic acid had positive effects on bone formation in response to sagittal suture expansion and decreased relapse. Ortega et al. (2012) demonstrated a single local dose of zoledronic acid in rats provided maximum anchorage and prevented significant bone loss. Hujaa et al. (2011) demonstrated zoledronic acid administration in dogs diminished, not abolished, the healing response which was represented by the turnover in mini implant supporting bone.

Intake of BPs poses a significant challenge for orthodontic treatment planning, because of the possible pharmacologic inhibition of tooth movement and the potential for the development of jaw osteonecrosis. The case reports published by Rinchuse et al. (2007) indicate that the high-dose BP produces a significant impediment to OTM and elicits a chance for the development of osteonecrosis as well. Case reports by Zahrowski (2009) reveal that decreased OTM can occur from low-dose BP. In a small retrospective cohort study, Lotwala et al. (2012) compared the effect of low dose BPs on OTM in women more than 50 years old. They found orthodontic extraction cases are associated with longer treatment times, increased odds of poor space closure, and increased odds of poor root parallelism. However, due to individual variation, it is difficult to predict the quantity of BP effect upon OTM. Intuitively, since BP accumulates within the bone, a higher dose or longer duration of use should cause a greater reduction in OTM. Concurrent BP administration during OTM is expected to deposit more BP within the bone surrounding the teeth which may further slow OTM. Theoretically, the BP effect on OTM may lessen 3 months after discontinuing the drug, after BP has cleared from the bone surface (Zahrowski, 2009). However, BP remaining integrated within the bone can continue to affect OTM for possibly decades, until the drug clears from the bone. A systematic review of seven articles reported orthodontic patients taking BP had compromised treatment results and longer treatment times (Zymperdikas et al., 2020). They also reported mild root resorption and radiographic changes, consisting of widened PDL spaces and sclerotic changes surrounding alveolar bone. Kaipatur et al. (2015) studied selective decortication in rats undergoing alendronate treatment. During selective decortication, alendronate slowed OTM with severe adverse effects of osteonecrotic bone loss interproximally and buccally to the molars.

Prior to and during mechanotherapy, the orthodontist should consider looking for Stage 0 signs and symptoms, which may suggest a more drug-induced decrease of OTM or increased risk of osteonecrosis (Zahrowski, 2009; Hellstein et al., 2011; AAOMS, 2014). Stage 0 signs and symptoms may be dental mobility, pain, tingling of teeth, and radiographic sclerosis of lamina dura or widened PDL. The clinician should note that BP and DN not only decrease bone resorption, but can also decrease bone formation, thereby making teeth more mobile.

Other antiresorptive drugs, which have been used to treat osteoporosis, are estrogens, raloxifene, and calcitonin. These agents have much less effect upon decreasing osteoclastic activity and therefore an anticipated smaller decrease of OTM, than BP or DN. Newer, strong antiresorptive drugs are in clinical trials required by the FDA, such as odanacatib, which prevents the osteoclast from secretion of cathepsin, an enzyme which breaks down the bone collagen matrix (Sirisoontorn et al., 2012). The orthodontist is encouraged to evaluate new antiresorptive drugs for their anticipated effect upon OTM based on: (i) how much the drug decreases osteoclastic activity and (ii) the duration of the drug action within the bone.

Implication
The antiresorptive drugs, BP and DN, have the potential to severely affect orthodontic treatment. More orthodontic research is needed for antiresorptive medications in order to evaluate systemic adverse OTM effects in humans and perhaps a beneficial effect by increasing anchorage through local injections. Clinically, the orthodontist should consider no extractions or no orthodontic treatment for patients taking high doses of BP or DN for bone cancer treatment due to decreased systemic immunity, higher risk of osteonecrosis, lack of OTM, and increased tooth mobility. For osteoporosis patients taking low dose BP or DN, extractions should be conservatively avoided due to the possible risk of osteonecrosis, increased risk of not ideally closing spaces, paralleling of roots, and resulting tooth mobility. Selective decortication techniques to increase OTM should be avoided during BP or DN treatment. Interproximal reduction should be considered as an alternative to extractions, if possible. Patients taking BP or DN should be informed that the OTM may slow or even stop before ideal tooth position is achieved and that tooth mobility may be increased. Orthodontics may be optimized by possibly delaying orthodontic treatment until 6 months after BP or DN can be stopped by the physician. This action would clear the BP from the bone surface and possibly allow more normalization of bone cells, osteoclasts, and osteoblasts. However, some BP will remain integrated within the bone with the possibility of OTM slowing for decades after the BP is stopped. DN does not accumulate within bone and its action to slow OTM should subside 6 months after the drug is stopped. Patients taking BP or DN should be monitored for clinical signs of osteonecrosis and Stage 0 signs and symptoms prior and during orthodontics. The physician should be consulted for the medical prognosis and the anticipated length of antiresorptive treatment in order to select the best timing to initiate and finish orthodontic treatment.

Asthma medications
Bronchial asthma is an episodic narrowing of the airways that result in breathing difficulties and wheezing (Sonis, 2004). The pulmonary distress developed by this disease can be debilitating and affect the quality of life of these patients. Simon et al. (2003) found higher incidence of this disease in Blacks (15.8%) followed by Whites (7.3%), Asians (6%), and Latinos (3.9%). Given the frequency of incidence, it is highly possible that orthodontists will encounter these patients in their clinical practice. For patients at low to moderate asthma severity, morning appointments with short waiting times are advised. Orthodontists should ascertain that the patient has taken adequate medications, and, if needed, has his/her inhaler available at the time of treatment appointments. These patients are sensitive to certain medications, such as erythromycin, aspirin, antihistamines, and local anesthetics with epinephrine (Sonis, 2004). Chronic use of inhalers with steroids by these patients may result in oral candidiasis. Appropriate measures to treat these conditions with topical antifungal agents and salivary substitutes may need to be performed before and during the orthodontic treatment period. The importance of aggressive oral hygiene measures and topical fluoride application should be emphasized to these patients (Sonis, 2004).

Elevated levels of immunoglobulin E (IgE) are always present in patients with asthma, atopy, and allergy. IgE-induced mast cell degranulation *in vivo* is often followed by a late-phase reaction, a second wave of hypersensitivity responses occurring many hours after the acute reaction, and is dependent upon the eosinophils. In asthmatics, this event manifests as a second wave of decreased airflow 4–8 hours after the initial allergen contact. It has been postulated that chronic airway symptoms result from persistent late-phase inflammatory responses in situations of perennial allergen exposure (Oettgen and Geha, 1999). Until recently, bronchospasm of the smooth airway musculature was considered to be a major cause of bronchial asthma, and beta-adrenergic agonists were used for its management. With recent research, it has become increasingly clear that ongoing chronic inflammation of the bronchial wall plays a prominent role in the disease process, with histamine as an important mediator. The late/delayed reaction is characterized by an inflammatory infiltration of the bronchial wall, notably by eosinophils and lymphocytes. A complex interplay of mediators, such as leukotrienes, PGs, and platelet activating factor (PAF) may lead to a chronic inflammation (Elsasser and Perruchoud, 1992). Based on this new disease concept, anti-inflammatory drugs, such as corticosteroids, are used in mild to moderate asthmatics. Asthmatic patients are often prescribed medications that block the leukotriene inflammation pathway, such as montelukast (Singulair), zafirlukast (Accolate), or zileuton (Zyflo) (Kastrup, 2010). Moura et al. (2014) showed leukotriene inhibitors, montelukast and zileuton, decreased bone resorption by reducing osteoclast differentiation and recruitment after strain-induced movement of molars in mice. Recently, Asaad et al. (2017) reported a slight delay in orthodontic movement and decreased osteoclast activity in the montelukast-treated group but the results were insignificant when compared with untreated controls.

The orthodontic literature is replete with data suggesting that there is an increase in the extent of external apical root resorption in patients with chronic asthma, once orthodontic force is applied (McNab et al., 1999; Davidovitch et al., 2000; Owman-Moll and Kurol, 2000; Nishioka et al., 2006). Patients with asthma have an imbalance between two groups of lymphocytes – the T helper 1 and the T helper 2 cells. The latter group of cells is responsible for the synthesis and release in the lung of many inflammatory mediators, such as interleukin (IL)-4, IL-5, IL-6, IL-10, and IL-13. These cytokines attract many inflammatory cells to the lung airways, including eosinophils, which secrete large amounts of histamines, PGs, and leukotrienes, causing blood vessels to leak, and lung tissues to swell and secrete large amounts of mucus. These signal molecules can enter the circulation and reach the PDL, where they can interact with target cells involved in tissue remodeling and OTM (Brodie et al., 1992). Recent systematic reviews have concluded that there is an association between bronchial asthma and periodontal disease, especially gingivitis with statistically significant changes in gingival bleeding, plaque index, and gingival index in comparison with control group patients (Moraschini et al., 2018; Ferreira et al., 2019). Mohammed et al. (1989) showed a decreased OTM in rats when given a leukotriene blocker. This statement makes it clear that the immune system of chronic asthmatic patients is always active, and there will be an increased production of osteoclasts and odontoclasts, both multinucleated cells involved in bone as well as root resorption respectively. Moreover, in asthmatic patients, the application of excessive orthodontic force often results in tissue compression and necrotic areas, which frequently contain odontoclasts engaged in resorbing the dental roots. Therefore, the clinician may consider deferring orthodontic treatment in patients who report symptomatic disease or who have frequent flare ups despite being adequately medicated.

Implication
Orthodontic therapy should be approached cautiously in asthmatic patients because the disease process may effect a negative outcome and routine medications may increase allergy or sensitivity. Oral asthmatic medications, such as leukotriene blockers, may decrease OTM. Beta-adrenergic agonists, as a rescue inhaler, remains an important drug for the relief of acute bronchospasm in the orthodontic office. Corticosteroids or antihistamines may also be taken chronically and may affect OTM as described further in this chapter.

Corticosteroids
The human body needs inflammation to survive, fight infections, and strengthen tissues from daily physical stress. If chronic inflammation becomes uncontrolled by the body, it can become destructive, leading to medical conditions, such as lupus, rheumatoid arthritis, or asthma. Corticosteroids, having one of the strongest anti-inflammatory actions, are sometimes given chronically for severe uncontrolled inflammatory diseases.

The anti-inflammatory activity of corticosteroids depends on the indirect blocking of phospholipase A2 and the suppression of the synthesis of both COX-1 and COX-2, leading to inhibition of the synthesis of PGs and leukotrienes (Bartzela et al., 2009). All the studies conducted in this regard conclude that the effect of corticosteroid therapy depends on the induction period and dosage (Ong et al., 2000; Kalia et al., 2004). Changes in the response of alveolar bone to acute and chronic systemic glucocorticoid administration in a rat model with and without orthodontic forces was studied by Kalia et al. (2004). They observed a noticeable change in the bone turnover rate and a differential response to short-term and long-term steroid therapy. In the group that was prescribed a short-duration drug therapy, OTM was not affected, but at a tissue level the remodeling process seemed delayed. In the chronic group, however, the OTM rate did increase, possibly as a result of the induction of a secondary hyperparathyroidism. Abtahi et al. (2014) demonstrated that after long-term treatment with the corticosteroid triamcinolone acetonide, tooth movement in rabbits was increased through increased resorptive activity in the alveolar bone. Comparison with various animal studies which evaluated the influence of corticosteroids using ARRIVE (Animal Research: Reporting of In Vivo Experiments) guidelines revealed that the role of corticosteroids on OTM is debatable. While two studies reported decreases in the magnitude of OTM, two studies showed no significant influence of corticosteroids on OTM, and two studies found that corticosteroids increase OTM. The data remains inconclusive (Michelogiannakis et al., 2018a).

In humans, chronic corticosteroid administration (commonly prednisone) for more than 3–6 months can cause severe bone resorption and osteoporosis (Longo et al., 2011). Often the primary treatment for corticosteroid-induced osteoporosis is BP therapy, which has the potential to severely decrease OTM.

Implication
When corticosteroids are used acutely for allergy reactions, usually for 1–2 weeks, a slower OTM may be noticed since these medications strongly decrease inflammation. However, when corticosteroids are used chronically over 3–6 months, many adverse catabolic events occur within the body, including break down of bones and possible osteoporosis. Since increased bone resorption has the potential to increase OTM, light forces are important during the orthodontic treatment. At the same time, the patients should be monitored for inclusion of new medications along with chronic corticosteroid use that may strongly hinder OTM, such as BP used to treat chronic corticosteroid-induced osteoporosis.

Antihistamines

Antihistamine medications are very commonly taken for allergies, asthma, or many other medical conditions and may be prescribed or purchased over the counter. Antihistamines are histamine 1 (H1) receptor antagonists. In regions where there is high bone turnover, histamine will promote formation of osteoclasts indirectly via H1 receptors on osteoblasts. Meh et al. (2011) demonstrated increased alveolar bone density in rats after administration of cetirizine along with orthodontic force application. They observed a reduction in tooth movement by indirectly blocking recruitment and differentiation of osteoclasts by blocking H1 receptors on osteoblasts. Therefore, animal research has suggested that antihistamines have the potential to slow OTM.

Cimetidine, ranitidine, and famotidine are histamine (H2) receptor agonists, medications that block stomach acid production. Sprogar et al. (2008) found that famotidine interfered with osteoclastic resorption in rats and OTM was decreased.

Implication

Antihistamines, both H1 (antihistamines) and H2 (decrease stomach acid) blockers, have the potential to decrease OTM by decreasing inflammation and decreasing bone resorption. OTM should be monitored during chronic antihistamine use.

Statins: cholesterol-lowering drugs

Mundy (2001) stated that statins are one of the most common and widely prescribed drugs for lowering high cholesterol levels with more than 3 million Americans taking statins daily. In their research on rodents, Maritz et al. (2001) found that osteoblasts and osteoclasts may differ in their sensitivities to various statins, and to different dosages. They evaluated the effects on bone mineral density (BMD), bone formation, and bone resorption of different dosages of simvastatin (1, 5, 10, and 20 mg/kg/day), as well as fixed doses of atorvastatin (2.5 mg/kg/day) and pravastatin (10 mg/kg/day) in female rats. After 12 weeks of administration, rats receiving atorvastatin, pravastatin, and simvastatin 1 mg/kg/day, demonstrated a significant decrease in BMD when compared with the control group. As the dosage of simvastatin was increased, it was noted that the rate of decrease of BMD was reduced. When evaluating bone remodeling in detail, the investigators discovered that the simvastatin 20 mg/kg/day group showed an increase in both resorption and deposition, with marked increases in osteoid volumes, osteoid surfaces, and osteoblast and osteoclast numbers. They observed an inverse correlation between higher dose and more decreased BMD. They noted a decrease in bone formation with an increase in bone resorption, resulting in a greater decrease in BMD when lower doses of simvastatin were administered to rodents. Reports in the orthodontic and periodontal literature (Yazawa et al., 2005; Wong and Rabie, 2006; Seto et al., 2008) have demonstrated anabolic effects of simvastatin on bone remodeling.

Animal experiments revealed that statins may play a dual role, in that in normal dosages they promote bone formation more than bone resorption, increasing the BMD, while in lower doses they are more catabolic than anabolic. Yazawa et al. (2005) demonstrated an increase in the proliferation and differentiation of human PDL cells in vitro while Seto et al. (2008) showed bone induction with simvastatin even in rats with periodontitis. Comparing the effects of collagen matrix carrier alone (water for injection, mixed with absorbable collagen sponge alone) and collagen matrix carrier combined with statin (simvastatin dissolved in water for injection, mixed with absorbable collagen sponge), Wong and Rabie (2006) demonstrated a 308% higher bone formation rate with the latter than the former, when grafted to bone defects. Immunolocalization studies demonstrated a marked increase in mRNA expression for bone morphogenetic protein-2 (BMP-2), vascular endothelial growth factor (VEGF), alkaline phosphatase, type I collagen, bone sialoprotein, and osteocalcin in nontransformed osteoblastic cells, indicating the role of statins in osteoblast differentiation (Maeda et al., 2004; Wong and Rabie, 2005; Han et al., 2010). Han et al. (2010) have illuminated the beneficial effects of simvastatin in preventing relapse after OTM, measured on plaster models as well as immunohistochemistry. Upon injecting rats with simvastatin, 2.5 mg/kg for 4 days post-OTM, they observed a reduction in bone-resorbing activity, while stimulating bone formation, probably by controlling the ratio of local osteoprotegerin to RANKL in the periodontal tissues. Dolci et al. (2017, 2018) showed that the long-term use of atorvastatin can significantly promote osteoclast inhibition and slow the OTM in the first week in rats, due to increased periodontal expression of osteoprotegerin. However, AlSwafeeri et al. (2018) found local administration of simvastatin reduced active bone resorption but did not significantly minimize post-treatment relapse in rabbits A recent systematic review found nine eligible studies (one clinical and eight animal studies) out of 265 identified studies, and concluded the debatable role of statins on OTM considering the high risk-of-bias and methodological inconsistencies among the included studies. They observed six experimental studies and one clinical study which reported reduction, while two experimental studies reported no effect of statin administration on OTM (Kommuri et al., 2020).

Implication

While research points to the beneficial effects of statins during the retention period by reducing bone resorption, the anabolic effects of statins might be a drawback during OTM. Most studies mentioned above were performed on animal models and human trials are underway in different institutions worldwide. Until further studies are performed, it may be hypothesized that orthodontic patients on statins might show reduced bone resorption, and the orthodontist may expect a slower pace of tooth movement in these patients.

Drugs inducing gingival enlargement

Gingival enlargement can slow OTM by creating a physical obstruction to space closure. Drug-induced enlargement usually appears as swollen gingiva without bleeding. It is thought that certain drugs cause fibroblast proliferation and can be augmented by poor oral hygiene. The chronic administration of certain drugs, such as phenytoin, nifedipine, cyclosporine A, and estrogen, usually for more than one year, has been noted to cause gingival enlargement (Kastrup, 2010; Brunton et al., 2011; Longo et al., 2011). Phenytoin, an anticonvulsant drug, is the medication that induces gingival enlargement most often. Gingival enlargement has also been noted with nifedipine and possibly other calcium blockers taken for cardiovascular problems, estrogen released during pregnancy or taken routinely as birth control pills, or cyclosporine A, used to suppress immunity after organ transplantation (Daley et al., 1991). Another gingival manifestation has been noted with valproic acid, usually taken to prevent seizures or bipolar disorders, which has the potential to induce gingival bleeding even with minor trauma, making orthodontic maneuvers difficult (Brodie, 2003). Meticulous oral hygiene should be implemented, as this has been noted to lessen gingival enlargement. The patient's physician should be consulted for possible alternative medications and/or a removal of braces to promote better oral hygiene. Gingival enlargement may decrease by 50% after the drug has been discontinued for 6–12 months. However, often a gingivectomy may be needed esthetically with the understanding that gingival enlargement may still reoccur after gingivectomy.

Should gingival enlargement and gingival bleeding be present after proper oral hygiene is confirmed and bodily bruises are noted by patient or parent, a physician referral should be considered to rule out possible leukemia.

Implication
In patients with gingival enlargement, the orthodontist should take a medical/drug history, monitor oral hygiene, OTM, gingival size and bleeding, question bodily bruising, and make an appropriate physician consultation or referral.

Anticholinergic drugs
Anticholinergic medications decrease salivary flow and dry oral mucous membranes. Anticholinergic drugs effects are usually typified by the drug, atropine. Anticholinergics, such as benzatropine, are typically given to decrease the extrapyramidal adverse effects from antipsychotic medications. However, there are many other medications that have anticholinergic action, such as certain antihistamines (diphenhydramine) or combination OTC medications to relieve cold or allergy symptoms. Atypical facial pain medications may also have anticholinergic properties such as muscle relaxants (cyclobenzaprine), tricyclic antidepressants (amitryptyline), or benzodiazepines (diazepam) (Luther, 2007). A side effect associated with all these drugs is xerostomia, which may be a significant condition in patients under orthodontic care. In these individuals, xerostomia can negatively affect proper maintenance of oral hygiene, increasing the risk for caries and periodontitis. Xerostomia might particularly increase the incidence of root surface caries or changes in oral tissues (Krishnan and Davidovitch, 2006b).

Implication
Anticholinergic drugs cause less salivary secretion, increasing the possibility of a dry mouth, higher caries potential. and changes in oral tissues.

Psychiatric drugs
Adolescents with psychiatric problems might be on medications which may have definite influences on dental, as well as orthodontic care. There are many psychiatric disorders, such as attention deficit/hyperactivity disorders, depression, eating disorders, anxiety disorders, and oppositional defiant/conduct disorders. The attention deficit/hyperactivity disorder is mainly treated with central nervous system stimulants, such as methylphenidate, dextroamphetamine, atomoxetine, buproprion, clonidine, and guanfacine. These drugs may have immediate impact on orthodontic treatment, related to problems with patient compliance and home care, as well as maintenance of oral hygiene (Goldman, 2004). Patients on antidepressants and mood stabilizers will be overly concerned about their appearance, while at the same time being noncompliant. Benzodiazepines used for anxiety disorders or psychological stress can raise undue concerns in the patients' minds; they will be more concerned about side effects and outcomes but will utilize every chance to disrupt office visits. Psychiatric disorders of developmental origin are treated with second-generation neuroleptics which often lead to challenging, unreasonable worries, inflexibility, odd behavior, and misbehavior with office staff. Orthodontists should keep in mind these behavioral changes in patients on drugs for proper management in the orthodontic offices (Goldman, 2004).

Psychological stress affects the hypothalamic–pituitary–adrenal (HPA) axis, and the immune system. Since osteoclasts and odontoclasts are derived from the immune system, modification of their function by psychological stress may impact the process of root resorption. A survey by Davidovitch et al. (2000) revealed a high risk for developing excessive root resorption during the course of orthodontic treatment in patients with psychological distress. Among the reasons for partial and total loss of scalp hair (alopecia areata and alopecia totalis) is psychological stress, probably through effects on the HPA axis. Davidovitch et al. (1999) reported a case of an adolescent orthodontic patient who developed alopecia totalis during orthodontic treatment. A review of the case revealed a normal medical background, with the presence of a persistent psychological stress perhaps intensified by orthodontic mechanotherapy. Siadat et al. (2017) demonstrated decrease in the rate of tooth movement and the percentages of bone formation and root resorption in dogs with systemic administration of amitriptyline although these changes were not statistically significant in comparison with the control group. They attributed this decrease to be related to anti-inflammatory and antiprostaglandin effects of amitriptyline.

Implication
Patients with psychological distress or being treated with psychiatric medications may exhibit different behaviors during orthodontic treatment, which may influence eating habits, physical appearance, more susceptibility to caries, and compliance which may affect proper orthodontic outcome and the patient's physical and mental health. Orthodontists should expect reduction in rate of tooth movement and bone remodeling in patients taking serotonergic and noradrenergic reuptake inhibitor (SNRI) medications used in the treatment of major depression and different types of pain due to its anti-inflammatory and antagonist effects on prostaglandin.

Hormonal influences on tooth movement

Thyroid hormones
Thyroid hormones play an essential role in the normal growth and development of vertebrates. These hormones enhance the response to growth hormone, stimulate cartilage growth and differentiation, and promote bone maturation and resorption (Gameiro et al., 2007) and are used in the treatment of hypothyroidism, other types of thyroid disorders (such as certain types of goiters, thyroid cancer), and also to test for thyroid function. In bone remodeling, these signal molecules act directly by stimulating the action of osteoclasts, along with an indirect effect through growth factors that are closely related to bone metabolism, such as insulin-like growth factor I (IGF-I) (Wakita et al., 1998). Reports on thyroid hormone administration in rats have revealed that there would be an increase in the rate of tooth movement but, interestingly, a decrease in the amount of root resorption (Vazquez-Landaverde et al., 2002). Seifi et al. (2015b) showed intraperitoneal injection of thyroid hormone and local submucosal injection of prostaglandin E_2 in rats increased OTM while decreasing root resorption. A recent systematic review

which included a total of nine human and 36 animal trials, which met the inclusion criteria, concluded that orthodontically induced inflammatory root resorption (OIIRR) was inhibited by fluoride (estimated treatment effects [ES] = -2.08 [-3.02, -1.14]), thyroxine (ES = -1.91 [-3.20, -0.61]), and steroids (ES = -2.79 [-4.26, -1.33]), while corticotomy (ES = 0.38 [0.05, 0.71]) significantly enhanced OIIRR (Haugland et al., 2018).

Implication
Thyroid hormone administration may accelerate OTM, but in clinical practice the orthodontist can expect normal OTM if patients have normal thyroid serum levels which are monitored by their physician. It is concluded that the amount of root resorption will be less in patient under thyroid hormone therapy. Consider monitoring OTM and anterior periapical radiographs since some patients may be noncompliant with their medication.

Parathyroid hormone and analogues
Parathyroid hormone (PTH), produced by the parathyroid glands, regulates serum calcium concentrations. PTH affects osteoblastic cellular metabolic activity, gene transcriptional activity, and multiple protease secretions (Gameiro et al., 2007; Jilka, 2007) and are used in those who are at high risk of fractures, most often postmenopausal women. Animal studies demonstrate that PTH induces an increase in bone turnover, thereby accelerating OTM (Soma et al., 2000). Salazar et al. (2011) evaluated the effects of teriparatide, a recombinant form of the active (1–34) fragment of PTH used to treat advanced osteoporosis, and suggested that it would be more beneficial for OTM than antiresorptive treatment. Souza-Silva et al. (2016) reported that a systematic review of teriparatide administration to animals demonstrated potential acceleration of OTM in Wistar rats depending on the drug concentration, drug administration, and time for drug release.

This drug reinstates bone density by increasing osteoblastic activity rather than decreasing osteoclastic activity. However, teriparatide (Forteo) treatment for osteoporosis is not for every patient because it is very expensive and can only rebuild bone for 2 years. After 2 years, teriparatide is stopped and an antiresorptive medication is usually prescribed to maintain the increased bone density.

Implication
Teriparatide treatment for osteoporosis during orthodontics should not negatively affect OTM. Orthodontists are encouraged to consult with a physician as to how long the patient will continue teriparatide treatment since teriparatide is usually given for 2 years. After teriparatide treatment is stopped, monitor for commonly given antiresorptive treatments that may decrease OTM such as a BP.

Growth hormone
Growth hormone is being used more by endocrinologists to increase the height of small children. It is common to have these children/teens treated with growth hormone during orthodontic treatment. Varble (2009) found OTM to increase in rats given growth hormone for 12 days. Funatsu et al. (2006) suggested that growth hormone increases facial growth of the maxilla and mandibular ramus. The important role played by growth hormone in compression side bone resorption through elevated expression of osteopontin was demonstrated through a male Wistar rat study (Ju and Cai, 2017). A recent systematic review by Makrygiannakis et al. (2019) revealed a reduction in root resorption in orthodontic patients treated with growth hormone

Implication
More research is needed to evaluate growth hormone effects upon OTM and facial growth. Clinically, the orthodontist should carefully monitor the maxillary and mandibular growth rates and perhaps anticipate a mild increase in OTM and reduced root resorption.

Estrogen
Estrogens have been used for many decades for birth control and to treat postmenopausal effects in women. Estrogen, an important hormone affecting bone metabolism in women, inhibits the production of cytokines involved in osteoclastic activation and bone resorption, such as IL-1β, IL-6, and TNF-α (Carlsten, 2005). The importance of estrogen receptor (ERα) in maintenance of the microarchitecture of maxillary alveolar bone and disruption of it resulting out of ERα deficiency is reported by Macari et al. (2016). Their experiments demonstrated lower levels of calcium in bone and increased expression of IL-33 (interleukin-33), TNF-α (tumor necrosis factor α), and IL-1β (interleukin-1β) and decreased expression of dentin matrix acidic phosphoprotein and alkaline phosphatase in periodontal tissues in ERKOα mice. The bone marrow cells obtained from these mice exhibited significantly higher levels of osteoclasts and osteoblasts.

Investigators proposed that the application of orthodontic force after each ovulation may promote tooth movement, thereby shortening the course of orthodontic treatment. Yamashiro and Takano-Yamamoto (2001) reported that estrogen deficiency would cause rapid OTM in rats. Celebi et al. (2013) confirmed that tooth movement will be slow in cats injected with estrogen in conjunction with orthodontic force application. Seifi et al. (2015a) through their study on ovariectomized female and orchiectomized male rats reported that lack of estrogen and progesterone as well as testosterone increased the rate of tooth movement and at the same time reduced the risk of orthodontic-induced root resorption. Wheat seeds, the natural material containing phytoestrogens with similar characteristics to estrogen, when administered to 40 male Sprague Dawley rats resulted in significantly higher OPG levels on days 1, 7, and 14, while the RANKL level was considerably lower on day 14. The researchers concluded that wheat seeds can decrease osteoclastogenesis and inhibit tooth movement (Suparwitri et al., 2019). Accordingly, women taking oral contraceptives might experience a reduced rate of tooth movement.

Raloxifene (Evista) is a selective estrogen receptor modulator (SERM), which is an antiresorptive used to treat osteoporosis in place of estrogen with possibly fewer medical adverse effects (Kastrup, 2010). Recently, the efficacy of raloxifene was evaluated in 15-week-old male Wistar rats by injecting 2.0 mg/kg/day subcutaneously after OTM during the retention period. The researchers reported a significant increase in bone volume fraction, tissue density, and a decrease in number of osteoclasts and RANKL expression with raloxifene injection for 14 days along with retention-preventing relapse tendencies (Azami et al., 2020).

Implication
Estrogens decrease bone turnover and may decrease OTM. Estrogens do have a short effect (one day) within the body. However, many patients have been on estrogens during orthodontics without many literature reports of adverse effects. It is advisable to monitor OTM, anticipate mild decreased OTM, and discuss with a physician should an observed decreased OTM affect orthodontic outcome.

Relaxin

Relaxin, a known pregnancy hormone, is released just before childbirth to loosen the pubic symphysis, in order for the relaxed suture to allow widening of the birth canal for parturition (Dschietzig et al., 2006). It is demonstrated through various studies that relaxin has stimulatory effects on PDL collagen metabolism and collagenase production, as reflected by elevated expression of MMP1 and MMP8, and increases collagen degradation activity in the PDL (Stewart et al., 2005; Takano et al. 2009; Swidi et al., 2018). Liu et al. (2005) observed that the administration of human relaxin in rats accelerated the early stages of OTM. Nicozisis et al. (2000) suggested that relaxin might be used: as an adjunct to orthodontic therapy, during or after tooth movement, for promotion of stability; for rapid remodeling of gingival tissue during extraction space closure; or for orthopedic expansion in nongrowing patients, by reducing the tension of the stretched soft-tissue envelope and after orthognathic surgery. Further experiments on relaxin by Takano et al. (2009) on stretched human PDL cells confirmed that relaxin did modulate collagen metabolism via the release and expression of COL-1 and MMP-1. They further proposed its use in preventing orthodontic relapse. However, casting doubt on all these findings were the results reported by McGorray et al. (2012) through their randomized, placebo-controlled clinical trial. They could observe no differences in tooth movement over 8 weeks of treatment, or relapse at 4 weeks after treatment, when comparing subjects who received weekly injections of relaxin with those who received a placebo.

Implication

Relaxin did not affect OTM in a human random controlled trial. No clinical effect on OTM is to be anticipated for relaxin analogs used for medical purposes.

Effects of vitamins, minerals, and diet on tooth movement

The various adverse effects on the body as a result of the lack of vitamins and essential minerals in the diet, led to their discovery. The role of vitamins, minerals, and other dietary components on collagen and bone remodeling processes has long been a subject of great interest for clinicians and researchers alike (Hercz, 2001). The findings led to the conclusion that certain elements found in the diet and in dietary supplements may find their way through the circulation, into the PDL, and may modulate the cellular response to mechanical loads.

Vitamins

Vitamins are a group of substances essential for normal metabolism, growth and development, and regulation of cell functions. Vitamins work in concert with enzymes, co-enzymes, and other substances necessary for a healthy life. There are 13 vitamins essential for bodily functions of which vitamin A, D, E, and K are fat soluble, and B-complex and vitamin C, which are water-soluble. Even though all vitamins are essential for maintenance of healthy teeth and paradental tissues, those that impact bone and PDL remodeling are discussed below.

Vitamin C

Vitamin C (ascorbic acid) is a co-factor required for the function of several hydroxylases and can only be obtained through the diet. The absence of vitamin C in the diet is responsible for the development of scurvy. The classical signs of scurvy include gingival hyperplasia, bleeding gums, and tooth mobility. The disease is typified by the synthesis of defective collagen due to the reduced function of prolyl hydroxylase. The absence of this essential vitamin is a risk factor for periodontitis (Touyz, 1997). Vitamin C induces stem cells to differentiate into osteoblasts through the synthesis of type I collagen, interaction with specific integrins, activation of a protein kinase pathway, and phosphorylation of osteoblast-specific transcription factors (Ishikawa et al., 2004).

About 30% of the total body protein consists of collagen, which is the main component of the organic matrix of dentin, cementum, alveolar bone, and PDL. About 10–15% of the collagen consists of hydroxyproline, which is required for crosslinking. Vitamin C is an important co-factor in hydroxyproline formation, and it also stimulates fibroblasts to produce collagen. McCanlies et al. (1961) showed rapid relapse in guinea pigs deficient in ascorbic acid, emphasizing its role in the retention of treated malocclusions. Miresmaeili et al. (2015) reported oral vitamin C increases OTM in rats with more osteoclast lacunae around roots in the pressure areas increasing the possibility of inducing root resorption. Motoji et al. (2020) also confirmed the acceleration in tooth movement observed with administration of vitamin C in 9-week-old male osteogenic disorder Shionogi rats and they also reported the synergistic effect it holds when administered along with egg shell membrane and attributed it to increased expression of type I and III collagen.

Implication

Normal dietary ingestion of vitamin C is needed for a healthy periodontium during orthodontics. Based on one animal study, vitamin C supplementation possibly increases OTM slightly. However, human trials are needed to evaluate the effect of vitamin C administration clinically.

Vitamin D

Another agent that has been identified as an important factor in OTM is 1, 25, dehydroxycholecalciferol (1, 25, DHCC) (Collins and Sinclair, 1988). This agent is a biologically active form of vitamin D and has a significant role in calcium homeostasis. A decrease in the serum calcium level stimulates secretion of PTH, which in turn increases excretion of PO_4^{3-}, reabsorption of calcium from the kidneys, and hydroxylation of 25, hydroxycholecaliferol to 1, 25, DHCC. The latter molecule has been shown to be a potent stimulator of bone resorption by inducing differentiation of osteoclasts from their precursors (Kale et al., 2004; Kawakami and Takano-Yamamoto, 2004). Kale et al. (2004) compared the effects of local administration of 1, 25, DHCC and PGE_2 on OTM and reported that both molecules enhance tooth movement significantly compared with a control group. In that study, 1, 25, DHCC was found to be more effective than PGE_2 in modulating bone turnover during OTM, because of its well-balanced effects on bone formation and resorption. Another study by Kawakami and Takano-Yamamoto et al. (2004) tried to determine the effect of 1, 25, DHCC on alveolar bone formation during OTM in rats. The researchers observed significant increases in the mineral appositional rate associated with an elevated osteoblast surface in PDL tension sites of teeth subjected to repeated injections of 1, 25, DHCC. They concluded that local applications of calcitriol could enhance the reestablishment of dental supporting tissues, especially alveolar bone, after OTM. Iosub Ciur et al. (2016) showed local administration of vitamin D_3 seemed to increase the rate of OTM of cuspids in a split-mouth controlled study. A recent systematic review in this regard has concluded that local injections of calcitriol, a vitamin D metabolite, were not shown to exert a statistically significant effect on the rate of OTM, but with a low level of confidence (Kaklamanos et al., 2020).

Implication
Orthodontic research has demonstrated that a local injection of vitamin D can increase OTM. However, it is more likely that the orthodontist might notice no effect or a mild increase in OTM during patient supplementation of vitamin D systemically.

Vitamin A
Vitamin A has important roles to play in bone remodeling and collagen metabolism, through its action on cell metabolism. Animal studies have demonstrated that supplementation of vitamin A increases the breaking strength of healing wounds along with enhanced collagen production (Togari et al., 1991). Retinol deficiency leads to inhibited processes of bone remodeling by decreasing the activity of osteoclasts and bone deformation. The basic adverse symptom of retinol excess in the body (vitamin A hypervitaminosis) is intensification of the bone tissue resorption processes. However, the research with OTM in rats receiving injections of different doses of vitamin A did not increase the rate of OTM and led to the conclusion that vitamin A has no role in OTM (Sodagar et al., 2008). Nishio et al. (2017) reported isotretinoin, a synthetic form of vitamin A used for severe acne, did not affect the OTM when injected into rats.

Implication
Vitamin A appears not to affect OTM clinically.

Minerals
Minerals, are important in collagen metabolism and calcified tissue maintenance and remodeling. Copper is important in crosslinking of collagen and elastin, deficiency of which can lead to decreased tensile strength of collagen, and osteoporotic-like bone lesions. The other mineral of importance is manganese, which is involved in several enzyme systems such as metalloenzymes pyruvate carboxylase and superoxide dismutase, and in protein and energy metabolism and glucose utilization. This element is implicated in playing a major role in bone remodeling. It was found to be associated with decreased bone resorption, production of labile bone, and decreased synthesis of organic matrix in rats deficient in manganese (Strause et al., 1987). Riordan (1997) reported that manganese and copper mean intakes were the only intakes to decrease significantly after orthodontic appliance adjustments. They attributed this effect to the decrease in intake of nuts, whole grains, and fruits and vegetables that can cause discomfort to pressure-sensitive teeth. It was suggested that bone remodeling in these patients occurs at a slower rate, and that this bone is less dense than normal. Moreover, these patients demonstrated a steady increase in calcium intake, and a 1:1 ratio between calcium and phosphorous intake was not being maintained because of an increase in the intake of phosphorus-rich soft drinks and fast food items. However, an increase in the consumption of dairy products after wearing orthodontic appliances has led to an increase in calcium intake from a pretreatment value of 0.76 to 0.87 (Sharma et al., 2011) during and after treatment. This effect may be beneficial for bone remodeling during OTM. Seifi et al. (2003) gave calcium supplementation to rats and found low blood concentrations of PTH and a mild decrease in OTM. Supplementation of these minerals at recommended daily allowance (RDA) levels should be maintained during orthodontic treatment.

Implication
Adequate vitamin and mineral uptake is important, so deficiencies should not occur and affect the patient's health. Calcium supplementation may possibly effect a mild decrease in OTM. However, the evidence regarding mineral supplementation has not been conclusive for effects upon OTM.

Fluoride
Fluoride is taken up by hydroxyapatite, making the enamel more impervious to breakdown by bacterial products. Fluoride may be ingested from drinking water, inadvertent swallowing of toothpaste, or taken by prescription. Fluoride is also deposited in the bone and may change bone resorption. Gonzales et al. (2011) showed a decreased OTM in rats after administering 10 ppm of fluoride in water for 12 weeks. However, Karadeniz et al. (2011) found an increase in OTM using high forces during 4 weeks in adult extraction patients who were ingesting high fluoride levels in drinking water (2 ppm). However, no increased tooth movement was seen with low forces and high fluoride when compared with drinking water with low fluoride levels (0.05 ppm). Zorlu et al. (2019), through their Wistar albino rat study, reported that even though fluoride significantly reduced the number of osteoclasts in the experimental groups, no difference was observed with respect to the amount of tooth movement between the fluoridated and nonfluoridated groups.

Implication
The small amount of fluoride ingested to decrease dental decay may have mild changes in OTM but needs further human study.

Lipids
Lipids play an important role in skeletal biology (Watkins et al., 2001a). Emerging evidence suggests that dietary intake of certain fatty acids influences bone modeling and remodeling by maintaining BMD in the elderly and increasing it in children (Watkins et al., 2001b). Lipids are thought to influence the process of bone metabolism, in part by altering the synthesis of PGs. Watkins et al. (2001b) reported that dietary lipids modulate *ex vivo* bone PGE_2 production and the concentration of IGF-1 in bone, leading to altered bone formation rates. Kokkinos et al. (1993) conducted experiments on rats and found that arachidonic acid and PGE_2 concentrations were significantly lower in alveolar bone of rats fed with n-3 rich fatty acids than in the group fed with a purified diet rich in n-6 fatty acids. The tooth movement was also significantly slower in the former group than in the latter, suggesting that PGE_2 levels in alveolar bone and OTM can be affected by the type of dietary fat. Riordan (1997) observed that, with orthodontic treatment, the total calorie intake by adolescents increased from a pretreatment value of 30% to 36.71%, but at the expense of carbohydrates, which dropped to 49.32% below the recommended 55%. He concluded that most of this increase came from an increase in saturated fat (14.32%) and monounsaturated fat with little change in polyunsaturated fat. The patients moved further away from the guidelines in all areas with a decrease in fiber, a decrease in percentage of calories from

carbohydrate, and an increase in percentage of calories from total fat and saturated fat. Iwami-Morimoto (1999) found a decreased OTM when feeding rats a diet high in omega 3,6 fatty acids. Ogrenim et al. (2019) investigated the effects of omega-3 fatty acids on OTM in male Wistar albino rats and concluded that systemic administration of the same resulted in antioxidant and anti-inflammatory effects and reduced the OTM.

Implication
Omega 3,6 fatty acids (fish oil, flax seed) in large amounts may mildly to moderately decrease OTM by blocking inflammation pathways. Orthodontics and especially combined orthodontic/orthognathic treatment may adversely affect eating habits by patients selecting poor food choices. Often a nutritionist may be of help in order to ensure that proper carbohydrates, proteins, lipids, essential vitamins and minerals are taken, and to keep our patients in a healthy state during and after orthodontic treatment.

Substance abuse and OTM

Alcohol use
Chronic alcohol consumption results in an osteopenic skeleton and an increased risk for osteoporosis. These patients are prone to delayed fracture healing when compared with nonalcoholics (Chakkalakal, 2005). Alcohol consumption during adolescence reduces peak bone mass and can result in relatively weak adult bones (Sampson, 1998). This occurs as a direct result of inhibited *Wnt* signaling and activation of peroxisome proliferator-activated receptor-γ (PPAR-γ) pathways in mesenchymal stem cells by fatty acids as the result of oxidative stress. This event will result in inhibited bone formation accompanied by increased bone-marrow adiposity. Alcohol-induced oxidative stress as the result of increased nicotinamide adenine dinucleotide phosphate oxidase (NADPH-oxidase) activity in bone cells also results in enhanced RANKL-RANK signaling to increase osteoclastogenesis (Ronis et al., 2011).

Orthodontists treating patients with chronic alcoholism should therefore be aware of the bone-remodeling response and take necessary precautions to avoid excessive force application leading to tooth mobility. In addition, Davidovitch et al. (1996) have found that chronic alcoholics receiving orthodontic treatment are at a high risk of developing severe root resorption during the course of orthodontic treatment. The effects of chronic alcoholism and ovariectomy in rats were studied on samples of alveolar bone crest to verify composition changes of hydroxyapatite by measuring the calcium and phosphorus (Ca/P) ratios with micro X-ray fluorescence spectrometry (Marchini et al., 2012). The ovariectomy/alcohol group presented lower values for Ca/P ratios (1.92 ± 0.06), being the only group statistically different ($P < 0.001$) from the control group. Ovariectomy associated with alcohol consumption significantly changed the stoichiometry composition of hydroxyapatite in the alveolar bone crest, leading to a reduction in Ca/P ratios. This type of bone may be prone to periodontal disease and excessive resorption during OTM. Schröder et al. (2019) showed that when compressive forces were placed on human periodontal fibroblasts during high ethanol levels, bone resorption increased and increased tooth movement could be expected.

Implication
Chronic alcohol ingestion can cause many medical, dental, social, and dietary problems for which the orthodontist should make the proper referrals. If the patient is considered a candidate for elective orthodontic treatment, light forces should be used since OTM may be increased.

Nicotine use
Cigarette smoking is an important risk factor in lung cancers and is implicated in the progression of atherosclerosis and cardiovascular diseases. Investigations of American students have shown that 8.1% of middle school students and 22.3% of high school students smoke cigarettes, and about 20% of American adults are smokers (US Centers for Disease Control and Prevention, 2005). Moreover, smoking has injurious intraoral effects, such as increases in the progression of periodontal disease, as well as carious lesions. Nicotine is a very addicting substance found within cigarette smoke and the vapor from electronic cigarettes. Vaping, use of electronic cigarettes, is becoming more popular in the younger generations. The nicotine content per puff in vaping can vary from low to a much higher nicotine level found in cigarettes. The increase in bone resorption observed with nicotine is mediated through the COX enzyme, which converts arachidonic acid to PGs (Baljoon et al., 2005). Nicotine causes an increase in the expression of the *COX-2* gene and PGE_2 release from human gingival fibroblasts, thereby increasing the pace of OTM in a time- and dose-dependent manner. This was proven to be true in rats, as daily administration of nicotine adversely affected the periodontal tissues in a dose-dependent manner (Sodagar et al., 2011). A systematic review (Michelogiannakis et al., 2018b) including six rat studies suggested nicotine exposure increases OTM by increasing alveolar bone loss with more root resorption also being noted. Araujo et al. (2018) evaluated the effect of acute administration of nicotine and ethanol on tooth movement in rats and concluded that nicotine and ethanol did not affect the tooth movement rate, regardless of induction of orthodontic movement. Nicotine influenced the number of osteoclasts by decreasing their quantity and when it was associated with ethanol, it interfered in the maturation of collagen fibers during orthodontic movement.

Implication
Orthodontists should be aware of patients that smoke or vape. They should encourage their patients to stop using tobacco due to its adverse effects on longevity, quality of life, and oral tissues. Patients that vape should understand that nicotine is a highly addictive substance and long-term adverse effects on the brain are unsure. Nicotine-replacement therapy, such as nicotine patches or nicotine gum, is beneficial to stop smoking. Nicotine has the potential to possibly increase OTM, therefore light orthodontic forces should be used. Root resorption may be more prevalent and should be monitored during nicotine use.

Conclusions
Human beings, in every culture and community on earth, consume a large variety of molecules, in the form of food ingredients, medications, drugs, and remedies. Medically related molecules are prescribed and/or provided by physicians, dentists, other healthcare providers, and the patients themselves. These medications are aimed at specific illnesses, but they always have systemic effects involving several systems, organs, tissues, and cells. Some of these systems, including the nervous, endocrine, immune, vascular, and skeletal systems, can respond readily to the presence of medically related molecules in the body and alter their functions. Such

alterations may profoundly affect the course and outcome of therapeutic procedures, such as orthodontic treatment. Tooth movement by mechanical forces during orthodontic treatment requires cellular inflammation and bone changes. Any medication that affects inflammation or bone turnover may affect orthodontic outcome to change tooth position.

Each year the FDA is approving many new drugs, such as monoclonal antibodies with a suffix '–mab.' These drugs effectively target a specific receptor site on a specific cell. For example, denosumab, an antiresorptive drug which effectively targets an area on osteoclasts causing them not to mature, severely decreases 80% of osteoclastic activity and thereby decreasing bone resorption. When osteoclastic activity is severely decreased within the body, bone production is also decreased by a subsequent 60% decrease in osteoblastic activity within 6 months. This drug, taken during normal orthodontic treatment, has the potential to severely change orthodontic outcome by severely decreasing tooth movement and leaving teeth mobile. Therefore, it is imperative that the orthodontist should obtain a comprehensive list of all the medications consumed by every patient both before and during the course of orthodontic treatment. Furthermore, the orthodontist should explore and understand the pharmacologic actions of each medication and utilize this information as a helpful tool in identifying, assessing, and predicting variables that may affect cellular and tissue responses, as well as treatment outcomes. Moreover, it is strongly recommended to seek a physician's advice before embarking on orthodontic treatment whenever it becomes evident that a patient is consuming medications or drugs capable of affecting systems and cells involved in the modeling or remodeling of paradental tissues during orthodontic treatment.

Dietary ingredients and supplements, when reaching the mechanically strained PDL and alveolar bone, may also interact with cells responding to the mechanical loads, modifying their responses to the orthodontic forces applied. Seeking the professional services of a nutritionist, pharmacist, or physician may help orthodontists gather valuable information about the biological background of each of their patient's needs. This knowledge may assist the orthodontist in crafting treatment plans tailored for the specific needs of each individual patient. Moreover, such information may enable the orthodontist to understand better the reasons for successful outcomes, as well as undesirable side effects, such as decreased OTM, severe root resorption, and rapid relapse of otherwise successfully treated malocclusions. At the present time we are entering the era of personalized medicine and dentistry, facilitated by a wave of technological advancements. The contents of this chapter illuminate the biological differences that occur between patients and raise hopes that the wave of innovations will bring us closer to accomplishing the goal of individualized orthodontics in a real biological sense. This goal may be attained by integrating the orthodontic specialty with the rest of medicine.

References

AAOMS (2014) American Association of Oral and Maxillofacial Surgeons Position Paper on Medication-Related Osteonecrosis of the Jaw – 2014 Update. *Journal of Oral and Maxillofacial Surgery* **7**, 1938–1956.

Abtahi, M., Shafaee, H., Saghravania, N. et al. (2014) Effect of corticosteroids on orthodontic tooth movement in a rabbit model. *Journal of Clinical and Pediatric Dentistry* **38**(3), 285–289.

Alatli, I., Hellsing, E. and Hammarström, L. (1996) Orthodontically induced root resorption in rat molars after 1-hydroxyethylidene-1,1-bisphosphonate injection. *Acta Odontologica Scandinavica* **54**, 102–108.

AlSwafeeri, H., ElKenany, W., Mowafy, M. and Karam, S. (2018) Effect of local administration of simvastatin on postorthodontic relapse in a rabbit model. *American Journal of Orthodontics and Dentofacial Orthopedics* **153**(6), 861–871.

Arantes, G. M., Arantes, V. M. N., Ashmawi, H. A. and Posso, I. P. (2009) Tenoxicam controls pain without altering orthodontic movement of maxillary canines. *Orthodontics and Craniofacial Research* **12**, 14–19.

Araujo, C. M. D., Rocha, A. C., Araujo, B. M. D. M. D. et al. (2018) Effect of acute administration of nicotine and ethanol on tooth movement in rats. *Brazilian Oral Research* **32**, e96.

Arias, O. R and Marquez-Orozco, M. C. (2006) Aspirin, acetaminophen, and ibuprofen: their effects on orthodontic tooth movement. *American Journal of Orthodontics and Dentofacial Orthopedics* **130**, 364–370.

Asaad, H., Al-Sabbagh, R., Al-Tabba, D. and Kujan, O. (2017) Effect of the leukotriene receptor antagonist montelukast on orthodontic tooth movement. *Journal of Oral Science* **59**(2), 297–302.

Azami, N., Chen, P. J., Mehta, S. et al. (2020) Raloxifene administration enhances retention in an orthodontic relapse model. *European Journal of Orthodontics*. doi: 10.1093/ejo/cjaa008

Baljoon, M., Natto, S. and Bergström, J. (2005) Long-term effect of smoking on vertical periodontal bone loss. *Journal of Clinical Periodontology* **32**, 789–797.

Bartzela, T., Turp, J. C., Motschall, E. and Maltha, J. C. (2009) Medication effects on the rate of orthodontic tooth movement. *American Journal of Orthodontics and Dentofacial Orthopedics* **135**, 16–26.

Black, D. M., Thompson, D. E., Bauer, D. C. et al. (2000) Fracture risk reduction with alendronate in women with osteoporosis: the Fracture Intervention Trial. FIT research group. *Journal of Clinical Endocrinology and Metabolism* **85**, 4118–4124.

Brodie, D. H., Lots, M., Cuomo, A. J. et al. (1992) Cytokines in symptomatic asthma airways. *Journal of Allergy and Clinical Immunology* **89**, 958–967.

Brodie, M. J. (2003) Building new understandings in epilepsy: maximizing patient outcomes without sacrificing seizure control. *Epilepsia* **44**, 1–2.

Brunton, L. L., Blumenthal, D. K., Murri, N. et al. (2011) *Goodman and Gilman's Pharmacological Basic of Therapeutics*, 12th edn. McGraw-Hill Medical, New York, NY.

Cağlaroğlu, M. and Erdem, A. (2012) Histopathologic investigation of the effects of prostaglandin E2 administered by different methods on tooth movement and bone metabolism. *Korean Journal of Orthodontics* **42**, 118–128.

Carlsten, H. (2005) Immune responses and bone loss: the estrogen connection. *Immunological Reviews* **208**, 194–206.

Celebi, A. A., Demirer, S., Catalbas, B. and Arikan, S. (2013) Effect of ovarian activity on orthodontic tooth movement and gingival crevicular fluid levels of interleukin-1β and prostaglandin E(2) in cats. *The Angle Orthodontist* **83**, 70–75.

Chakkalakal, D. A. (2005) Alcohol-induced bone loss and deficient bone repair. *Alcohol Clinical and Experimental Research* **29**, 2077–2090.

Chumbley, A. B. and Tuncay, O. C. (1986) The effect of indomethacin (an aspirin like drug) on the rate of orthodontic tooth movement. *American Journal of Orthodontics and Dentofacial Orthopedics* **89**, 312–314.

Collins, M. and Sinclair, P. M. (1988) The local use of vitamin D to increase rate of orthodontic tooth movement. *American Journal of Orthodontics and Dentofacial Orthopedics* **94**, 278–284.

Consolaro, A., Maldonado, V. B., Santamaria, M. Jr. and Consolaro, M. F. (2010) Sources of controversies over analgesics prescribed after activation of orthodontic appliances: acetylsalicylic acid or acetaminophen? *Dental Press Journal of Orthodontics* **15**, 16–24.

Correa, A. S., Almeida, V. L., Lopes, B. et al. (2017) The influence of non-steroidal anti-inflammatory drugs and paracetamol used for pain control of orthodontic tooth movement: a systematic review. *Anais da Academia Brasileira de Ciências* **89**(4), 2851–2863.

Cremers, S., Sparidans, H., den Hartigh, J. et al. (2002) A pharmacokinetic and pharmacodynamic model for intravenous bisphosphonate (pamidronate) in osteoporosis. *European Journal of Clinical Pharmacology* **57**, 883–890.

Cummings, S. R., San Martin, J., McClung, M. R. et al. (2009) Denosumab for prevention of fractures in postmenopausal women with osteoporosis. *New England Journal of Medicine* **361**, 756–765.

Daley, T. D., Wysocki, G. P. and Mamandras, A. H. (1991) Orthodontic therapy in the patient treated with cyclosporine. *American Journal of Orthodontics and Dentofacial Orthopedics* **100**, 537–541.

Davidovitch, Z., Godwin, S. L., Park, Y. G. et al. (1996) The etiology of root resorption, in *Orthodontic Treatment: The Management of Unfavorable Sequelae* (eds. J. A. McNamara and C. A. Trotman) University of Michigan Press, Ann Arbor, MI, pp. 93–117.

Davidovitch, Z., Lee, Y. J., Chung, K. R. et al. (1999) Alopecia: an unexpected effect of orthodontic treatment. *Korean Journal of Orthodontics* **29**, 663–672.

Davidovitch, Z., Lee, Y. J., Counts, A. L. et al. (2000) The immune system possibly modulates orthodontic root resorption, in *Biological Mechanisms of Tooth Movement* and *Craniofacial Adaptation* (eds. Z. Davidovitch and J. Mah). Harvard Society for the Advancement of Orthodontics, Boston, MA, pp. 207–217.

de Carlos, F., Cobo, J., Perillan, C. et al. (2007) Orthodontic tooth movement after different coxib therapies. *European Journal of Orthodontics* 29(6), 596–599.

Dolci, G. S., Ballarini, A., Gameiro, G.H. et al. (2018) Atorvastatin inhibits osteoclastogenesis and arrests tooth movement. *American Journal of Orthodontics and Dentofacial Orthopedics* 153(6), 872–882.

Dolci, G. S., Portela, L. V., de Souza, D. O. and Fossati, A. C. M. (2017) Atorvastatin-induced osteoclast inhibition reduces orthodontic relapse. *American Journal of Orthodontics and Dentofacial Orthopedics* 151(3), 528–538.

Dschietzig, T., Bartsch, C., Baumann, G. and Stangl, K. (2006) Relaxin – a pleiotropic hormone and its emerging role for experimental and clinical therapeutics. *Pharmacology and Therapeutics* 112, 38–56.

Elsasser, S. and Perruchoud, A. P. (1992) Pathophysiology of bronchial asthma. *Schweizerische Rundschau fur Medizin Praxis* 81, 346–349.

Fernández-González, F. J., López-Caballo, J. L., Cañigral, A. et al. (2016) Osteoprotegerin and zoledronate bone effects during orthodontic tooth movement. *Orthodontics and Craniofacial Research* 19(1), 54–64.

Ferreira, M. K. M., de Oliveira Ferreira, R., Castro, M. M. L. et al. (2019) Is there an association between asthma and periodontal disease among adults? Systematic review and meta-analysis. *Life Sciences* 223, 74–87.

Fizazi, K., Carducci, M., Smith, M. et al. (2011) Denosumab versus zoledronic acid for the treatment of bone metastases in men with castration-resistant prostate cancer: a randomized, double-blind study. *Lancet* 377, 813–822.

Funatsu, M., Saito, K. and Mitani, H. (2006) Effects of growth hormone on craniofacial growth. *The Angle Orthodontist* 76, 970–977.

Gameiro, G. H., Pereira-Neto, J. S., Magnani, M. B. and Nouer, D. F. (2007) The influence of drugs and systemic factors on orthodontic tooth movement. *Journal of Clinical Orthodontics* 41, 73–78.

Goldman, S. J. (2004) Practical approaches to psychiatric issues in the orthodontic patient. *Seminars in Orthodontics* 10, 259–265.

Gonzales, C., Hotokezaka, H., Karadeniz, E. I. et al. (2011) Effects of fluoride intake on orthodontic tooth movement and orthodontically induced root resorption. *American Journal of Orthodontics and Dentofacial Orthopedics* 139, 196–205.

Gurton, A. U., Akin, E., Sagdic, D. and Olmez, H. (2004) Effects of PGI2 and TxA2 analogs and inhibitors in orthodontic tooth movement. *The Angle Orthodontist* 74, 526–532.

Gustafson, T., Eckerdal, O., Leever, D. L. et al. (1977) Prostaglandin E2 (PGE2) levels in alveolar bone of orthodontically treated cats. *Journal of Dental Research* 56, 407–415.

Han, G., Chen, Y., Hou, J. et al. (2010) Effects of simvastatin on relapse and remodeling of periodontal tissues after tooth movement in rats. *American Journal of Orthodontics and Dentofacial Orthopedics* 138, 550.e1–557.

Haugland, L., Kristensen, K. D., Lie, S. A. and Vandevska-Radunovic, V. (2018) The effect of biologic factors and adjunctive therapies on orthodontically induced inflammatory root resorption: a systematic review and meta-analysis. *European Journal of Orthodontics* 40, 326–336.

Hellstein, J. W., Adler, R. A., Edwards, B. et al. (2011) Managing the care of patients receiving anti-resorptive therapy for prevention and treatment of osteoporosis: Executive summary of recommendations from the American Dental Association Council on Scientific Affairs. *Journal of American Dental Association* 142, 1243–1251.

Henry, D. H., Costa, L., Goldwasser, F. et al. (2011) Randomized, double-blind study of denosumab versus zoledronic acid in the treatment of bone metastases in patients with advanced cancer (excluding breast and prostate cancer) or multiple myeloma. *Journal of Clinical Oncology* 29, 1125–1132.

Hercz, G. (2001) Regulation of bone remodeling: impact of novel therapies. *Seminars in Dialysis* 14, 55–60.

Hokugo, A., Kanayama, K., Sun, S. et al. (2019) Rescue bisphosphonate treatment of alveolar bone improves extraction socket healing and reduces osteonecrosis in zoledronate-treated mice. *Bone* 123, 115–128.

Hujaa, S. S., Kayab, B., Moc, X. et al. (2011) Effect of zoledronic acid on bone healing subsequent to mini-implant insertion. *The Angle Orthodontist* 81, 363–369.

Iglesias-Linares A., Yáñez-Vico, R. M., Solano-Reina, E. et al. (2010) Influence of bisphosphonates in orthodontic therapy: systematic review. *Journal of Dentistry* 38, 603–611.

Iosub Ciur, M.D., Zetu, I.N., Haba, D. et al. (2016) Evaluation of the influence of local administration of vitamin D on the rate of orthodontic tooth movement. *Revista Medico-Chirurgicala A Societatii De Medici Si Naturalisti Din Iasi* 20(3), 694–699.

Ishikawa, S., Iwasaki, K., Komaki, M. and Ishikawa, I. (2004) Role of ascorbic acid in periodontal ligament cell differentiation. *Journal of Periodontology* 75, 709–716.

Iwami-Morimoto, Y., Yamaguchi, K. and Tanne, K. (1999) Influence of dietary n-3 polyunsaturated fatty acid on experimental tooth movement in rats. *The Angle Orthodontist* 69, 365–371.

Jilka, R. L. (2007) Molecular and cellular mechanisms of the anabolic effect of intermittent PTH. *Bone* 40, 1434–1446.

Kaipatur, N., Major, P., Stevenson, T. et al. (2015) Impact of selective alveolar decortication on bisphosphonate burdened alveolar bone during orthodontic tooth movement. *Archives of Oral Biology* 60(11), 1681–1689.

Kale, S., Kocadereli, I., Atilla, P. and Asan, E. (2004) Comparison of the effects of 1,25 dihydroxycholciferol and prostaglandin E2 on orthodontic tooth movement. *American Journal of Orthodontics and Dentofacial Orthopedics* 125, 607–614.

Kalia, S., Melsen, B. and Verna, C. (2004) Tissue reaction to orthodontic tooth movement in acute and chronic corticosteroid treatment. *Orthodontics and Craniofacial Research* 7, 26–34.

Kaklamanos, E. G., Makrygiannakis, M. A. and Athanasiou, A. E. (2020) Does medication administration affect the rate of orthodontic tooth movement and root resorption development in humans? A systematic review. *European Journal of Orthodontics* 42, 407–414.

Karadeniz, E. I., Gonzales, C., Elekdag-Turk, S. et al. (2011) The effect of fluoride on orthodontic tooth movement in humans. A two- and three-dimensional evaluation. *Australian Orthodontic Journal* 27, 94–101.

Kastrup, E. K. (eds.) (2010) *Facts and Comparisons*. Wolters Kluwer, St. Louis, MO.

Kawakami, M. and Takano-Yamamoto, T. (2004) Local injection of 1,25-dihydroxyvitamin D3 enhanced bone formation for tooth stabilization after experimental tooth movement in rats. *Journal of Bone and Mineral Metabolism* 22, 541–546.

Kehoe, M. J., Cohen, S. M., Zarrinnia, K. and Cowan, A. (1996) The effect of acetaminophen, ibuprofen and misoprotol on prostaglandin E2 synthesis and the degree and rate of orthodontic tooth movement. *The Angle Orthodontist* 66, 339–350.

Kim, T., Yoshida, Y., Yokoya, K. and Sasaki, T. (1999) An ultrastructural study of the effects of bisphosphonates administration on osteoclastic bone resorption during relapse of experimentally moved rat molars. *American Journal of Orthodontics and Dentofacial Orthopedics* 115, 645–653.

Knop, L. A., Shintcovsk, R. L., Retamoso, L. B. et al. (2012) Non-steroidal and steroidal anti-inflammatory use in the context of orthodontic movement. *European Journal of Orthodontics* 34(5), 531–535.

Kohli, V. S. and Kohli, S. S. (2011) Effectiveness of piroxicam and ibuprofen premedication on orthodontic patients' pain experiences: a randomized control trial. *The Angle Orthodontist* 81, 1097–1102.

Kokkinos, P. P., Shaye, R., Alam, B. S. and Alam, S. Q. (1993) Dietary lipids, prostaglandin E2 levels, and tooth movement in alveolar bone of rats. *Calcified Tissue International* 53, 333–337.

Kommuri, K., Javed, F., Akram, Z. and Khan, J. (2020) Effect of statins on orthodontic tooth movement: a systematic review of animal and clinical studies. *Archives of Oral Biology*, 104665.

Krishnan, V. and Davidovitch, Z. (2006a) Cellular, molecular, and tissue-level reactions to orthodontic force. *American Journal of Orthodontics and Dentofacial Orthopedics* 129, 469.e1–32.

Krishnan, V. and Davidovitch, Z. (2006b) The effect of drugs on orthodontic tooth movement. *Orthodontics and Craniofacial Research* 9, 163–171.

Krishnan, V. and Davidovitch, Z. (2009) On a path to unfolding the biological mechanisms of orthodontic tooth movement. *Journal of Dental Research* 88, 597–608.

Kyrkanides, S., Banion, K. O. and Subtelny, D. J. (2000) Non-steroidal anti-inflammatory drugs in orthodontic tooth movement – metalloproteinase activity and collagen synthesis by endothelial cells. *American Journal of Orthodontics and Dentofacial Orthopedics* 118, 203–209.

Leiker, B. J., Nanda, R. S., Currier, G. F. et al. (1995) The effects of exogenous prostaglandins on orthodontic tooth movement in rats. *American Journal of Orthodontics and Dentofacial Orthopedics* 108(4), 380–388.

Licata, A. A. (2005) Discovery, clinical development, and therapeutic uses of bisphosphonates. *The Annals of Pharmacotherapy* 39, 668–677.

Lin, J. H., Russell, G. and Gertz, B. (1999) Pharmacokinetics of alendronate: an overview. *International Journal of Clinical Practice* 101(suppl.), 18–26.

Liu, L., Igarashi, K., Haruyama, N. et al. (2004) Effects of local administration of clodronate on orthodontic tooth movement and root resorption in rats. *European Journal of Orthodontics* 26, 469–473.

Liu, Z. J., King, G. J., Gu, G. M. et al. (2005) Does human relaxin accelerate orthodontic tooth movement in rats? *Annals of New York Academy of Sciences* 1041, 388–394.

Lo, J. C., O'Ryan, F. S., Gordon, N. P. et al. (2010) Prevalence of osteonecrosis of the jaw in patients with oral bisphosphonate exposure. *Journal of Oral and Maxillofacial Surgery* 68, 243–253.

Longo, D. L., Fauci, A., Kasper, D. et al. (2011) *Harrison's Principles of Internal Medicine*, 18th edn. McGraw-Hill, New York, NY.

Lotwala, R. B., Greenlee, G. M., Ott, S. M. et al. (2012) Bisphosphonates as a risk factor for adverse orthodontic outcomes: a retrospective cohort study. *American Journal of Orthodontics and Dentofacial Orthopedics* 142(5), 625–634.

Luther, F. (2007) TMD and occlusion part I. Damned if we do? Occlusion: the interface of dentistry and orthodontics. *British Dental Journal* 202, E2.

Macari, S., Ajay Sharma, L., Wyatt, A. et al. (2016) Osteoprotective effects of estrogen in the maxillary bone depend on ERα. *Journal of Dental Research* **95**(6), 689–696.

Maeda, T., Matsunuma, A., Kurahashi, I. et al. (2004) Induction of osteoblast differentiation indices by statins in MC3T3-E1 cells. *Journal of Cellular Biochemistry* **92**, 458–471.

Marchini, A. M., Deco, C. P., Lodi, K. B. et al. (2012) Influence of chronic alcoholism and oestrogen deficiency on the variation of stoichiometry of hydroxyapatite within alveolar bone crest of rats. *Archives of Oral Biology* **57**(10), 1385–1394.

Martin, C. B., Hales, C.M., Gu, Q. and Ogden, C. L. (2019) Prescription drug use in the United States, 2015–2016. NCHS Data Brief, no 334. National Center for Health Statistics, Hyattsville, MD.

Maritz, F. J., Conradie, M. M., Hulley, P. A. et al. (2001) Effect of statins on bone mineral density and bone histomorphometry in rodents. *Arteriosclerosis, Thrombosis and Vascular Biology* **21**, 636–641.

Makrygiannakis, M. A., Kaklamanos, E. G. and Athanasiou, A. E. (2019) Effects of systemic medication on root resorption associated with orthodontic tooth movement: a systematic review of animal studies. *European Journal of Orthodontics* **41**(4), 346–359.

McCanlies, J. M., Alexander, C. M., Robnett, J. H. and Magness, W. B. (1961) Effect of vitamin C on the mobility and stability of guinea pig incisors under the influence of orthodontic force. *The Angle Orthodontist* **31**, 257–263.

McGorray, S. P., Dolce, C., Kramer, S. et al. (2012) A randomized, placebo-controlled clinical trial on the effects of recombinant human relaxin on tooth movement and short-term stability. *American Journal of Orthodontics and Dentofacial Orthopedics* **141**, 196–203.

McNab, S., Battistutta, D., Taverne, A. and Symons, A. L. (1999) External apical root resorption of posterior teeth in asthmatics after orthodontic treatment. *American Journal of Orthodontics and Dentofacial Orthopedics* **116**, 545–551.

Meh, A., Sprogar, S., Vaupotic, T. et al. (2011) Effect of cetirizine, a histamine (H(1)) receptor antagonist, on bone modeling during orthodontictooth movement in rats. *American Journal of Orthodontics and Dentofacial Orthopedics* **139**, e323–329.

Meikle, M. C. (2006) The tissue, cellular, and molecular regulation of orthodontic tooth movement: 100 years after Carl Sandstedt. *European Journal of Orthodontics* **28**, 221–240.

Mhaskar, R., Kumar, A., Miladinovic, B. and Djulbegovic, B. (2017) Bisphosphonates in multiple myeloma: an updated network meta-analysis. *Cochrane Database of Systematic Reviews* **12**, CD003188

Michelogiannakis, D., Al-Shammery, D., Rossouw, P. E. et al. (2018a) Influence of corticosteroid therapy on orthodontic tooth movement: a narrative review of studies in animal-models. *Orthodontics and Craniofacial Research* **21**(4), 216–224.

Michelogiannakis, D., Rossouw, P.E., Al-Shammery, D. et al. (2018b) Influence of nicotine on orthodontic tooth movement: a systematic review of experimental studies in rats. *Archives of Oral Biology* **93**, 66–73.

Migliorati, C. A., Saunders, D., Conlon, M. S. et al. (2013) Assessing the association between bisphosphonate exposure and delayed mucosal healing after tooth extraction. *Journal of American Dental Association* **144**, 406–414.

Migliorati, C. A., Woo, S. B., Hewson, I. et al. (2010) A systematic review of bisphosphonate osteonecrosis (BON) in cancer. *Support Care Cancer* **18**, 1099–1106.

Miresmaeili, A., Mollaei, N., Azar, R. et al. (2015) Effect of dietary vitamin C on orthodontic tooth movement in rats. *Journal of Dentistry (Tehran)* **12**(6), 409–413.

Mohammed, A. H., Tatakis, D. N. and Dziak, R. (1989) Leukotrienes in orthodontic tooth movement. *American Journal of Orthodontics and Dentofacial Orthopedics* **95**, 231–237.

Monk, A. B., Harrison, J. E., Worthington, H. V. and Teague, A. (2017) Pharmacological interventions for pain relief during orthodontic treatment. *Cochrane Database of Systematic Reviews* **11**, CD003976.

Moraschini, V., Calasans-Maia, J. D. A. and Calasans-Maia, M. D. (2018) Association between asthma and periodontal disease: a systematic review and meta-analysis. *Journal of Periodontology*, **89**(4), 440–455.

Motoji, H., To, M., Hidaka, K. and Matsuo, M. (2020) Vitamin C and eggshell membrane facilitate orthodontic tooth movement and induce histological changes in the periodontal tissue. *Journal of Oral Biosciences* **62**, 80–87.

Moura, A. P., Taddei, S. R., Queiroz-Junior, C. M, et al. (2014) The relevance of leukotrienes for bone resorption induced by mechanical loading. *Bone* **69**, 133–138.

Mundy, G. (2001) Statins and their potential for osteoporosis. *Bone* **29**, 495–497.

Ngan, P., Wilson, S., Shanfeld, J. and Amini, H. (1994) The effect of ibuprofen on the level of discomfort in patients undergoing orthodontic treatment. *American Journal of Orthodontics and Dentofacial Orthopedics* **106**, 88–95.

Nicozisis, J. L., Nah-Cederquist, H. D. and Tuncay, O. C. (2000) Relaxin affects the dentofacialsutural tissues. *Clinical Orthodontics and Research* **3**, 192–201.

Nishioka, M., Ioi, H., Nakata, S. et al. (2006) Root resorption and immune system factors in the Japanese. *The Angle Orthodontist* **76**, 103–108.

Nishio, C., Rompré, P. and Moldovan, F. (2017) Effect of exogenous retinoic acid on tooth movement and periodontium healing following tooth extraction in a rat model. *Orthodontic and Craniofacial Research* **20**(Suppl 1), 77–82.

Oettgen, H. C. and Geha, R. S. (1999) IgE in asthma and atopy: cellular and molecular connections. *Journal of Clinical Investigation* **104**, 829–835.

Oizumi T, Yamaguchi K, Sato K et al. (2016) A strategy against the osteonecrosis of the jaw associated with nitrogen-containing bisphosphonates (N-BPs): attempts to replace N-BPs with the non-N-BP etidronate. *Biological and Pharmaceutical Bulletin* **39**, 1549–1554.

Ong, C. K., Walsh, L. J., Harbrow, D. et al. (2000) Orthodontic tooth movement in the prednisolone-treated rat. *The Angle Orthodontist* **70**, 118–125.

Ogrenim, G., Cesur, M. G., Onal, T. et al. (2019) Influence of omega-3 fatty acid on orthodontic tooth movement in rats: A biochemical, histological, immunohistochemical and gene expression study. *Orthodontics and Craniofacial Research* **22**(1), 24–31.

Ortega, A. J., Campbell, P. M., Hinton, R. et al. (2012) Local application of zoledronate for maximum anchorage during space closure. *American Journal of Orthodontics and Dentofacial Orthopedics* **142**, 780–791.

Owman-Moll, P. and Kurol, J. (2000) Root resorption after orthodontic treatment in high- and low risk patients: analysis of allergy as a possible predisposing factor. *European Journal of Orthodontics* **22**, 657–663.

Oztürk, F., Babacan, H., Inan, S. and Gümüş, C. (2011) Effects of bisphosphonates on sutural bone formation and relapse: a histologic and immunohistochemical study. *American Journal of Orthodontics and Dentofacial Orthopedics* **140**, e31–e41.

Padisar, P., Nasseh, R., Khorasani, M. and Assl, M. N. (2009) A study on efficacy of NSAIDs in control of pains after orthodontic. *Research Journal of Biological Sciences* **4**, 404–408.

Paganelli, C. (1993) Pharmacological support during orthodontic therapy with a topical anti-inflammatory. *Minerva Stomatologica* **42**, 271–274.

Patil, A. K., Keluskar, K. M. and Gaitonde, S.D. (2005) The clinical application of prostaglandin E1 on orthodontic tooth movement. *Journal of the Indian Orthodontic Society* **38**, 91–98.

Polat, O. and Karaman, A. I. (2005) Pain control during fixed orthodontic appliance therapy. *The Angle Orthodontist* **75**, 214–219.

Polat, O., Karaman, A. I. and Durmus, E. (2005) Effects of preoperative ibuprofen and naproxen sodium on orthodontic pain. *The Angle Orthodontist* **75**, 791–796.

Retamoso, L., Knop, L., Shintcovsk, R. et al. (2011) Influence of anti-inflammatory administration in collagen maturation process during orthodontic tooth movement. *Microscopy Research and Technique* **74**(8), 709–713.

Rinchuse, D. J., Rinchuse, D. J., Sosovicka, M. F. et al. (2007) Orthodontic treatment of patients using bisphosphonates: a report of 2 cases. *American Journal of Orthodontics and Dentofacial Orthopedics* **131**, 321–326.

Riordan, D. J. (1997) Effects of orthodontic treatment on nutrient intake. *American Journal of Orthodontics and Dentofacial Orthopedics* **111**, 554–561.

Roberts-Harry, D. and Sandy, J. (2004) Orthodontics. Part 10: Impacted teeth. *British Dental Journal* **196**, 319–327.

Ronis, M. J., Mercer, K. and Chen, J. R. (2011) Effects of nutrition and alcohol consumption on bone loss. *Current Osteoporosis Reports* **9**, 53–59.

Rosen, C. (2005) Postmenopausal osteoporosis. *New England Journal of Medicine* **353**, 595–603.

Salazar, M., Hernandes, L., Ramos, A. L. et al. (2011) Effect of teriparatide on induced tooth displacement in ovariectomized rats: a histomorphometric analysis. *American Journal of Orthodontics and Dentofacial Orthopedics* **139**, e337–344.

Salvi, G. E. and Lang, N. P. (2005) The effects of non-steroidal anti-inflammatory drugs (selective and non-selective on the treatment of periodontal diseases). *Current Pharmaceutical Design* **11**, 1757–1769.

Sampson, H. W. (1998) Alcohol's harmful effects on bone. *Alcohol Health and Research World* **22**, 190–194.

Sari, E., Olmez, H. and Gurton, A. V. (2004) Comparison of some effect of acetylsalicylic acid and rofecoxib during orthodontic tooth movement. *American Journal of Orthodontics and Dentofacial Orthopedics* **25**, 310–315.

Schröder, A., Küchler, E. C., Omori, M. et al. (2019) Effects of ethanol on human periodontal ligament fibroblasts subjected to static compressive force. *Alcohol* **77**, 59–70.

Seifi, M., Eslami, B. and Saffar, A. S. (2003) The effect of prostaglandin E2 and calcium gluconate on orthodontic tooth movement and root resorption in rats. *European Journal of Orthodontics* **25**, 199–204.

Seifi, M., Ezzati, B., Saedi, S. and Hedayati, M. (2015a) The effect of ovariectomy and orchiectomy on orthodontic tooth movement and root resorption in Wistar rats. *Journal of Dentistry (Shiraz)* **16**(4), 302–309.

Seifi, M., Hamedi, R. and Khavandegar, Z. (2015b) The effect of thyroid hormone, prostaglandin E2, and calcium gluconate on orthodontic tooth movement and root resorption in rats. *Journal of Dentistry (Shiraz)* **16**(1 Suppl), 35–42.

Seto, H., Ohba, H., Tokunaga, K. *et al.* (2008) Topical administration of simvastatin recovers alveolar bone loss in rats. *Journal of Periodontal Research* **43**, 261–267.

Sharma, R., Singla, A., Mittal, S. and Grover, V. (2011) Effect of orthodontic treatment on nutrient intake – a clinical study. *Journal of Innovative Dentistry* **1**(2), journal. pdmdcri.com/issue2/originalarticle/article1.pdf (accessed September 10, 2020).

Shetty, N., Patil, A.K., Ganeshkar, S.V. and Hegde, S. (2013) Comparison of the effects of ibuprofen and acetaminophen on PGE2 levels in the GCF during orthodontic tooth movement: a human study. *Progress in Orthodontics* **14**(6), 6.

Siadat, S., Sadeghian, S., Heidarpour, M. *et al.* (2017) The effects of systemic prescription of amitriptyline on orthodontic tooth movement rate, root resorption and alveolar bone remodeling in dog. *Biomedical and Pharmacology Journal* **10**(3), 1537–1544.

Simmons, K. E. and Brandt, M. (1992) Control of orthodontic pain. *Journal of Indiana Dental Association* **71**, 8–10.

Simon, P. A., Zeng, Z., Wold, C. M. *et al.* (2003) Prevalence of childhood asthma and associated morbidity in Los Angeles County: Impacts of race/ethnicity and income. *Journal of Asthma* **40**, 535–543.

Sirisoontorn, I., Hotokezaka, H., Hashimoto, M. *et al.* (2012) Orthodontic tooth movement and root resorption in ovariectomized rats treated by systemic administration of zoledronic acid. *American Journal of Orthodontics and Dentofacial Orthopedics* **141**, 563–573.

Sodagar, A., Donyavi, Z., Arab, S. and Kharrazifard, M. J. (2011) Effect of nicotine on orthodontic tooth movement in rats. *American Journal of Orthodontics and Dentofacial Orthopedics* **139**, e261–265.

Sodagar, A., Ghahramani, M., Motahhari, P. and Zahedpasha, S. (2008) The effect of vitamin A on orthodontic tooth movement in male rat. *The Journal of the Islamic Dental Association of Iran* **19**, 8–17.

Soma, S., Matsumoto, S., Higuchi, Y. *et al.* (2000) Local and chronic application of PTH accelerates tooth movement in rats. *Journal of Dental Research* **79**, 1717–1724.

Sonis, S. T. (2004) Orthodontic management of selected medically compromised patients: cardiac disease, bleeding disorders and asthma. *Seminars in Orthodontics* **10**, 277–280.

Sprogar, S., Kriznar, I., Drevensek, M. *et al.* (2008) Famotidine, a H2 receptor antagonist, decreases the late phase of orthodontic tooth movement in rats. *Inflammation Research* **57**(Suppl. 1), S31–32.

Stewart, D. R., Sherick, P., Kramer, S. and Breining, P. (2005) Use of relaxin in orthodontics. *Annals of the New York Academy of Sciences* **1041**(1), 379–387.

Stopeck, A. T., Lipton, A., Body, J. J. *et al.* (2010) Denosumab compared with zoledronic acid for the treatment of bone metastases in patients with advanced breast cancer: a randomized, double-blind study. *Journal of Clinical Oncology* **28**, 5132–5139.

Strause, L., Saltman, P. and Glowacki, J. (1987) The effect of deficiencies of manganese and copper on osteoinduction and on resorption of bone particles in rats. *Calcified Tissue International* **41**, 145–150.

Souza-Silva, B. N., Rodrigues, J.A., Moreira, J.C. *et al.* (2016) The influence of teriparatide in induced tooth movement: a systematic review. *Journal of Clinical and Experimental Dentistry* **8**(5), e615–e621

Suparwitri, S., Rosyida, N. F. and Alhasyimi, A. A. (2019) Wheat seeds can delay orthodontic tooth movement by blocking osteoclastogenesis in rats. *Clinical, Cosmetic and Investigational Dentistry* **11**, 243.

Swidi, A. J., Taylor, R. W., Tadlock, L. P. and Buschang, P. H. (2018) Recent advances in orthodontic retention methods: a review article. *Journal of the World Federation of Orthodontists* **7**(1), 6–12.

Takano, M., Yamaguchi, M., Nakajima, R. *et al.* (2009) Effects of relaxin on collagen type I released by stretched human periodontal ligament cells. *Orthodontics and Craniofacial Research* **12**, 282–288.

Togari, A., Kondo, M., Arai, M. and Matsumoto, S. (1991) Effects of retinoic acid on bone formation and resorption in cultured mouse calvaria. *General Pharmacology* **22**, 287–292.

Touyz, L. Z. (1997) Oral scurvy and periodontal disease. *Journal of Canadian Dental Association* **63**, 837–845.

Turpin, D. L. (2009) Editorial: medications weigh in-on tooth movement. *Amercian Journal of Orthodontics and Dentofacial Orthopedics* **135**, 139–140.

Urade, M., Tanaka, N., Furusawa, K. *et al.* (2011) Nationwide survey for bisphosphonate-related osteonecrosis of the jaws in Japan. *Journal of Oral and Maxillofacial Surgery* **69**, e364–371.

US Centers for Disease Control and Prevention (2005) Tobacco use, access, and exposure to tobacco in media among middle and high school students: United States, 2004, *Morbidity and Mortality Weekly Report* **54**, 297–301.

Varble, Z. L. (2009) *The Effect of Growth Hormone on Tooth Movement in Rats*. Master thesis. University of St. Louis (unpublished).

Vazquez-Landaverde, L. A., Rojas-Huidobro, R., Alonso Gallegos-Corona, M. and Aceves, C. (2002) Periodontal 5'-deiodination on forced-induced root resorption – the protective effect of thyroid hormone administration. *European Journal of Orthodontics* **24**, 363–369.

Wakita, R., Izumi, T. and Itoman, M. (1998) Thyroid hormone-induced chondrocyte terminal differentiation in rat femur organ culture. *Cell and Tissue Research* **293**, 357–364.

Watkins, B. A., Li, Y., Lippman, H. E. and Seifert, M. F. (2001a) Omega-3 polyunsaturated fatty acids and skeletal health. *Experimental Biology and Medicine* **226**, 485–497.

Watkins, B. A., Li, Y. and Seifert, M. F. (2001b) Nutraceutical fatty acids as biochemical and molecular modulators of skeletal biology. *Journal of the American College of Nutrition* **20**, 410S–416S.

Wong, R. W. and Rabie, A. B. (2005) Early healing pattern of statin-induced osteogenesis. *British Journal of Oral and Maxillofacial Surgery* **43**, 46–50.

Wong, R. W. and Rabie, A. B. (2006) Statin-induced osteogenesis uses in orthodontics: a scientific review. *World Journal of Orthodontics* **7**, 35–40.

Yamaguchi, K., Oizumi, T., Funayama, H. *et al.* (2010) Osteonecrosis of the jawbones in 2 osteoporosis patients treated with nitrogen-containing bisphosphonates: osteonecrosis reduction replacing NBP with non-NBP (etidronate) and rationale. *Journal of Oral and Maxillofacial Surgery* **68**, 889–897.

Yamasaki, K., Shibata, Y. and Furihara, T. (1982) The effect of prostaglandins on experimental tooth movement in monkeys (Macaca fuscata). *Journal of Dental Research* **61**, 1444–1446.

Yamasaki, K., Shibata, Y., Imai, S. *et al.* (1984) Clinical application of prostaglandin E1 (PGE1) upon orthodontic tooth movement. *American Journal of Orthodontics and Dentofacial Orthopedics* **85**, 508–518.

Yamashiro, T. and Takano-Yamamoto, T. (2001) Influences of ovariectomy on experimental tooth movement in the rat. *Journal of Dental Research* **80**, 1858–1861.

Yazawa, H., Zimmermann, B., Asami, Y. and Bernimoulin, J. P. (2005) Simvastatin promotes cell metabolism, proliferation and osteoblastic differentiation in human periodontal ligament cells. *Journal of Periodontology* **76**, 295–302.

Zhong, W., Maradit-Kremers, H., St Sauver, J.L. *et al.* (2013) Age and sex patterns of drug prescribing in a defined american population. *Mayo Clinic Proceedings* **88** (7), 697–707.

Zahrowski, J. J. (2007) Bisphosphonate treatment: an orthodontic concern calling for a proactive approach. *American Journal of Orthodontics and Dentofacial Orthopedics* **131**, 311–320.

Zahrowski, J. J. (2009) Optimizing orthodontics during bisphosphonate treatment for osteoporosis. *American Journal of Orthodontics and Dentofacial Orthopedics* **135**, 361–374.

Zorlu, F. Y., Darici, H. and Turkkahraman, H. (2019) Histomorphometric and histopathologic evaluation of the effects of systemic fluoride intake on orthodontic tooth movement. *European Journal of Dentistry* **13**(3), 361–369.

Zymperdikas, V. F., Yavropoulou, M.P., Kaklamanos, E.G. and Papadopoulos, M.A. (2020) Effects of systematic bisphosphonate use in patients under orthodontic treatment: a systematic review. *European Journal of Orthodontics* **42**, 60–71.

PART 5

Rapid Orthodontics

CHAPTER 15
Biological Orthodontics: Methods to Accelerate or Decelerate Orthodontic Tooth Movement

Vinod Krishnan, Ze'ev Davidovitch, and Anne Marie Kuijpers-Jagtman

> **Summary**
>
> From the outset, orthodontists wished they could increase the velocity of tooth movement, for the benefit of their patients, and for their own sake. Expanding knowledge about cell physiology enabled researchers to explore methods for the acceleration of tooth movement. The cells in and around teeth are being used as keys to accelerated orthodontics. Some of the main cell types, whose biological responses are used as yardsticks for estimation of the degree of their involvement in the acceleration process, are osteoclasts, osteoblasts, osteocytes, and cells of the nervous, immune, and endocrine systems. This chapter reviews the ability of biochemical and physical agents to evoke cellular responses that lead to accelerated orthodontic tooth movement. The list of participating molecules includes cytokines, prostaglandins, RANKL and macrophage colony stimulating factor, parathyroid hormone, vitamin D_3, relaxin, corticosteroids, osteocalcin, and vascular endothelial growth factor. The physical entities used to stimulate the target dental and paradental cells are low level lasers, direct electric currents, pulsed electromagnetic fields, vibrations, light, and surgical interventions. This review evaluates the advantages and shortcomings of each of the methods that have been proposed for reaching the goal of shortening the duration of orthodontic treatment. Additionally, this chapter discusses a few methods for slowing down the rate of tooth movement, pertaining to anchorage and relapse situations.

Introduction

Orthodontic treatment depends upon the development of force-induced mechanical strain in the paradental tissues, where the cells respond to changes in their environment. The deformation of the extracellular matrix (ECM) by mechanical forces is capable of altering the neutral state activity of each cell, be it a bone cell, periodontal ligament (PDL) fibroblast, neural or blood vessel wall cell, by changing the architecture of the cell membrane and its attachment foci, crystallizing its cytoskeleton, nuclear protein matrix and, ultimately, reaching the genome. The induced genomic changes are always capable of altering the cell viability, proliferation, and differentiation, which form the biomechanical basis of orthodontic mechanics.

According to Buschang et al. (2012), orthodontic treatment differs from patient to patient, based on individual characteristics, but on average lasts from 21 to 27 months for nonextraction treatment, and 25 to 35 months for extraction treatment. A systematic review by Tsichlaki et al. (2016) has concluded, based on 22 studies, that the average orthodontic treatment lasts for fewer than 24 months with a mean of 19.9 months. According to them, the most significant arbiter of treatment duration appears to be the operator, with his or her treatment planning decisions, standards, and finishing practices. The duration is also determined by severity of the malocclusion, patient compliance, such as missing appointments, bracket breakage, poor oral hygiene, and anchorage problems. With increase in awareness of available cosmetic dental procedures and the apprehension towards social judgement regarding facial appearances with aging, nowadays there is a growing uptake of orthodontic treatment among the adult population. But sometimes, prolonged periods of wearing oral braces, particularly noncosmetic appliances, tend to keep patients, especially adults, away from seeking treatment, even when it is clearly indicated. Moreover, longer treatment durations are expensive for both the patient and the orthodontist. Therefore, one of the best ways to overcome this problem is to speed up the velocity of tooth movement from its usual rate of 0.8–1.2 mm/month (when continuous forces are applied) (Buschang et al., 2012).

Early attempts to accelerate tooth movement

The finding that cells can respond biologically to two or more signals, be they physical or chemical, which are applied simultaneously, has initiated a new wave of experiments to increase the pace of tooth movement. As early as 1888, Farrar advocated the use of heavy forces to move teeth, because he surmised that orthodontic

---

Biological Mechanisms of Tooth Movement, Third Edition. Edited by Vinod Krishnan, Anne Marie Kuijpers-Jagtman and Ze'ev Davidovitch.
© 2021 John Wiley & Sons Ltd. Published 2021 by John Wiley & Sons Ltd.

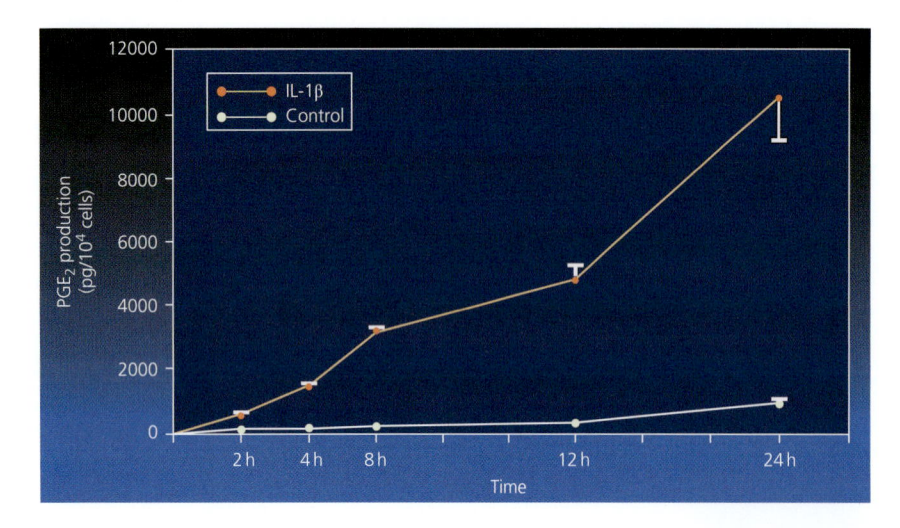

Figure 15.1 In this experiment by Saito et al. (1991), human PDL fibroblasts, obtained from teeth extracted from an adolescent patient, were incubated for 24 hours, with or without an addition of interleukin-1β (IL-1β), 1 ng/mL. In the absence of the cytokine IL-1β (control), the fibroblasts synthesized and secreted a minimal amount of prostaglandin E_2 (PGE_2) into the incubation medium. However, in the presence of IL-1β, the cells displayed a sharp increase in the production of PGE_2. (Source: Based on Saito, 1991.)

forces bend the alveolar bone, and the more the bone is bent, the further the teeth would move. However, this principle was proven hazardous, because the application of extremely high forces resulted frequently in fractures of the alveolar bone. Consequently, applying very heavy forces in orthodontics faded away at the end of the nineteenth century. It was not until 1969 that Baumrind reported that orthodontic forces do strain the alveolar bone, causing teeth to move a greater distance than the width of their PDL. This finding was preceded by numerous reports on the generation of electric potentials in bent long bones (Basset and Becker, 1962; Zengo et al., 1973), and subsequent reports on similar reactions in alveolar bone subjected to mechanical forces. These reports highlighted two points: firstly, that bone can be bent and, secondly, that bending of bone generates electric potentials. These facts led to applications of minute electric currents to non-union fractures, to induce and enhance osteogenesis (Borgens, 1984).

Following these principles, attempts to increase the pace of tooth movement were conducted by Davidovitch et al. (1980a, b), who applied direct electrical current to cat gingivae near maxillary canines, while these teeth were being pulled distally. This experiment demonstrated enhanced tooth movement, accompanied by increases in the cellular concentrations of the second messenger adenosine 3′, 5′ monophosphate (cyclic AMP, cAMP) in the paradental tissues.

In the following years, other researchers started marching on the road to the target of discovering efficient ways of enhancing the velocity of orthodontic tooth movement (OTM). Successful results of experiments in animals and humans, with periodical local injections of prostaglandin E_1 or E_2 during orthodontic treatment, doubled the rate of tooth movement (Yamasaki et al., 1982, 1984). They did not observe any side effects either clinically or radiographically with this procedure, except for a slight pain reaction expressed by the patients. A 60% increase in tooth movement was demonstrated by Collins and Sinclair (1988) after intraligamentous injections of a vitamin D metabolite, 1,25-dihydroxycholecalciferol in cats. They also could not observe any obvious clinical and biochemical side effects and reported finding increased osteoclast recruitment with this injection in the PDL pressure sites, augmenting bone resorption. Saito et al. (1990a, b) demonstrated the ability of cells to respond at the same time to two or more kinds of stimuli (Figures 15.1 and 15.2). They demonstrated minimal release of prostaglandin E_2 (PGE_2) into the incubation medium by fibroblasts in the absence of the cytokine IL-1β (control), while in the presence of IL-1β the cells displayed a sharp increase in the production of PGE_2. Following this, PDL

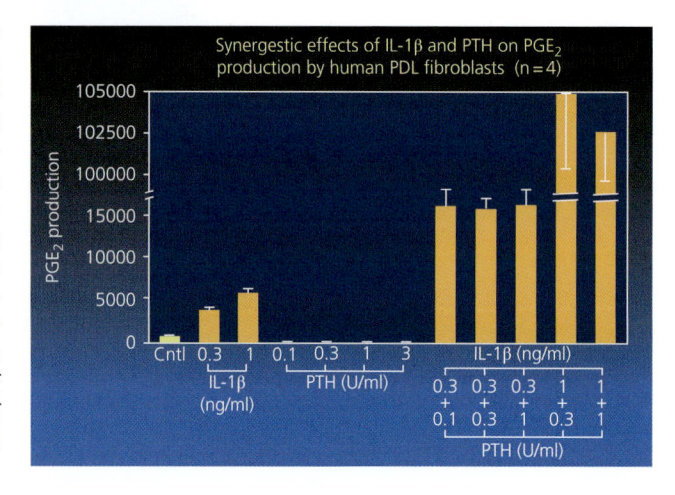

Figure 15.2 Human PDL fibroblasts were incubated without any added stimulating substance (control), with added IL-1β, with added PTH, or with the addition of both agents simultaneously. The combined group, which was subjected to a simultaneous exposure to both signals, reacted synergistically in terms of PGE_2 production. A noteworthy finding is that just a minimal amount of each signal is required to attain a synergistic effect (Ngan et al., 1988). (Source: Based on Saito, 1991.)

fibroblasts were incubated without any added stimulating substance (control), with added IL-1β, with added parathyroid hormone (PTH), or with the addition of both agents simultaneously (Figure 15.2). The latter group, which was subjected to a simultaneous exposure to both signals, reacted synergistically in terms of PGE_2 production. A noteworthy finding is that just a minimal amount of each signal is required for attaining a synergistic effect.

If these observations are extrapolated to the orthodontic patient, it means that when a mechanical force is applied to teeth, in the presence of certain signals known to affect cells of nonmineralized or mineralized connective tissues, the cellular response and the resulting tissue remodeling will be accelerated and, consequently, the teeth will move faster to their new positions. The goal of follow-up experiments along this line of research was to elucidate factors capable of augmenting the effects of mechanical force on tissues and cells involved in tooth movement. A brief review follows of techniques evolved through experiments in animal models, clinical trials, and case reports, on various modalities for increasing or decreasing the pace of tooth movement.

Accelerating tooth movement: pharmacological approaches

Local cytokine delivery

Cytokines are extracellular signaling proteins directly involved in bone remodeling, and in inflammatory reactions, two key events that facilitate OTM. This activity is also known to facilitate PDL cell differentiation, activation, as well as apoptosis (Krishnan and Davidovitch, 2006). This statement stands true with the elevated levels of cytokines such as interleukins, tumor necrosis factor-alpha, and RANKL during tooth movement. The actions of interleukins are mediated through increases in the production of PGE_2 and macrophage colony stimulating factor (M-CSF), which facilitate differentiation of osteoclasts (Krishnan and Davidovitch, 2006).

Prostaglandins

The prostaglandins (PGs) are a group of lipid compounds that are derived enzymatically by cyclooxygenase (COX) from fatty acids in the cell membrane but are not stored in cells. Every prostaglandin contains 20 carbon atoms, including a 5-carbon ring. They are mediators and have a variety of strong physiological effects, such as regulating the contraction and relaxation of smooth muscles, and bone remodeling. Prostaglandins function as autocrines or paracrines, which are locally acting messenger molecules. They differ from hormones in that they are not produced at a discrete site but in many places throughout the human body. Their target cells are present in the immediate vicinity of the site of their secretion. The PGs, together with the thromboxanes and prostacyclins, form the prostanoid class of fatty-acid derivatives, a subclass of eicosanoids.

In 1970, Klein and Raisz demonstrated the bone resorptive activity of PGs by their capability of inducing osteoclastic hyperplasia. With this background, Yamasaki et al. (1980) found it to be a major mediator of bone resorption following orthodontic force application and injected it locally in monkeys (1982) and humans (1984). They could observe double the amount of tooth movement in comparison to conventional orthodontic mechanics without any evident clinical or biochemical side effects except for pain. Lee (1990) conducted a histological evaluation of paradental tissues after administering PGE_1 and observed the presence of osteoclasts within 6 hours of force application, reaching peak levels within 3 days. Brudvik and Rygh (1991) pointed out the tendency towards root resorption in rats who received PGE_2 injection locally, elucidating a possible side effect.

Leiker et al. (1995) through their experiments in rats concluded that low concentrations (0.1–1.0 µg) of PGE_2 injection produced a statistically significant acceleration of tooth movement, and that a single injection is all that is needed, as repeated injections have no effect on the process. To reduce the incidence of root resorption that is associated with PG application, Seifi et al. (2003), in an experiment in rats, combined calcium gluconate along with PGE_2 but could not observe any statistically significant reduction in the root resorption process. However, they could observe a reduction in the rate of tooth movement in the combined group in comparison to the PGE_2 alone group, and a nonsignificant increase in relation to the control group, where no PGE_2 injection was performed. In line with Yamasaki et al. (1984), Patil et al. (2005) conducted a human clinical trial on 15 patients (13–25 years) with local injection of PGE_1, in low dose of 1.0 µg along with lignocaine as a vehicle (which can reduce painful sensations), and reported finding a statistically significant increase (1.7:1) in the rate of distal canine retraction. They could also observe no root resorption phenomena evident upon evaluation of follow-up radiographs.

Recent systematic reviews regarding the effect of prostaglandin on accelerating tooth movement are not encouraging. While Spoerri et al. (2018) reported no effect of prostaglandin injections on the root resorption process, Eltimamy et al. (2019) concluded that there exists inconclusive evidence regarding acceleration of tooth movement with prostaglandin. More well-conducted clinical research is needed as the evidence currently available is incomplete and scarce.

RANKL

Receptor activator of nuclear factor kappa-B ligand (RANKL) is a molecule critical for adequate bone metabolism. Osteoclastic activity is triggered via the osteoblasts' surface-bound RANKL activating the osteoclasts' surface-bound receptor activator of nuclear factor kappa-B (RANK). Overproduction of RANKL is implicated in a variety of degenerative bone diseases, such as rheumatoid arthritis and psoriatic arthritis. The first FDA-approved RANKL inhibitor was denosumab (to treat osteoporosis in postmenopausal women).

As a method to accelerate tooth movement, Kanzaki et al. (2006), with the help of HVJ (hemagglutinating-virus of Japan) envelope vector containing pcDNA-mRANKL, transfected the PDL of male Wistar rats with the RANKL gene. They observed a 30–40% increase in the rate of tooth movement, and a high number of osteoclasts at day 2 after RANKL gene transfer (Figure 15.3). In order to avoid the viral recombination, neoplastic transformation, and high toxicity, the follow-up experiment by Iglesias-Linares et al. (2011) used a mixed nonviral system to transfect RANKL to the PDL and observed a higher number of osteoclasts. Their experiments with local gene transfer in comparison to corticotomies revealed above 40% and 20% acceleration in tooth movement rate respectively in comparison with conventional mechanics and concluded that local gene transfer could be superior to mere corticotomies (Figure 15.4). They explained it with the help of reduction in RANKL after the initial rise (soon after the surgical procedure) while local gene transfer with RANKL continues to release the same over a long period. Li et al. (2019a) investigated the effect of local injection of RANKL in mice and observed a reversible transitional acceleration of bone resorption, wherein there is increased osteoclastic activity facilitating tooth movement initially, followed by subsequent alveolar bone formation. Chang et al. (2020) developed a sustained-release RANKL formulation from 100 µL of 100 µg/mL RANKL adsorbed on 10 mg of poly(lactic acid-co-glycolic acid) microspheres embedded in a 10 wt% aqueous hydroxyethyl cellulose carrier gel. They observed a sustained release for 30 days with a positive effect on mice osteoclast precursor cells. In a further in vivo experiment in 15-week-old male Wistar rats they observed, corresponding with increased TRAP activity, 129.2% more tooth movement than no formulation and 71.8% more than placebo formulation.

Hormones promoting tooth movement
Parathyroid hormone

PTH is secreted by the parathyroid glands which are located close to the thyroid. Its main effect is an increase of blood calcium concentration; consequently, it stimulates bone resorption. The initial report on the effect of PTH on tooth movement was published by Kamata (1972), where he encountered difficulties in moving teeth after parathyroidectomy in rats, which was overcome by injecting parathyroid extract (as cited in Soma et al., 1999). Davidovitch et al. (1972) compared the effect of systemic administration of PTH and cortisone acetate in cats and observed a greater rate of tooth

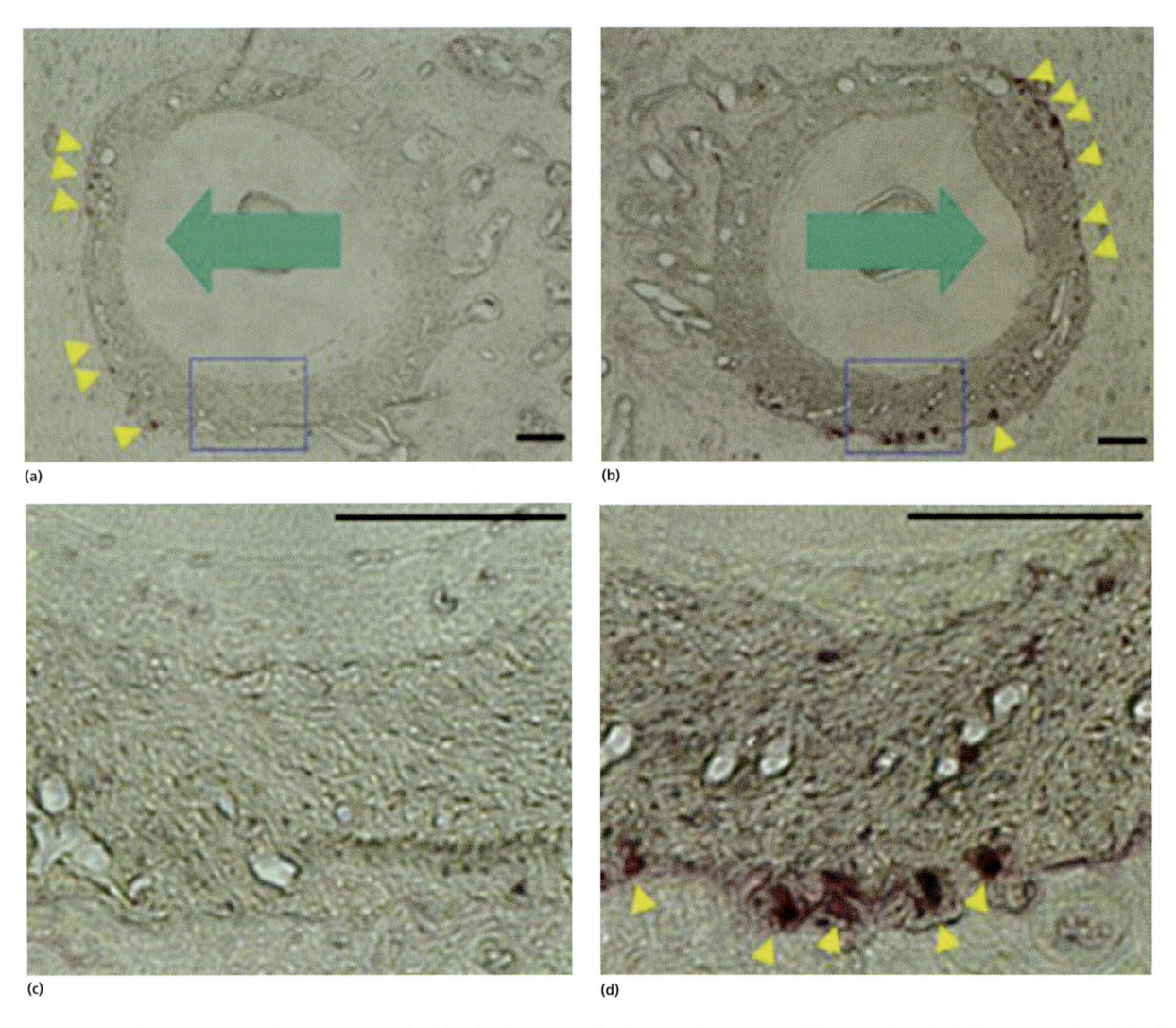

Figure 15.3 Osteoclasts in the periodontium in 6-week-old male Wistar rats after force application. (a, c) Photograph of the PBS injected side and (b, d) RANKL-transfected side. The green arrow indicates the force direction and yellow arrows indicate osteoclasts. Bar 100 μm (c, d) shows enlarged images indicated by the blue box in (a, b). (Source: Kanzaki et al., 2006. Reproduced with permission of Nature Publishing Group.)

movement with PTH (50 μm daily) followed by the control and cortisone groups. Histologic examination of the cat jaws revealed intense osteoclastic activity in the PDL, with the highest levels of both resorptive and formative activities found in the PTH group, while these were least evident in the cortisone-treated group.

Considering the fact that bone remodeling is essential for tooth movement, and following the experiments by Davidovitch et al. (1980a, b) accelerating bone remodeling with exogenous electric current application locally, Midgett et al. (1981) put forward a pertinent question: will the rate of tooth movement be elevated in patients with disease conditions having elevated bone metabolism? To answer this question, they induced nutritional hyperparathyroidism in male beagle dogs, with a high phosphorous and low calcium diet, resulting in higher serum PTH concentrations. Interestingly at the end of the treatment period they recorded 15.2 ± 1.4 mm tooth movement in the experimental group, in comparison to 10.3 ± 1.9 mm in the control group, demonstrating evident acceleration. Soma et al. (1999) concluded that continuous rather than intermittent infusion of PTH will increase the bone metabolism rate without creating bone loss in adjacent areas. To effect a continuous infusion, a follow-up experiment by the same group (Soma et al., 2000) used methylcellulose gel (MC 2%) as a carrier for slow release of PTH, and injected it subperiosteally in the mesio-palatal region of first molars in rats. They observed a 1.6 times increase in the rate of tooth movement with this method, while injection of PTH dissolved in saline could not induce such an effect (Figure 15.5). Shirazi et al. (2001) demonstrated a statistically significant increase in the rate of tooth movement in renal insufficiency induced rats and attributed it to the elevated levels of PTH, as part of a secondary hyperparathyroidism induced by associated hyperphosphatemia and hypocalcemia. Salazar et al. (2011) revealed an increase in the number of osteoclasts and an associated increase in the rate of tooth movement along with normal bone density through histomorphometric analysis of paradental tissues related to maxillary first molar in ovariectomized rats after injection with teriparatide (portion of human PTH). Li et al. (2013) evaluated the effect of PTH injection on the RANKL/osteoprotegerin (OPG) mechanism, and on insulin-like growth factor IGF-1 in male Wistar rats, and reported accelerated tooth movement but only after 9 days of force application. They attributed this delay to

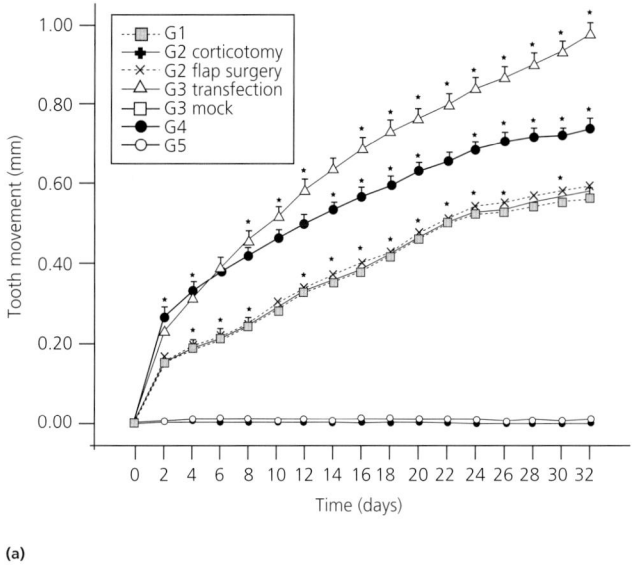

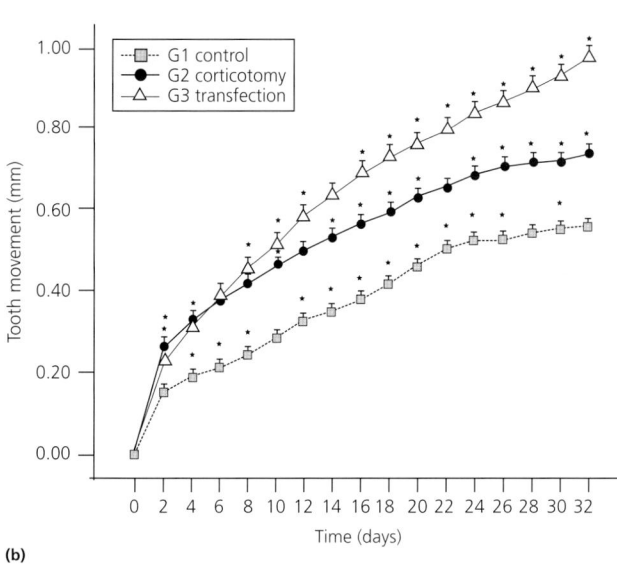

Figure 15.4 (a) Clinical tooth movement data registered on the hemimaxillae of five groups of 7-week-old Wistar rats comparing corticotomy, flap surgery, and RANKL transfection. To simplify, groups 1, 4, and 5 were summarized as one line (G1), because almost identical clinical results were obtained. (b) Statistical comparison of tooth movement measurements registered for the groups with the highest final tooth movement rate – G2 corticotomy and G3 transfection – and the external control group (G1). (Source: Iglesias-Linares et al., 2011. Reproduced with permission of John Wiley & Sons.)

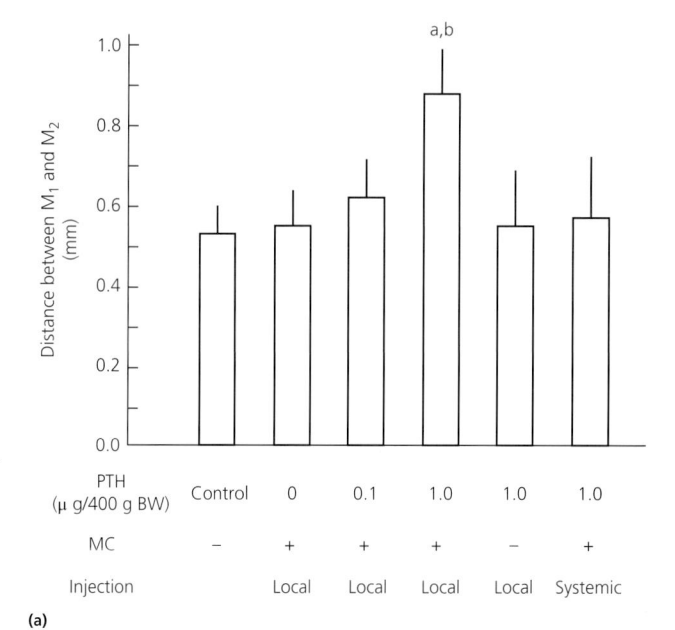

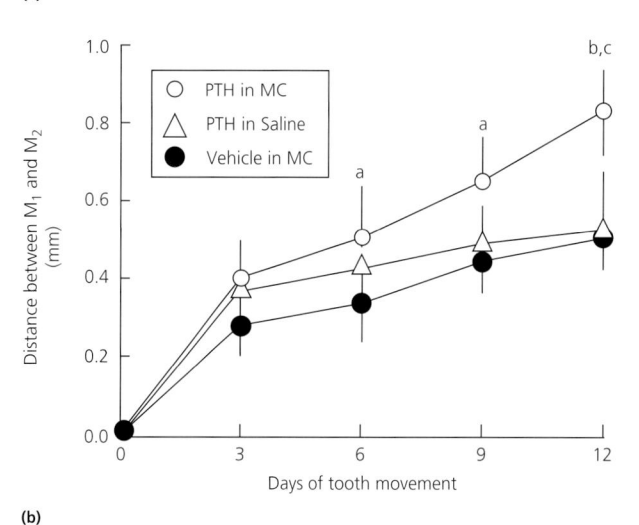

Figure 15.5 Effects of local injection of PTH on OTM. (a) In rats the right maxillary first molar (M_1) was moved mesially after subperiosteal injection of vehicle or PTH in the mesio-palatal region. The systemic injection group received a subcutaneous injection of 1.0 µg PTH-containing methylcellulose (MC) gel in the dorso-cervical area. The distance between M_1 and M_2 was measured on day 12 of tooth movement. (b) Time course of the effects of local injection of PTH on OTM. Each animal received a local injection of MC gel (vehicle in MC), 1.0 µg PTH containing MC gel (PTH in MC), or 1 µg PTH-containing saline (PTH in saline). The distance between M_1 and M_2 was measured on the indicated days of tooth movement. (Source: Soma et al., 2000. Reproduced with permission of SAGE Publishing.)

the time taken for accumulation of PTH for reaching a pharmacologically effective dose. Moreover, this study demonstrated the biphasic activity of PTH, as evidenced by increased expression of both RANKL and IGF-1, showing both osteoclastogenic and osteoblastogenic activities. Recently, Li et al. (2019b) observed significantly higher *RANKL* mRNA levels (enhanced osteoclast activity) on the compression side of the alveolar bone promoting rapid OTM and lower *RUNX2* mRNA levels (indicative of osteoblastic activity) on the compression side of the periodontal tissues in rabbits who were injected with PTH in conjunction with mandibular ramus osteotomy.

1,25-Dihydroxycholecalciferol (1,25-$(OH)_2D_3$) (Vitamin D_3)

1,25-$(OH)_2D_3$ is a systemic calcium-regulating steroid hormone having a major role in mineral homeostasis through calcium absorption from the intestine and mobilization of minerals out of bone. It acts on precursors of both osteoclasts and osteoblasts, promoting their differentiation, to increase the number of mature osteoclasts involved in bone resorption (Merke et al., 1986). Taking into consideration the fact that low systemic doses of $1,25\text{-}(OH)_2D_3$ are capable of activating osteoclastic activity, Collins and Sinclair (1988) tried it as a local injection at the site of canine retraction in cats and observed a 60% increase in the rate of tooth movement. They could not observe any systemic side effects when serum profiles of the cats were studied after the injection. Kawakami (1990) replicated in rats the experiment of Collins and Sinclair (1988) and reported that a local application of 10^{-10} mol/L of $1,25\text{-}(OH)_2D_3$ tends to prevent mineral apposition at the alveolar bone during OTM. Takano-Yamamoto et al. (1992) tried submucosal injection of $1,25\text{-}(OH)_2D_3$ into the palatal area of the bifurcation of the first molar in rats and demonstrated a dose-dependent increase in the number of osteoclasts and bone resorption when used along with orthodontic forces. The study demonstrated a synergistic effect for tooth movement in high doses (10^{-8} and 10^{-7} mol/L) while lower doses (10^{-10} mol/L) showed an additive effect.

Kale et al. (2004) compared the effects of local application of PGE_2 and $1,25\text{-}(OH)_2D_3$ in rats). They concluded that $1,25\text{-}(OH)_2D_3$ promotes better coupling of bone formation and resorption, leading to better alveolar bone remodeling than PGE_2. Although they observed only a minute difference between these two agents in accelerating tooth movement (2.11 ± 0.04 and 2.16 ± 0.6 with $1,25\text{-}(OH)_2D_2$ and PGE_2 respectively), they favored the use of $1,25\text{-}(OH)_2D_3$ as it promotes production of an increased number of osteoblasts, which in turn promote the differentiation of osteoclasts, while not disturbing the coupling system of bone remodeling. Al-Hasani (2011) conducted the first human clinical trial on vitamin D by injecting calcitrol (15, 25, or 40 pg/0.2 mL calcitrol diluted with 10% dimethyl sulphide) to 15 patients (17–28 years). They observed around 51% increases in tooth movement with the 25 pg group while the other two groups exhibited 10% acceleration. Radiographic evaluation of the dental and paradental tissues revealed no side effects with calcitrol injection. Further, Iosub Ciur et al. (2016) conducted a split mouth approach to study effects of Vitamin D_3 on tooth movement and root resorption and observed 70% increase in the rate of tooth movement in relation to the control side. Cone beam computed tomography evaluation of dental roots revealed no signs of root resorption.

Relaxin
Relaxin, a member of the insulin/relaxin family, is produced during pregnancy for cervical softening and elongation of interpubic ligaments. This effect is materialized by altering the physiologic processes associated with collagen turnover, angiogenesis, and angiofibrosis. Considering its role in collagen turnover, Stewart et al. (2005) injected relaxin locally in a dog model and found it to stimulate collagen production by gingival fibroblasts and accelerate tooth movement. Following this result, Liu et al. (2006) successfully accelerated tooth movement in rats by administration of relaxin through either mini pumps or subcutaneous injections. However, these results could not be replicated in a detailed experiment performed on 120 male rats by Madan et al. (2007). They stated that relaxin does not affect either the rate or amount of tooth movement. Investigating the controversial finding of Madan et al. (2007), Henneman et al. (2008) concluded that relaxin produces a dose-dependent increase in matrix metalloproteinase (MMP)-2, but it does not affect total MMP activity in human PDL cells. These investigators were able to stimulate alpha-smooth muscle actin, but its role in accelerating tooth movement remains questionable. A randomized placebo-controlled trial in humans by McGorray et al. (2012) could also not detect any difference in tooth movement over a period of 8 weeks after weekly injections of relaxin (50 μg). Two systematic reviews published recently supported this finding to state that relaxin has no effect on OTM (Yi et al., 2017; Eltimamy et al., 2019).

Corticosteroids
Corticosteroids are a class of chemicals that includes steroid hormones naturally produced in the adrenal cortex, and their analogues, which are synthesized in laboratories. Corticosteroids are involved in a wide range of physiological processes, including stress response, immune response, and regulation of inflammation, carbohydrate metabolism, protein catabolism, blood electrolyte levels, and behavior. Chronic administration of corticosteroids induces bone resorption, as well as osteoporosis, due to its uncoupling effect on bone remodeling. It induces direct inhibition of osteoblastic activity, indirectly favoring osteoclastic activity (Ashcraft et al., 1992).

Storey (1958) was the first to evaluate the effect of cortisone and adrenocorticotropic hormone (ACTH) on the rate of tooth movement in rabbits and guinea pigs. He found an increase in the amount of bone and connective tissue resorption following cortisone administration in rabbits, which could not be observed with ACTH. Interestingly, he could not duplicate these results in guinea pigs, where both these agents showed no effect on bone resorption. Davidovitch et al. (1972), while evaluating in cats the role of cortisone acetate in tooth movement, found no accelerating effect on tooth movement following a short-term administration. Ashcraft et al. (1992) studied the effect of cortisone acetate-induced osteoporosis in rabbits and found that the teeth in the experimental group moved approximately three to four times faster than in the control group. Ong et al. (2000) evaluated the effect of prednisolone (1 mg/kg) administered for a period of 23 days in rats and concluded that it does not affect the rate of tooth movement. Michelogiannakis et al. (2018) pointed out the debatable role that corticosteroids have on OTM. Their review could identify two studies which reported decrease of OTM, two studies showing no significant influence, and two studies showing increase in OTM with corticosteroids. They reported that corticosteroids significantly decrease bone density and increase bone resorption during OTM. Further they reported that corticosteroids decrease orthodontically induced root resorption, which is supported by the systematic review and meta-analysis conducted by Haugland et al. (2018). The impression that we get from these studies is that corticosteroids, when administered short term, will not affect the magnitude of tooth movement, whereas long-term administration tends to induce bone resorption and accelerate tooth movement.

Conclusion
Whether it is local injection or local gene transfer, all the methods are aiming at release of injected agents over a period of time, inducing inflammatory reactions or protein expression respectively. All these experiments have shown promising results in laboratory or controlled clinical settings, but clinical applicability and routine use have not been validated. Until then, these results have to be viewed cautiously. Clinical application is not yet possible, and unwanted side effects also need further attention.

Accelerating tooth movement: physical stimuli

Direct electric currents and pulsed electromagnetic fields
Beeson et al. (1975) were the first to try application of constant direct electric current (10 μA) in cats for 5 weeks during OTM but were unsuccessful in increasing the rate of tooth movement. The

concept was revived by Davidovitch et al. (1980a, b), who investigated the levels of cyclic nucleotides in cats in the PDL and alveolar bone and observed enhanced phosphorylation activities in these tissues during tooth movement. They proposed the application of direct current for 7 and 14 days and showed that electricity can serve as a modality for accelerating tooth movement.

Based on the piezoelectric theory Stark and Sinclair (1987) studied the effect of pulsed electromagnetic fields (PEMF) in guinea pigs and observed almost double the rate of tooth movement (0.42 ± 0.17 mm) in comparison with the control group (0.28 ± 0.08 mm). They also recorded significant increases in the number of osteoclasts and raised levels of uric acid, creatinine, and creatinine phosphokinase, indicating increased protein metabolism in the experimental group.

Research following this report by other groups revealed increases in intracellular ionic calcium concentrations with PEMF in human PDL fibroblasts (499 ± 115.5 nM) in comparison with controls (232.7 ± 25 nM) (Satake et al., 1990), and also an increase in number of active osteoclasts (Chen, 1991). Darendeliler et al. (1995, 2007) demonstrated in rats that PEMF vibrations produced by either samarium cobalt or neodymium-iron-boron magnets induced a greater amount of tooth movement when used along with coil springs than when a coil spring was used alone. These results were duplicated in a study on 10 patients (mean age 23.0 ± 3.3 years) by Showkatbakhsh et al. (2010). Through their experiments with male Wistar rats, Spadari et al. (2016) observed that electrical stimulation ($10 \mu A/5$ min) along with orthodontic force application enhanced tissue responses, reducing the number of granulocytes and increasing the number of fibroblasts, blood vessels, and osteoclasts while modulating the expression of TGF-β1, VEFG, and bFGF.

In recent years hardly any primary studies have been published in orthodontics about the topic. The systematic reviews conducted in this regard (Long et al., 2013; Kalemaj et al., 2015; Yi et al., 2017) have pointed out the very low quality evidence to promote this modality for routine clinical use and emphasized that high quality trials must be conducted to substantiate the claim of accelerating tooth movement with either direct electric currents or pulsed electromagnetic fields.

Vibratory stimulus

The credits for the initial efforts to accelerate tooth movement with a vibratory stimulus goes to Krishtab et al. (1986) following which, Ohmae et al. (2001) successfully increased the rate of tooth movement with ultrasonic vibration. Nishimura et al. (2008) developed a vibration-imposed system through which a vibratory stimulus (61.02 ± 8.375 Hz) could be added to an expansive force applied on maxillary molars of male Wistar rats. They observed a significant increase in the rate of tooth movement with resonance vibration (Figure 15.6), and a greater number of osteoclasts in comparison with the control group, thus providing a solid foundation to the efficacy of vibrational stimulation. Immunohistochemistry revealed increased RANKL expression in the resonance vibration group, indicating an increase in osteoclast formation, function, and survival (Figure 15.7). Root resorption in the experimental group was not significantly greater in comparison with the control group.

Contradictory results were reported by Miles et al. (2012) in humans (sample size: 66 patients), who were instructed to wear a vibrational appliance for a minimum of 20 minutes per day, along with fixed-appliance treatment. During the 10-week study period, they recorded a 65% reduction in mandibular crowding in the experimental group, while in the control group it was 69%, questioning the efficacy of the appliance. These results were confirmed in a three-center randomized controlled trial that also found no

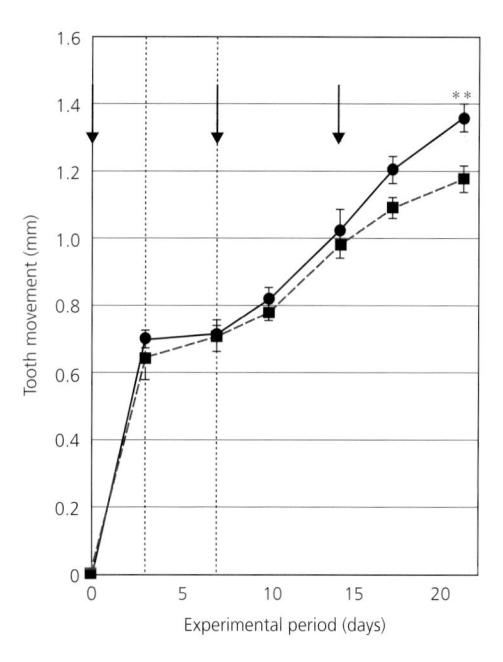

Figure 15.6 Time–displacement curve of the maxillary first molars of 6-week-old male Wistar rats that were expanded buccally for 21 days. In the experimental group additionally vibration was applied to the first molars during OTM (line with black circles). In the control group only an expansive force was applied (line with black squares). Tooth movement in both groups was divided into three phases. The extent of tooth movement in the vibration group was significantly higher than in the control group. (Source: Nishimura et al., 2008. Reproduced with permission of Elsevier.)

evidence that supplemental vibration could reduce the time needed for mandibular alignment and total treatment duration (Woodhouse et al., 2015; DiBiase et al., 2018). A concordant result to this was reported by Dobie (2013), who could not find any significant rise in the rate of tooth movement after application of either 5 Hz, 10 Hz, or 20 Hz vibration in conjunction with NiTi coil springs for space closure in mice. They also did not find any significant change in bone mineral density and volume between the experimental and control groups. Recently Chatmahamongko et al. (2019) could not find any difference in expression of IL-1β, IL-6, RANKL, and OPG in compressed human alveolar bone osteoblasts subjected to vibratory stimulus in comparison with a control group who experienced no vibration.

Systematic reviews conducted in this regard also provided no encouraging conclusions and pointed towards the need for higher level of evidence (Jing et al., 2017; Uribe et al., 2017). Interestingly, Jing et al. (2017) concluded that even though weak evidence exists, vibrational stimulus is effective for accelerating canine retraction but not for alignment. The effects of vibration on pain intensity and root resorption during orthodontic treatment are inconclusive.

Photobiomodulation

Photobiomodulation is defined as the ability to stimulate or inhibit cellular functions by using light at specific wavelengths, intensities, and irradiation regimens. Photobiomodulation therapy has been described to accelerate tooth movement, to diminish pain related to orthodontic treatment with fixed appliances, and to prevent orthodontic relapse (Sonesson et al., 2016). Interest in low-level laser therapy (LLLT) and the use of light-emitting diode (LED) devices as adjunctive tools during orthodontic treatment has increased over the past 20 years.

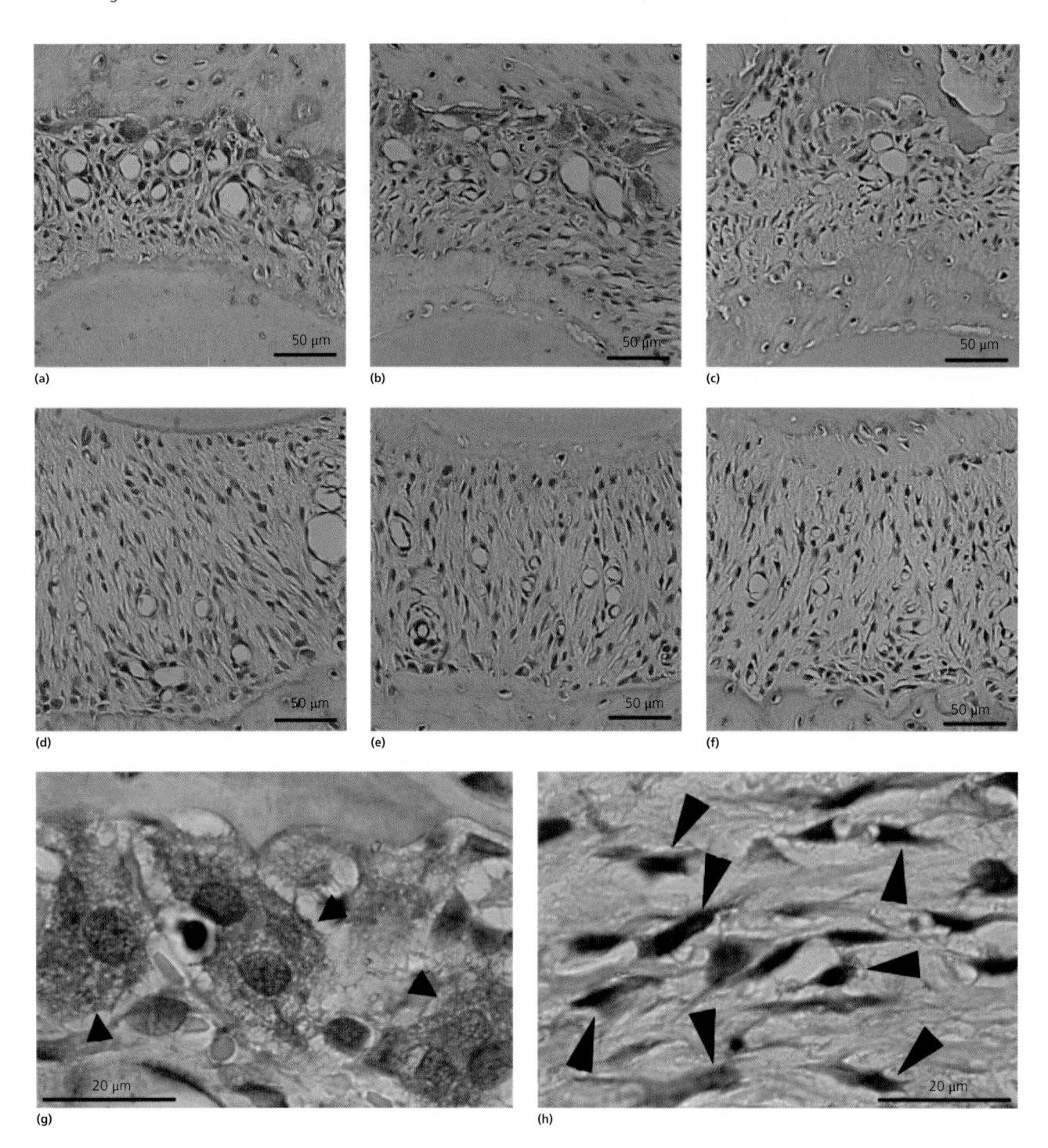

Figure 15.7 Comparison of RANKL distribution in rat PDLs with or without intermittent stimulation by resonance vibration. Strong RANKL expression was observed on day 3 in the PDL cells of the resonance vibration (RV) group. (a) RANKL immunostaining in the PDL tissue at the compressed side of the control (C) group on day 3; (b) and (g) RANKL immunostaining in the PDL tissue at the compressed side of the RV group on day 3; (c) and (f) negative control (secondary antibody only); (d) RANKL immunostaining in the PDL tissue at the tension side of the C group on day 3; (e) and (h) RANKL immunostaining in the PDL tissue at the tension side of the RV-group on day 3. *Small arrows*, RANKL immunostaining of osteoclasts; *large arrows*, RANKL immunostaining of PDL fibroblasts. (Source: Nishimura *et al.*, 2008. Reproduced with permission of Elsevier.)

Low-level laser therapy

Because low-level laser irradiation can augment bone fracture healing, as well as wound healing, Saito and Shimizu (1997) tried it in rats along with rapid maxillary expansion and observed augmented bone regeneration. Further experiments on the effects of low-level laser on the speed of tooth movement and bone remodeling in the rat model (Kawasaki and Shimizu, 2000) showed a 1.3 times increase, and an augmented response in both osteoblasts and osteoclasts in bone remodeling. Following this report, a study comprising 12 adult young patients (mean age 20.11 ± 3.4 years) was performed by Limpanichkul *et al.* (2006), who found no significant difference in tooth movement between experimental and control groups during the 3-month observation period. They suggested that the low dosage (25 J/cm^2) used might be the reason for this. Seifi et al. (2007) experimented with two types (continuous 630 nm and pulsed 850 nm) of laser irradiation in rabbits and discovered that it reduced the rate of tooth movement. They concluded that further increases in dosage might be necessary to obtain the results as proposed by Saito and Shimizu (1997). Contradictory to this, the results of a human study published by Youssef et al. (2008) with the application of the GaAlAs diode laser (809 nm, 100 mW) resulted in a greater amount of tooth movement in comparison with the nonirradiated group, regaining further interest in laser application.

Investigating the laser's mechanism of action, Yamaguchi et al. (2007) concluded that the *M-CSF/c-fms* pathway is activated, through which laser irradiation produces osteoclastogenesis and increased bone remodeling (Figure 15.8). Additionally, the role of RANK-RANKL in the process was reported by Fujita et al. (2008), with the help of immunohistochemistry comparing laser irradiation, LED irradiation, and controls in rats (Figures 15.9 and 15.10). In further research on the mechanism behind the acceleration of tooth movement with low-level lasers, the role of many molecules has been elucidated, including an increase in fibronectin and collagen type I turnover (Kim et al., 2010), elevated expression of MMP-9, cathepsin K and alpha (v) beta (3) integrins (Yamaguchi et al., 2010), and even statistically significant increases in the release of RANKL and OPG in the GCF (Dominiquez et al., 2013). Recent research with laser irradiation reported increased levels of interleukins (IL-6, IL-8, and IL-1β) helping to increase bone remodeling associated with orthodontic forces (Varella et al., 2018; Fernandes et al., 2019).

The number of publications pertaining to the acceleratory effect of a low-level laser has accumulated in such a way that many investigators have been able to perform systematic reviews of the subject (Long et al., 2013, 2015; Carvalho-Lobato et al., 2014; Ge et al., 2014; Kalemaj et al., 2015; Sonesson et al., 2016; Yi et al., 2017; Cronshaw et al., 2019). All the reviews to date point to the low-level evidence stating that laser irradiation can result in accelerated tooth movement. They all agree that an acceleration is observed in the initial stages of laser application, but the data are too weak to perform an evidence-based analysis. This indicates that there is a need for high-quality trials which can suggest optimal application protocols as well as monitor long-term effects before it is made a routine adjunct in orthodontic practices.

Light emitting diode (LED) therapy

Ekizer et al. (2013) tried light emitting diode (LED) mediated photobiomodulation therapy in rats and found tooth movement in the experimental group to be 1.55 ± 0.33 mm, in comparison with 1.06 ± 0.35 mm in the control group. The main advantage was the smaller amount of root resorption in the experimental group. At the same time, Kau et al. (2013) evaluated the efficacy of near infrared light with 850 nm wavelength, which was applied through a device with a set of LEDs worn by the patient at home for 20–30 min/day in 90 subjects (73 test subjects and 17 controls). They also observed significantly faster crowding resolution (1.12 mm/week) in comparison to 0.49 mm/week in the control group. However, this study was at high risk of bias as it lacked appropriate and complete reporting (Gkantidis et al., 2014). In contrast, Chung et al. (2015) could not find any significant acceleration in the LED-activated side in their split mouth randomized clinical trial in human subjects. Encouragingly, Fernandes et al. (2019) reported intrusion velocity of 0.26 mm/month in the irradiated group in comparison with 0.17 mm/month for the non-irradiated group within a period of 8 months. Additionally, the levels of cytokines (IL-6, IL-8, and IL-1β) were increased significantly in the photombiomodulation group when compared with the control group (G1),

All these approaches show convincing results in animal models, but in humans the results remain questionable. Extrapolating results of animal research to humans will require further biological research, both basic and clinical, before adding either lower level lasers, direct electric currents, vibratory stimulus, or photobiomodulation to our cache of reliable methods for acceleration of the pace of tooth movement.

Surgical approaches

The first efforts to move teeth with combined orthodontics and surgery are credited to Kole (1959a, b, c) who described corticotomy in a three-part article. He identified the main tissue layer to resist tooth movement as the cortical bone, and corticotomies as the means to move teeth faster. He advocated the use of labial as well as lingual/palatal surgical cuts, extending to the entire alveolar height, sparing or leaving the spongiosa intact. This procedure allows proper nutritional supply to the bone which is denuded of its periosteum. He also suggested horizontally osteotomizing the bone well above the apex, which can further enhance the tooth movement process (Figure 15.11). Duker (1975) tried corticotomies successfully in beagle dogs and reported that the procedure will neither damage the blood supply to the pulpal tissues, nor the vitality of periodontal tissues. After a long pause, the revival of the technique can be credited to Suya (1991), who tried it on 395 adult Japanese patients. Suya replaced the horizontal osteotomy of Kole with a corticotomy cut alone, and all reported cases were completed within 6–12 months. He reported this technique to be less painful, and at the same time causing less root resorption and relapse. Thereafter, a plethora of case reports have been published, proposing it as a valuable technique augmenting the rate of tooth movement. Through a series of publications, Wilcko et al. (2000, 2001, 2003, 2008) propagated alveolar augmentation with corticotomy and named it as accelerated osteogenic orthodontics or periodontally accelerated osteogenic orthodontics (AOO/PAOO). Case reports describe using this technique successfully, reducing treatment time with no evidence of root resorption (Wilcko et al., 2008). A detailed essay on the evolution, applicability, and the evidence-based answers on surgically facilitated orthodontic treatment with corticotomies and alveolar bone augmentation follows this chapter, limiting the scope of this discussion here.

The first efforts to study the histological reactions at the corticotomy site were performed by Kawakami et al. (1996). They observed irregular arrangement of cells and fibers and an increase in the number of bone remodeling cells and enlargement of suture width. They observed more bone loss and root resorption in the control than in the experimental group. At the cellular level, the corticotomy-induced acceleration of OTM is at least partly through stimulating macrophage infiltration and regulating their polarization into M1 and M2 phenotypes via NF-κB and JAK/STAT3 pathways, at early and late phases respectively (Wang et al., 2018).

Recent reports are questioning the validity of this technique in accelerating tooth movement. As stated previously in this chapter, Iglesias-Linares et al. (2011) have shown RANKL gene therapy to be far superior to corticotomies in increasing the rate of tooth movement. Mathews and Kokich (2013) pointed out, based on previous studies, that the regional acceleratory phenomenon (RAP) will last

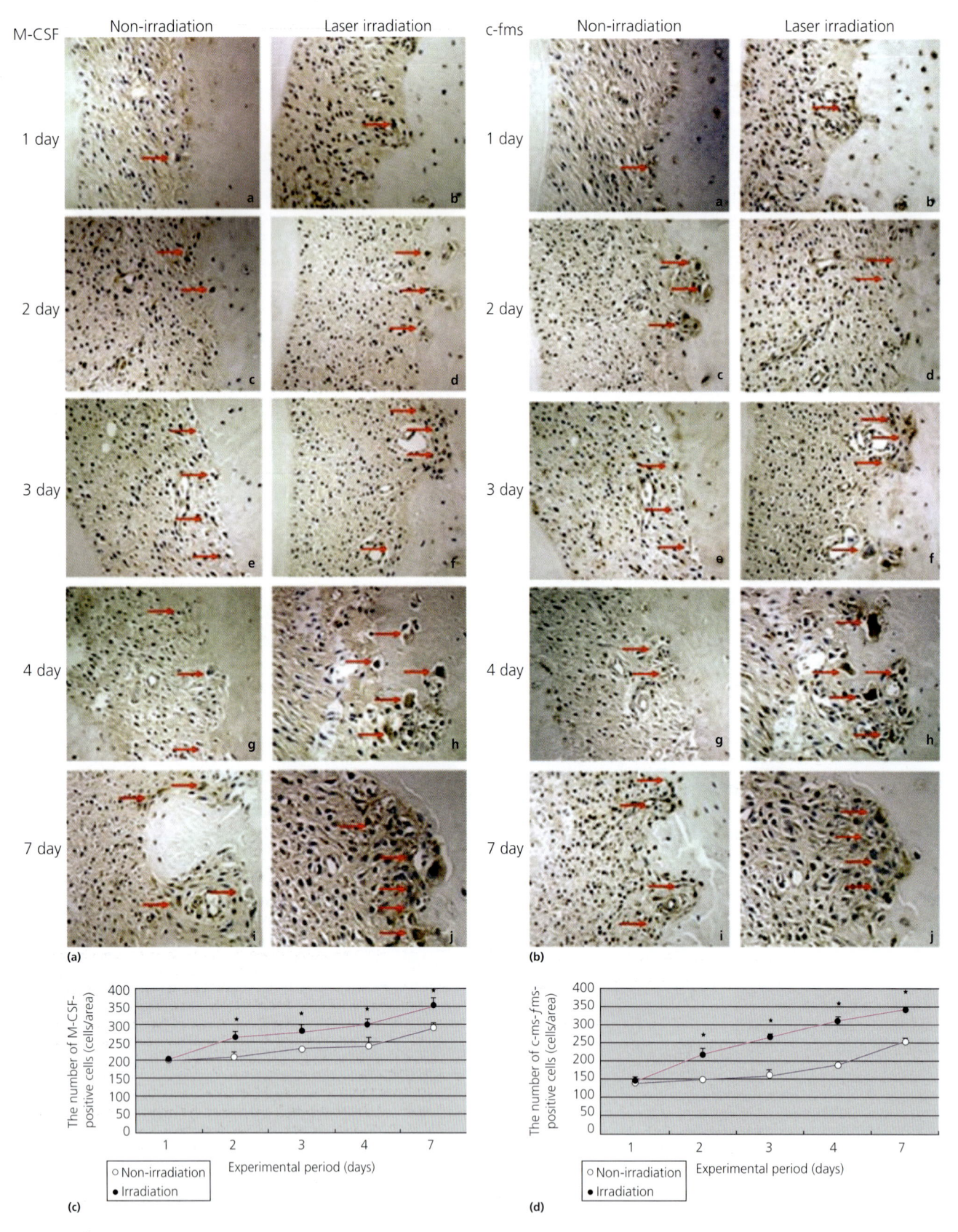

Figure 15.8 Effects of laser irradiation on M-CSF and *c-fms* positive osteoclasts in rats as shown by immunohistochemistry. M-CSF and *c-fms* immunoreactions were observed in osteoclasts on the alveolar bone surface in the irradiation group on days 2, 3, 4, and 7 (A: d, f, h, and j; B: d, f, h, and j). Further, those of M-CSF and *c-fms* were detected on days 3, 4, and 7 (A: e, g, and i; B: e, g, and i) in the non-irradiation group. The numbers of M-CSF and *c-fms* positive osteoclasts in the irradiation group were greater than those in the non-irradiation group on days 2, 3, 4, and 7. *$P < 0.05$ (graph C and D). Values are shown as the mean ± SD of five rats. (Source: Yamaguchi *et al.*, 2007. Reproduced with permission of Elsevier.)

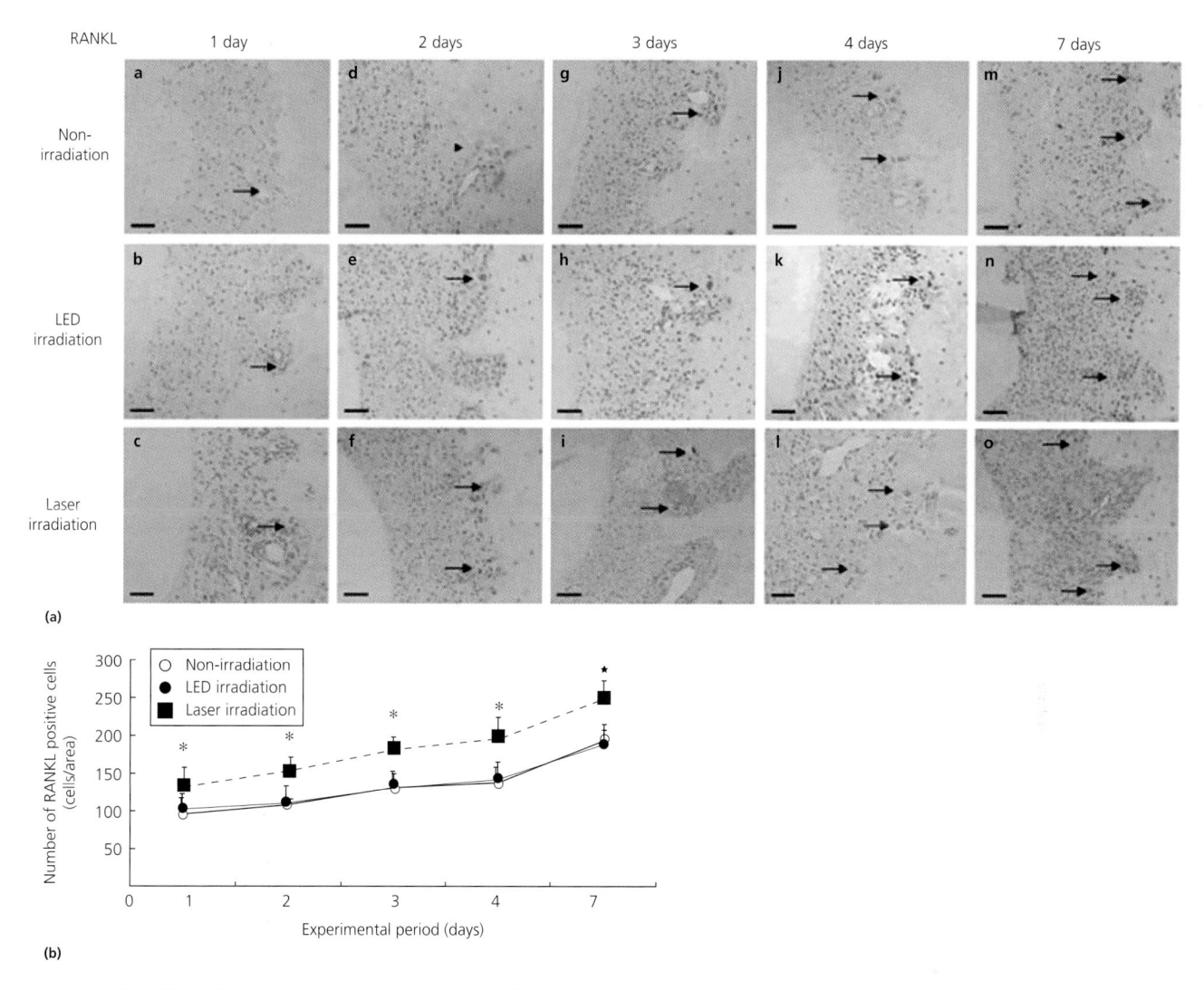

Figure 15.9 (A) Effects of laser irradiation on RANKL positive cells as shown by immunohistochemistry in rats (bar: 50 μm). RANKL immunoreactivity was observed in osteoclasts on the alveolar bone surface of the pressure side in the laser irradiation group (f, i, l, and o) on days 2, 3, 4, and 7, while both RANKL and RANK were detected on days 3, 4, and 7 (g–h, j–k, and m–n) in the non-irradiation and LED irradiation groups. (B) The number of RANKL and RANK positive cells in the laser irradiation group was greater than that in the non-irradiation and LED irradiation groups on days 2, 3, 4, and 7. *indicates $P < 0.05$. Values are shown as the mean ± SD of five rats. (Source: Fujita et al., 2008. Reproduced with permission of John Wiley & Sons.)

only for 4 months, and the same is the case with corticotomy-facilitated orthodontics. They stressed the need for further analysis of the technique in at least two matched cohorts before finalizing a conclusion. Moreover, the systematic review by Hoogeveen et al. (2014) has concluded that there exists only low to moderate quality evidence to suggest that corticotomy is a safe technique. A temporary phase of acceleration occurs, due to activation of RAP, which can effectively shorten the treatment time without any evidence of loss of vitality, bone loss, or root resorption. The same result was upheld by Dab et al. (2019), through their recent systematic review, in which they found an increase in bone thickness of 0.68 mm with bone graft use and a significant reduction in the overall treatment time by 2.8 months, which mainly occurs during the first few months of treatment. However, statistically insignificant differences existed for values of root resorption (0.24 mm), anchorage loss (0.49 mm), worsening of periodontal parameters (gingival index, 0.30), and mean increase in bone density of 7.07% on the corticotomy side at 6 months. Briefly, although corticotomies show reduction in treatment time, at least initially, the methodological quality of the published studies is low, with only low to moderate scientific evidence to support its routine clinical use.

Other than corticotomies, many other surgical techniques prevail, with much less evidence to substantiate their use. Dentoalveolar distraction, for rapid canine movement, was successfully performed in 15 patients by Liou and Huang (1998), who observed 6.5 mm of canine movement within 3 weeks with no (73%) or less (27%; less than 0.5 mm) forward movement of molars. Wang et al. (2004), who evaluated the area histologically, observed abundant vascularity with the presence of plenty of fibroblasts and osteoblasts in the site, indicative of bone and PDL remodeling. The lack of unfavorable gingival effects, with no alteration in the width of keratinized gingiva (Gürgan et al., 2005), as well as periodontal side effects (Lv et al., 2009) were demonstrated in the follow-up experiments. El Sharaby et al. (2011) reported, based on their histological study in a dog model, that at least a 6-week consolidation period should be allowed, to form a proper regenerate to which the tooth can be safely moved. It is encouraging to see that long-term results, showing stability and a lack of periodontal side effects, have started

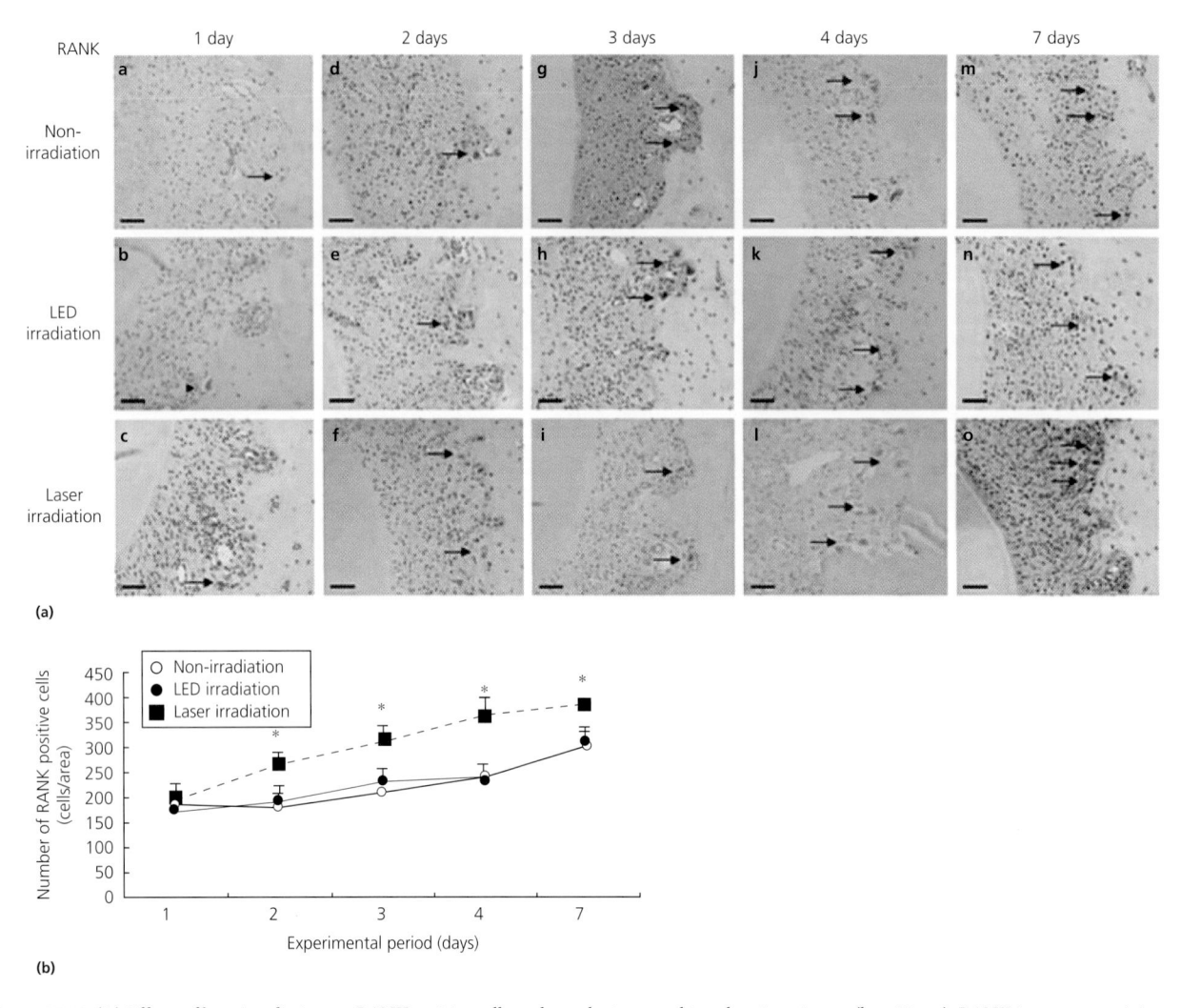

Figure 15.10 (A) Effects of laser irradiation on RANK positive cells as shown by immunohistochemistry in rats (bar: 50 μm). RANK immunoreactivity was observed in osteoclasts on the alveolar bone surface of the pressure side in the laser irradiation group (f, i, l, and o) on days 2, 3, 4, and 7, as well as on days 3, 4, and 7 (g–h, j–k, and m–n) in the non-irradiation and LED irradiation groups. (B) The number of RANK positive cells in the laser irradiation group was greater than that in the non-irradiation and LED irradiation groups on days 2, 3, 4, and 7. *Indicates $P < 0.05$. Values are shown as the mean ± SD of five rats. (Source: Fujita et al., 2008. Reproduced with permission of John Wiley & Sons.)

to appear in the literature in recent years (Allgayer et al., 2013; Kateel et al., 2016; Kurt et al., 2017).

In 2009, two more surgical techniques were introduced, which are modifications of corticotomy: corticision (Kim et al., 2009) and piezocision (Dibart et al., 2009). The first report of piezosurgery permitting microsurgical corticotomy was performed by Vercellotti and Podesta (2007) but with flap elevation and osseous surgery. Dibart et al. (2009, 2010) introduced a minimally invasive procedure combining microincisions with selective tunneling, followed by piezoelectric incisions and hard or soft tissue grafting. The same research group (Keser and Dibart, 2013) reported sequential piezocision, which involves a staged approach in which selected areas or segments of the arch are demineralized at different times to achieve desired results. Through this approach they have demonstrated a correction of Class III malocclusion, achieved with a treatment time of 8 months, and a follow up at 15 months, which revealed only a mild relapse. Several systematic reviews (Yi et al., 2017; Viwattanatipa and Charnchairerk, 2018; Rekhi et al., 2020) concluded that corticotomy (with a flap design avoiding marginal bone incision) or flapless piezocision procedures were not detrimental to periodontal health and the rate of canine movement after the latter was almost comparable to that of former. Nevertheless, piezocision resulted in higher levels of patient satisfaction.

Although Park (2006) proposed corticision through a local publication, this technique received greater attention in 2009, when the experiment in cats was published in *The Angle Orthodontist* (Kim et al., 2009). They used a reinforced scalpel as a thin chisel to separate the interproximal cortices transmucosally without flap reflection (Figure 15.12). Histologic analysis at day 14 revealed large resorption cavities filled with osteoclasts, which accelerated tooth movement, and the healing process was initiated at this site by day 21, suggesting a catabolic remodeling of bone with this procedure. In line with these publications, Safavi et al. (2012) suggested flapless bur decortications, in which small holes are made along the buccal bone of the tooth, using a fine surgical fissure bur. In a study performed in male dogs, they have concluded that although efficient in the initial stages, flapless bur corticotomy has an inhibitory effect on tooth movement in later stages, which can be attributed to the

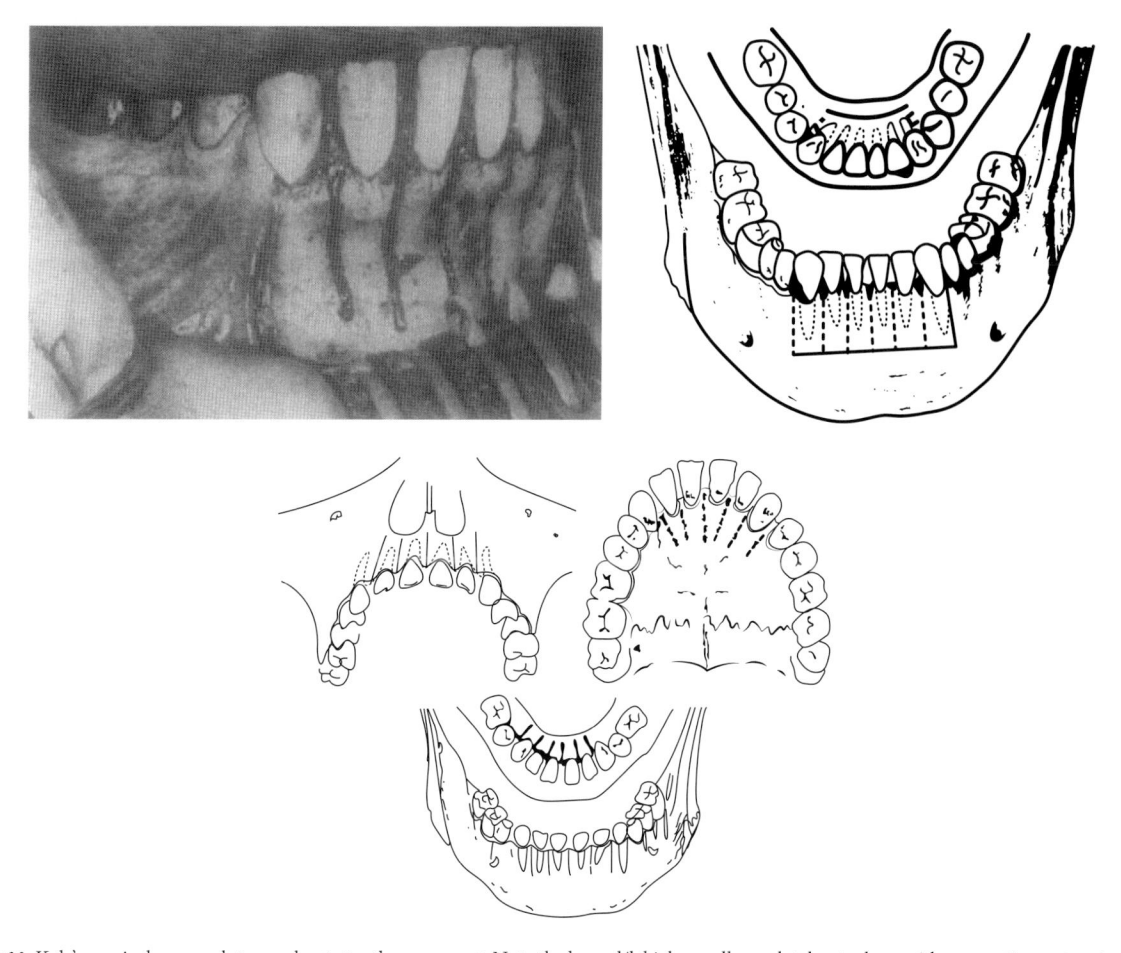

Figure 15.11 Kole's surgical approach to accelerate tooth movement. Note the buccal/labial as well as palatal cuts along with connecting cuts apical to tooth roots. (Source: Kole, 1959a. Reproduced with permission of Elsevier.)

maturation of newly formed bone. The existence of limited evidence about the effectiveness of minimally invasive surgically accelerated orthodontics is reported through recent systematic reviews (Alfawal et al., 2016; Fu et al., 2019). Fu et al. (2019) has observed no accelerated tooth movement with micro-osteoperforation and a mean treatment time reduction of 68.42 days with piezocision. No additional pain, changes in periodontal parameters, or root resorption was observed with minimally invasive surgical approaches to accelerate tooth movement.

The purpose of any surgical manipulation is to induce trauma, and evoke an osteopenic state, stimulating RAP, which in itself is an anabolic process. Regarding the finding that the RAP will only last for a maximum of 6 months, methods to reactivate the site must be the next research direction. If we can activate these sites successfully, without creating patient discomfort and additional cost, the acceptability of this technique has a chance to become widespread. It should be remembered that sufficient evidence to support these as routine clinical procedures is still lacking. Although there is a high experimental heterogeneity between studies, because of the poor quality of these studies, which generally have small sample sizes, the generation of conclusions becomes difficult. This points to the need for additional rigorously designed randomized controlled trials to validate the claims of the proponents of minimally invasive surgical approaches for accelerating tooth movement.

Methods to decelerate tooth movement

Drugs

Regulation of the functions of osteoclasts by either reducing their numbers or differentiation from preosteoclasts, can lead to reduced bone resorption, thereby reducing the rate of tooth movement. It has been established that nonsteroidal anti-inflammatory drugs, which inhibit prostaglandin synthesis, and bisphosphonates, which reduce osteoclastic activity, have definite tendencies to reduce tooth movement. Readers are referred to Chapter 14 for further information on drugs that have an inhibitory effect on tooth movement. We also would like to refer to the excellent overview of the topic by Swidi et al. (2018). In their paper they discuss the biological action mechanisms of various substances, focusing on their potential orthodontic applicability for orthodontic retention, which is the ultimate effort to decelerate OTM (see Table 15.1).

The class of drugs not discussed in Chapter 14 is chemically modified tetracyclins, which can induce apoptosis of osteoclasts and prevent their migration in rats (Bildt et al., 2007). Chemically modified tetracyclins have a definite role in inhibiting MMP activity (Figure 15.13) and may have a valuable role in preventing orthodontic relapse. Another study demonstrated the decreased osteoclast volume density expressed by cetirizine, a histamine-1 receptor antagonist, which will lead to an increase in alveolar bone density and reduced rate of tooth movement in

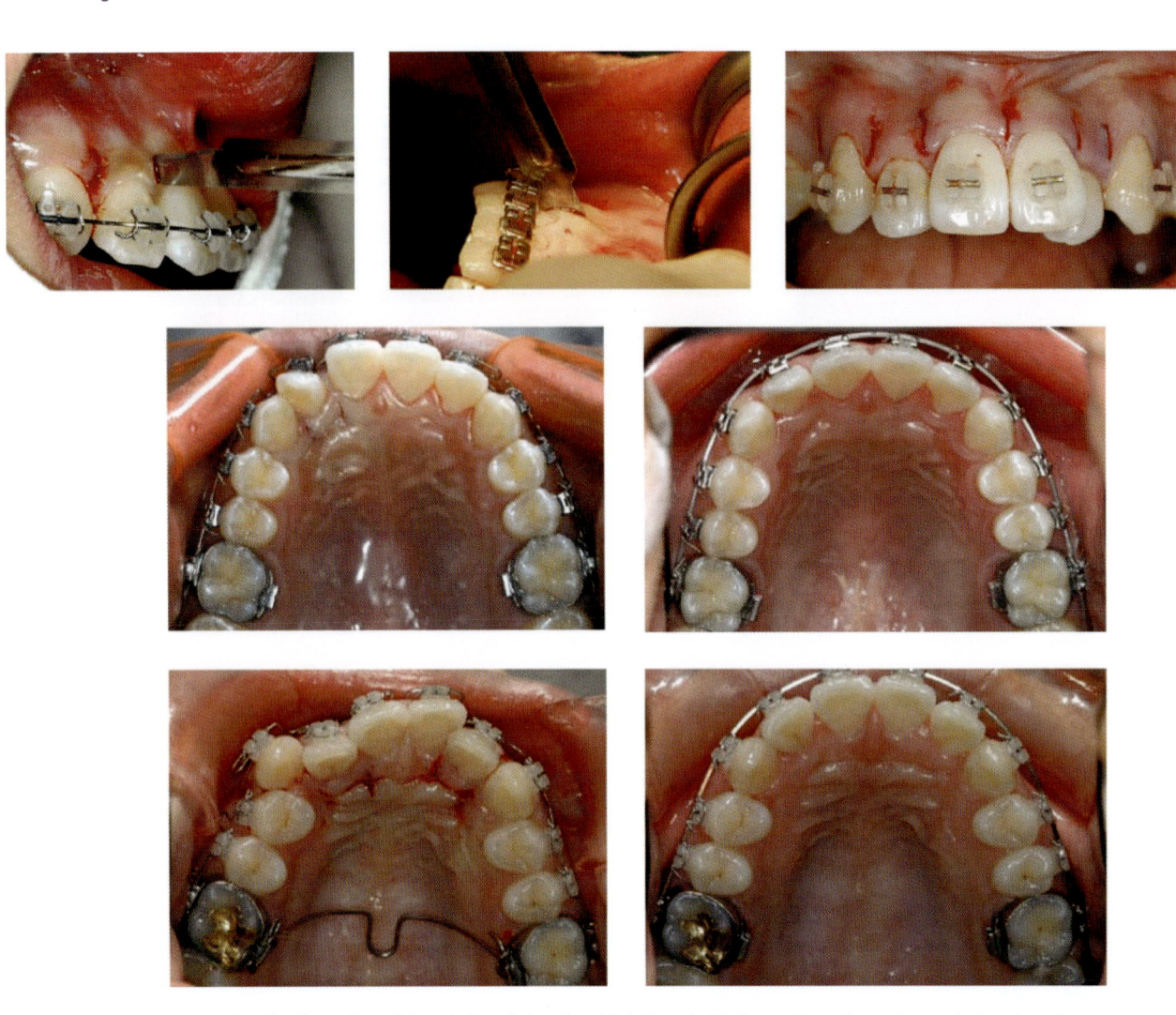

Figure 15.12 Corticision as described by Park et al. (2006). (Top, left and middle) Place the blade at right angles to the gingival surface, then turn obliquely at 45–60° down toward the apex, which helps the longer cut into the medullary bone with minimal gingival injury. The scalpel penetrates about 10 mm in depth to obtain cortical bone as well as cancellous bone cut. The corticision cut begins at 5 mm down to the papillary gingiva to keep papillary gingiva intact. (Top, right) Note there is no conspicuous postoperative bleeding immediately after the corticision. (Middle and bottom) Intraoral photos before and after the corticision. The mild crowding was completely relieved in 3 weeks, while moderate crowding took 9 weeks for complete alleviation. (Source: Dr. Young Guk Park, Kyung Hee University, South Korea. Reproduced with permission of Dr. Park.)

Table 15.1 Effects of various substances on bone and the PDL and the effect on OTM. (Source: Modified from Swidi et al., 2018.)

Biomedical substance	Biological effect	Effect on tooth movement	Suitable for human application
Osteoprotegerin	Inhibits bone resorption and accelerates PDL maturation	Decrease	No
Biphosphonates	Inhibit bone resorption	Decrease	Further research needed
Bone morphogenetic proteins	Stimulate bone and PDL formation	Decrease	Further research needed
Relaxin	Stimulates PDL turnover	No effect	No
Simvastatin	Stimulates bone formation	Decrease	No
Strontium ranelate	Stimulates bone formation and inhibits bone resorption	Decrease	No

rats (Meh et al., 2011). These researchers could not identify any effect on osteoclast function, osteoblast activity, or osteoblast volume density for this drug. Kondo et al. (2013) demonstrated that blockage of sympathetic signaling can reduce the rate of tooth movement. To demonstrate this effect, mice were injected intraperitoneally with propranolol (20 µg/g of body weight), isoproterenol (10 µg/g of body weight), or vehicle (0.9% saline); the propranolol-treated group showed the least amount of tooth movement in comparison with both the vehicle and isoproterenol group (Figure 15.14). Recently, Al Swafeeri et al. (2019) showed significant reduction in the numbers of osteoclasts and areas of active bone-resorptive lacunae hindering bone resorption processes resulting in reduction in tooth movement with local application of simvastatin.

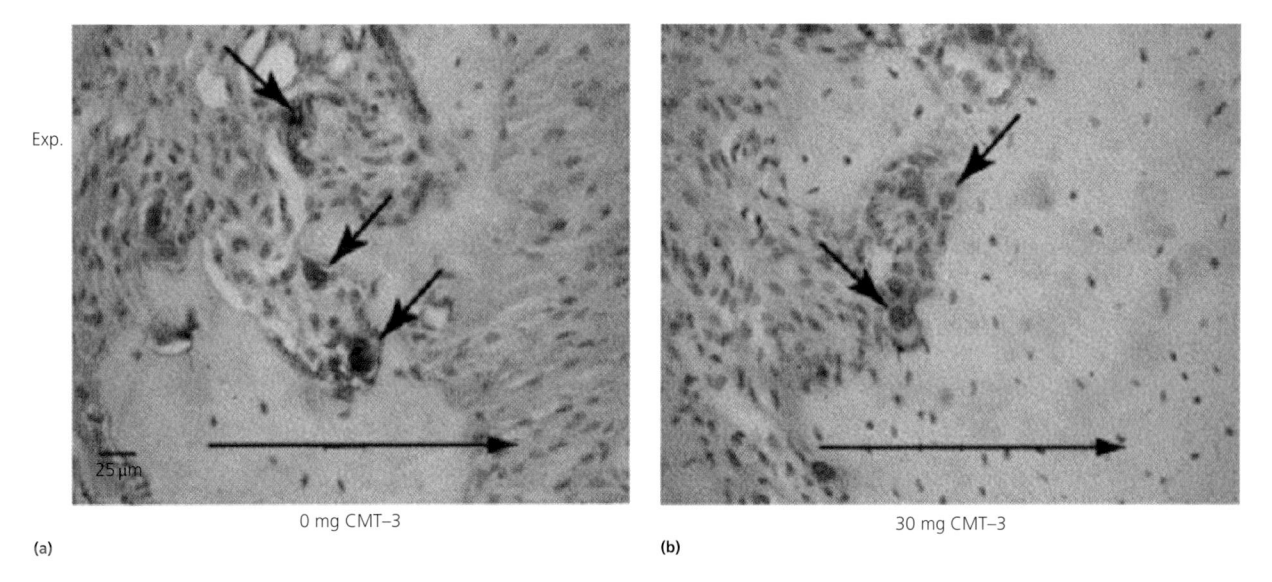

Figure 15.13 Immunohistochemical staining for MMP-9 after administration of chemically modified tetracyclins in adult Wistar rats. The figure shows the mesial side of the experimental roots. Tooth movement is in the direction of the arrow. Osteoclasts are visible as brown cells lining the alveolar bone surface. The osteoclasts in the 30 mg/kg group (b) seemed to stain less for MMP-9 compared with the 0 mg/kg group (a). (Source: Bildt et al., 2007. Reproduced with permission of Elsevier.)

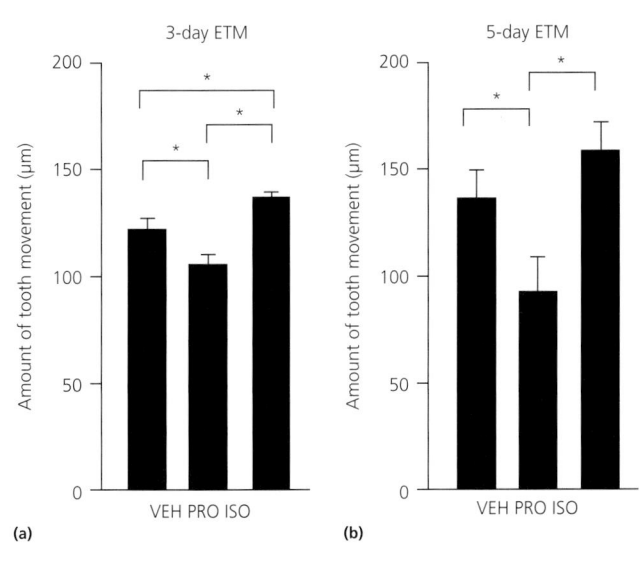

Figure 15.14 Experimental tooth movement was suppressed in mice by β-antagonists and increased by β-agonists. An elastic band was inserted between M1 and M2 for 3 days (3-day ETM) and 5 days (5-day ETM). ETM, experimental tooth movement; VEH, vehicle-treated group; PRO, propranolol (20 µg/g body weight/day)-treated group; ISO, isoproterenol (10 µg/g body weight/day)-treated group. Bars represent the mean ± SEM of $n = 8$ mice per group. *Indicates $P < 0.05$. (Source: Kondo et al., 2013. Reproduced with permission of Elsevier.)

Local MMP inhibitors and osteoprotegerin transfer

Considering the important role played by MMPs in bone remodeling associated with OTM, Holliday et al. (2003) locally injected ilomastat, a general MMP inhibitor, with ELVAX-40, a nonbiodegradable, noninflammatory sustained-release polymer in Sprague–Dawley rats. They observed tooth movement to be blocked between days 7 and 10, indicating its role in blocking bone resorption. Following this finding, Kanzaki et al. (2004) injected inactivated HVJ envelope containing pcDNA3.1(+)-mOPG into the palatal periodontal tissue of the maxillary first molar in Wistar rats. They observed a significant reduction of tooth movement in the OPG group (0.277 ± 0.034 mm) in comparison with the control group (0.531 ± 0.036 mm) after 21 days. A greater (93%) inhibition was observed by them at day 3, indicating long-term activity for transferred OPG in controlling the rate of tooth movement. Dunn et al. (2007) demonstrated in rats a dose dependent reduction in tooth movement with a higher dose of OPG (5 mg/kg), showing more potent action in comparison with low dose (0.5 mg/kg) during their observation periods of 7, 14, and 21 days (Figure 15.15). Research by other workers in animal models confirmed these findings (Hudson et al., 2012; Zhao et al., 2012), but clinical applicability of this procedure in humans is yet to be demonstrated. Schneider et al. (2015) and Baxter et al. (2019) showed in their study in male Sprague–Dawley rats that a single local injection of recombinant OPG effectively inhibits orthodontic relapse, with minimal systemic bone metabolic effects. This was the conclusion of the study by Fernández-González et al. (2016) and their systematic review in 2015 (Fernández-González et al., 2015) which concludes that compared with zoledronic acid, OPG is the most effective molecule in blocking the action of osteoclasts, thereby reducing undesired movements. Sydorak et al. (2019) encapsulated OPG in polymer microspheres and showed that a controlled drug release is possible, enhancing site-specific orthodontic anchorage without systemic side effects.

Estrogen

The possible variation in the rate of tooth movement during pregnancy was evaluated by Hellsing and Hammarström (1991) in adult female Sprague–Dawley rats. A significant increase in the pace of tooth movement was observed in pregnant animals in comparison with the control group. Investigating the rate of tooth movement during the estrous cycle in rats, Haruyama et al. (2002) reported that orthodontic treatment was faster in rats receiving orthodontic

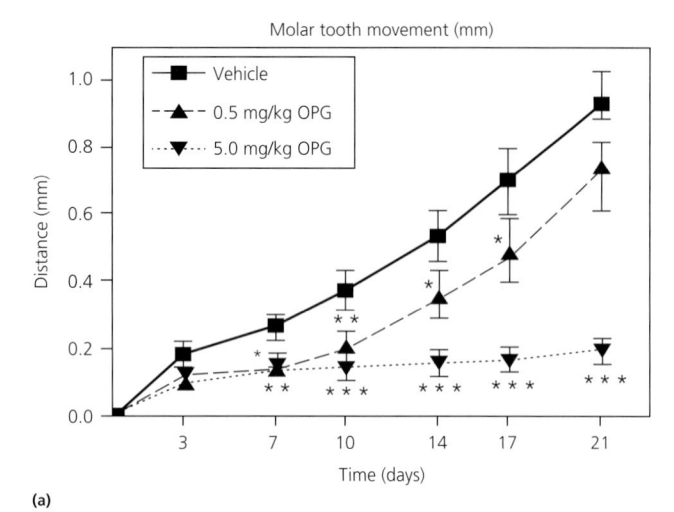

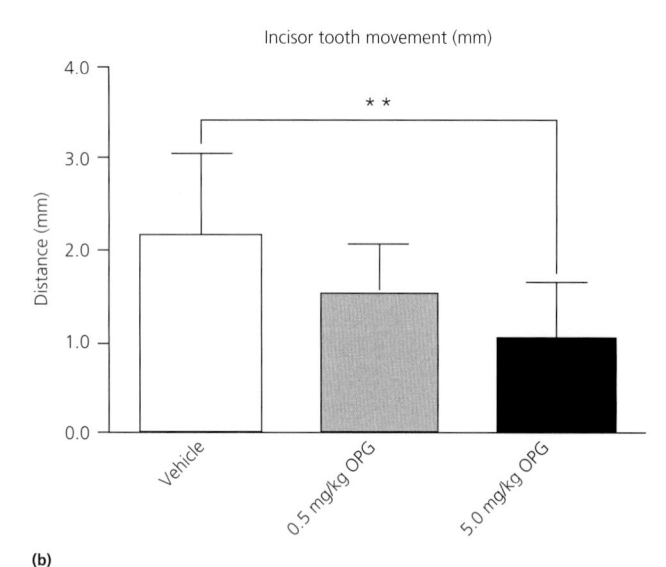

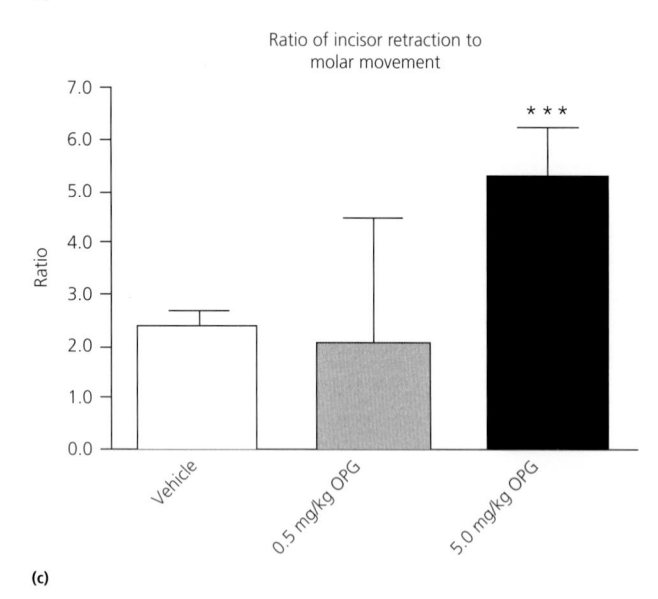

Figure 15.15 Inhibition of tooth movement by local delivery of OPG-Fc in rats. (a) Molar tooth movement over the course of time in vehicle (0.9% saline), 0.5 mg/kg OPG-Fc, and 5.0 mg/kg OPG-Fc injected groups. (b) Incisor retraction measured at day 21. (c) Ratio of incisor retraction to molar tooth movement at day 21. All results are expressed as the mean ± SEM, $n = 10$: $*P < 0.05$; $**P < 0.01$; $***P < 0.001$. Comparisons made versus time-matched vehicle groups. (Source: Dunn et al., 2007. Reproduced with permission of Elsevier.)

force during the estrous cycle than in those in the pre-estrous stage. This variation was due to the fact that serum estradiol retains a peak value during the pre-estrous stage, and keeps a low value during the estrous stage, suggesting that estrogen is anabolic in nature as far as bone remodeling is concerned. This was corroborated by the finding that Ghajar et al. (2013) reported in pregnant Wistar rats. They observed a decrease in tooth movement during pregnancy due to increased levels of estrogen and attributed it to the decrease in the number of osteoclasts. Olyaee et al. (2013) evaluated the effect of oral contraceptives containing ethinylestradiol/norgestrel in a rat model and found them to reduce the rate of tooth movement and the number of osteoclasts. It is clear that the effect of estrogen on alveolar bone turnover is the same as that of other bones, and it acts via the RANK/RANKL/OPG mechanism, at the same time reducing the amount of proinflammatory cytokines such as IL-1 and IL-6 (Syed and Khosla, 2005).

Conclusions

The cells which respond to orthodontic forces are capable of simultaneously responding to other stimuli, chemical and/or physical. The combined cellular response can be inhibitory, additive, or synergistic, depending on the type of stimulating agent. Clinically, there seems to be a choice between agents that increase the velocity of tooth movement, and those that can slow it down.

Research related to reducing the rate of tooth movement is in its initial stages as it reached only phase II evaluation with little evidence from human studies until now. Moreover, few reports regarding the adverse effects of these locally delivered agents have been published, warranting further studies so that harmful results are not generated. In any case, most proposed methods to alter tooth velocity apparently need a broader scientific basis, and to be derived from comprehensive prospective studies.

References

Alfawal, A. M., Hajeer, M. Y., Ajaj, M. A. et al. (2016) Effectiveness of minimally invasive surgical procedures in the acceleration of tooth movement: a systematic review and meta-analysis. *Progress in Orthodontics* **17**(1), 33.

Al Swafeeri, H., El Kenany, W., Mowafy, M. and Karam, S. (2019) Effect of local administration of simvastatin on orthodontic tooth movement in rabbits. *American Journal of Orthodontics and Dentofacial Orthopedics* **156**(1), 75–86.

Al-Hasani, N. R., Al-Bustani, A. I., Ghareeb, M. M. and Hussain, S. A. (2011) Clinical efficacy of locally injected calcitriol in orthodontic tooth movement. *International Journal of Pharmacy and Pharmaceutical Sciences* **3**, 139–143.

Allgayer, S., Rosenbach, G., Tavares, C. A. E. and Polido, W. D. (2013) Periodontal ligament distraction: Esthetics and occlusal stability at the 2-year follow-up. *American Journal of Orthodontics and Dentofacial Orthopedics* **143**, 535–546.

Ashcraft, M. B., Southard, K. A. and Tolley, E. A. (1992) The effect of corticosteroid-induced osteoporosis on orthodontic tooth movement. *American Journal of Orthodontics and Dentofacial Orthopedics* **102**, 310–319.

Basset, C. A. L. and Becker, R. O. (1962) Generation of electric potentials by bone in response to mechanical stress. *Science* **137**, 1063–1065.

Baxter, S. J., Sydorak, I., Ma, P. X. and Hatch, N. E. (2019) Impact of pharmacologic inhibition of tooth movement on periodontal and tooth root tissues during orthodontic force application. *Orthodontics and Craniofacial Research* **23**(1), 35–43.

Beeson, D. C., Johnston, L. E. and Wisotzky, J. (1975) Effect of constant currents on orthodontic tooth movement in the cat. *Journal of Dental Research* **54**, 251–254.

Bildt, M. M., Henneman, S., Maltha, J. C. et al. (2007) CMT-3 inhibits orthodontic tooth displacement in the rat. *Archives of Oral Biology* **52**, 571–578.

Borgens, R. B. (1984) Endogenous ionic currents traverse intact and damaged bone. *Science* **225**, 478–482.

Brudvik, P. and Rygh, P. (1991) Root resorption after local injection of prostaglandin E2 during experimental tooth movement. *European Journal of Orthodontics* **13**, 255–263.

Buschang, P. H., Campbell, P. M. and Ruso, S. (2012) Accelerating tooth movement with corticotomies: is it possible and desirable? *Seminars in Orthodontics* **16**, 286–294.

Carvalho-Lobato, P., Garcia, V. J., Kasem, K. et al. (2014) Tooth movement in orthodontic treatment with low-level laser therapy: a systematic review of human and animal studies. *Photomedicine and Laser Surgery* **32**, 302–9

Chang, J. H., Chen, P. J., Arul, M. R. et al. (2020) Injectable RANKL sustained release formulations to accelerate orthodontic tooth movement. *European Journal of Orthodontics* **42**, 317–325.

Chatmahamongkol, C., Pravitharangul, A., Suttapreyasri, S. and Leethanakul, C. (2019) The effect of compressive force combined with mechanical vibration on human alveolar bone osteoblasts. *Journal of Oral Biology and Craniofacial Research* **9**(1), 81–85.

Chen, Q. (1991) Effect of pulsed electromagnetic field on orthodontic tooth movement through transmission electromicroscopy. *Zhonghua Kou Qiang Yi Xue Za Zhi* **26**, 7–10, 61.

Chung, S. E., Tompson, B. and Gong, S. G. (2015) The effect of light emitting diode phototherapy on rate of orthodontic tooth movement: a split mouth, controlled clinical trial. *Journal of Orthodontics* **42**(4), 274–283.

Collins, M. K. and Sinclair, P. M. (1988) The local use of vitamin D to increase the rate of orthodontic tooth movement. *American Journal of Orthodontics and Dentofacial Orthopedics* **94**, 278–284.

Cronshaw, M., Parker, S., Anagnostaki, E. and Lynch, E. (2019) Systematic review of orthodontic treatment management with photobiomodulation therapy. *Photobiomodulation, Photomedicine, and Laser Surgery* **37**, 862–868.

Dab, S., Chen, K. and Flores-Mir, C. (2019) Short-and long-term potential effects of accelerated osteogenic orthodontic treatment: a systematic review and meta-analysis. *Orthodontics and Craniofacial Research* **22**(2), 61–68.

Darendeliler, M. A., Sinclair, P. M. and Kusy, R. P. (1995) The effects of samariumcobalt magnets and pulsed electromagnetic fields on tooth movement. *American Journal of Orthodontics and Dentofacial Orthopedics* **107**, 578–588.

Darendeliler, M. A., Zea, A., Shen, G. and Zoellner, H. (2007) Effects of pulsed electromagnetic field vibration on tooth movement induced by magnetic and mechanical forces: a preliminary study. *Australian Dental Journal* **52**, 282–287.

Davidovitch, Z., Finkelson, M. D., Steigman, S. et al. (1980a) Electric currents, bone remodeling, and orthodontic tooth movement. I. The effect of electric currents on periodontal cyclic nucleotides. *American Journal of Orthodontics* **77**(1), 14–32.

Davidovitch, Z., Finkelson, M. D., Steigman, S. et al. (1980b) Electric currents, bone remodeling, and orthodontic tooth movement. II. Increase in rate of tooth movement and periodontal cyclic nucleotide levels by combined force and electric current. *American Journal of Orthodontics* **77**, 33–47.

Davidovitch, Z., Musich, D. and Doyle, M. (1972) Hormonal effects on orthodontic tooth movement in cats – a pilot study. *American Journal of Orthodontics* **62**, 95–96.

Dibart, S., Sebaoun, J. D. and Surmenian, J. (2009) Piezocision: a minimally invasive, periodontally accelerated orthodontic tooth movement procedure. *Compendium of Continuing Education in Dentistry* **30**, 342–4, 346, 348–50.

Dibart, S., Surmenian, J., Sebaoun, J. D. and Montesani, L. (2010) Rapid treatment of Class II malocclusion with piezocision: two case reports. *International Journal of Periodontics and Restorative Dentistry* **30**, 487–493.

DiBiase, A.T., Woodhouse, N.R., Papageorgiou, S.N. et al. (2018) Effects of supplemental vibrational force on space closure, treatment duration, and occlusal outcome: a multicenter randomized clinical trial. *American Journal of Orthodontics and Dentofacial Orthopedics* **153**(4), 469–480.e4.

Dobie, T. G. (2013) The effect of varying frequencies of mechanical vibration on the rate of orthodontic tooth movement in mice. Master's Thesis, University of Connecticut, http://digitalcommons.uconn.edu/gs_theses/523 ((accessed September 10, 2020))

Dominiquez, A., Gómez, C. and Palma, J. C. (2013) Effects of low-level laser therapy on orthodontics: rate of tooth movement, pain, and release of RANKL and OPG in GCF. *Lasers in Medical Science* **30**, 915–923.

Duker, J. (1975) Experimental animal research into segmental alveolar movement after corticotomy. *Journal of Maxillofacial Surgery* **3**, 81–84.

Dunn, M. D., Park, C. H., Kostenuik, P. J. et al. (2007) Local delivery of osteoprotegerin inhibits mechanically mediated bone modeling in orthodontic tooth movement. *Bone* **41**, 446–455.

Ekizer, A., Uysal, T., Güray, E. and Akkuş, D. (2013) Effect of LED-mediated-photobiomodulation therapy on orthodontic tooth movement and root resorption in rats. *Lasers in Medical Science* **30**, 779–785.

El Sharaby, F. A., El Bokle, N. N., El Boghdad, D. M. and Mostafa, Y. A. (2011) Tooth movement into distraction regenerate: when should we start? *American Journal of Orthodontics and Dentofacial Orthopedics* **139**, 482–494.

Eltimamy, A., El-Sharaby, F. A., Eid, F. H. and El-Dakrory, A. E. (2019) The effect of local pharmacological agents in acceleration of orthodontic tooth movement: a systematic review. *Open Access Macedonian Journal of Medical Sciences* **7**(5), 882.

Fernandes, M. R., Suzuki, S. S., Suzuki, H. et al. (2019) Photobiomodulation increases intrusion tooth movement and modulates IL-6, IL-8 and IL-1β expression during orthodontically bone remodeling. *Journal of Biophotonics*, e201800311.

Fernández-González, F. J., Cañigral, A., Balbontín-Ayala, F. et al. (2015) Experimental evidence of pharmacological management of anchorage in Orthodontics: a systematic review. *Dental Press Journal of Orthodontics* **20**(5), 58–65.

Fernández-González, F. J., López-Caballo, J. L., Cañigral, A. et al. (2016) Osteoprotegerin and zoledronate bone effects during orthodontic tooth movement. *Orthodontics and Craniofacial Research* **19**(1), 54–64.

Fu, T., Liu, S., Zhao, H. et al. (2019) Effectiveness and safety of minimally invasive orthodontic tooth movement acceleration: a systematic review and meta-analysis. *Journal of Dental Research* **98**, 1469–1479.

Fujita, S., Yamaguchi, Y., Utsunomiya, T. et al. (2008) Low-energy laser irradiation stimulates tooth movement velocity via expression of RANK and RANKL. *Orthodontics and Craniofacial Research* **11**, 143–155.

Ge, M. K., He, W. L., Chen, J. et al. (2014) Efficacy of low-level laser therapy for accelerating tooth movement during orthodontic treatment: a systematic review and meta-analysis. *Lasers in Medical Science* **30**, 1609–1618.

Ghajar, K., Olyaee, P., Mirzakouchaki, B. et al. (2013) The effect of pregnancy on orthodontic tooth movement in rats. *Medicina Oral Patologia Oral y Cirugia Bucal* **18**, e351–355.

Gkantidis, N., Mistakidis, I., Kouskoura, T. and Pandis, N. (2014) Effectiveness of non-conventional methods for accelerated orthodontic tooth movement: a systematic review and meta-analysis. *Journal of Dental Research* **42**(10), 1300–1319.

Gürgan, C. A., Işeri, H. and Kişnişci, R. (2005) Alterations in gingival dimensions following rapid canine retraction using dentoalveolar distractionosteogenesis. *European Journal of Orthodontics* **27**, 324–332.

Haruyama, N., Igarashi, K., Saeki, S. et al. (2002) Estrous-cycle-dependent variation in orthodontic tooth movement. *Journal of Dental Research* **81**, 406–410.

Haugland, L., Kristensen, K. D., Lie, S. A. and Vandevska-Radunovic, V. (2018) The effect of biologic factors and adjunctive therapies on orthodontically induced inflammatory root resorption: a systematic review and meta-analysis. *European Journal of Orthodontics* **40**(3), 326–336.

Hellsing, E. and Hammarström, L. (1991) The effects of pregnancy and fluoride on orthodontic tooth movements in rats. *European Journal of Orthodontics* **13**, 223–230.

Henneman, S., Bildt, M. M., DeGroot, J. et al. (2008) Relaxin stimulates MMP-2 and α-smooth muscle actin expression by human periodontal ligament cells. *Archives of Oral Biology* **53**, 161–167.

Holliday, S., Vakani, A., Archer, L. and Dolce, C. (2003) Effects of matrix metalloproteinase inhibitors on bone resorption and orthodontic tooth movement. *Journal of Dental Research* **82**, 9687–9691.

Hoogeveen, E. J., Jansma, J. and Ren, Y. (2014) Surgically facilitated orthodontic treatment: a systematic review. *American Journal of Orthodontics and Dentofacial Orthopedics* **145**, S51–64.

Hudson, J. B., Hatch, N., Hayami, T. et al. (2012) Local delivery of recombinant osteoprotegerin enhances post-orthodontic tooth stability. *Calcified Tissue International* **90**, 330–342.

Iglesias-Linares, A., Moreno-Fernandez, A. M., Yañez-Vico, R. et al. (2011) The use of gene therapy vs. corticotomy surgery in accelerating orthodontic tooth movement. *Orthodontics and Craniofacial Research* **14**, 138–148.

Iosub Ciur, M., Zetu, I. N., Haba, D. et al. (2016) Evaluation of the influence of local administration of vitamin d on the rate of orthodontic tooth movement. *Revista medico-chirurgicala a Societatii de Medici si Naturalisti din Iasi* **120**(3), 694–699.

Jing, D., Xiao, J., Li, X. et al. (2017) The effectiveness of vibrational stimulus to accelerate orthodontic tooth movement: a systematic review. *BMC Oral Health* **17**(1), 143.

Kale, S., Kocadereli, I., Atilla, P. and Aşan, E. (2004) Comparison of the effects of 1,25 dihydroxycholecalciferol and prostaglandin E2 on orthodontic tooth movement. *American Journal of Orthodontics and Dentofacial Orthopedics* **125**, 607–614.

Kalemaj, Z., DebernardI, C. L. and Buti, J. (2015) Efficacy of surgical and non-surgical interventions on accelerating orthodontic tooth movement: a systematic review. *European Journal of Oral Implantology* **8**(1), 9–24

Kamata, M. (1972) Effect of parathyroid hormone on tooth movement in rats. *Bulletin of Tokyo Medical and Dental University* **19**, 411–425.

Kanzaki, H., Chiba, M., Arai, K. et al. (2006) Local RANKL gene transfer to the periodontal tissue accelerates orthodontic tooth movement. *Gene Therapy* **13**, 678–685.

Kanzaki, H., Chiba, M., Takahashi, I. et al. (2004) Local OPG transfer to periodontal tissues inhibits orthodontic tooth movement. *Journal of Dental Research* **83**, 920–925.

Kateel, S. K., Agarwal, A., Kharae, G. et al. (2016) A comparative study of canine retraction by distraction of the periodontal ligament and dentoalveolar distraction methods. *Journal of Maxillofacial and Oral Surgery* **15**(2), 144–155.

Kau, C. H., Kantarci, A., Shaughnessy, T. et al. (2013) Photobiomodulation accelerates orthodontic alignment in the early phase of treatment. *Progress in Orthodontics* **14**, 30.

Kawakami, M. (1990) Effects of local application of 1,25 (OH)2D3 on experimental tooth movement in rats. *Osaka Daigaku Shigaku Zasshi* **35**, 128–146.

Kawakami, T., Nishimoto, M., Matsuda, Y. et al. (1996) Histological suture changes following retraction of the maxillary anterior bone segment after corticotomy. *Endodontics and Dental Traumatology* **12**, 38–43.

Kawasaki, K. and Shimizu, N. (2000) Effects of low-energy laser irradiation on bone remodeling during experimental tooth movement in rats. *Lasers in Surgery and Medicine* **26**, 282–291.

Keser, E. L. and Dibart, S. (2013) Sequential piezocision: a novel approach to accelerated orthodontic treatment. *American Journal of Orthodontics and Dentofacial Orthopedics* **144**, 879–889.

Kim, S. J., Park, Y. G. and Kang, S. G. (2009) Effects of corticision on paradental remodeling in orthodontic tooth movement. *The Angle Orthodontist* **79**, 284–291.

Kim, Y. D., Kim, S. S., Kim, S. J. et al. (2010) Low-level laser irradiation facilitates fibronectin and collagen type I turnover during tooth movement in rats. *Lasers in Medical Science* **25**, 25–31.

Klein, D. C. and Raisz, L. G. (1970) Prostaglandins: stimulation of bone resorption in tissue culture. *Endocrinology* **86**, 1436–1440.

Kole, H. (1959a) Surgical operations on the alveolar ridge to correct occlusal abnormalities. *Oral Surgery, Oral Medicine, Oral Pathology* **12**, 277–288.

Kole, H. (1959b) Surgical operations on the alveolar ridge to correct occlusal abnormalities. *Oral Surgery, Oral Medicine, Oral Pathology* **12**, 413–420.

Kole, H. (1959c) Surgical operations on the alveolar ridge to correct occlusal abnormalities. *Oral Surgery, Oral Medicine, Oral Pathology* **12**, 515–529.

Kondo, M., Kondo, H., Miyazawa, K. et al. (2013) Experimental tooth movement-induced osteoclast activation is regulated by sympathetic signaling. *Bone* **52**(1), 39–47.

Krishnan, V. and Davidovitch, Z. (2006) Cellular, molecular, and tissue-level reactions to orthodontic force. *American Journal of Orthodontics and Dentofacial Orthopedics* **129**, 469.e1–32.

Krishtab, S. I., Doroshenko, S. I. and Liutik, G. I. (1986) Use of vibratory action on the teeth to accelerate orthodontic treatment. *Stomatologiia (Mosk)* **65**, 61–63.

Kurt, G., İşeri, H., Kişnişci, R. and Özkaynak, Ö. (2017) Rate of tooth movement and dentoskeletal effects of rapid canine retraction by dentoalveolar distraction osteogenesis: a prospective study. *American Journal of Orthodontics and Dentofacial Orthopedics* **152**(2), 204–213.

Lee, W. C. (1990) Experimental study of the effect of prostaglandin administration on tooth movement – with particular emphasis on the relationship to the method of PGE1 administration. *American Journal of Orthodontics and Dentofacial Orthopedics* **98**, 31–41.

Leiker, B. J., Nanda, R. S., Currier, G. F. et al. (1995) The effects of exogenous prostaglandins on orthodontic tooth movement in rats. *American Journal of Orthodontics and Dentofacial Orthopedics* **108**, 380–388.

Li, F., Li, G., Hu, H. et al. (2013) Effect of parathyroid hormone on experimental tooth movement in rats. *American Journal of Orthodontics and Dentofacial Orthopedics* **144**, 523–532.

Li, C., Chung, C. J., Hwang, C. J. and Lee, K. J. (2019a) Local injection of RANKL facilitates tooth movement and alveolar bone remodelling. *Oral Diseases* **25**(2), 550–560.

Li, Y., Chen, X. Y., Tang, Z. L. et al. (2019b) Differences in accelerated tooth movement promoted by recombinant human parathyroid hormone after mandibular ramus osteotomy. *American Journal of Orthodontics and Dentofacial Orthopedics* **155**(5), 670–680.

Limpanichkul, W., Godfrey, K., Srisuk, N. and Rattanayatikul, C. (2006) Effects of low-level laser therapy on the rate of orthodontic tooth movement. *Orthodontics and Craniofacial Research* **9**, 38–43.

Liou, E. J. and Huang, C. S. (1998) Rapid canine retraction through distraction of the periodontal ligament. *American Journal of Orthodontics and Dentofacial Orthopedics* **114**, 372–382.

Liu, Z. J., King, G. J., Gu, G. M. et al. (2006) Does human relaxin accelerate orthodontic tooth movement in rats? *Annals of New York Academy of Science* **1041**, 388–394.

Long, H., Pyakurel, U., Wang, Y. et al. (2013) Interventions for accelerating orthodontic tooth movement: a systematic review. *The Angle Orthodontist* **83**, 164–171.

Long, H., Zhou, Y., Xue, J. et al. (2015) The effectiveness of low-level laser therapy in accelerating orthodontic tooth movement: a meta-analysis. *Lasers in Medical Science* **30**, 1161–1170.

Lv, T., Kang, N., Wang, C. et al. (2009) Biologic response of rapid tooth movement with periodontal ligament distraction. *American Journal of Orthodontics and Dentofacial Orthopedics* **136**, 401–411.

Madan, M. S., Liu, Z. J., Gu, G. M. and King, G. J. (2007) Effects of human relaxin on orthodontic tooth movement and periodontal ligaments in rats. *American Journal of Orthodontics and Dentofacial Orthopedics* **131**, 8.e1–10.

Mathews, D. P. and Kokich, V. G. (2013) Accelerating tooth movement: the case against corticotomy-induced orthodontics. *American Journal of Orthodontics and Dentofacial Orthopedics* **144**, 5–13.

McGorray, S. P., Dolce, C., Kramer, S. et al. (2012) A randomized, placebo-controlled clinical trial on the effects of recombinant human relaxin on tooth movement and short-term stability. *American Journal of Orthodontics and Dentofacial Orthopedics* **141**, 196–203.

Meh, A., Sprogar, S., Vaupotic, T. et al. (2011) Effect of cetirizine, a histamine (H(1)) receptor antagonist, on bone modeling during orthodontic tooth movement in rats. *American Journal of Orthodontics and Dentofacial Orthopedics* **139**, e323–329.

Merke, J., Klaus, G., Hügel, U. et al. (1986) No 1,25-dihydroxyvitamin D3 receptors on osteoclasts of calcium-deficient chicken despite demonstrable receptors on circulating monocytes. *Journal of Clinical Investigation* **77**, 312–314.

Michelogiannakis, D., Al-Shammery, D., Rossouw, P. E. et al. (2018) Influence of corticosteroid therapy on orthodontic tooth movement: a narrative review of studies in animal-models. *Orthodontics and Craniofacial Research* **21**(4), 216–224.

Midgett, R. J., Shaye, R. and Fruge, J. F. Jr. (1981) The effect of altered bone metabolism on orthodontic tooth movement. *American Journal of Orthodontics* **80**, 256–262.

Miles, P., Smith, H., Weyant, R. and Rinchuse, D. J. (2012) The effects of a vibrational appliance on tooth movement and patient discomfort: a prospective randomized clinical trial. *Australian Orthodontic Journal* **28**, 213–218.

Ngan, P.W., Zadeh, Y.Z., Shanfeld, J. and Davidovitch, Z. (1988) The effect of interleukin-113 and parathyroid hormone on cyclic nucleotide and prostaglandin levels in human periodontal ligament fibroblasts in vitro, in *The Biological Mechanisms of Tooth Eruption and Root Resorption* (ed. Z. Davidovitch). EBSCO Media, Birmingham, pp. 261–267.

Nishimura, M., Chiba, M., Ohashi, T. et al. (2008) Periodontal tissue activation by vibration: intermittent stimulation by resonance vibration accelerates experimental tooth movement in rats. *American Journal of Orthodontics and Dentofacial Orthopedics* **133**, 572–583.

Ohmae, M., Saito, S., Morohashi, T. et al. (2001) Biomechanical acceleration of experimental tooth movement by ultrasonic vibration in vivo – part 1: homo-directional application of ultrasonication to orthodontic force. *Orthodontic Waves* **60**, 201–212.

Olyaee, P., Mirzakouchaki, B., Ghajar, K. et al. (2013) The effect of oral contraceptives on orthodontic tooth movement in rat. *Medicina Oral Patologia Oral y Cirugia Bucal* **18**, 146–150.

Ong, C. K. L., Walsh, L. J., Harbrow, D. et al. (2000) Orthodontic tooth movement in the prednisolone-treated rat. *The Angle Orthodontist* **70**, 118–125.

Park, Y. G., Kang, S. G. and Kim, S. J. (2006) Accelerated tooth movement by corticision as an osseous orthodontic paradigm. *Kinki Tokai Kyosei Shika Gakkai Gakujyutsu Taikai, Sokai* **48**, 6.

Patil, A. K., Keluskar, K. M. and Gaitonde, S. D. (2005) The clinical application of prostaglandin E1 on orthodontic tooth movement – a clinical trial. *Journal of the Indian Orthodontic Society* **38**, 91–98.

Rekhi, U., Catunda, R.Q. and Gibson, M.P. (2020) Surgically accelerated orthodontic techniques and periodontal response: a systematic review. *European Journal of Orthodontics* Jan 15. doi: 10.1093/ejo/cjz103. [Epub ahead of print]

Safavi, S. M., Heidarpour, M., Izadi, S. S. and Heidarpour, M. (2012) Effect of flapless bur decortications on movement velocity of dog's teeth. *Dental Research Journal* **96**, 273–289.

Saito, S., Ngan, P., Saito, M. et al. (1990a) Effects of cytokines on prostaglandin E and CAMP levels in human periodontal ligament fibroblasts in vitro. *Archives in Oral Biology* **35**, 387–395.

Saito, S., Rosol, T. J., Saito, M. et al. (1990b) Bone resorbing activity and prostaglandin E produced by human periodontal ligament cells in vitro. *Journal of Bone and Mineral Research* **5**, 1013–1018.

Saito, M., Saito, S., Ngan, P. W. et al. (1991) Interleukin 1 beta and prostaglandin E are involved in the response of periodontal cells to mechanical stress in vivo and in vitro. *American Journal of Orthodontics and Dentofacial Orthopedics* **99**(3), 226–240.

Saito, S. and Shimizu, N. (1997) Stimulatory effects of low-power laser irradiation on bone regeneration in mid-palatal suture during expansion in rat. *American Journal of Orthodontics and Dentofacial Orthopedics* **111**, 525–532.

Salazar, M., Hernandes, L., Ramos, A. L. et al. (2011) Effect of teriparatide on induced tooth displacement in ovariectomized rats: a histomorphometric analysis. *American Journal of Orthodontics and Dentofacial Orthopedics* **139**, e337–344.

Satake, T., Yasu, N., Kakai, Y. et al. (1990) Effect of pulsed electromagnetic fields (PEMF) on human periodontal ligament in vitro. Alterations of intracellular Ca2+. *Kanagawa Shigaku* **24**, 735–742.

Schneider, D. A., Smith, S. M., Campbell, C. et al. (2015) Locally limited inhibition of bone resorption and orthodontic relapse by recombinant osteoprotegerin protein. *Orthodontics and Craniofacial Research* **18**, 187–195.

Seifi, M., Eslami, B. and Saffar, A. S. (2003) The effect of prostaglandin E2 and calcium gluconate on orthodontic tooth movement and root resorption in rats. *European Journal of Orthodontics* **25**, 199–204.

Seifi, M., Shafeei, H. A., Daneshdoost, S. and Mir, M. (2007) Effects of two types of low-level laser wave lengths (850 and 630 nm) on the orthodontic tooth movements in rabbits. *Lasers in Medical Science* **22**, 261–264.

Shirazi, M., Khosrowshahi, M. and Dehpour, A. R. (2001) The effect of chronic renal insufficiency on orthodontic tooth movement in rats. *The Angle Orthodontist* **71**(6), 494–498.

Showkatbakhsh, R., Jamilian, A. and Showkatbakhsh, M. (2010) The effect of pulsed electromagnetic fields on the acceleration of tooth movement. *World Journal of Orthodontics* **11**, e52–56.

Soma, S., Iwamoto, M., Higuchi, Y. and Kurisu, K. (1999) Effects of continuous infusion of PTH on experimental tooth movement in rats. *Journal of Bone and Mineral Research* **14**, 546–554.

Soma, S., Matsumoto, S., Higuchi, Y. et al. (2000) Local and chronic application of PTH accelerates tooth movement in rats. *Journal of Dental Research* **79**, 1717–1724.

Sonesson, M., De Geer, E., Subraian, J. and Petrén, S. (2016) Efficacy of low-level laser therapy in accelerating tooth movement, preventing relapse and managing acute pain during orthodontic treatment in humans: a systematic review. *BMC Oral Health* **17**(1), 11.

Spadari, G. S., Zaniboni, E., Vedovello, S. A. S. et al. (2017) Electrical stimulation enhances tissue reorganization during orthodontic tooth movement in rats. *Clinical Oral Investigations* **21**(1), 111–120.

Spoerri, A., Koletsi, D. and Eliades, T. (2018) Intrinsic hormone-like molecules and external root resorption during orthodontic tooth movement. a systematic review and meta-analysis in preclinical in-vivo research. *Frontiers in Physiology* **9**, 303.

Stark, T. M. and Sinclair, P. M. (1987) Effect of pulsed electromagnetic fields on orthodontic tooth movement. *American Journal of Orthodontics and Dentofacial Orthopedics* **91**, 91–104.

Stewart, D. R., Sherick, P., Kramer, S. and Breining, P. (2005) Use of relaxin in orthodontics. *Annals of New York Academy of Science* **1041**, 379–387.

Storey, E. (1958) The influence of cortisone and ACTH on bone subjected to mechanical stress (tooth movement). *Journal of Bone and Joint Surgery* **40B**, 558–573.

Suya, H. (1991) Corticotomy in orthodontics, in *Mechanical and Biological Basis in Orthodontic Therapy* (eds. E. Hosl and A. Bauldhauf). Huthig Book Verlag GmbH, Heidelberg, pp. 207–226.

Swidi, A.J., Taylor, R.W., Tadlock, L.P. and Buschang, P.H. (2018) Recent advances in orthodontic retention methods: a review article. *Journal of the World Federation of Orthodontists* **7**, 6–12.

Sydorak, I., Dang, M., Baxter, S. J. et al. (2019) Microsphere controlled drug delivery for local control of tooth movement. *European Journal of Orthodontics* **41**(1), 1–8.

Syed, F. and Khosla, S. (2005) Mechanisms of sex steroid effects on bone. *Biochemical and Biophysical Research Communications* **328**, 688–696.

Takano-Yamamoto, T., Kawakami, M., Kobayashi, Y. et al. (1992) The effect of local application of 1,25-dihydroxycholecalciferol on osteoclast numbers in orthodontically treated rats. *Journal of Dental Research* **71**, 53–59.

Tsichlaki, A., Chin, S. Y., Pandis, N. and Fleming, P. S. (2016) How long does treatment with fixed orthodontic appliances last? A systematic review. *American Journal of Orthodontics and Dentofacial Orthopedics* **149**(3), 308–318.

Uribe, F., Dutra, E. and Chandhoke, T. (2017) Effect of cyclical forces on orthodontic tooth movement, from animals to humans. *Orthodontics and Craniofacial Research* **20**, 68–71.

Varella, A. M., Revankar, A. V. and Patil, A. K. (2018) Low-level laser therapy increases interleukin-1β in gingival crevicular fluid and enhances the rate of orthodontic tooth movement. *American Journal of Orthodontics and Dentofacial Orthopedics* **154**(4), 535–544.

Vercellotti, T. and Podesta, A. (2007) Orthodontic microsurgery: a new surgically guided technique for dental movement. *International Journal of Periodontics and Restorative Dentistry* **27**, 325–331.

Viwattanatipa, N. and Charnchairerk, S. (2018) The effectiveness of corticotomy and piezocision on canine retraction: a systematic review. *The Korean Journal of Orthodontics* **48**(3), 200–211.

Wang, S., Ye, X. Y., Zhou, H. and Feng, P. X. (2004) Histological changes on the stress side in orthodontic rapid tooth movement through distraction osteogenesis of the periodontal ligament on dogs. *Shanghai Kou Qiang Yi Xue* **13**, 312–314.

Wang, Y., Zhang, H., Sun, W. et al. (2018) Macrophages mediate corticotomy-accelerated orthodontic tooth movement. *Scientific Reports* **8**(1), 16788.

Wilcko, M. T., Wilcko, W. M. and Bissada, N. F. (2008) An evidence-based analysis of periodontally accelerated orthodontic and osteogenic techniques: a synthesis of scientific perspective. *Seminars in Orthodontics* **14**, 305–316.

Wilcko, W. M., Ferguson, D. J., Bouquot, J. E. and Wilcko, M. T. (2003) Rapid orthodontic decrowding with alveolar augmentation: case report. *World Journal of Orthodontics* **4**, 197–205.

Wilcko, W. M., Wilcko, M. T., Bouquot, J. E. and Ferguson, D. J. (2000) Accelerated orthodontics with alveolar reshaping. *Journal of Orthodontic Practice* **10**, 63–70.

Wilcko, W. M., Wilcko, M. T., Bouquot, J. E. and Ferguson, D. J. (2001) Rapid orthodontics with alveolar reshaping: two case reports of decrowding. *International Journal of Periodontics and Restorative Dentistry* **21**, 9–19.

Woodhouse, N.R., DiBiase, A.T., Johnson, N. et al. (2015) Supplemental vibrational force during orthodontic alignment: a randomized trial. *Journal of Dental Research* **94**(5), 682–689.

Yamaguchi, M., Fujita, S., Yoshida, T. et al. (2007) Low-energy laser irradiation stimulates the tooth movement velocity via expression of M-CSF and c-fms. *Orthodontic Waves* **66**, 139–148.

Yamaguchi, M., Hayashi, M., Fujita, S. et al. (2010) Low-energy laser irradiation facilitates the velocity of tooth movement and the expressions of matrix metalloproteinase-9, cathepsin K, and alpha(v) beta(3) integrin in rats. *European Journal of Orthodontics* **32**, 131–139.

Yamasaki, K., Miura, F. and Suda, T. (1980) Prostaglandin as a mediator of bone resorption induced by experimental tooth movement in rats. *Journal of Dental Research* **59**, 1635–1642.

Yamasaki, K., Shibasaki, Y. and Fukuhara, T. (1982) The effect of prostaglandins on experimental tooth movement in monkeys (Macaca fuscata). *Journal of Dental Research* **61**, 1444–1446.

Yamasaki, K., Shibata, Y., Imai, S. et al. (1984) Clinical application of prostaglandin E1 (PGE1) upon orthodontic tooth movement. *American Journal of Orthodontics* **85**, 508–518.

Yi, J., Xiao, J., Li, H. et al. (2017) Effectiveness of adjunctive interventions for accelerating orthodontic tooth movement: a systematic review of systematic reviews. *Journal of Oral Rehabilitation* **44**(8), 636–654.

Youssef, M., Ashkar, S., Hamade, E. et al. (2008) The effect of low-level laser therapy during orthodontic movement: a preliminary study. *Lasers in Medical Science* **23**(1), 27–33.

Zengo, A. N., Pawluk, R. J. and Bassett, C. A. (1973) Stress induced bioelectric potentials in the dentoalveolar complex. *American Journal of Orthodontics* **64**, 17–27.

Zhao, N., Lin, J., Kanzaki, H. et al. (2012) Local osteoprotegerin gene transfer inhibits relapse of orthodontic tooth movement. *American Journal of Orthodontics and Dentofacial Orthopedics* **141**, 30–40.

CHAPTER 16
Surgically Assisted Tooth Movement: Biological Application

Carlalberta Verna, Raffaele Spena, Michel Dalstra, Paolo M. Cattaneo, and Judith V. Ball

> **Summary**
>
> A main consideration for patients seeking orthodontic treatment is its duration. The desire for a reduction in treatment time is shared both by the patient and the orthodontist. In recent years various methods to achieve this have been proposed and among them corticotomy has been a popular option. In this chapter, the biological principles, the various surgically assisted approaches, and the biomechanical considerations will be presented and discussed in relation to state-of-the-art evidence. The potential benefit of a reduction in treatment time will also be reviewed with respect to the treatment of cases with severe malocclusions, especially adult patients, where a shorter treatment time would be particularly beneficial. Because the acceleration phenomenon seen with corticotomy lasts between 4 and 6 months, the benefits to treatment last for a limited time period, and also the area where it can be applied is spatially restricted. Therefore, the use of corticotomy must be carefully evaluated with respect to the additional biological and economic burdens incurred. On the other hand, corticotomy-assisted orthodontic treatment could be beneficial if an enhanced biological response is needed to support treatment especially in extremely complex cases.

Introduction

One of the most burning questions from our patients, even before starting orthodontic treatment, is "How long will the treatment take?". In general, patients prefer treatments which take a short period of time using simple, less visible appliances (Pacheco-Pereira et al., 2015). For these reasons, the key considerations in the last two decades have been to improve efficiency and reduce treatment time. The most recent developments include appliances with improved designs, new archwire alloys, precise and effective force delivering auxiliaries, reliable and user-friendly temporary anchorage devices, aligners with better aesthetic, biomechanical and clinical properties, and surgical and nonsurgical manipulation of the alveolar bone metabolism.

Orthodontic treatment is no longer limited to growing patients; increasing numbers of adults seek orthodontic treatment. Adult patients can benefit considerably from the latest advances in the field. The treatment of adult patients is much more challenging than treating young growing patients because growth compensation cannot be anticipated, periodontal complications are more likely, and often the treatment is part of a more complex interdisciplinary treatment plan. In adults, the cellular activation following the application of an orthodontic force takes longer to be initiated than in growing subjects, and tooth movement in adults seems to be slower (Ren et al., 2003; Iwasaki et al., 2017; Alikhani et al., 2018). Moreover, concerns relating to facial and dental aesthetics, the type of orthodontic appliances, and the duration of treatment are more challenging than for growing patients.

The predicted treatment time of a malocclusion treated with conventional orthodontics is on average 19.9 months, although there is a huge variation ranging from 14 to 33 months (Tsichlaki et al., 2016). However, today the mean duration is less than in earlier times. We recognize that numerous variables affect the duration of orthodontic treatment (Mavreas and Athanasiou, 2008): the initial complexity of the malocclusion and severity of tooth malposition; the age of the patient; the variability of the individual's response to the treatment; the quality of the end result and finally the patient's compliance.

A shorter treatment time is not only desirable for the patient's acceptance and compliance, but also for biological reasons, because long treatments are often associated with an increased risk for orthodontically induced root resorption (Roscoe et al., 2015). Also, a long treatment time increases the exposure to biofilms which, if not removed, can lead to dental decalcification (Richter et al., 2011). The duration of treatment as mentioned above is related to the

---

Biological Mechanisms of Tooth Movement, Third Edition. Edited by Vinod Krishnan, Anne Marie Kuijpers-Jagtman and Ze'ev Davidovitch.
© 2021 John Wiley & Sons Ltd. Published 2021 by John Wiley & Sons Ltd.

severity of the malocclusion which influences the clinical scenario (Mavreas and Athanasiou, 2008). An adjunctive tool with potential to facilitate more rapid correction of severe malocclusions and shorten treatment time would be beneficial to the orthodontist.

Surgically assisted tooth movement

The final orthodontic outcome is always the result of the interaction between the planned force system which is applied by the clinician and the individual response of the patient (Pilon et al., 1996). Both clinician- and patient-related variables therefore influence the final result of treatment. The mechanisms available to the orthodontist to avoid undesired tooth movement and control treatment duration reside basically in correct treatment planning and efficient handling of the biomechanical systems delivering the forces. Today we also have the possibility of digital 3D planning to optimize the planning of the desired tooth movement and in selected cases we can also assess the quality of the supporting tissues and thus avoid undesired round tripping. Digital 3D planning aids the choices made by the clinician in order to optimize the treatment duration, particularly in mild cases (Alford et al., 2011; Hou et al., 2020). Self-ligating brackets have been exhorted to shorten treatment time but this has not as yet been confirmed (Dehbi et al., 2017). The introduction of intraoral bone anchorage in the form of mini-implants or mini-plates, has considerably broadened the spectrum of treatment possibilities, facilitating tooth movements previously found to be difficult or impossible with conventional orthodontic appliances (Jambi et al., 2014; Alharbi et al., 2019).

Anatomical and biological variables relating to the patient influence the velocity of tooth movement. Since bone turnover is slower in cortical than in cancellous bone, teeth that must be moved towards cortical bone will move more slowly than teeth that are well placed within cancellous bone. This is because with in cancellous bone more surfaces are covered by bone marrow, and consequently there is greater availability of bone resorbing cells and a more rapid response to bone resorption.

The adjunctive procedures influencing a patient's biological response and thus to accelerate tooth movement can be divided into surgical and nonsurgical techniques (Almpani and Kantarci, 2016a, b).

Nonsurgical techniques include pharmacological approaches, low-intensity laser irradiation, resonance vibration, pulsed electromagnetic fields, and electrical currents. Within this group, there is a low level of evidence that low-intensity laser irradiation therapy accelerates the rate of tooth movement (Gkantidis et al., 2014), whereas there is no evidence that vibrational forces have any influence on the rate of tooth movement (Lyu et al., 2019).

The surgically assisted approach, which will be extensively described in the following sections of this chapter, is particularly interesting for the orthodontist, with various approaches being discussed, from the less invasive fiberotomy, to more aggressive procedures such as distraction osteogenesis and alveolar surgical procedures. Compared with the nonsurgically assisted accelerated tooth movement, these approaches allow customized local interventions, therefore enabling a more rational approach to anchorage control. Although there is a low level of evidence, meta-analysis has shown that corticotomies, corticotomy-assisted osteogenic treatment, piezocision, and micro-osteo-perforation (MOP) are all able to increase significantly the rate of tooth movement, without creating root resorption or periodontal injury (Abdallah and Flores-Mir, 2014; Dab et al., 2019; Mheissen et al., 2020; Shahabee et al., 2020). When combined with soft or hard tissue augmentation the corticotomy-assisted tooth movement appears to improve periodontal support (Wang et al., 2020). As expected, the acceleration lasts between 4 and 6 months, and therefore the benefit to treatment time must be questioned because of the incurring additional costs. Despite it being an invasive approach with related side effects, the procedure seems to be well accepted by patients (Charavet et al., 2019; Dab et al., 2019).

Biological principles and biomechanical considerations

The regional acceleratory phenomenon

Any local noxious stimulus can evoke a regional acceleratory phenomenon (RAP) characterized by an acceleration of normal regulatory tissue processes, which involves both soft and hard tissues, first described by Harold Frost (Frost, 1983). The metabolism and the activities of the differentiated cells and the precursor cells, the differentiation of cells, the longitudinal and transversal growth of bone and cartilage, together with bone remodeling are all activities affected by RAP. This process affects all types of bone tissues, such as woven bone, lamellar bone, cancellous bone, and compact bone (Frost, 1983). The group of cells responsible for the bone remodeling cycle form the so-called bone multicellular unit (BMU). The RAP should be seen as an "SOS" mechanism that facilitates healing and induces local tissue defense activities against infection and mechanical abuse necessary for the species to survive in a competitive environment. Therefore, RAP is an essential step in normal bone healing and any failure in RAP will cause a delay in healing and may promote a higher rate of infection (Frost, 1994).

In the mandible and in the maxilla, RAP occurs after tooth extraction, following fractures, surgical procedures and implant placement, in periodontal disease and following orthodontic loading. In all the abovementioned situations the alveolar or basal bones are submitted to noxious stimuli, whether mechanical or infectious. The acceleration of local bone turnover can be macroscopically visualized by an increased uptake of bone-seeking isotopes and radiographically by areas of reduced bone density. Histologically, the increased number of BMUs activated per unit of time is reflected by a larger area of bone surface covered by active bone resorptive and formative cells. Orthodontic loading causes a strain-generated RAP phenomenon resulting in increased apposition of cancellous bone which can be observed in the interradicular area and at the front of the alveolar socket in the direction of the applied force (Figure 16.1) (Verna et al., 1999). The cancellous bone formed is then reorganized over time into lamellar bone.

The duration of the RAP depends firstly on the tissue type and secondly on the form of the noxious stimulus; in the bone of healthy subjects the typical duration is 4 months, while in soft tissues the duration is usually shorter. After excessive stimuli the RAP may last longer than the following mild stimuli and is longer for adults than in growing patients. According to Frost, the area of the affected region and the intensity of the response varies directly with the magnitude of the stimulus, although to varying degrees in different individuals (Frost, 1983). Figure 16.2 portrays the intensity of RAP with different procedures. The clinical consequence of this is that the clinician's decision on the type of surgical intervention to be carried out can be adjusted according to the individual's need. Bone turnover is faster in cancellous than in cortical bone and therefore less invasive surgery may be needed in anatomical regions

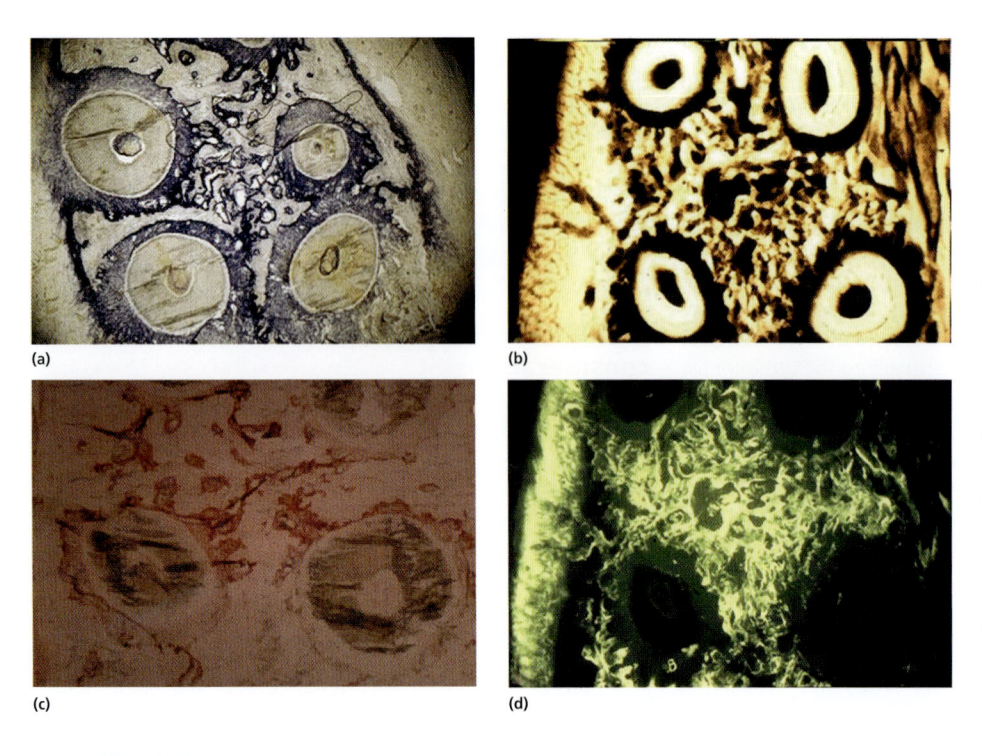

Figure 16.1 Alkaline (a) and acid (c) phosphatase staining of an interradicular specimen from a rat molar after the application of an orthodontic load of 25 g for 2 weeks. The 10 μm thick sections were taken consecutively. It is important to note the positive staining for both anabolic (a) and catabolic (c) activities, supporting the presence of a RAP after the application of the orthodontic load. The microradiographic image of the same samples (b) reveal decreased bone density and the formation of cancellous bone. The intensity of bone activity in forming cancellous bone is detected by the uptake of tetracycline labeling, as depicted in (d). (Source: Dr. C. Verna.)

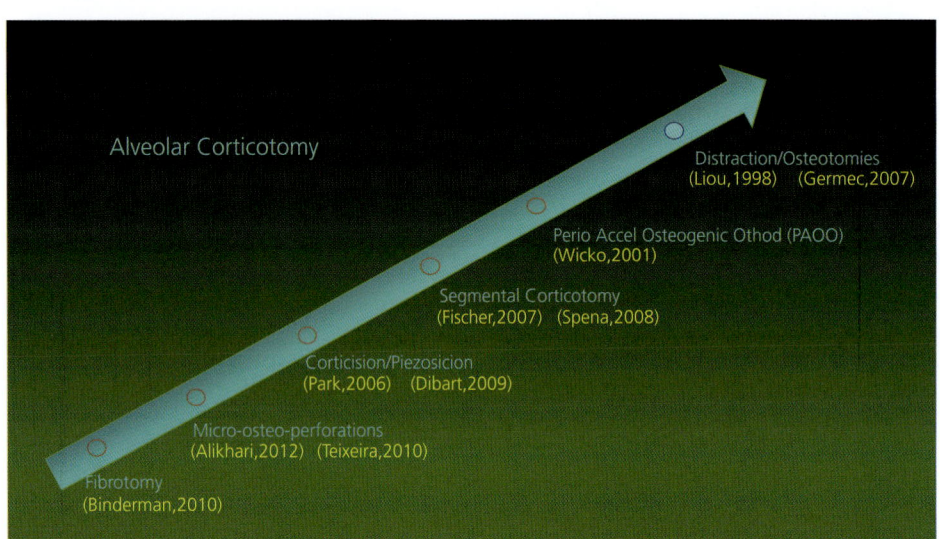

Figure 16.2 RAP intensity in relationship to the surgical procedure.

where more cancellous bone is present, such as the maxilla. On the other hand, a more aggressive surgical approach is required in cases where tooth movement must be performed in areas where the ratio between cortical and trabecular bone is very high, such as in the symphysis. Since the turnover of cortical bone is less than trabecular bone, the "SOS" mechanism of RAP may be less effective with a higher risk of a lack of coordination between resorption and formation, and supplemental grafting may be needed.

Moreover, the bone remodeling rate seems to be faster in the maxilla than in the mandible, independent of the ratio of cortical to cancellous bone (Deguchi et al., 2008). Therefore, a more invasive surgical approach may more often be indicated for the mandible compared with the maxilla. The intensity of the response gradually decreases as the distance from the affected site increases. Verna and co-workers found, in an animal study, that the RAP occurs not only around the teeth directly loaded by the orthodontic appliance but also at sites some distance away (Verna et al., 1999; Sebaoun et al., 2008; McBride et al., 2014).

Finite element analysis of surgically assisted tooth movement

A simple fiberotomy of the dento-gingival and interdental fibers has been found, in an animal study, to modify tooth movement rate and shift the center of rotation of a tipping movement toward the apex (Glenn et al., 1983). By performing a corticotomy, the mechanical support of the alveolar wall is undermined, which can potentially affect the location of the centre of resistance (CR) of the affected tooth. For a comprehensive assessment of the various aspects of the CR and the consequences for orthodontic tooth movement (OTM), please see Chapter 9. Although, the intention of a corticotomy is to trigger a RAP for an accelerated biological response to the orthodontic loading (Fu et al., 2019), the relocation

Figure 16.3 Influence of a buccal corticotomy on the alveolar load transfer. The stress intensity (von Mises stress) in the alveolar bone increases along the internal lingual marginal edge of the canine and the external buccal edge of the first premolar with both teeth tipping when compared with the non-corticotomized case. Also note the increase in the area of low range stresses along the buccal wall of the canine. (Source: Dr. C. Verna.)

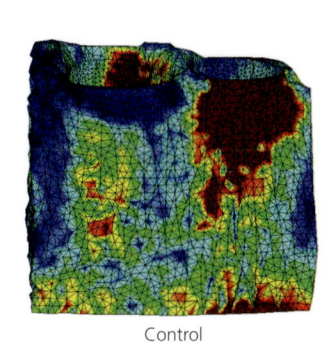

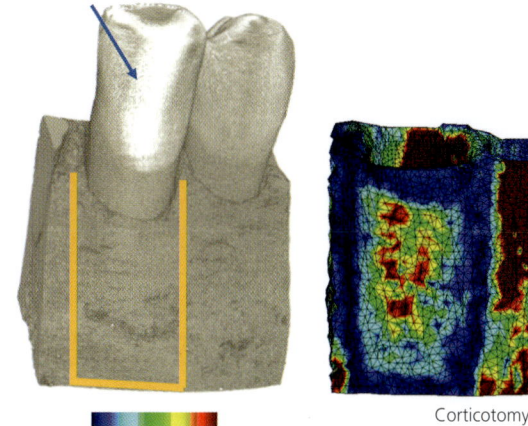

of the CR will also have mechanical consequences. It is known that a corticotomy changes the bone density considerably, with authors reporting around a 60% decrease in animal models (Baloul et al., 2011). This decrease certainly has quite an influence on the mechanical properties of the bone components within the alveolar bone structures since bone strength is strongly correlated to bone density (Carter and Hayes, 1977; Rice et al., 1988; Schaffler and Burr, 1988).

Different corticotomy techniques have been proposed, where the type, extension, and location of the incision varies. According to the technique used, the biomechanical response to the applied force system at the bracket will be quite different, with variable mechanical effects on the teeth, periodontal ligament (PDL), trabecular as well as alveolar bone. On the other hand, most corticotomies typically produce relatively little damage to the bone, with most of the original alveolar bone remaining intact. Based on this knowledge, it could be anticipated that changes in bone stiffness and therefore the initial tooth movement when an orthodontic load is applied would only be minimal (Verna, 2008).

A series of 3-dimensional Finite Element (FE) analyses were made, using an FE model of a lateral incisor with its supporting tissues, with the intention of studying the effect of a corticotomy on OTM. In the first simulation, only damage produced by the corticotomy was introduced with different loads and moment-to-force (M/F) ratios at the bracket. The results corroborated what was anticipated: only minor changes were observed in the PDL and little or no change could be detected in the location of the center of resistance (Figure 16.3). In contrast, when the FE model simulated incisions around all the teeth in the upper anterior region, the best location for retraction of the anterior teeth seems to be where the incision is close to the margins of the apical area (Liu et al., 2020).

In a second series of FE analyses it was assumed that the corticotomy greatly reduced the mechanical resilience of the buccal alveolar wall, which was expressed as a significantly lower Young's modulus of the elements in the site under investigation (Verna et al., 2018). Once again, various loadings with different M/F ratios at the bracket were simulated. It was found that both the mode and magnitude of the movement were affected; in addition, the calculated tooth movements were graphically represented according to the method of Burstone and Pryputniewicz (1980). This showed that a pure translation, which is normally associated with an M/F-ratio of 10 mm, already occurred at a M/F ratio of only 8 mm. (Figure 16.4) This means that orthodontists need to be aware of this

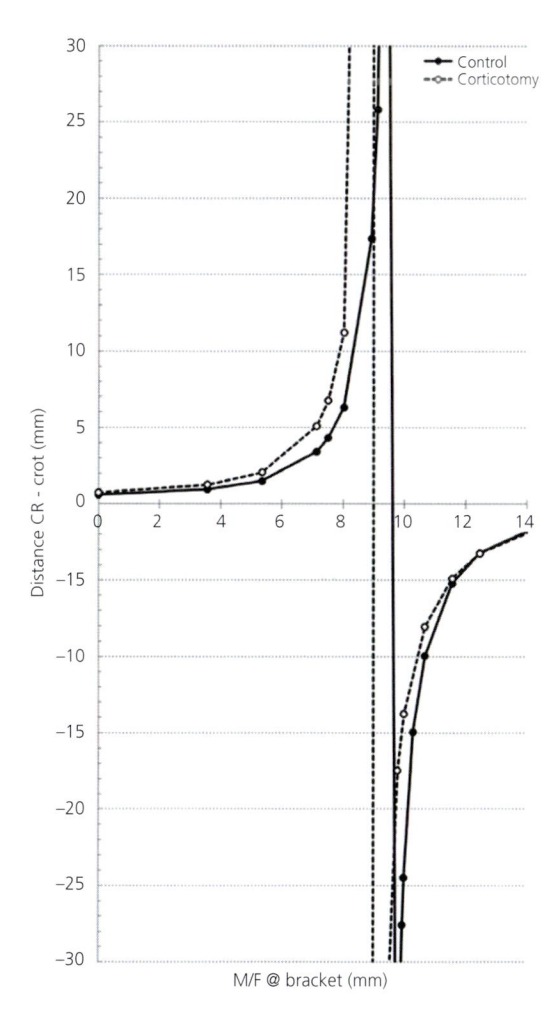

Figure 16.4 The "Burstone and Pryputniewicz" curves showing the dependency of the distance between CR and Crot of the lateral incisor and the applied M/F ratio for both the control and corticotomized models. (Source: Modified from Burstone and Pryputniewicz, 1980.)

shift for treatment planning and consequently modification of the orthodontic appliance is required. Furthermore, with less alveolar bone to resist tooth displacement, the amount of tooth movement, in particular tipping and root torque, was increased by corticotomy by up to 30% and the PDL showed fewer compressive stresses

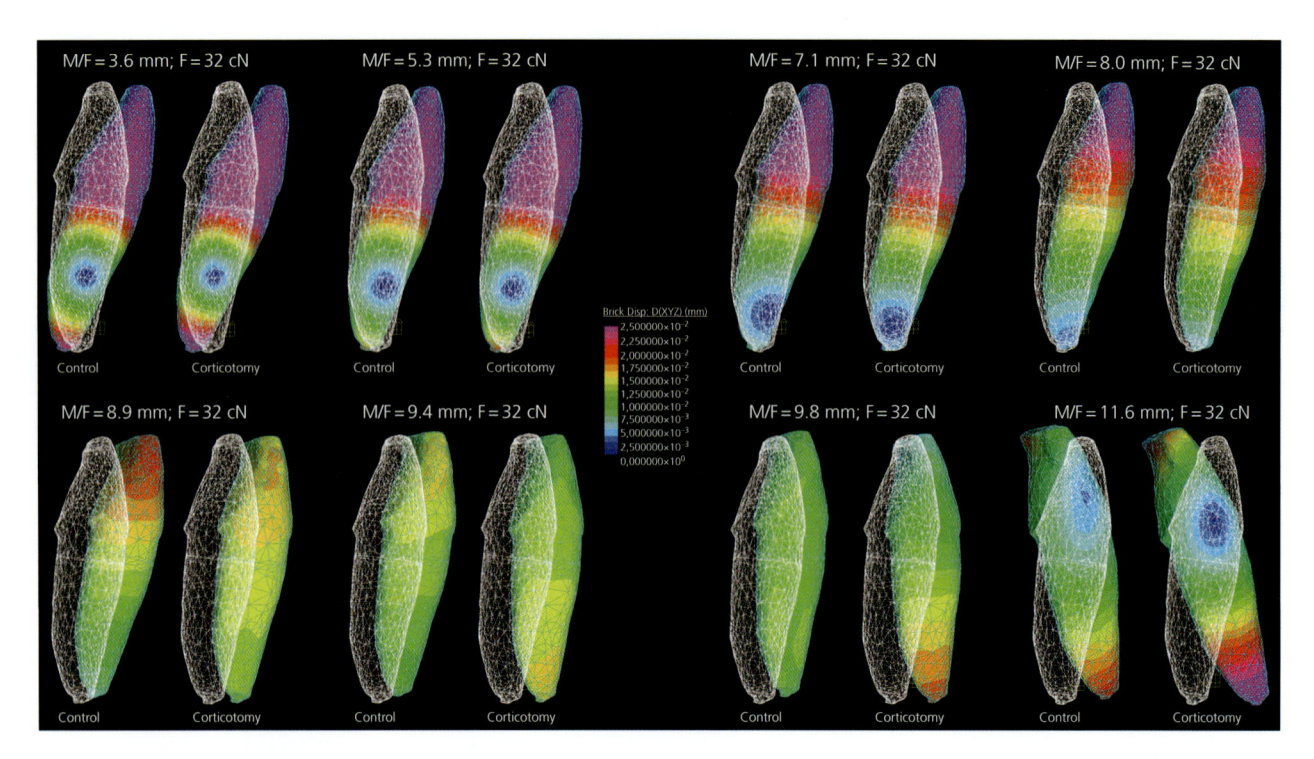

Figure 16.5 The pattern of movement for a lateral incisor under various moment to force (M/F) ratios following the application of a force (F) at the crown of 32 cN (F = 32 cN). Note how the centre of rotation (blue spot) first moves apically with an increasing M/F ratio. Around a M/F of 9 mm, pure translation occurs; for the control case this occurs at 8.9 mm; for the corticotomy case at 9.4 mm. (Source: Dr. C. Verna.)

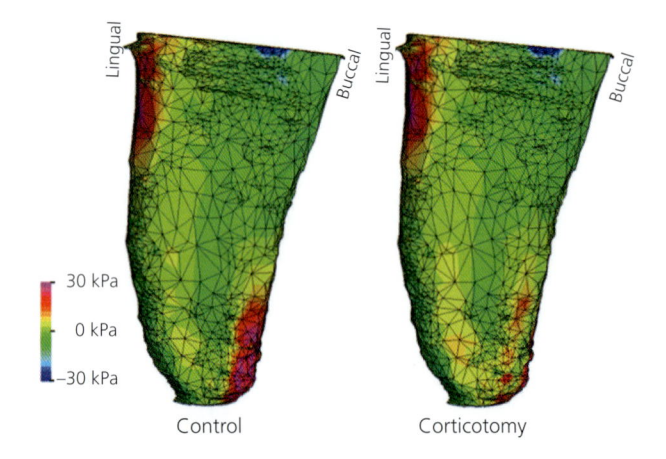

Figure 16.6 The buccolingual stresses in the PDL of the lateral incisor in the case of an uncontrolled tipping (M/F = 0) for both the control and corticotomized models. Note that the control PDL demonstrates tensile stresses both at the lingual cervical area and the buccal apical area, while for the corticotomized PDL the stresses in the lingual cervical area are increased but in the buccal apical area they are reduced. The control PDL also features higher compressive stresses along its buccal cervical edge than the corticotomized PDL.

(Figures 16.5 and 16.6).The outcome of this study was in general confirmed by the results from the study by Ouejiaraphant et al. (2018) although they raised the question as to whether the shift in M/F ratio would actually be clinically detectable.

In a follow-up study, the model was extended to the neighboring central incisor (also subject to the corticotomy) and with the variation of applying a corticotomy to the lingual alveolar wall (Vidovic et al., 2017). Here, it was found that the presence of a corticotomy of the alveolar wall of one tooth did not have a noticeable effect on the OTM of the non-corticotomized neighboring tooth, at least not mechanically. In reality, the biological markers induced by the RAP will obviously not only be limited to the corticotomy site and will diffuse throughout the surrounding tissues, thus a decreased bone density could be expected. Furthermore, a difference was seen according to whether the corticotomy was applied to the buccal or lingual side of the alveolar wall. Depending on the direction of movement, the largest deviation in the M/F ratio was for pure translation, compared with the non-corticotomized control case, and occurred when the corticotomy had been performed on the side facing the direction of translation. So, a buccal corticotomy at the alveolar wall of a tooth translating lingually would require almost the same M/F ratio as the non-corticotomized case, and to obtain a buccal translation a higher M/F ratio would need to be applied. This can be achieved using a slightly longer power arm (0.5–1 mm) at the bracket or using a bracket with a larger pre-angulation. Moreover, the presence of reduced bone support becomes more relevant as the forces applied increase in magnitude.

The influence of the shape and extent of the corticotomy on the orthodontic load transfer was studied by Pacheco et al. (2016). They looked specifically at the stress distribution in the PDL with (a) no corticotomy, (b) a box-shaped corticotomy and perforations in the cortical bone of the canine (CVC), and (c) CVC and a circular-shaped corticotomy in the cortical bone of the edentulous space of the first premolar. Interestingly, they did not find any noticeable differences in the stress distributions between the three analysed cases. However, in this study the authors used a linear, elastic, and symmetric formulation for the material properties of the PDL, which certainly influenced the results of their FE simulation, as clearly demonstrated in previous publications (Cattaneo et al., 2005; McCormack et al., 2017). In the authors' study, however, the maximal tensile stresses in the PDL were about 20% higher compared with the non-corticotomized case, while the maximal compressive stresses remained largely unaffected (Verna et al., 2018).

Historical background

Previously, cortical bone was considered the major barrier in resisting OTM. The assumption was made that by simply removing or simply cutting it (corticotomy), a more efficient acceleration of the OTM would occur along with the benefits of a reduced risk of side effects such as root resorption, loss of vitality, and periodontal damage. This has subsequently led to several surgical protocols prior or during the orthodontic therapy being introduced as adjunctive therapy.

The evolution of alveolar decortication may be split in two distinct phases:

1. The pre-RAP phase follows the idea that vertical interdental and horizontal sub-apical surgical cuts create independent blocks of bone and teeth which can be rapidly moved in the first 3–4 months following the surgery before the blocks fuse (bone healing). Suya modified the surgery described by Kole by eliminating the luxation of the blocks and changing the horizontal cut to a corticotomy rather than an osteotomy (Kole, 1959; Suya, 1991).
2. The post-RAP phase is described in a case report by Wilcko et al. who found that surgical insult increases bone metabolism with a transient and local reduction of bone density (osteopenia) followed by healing, similar to the postfracture cascade of events described by Frost and defined as the regional acceleratory mechanism or simply RAP reaction (Frost, 1983). In this key case report, two adult patients received a selective corticotomy and additionally alloplastic resorbable grafts to increase the bone levels and avoid the risk of recessions. Following full thickness labial and lingual flaps, vertical interproximal cuts and numerous holes on the cortical bone were made using surgical rotating burs to promote significant bleeding. An accurate evaluation with CT scans before and after treatment, and in one case histological sections allowed the authors to formulate a new hypothesis about what really happens at the bone level after corticotomy (Wilcko et al., 2001).

We are now moving from a purely mechanical to a more biological and physiological concept of alveolar corticotomy.

The original surgical protocols were both invasive and extensive, requiring full mucoperiosteal flaps and significant amounts of grafting. The increased risks of complications such as pain, swelling, periodontal problems, and damage to the teeth plus the increased cost may reduce acceptance by the patient and exclude these procedures from routine practice. Thus, different surgical procedures to minimize the invasiveness while trying to maintain clinical efficacy have been proposed.

Wilcko et al. patented their surgical protocol as periodontally accelerated osteogenic orthodontics (PAOO) or Wilckodontics and claimed as the benefits:

1. Accelerated tooth movement with reduction of the total treatment time.
2. Osteogenic modification with relocation of the bony matrix resulting in an improvement of hard and soft tissue support for the treated orthodontically teeth.
3. Better short- and long-term stability of the orthodontic treatment (Wilcko et al., 2008).

A large number of studies have been undertaken to validate these effects but, despite the lack of strong scientific evidence to support the benefits, many clinicians still consider alveolar corticotomy an aid to accelerate OTM and reduce treatment time: these beneficial effects are very attractive for patients, especially adults, making this surgery more acceptable. We strongly believe, even though there is a low level of evidence to date, that alveolar corticotomy should be reconsidered as part of the armamentarium for the orthodontic speciality.

A different perspective: six rules for effective alveolar corticotomy

Based on available research and clinical findings, and after more than 15 years of clinical experience, we have found six basic rules to be followed for effective and safe alveolar corticotomy, enabling positive effects to be delivered for orthodontic treatment which justify its use in this field (Spena, 2018). The six rules are:

1. Alveolar corticotomy is to facilitate OTM.
2. Alveolar corticotomy has a limited effect in time.
3. Alveolar corticotomy has limited effects in space.
4. Alveolar corticotomy needs a proper surgical protocol.
5. Alveolar corticotomy needs correct orthodontic management postsurgery.
6. Alveolar corticotomy needs a proper selection of patients.
A detailed description of these rules follows.

1. Alveolar corticotomy is to facilitate OTM

When evaluating the rate of tooth movement, we must recognize that there is a great variability in our patients. Studies have shown that speed of OTM is influenced by bone turnover and the individual's response to mechanical forces, but is not related to the level of the forces (Pilon et al., 1996; Verna et al., 2000; Von Bohl et al., 2004). Shorter treatment time is one the major objectives for both clinicians and patients. Numerous case reports have been published showing how corticotomy may reduce treatment time. Case reports, however, provide limited scientific evidence. Systematic reviews and meta-analysis have shown that alveolar corticotomy can reduce treatment time, saving a few months of treatment, but with a very low level of evidence (Abdallah and Flores-Mir, 2014; Dab et al., 2019; Mheissen et al., 2020; Shahabee et al., 2020). This is because the ideal randomized controlled trial in which similar malocclusions are treated, with or without corticotomy, using the same appliance, and reaching the same quality of treatment result, is difficult to be realized and has not been performed yet.

As mentioned above, alveolar corticotomy accelerates OTM but for a very short period of time. The rate of tooth movement returns to a normal pace once the RAP reaction is over. Dibart and Murphy claimed that, by maintaining a constant mechanical stimulation with constantly activated appliances, the transient osteopenia and the period during which teeth can be moved rapidly may be almost indefinitely prolonged (Murphy et al., 2009; Dibart et al., 2014). In their meta-analysis, Shahabee and coworkers concluded that the difference in the rate of canine retraction after performing the MOP was statistically significant but clinically not really relevant, with a 0.45 mm increase in a month (Shahabee et al., 2020).

Keser and Dibart (2013) proposed repeating the surgical intervention during the 8-month treatment of a patient with Class III malocclusion with two alveolar corticotomies. However, the approach was limited to one case, and therefore cannot be used to justify this method as a standardized protocol (Keser and Dibart, 2013). Sanjideh et al. in a split-mouth research on foxhounds where premolar spaces were closed after corticotomy on only one side, found that maxillary tooth movement peaked between 22 and 25 days. At the peak, the rate of tooth movement on the experimental side was 85% faster and the total tooth movement was twice that of the control side. Over time the rates became progressively similar on both sides. In the mandible, where a second corticotomy was performed on one side after 28 days, the higher rate of tooth movement was prolonged but resulted in only a slightly increased total tooth movement (Sanjideh et al., 2010). Therefore, a second surgery to prolong acceleration of OTM may be not justifiable considering the limited effects, added expense, time, and risks.

Reduction of treatment time should not be made at the expense of a good quality end result: quality is always more important than speed. So, why use a corticotomy?

Corticotomy should be considered as facilitating OTM in order to reduce anchorage challenges, not as an accelerating tool. Animal studies have shown that the surgical insult, which increases the activation rate of the BMUs, creates a transient reduced regional bone density (osteopenia) and reduces indirect resorption and hyalinization (Yaffe *et al.*, 1994; Iino *et al.*, 2007; Lee *et al.*, 2008; Sebaoun *et al.*, 2008; Mostafa *et al.*, 2009; Wang *et al.*, 2009; Teixeira *et al.*, 2010; Baloul *et al.*, 2011). Consequently, the limitations and variability of the patient's response to orthodontic treatment are overcome. The decorticated tooth is less resistant to orthodontic forces, easier to move, and therefore will require less anchorage.

When decortication is not extended to an entire arch or quadrant but limited to the active unit (teeth to move), the reactive unit (anchor teeth) can be managed, with the RAP reaction contributing to optimize the biomechanics of complex OTM. This effect may be enhanced by the use of temporary anchorage devices (TADs): the alveolar corticotomy reduces tooth resistance to orthodontic forces while the TADs enhance the anchorage.

Spena *et al.*, in two studies on a total of 12 adult patients with Class II malocclusions treated with distalization of the upper molars, showed how upper molars could be bodily distalized using simple buccal mechanics and no anterior anchorage. A corticotomy was only performed on the teeth to be moved (segmental corticotomy) thus reducing their resistance to distalizing forces and consequently the demands on anchorage (Figure 16.7) (Spena *et al.*, 2007; Spena and Garganese, 2015).

Canine and incisor retraction in extraction cases (Germec *et al.*, 2006; Lee *et al.*, 2007; Aboul-Ela *et al.*, 2011), molar and premolar intrusion to treat vertical problems (Moon *et al.*, 2007; Oliveira *et al.*, 2008; Akay *et al.*, 2009), impacted canines (Fischer, 2007), and decompensation of incisors in surgical Class III malocclusions (Ahn *et al.*, 2012), represent just a few clinical examples where segmental alveolar corticotomy, alone or in combination with TADs, have been found to be useful.

Alveolar corticotomy can be considered as a procedure that allows treatment alternatives in the case of high risk tooth movement, such as thin alveolar bone and gingival biotype, or when movements like expansion, labial proclination, or anteroposterior movements within reduced bone volumes are necessary. In such cases alveolar corticotomy is complemented with extensive grafting to increase the volume of bone, reduce/eliminate fenestrations and dehiscences, create additional support for the roots, and improve final esthetics and stability (Wang *et al.*, 2020).

In conclusion, alveolar corticotomy should be considered as a way of enhancing orthodontic movement to reduce the complexity of an orthodontic treatment, allowing an alternative option to traditional orthodontics and improve the final result. A faster treatment may be considered a secondary unpredictable "bonus" which is only relevant for "simple" orthodontic cases that anyway require a short treatment time to be resolved.

2. Alveolar corticotomy has a limited effect in time

The modeling and remodeling of the alveolar bone following the application of an orthodontic load is the response of bone to a mechanical disturbance. Once the mechanical equilibrium has been reached and no further loading is applied, tooth movement ceases. The same is true following a corticotomy, where the surgical intervention undermines the metabolic balance and bone healing needs to occur. The increased activation of the BMUs that peaks at 1–2 months, ceases after 4–6 months, which in humans is the normal duration of a remodeling cycle (Eriksen, 2010). The accelerated/facilitated movement lasts as long as there is this reaction.

The timing of surgery is critical: an alveolar corticotomy should be planned and performed when the RAP reaction is clinically and biomechanically needed. The precise management of the orthodontic movements following surgery is also fundamental to success (see in Rule 5). The benefits from a corticotomy when performed during another surgery (i.e., exposure of impacted teeth) (Fischer, 2007) or orthognathic surgery (Hernandez-Alfaro and Guijarro-Martinez, 2012) should be considered. In these situations there is no additional cost or risk for the patient and the procedure may aid orthodontic therapy.

3. Alveolar corticotomy has limited effects in space

Alveolar corticotomy cannot be standardized but should be planned by both the orthodontist and the surgeon based upon an individual

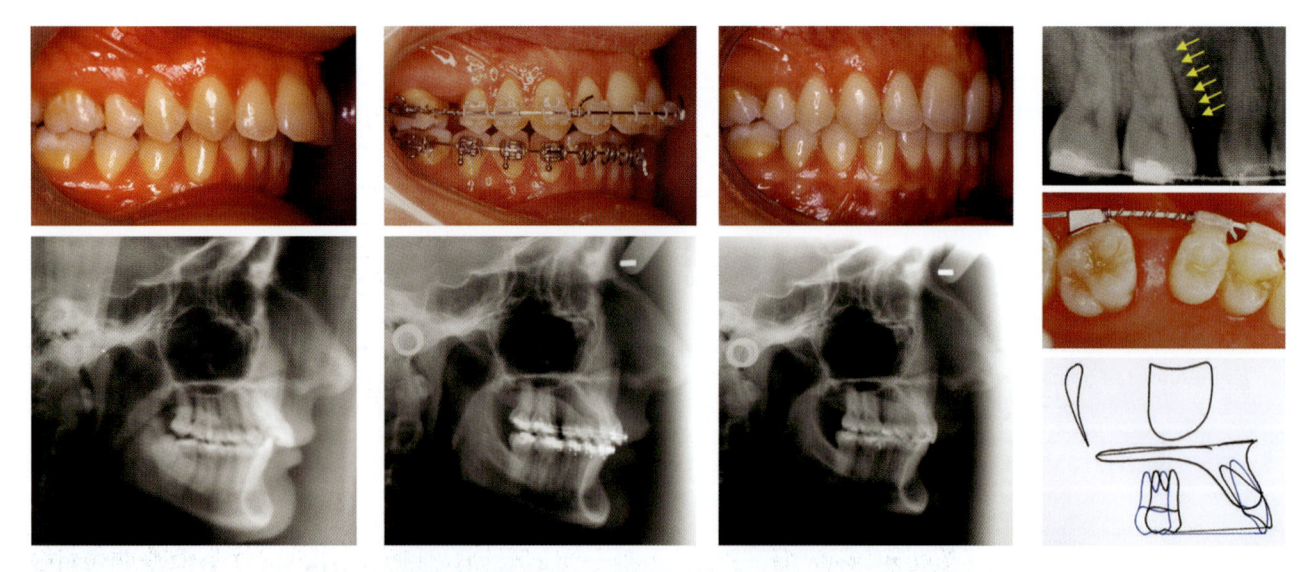

Figure 16.7 Adult patients with a Class II malocclusion treated with corticotomy. Note how the anterior anchorage was maintained while the molars were bodily distalized, with new bone formation evident. (Source: Dr. Raffaele Spena.)

patient's needs such as the initial periodontal status and biomechanical and biological considerations because the type of surgery may influence the resulting OTM.

The effects of decortication are localized to the area immediately adjacent to the site of injury (Sebaoun et al., 2008; McBride et al., 2014). In adult rats, perforation of the buccal and lingual cortical plates caused a large increase in osteoclast numbers and bone apposition rate around the surface of the PDL of the roots of the teeth along with a decrease of calcified spongiosa in the region of the surgical insult. This finding is of utmost importance.

If the surgical insult is limited to a specific area of the alveolar bone (i.e., middle coronal third and buccal surface only) (Figure 16.8), the RAP reaction most likely will not extend to the entire root area. The modifications at bone level (osteopenia) will be limited to the area of the decortication, and the apical and lingual sides will not be affected as desired.

There is a directly proportional relationship between the intensity of the injury and the amount of RAP reaction (McBride et al., 2014). In a study on foxhound dogs, increasing the surgical insult resulted in less dense and mature bone but had no effect on bone volume at 9 weeks after surgery. In a study on rats, it has been found that increasing the surgical insult speeds up the rate of OTM and causes a decrease in both bone volume and tissue density (Chang et al., 2019).

Both biomechanical and clinical needs determine the type of procedure with both open flap and flapless surgery (see Rule 4). As a general rule, if enhanced bodily movement or a better control of the apical area are the biomechanical requirements for the OTM (i.e., intrusion/extrusion and distalization/mesialization), then decortication should be extended over the entire alveolar bone surrounding the roots of the tooth, buccal, and lingual (Figure 16.9). If a bodily movement is not desired or if anatomical limitations of the surgical site prevent an extended decortication, the surgical intervention may be limited to the direction of the OTM (Figure 16.10).

4. Alveolar corticotomy needs a proper surgical protocol

Several surgical procedures have been proposed for the decortication of alveolar bone and vary in the level of invasiveness and cost. Hard and soft tissue grafting may or may not be required. The types of surgery can be divided into two groups: open flap and flapless surgery (Table 16.1). Each one of them follow well described protocols, indications (Table 16.2) and contraindications, advantages and disadvantages.

The open flap corticotomy and grafting

The first corticotomies were performed by raising a flap. Open flap surgery is still the preferred choice when an extended or critical area of decortication has to be managed, when a large area of grafting is planned, or when the corticotomy is simply part of another open flap surgery. A description of the surgical protocols and the hard and soft tissue grafting follows.

The *open flap corticotomy procedure* is indicated and routinely used during orthognathic surgery and particularly in primary surgical procedures, exposure of impacted teeth, expansion for the correction of transverse maxillary deficiencies, anterior expansion in Class II and Class III malocclusions, and complex OTM in periodontally involved cases (Table 16.2). The two primary goals of the surgery are to provide: (i) optimal access to the area of decortication and (ii) effective placement and coverage of the graft material. On the buccal side, the flap is designed according to the periodontal characteristics of the site, and it may or may not include the interdental papillae. A full-thickness flap is raised from the coronal side to 2–3 mm beyond the apical area (area that will be decorticated) and a split-thickness flap in the remaining area to allow mobility and sufficient blood supply to the flap. Following surgery, a tension-free flap closure with Gore-Tex non-resorbable sutures must be achieved to provide optimal coverage of the decorticated area and the grafted material. Sutures remain for at least 14–21 days.

Decortication of the alveolar bone may be performed with surgical burs or with piezo blades/microsaws. Piezosurgery has recently become more widely used in periodontal and maxillofacial surgery because of its advantages (Vercellotti et al., 2005; Gulnahar et al., 2013; Thind et al., 2018). The calibrated blades cut the bone with low-frequency ultrasonic waves and allow very precise micrometric cuts, reducing the risk of damaging the soft tissues or cutting vessels and nerves. The cavitation effect created by the oscillating tip along with ample irrigation help avoid the creation of heated and necrotic areas resulting in less oxidative stress and inflammation at cellular level. Studies on animal models (Preti et al., 2007; Gulnahar et al., 2013) have shown that alveolar osteotomies with piezo blades

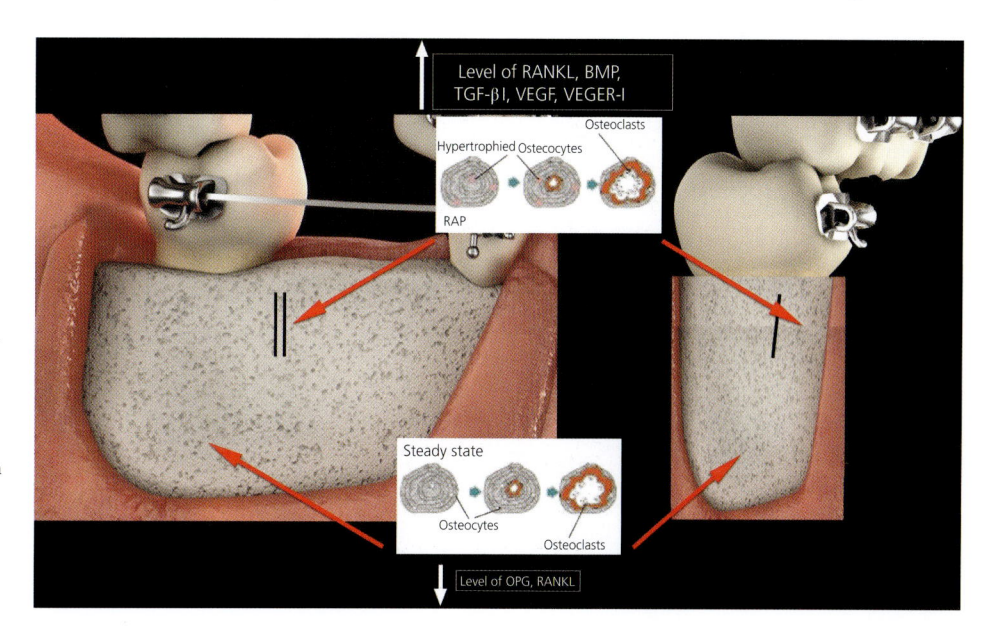

Figure 16.8 Limiting the area of surgical insult reduces the extension of the regional accelleratory phenomenon (RAP) reaction around the teeth to be moved. BMP, bone morphogenetic protein; OPG, osteoprotegerin; RANKL, receptor activator of nuclear factor kappa B ligand; TGF-b1, transforming growth factor-beta1; VEGF, vascular endothelial growth factor; VEGFR-1 vascular endothelial growth factor receptor-1. (Source: Dr. Raffaele Spena.)

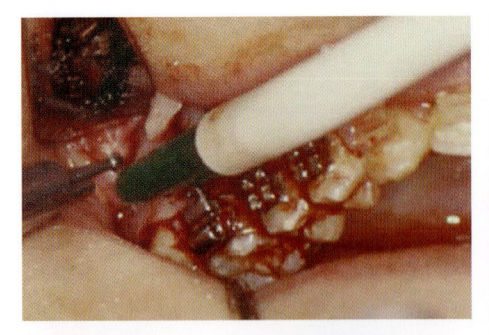

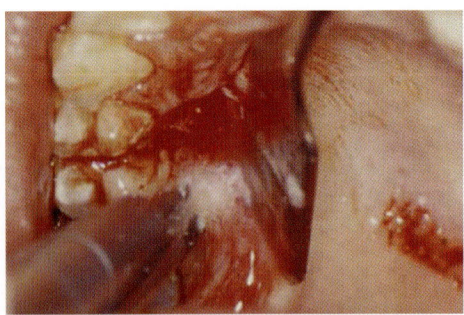

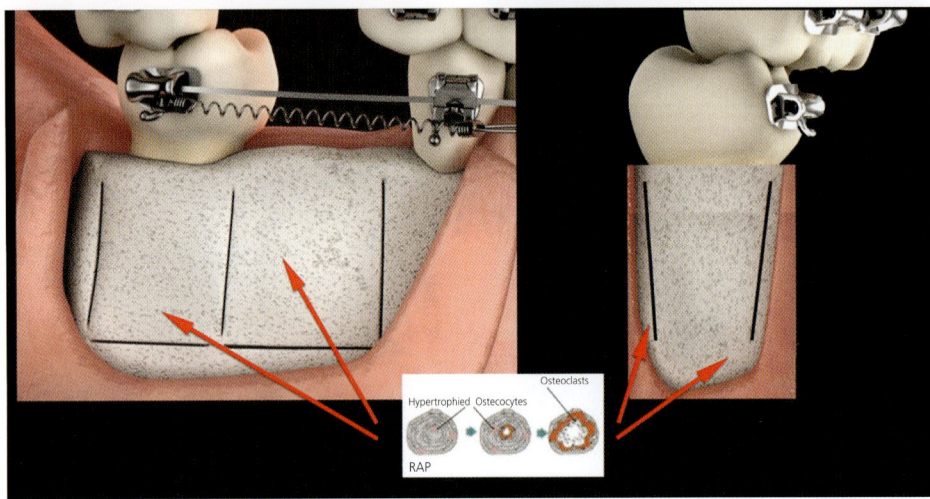

Figure 16.9 Extending the area of surgical insult helps produce a regional acceleratory phenomenon (RAP) reaction in the entire alveolus around the teeth to be moved and in the alveolar bone where movement is directed. (Source: Dr. Raffaele Spena.)

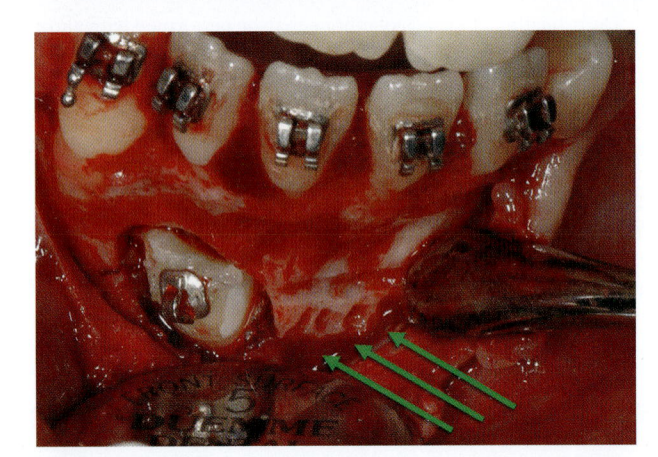

Figure 16.10 Alveolar corticotomy in the direction of the movement on a transmigrated lower canine. (Source: Dr. Raffaele Spena.)

Table 16.1 Different types of corticotomy

Open flap	Flapless
• Periodontally Accelerated Osteogenic Orthodontics (PAOO; Wilckodontics) • Segmental corticotomy • Any surgery requiring a flap with associated corticotomy	• Cortocision • Discision • Piezocision • Micro-Osteo-Perforations (MOP)

Table 16.2 Indications for open flap technique and MOPs

Open Flap ± Grafting	Micro-Osteo-Perforations
• Impacted teeth (without grafting) • Orthognathic surgery • Molar movement (grafting if atrophic bone) • Complex space closures • Expansion	• Cases without periodontal problems • Economical limitations • Complex treatments with aligners • RPE in adults • Complex movements (in adults)

stimulate more active osteogenesis and ingrowth of vital bone-forming tissue when compared with rotating burs. An evaluation of a large number of patients has shown that significantly less fenestrations and dehiscences were present after piezoelectric decortication (Kim et al., 2011). Finally, piezosurgery is less traumatic and better accepted by the patient.

Decortication (interproximal vertical cuts from 2 mm below the alveolar crest to 1–2 mm beyond the root apices connected with horizontal cuts in the supra-apical area) is used only on the teeth that need enhanced movement (Figure 16.11). The depth of the cuts is approximately 2–3 mm, extending slightly into the medullary bone. Light scraping of the cortex in between the cuts (instead of the numerous holes previously made when using burs) stimulates a pronounced RAP reaction and creates a bleeding bed that will eventually host the graft (Figure 16.12).

Grafting may be combined with alveolar corticotomy. It is usually planned before surgery based on initial clinical and radiological evaluation, desired OTM and short- and long-term periodontal considerations (Figure 16.13). Grafting may include hard tissue, soft tissue, and autologous growth factors (Marx et al., 1998; Gapski et al., 2005; Nowzari et al., 2008). The quality and quantity may be determined at the time of surgery depending on the clinical conditions of the surgical site and the subsequent OTM.

Bone for grafting can have different origins (Table 16.3). As a general rule, a mixture of different bone materials is preferred

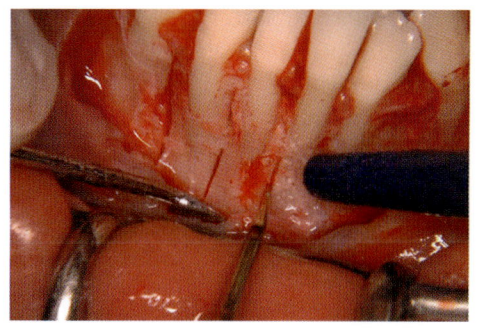

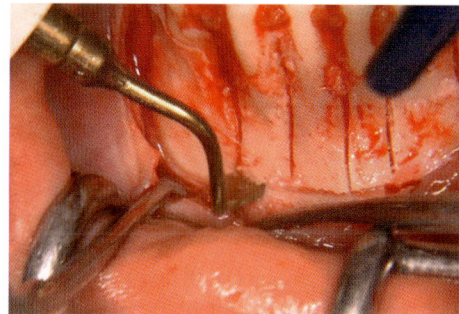

Figure 16.11 Interdental vertical corticotomies (left) and sub-apical horizontal corticotomies (right). (Source: Dr. Raffaele Spena.)

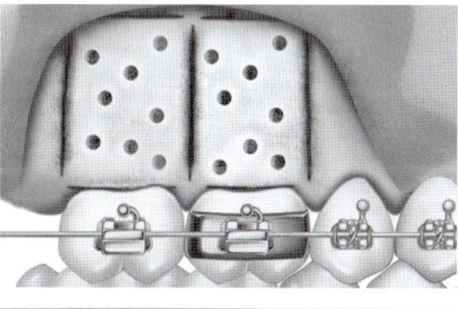

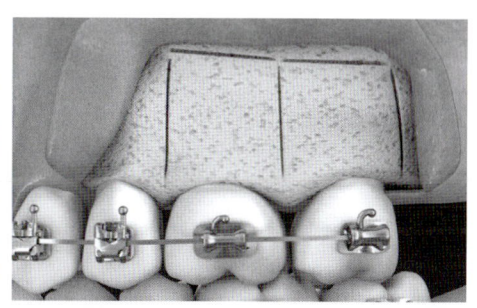

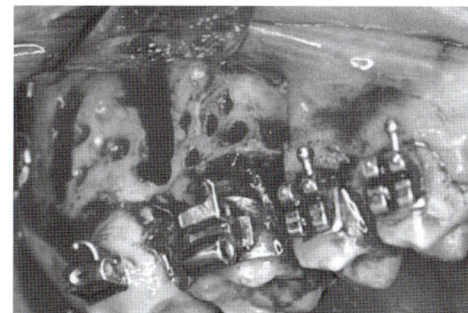

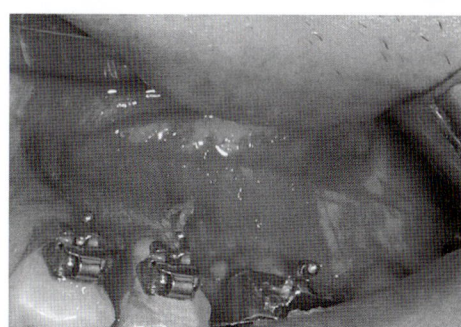

Figure 16.12 Alveolar corticotomy: rotating burs versus piezosurgery. (Source: Dr. Raffaele Spena.)

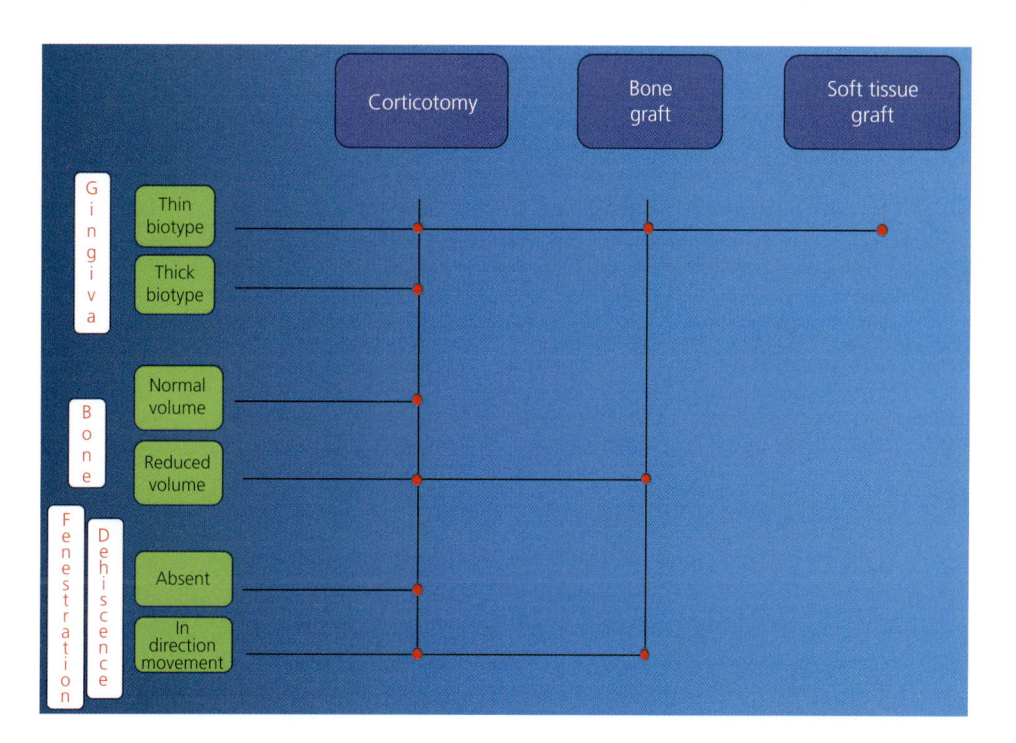

Figure 16.13 Flow chart depicting selection criteria for the choice of bone or soft tissue graft in combination with corticotomy.

(Figure 16.14). When performing a corticotomy, with composite grafting, the minimal portion of autologous bone collected from the cuts and the scraping is combined with allogenic bone (in chips that are freeze-dried to reduce antigenicity and demineralized to expose the underlying collagen and its growth factors, such as BMP) with osteoinductive properties and to xenogenic bone (in chips, providing a physical matrix or scaffold suitable for deposition of new bone and preventing its rapid resorption) with osteoconductive properties.

Soft tissue grafts are placed over the bone graft when a thin biotype or gingival recessions are present. An autologous connective tissue graft is the gold standard when the area to regenerate is small. When combined with coronally advanced flaps, it is the most effective procedure to treat a single tooth recession (Cairo et al., 2014).

Allogenic, human, acellular dermal matrices, available in different sizes and thicknesses, may be used with similar results and avoid the necessity for a second surgical site when large areas need to be managed (Figure 16.15) (Tatakis et al., 2015; Tonetti et al., 2018).

Both bone and soft tissue grafts may be coupled with autologous growth factors. The number of stem cells, crucial for the healing process, rapidly decreases with age. Studies have shown that growth factors from platelet-concentrated plasma (platelet-derived growth factor, vascular endothelial growth factor, transforming growth factor $TGF-\beta_1$ and $TGF-\beta_2$) may rapidly increase the number of the available stem cells, stimulate their activity, as well as reduce post-surgical inflammation, swelling, and pain (Marx et al., 1998). The platelet-rich fibrin (PRF) developed by Chokroun et al. (2006) and the platelet-rich growth factors (PRGF) proposed by Anituaare et al. (2001) are two different protocols where blood centrifugation allows separation of the plasma platelets from the white and red cells. PRF contains platelets and fractions of leukocytes and allows, with a light compression of the centrifuged fraction, production of membranes that are usually placed above the layer of the bone grafts (Figure 16.16). PRGF produces three fractions with different concentrations of platelets: some of them may be mixed with the bone graft increasing its viscosity and adherence to the surgical site thus making the application of both the bone graft and allogenic dermal graft easier, while other fractions may be used to produce clots/membranes of fibrin that are placed on the bone graft (Figures 16.17 and 16.18).

At the end of the surgery, when a graft is applied to the alveolar corticotomy, a tension-free flap closure must be achieved to provide optimal coverage of the decorticated and grafted area and to enhance final soft-tissue healing. Nonresorbable Gore-Tex sutures are left *in situ* for at least 14–21 days.

Table 16.3 Different types of bone grafts

Autograft	Allograft	Xenograft
from the same patient in blocks or chips	from human cadavers in blocks or chips	from animals in blocks or chips
Properties		
Osteogenic		
Osteo-inductive	Not osteo-inductive	Not osteo-inductive
Osteoconductive	Osteoconductive	Osteoconductive
No antigenicity		
Histocompatibility		
Resorption	Resorption	No resorption
Remodeling	Remodeling	No remodeling
Disadvantages		
Second surgical site	Possible antigenicity	Possible antigenicity
Limited quantities	Possible risk of infection (rare)	Possible risk of infection (rare)

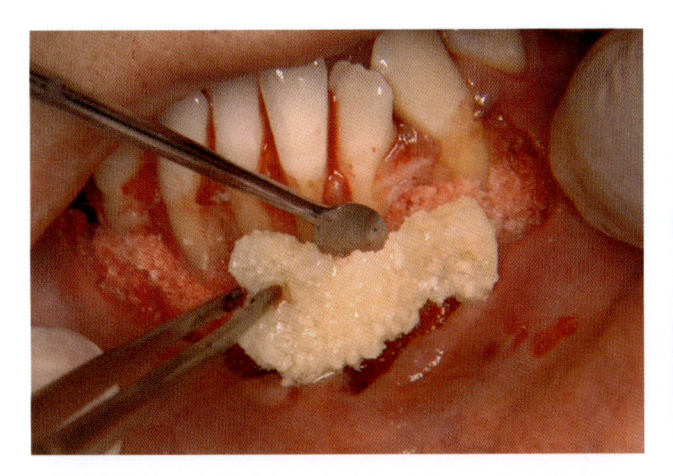

Figure 16.14 A mix of bone grafting with PRGF. (Source: Dr. Raffaele Spena.)

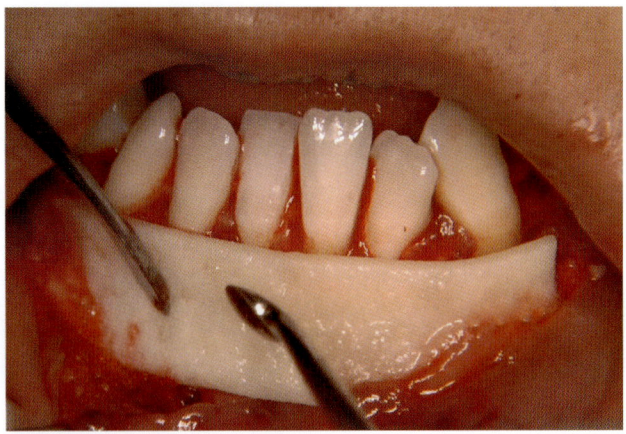

Figure 16.15 An allogenic membrane used to graft a large area of decortication. (Source: Dr. Raffaele Spena.)

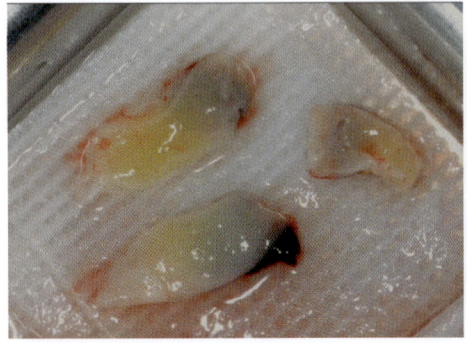

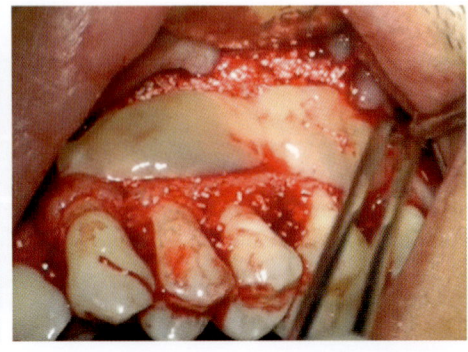

Figure 16.16 Membranes of PRF. (Source: Dr. Raffaele Spena.)

The flapless corticotomy

Flapless corticotomies are surgeries that allow bone intervention via the alveolar mucosae without the need for raising a flap. Several alternative surgeries have been proposed to reduce the invasiveness of the open flap decortication, the potential periodontal damage, and postoperative discomfort: corticision with a reinforced scalpel and mallet (Kim *et al.*, 2009), corticision with piezosaws, piezocision (Dibart *et al.*, 2009), piezopuncture (Kim *et al.*, 2013), and discision (Yavuz *et al.*, 2018). Although attractive, they have shown both surgical and biomechanical limitations (Abbas *et al.*, 2016). The surgical limitations include a risk of root damage (Patterson *et al.*, 2017) in crowded arches, limited visibility when cutting, restriction of the cuts in the interproximal areas and the middle third of the roots, need for an optimal extension of the attached gingiva in the area of decortication and difficulty controlling the graft placement in the apico-coronal direction. In addition, some procedures are difficult for the patient to handle who may experience dizziness and vertigo.

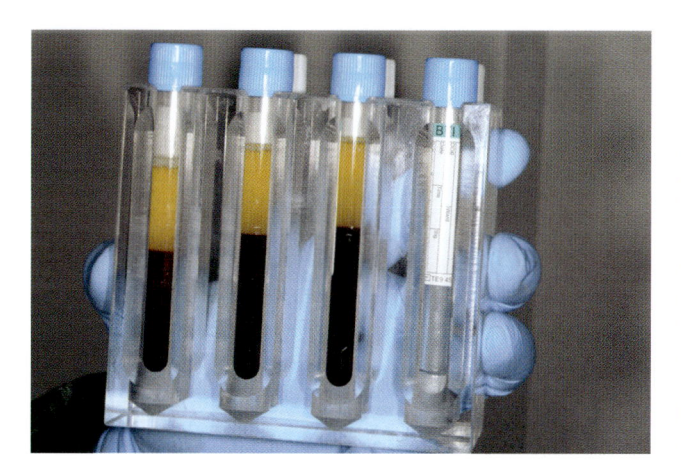

Figure 16.17 Centrifugated blood with the PRGF protocol. (Source: Dr. Raffaele Spena.)

The biomechanical drawbacks are related to the fact that the cuts are usually restricted to the buccal side and middle third of the roots. Although it has been claimed that flapless surgeries can produce modifications of the OTM similar to the open flap corticotomies, restricting the surgical insult to small portions of the alveolar bone (see Rule 3) may produce only small areas of RAP reaction which limits the resulting benefits to the OTM (Abbas *et al.*, 2016).

Most flapless corticotomies are certainly not minimally invasive surgeries as claimed by the authors and are quite expensive for the patient since only an expert periodontist/oral surgeon can perform them and they often need complex planning with 3D digitally fabricated surgical guides (Figure 16.19) (Cassetta *et al.*, 2016).

The MOPs described by Alikhani *et al.* (2013) and Teixeira *et al.* (2010) seem to be the least invasive way of producing insult to the cortical alveolar bone and still positively influence OTM (Teixeira *et al.*, 2010; Alikhani *et al.*, 2013; Cheung *et al.*, 2016). MOPs are numerous punctures made in both the distal and mesial interproximal areas which extend into the cortex for 1–2 mm in depth. Since the effect of a corticotomy does not extend in space it is advisable to introduce as many MOPs as possible in each interproximal area of the teeth from the apical to the coronal thirds and both buccally and lingually (Figure 16.20) to be sure that the metabolic changes extend around the entire radicular alveolar bone of the tooth to be moved. A detailed discussion on this procedure is provided in the Chapter 17 by the inventors of the technique (Drs. Alikhani and Teixeira).

In most patients, instead of traditional local anesthesia with needles, a strong anesthetic gel placed on the mucosa for 3 minutes is sufficient to control the patient's pain and discomfort during the procedure. The MOPs may be made by one of two techniques: with manual instruments (Ex-cellerator by Propel) (Figure 16.20) or with dedicated burs on a reduced speed-torque control electric handpiece. In most cases the second option is preferable. If close to critical areas, simple surgical guides may help to reduce the risks and complications. The procedure and the precautions to be aware of are similar to the insertion of miniscrews. The tip of the bur

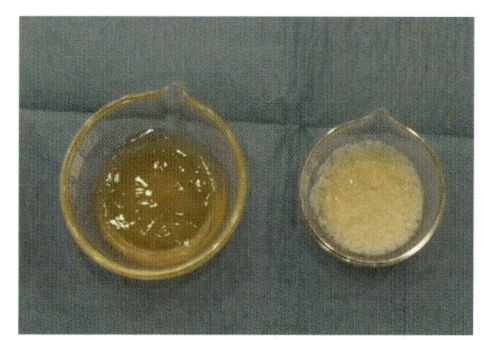

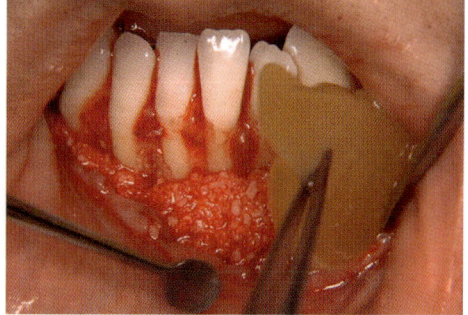

Figure 16.18 Membranes of PRGF. (Source: Dr. Raffaele Spena.)

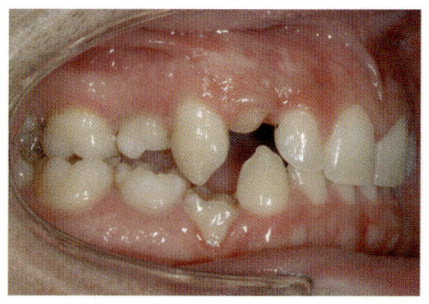

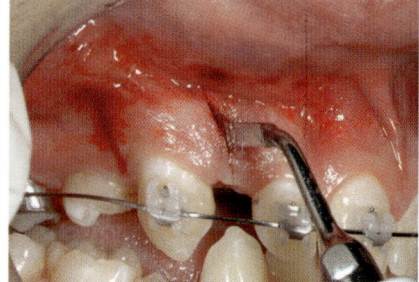

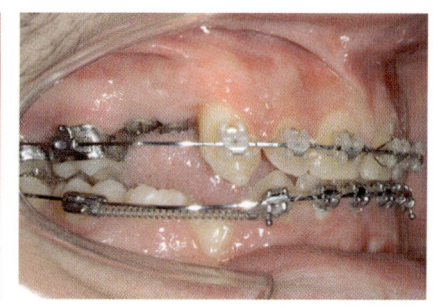

Figure 16.19 Piezocision performed on an upper canine to be mesialized. Note the mesial inclination of the canine at the end of the movement. (Source: Dr. Raffaele Spena.)

should be inserted and removed perpendicular to the bone surface keeping away from dental roots. Manual MOPs are usually made in the frontal areas whereas drilled MOPs are usually made in the posterior and lingual areas (Figure 16.21). Orthodontists can easily perform MOPs at the chairside; they can even be repeated during treatment if additional bone stimulation is needed, and the cost is affordable for the patient. No surgical packing or sutures are necessary after MOPs. Additional grafting is not an option, and this limits MOPs to patients with no periodontal pathology and good gingival biotypes.

This low cost, and clinician-friendly procedure with good acceptance by the patient has been extensively used in clinical practice. The possible clinical indications are listed in Table 16.2.

5. Alveolar corticotomy needs correct orthodontic management postsurgery

Alveolar corticotomy can complement orthodontic treatment carried out with any fixed or removable appliances. The use of 3D software may help to carefully design the positioning/manufacturing of the appliance, the biomechanics, and the delivery of the exact desired OTM.

As already mentioned, the timing of the surgical decortication must be carefully planned to profit from the RAP-induced enhanced tooth movement at the desired time point.

When using fixed appliances, the management and wire changes are similar to any orthodontic case. The timing of bonding and the application of the forces changes according to the specific requirements of the case.

When expanding (see the Cases 1, 2, and 7), corticotomy is usually combined with extensive grafting. One week after surgery the appliance is bonded and the initial archwires are inserted. Three weeks after surgery (2 weeks after the initial loadings), usually the tension of the flap is reduced, and the sutures may be removed. The appointments for appliance activations are planned every 2 weeks instead of the usual 6–8 week interval until tooth movement is clearly enhanced.

When distalizing or mesializing molars or repositioning impacted teeth, the alveolar corticotomy is performed when the movement can be started: according to different situations it may occur at the beginning of the treatment (see Cases 4 and 6) or after levelling and insertion of a stiff working wire (see Case 3 and 5).

When a corticotomy is associated with aligner treatment, the frequency of appliance changes after the surgery should reduce to every 3–4 days.

As mentioned, the advantages offered by facilitated tooth movement through alveolar corticotomy may be reinforced using temporary skeletal anchorage devices. This combination ensures the achievement of a high biomechanical effectiveness.

6. Alveolar corticotomy needs a proper selection of patients

Alveolar corticotomy is not indicated in every case. In Table 16.2, possible indications for both open flap and flapless corticotomies have been listed.

Clinical examples

In the following examples, cases treated with both procedures are described. The cases are categorized into four groups. The first two cases are a Class I open bite malocclusion and a Class III skeletal malocclusion. They have in common an open flap corticotomy with extensive grafting on the lower six anterior teeth. The third and the fourth cases present a lower canine transmigration and an upper transposition between a canine and the lateral incisor. Cases 5 and 6 present lower second permanent molars mesialized into the space of the extracted first permanent molars. The last two cases are adult patients with asymmetric malocclusions that needed expansion of the upper arch.

Patient 1 (Figure 16.22)

The first patient is a 20-year-old female with two previous unsuccessful treatments and a Class I open bite malocclusion. The initial lateral cephalograms shows a skeletal Class II and hyperdivergent facial pattern. The initial panoramic radiograph reveals periodontal bone loss present on all the upper posterior teeth, preventing any possible intrusion therapy. The patient refused the ideal treatment of preference (orthognathic surgery) and accepted being treated with an open flap corticotomy with extensive grafting in the lower anterior region, stripping, and coordination of the arches. At the end of treatment optimal dental and occlusal relationships are achieved, with significant

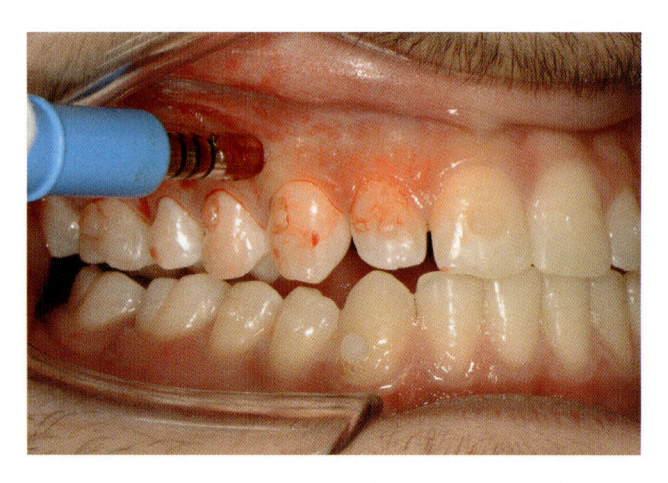

Figure 16.20 MOPs created with a manual Excellerator. (Source: Dr. Raffaele Spena.)

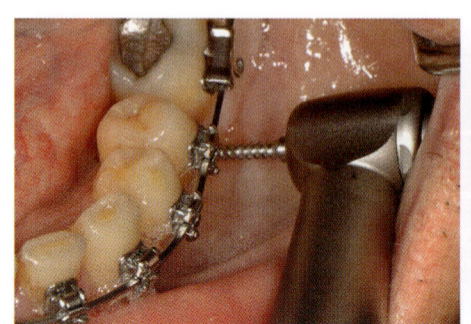

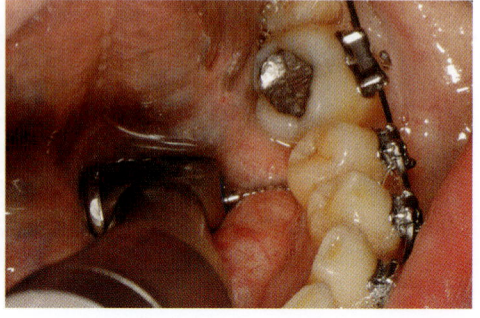

Figure 16.21 MOPs performed with a bur and dedicated handpiece. (Source: Dr. Raffaele Spena.)

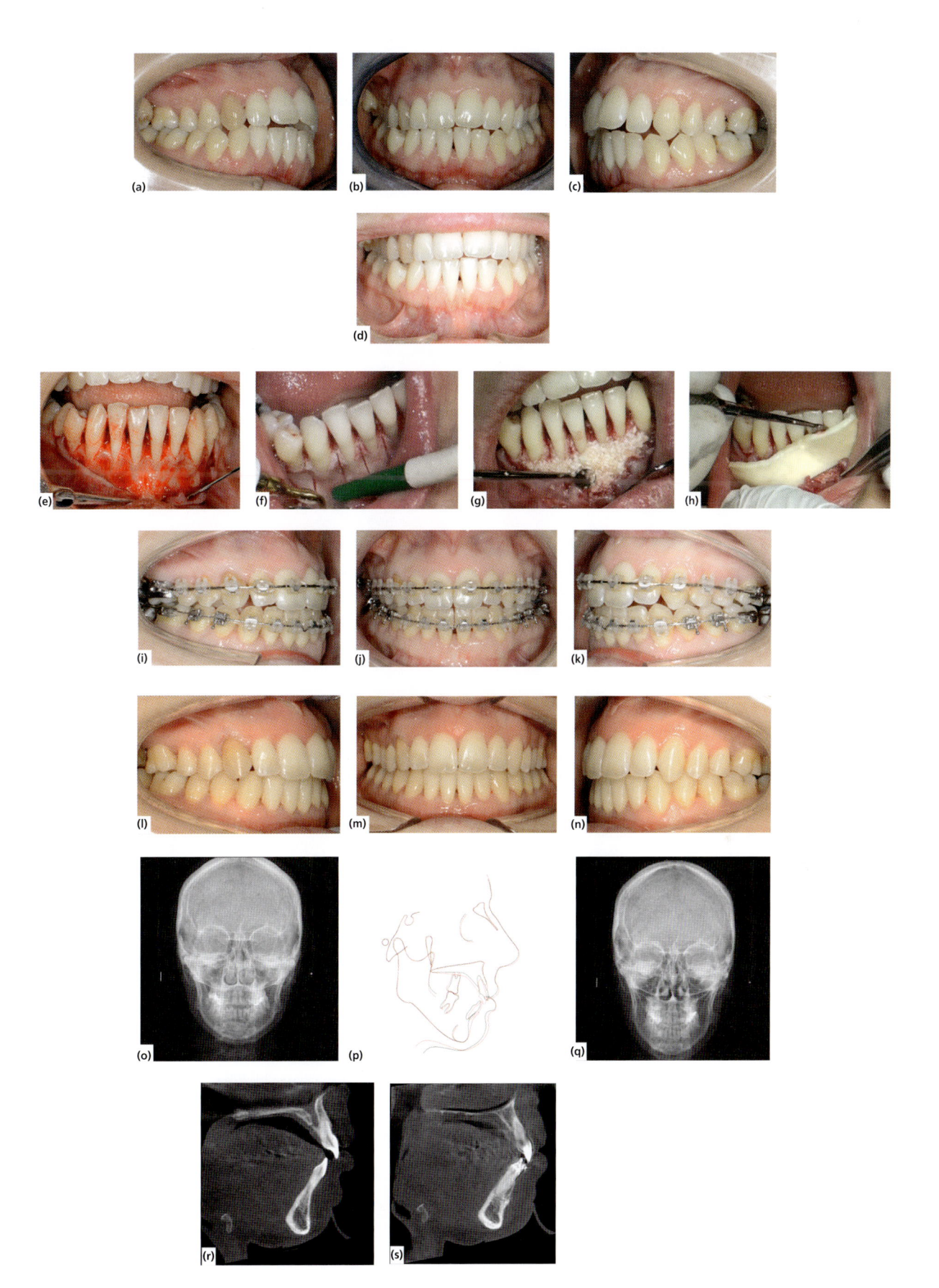

Figure 16.22 A 20-year-old woman with an open bite, thin biotype, and gingival recession in the lower front (a, b, c, and d). Alveolar corticotomy followed by hard and soft tissue grafts was performed to improve the supporting tissue (e, f, g and h). Arch coordination was undertaken with fixed appliances (i, j, and k). At the end of the treatment a neutral occlusion, correct overbite, and overjet were achieved, with good periodontal support and absence of any gingival recession (l, m, and n). The dental compensation of the skeletal open bite was confirmed by the antero-posterior radiographic head film and the superimposition of the lateral head films (o, p, and q). The alveolar corticotomy with a graft improved the bone volume to allow forward tooth movement, as shown by the cbct before and after treatment (r and s). (Source: Dr. Raffaele Spena.)

periodontal improvement around the lower teeth. The superimposition of the lateral cephalograms taken before the end of treatment and 2 years after the end of treatment shows minor changes.

The digital cuts from the cone beam computed tomography (CBCT) scan taken before and at the end of treatment show the changes in both the form and volume of the mandibular symphysis. This was thanks to the alveolar corticotomy combined with grafting and helped with the correction of the anterior open bite and the large overjet.

Patient 2 (Figure 16.23)

This patient is a 22-year-old female with a skeletal Class III malocclusion and missing upper lateral incisors, a very thin mandibular

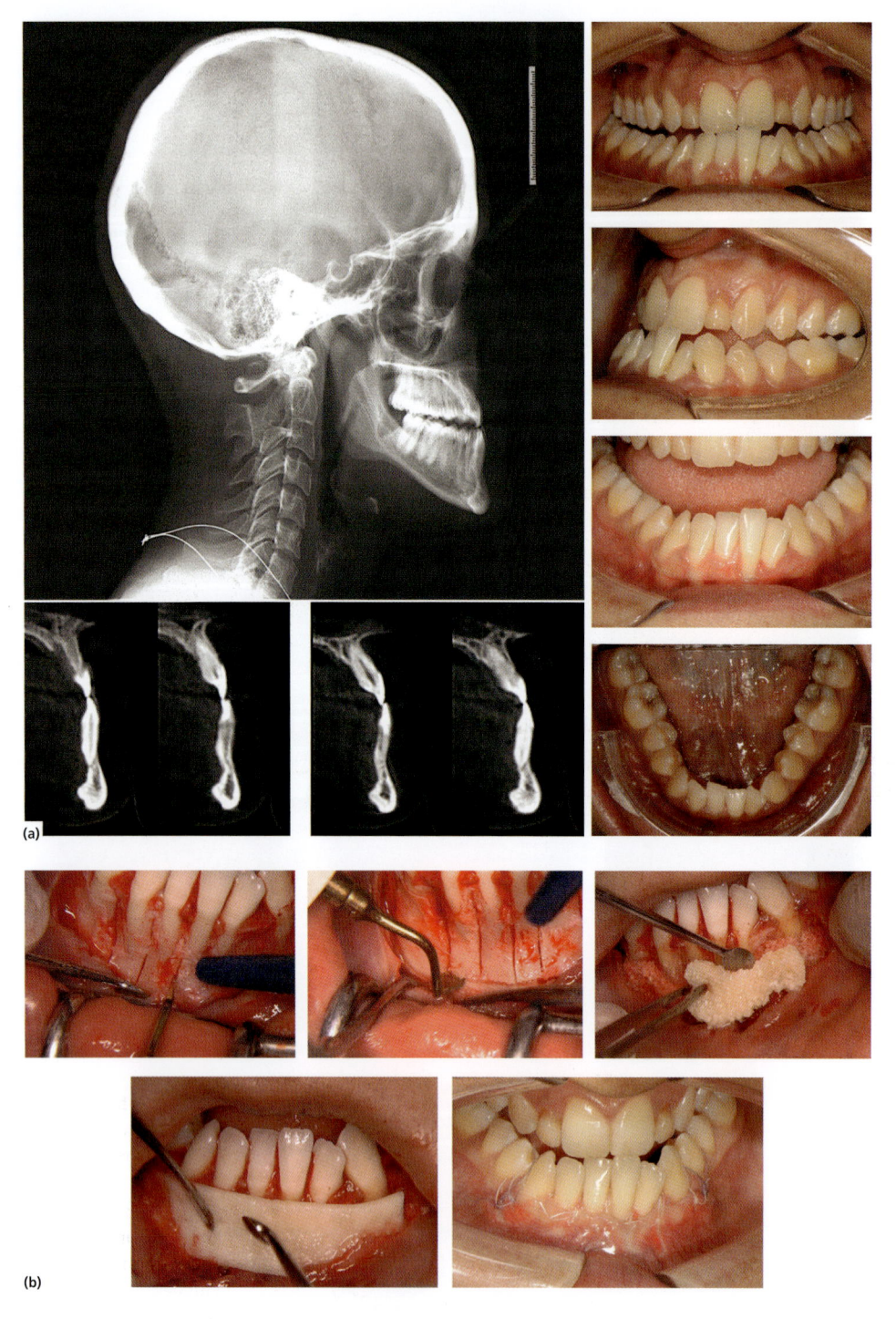

Figure 16.23 A 22-year-old female with a skeletal Class III, narrow maxilla, thin biotype, and gingival recession. The details of the CBCT showed thin alveolar bone in the lower anterior region with thin cortical plates. (a) The extended alveolar corticotomy was performed through interdental and apical cuts, complemented by both hard and soft tissue grafts. (b) At the end of the presurgical fixed appliance phase, the Class III was decompensated, with the lower incisors in the correct position relative to the alveolar bone in the anteroposterior plane. The corticotomy with graft ensured enough bone volume to allow forward movement of the lower incisors. (c and d) At the end of the surgical treatment optimal intercuspation was reached, without gingival recession and good periodontal support. (Source: Dr. Raffaele Spena.)

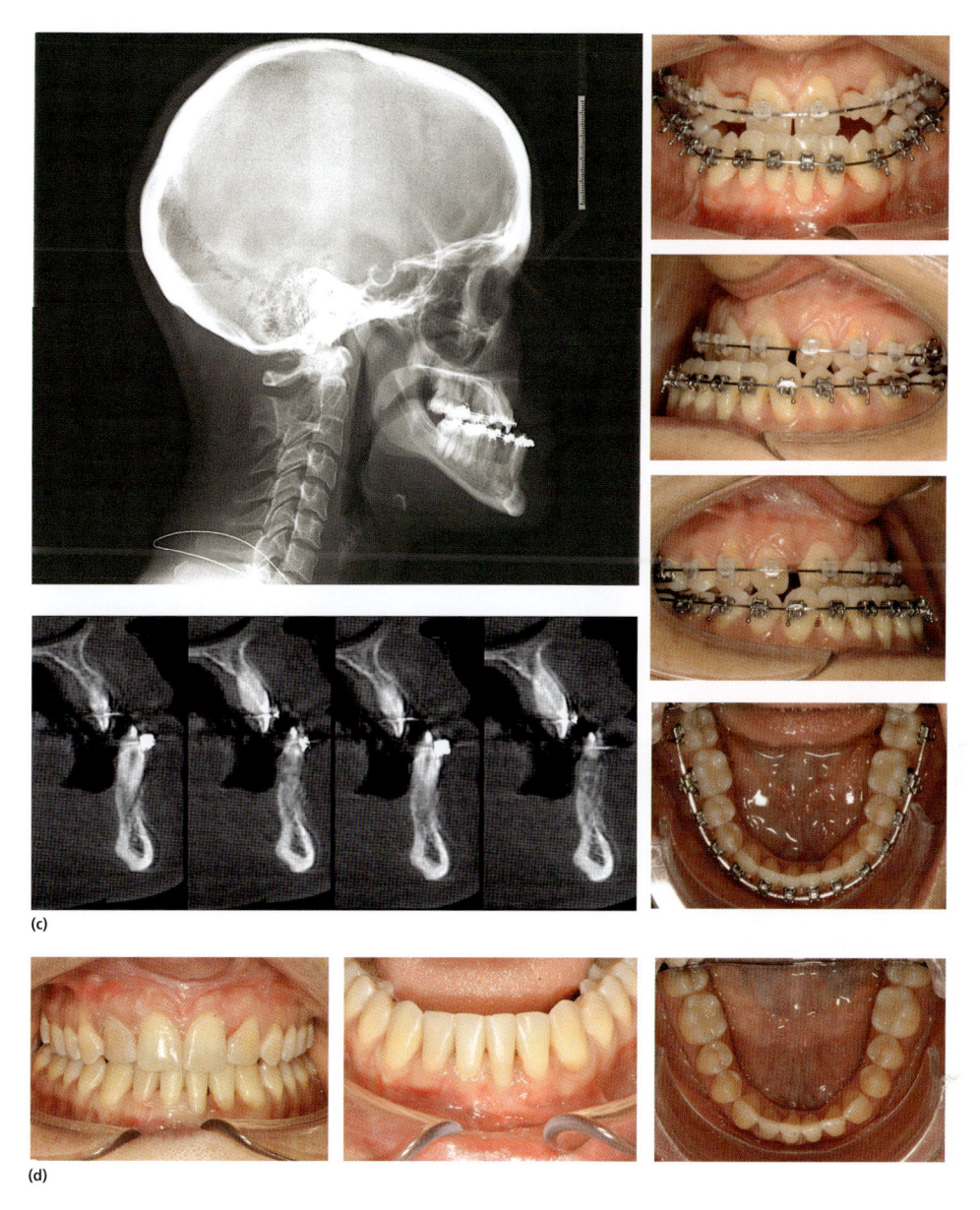

Figure 16.23 (Continued)

symphysis, thin gingival biotype, and recessions on the lower incisors.

In order to allow the lower incisor decompensation to take place despite the presence of periodontal limitations, alveolar corticotomy with an extended hard and soft tissue grafting was performed on the lower anterior area. Bonding was made a week after the surgery and sutures where removed after 3 weeks at the second orthodontic control.

At the end of the presurgical preparation a correct up righting of the teeth on the alveolar bone has been reached, without the loss of periodontal support, as shown by the presurgical lateral cephalogram. Detailed analysis from the CBCT scan shows a significantly improved volume of the symphysis. At the end of treatment, the final results show an optimal occlusion, good esthetics, and periodontal support.

Patient 3 (Figure 16.24)

A 12-year-old patient presented with a lower right canine with a buccal transmigration. The canine exposure with extensive corticotomy in the direction of the planned disinclusion was performed, as shown in Figure 16.10.

The correction of the transmigration was achieved using a simple biomechanical system to keep the canine low in the vestibule during the movement toward its final position in the arch. Finally, the canine reached its position in the dental arch with good periodontal support and good root parallelism.

Patient 4 (Figure 16.25)

The patient, a 12-year-old girl, had a transposition of the upper right canine and lateral incisor.

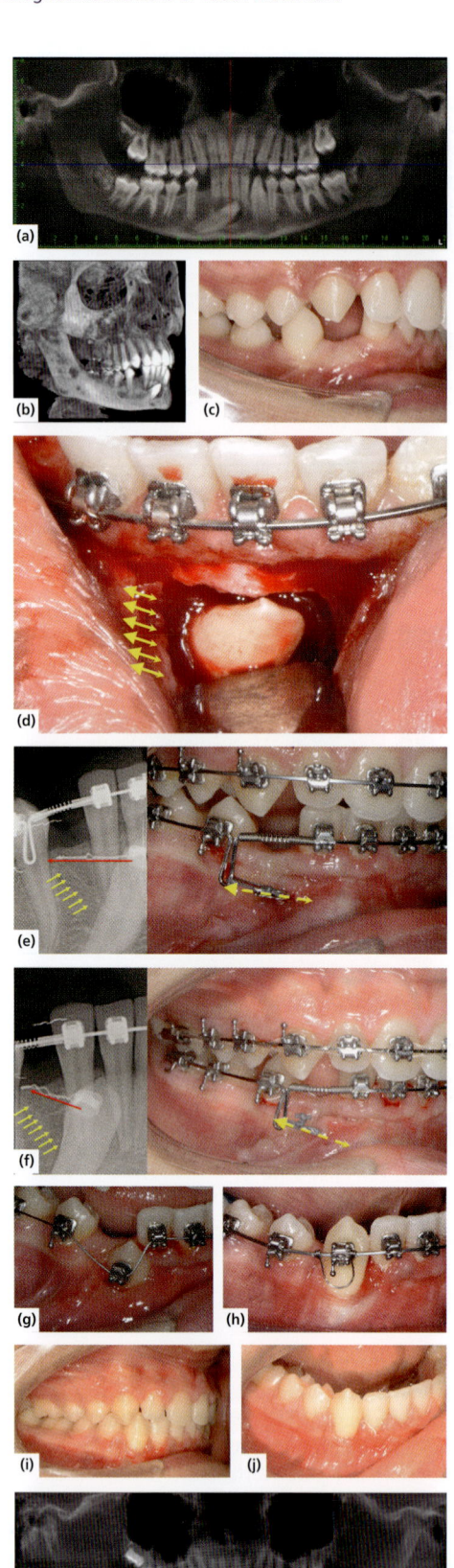

After exposure of the transposed canine, selective decortication was performed on the mesial and on the distal aspects of the impacted tooth.

The disimpaction and the resolution of the transposition was carried out, maintaining the canine high in the vestibule while correcting the transposition before applying any force toward the occlusal plane.

Patient 5 (Figure 16.26)

A 23-year-old woman presented with a Class II division 2 asymmetrical malocclusion, bimaxillary protrusion, lower midline deviation toward the right, missing lower right first permanent molar and a transverse cant of the occlusal plane (low on the right). Her chief wish was to correct the malocclusion but without an implant. The treatment plan included two upper first premolars extractions, interproximal reduction in the lower left quadrant, mesialization of the lower second and third permanent molars supported by MOPs, and no anterior skeletal anchorage.

After the initial stages of treatment consisting of levelling and alignment, the upper first premolars were extracted.

The CBCT of the lower right segment in the region where the lower first permanent molar was absent showed the presence of thick cortical bone on both buccal and lingual sides. MOPs were performed around the second and third molars to facilitate the mesialization through sliding mechanics. The final documentation shows complete space closure brought about through bodily movement and optimal interdigitation.

Patient 6 (Figure 16.27)

A young patient had four first permanent molars extracted when younger and several dental pathologies. He was treated with an open flap corticotomy and bone graft in the lower quadrants followed by conventional mechanics with no anterior skeletal anchorage. The only trick in reinforcing anterior anchorage was to rotate the lower incisor brackets 180° to convert the torque from -6° to +6°. The corticotomy notably reduced the resistance of the lower molars to the mesializing forces.

Patient 7 (Figure 16.28)

This patient was an adult with two unsuccessful past treatments. He had a Class II division 1 malocclusion with an asymmetrical open bite, constricted upper arch, and generalized recessions in a thin gingival biotype. The treatment included an open flap corticotomy with hard and soft tissue grafting over the entire upper arch followed by multibracket appliance and sequential archwires to coordinate the arches. Interproximal reduction helped to control the position of the upper and lower anterior teeth.

Figure 16.24 Buccal transmigration of the lower right canine over the midline, as demonstrated by the CBCT (a, b, and c). The alveolar corticotomy was extended in the direction of the planned movement (d, arrows). The force was applied to produce movement through the corticotomized bone (e and f, arrows). The canine was maintained inferiorly in the alveolus until it reached the correct anteroposterior position and only then was moved vertically (g and h). The canine reached its position in the dental arch with good periodontal support and good root parallelism (i, j, and k). (Source: Dr. Raffaele Spena.)

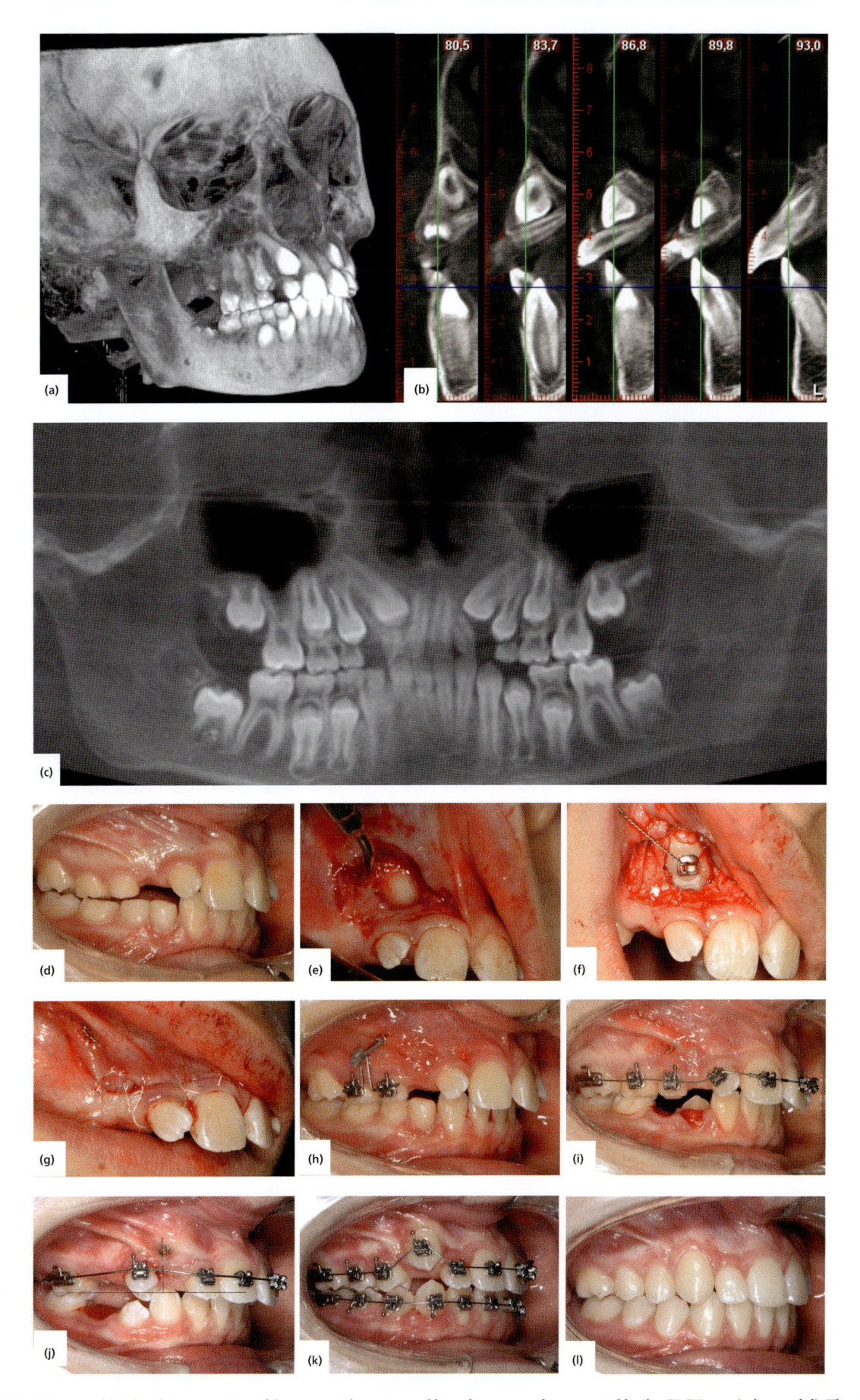

Figure 16.25 A 12-year-old girl with transposition of the upper right canine and lateral incisor, as demonstrated by the CBCT scan (a, b, c, and d). The alveolar bone was corticotomized mesially and distally, and the flap sutured (e, f, and g). Traction was applied through the mucosa to allow a horizontal and distal movement initially using the deciduous molars as anchorage (h) and then subsequently moved vertically (i). Once all the permanent teeth were erupted, arch coordination through continuous arch mechanics was performed (j and k) until optimal interdigitation was attained (l). (Source: Dr. Raffaele Spena.)

256 Biological Mechanisms of Tooth Movement

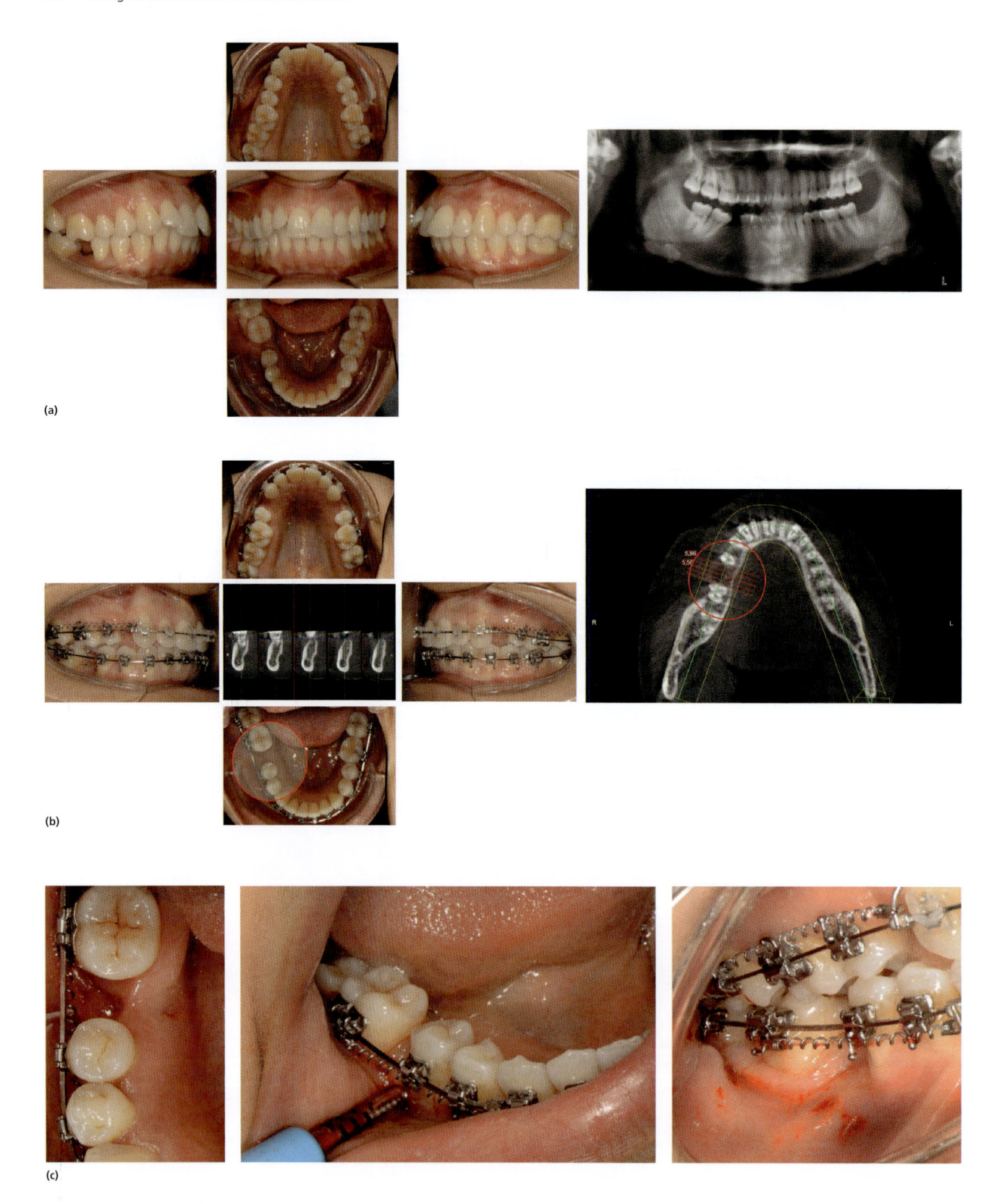

Figure 16.26 A 23-year-old woman with a Class II Division 1 asymmetric occlusion whose treatment plan included mesialization of the lower second and third molars and extraction of the first upper premolars (a). The CBCT showed that the alveolar bone towards which the molars had to move was thick cortical bone on both the buccal and the lingual aspects, thus potentially slowing down the movement and challenging the anchorage (b). Micro-osteo-perforations were performed buccally and lingually during the mesialization (c). The final results showed optimal intercuspation and bodily tooth movement (d). The superimposition showed mesialization and uprighting of the second and third lower right molars without anchorage loss (e). (Source: Dr. Raffaele Spena.)

(d)

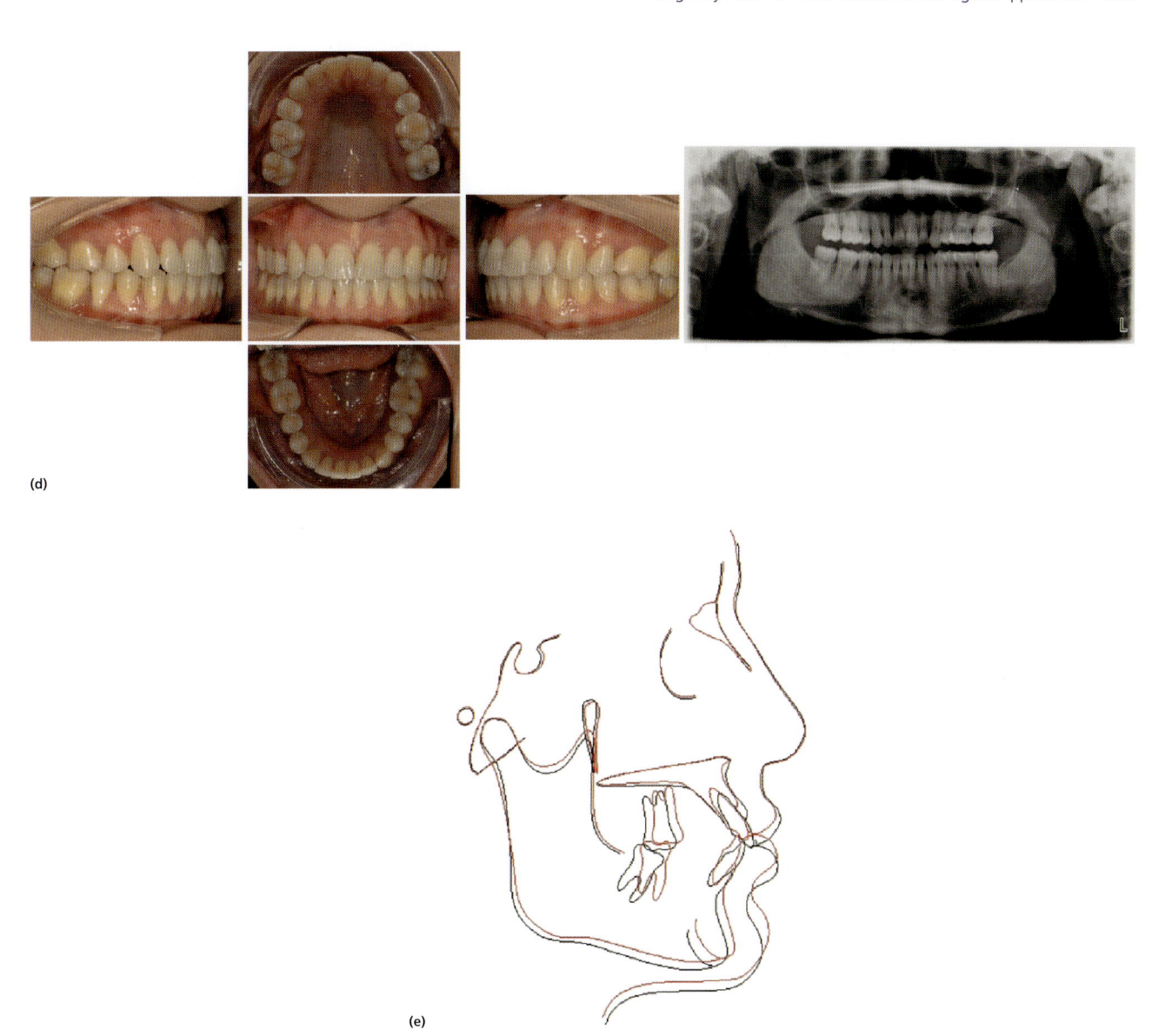

(e)

Figure 16.26 (Continued)

A good cusp to fossa relationship was established in the buccal segments and both the sagittal relationship and the open bite were resolved.

Patient 8 (Figure 16.29)

This young adult female patient had a severe skeletal asymmetry, a constricted maxillary arch and upper and lower arch crowding. The treatment started with an orthopedic expansion of the maxilla with a bone-borne expander. Osteo-perforations were performed along the entire maxillary suture at the start of expansion. This ensured a purely parallel expansion of the suture. The treatment continued with a multibracket appliance, complemented by upper and lower interproximal reduction, and temporary anchorage devices in the upper right quadrant to intrude the molar and premolars thus correcting the cant of the occlusal plane. At the end of treatment, the asymmetry was notably reduced.

Conclusions

The *efficacy* of alveolar corticotomy in terms of temporarily accelerating OTM has been demonstrated, and among the tools available to influence patients' treatment response seem to be the most reliable for clinical applications. This specific type of periodontal surgery, when combined with bone and soft tissue grafts, and precise mechanical loading, widens the spectrum of treatment possibilities in challenging situations.

If we consider surgically assisted tooth movement in terms of *efficiency* in reducing treatment time, it has to be observed that, if the goal is to achieve optimal treatment results, the real total time gain is relatively limited and therefore may not be clinically significant. The use of this technique to speed up tooth movement in easy cases, which only require a proper biomechanical plan to be accomplished in a short time, is not warranted, and may be of minimal benefit to the patients but primarily for the

(a)

(b)

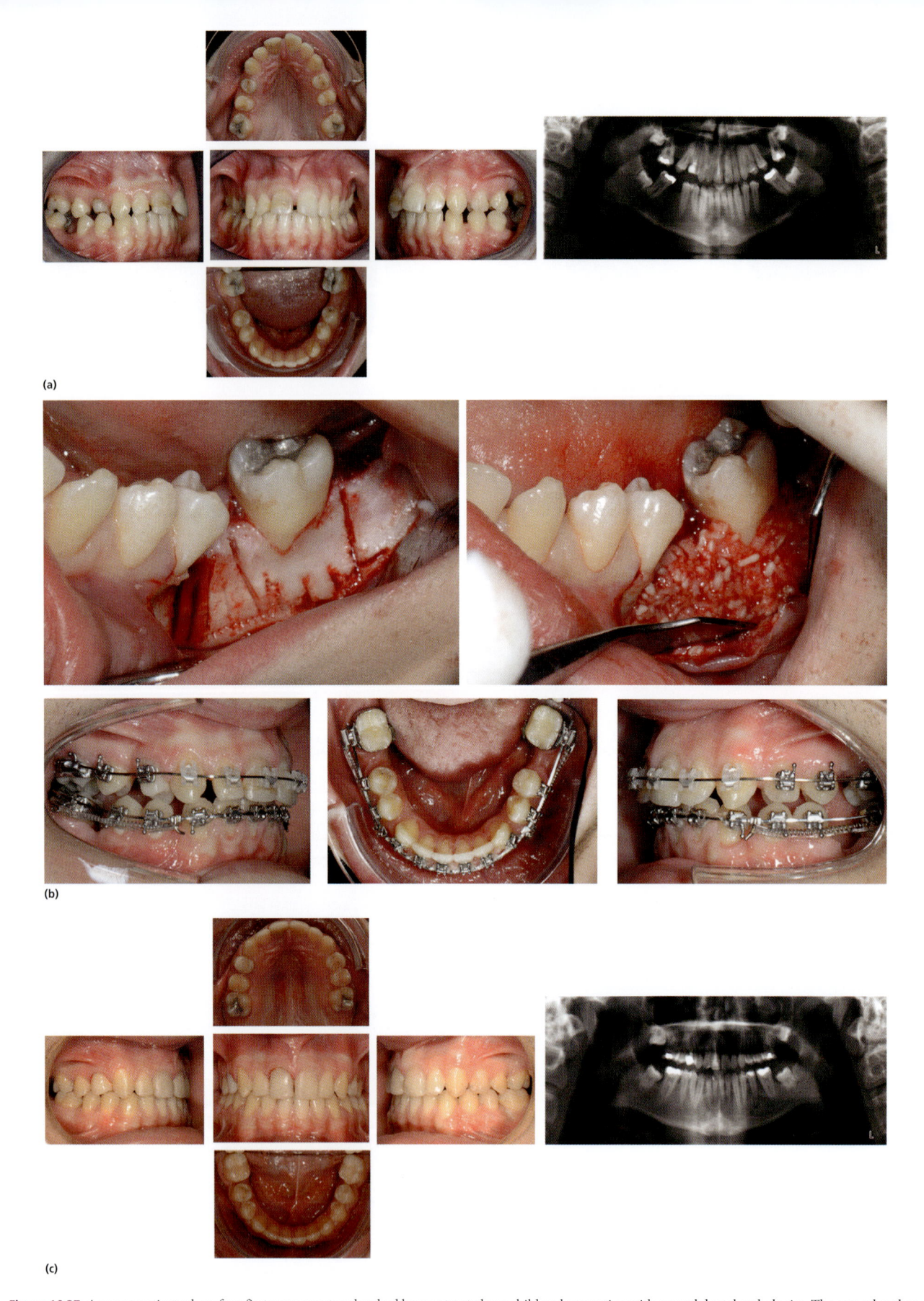

(c)

Figure 16.27 A young patient where four first permanent molars had been extracted as a child and presenting with several dental pathologies. The second molars tipped mesially towards the atrophic alveolus and the second premolars had moved distally (a). Space closure with total mesialization of the second molars was planned (C-Anchorage). The distal tip of the second premolars was not favorable for the mesial movement of the lower molars. He was treated with an open flap corticotomy and bone graft in the lower quadrants followed by conventional mechanics with no anterior skeletal anchorage (b). The only trick to reinforce anterior anchorage was to rotate the lower incisor brackets 180° to convert the torque from -6° to +6°. The corticotomy notably reduced the resistance of the lower molars to the mesializing forces. At the end of treatment an optimal occlusion was reached with correct root parallelism (c). (Source: Dr. Raffaele Spena.)

Surgically Assisted Tooth Movement: Biological Application   259

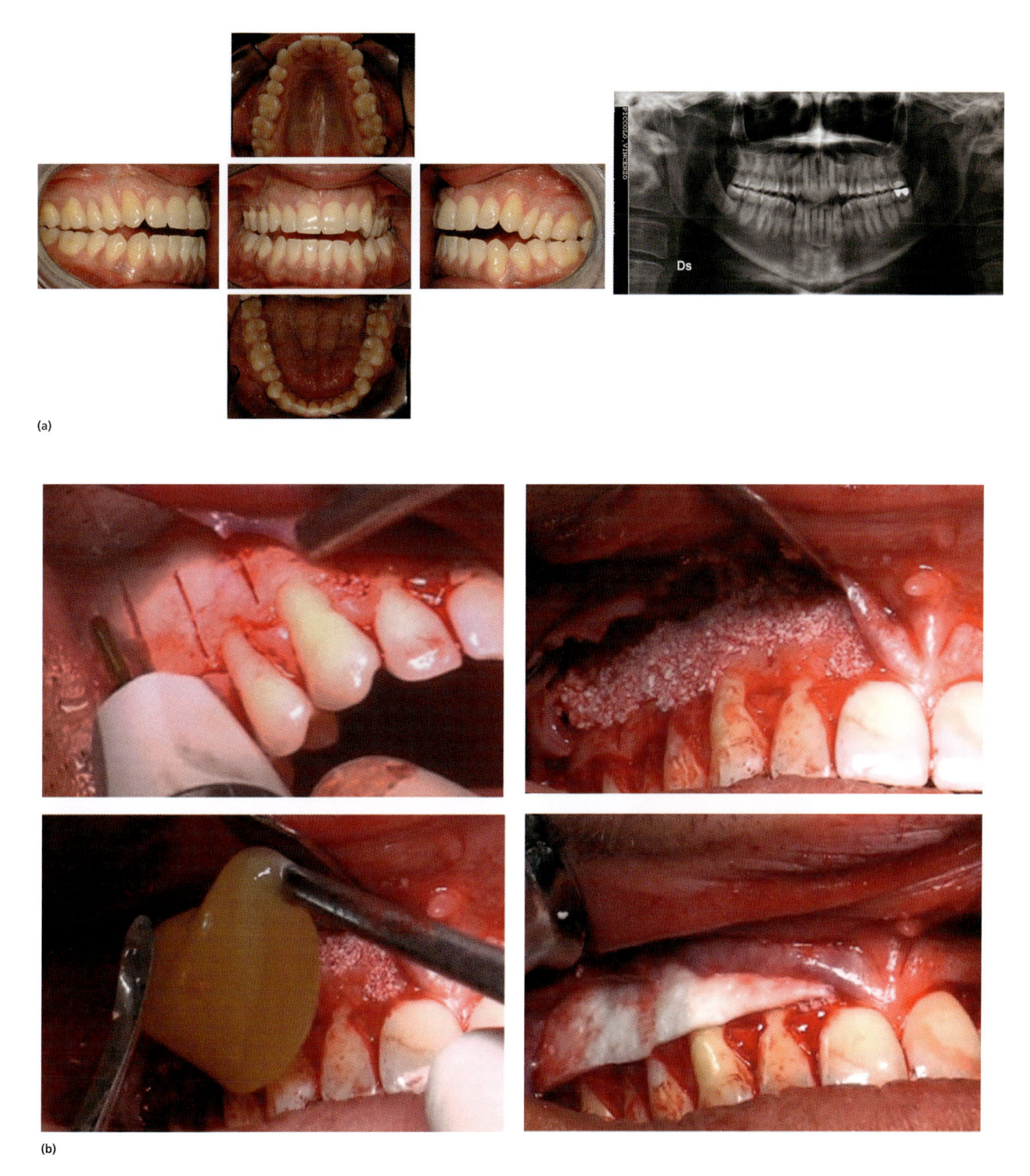

Figure 16.28 Adult patient with two unsuccessful past treatments who presented with a Class II Division 1 malocclusion, asymmetrical open bite, constricted upper arch, and generalized recessions in a thin gingival biotype (a). The treatment included an open flap corticotomy with hard and soft tissue grafting over the entire upper arch followed by a multibracket appliance and sequential archwires to coordinate the arches (b and c). Interproximal reduction helped control the position of the upper and lower anterior teeth. With a good cusp to fossa relationship in the buccal segments, the open bite was resolved in addition to correction of the sagittal relationship (d). The CBCT and anteroposterior headfilms after treatment showed a substantial increase of buccal alveolar bone and a harmonious transverse relationship (e). (Source: Dr. Raffaele Spena.)

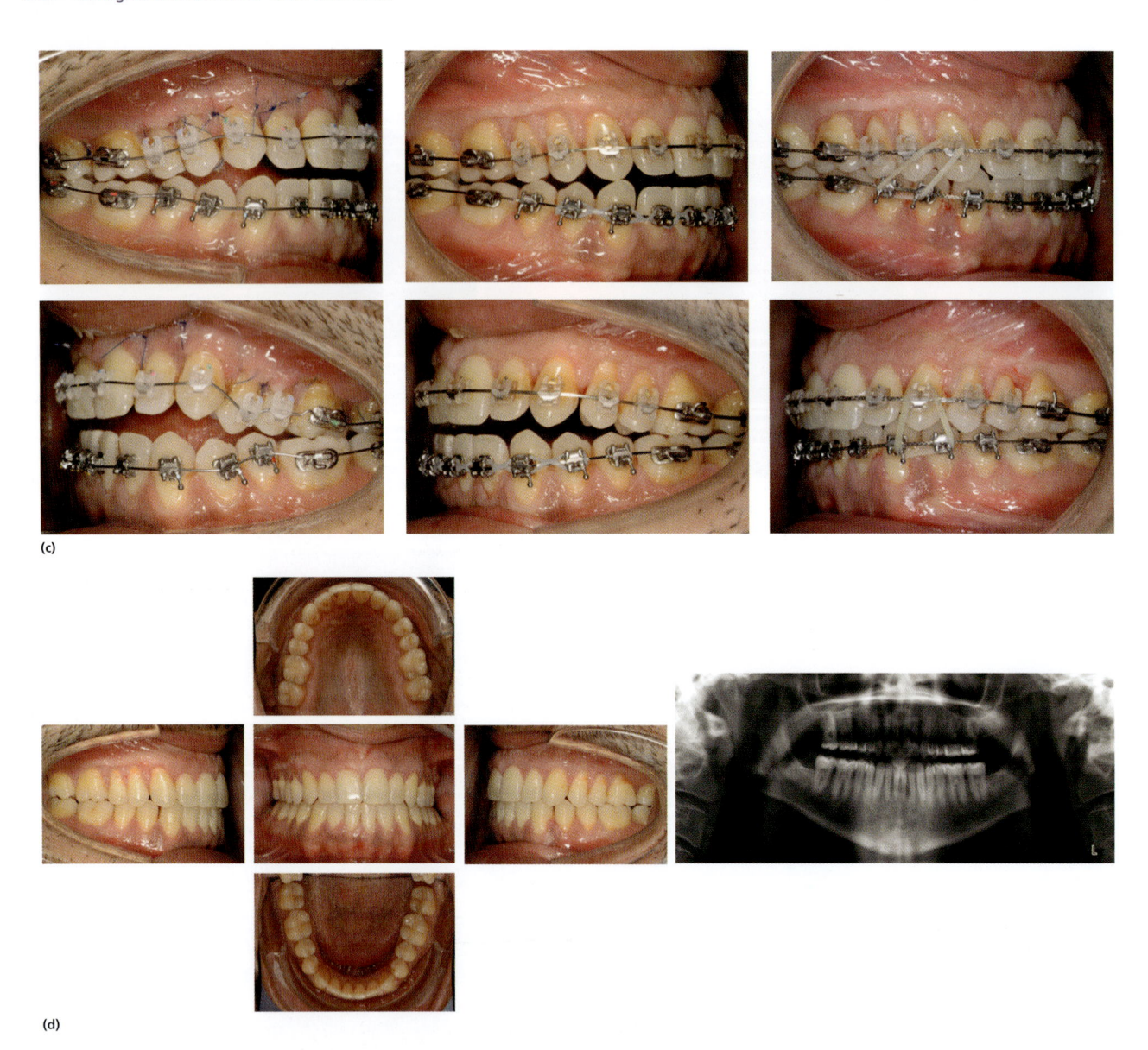

Figure 16.28 (Continued)

purpose of marketing the orthodontic practice. Any surgical procedure carries with it some morbidity and should not be recommended in cases which can be adequately achieved by conventional orthodontics.

Since highly controlled trials demonstrating equality in the quality of the final treatment relative to the time of treatment are not available, we should see the primary indications for this approach, instead, as the possibility to treat patients with complex OTM, unfavourable anatomy, and periodontal support with fewer complications.

The utilization of corticotomies in orthodontics should be considered therefore for their *effectiveness* in delivering excellent clinical results for the individual patient with complex treatment needs while keeping in mind the available evidence and the possible challenges (Table 16.4). The advantages given by the increased remodeling rate have to be seen in the framework of the individual patients' need and conditions. The patient specific treatment must be evaluated in relation to the biological, social, and economic characteristics of the patient, following the principle of patient-centered orthodontics, because only then is the use of the technique justified.

The corticotomy-assisted approach should be seen as a biological reinforcement of the segmented arch biomechanics approach. It allows a clear distinction to be made between the unit to be moved, the corticotomized unit, and the unit to be stabilized, although the anchorage unit can be reinforced with TADs. The advantage is the ability to find solutions for extremely complex cases and still achieve excellence in the quality of the results with the additional benefit of a reduced treatment time.

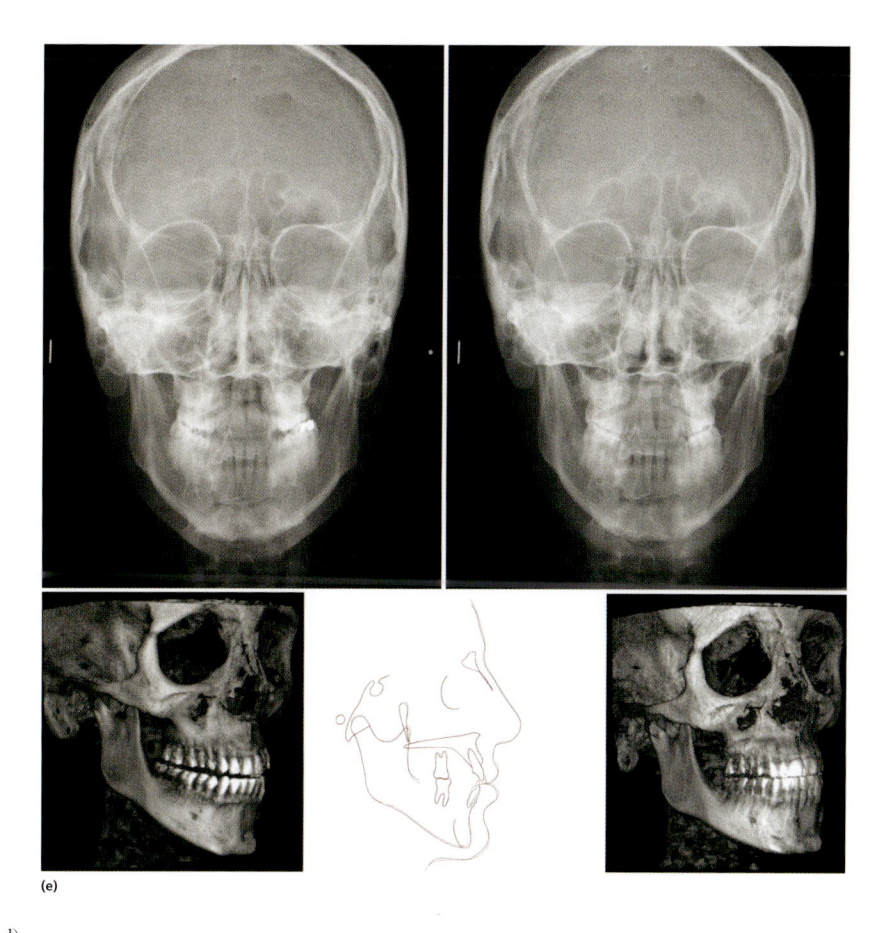

Figure 16.28 (Continued)

Figure 16.29 Young adult female patient with a severe skeletal asymmetry, constricted upper arch, cross bite, and upper and lower crowding, as shown by the initial records (a). The treatment started with an orthopedic expansion of the maxilla with a bone-borne expander. Osteo-perforations were performed along the entire maxillary suture at the beginning of the expansion (b). This allowed a perfect expansion of the suture with parallel margins, as depicted by the CBCT (c). The treatment continued with a multibracket appliance, complemented by upper and lower interproximal reduction, and temporary anchorage devices in the upper right quadrant to intrude the molar and premolars to correct the cant of the occlusal plane (d). At the end of treatment, the asymmetry was notably reduced (e).

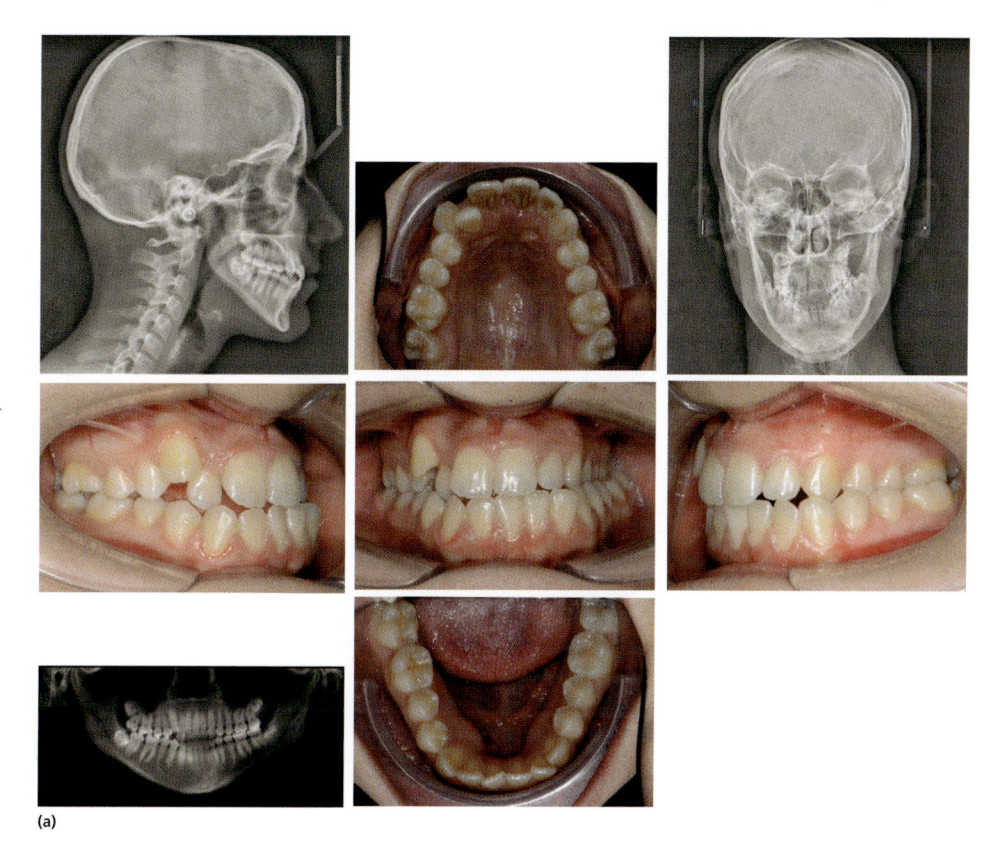

262 Biological Mechanisms of Tooth Movement

(b)

(c)

(d)

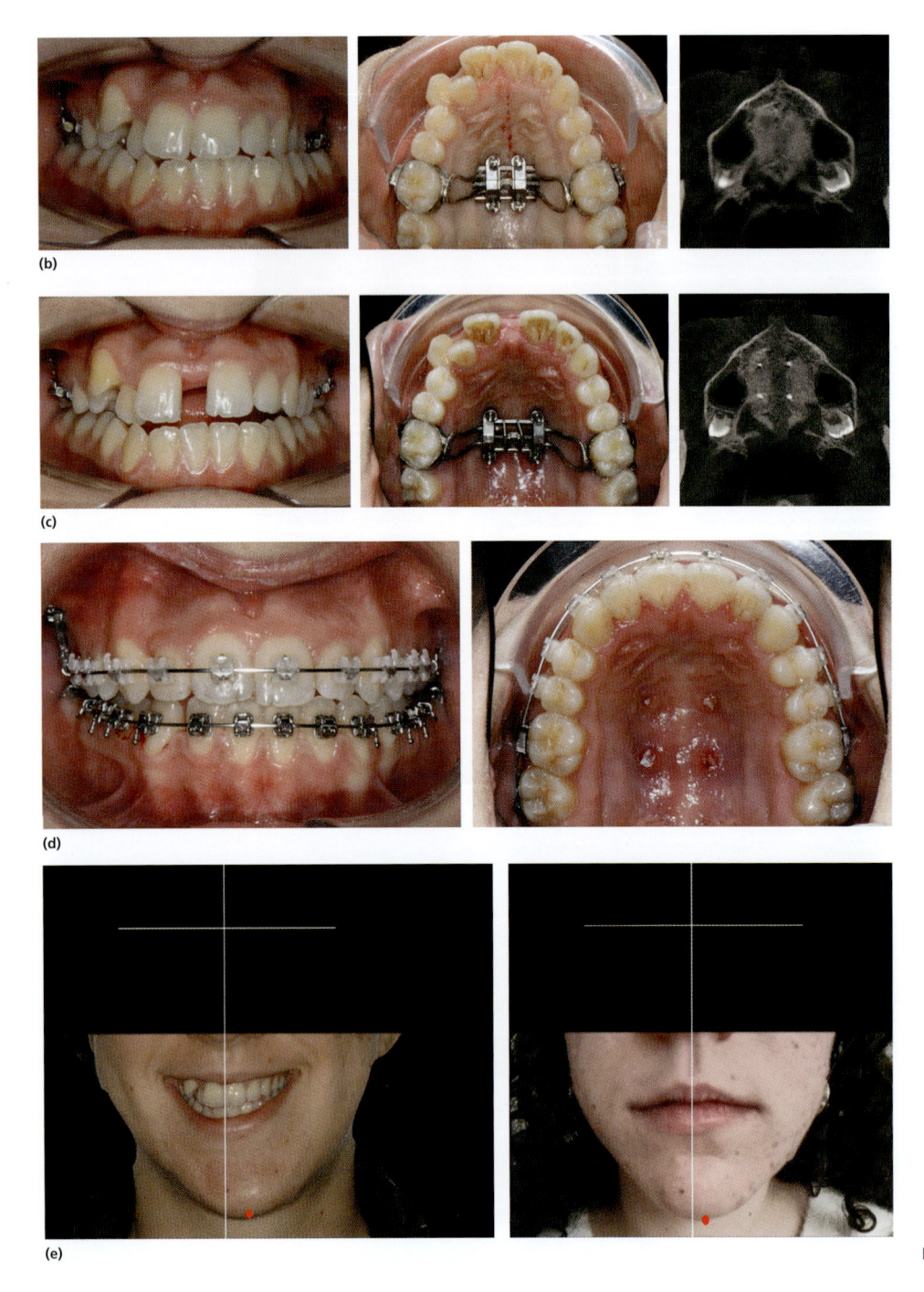

(e)

Figure 16.29 (Continued)

Table 16.4 Facts and challenges with corticotomies.

Facts	Challenges
• Facilitates individual tooth movement • Improves periodontal support when combined with grafts • Reduces anchorage demands • Expand interdisciplinary treatment possibilities	• Limited time window to operate • Questionable significantly shorter total treatment duration, provided good treatment results • Additional costs

References

Abbas, N. H., Sabet, N. E. and Hassan, I. T. (2016) Evaluation of corticotomy-facilitated orthodontics and piezocision in rapid canine retraction. *American Journal of Orthodontics and Dentofacial Orthopedics* **149**, 473–480.

Abdallah, M. N. and Flores-Mir, C. (2014) Are interventions for accelerating orthodontic tooth movement effective? *Evidence Based Dentistry* **15**, 116–117.

Aboul-Ela, S. M., El-Beialy, A. R., El-Sayed, K. M. *et al.* (2011) Miniscrew implant-supported maxillary canine retraction with and without corticotomy-facilitated orthodontics. *American Journal of Orthodontics and Dentofacial Orthopedics* **139**, 252–259.

Ahn, H. W., Lee, D. Y., Park, Y. G. et al. (2012) Accelerated decompensation of mandibular incisors in surgical skeletal class III patients by using augmented corticotomy: a preliminary study. *American Journal of Orthodontics and Dentofacial Orthopedics* **142**, 199–206.

Akay, M. C., Aras A., Gunbay, T. et al. (2009) Enhanced effect of combined treatment with corticotomy and skeletal anchorage in open bite correction. *Journal of Oral and Maxillofacial Surgery* **67**, 563–569.

Alford, T. J., Roberts, W. E., Hartsfield, J. K., Jr. et al. (2011) Clinical outcomes for patients finished with the SureSmile method compared with conventional fixed orthodontic therapy. *The Angle Orthodontist* **81**, 383–388.

Alharbi, F., Almuzian, M. and Bearn, D. (2019) Anchorage effectiveness of orthodontic miniscrews compared to headgear and transpalatal arches: a systematic review and meta-analysis. *Acta Odontologica Scandinavica* **77**, 88–98.

Alikhani, M., Chou, M. Y., Khoo, E. et al. (2018) Age-dependent biologic response to orthodontic forces. *American Journal of Orthodontics and Dentofacial Orthopedics* **153**, 632–644.

Alikhani, M., Raptis, M., Zoldan, B. et al. (2013) Effect of micro-osteoperforations on the rate of tooth movement. *American Journal of Orthodontics and Dentofacial Orthopedics* **144**, 639–648.

Almpani, K. and Kantarci, A. (2016a) Nonsurgical methods for the acceleration of the orthodontic tooth movement. *Frontiers in Oral Biology* **18**, 80–91.

Almpani, K. and Kantarci, A. (2016b) Surgical methods for the acceleration of the orthodontic tooth movement. *Frontiers in Oral Biology* **18**, 92–101.

Anitua, E. (2001) The use of plasma-rich growth factors (PRGF) in oral surgery. *Practical Procedures & Aesthetic Dentistry* **13**, 487–493.

Baloul, S. S., Gerstenfeld, L. C., Morgan, E.F. et al. (2011) Mechanism of action and morphologic changes in the alveolar bone in response to selective alveolar decortication-facilitated tooth movement. *American Journal of Orthodontics and Dentofacial Orthopedics* **139**, S83–101.

Burstone, C.J. and Pryputniewicz, R.J. (1980) Holographic determination of centers of rotation produced by orthodontic forces. *American Journal of Orthodontics* **77**, 396–409.

Cairo, F., Nieri, M. and Pagliaro, U. (2014) Efficacy of periodontal plastic surgery procedures in the treatment of localized facial gingival recessions. A systematic review. *Journal of Clinical Periodontology* **41**(Suppl. 15), S44–62.

Carter, D. R. and Hayes, W.C. (1977) The compressive behavior of bone as a two-phase porous structure. *Journal of Bone and Joint Surgery (America)* **59**, 954–962.

Cassetta, M., Giansanti, M., Di Mambro, A. et al. (2016) Minimally invasive corticotomy in orthodontics using a three-dimensional printed CAD/CAM surgical guide. *International Journal of Oral and Maxillofacial Surgery* **45**, 1059–1064.

Cattaneo, P. M., Dalstra, M. and Melsen, B. (2005) The finite element method: a tool to study orthodontic tooth movement. *Journal of Dental Research* **84**, 428–433.

Chang, J., Chen, P.J., Dutra, E.H. et al. (2019) The effect of the extent of surgical insult on orthodontic tooth movement. *European Journal of Orthodontics* **41**, 601–608.

Charavet, C., Lecloux, G., Jackers, N. et al. (2019) Patient-reported outcomes measures (PROMs) following a piezocision-assisted versus conventional orthodontic treatments: a randomized controlled trial in adults. *Clinical and Oral Investigation* **23**, 4355–4363.

Cheung, T., Park, J., Lee, D., Kim, C. et al. (2016) Ability of mini-implant-facilitated micro-osteoperforations to accelerate tooth movement in rats. *American Journal of Orthodontics and Dentofacial Orthopedics* **150**, 958–967.

Choukroun, J., Diss, A., Simonpieri, et al. (2006) Platelet-rich fibrin (PRF): a second-generation platelet concentrate. Part IV: clinical effects on tissue healing. *Oral Surgery, Oral Medicine, Oral Pathology, Oral Radiology, and Endodontology* **101**, e56–60.

Dab, S., Chen, K. and Flores-Mir, C. (2019) Short- and long-term potential effects of accelerated osteogenic orthodontic treatment: a systematic review and meta-analysis. *Orthodontics and Craniofacial Research* **22**, 61–68.

Deguchi, T., Takano-Yamamoto, T., Yabuuchi T et al. (2008) Histomorphometric evaluation of alveolar bone turnover between the maxilla and the mandible during experimental tooth movement in dogs. *American Journal of Orthodontics and Dentofacial Orthopedics* **133**, 889–897.

Dehbi, H., Azaroual, M. F., Zaoui, F. et al. (2017) Therapeutic efficacy of self-ligating brackets: A systematic review. *Internation Orthodontics* **15**, 297–311.

Dibart, S., Sebaoun, J.D. and Surmenian, J. (2009) Piezocision: a minimally invasive, periodontally accelerated orthodontic tooth movement procedure. *Compendium of Continuing Education in Dentistry* **30**, 342–344, 346, 348–350.

Dibart, S., Yee, C., Surmenian, J., Sebaoun, J. D. et al. (2014) Tissue response during Piezocision-assisted tooth movement: a histological study in rats. *European Journal of Orthodontics* **36**, 457–464.

Eriksen, E. F. (2010) Cellular mechanisms of bone remodeling. *Reviews in Endocrine and Metabolic Disorders* **11**, 219–227.

Fischer, T.J. (2007) Orthodontic treatment acceleration with corticotomy-assisted exposure of palatally impacted canines. *The Angle Orthodontist* **77**, 417–420.

Frost, H. M. (1983) The regional accelerating phenomenon: a review. *Henry Ford Hospital Medical Journal* **31**, 3–9.

Frost, H.M. (1994) Wolff's Law and bone's structural adaptations to mechanical usage: an overview for clinicians. *The Angle Orthodontist* **64**, 175–188.

Fu, T., Liu, S., Zhao, H. et al. (2019) Effectiveness and safety of minimally invasive orthodontic tooth movement acceleration: a systematic review and meta-analysis. *Journal of Dental Research* **98**, 1469–1479.

Gapski, R., Parks, C. A. and Wang, H. L. (2005) Acellular dermal matrix for mucogingival surgery: a meta-analysis. *Journal of Periodontology* **76**, 1814–1822.

Germec, D., Giray, B., Kocadereli, I. and Enacar, A. (2006) Lower incisor retraction with a modified corticotomy. *The Angle Orthodontist* **76**, 882–890.

Gkantidis, N., Mistakidis, I., Kouskoura, T. and Pandis, N. (2014) Effectiveness of non-conventional methods for accelerated orthodontic tooth movement: a systematic review and meta-analysis. *Journal of Dentistry* **42**, 1300–1319.

Glenn, R.W., Weimer, A.D., Wentz, F.M. and Krejci, R.F. (1983) The effect of gingival fiberotomy on orthodontic cuspid retraction in cats. *The Angle Orthodontist* **53**, 320–328.

Gulnahar, Y., Huseyin Kosger, H. and Tutar, Y. (2013) A comparison of piezosurgery and conventional surgery by heat shock protein 70 expression. *International Journal of Oral and Maxillofacial Surgery* **42**, 508–510.

Hernandez-Alfaro, F. and Guijarro-Martinez, R. (2012) Endoscopically assisted tunnel approach for minimally invasive corticotomies: a preliminary report. *Journal of Periodontology* **83**, 574–580.

Hou, D., Capote, R., Bayirli, B. et al. (2020) The effect of digital diagnostic setups on orthodontic treatment planning. *American Journal of Orthodontics and Dentofacial Orthopedics* **157**, 542–549.

Iino, S., Sakoda, S., Ito, G. et al. (2007) Acceleration of orthodontic tooth movement by alveolar corticotomy in the dog. *American Journal of Orthodontics and Dentofacial Orthopedics* **131**, 448 e441–448.

Iwasaki, L.R., Liu, Y., Liu, H. and Nickel, J. C. (2017) Speed of human tooth movement in growers and non-growers: Selection of applied stress matters. *Orthodontic and Craniofacial Research* **20**(Suppl. 1), 63–67.

Jambi, S., Walsh, T., Sandler, J. et al. (2014) Reinforcement of anchorage during orthodontic brace treatment with implants or other surgical methods. *Cochrane Database Systematic Review*:CD005098.

Keser, E. I. and Dibart, S. (2013) Sequential piezocision: a novel approach to accelerated orthodontic treatment. *American Journal of Orthodontics and Dentofacial Orthopedics* **144**, 879–889.

Kim, S. H., Kim, I., Jeong, D. M. et al. (2011) Corticotomy-assisted decompensation for augmentation of the mandibular anterior ridge. *American Journal of Orthodontics and Dentofacial Orthopedics* **140**, 720–731.

Kim, S. J., Park, Y. G. and Kang, S. G. (2009) Effects of corticision on paradental remodeling in orthodontic tooth movement. *The Angle Orthodontist* **79**, 284–291.

Kim, Y.S., Kim, S.J., Yoon, H.J. et al. (2013) Effect of piezopuncture on tooth movement and bone remodeling in dogs. *American Journal of Orthodontics and Dentofacial Orthopedics* **144**, 23–31.

Kole, H. (1959) Surgical operations on the alveolar ridge to correct occlusal abnormalities. *Oral Surgery, Oral Medicine, Oral Pathology, and Oral Radiology* **12**, 515–529.

Lee, J. K., Chung, K. R. and Baek, S. H. (2007) Treatment outcomes of orthodontic treatment, corticotomy-assisted orthodontic treatment, and anterior segmental osteotomy for bimaxillary dentoalveolar protrusion. *Plastic and Reconstructive Surgery* **120**, 1027–1036.

Lee, W., Karapetyan, G., Moats, R. et al. (2008) Corticotomy-/osteotomy-assisted tooth movement microCTs differ. *Journal of Dental Research* **87**, 861–867.

Liu, Y., Wu, Y., Yang, C. et al. (2020) Biomechanical effects of corticotomy facilitated orthodontic anterior retraction: a 3-dimensional finite element analysis. *Computer Methods in Biomechanics and Biomedical Engineering* **23**, 295–302.

Lyu, C., Zhang, L. and Zou, S. (2019) The effectiveness of supplemental vibrational force on enhancing orthodontic treatment. A systematic review. *European Journal of Orthodontics* **41**, 502–512.

Marx, R.E., Carlson, E.R., Eichstaedt, R.M. et al. (1998) Platelet-rich plasma: *growth factor enhancement for bone grafts*. Oral Surgery, Oral Medicine, Oral Pathology, and Oral Radiology **85**, 638–646.

Mavreas, D. and Athanasiou, A. E. (2008) Factors affecting the duration of orthodontic treatment: a systematic review. European Journal of Orthodontics **30**, 386–395.

McBride, M. D., Campbell, P. M., Opperman, L.A. et al. (2014) How does the amount of surgical insult affect bone around moving teeth? American Journal of Orthodontics and Dentofacial Orthopedics **145**, S92–99.

McCormack, S.W., Witzel, U., Watson, P. J. et al. (2017) Inclusion of periodontal ligament fibres in mandibular finite element models leads to an increase in alveolar bone strains. PLoS One **12**, e0188707.

Mheissen, S., Khan, H. and Samawi, S. (2020) Is Piezocision effective in accelerating orthodontic tooth movement: a systematic review and meta-analysis. PLoS One **15**, e0231492.

Moon, C. H., Wee, J. U. and Lee, H.S. (2007) Intrusion of overerupted molars by corticotomy and orthodontic skeletal anchorage. The Angle Orthodontist **77**, 1119–1125.

Mostafa, Y.A., Mohamed Salah Fayed, M., Mehanni, S. et al. (2009) Comparison of corticotomy-facilitated vs standard tooth-movement techniques in dogs with mini-screws as anchor units. American Journal of Orthodontics and Dentofacial Orthopedics **136**, 570–577.

Murphy, K.G., Wilcko, M.T., Wilcko, W.M. and Ferguson, D.J. (2009) Periodontal accelerated osteogenic orthodontics: a description of the surgical technique. Journal of Oral and Maxillofacial Surgery **67**, 2160–2166.

Nowzari, H., Yorita, F.K. and Chang, H.C. (2008) Periodontally accelerated osteogenic orthodontics combined with autogenous bone grafting. Compendium of Continuing Education in Dentistry **29**, 200–206; quiz 207, 218.

Oliveira, D. D., de Oliveira, B. F., de Araujo Brito, H. H. et al. (2008) Selective alveolar corticotomy to intrude overerupted molars. American Journal of Orthodontics and Dentofacial Orthopedics **133**, 902–908.

Ouejiaraphant, T., Samruajbenjakun, B. and Chaichanasiri, E. (2018) Determination of the centre of resistance during en masse retraction combined with corticotomy: finite element analysis. Journal of Orthodontics **45**, 11–15.

Pacheco, A. A., Saga, A. Y., de Lima, K. F. et al. (2016) Stress distribution evaluation of the periodontal ligament in the maxillary canine for retraction by different alveolar corticotomy techniques: a three-dimensional finite element analysis. Journal of Contemporary Dental Practice **17**, 32–37.

Pacheco-Pereira, C., Pereira, J.R., Dick, B.D. et al. (2015) Factors associated with patient and parent satisfaction after orthodontic treatment: a systematic review. American Journal of Orthodontics and Dentofacial Orthopedics **148**, 652–659.

Patterson, B. M., Dalci, O., Papadopoulou, A. K. et al. (2017) Effect of piezocision on root resorption associated with orthodontic force: a microcomputed tomography study. American Journal of Orthodontics and Dentofacial Orthopedics **151**, 53–62.

Pilon, J. J., Kuijpers-Jagtman, A. M. and Maltha, J. C. (1996) Magnitude of orthodontic forces and rate of bodily tooth movement. An experimental study. American Journal of Orthodontics and Dentofacial Orthopedics **110**, 16–23.

Preti, G., Martinasso, G., Peirone, B. et al. (2007) Cytokines and growth factors involved in the osseointegration of oral titanium implants positioned using piezoelectric bone surgery versus a drill technique: a pilot study in minipigs. Journal of Periodontology **78**, 716–722.

Ren, Y., Maltha, J. C., Van 't Hof, M. A. and Kuijpers-Jagtman, A. M. (2003) Age effect on orthodontic tooth movement in rats. Journal of Dental Research **82**, 38–42.

Rice, J. C., Cowin, S. C. and Bowman, J. A. (1988) On the dependence of the elasticity and strength of cancellous bone on apparent density. Journal of Biomechanics **21**, 155–168.

Richter, A. E., Arruda, A. O., Peters, M. C. and Sohn, W. (2011) Incidence of caries lesions among patients treated with comprehensive orthodontics. American Journal of Orthodontics and Dentofacial Orthopedics **139**, 657–664.

Roscoe, MG., Meira, J. B. and Cattaneo, P. M. (2015) Association of orthodontic force system and root resorption: a systematic review. American Journal of Orthodontics and Dentofacial Orthopedics **147**, 610–626.

Sanjideh, P. A., Rossouw, P. E., Campbell, P. M. et al. (2010) Tooth movements in foxhounds after one or two alveolar corticotomies. European Journal of Orthodontics **32**, 106–113.

Schaffler, M. B. and Burr, D. B. (1988) Stiffness of compact bone: effects of porosity and density. Journal of Biomechanics **21**, 13–16.

Sebaoun, J. D., Kantarci, A., Turner, J. W. et al. (2008) Modeling of trabecular bone and lamina dura following selective alveolar decortication in rats. Journal of Periodontology **79**, 1679–1688.

Shahabee, M., Shafaee, H., Abtahi, M. et al. (2020) Effect of micro-osteoperforation on the rate of orthodontic tooth movement-a systematic review and a meta-analysis. European Journal of Orthodontics **42**, 211–221.

Spena, R. (2018) Alveolar corticotomy: are we looking at it in the right way? Revista Española de Ortodoncia **48**, 112–126.

Spena, R., Caiazzo, A., Gracco, A. and Siciliani, G. (2007) The use of segmental corticotomy to enhance molar distalization. Journal of Clincal Orthodontics **41**, 693–699.

Spena, R. and Garganese, D. (2015) Parodontal unterstützte Kieferorthopädie – ein neuer Blick auf die Kortikotomie des Alveolarfortsatzes. Informationen aus Orthodontie und Kieferorthopädie **47**, 3–27.

Suya, H. (1991) Corticotomy in orthodontics, in Mechanical and Biological Basics in Orthodontic Therapy (eds. E. Hoesl and A. Baldauf). Huthig Buch Verlag, Heidelberg, Germany, p. 207–226.

Tatakis, D. N., Chambrone, L., Allen, E. P. et al. (2015) Periodontal soft tissue root coverage procedures: a consensus report from the AAP Regeneration Workshop. Journal of Periodontology **86**, S52–55.

Teixeira, C. C., Khoo, E., Tran, J. et al. (2010) Cytokine expression and accelerated tooth movement. Journal of Dental Research **89**, 1135–1141.

Thind, S. K., Chatterjee, A., Arshad, F. et al. (2018) A clinical comparative evaluation of periodontally accelerated osteogenic orthodontics with piezo and surgical bur: an interdisciplinary approach. Journal of the Indian Society of Periodontology **22**, 328–333.

Tonetti, M. S., Cortellini, P., Pellegrini, G. et al. (2018) Xenogenic collagen matrix or autologous connective tissue graft as adjunct to coronally advanced flaps for coverage of multiple adjacent gingival recession: randomized trial assessing non-inferiority in root coverage and superiority in oral health-related quality of life. Journal of Clinical Periodontology **45**, 78–88.

Tsichlaki, A., Chin, S. Y., Pandis, N. and Fleming, P.S. (2016) How long does treatment with fixed orthodontic appliances last? A systematic review. American Journal of Orthodontics and Dentofacial Orthopedics **149**, 308–318.

Vercellotti, T., Nevins, M. L., Kim, D. M. et al. (2005) Osseous response following resective therapy with piezosurgery. International Journal of Periodontics and Restorative Dentistry **25**, 543–549.

Verna, C., Cattaneo, P. M. and Dalstra, M. (2018) Corticotomy affects both the modus and magnitude of orthodontic tooth movement. European Journal of Orthodontics **40**, 107–112.

Verna, C., Dalstra, M. and Melsen, B. (2000) The rate and the type of orthodontic tooth movement is influenced by bone turnover in a rat model. European Journal of Orthodontics **22**, 343–352.

Verna, C., Zaffe, D. and Siciliani, G. (1999) Histomorphometric study of bone reactions during orthodontic tooth movement in rats. Bone **24**, 371–379.

Verna, C. (2008) Does corticotomy affect load transfer during orthodontic tooth movement? In: COAST Conference on Orthodontic Advances in Science and Technology. Monterey, CA, USA.

Vidovic, V. D., Dalstra, M. and Verna, C. (2017) Corticotomy of the buccal and lingual alveolar walls and its influence on orthodontic tooth displacement using finite element analysis. In: 93rd Congress of the European Orthodontic Society, Montreaux, Switzerland.

Von Böhl, M., Maltha, J., Von den Hoff, H. and Kuijpers-Jagtman, A. M. (2004) Changes in the periodontal ligament after experimental tooth movement using high and low continuous forces in beagle dogs. The Angle Orthodontist **74**, 16–25.

Wang, C. W., Yu, S. H., Mandelaris, G. A. and Wang, H. L. (2020) Is periodontal phenotype modification therapy beneficial for patients receiving orthodontic treatment? An American Academy of Periodontology best evidence review. Journal of Periodontology **91**, 299–310.

Wang, L., Lee, W., Lei, D.L. et al. (2009) Tisssue responses in corticotomy- and osteotomy-assisted tooth movements in rats: histology and immunostaining. American Journal of Orthodontics and Dentofacial Orthopedics **136**, 770 e771–711; discussion 770–771.

Wilcko, M. T., Wilcko, W. M. and Bissada, N. F. (2008) An evidence-based analysis of periodontally accelerated orthodontic and osteogenic techniques: a synthesis of scientific perspectives. Seminars in Orthodontics **14**, 305–316.

Wilcko, W. M., Wilcko, T., Bouquot, J. E. and Ferguson, D. J. (2001) Rapid orthodontics with alveolar reshaping: two case reports of decrowding. International Journal of Periodontics and Restorative Dentistry **21**, 9–19.

Yaffe, A., Fine, N. and Binderman, I. (1994) Regional accelerated phenomenon in the mandible following mucoperiosteal flap surgery. Journal of Periodontology **65**, 79–83.

Yavuz, M.C., Sunar, O., Buyuk, S. K. and Kantarci, A. (2018) Comparison of piezocision and discision methods in orthodontic treatment. Progress in Orthodontics **19**, 44.

CHAPTER 17
Precision Accelerated Orthodontics: How Micro-osteoperforations and Vibration Trigger Inflammation to Optimize Tooth Movement

Mani Alikhani, Jeanne M. Nervina, and Cristina C. Teixeira

> **Summary**
>
> In this chapter, we take you on our journey through the latest scientific evidence on bone remodeling and orthodontic tooth movement that led to the development of the biphasic theory of tooth movement and how we translated this new understanding into clinically useful tools to optimize and accelerate orthodontic tooth movement. According to the biphasic theory, an orthodontic force causes two sequential phases of bone remodeling, the catabolic phase, followed by the anabolic phase. In this chapter, we discuss how we were able to stimulate and harness this bone remodeling system to accelerate orthodontic tooth movement precisely, create biological anchorage, optimize the type of movement, and move teeth into areas of atrophic bone. Our journey from basic science to the clinic is chronicled by our development of micro-osteoperforations and vibration protocols that demonstrate how a sound understanding of the biology of teeth movement is translated into safe, minimally invasive, and predictable protocols for precision accelerated orthodontics.

Introduction

Advances in biomedical technologies are allowing us to peer deep into tissues, cells, and molecules to unravel biological mysteries of importance to orthodontists. The result is that we have a mountain of data on the biology of orthodontic tooth movement (OTM). The challenge we face now is mining that mountain for biological targets we can manipulate to increase orthodontic treatment efficacy. In this chapter, we recount the journey we have taken to address this challenge. Experienced clinicians and novice students alike, will see how we use the power of translational biomedical research to develop precision accelerated orthodontics for the benefit of our patients.

Sculpting biphasic theory from the bedrock of data

Having the clearest, most accurate picture of how the dentoalveolar complex responds to orthodontic force is critical for designing targeted treatment approaches. Interestingly, a careful reading of the literature going back to the earliest histological, cellular, and molecular studies (some dating back to the late 1800s) demonstrates considerable, but often dismissed, disagreement regarding the precise mechanism of OTM. The result is that the pressure–tension theory (Proffit et al., 2013), credited to Schwarz (Baumrind, 1969), is still a prevailing model of tooth movement.

The pressure–tension theory posits that heavy and light orthodontic forces displace the tooth in the alveolus, thereby simultaneously creating a region of pressure in the periodontal ligament (PDL)–alveolar bone on the side downstream of the force and tension in the PDL complex on the upstream side of the force. The focus of this model is on the pressure side of the tooth, which undergoes hypoxia-driven inflammation and osteoclastic resorption of the lamina dura (also referred to as undermining resorption), thereby creating the space into which the tooth will move. Less well studied is what happens on the tension side, where the consensus is that tension in the PDL accounts for a strong anabolic response in the alveolar bone. Thus, in the pressure–tension theory, the net result of orthodontic force is simultaneous bone resorption on the pressure side and bone formation on the tension side of the tooth.

As bone biologists, we questioned the validity of the pressure–tension theory because it failed to explain how tension in the PDL would trigger osteogenesis. If pressure decreases blood flow in the PDL by compressing blood vessels, tension will likewise decrease blood flow by flattening the blood vessels, with the net result being hypoxia in both the pressure and tension sides. This should trigger the same immunologically driven osteoclast-mediated bone resorption. Equally puzzling is how a tooth could move if bone is *simultaneously* resorbed on the pressure side and formed on the tension side. This scenario begs the question, if bone formation, rather than bone resorption, occurs on the tension side, why don't we see thickening of the lamina dura, decreased PDL width and, eventually, ankylosis on the tension side? These flaws in the pressure–tension theory's logic forced us to reexamine what is happening in the PDL–alveolar bone complex when an orthodontic force is applied to a tooth.

Since our major objection to the pressure–tension theory is its postulate that tooth movement requires restricted and site-specific bone resorption and formation on the pressure and tension sides, respectively, we first needed to describe accurately the histological and molecular events that occur all around the roots during tooth movement. Using the molar mesialization model in rats, we did not find any simultaneous differences in the pressure and tension responses in the PDL–alveolar bone complex, as proposed by the pressure–tension theory. Instead, we found that orthodontic force produces uniform histological and molecular responses around the entire tooth (Alikhani *et al.*, 2018b). Initially, orthodontic force changes the PDL morphology – compressing on the pressure side and stretching on the tension side – which triggers an inflammatory response around the entire root. This is evidenced by the time course of inflammatory markers in the gingival crevicular fluid (GCF), which peak within hours of force application and remain elevated until the force level dissipates due to tooth movement (Figure 17.1a). Histologically, bone resorbing osteoclasts appear on both the pressure and tension sides of the root (Figure 17.1b), and microCT data clearly shows the resulting decrease in bone density all around the roots of the moving tooth (Figure 17.1c). Most importantly, osteogenic markers do not appear until the osteolytic markers have decreased (Figure 17.1a). Thus, orthodontic forces produce tooth movement by activating an initial catabolic phase followed by an anabolic response, providing strong support for what we call the *biphasic theory of tooth movement* (Figure 17.2).

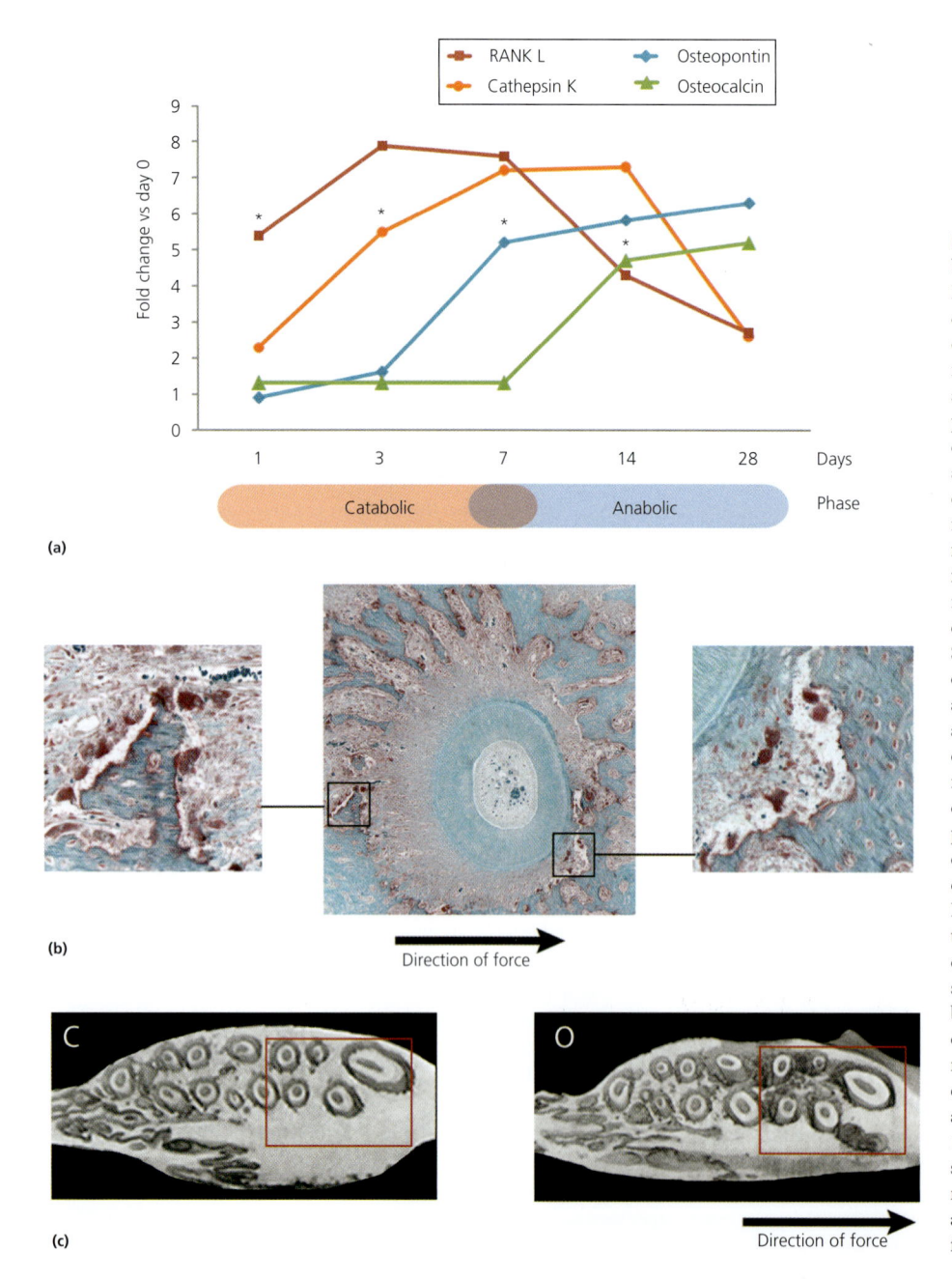

Figure 17.1 Evidence supporting the biphasic theory of tooth movement. Rat hemimaxillae were collected at different time points after application of force (25 cN) to mesialize the first molar. Control animals did not receive any force. (a) Reverse transcription polymerase chain reaction analysis of osteoclast (RANKL and cathepsin-K) and osteoblast (osteocalcin and osteopontin) markers in the hemimaxilla of rats at different time points after force activation. Data are presented as fold increase in gene expression in response to orthodontic force compared with day 0, and as mean ± SEM of three experiments. The onset of significant differences in RANKL and cathepsin-K was observed at day 1 and 3, and for osteopontin and osteocalcin at days 7 and 14, respectively, supporting that the catabolic phase precedes the anabolic phase during tooth movement. *Onset of statistically significant differences in comparison with day 0 ($P<0.05$). (b) Immunohistochemical staining for tartrate-resistant acid phosphatase 3 days after force application. Axial section shows osteoclasts (red cells) in both the tension and compression side of the moving mesiopalatal root of the maxillary first molar. (c) μCT images of maxillary right molars of control (c) and orthodontic force (o) animals, 14 days after application of force show significant osteopenia surrounding the moving first molar (red rectangular area). (Source: Used with permission from Alikhani *et al.*, 2018b.)

Indeed, both compression and tension damage the PDL (Figure 17.2a), stimulating an aseptic inflammatory response that generates a perimeter of osteoclastogenesis around the whole root (Figure 17.2b). The tooth then moves into the space created by osteoclasts in the direction of the orthodontic force vector. Importantly, the perimeter of osteoclastogenesis simultaneously drifts in the direction of the force during this catabolic phase. As the catabolic phase dissipates, the anabolic phase ensues with osteoblasts creating a perimeter of osteogenesis (Figure 17.2c). The osteoclastogenesis perimeter is a prerequisite for activation of the osteogenic perimeter. This observation agrees with existing data suggesting that osteoclasts are the principle osteoblast regulators (Matsuo and Irie, 2008). It is important to note that in considering the histological evidence for the biphasic theory, it may appear that the two phases are independent events. However, histological sections are deceiving because they are static representations of a dynamic process. Instead, the evidence on osteoresorptive and osteogenic marker expression clearly supports the temporal relationship that we propose in the biphasic theory of OTM.

Saturation of the biological response: more does not mean faster

We know that inflammatory markers play a critical role in OTM by controlling the rate of osteoclastic bone resorption. It logically follows that increasing the magnitude of orthodontic forces would increase inflammatory marker expression and osteoclastogenesis resulting in faster tooth movement. Surprisingly, there is a major controversy regarding the relation between force magnitude and the rate of tooth movement. Some studies show that higher force does not increase the rate of tooth movement (Quinn and Yoshikawa, 1985; Van Leeuwen et al., 2010), while others argue the opposite (Yee et al., 2009). This controversy exists because researchers inappropriately equate the distance teeth move with the rate that teeth move for a given magnitude of force. This difference is not trivial considering how many factors may affect this distance. While we want to know the distance teeth move in response to a given force magnitude, what we actually should be focusing on is the relation between force magnitude and the biological response, because it is the biological response that regulates the rate of tooth movement.

Using the molar mesialization model in rats, we found that increasing the magnitude of orthodontic force increases inflammatory marker levels (Figure 17.3a), osteoclast recruitment and formation (Figure 17.3b), alveolar bone resorption, and the rate of tooth movement (Figure 17.3c). Unexpectedly, we also found that there is a force magnitude above which no further biological responses are induced (Figure 17.3). Thus, the cytokine release produced by orthodontic forces has an upper limit and consequently the osteoclast activity initiated by orthodontic forces has a saturation point (Alikhani et al., 2015). While the saturation point varies with the type of tooth movement, patient anatomy, bone density, and duration of treatment, the range of this variation is limited and therefore, the rate of tooth movement is usually predictable.

If application of higher forces does not increase the activity of inflammatory markers and the cascade of molecular and cellular events that follows, then application of higher forces cannot increase the rate of tooth movement and can only expose the tooth to increased risk of side effects such as root resorption, and produce increased pain for the patient (Theodorou et al., 2019). Coupling our understanding of these limitations with our now well-described

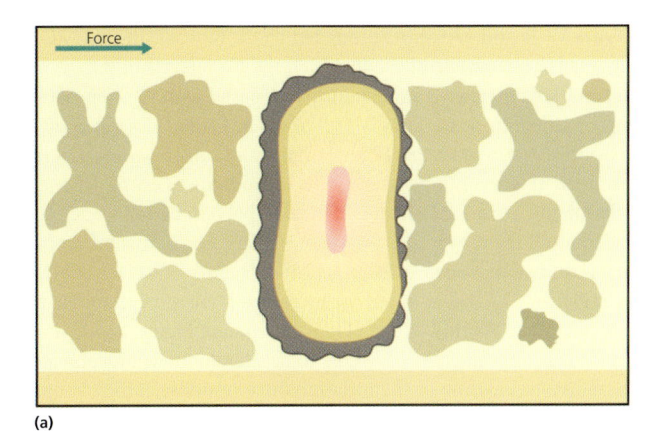

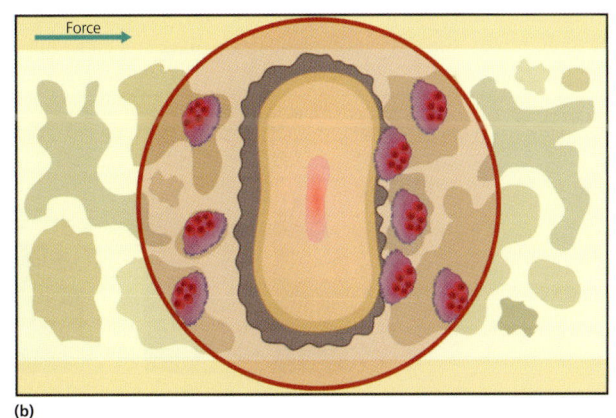

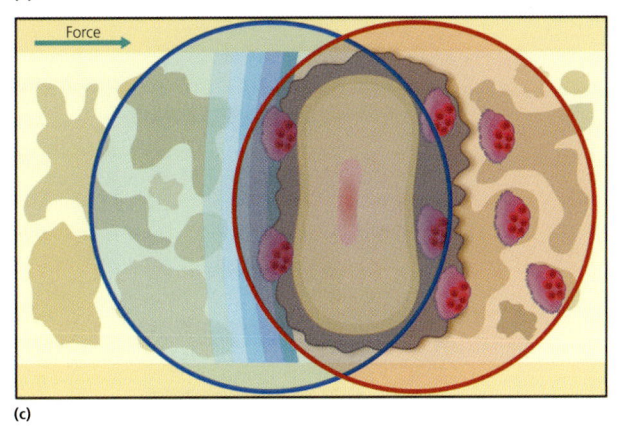

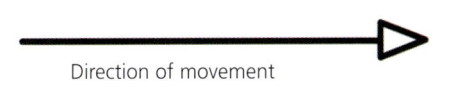

Figure 17.2 Schematic of biphasic theory of tooth movement. The biologic response during tooth movement comprises two clearly separated phases. After application of an orthodontic force (a) both the compression and tensile stresses generated by displacement of the tooth cause damage to the PDL, stimulating a perimeter of osteoclastogenesis (red circle in b). Once the tooth moves in the direction of the orthodontic force into the space created by osteoclast activity (c), the resulting perimeter of resorbed bone around the entire root (red circle) transitions into its anabolic phase, with a perimeter of osteogenesis arising in roughly the same area of the alveolar bone where the catabolic response took place (blue circle in c). Histological observation at this stage, led to erroneous interpretation of site-specific bone formation on the tension side (shaded blue bars), bone resorption on the pressure side (osteoclasts on the periodontal space), and to the proposal of the tension and pressure theory of tooth movement. (Source: Used with permission from Alikhani et al., 2018b.)

biological response to orthodontic force, we began developing methods to harness and stimulate the biological response in specific locations where tooth movement is desired. These methods include micro-osteoperforations (MOPs) and high-frequency acceleration (vibration)

MOPs: hyperlocalized inflammation for safe, minimally invasive accelerated tooth movement

Knowing that the catabolic phase is the initial response of the alveolar bone–PDL–tooth complex to orthodontic forces and that this response reaches a saturation point, we hypothesized that a novel approach to accelerated orthodontics treatment would be to safely boost catabolism beyond the saturation point at specific, or hyperlocalized, areas. Ideally, this approach should allow us to control both the level and location of inflammation, giving orthodontists the ability to move specific teeth as needed, while preserving anchorage and preventing negative side effects. This approach gives us the power to provide efficient, safe, individualized treatment for each patient.

Since controlled, hyperlocalized inflammation that produces safe accelerated tooth movement was our objective, we considered the model of microtrauma-triggered bone remodeling. Normal, healthy adaptive bone remodeling is often triggered by microfractures (e.g., stress fractures) (Hughes et al., 2017), which uses the direction and magnitude of force as a guide for bone remodeling that will withstand future force application at the site of microinjury. To mimic such a hyperlocalized inflammatory reaction, we proposed the use of transgingival MOPs in the alveolar bone when and where needed to overcome the biological saturation of an orthodontic force (Teixeira et al., 2010).

MOPs are small "dimples" placed in cortical alveolar bone under local anesthesia (see Alikhani, 2017, for a complete overview of the clinical application of MOPs). These microinjuries trigger the bone remodeling cascade as described by the biphasic theory (Figure 17.2). To verify and validate the safety and efficacy of MOPs treatment to accelerate tooth movement we tested our MOPs protocol in rats (Teixeira et al., 2010) (Figure 17.4) and humans (Alikhani et al., 2013) (Figure 17.5) undergoing orthodontic treatment. In each model, MOPs were placed in the alveolus on the side of the tooth toward which the desired tooth movement was planned

(Figure 17.4a and 17.5a). As predicted by the biphasic theory, MOPs triggered the catabolic phase in which the GCF levels of inflammatory markers increased significantly compared with the non-MOPs treated GCF (compare O to MOP group in Figure 17.4c and MOP to Control group in Figure 17.5b). Importantly, the response was not sustained (Figure 17.5b), giving the orthodontist control over the inflammatory process, which is critical to prevent pathological bone resorption if the response is too strong or sustained. This inflammatory response increases osteoclasts in the region of MOPs application (Figure 17.4d), leading to the increased bone resorption needed to accelerate tooth movement (Figure 17.4b and Figure 17.5 c, d).

Critical to the success of MOPs to accelerate tooth movement is the return to baseline of the inflammatory response, which is not a trivial response. As inflammation and catabolism increase, the tooth has the freedom to move in the direction of the applied force. As the tooth moves, the force level dissipates leading to a concomitant

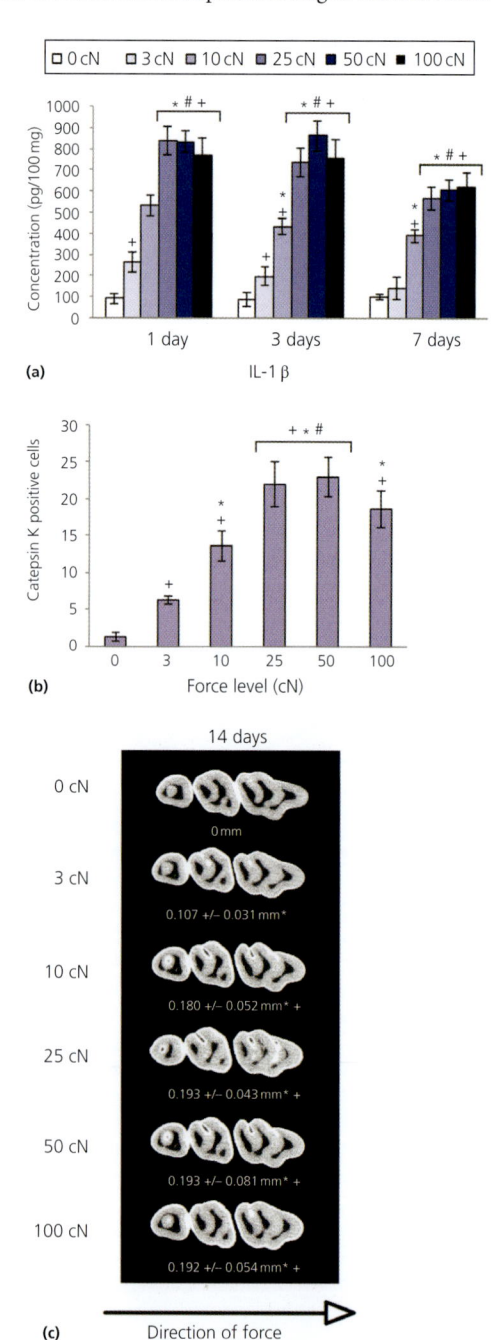

Figure 17.3 Saturation of biological response with increased orthodontic forces. The upper right maxillary molar of rats was exposed to different magnitude of forces (0–100 cN) and the hemimaxilla was collected for analyses at different time points. (a) IL-1β was evaluated by enzyme-linked immunosorbent-based assay after 1, 3, and 7 days of force applications. Data expressed as the mean ± SEM of concentration in picograms per 100 mg of tissue. +, Significantly different from 0 cN at same time point; *, significantly different from 3 cN at same time point; #, significantly different from 10 cN at same time point. $P < 0.05$. (b) Mean numbers of osteoclasts in the PDL and adjacent alveolar bone of the mesiopalatal root of the maxillary molar 7 days after application of force. Osteoclasts were identified as cathepsin K–positive cells in immunohistochemical stained sections (brown cells) from different force groups. Each value represents the mean ± SEM of five animals. +, Significantly different from 0 cN; *, significantly different from cN; #, significantly different from 10 cN. $P < 0.05$. (c) Micro-CT images of right maxillary molars of control and different experimental groups 14 days after application of force. Each value represents the mean ± SEM of the average distance between first and second molar measured at the height of contour of the posterior teeth in five animals. *, Significantly different from 0 cN; +, significantly different from 3 cN. $P < 0.05$. (Source: Modified from Alikhani et al., 2015.)

dissipation of inflammation and catabolism. Without this predictable and reliable return to baseline of the inflammatory response, MOPs as any other bone trauma, could potentially lead to persistent inflammation and unwanted bone and root resorption. Depending on the indication, the frequency of MOPs application can be adjusted to allow for sufficient inflammation to achieve the desired tooth movement. In general, it is wise to use MOPs either every visit or every other visit (with 4-week intervals between visits), which is the equivalent of every 28–56 days until movement is completed or forces have been stopped.

Importantly, any reactivation of orthodontic forces will stimulate cytokine release and further activation of osteoclasts. Therefore, while MOPs can cause a peak in osteoclast activation, shorter force reactivation intervals may prolong the effect of MOPs by preventing the drop in the level of cytokines. If the clinician plans to apply MOPs to accelerate the rate of tooth movement, we recommend seeing the patient more often to reactivate the appliances and forces. This approach will decrease the need for frequent MOPs application while ensuring that the rate of tooth movement will increase.

Clinical considerations for MOPs application

Orthodontic treatment has many stages and treatment mechanics divide the dentition into two groups: target teeth that should be moved and anchor teeth that should not be moved. While in one stage of treatment some teeth act as anchor units, in another stage of treatment the same teeth may become the target units. Therefore, simultaneously enhancing the biological response around all the teeth without proper planning for each tooth (as can happen when engaging a continuous archwire), is most likely unnecessary or even counterproductive. It should be emphasized that the principles of physics and mechanics are not affected by the rate of tooth movement. While MOPs can accelerate the rate of tooth movement, for every movement in the desired direction there is still a side effect movement that should be controlled. Therefore, treatment duration is not determined by how fast we move teeth but how wisely we plan each stage of treatment and take advantage of biology and physics to maximize our efficiency in achieving the goals of that stage. With the proper mechanical design, MOPs can be incorporated in clinical practice to accomplish the following objectives:

1. Accelerate the movement of target teeth.
2. Facilitate the desired type of tooth movement.
3. Develop biological anchorage.
4. Decrease the possibility of root resorption.
5. Moving teeth through atrophic bone.

1. Accelerate the movement of target teeth

The most common use of MOPs is to accelerate tooth movement (Alikhani et al., 2013). For this application, MOPs should be applied close to the target tooth only at the time when that target tooth is

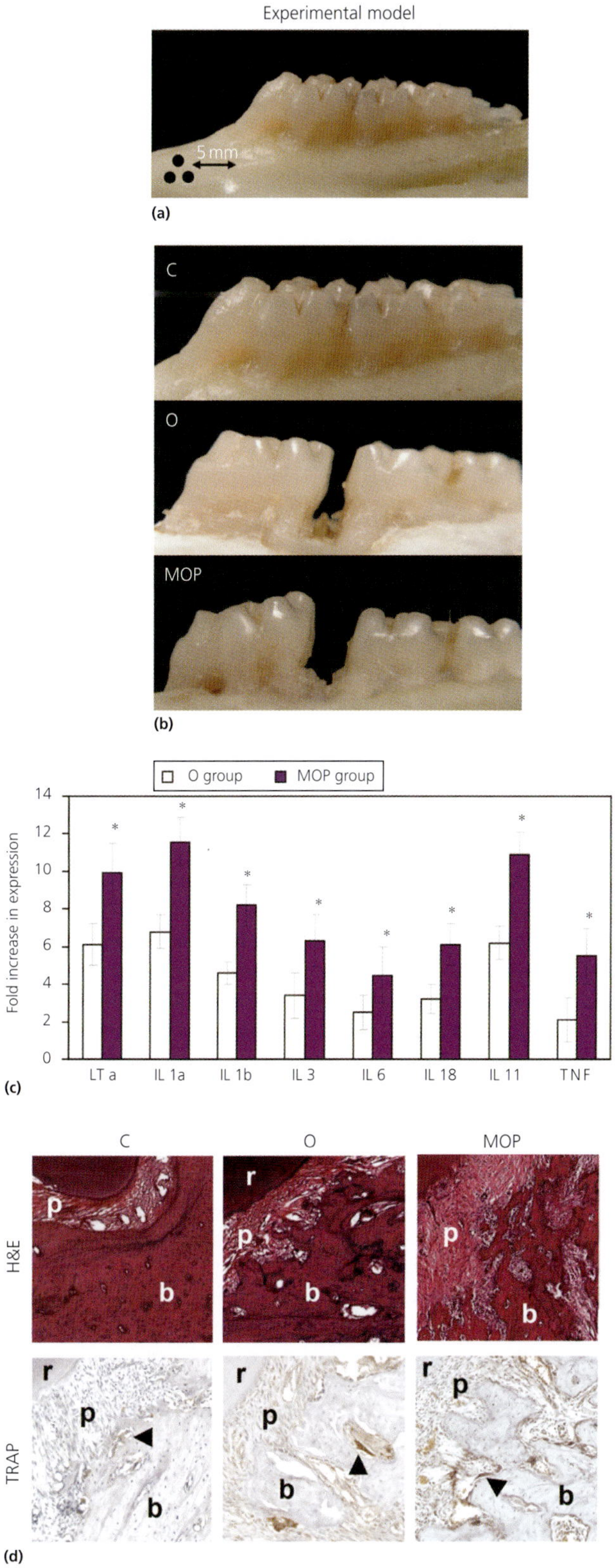

Figure 17.4 MOPs accelerate tooth movement in rats. (a) Rat hemimaxilla showing the location of three MOPs placed 5 mm mesial to the first molar. (b) Comparison of the magnitude of tooth movement after 28 days of orthodontic force application (C, control; O, orthodontic force only; MOP, orthodontic force + micro-osteoperforations). MOP shows greater magnitude of movement. (c) Reverse transcription polymerase chain reaction analysis of cytokine gene expression. Data is presented as fold increase in cytokine expression in the O and MOP groups in comparison with control group (IL, interleukins; LT, lymphotoxin alpha; TNF, tumor necrosis factor alpha). Data shown is mean ± SEM of three experiments. (d) Histological sections stained with hematoxylin and eosin (H & E, top panels) show increase of periodontal space (p) thickness around the mesiopalatal root (r) of the first molar and increase in bone (b) resorption both in the O and MOP groups. Immunohistochemical staining (bottom panels) shows an increase in the number of tartrate-resistant acid phosphatase (TRAP)-positive osteoclasts (brown cells, arrowhead) in both the O and MOP groups. (Source: Modified from Teixeira et al., 2010.)

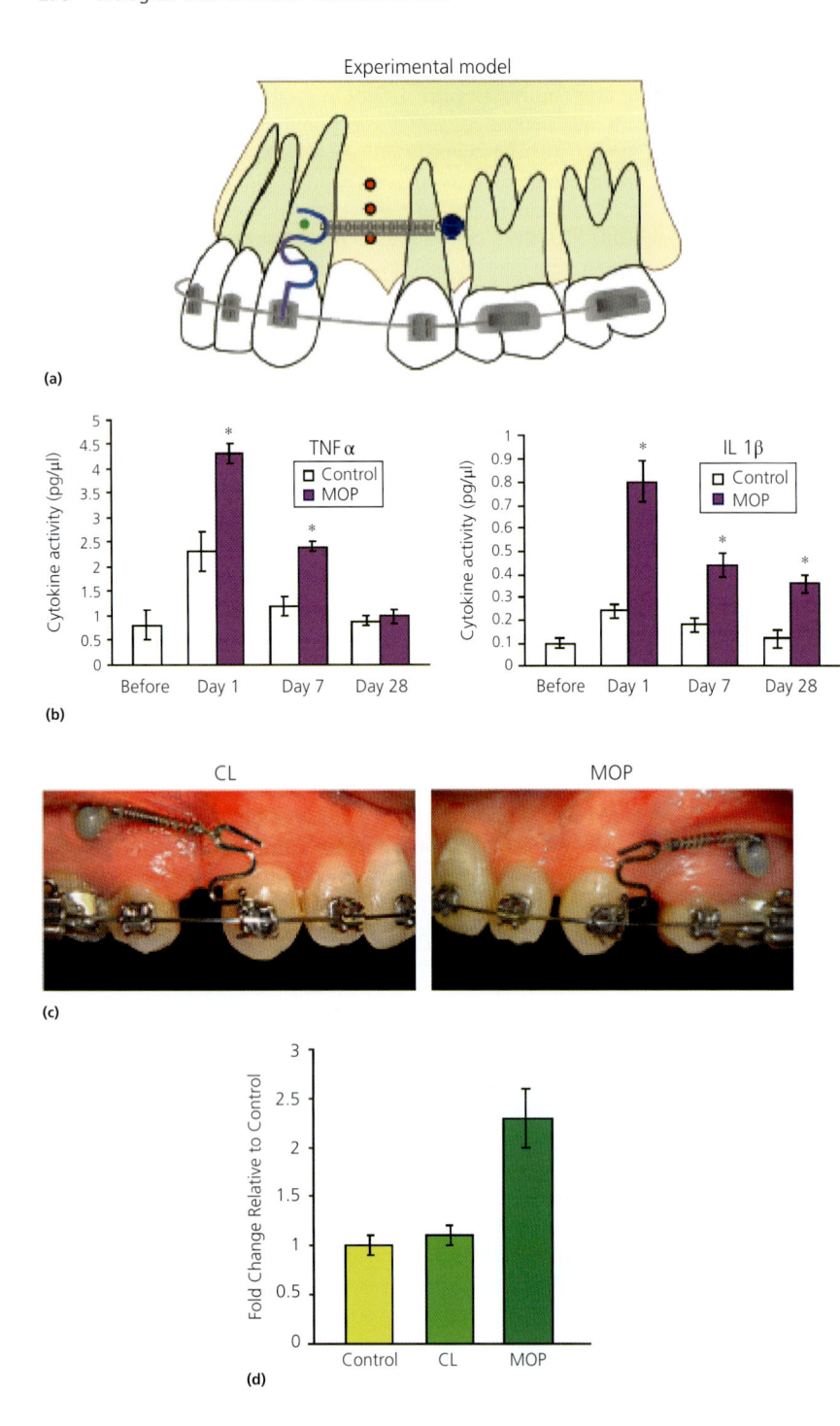

Figure 17.5 MOPs accelerate canine retraction in a human clinical study. In this study patients were assigned to a control group - C - and an experimental group, which received MOPs only on one side – MOP. The contralateral - CL - side of the experimental group functioned as an additional control. (a) Orthodontic setup during canine retraction. A power arm extending from the vertical slot of the canine bracket to the level of the center of resistance (CR, green dot) is connected to a temporary anchorage device (blue dot), placed between the second premolar and the first molar at the level of the CR of the canine, by a NiTi coil that exerts a continuous force of 50 cN. Three MOPs (red dots) were placed between the canine and the second premolar only on one side of the maxilla of the experimental group prior to retraction of left and right canines. The control group received the same retraction set up without MOPs application. (b) Expression of inflammatory markers in the GCF – as measured by enzyme-linked immunosorbent-based assay before retraction and 24 hours, 7 days, and 28 days after force application – shows significantly higher levels in the MOP side than in the control group. Data is presented as pg/uL. *Significantly higher than control ($P < 0.05$). (c) After 28 days of force application, the canine retraction is visibly greater in the MOP side than in the CL side (orthodontic force alone) of the experimental group. (d) Canine retraction in the MOP group increased by 2.3-fold after 28 days of retraction compared with the control group and the contralateral side (CL) of the experimental group. *Significantly different from control and contralateral side groups, $P < 0.05$). (Source: Modified from Alikhani et al., 2013; Alansari et al., 2017.)

ready to be moved. To accelerate the rate of movement, MOPs should be applied mostly in the direction of movement. However, the catabolic effects of MOPs are not limited to the point of application and can spread into the adjacent bone. This provides some leeway when attempting to find an adequate location for MOPs application.

2. Facilitate the desired type of tooth movement

MOPs not only affect the rate of tooth movement, they also can affect the type of tooth movement (Alikhani, 2017). The type of tooth movement depends on the relation between the force and the center of resistance of the tooth, which is determined by the surrounding bone. In denser bone, the center of resistance moves apically, which increases the distance between the point of force application (on the crown) and the center of resistance (on the root). Therefore, producing the desired bodily tooth movement requires a larger couple, to cancel the unwanted moments. However, when the bone density is low, the center of resistance moves occlusally towards the alveolar crest, which decreases the distance between the orthodontic force and the center of resistance, thereby reducing the couple required to overcome the unwanted moments (lower couple to force ratio) (Figure 17.6a). Thus, MOPs can help achieve the desired type of tooth movement by biologically changing the position of the center of resistance to a more favorable location, therefore facilitating difficult movements such as bodily movement.

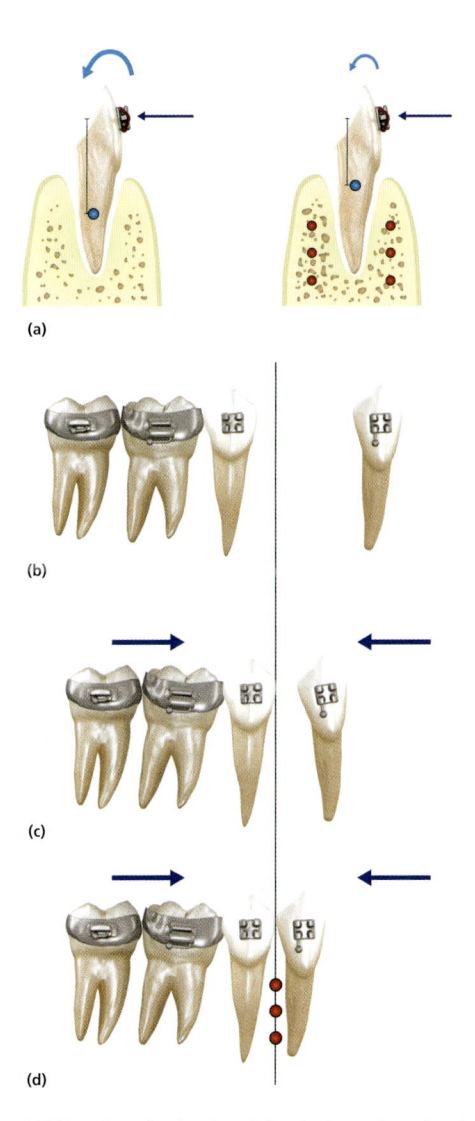

Figure 17.6 MOPs reduce the density of alveolar bone changing the response to orthodontic forces during tooth movement. (a) MOPS (red dots) reduces the density of alveolar bone, and as a result the center of resistance of a tooth (blue dot) moves occlusally, decreasing the moment generated by force application to the crown (curved blue arrow). MOPs could function as biological anchorage, by changing the density of alveolar bone surrounding the moving teeth. (b) Position of canine and posterior teeth before canine retraction. (c) During canine retraction, posterior teeth move mesially, while the canine moves distally. (d) After application of MOPs (red dots) posterior teeth move mesially, like (b), but the canine retraction and bodily movement increases during the same period. The increased distance travelled by the canine during retraction is not accompanied by additional movement of the anchor teeth, and it is accomplished by biological anchorage. (Source: Modified from Alikhani, 2017.)

3. Develop biological anchorage

During protraction or retraction of one tooth or a segment of teeth, the main concern in current mechanotherapy is how to minimize the movement of anchor teeth. The most common approach focuses on decreasing the rate of movement of the anchor tooth or teeth by increasing the size of the anchor unit. This approach assumes that the larger the anchorage mass, the slower or smaller the movement will be. This can be achieved by connecting the anchor teeth together through a transpalatal arch (TPA) or Nance appliance, adding second molars, interarch elastics, and other similar approaches designed to oppose a large number of anchor teeth against a smaller number of target teeth. While this is a good approach, similar results can be achieved by increasing the rate of movement of the target unit. By increasing the speed of target teeth movement through decreasing surrounding bone density, while preserving the bone density around the anchor unit, it is possible to add a biological component to the anchorage preparation (Figure 17.6b–d; Alikhani, 2017). With this understanding of anchor and target teeth, we can now easily define the area for application of MOPs. For example, for canine retraction or anterior teeth retraction, MOPs should be applied adjacent to the canine or anterior teeth. Conversely, to increase anterior anchorage during posterior protraction, MOPs should be applied around the posterior teeth.

4. Decrease the possibility of root resorption

In patients with very dense alveolar bone, any tooth movement may result in significant root resorption (Iglesias-Linares *et al.*, 2016). This is especially more likely in those movements that produce concentrated stress on a small area of the root, such as the apex. This can occur during intrusion or torqueing. However, even during movements that distribute stress over larger areas of root, if dense bone prevents quick bone clearance by osteoclasts along the path of movement, these osteoclasts will stay in the area for a long time, which allows them to attack the alveolar bone and adjacent roots. By applying MOPs, it is possible to increase the number of osteoclasts significantly along the path of movement compared with non-MOPs treatment, which increases the rate of bone resorption and tooth movement. Therefore, osteoclasts will not linger in one area long enough to attack the root(s) of the target tooth which rapidly move through the less dense bone of the MOPs site, allowing for faster tooth movement without root resorption (Aboalnaga *et al.*, 2019).

5. Moving teeth through atrophic bone

One of the challenges of orthodontic treatment is moving teeth in areas of significant bone loss, such as the residual alveolar ridge of an old extraction. These areas can also develop due to traumatic extraction, or lack of development of alveolar bone around an ankylosed tooth. MOPs in the area not only facilitate movement of teeth, but also stimulate bone formation, which helps keep the integrity of alveolar bone around the tooth moving into the atrophic bone area (Lee *et al.*, 2018).

In conclusion, MOPs are indicated not only to accelerate tooth movement but also in many orthodontics applications, including to move teeth for large distances to close spaces or into areas of atrophic bone, for intrusion of a tooth or segment of teeth, severe rotations, molar uprighting, root torque, and all clinical situations when reduced bone density can facilitate the proper type of tooth movement, and lessen the possibility of root resorption.

Good vibrations: catabolic response during OTM

Applying vibration in the form of high frequency acceleration (HFA) in the absence of any pathology or inflammation has an osteogenic effect on long bones and craniofacial bones, specifically alveolar bone (Garman *et al.*, 2007; Alikhani *et al.*, 2012). Likewise, applying HFA to healing bones, after the source of pathology has been eliminated, prevents extensive bone resorption and stimulates bone formation (Omar et al., 2008; Goodship et al., 2009; Alikhani et al., 2015). In both situations, HFA applied directly to the target site or indirectly to an adjacent site, does not induce any inflammatory mediators or increase the number of osteoclasts.

Several prospective randomized controlled clinical trials, pilot studies, or animal studies have recently investigated the effect of vibration on OTM (Miles et al., 2012; Pavlin et al., 2015; Yadav et al., 2015; Yang and Li, 2015; Liao et al., 2017). The differences in these treatment outcomes are controversial and still unclear, as some of these studies report that vibration increases the rate of tooth movement, while others found no effect. Moreover, these studies have not identified isolated effects of vibration characteristics, such as different acceleration, resultant load, frequency, and duration of applied load, thus making data interpretation and drawing definitive, clinically important conclusions exceedingly difficult. Recent systematic reviews reinforce the need for further study to resolve conflicting data in this area (Aljabaa et al., 2018; Lyu et al., 2019).

Given the strong anabolic effect of HFA on healthy and healing bones, one would hypothesize that HFA (vibration) application would inhibit any process that is inflammation-dependent, such as OTM. However, this hypothesis must be evaluated carefully. It is critical to recognize that conditions under which HFA is anabolic (i.e., when inflammatory mediators are at baseline or slightly above baseline and declining) are significantly different from conditions under which OTM occurs (i.e., when inflammatory mediators are significantly elevated).

When we applied HFA (0.05 g, 120 Hz, 5 min a day), during OTM in rats (Alikhani et al., 2018a), we observed an 2.3-fold increase in the rate of tooth movement compared with orthodontic force alone (Figure 17.7a, b). In addition, both an increase in the acceleration and frequency (Figure 17.7c) resulted in an increase in the rate of tooth movement. Interestingly, the effect of HFA on tooth movement was only observed when the vibration was applied to the tooth receiving the orthodontic force and not the adjacent teeth, suggesting the effect is mediated by the PDL. Indeed, application of HFA to the moving tooth significantly increased the levels of inflammatory markers in the tissues surrounding the tooth (Figure 17.8a), increased the number of osteoclasts around the roots of the moving teeth (Figure 17.8b), and decreased the bone density measured by microCT (Figure 17.8c).

While the anabolic effects of HFA are consistently observed in tissues that are healthy or in a repair phase (Garman et al., 2007; Omar et al., 2008; Goodship et al., 2009; Alikhani et al., 2012; Alikhani et al., 2015), in the presence of elevated levels of inflammatory mediators, HFA intensified the existing inflammation. In fact, without orthodontic forces – and the inflammation that accompanies them – no HFA-induced increase in inflammatory markers was observed (Alikhani et al., 2018a). Furthermore, the inflammatory markers are not only necessary for OTM, they are the main mechanism through which HFA increased the rate of tooth movement because treatment with NSAIDs decreased the rate of HFA-accelerated tooth movement.

Our studies demonstrated that different characteristics of vibration can significantly affect the rate of tooth movement in rats. In this regard, acceleration plays a significant role in the rate of tooth movement. However, from a practical point of view,

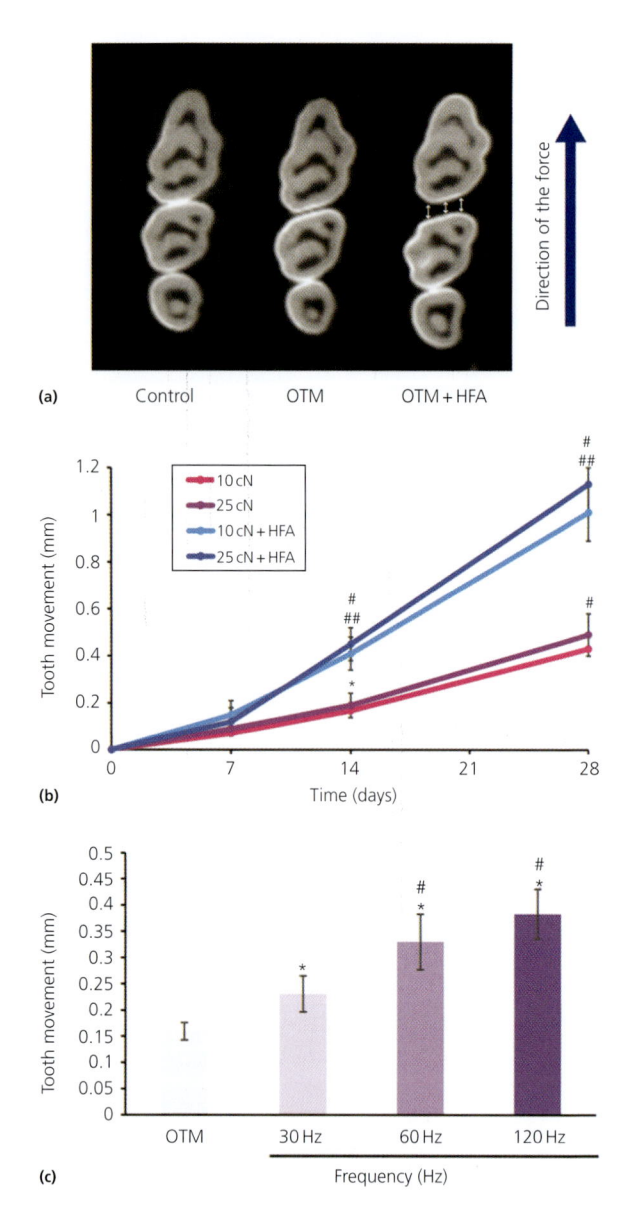

Figure 17.7 Vibration in the form of high frequency acceleration (HFA) stimulates the rate of OTM. Adult rats were exposed to orthodontic force alone or in combination with direct application of different HFA on the occlusal surface of maxillary right first molar. (a) Tooth movement was measured in the axial slice from the microCT scan of maxillary right molars at the level maximum convexity (height of contour) for control (no movement), orthodontic tooth movement (OTM) and OTM + HFA shown here for 14 days treatment with 10 cN force and HFA (120 Hz, 0.05 g for 5 min a day). (b) Rate of tooth movement on day 7, 14, and 28 after application of 10 cN or 25 cN orthodontic forces in the absence or presence of HFA for 5 min a day. Each value represents the mean ± SEM of four samples. (*Significantly different from day 0 for both forces, # significantly different from day 7 for both forces, ## significantly different from OTM group at same time point for both forces.) (c) Effect of different frequencies on the rate of tooth movement under 0.05 g acceleration for 5 minutes per day for 14 days in the presence of 10 cN orthodontic force (* Significantly different from OTM; # significantly different from 30 Hz, $P < 0.05$.) (Source: Modified from Alikhani et al., 2018a.)

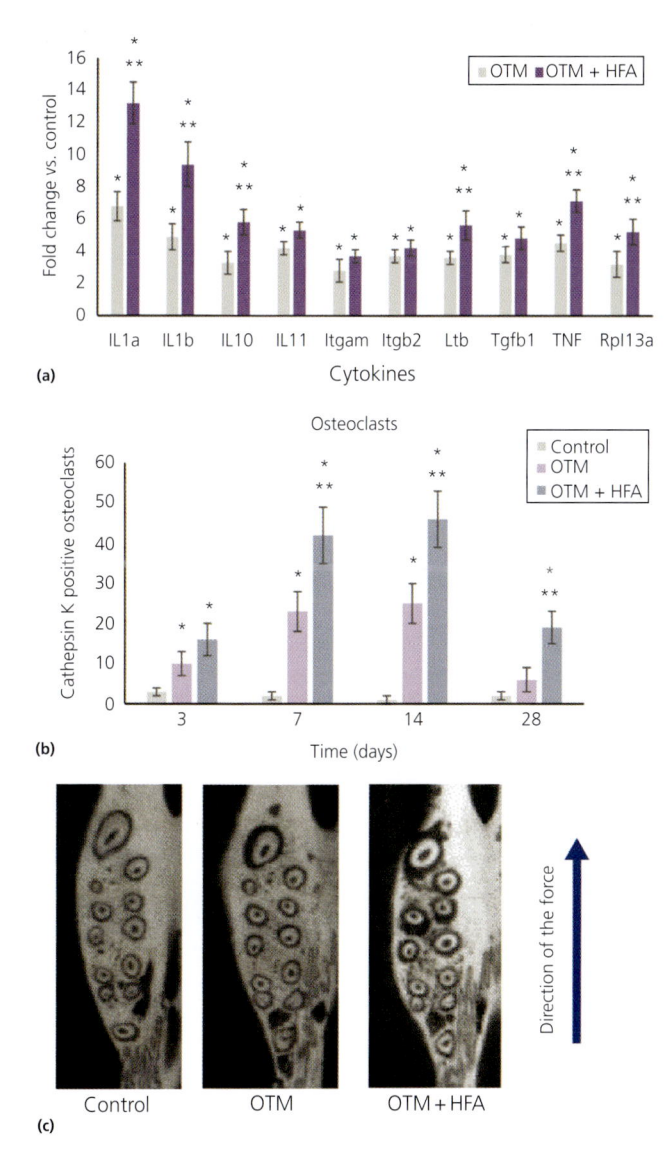

Figure 17.8 Vibration increases inflammatory markers and the number and activity of osteoclasts during tooth movement. (a) Cytokines (IL1a or interleukin-1alpha, IL1b or interleukin-1beta, IL10 or interleukin-10, IL11 or interleukin-11, Itgam or integrin sub-unit alpha M, Itgb2 or integrin beta 2, Ltb or lymphotoxin beta, Tgfb1 or transforming growth factor beta 1, TNF or tumor necrosis factor, and Rpl 13a or Ribosomal protein L 13a) were quantified by real time RT-PCR in maxillary right alveolar bone 24 hours after application of orthodontic force in the presence or absence of HFA (120 Hz, 0.05 g) stimulation. Data expressed as fold change in comparison with control (no movement) and as the mean ± SEM of five samples (*significantly different from control; **significantly different from OTM, $P < 0.05$). (b) We evaluated the number of cathepsin K–positive osteoclasts in immunohistochemically stained sections of the maxilla. Mean number of osteoclasts at different time points, in PDL, and adjacent alveolar bone of the mesiopalatal root of the maxillary first molar. Each value represents the mean ± SEM of four animals (*significantly different from control; **significantly different from OTM group, $P < 0.05$). (c) Representative axial microCT sections showing decrease in bone density in OTM+ HFA at 14 days. Arrow demonstrates the direction of force application. (Source: Modified from Alikhani et al., 2018b.)

there is a limit to how much we can increase acceleration, since an increase in acceleration is accompanied by an increase in loading of the PDL and alveolar bone, which can be uncomfortable for the patient. Under clinically acceptable acceleration, increasing vibrational frequency can increase the rate of tooth movement. However, after a certain frequency magnitude and duration, the effect plateaus and no further increase in the rate of tooth movement is observed (Alikhani et al., 2018a). This observation demonstrates that, like constant orthodontic forces, dynamic stimulation may also reach a biological saturation point, which requires further clarification. Therefore, based on these results, the physical characteristics of vibration should be more clearly defined before we can compare the results of different studies and reach conclusions on the effectiveness of the clinical application of this procedure. For example, some of the previous animal studies, which concluded that vibration cannot increase the rate of tooth movement, have used lower acceleration and lower frequencies (Miles et al., 2012; Yadav et al., 2015). Our study confirmed that lower acceleration and lower frequency are not very effective in increasing the rate of tooth movement (Alikhani et al., 2018a).

Conclusion

Evidence now exists that clarifies what happens when orthodontic force is applied to teeth (Figure 17.9). Inflammatory cells inundate the surrounding PDL space and release an array of powerful chemokines and cytokines that trigger osteoclastogenesis and osteoclast activity in the catabolic phase of the biphasic theory. Critically, this response occurs around the entire root, thereby freeing the tooth and PDL to move in the direction of the orthodontic force. As the tooth moves, the magnitude of the force dissipates, decreasing the inflammatory response. Reactivating the force reactivates the inflammatory response, allowing for continued tooth movement. In an otherwise healthy individual, increasing inflammation locally MOPs (MOPs in Figure 17.9) or vibration (HFA in Figure 17.9) enhances bone resorption by osteoclasts, decreasing bone density, and allowing clinicians to move teeth more easily. The catabolic phase is followed by the anabolic phase, in which osteoblasts regenerate bone to begin the process of stabilizing the tooth, PDL, and alveolar bone complex in its new configuration.

A deep understanding of the biology of tooth movement is as critical for successful development of innovative approaches to orthodontics treatment as it is for a successful orthodontic therapy in our daily practices. Knowledge of biomechanical principles is one half of designing a successful orthodontic therapy, while understanding the biological response to our force systems is the other half and as important in producing the desired treatment outcome. In this chapter we demonstrate how our critical review of existing data combined with our own data on bone remodeling under orthodontic forces, guided the development of the biphasic theory of tooth movement, and revolutionized our approach to precision accelerated orthodontics using MOPs and vibration. Our hope is that our success will inspire more clinicians and/or scientists to contribute to advances in orthodontics treatment using sound translational orthodontics research methodologies.

274 Biological Mechanisms of Tooth Movement

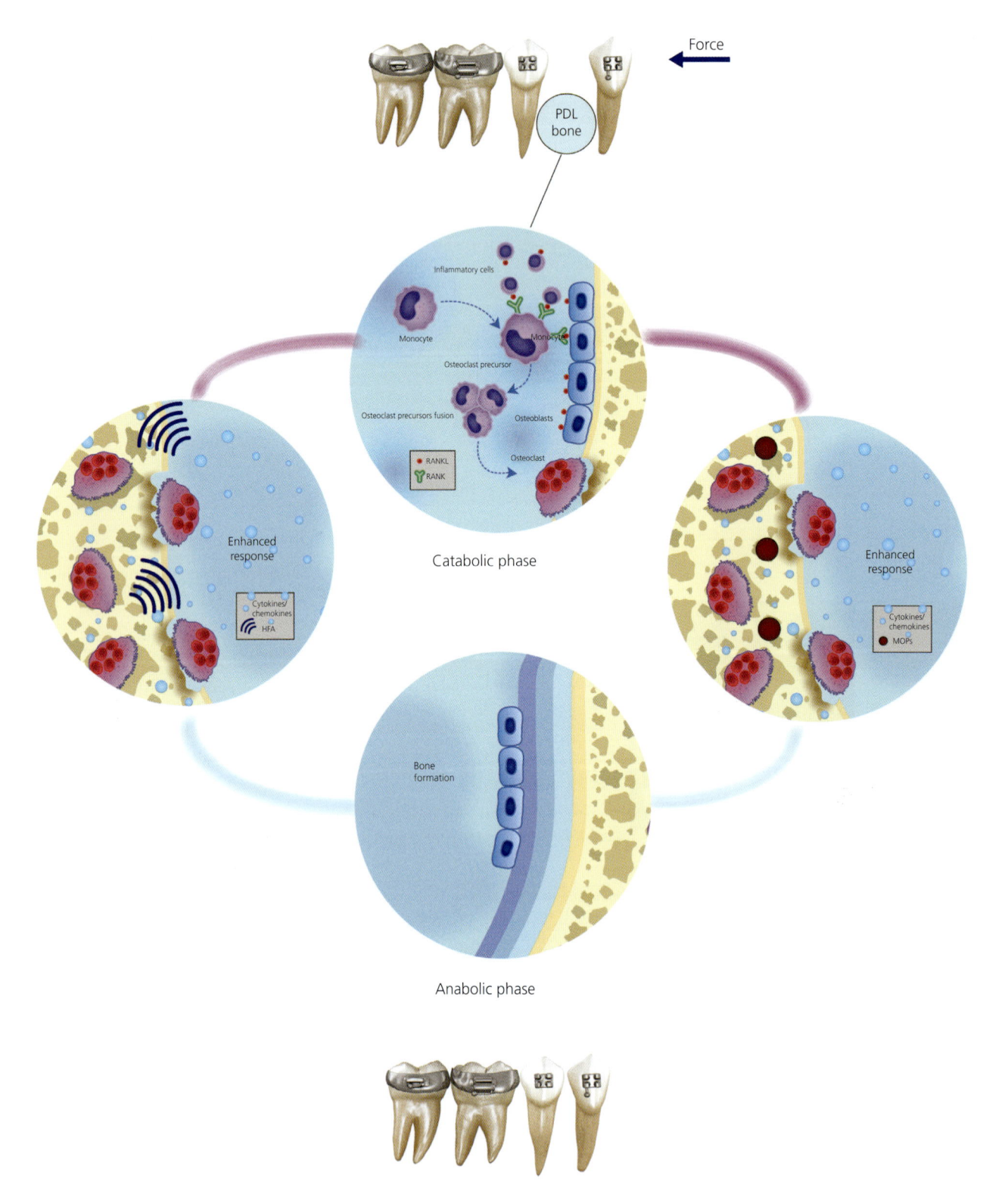

Figure 17.9 Harnessing inflammation to deliver precision-accelerated tooth movement: practical application of the biphasic theory. Applying orthodontic force to teeth triggers a robust, predictable, and controllable inflammatory response during the catabolic phase of tooth movement. Local inflammatory cells release an array of powerful cytokines and chemokines that attracts additional inflammatory cells to the site and trigger osteoclast differentiation and activation. Localized bone resorption around the whole tooth allows the tooth to move, and PDL and alveolar bone to remodel in the direction of the orthodontic force. Increasing inflammation locally through MOPs or vibration (HFA) enhances bone resorption by osteoclasts, decreasing bone density, allowing to move teeth more easily. As the force dissipates, the catabolic phase also dissipates due to declining inflammatory cell and osteoclast activity. If the orthodontic force is not reactivated, the catabolic phase gives way to the anabolic phase, during which osteoblasts regenerate bone around the whole root and the PDL remodels allowing the tooth, PDL, and alveolar bone complex to stabilize around the new tooth position. This process is time consuming, requiring retention once the orthodontics appliance is removed to ensure stability of the final occlusion. (Source: Drs. Alikhani, Nervina and Teixeira.)

References

Aboalnaga, A. A., Fayed, M. M. S., El-Ashmawi, N. A. and Soliman, S. A. (2019) Effect of micro-osteoperforation on the rate of canine retraction: a split-mouth randomized controlled trial. *Progress in Orthodontics* **20**, 21.

Alansari, S., Teixeira, C. C., Sangsuwon, C. and Alikhani, M. (2017) Introduction to micro-osteoperforations, in *Clinical Guide to Accelerated Orthodontics: With a Focus on Micro-Osteoperforations* (ed. M. Alikhani). Springer, New York, pp. 33–42.

Alikhani, M. (Ed.) (2017) *Clinical Guide to Accelerated Orthodontics: With a Focus on Micro-Osteoperforations*. Springer, New York.

Alikhani, M., Alansari, S., Hamidaddin, M. A. *et al.* (2018a) Vibration paradox in orthodontics: anabolic and catabolic effects. *PLoS One* **13**(5), e0196540.

Alikhani, M., Alyami, B., Lee, I. S. *et al.* (2015) Saturation of the biological response to orthodontic forces and its effect on the rate of tooth movement. *Orthodontic and Craniofacial Research* **18**(Suppl. 1), 8–17.

Alikhani, M., Khoo, E., Alyami, B. *et al.* (2012) Osteogenic effect of high-frequency acceleration on alveolar bone. *Journal of Dental Research* **91**(4), 413–419.

Alikhani, M., Sangsuwon, C., Alansari, S. *et al.* (2018b). Biphasic theory: breakthrough understanding of tooth movement. *Journal of the World Federation of Orthodontists* **7**(3), 82–88.

Alikhani, M., Raptis, M., Zodan B. *et al.* (2013) Effect of micro-osteoperforations on the rate of tooth movement. *American Journal of Orthodontics and Dentofacial Orthopedics* **144**(5), 639–648.

Aljabaa, A., Almoammar, K., Aldrees, A. and Huang, G. (2018) Effects of vibrational devices on orthodontic tooth movement: a systematic review. *American Journal of Orthodontics and Dentofacial Orthopedics* **154**(6), 768–779.

Baumrind, S. (1969) A reconsideration of the propiety of the "pressure-tension" hypothesis. *American Journal of Orthodontics* **55**(1), 12–22.

Garman, R., Rubin, C. and Judex, S. (2007) Small oscillatory accelerations, independent of matrix deformations, increase osteoblast activity and enhance bone morphology. *PLoS One* **2**(7), e653.

Goodship, A. E., Lawes, T. J. and Rubin, C. T. (2009) Low-magnitude high-frequency mechanical signals accelerate and augment endochondral bone repair: preliminary evidence of efficacy. *Journal of Orthopedic Research* **27**(7), 922–930.

Hughes, J. M., Popp, K. L., Yanovich, R. *et al.* (2017) The role of adaptive bone formation in the etiology of stress fracture. *Experimental and Biological Medicine (Maywood)* **242**(9), 897–906.

Iglesias-Linares, A., Morford, L. A. and Hartsfield, J.K., Jr. (2016) Bone density and dental external root resorption. *Current Osteoporosis Reports* **14**(6), 292–309.

Lee, J.-W., Cha, J.-Y., Park, K.-H. *et al.* (2018) Effect of flapless osteoperforation-assisted tooth movement on atrophic alveolar ridge: histomorphometric and gene-enrichment analysis. *The Angle Orthodontist* **88**(1), 82–90.

Liao, Z., Elekdag-Turk, S., Turk, T. *et al.* (2017) Computational and clinical investigation on the role of mechanical vibration on orthodontic tooth movement. *Journal of Biomechanics* **60**, 57–64.

Lyu, C., Zhang, L. and Zou, S. (2019) The effectiveness of supplemental vibrational force on enhancing orthodontic treatment. A systematic review. *European Journal of Orthodontics* **41**(5), 502–512.

Matsuo, K. and Irie, N. (2008) Osteoclast-osteoblast communication. *Archives of Biochemistry and Biophysics* **473**(2), 201–209.

Miles, P., Smith, H., Weyant, R. and Rinchuse, D. J. (2012) The effects of a vibrational appliance on tooth movement and patient discomfort: a prospective randomised clinical trial. *Australian Orthodontic Journal* **28**(2), 213–218.

Omar, H., Shen, G., Jones, A. S. *et al.* (2008) Effect of low magnitude and high frequency mechanical stimuli on defects healing in cranial bones. *Journal of Oral and Maxillofacial Surgery* **66**(6), 1104–1111.

Pavlin, D., Anthony, R., Raj, V. and Gakunga, P. T. (2015) Cyclic loading (vibration) accelerates tooth movement in orthodontic patients: a double-blind, randomized controlled trial. *Seminars in Orthodontics* **21**(3), 187–194.

Proffit, W. R., Fields, H. W., Sarver, D. M. and Ackerman, J. L. (Eds.). (2013) *Contemporary Orthodontics*, 5th edn. Elsevier, St. Louis, MO.

Quinn, R. S. and Yoshikawa, D. K. (1985) A reassessment of force magnitude in orthodontics. *American Journal of Orthodontics* **88**(3), 252–260.

Teixeira, C. C., Khoo, E., Tran, J. *et al.* (2010) Cytokine expression and accelerated tooth movement. *Journal of Dental Research* **89**(10), 1135–1141.

Theodorou, C. I., Kuijpers-Jagtman, A. M., Bronkhorst, E. M. and Wagener, F. A. D. T.G. (2019) Optimal force magnitude for bodily orthodontic tooth movement with fixed appliances: a systematic review. *American Journal of Orthodontics and Dentofacial Orthopedics* **156**(5), 582–592.

Van Leeuwen, E. J., Kuijpers-Jagtman, A. M., Von den Hoff, J. W. *et al.* (2010) Rate of orthodontic tooth movement after changing the force magnitude: an experimental study in beagle dogs. *Orthodontic and Craniofacial Research* **13**(4), 238–245.

Yadav, S., Dobie, T., Assefnia, A. *et al.* (2015) Effect of low-frequency mechanical vibration on orthodontic tooth movement. *American Journal of Orthodontics and Dentofacial Orthopedics* **148**(3), 440–449.

Yang, Y. and Li, Y. (2015) Re: Vibratory stimulation increases interleukin-1 beta secretion during orthodontic tooth movement. Chidchanok Leethanakul; Sumit Suamphan; Suwanna Jitpukdeebodintra; Udom Thongudomporn; Chairat Charoemratrote. 2015, Online Early. *The Angle Orthodontist* **85**(5), 899.

Yee, J. A., Turk, T., Elekdag-Turk, S. *et al.* (2009) Rate of tooth movement under heavy and light continuous orthodontic forces. *American Journal of Orthodontics and Dentofacial Orthopedics* **136**(2), 150 e151–159; discussion 150–151.

PART 6

Long-term Effects of Tooth-moving Forces

CHAPTER 18
Mechanical and Biological Determinants of Iatrogenic Injuries in Orthodontics

Vinod Krishnan, Ambili Renjithkumar, and Ze'ev Davidovitch

> **Summary**
>
> Orthodontic treatment affects not only the teeth and their surrounding tissues but also the extraoral tissues, psychological status, and the systemic health of the patient. If orthodontic treatment is to benefit the patient, the advantage it offers should outweigh the potential damage it might create. Although most orthodontically treated cases are successful, failures, imperfections, and difficulties do occur sometimes. To reduce and minimize the prevalence and extent of these negative outcomes, it is strongly recommended that all practicing orthodontists, as well as residents, be keenly aware and thoroughly familiar with the etiology of all possible untoward effects of the treatment mechanics they render, because of their legal and ethical implications. This chapter is aimed at discussing the iatrogenic or untoward effects that can follow orthodontic force application and possible ways to manage them as and when they appear. It is useful to generate proper communication with the patient to promote trust and improved oral hygiene habits, which will definitely help to increase patient compliance. At times, when iatrogenic damage is observed, proper consultation with the pertinent specialist should be sought without hesitation, to avoid complicating matters, benefiting the patients as well as our own clinical practice.

Introduction

Orthodontic forces, the prescription for correcting malocclusions, can be considered to have a multi-potential nature. To effect tooth movement, these forces depend on tissue and cellular reactions because of alterations of the stress-strain distributions in paradental tissues. Various systems of force application are capable of evoking different responses, both favorable and unfavorable, as evidenced by numerous studies. In general, orthodontics should not result in any appreciable damage to the dental and paradental tissues, if proper care is taken in diagnosis, treatment planning and treatment. It is prudent to note that when these principles are neglected or circumvented, the damage produced by the mechanics may become considerable, outweighing the potential benefits of treatment (Shaw *et al.*, 1991).

Iatrogenic damage is defined as "any adverse condition in a patient resulting from treatment by a physician, nurse, or allied health professional" (http://www.encyclo. co.uk/define/iatrogenic, accessed May 17, 2020). Every aspect of medical and dental treatment has a possibility of success or failure. Orthodontics is no exception to this rule. Although success is prevalent in most orthodontically treated cases, failures, imperfections, and difficulties do sometimes occur. Experienced clinicians may unwillingly engender such untoward effects, and then proceed to report these outcomes in the literature. To reduce and minimize the prevalence and extent of these negative outcomes, it is strongly recommended that all practicing orthodontists, as well as residents, be keenly aware and thoroughly familiar with the etiology of all possible untoward effects of the treatment mechanics they render, because of their potential legal consequences and ethical implications.

According to Behrents (1996), iatrogenic effects of orthodontic treatment can be avoided if the orthodontist routinely adopts the following steps:

1. Formulate a correct and comprehensive diagnosis.
2. Consult with the appropriate general practitioner.
3. Refer appropriately to specialists in other areas of medicine and dentistry.
4. Refrain from adopting an incorrect or dangerous treatment strategy.
5. Perform treatment at the appropriate time.
6. Alter the original treatment plan in mid-treatment if there are unforeseen developments.
7. Successfully resolve the malocclusion.
8. Establish proper communication with the patient.
9. Provide proper follow-up care.

Biological Mechanisms of Tooth Movement, Third Edition. Edited by Vinod Krishnan, Anne Marie Kuijpers-Jagtman and Ze'ev Davidovitch.
© 2021 John Wiley & Sons Ltd. Published 2021 by John Wiley & Sons Ltd.

Table 18.1 Iatrogenic effects of orthodontic force application and mechanics.

Tissue affected	Effect
Intraoral effects	
Gingiva and periodontal ligament	Gingivitis
	Periodontitis
	Gingival recession
	Dark triangles
	Poor gingival contours
Alveolar bone	Crestal bone resorption
Dental roots	Root resorption
	Early closure of the apex
Enamel	Decalcification
	Damage or fracture
	Excessive wear
Pulp	(Ir)reversible pulp damage
	Internal root resorption
Soft tissues (buccal and labial mucosa)	Ulcerations due to appliances
	Direct trauma
	Effect of clumsy instrumentation
Pain and discomfort	Soft tissue cleft formation
Extraoral effects	
Face	Headgear injuries (direct trauma and eye damage)
	Chemical burn from etchant
	Thermal burns from overheated instruments
	Nickel-induced sensitivity
	Allergy
	Cytotoxicity
	Unfavorable profile change
Temporomandibular joint	Dysfunction
	Condylar resorption
Systemic risks	
Heart	Infective endocarditis
Gastrointestinal/respiratory tract	Inhalation/swallowing of small parts
Systemic diseases	Bone, blood or endocrine diseases
Cross infection	Operator to patient
	Patient to operator
Growth	Unfavorable growth direction and/or amount
Psychological effects	
Effect	Depression
	Teasing
	Abnormal/patient/parent behavior
	Poor cooperation
Treatment results	
Effects	Non-ideal results
	Unable to maintain results
	Failed treatment
	Prolonged treatment duration

Orthodontic therapy affects not only the teeth and their surrounding tissues but also extraoral tissues that serve as anchorage sources for tooth movement. In addition, the mechanics and the subsequent inflammatory reactions can affect the psychological status, as well as the systemic health, of the patient. Hence, it seems reasonable to postulate that orthodontic treatment may have a profound influence on patients' dentofacial and general health. This chapter outlines and discusses the iatrogenic or untoward effects that can follow orthodontic force application. A classification system for the iatrogenic effects observed as part of orthodontic mechanotherapy is provided in Table 18.1.

Intraoral iatrogenic effects

The sequential events following force application leading to tooth movement have been elucidated and it has been concluded that inflammation is a process of significant importance in force-induced tissue remodeling (see Chapters 3 and 4 of this book). Force application, its duration, direction, and magnitude determine the nature of inflammatory changes that occur during treatment. Research has also shed light on the elevated levels of signaling molecules in the gingival crevicular fluid of moving teeth, both useful and harmful to the human body. Inappropriate mechanics, poor oral hygiene, and abnormal force application can lead to intraoral iatrogenic damage to teeth and paradental tissues (Travess et al., 2004). These effects may affect all components of the craniofacial complex, including the dental enamel, pulp, cementum, gingiva, periodontal ligament (PDL), bone, cartilage, and muscle. The susceptibility to adverse responses to applied mechanical forces and the extent of the damage is determined, at least in part, by the genetic composition of the individual (see Chapter 12).

Gingival effects

The introduction of fixed orthodontic appliances into the oral cavity in the form of orthodontic bands and resin-bonded attachments often evokes a local soft-tissue response inconsistent with health or esthetic treatment goals. The proximity of these attachments to the gingival sulcus, plaque accumulation, and the impediments they pose to oral hygiene habits further complicate the process of efficient salutary orthodontic care (Zachrisson, 1972; Zachrisson and Alnaes, 1973). The effects seen clinically following the insertion of orthodontic appliances into the oral cavity can contribute to chronic infection, inflammatory hyperplasia, gingival recession, irreversible loss of attachment (permanent bone loss), and excessive accumulation of gingival tissue, inhibiting complete closure of extraction spaces.

Clinically visible changes

Orthodontic mechanotherapy can produce local changes in the oral microbial ecosystem and alter the composition of the bacterial plaque, tipping the scale toward the inflammatory process. This trend is evident by the increased severity of gingival inflammation observed immediately after fixed appliance placement. Fixed appliances frequently encroach upon the gingival sulcus, inhibiting effective oral hygiene maintenance (Anderson et al., 1997). Zachrisson and Zachrisson (1972) reported that even after maintaining seemingly excellent oral hygiene, patients usually experience mild to moderate gingivitis within one to two months of appliance placement. Virtually all studies have reported that orthodontic appliances act as protective havens for bacterial plaque accumulation, providing an encumbrance to oral hygiene procedures, leading to gingival inflammation, bleeding on probing, and even destructive periodontal diseases.

Kloehn and Pfeifer (1974) reported that the average incidence of gingival enlargement was four times greater around posterior teeth compared with incisors and canines in orthodontic patients (Figures 18.1 and 18.2). They listed the following causes:
- mechanical irritation by bands, more on posterior than on anterior teeth;
- chemical irritation produced by cements used for banding;
- food impaction, because of the proximity of the archwires to the soft tissues; and
- less efficient oral hygiene maintenance.

They reported greater incidence of gingival enlargement at the interdental region, while Zachrisson (1972) found that the mandibular incisor region harbors the highest risk for the development of gingival hyperplasia. It was demonstrated that there would be a

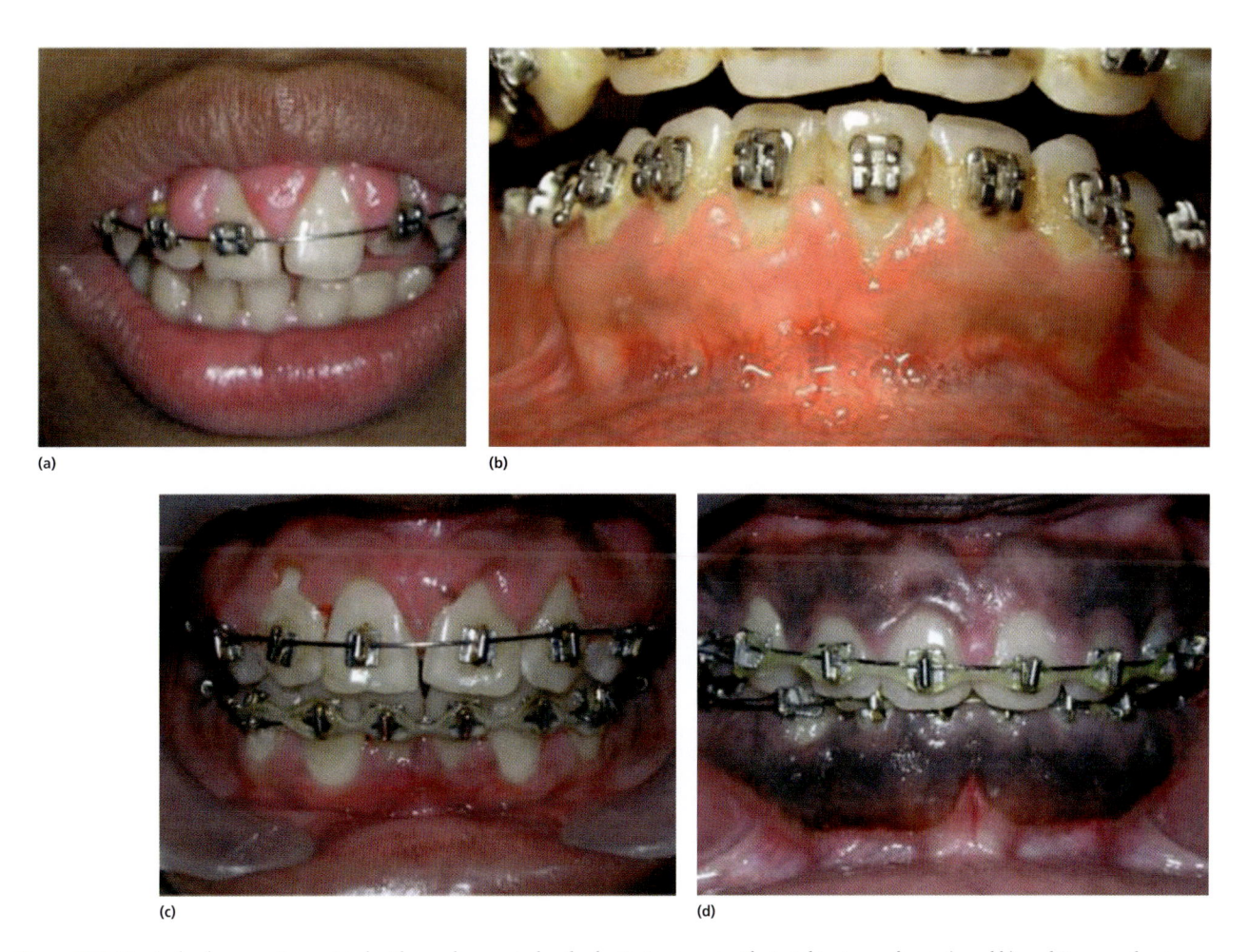

Figure 18.1 Gingival enlargement associated with poorly executed orthodontic treatment with straight wire appliance (a and b), and Begg mechanics (c and d). (a) Patient with mouth breathing and plaque accumulation, with an orthodontic appliance as a plaque-harboring area, leading to gingival enlargement. Note improper use of elastomeric chain in Begg mechanotherapy promoting food entrapment, plaque accumulation, and gingival inflammation and enlargement. (Source: Dr. Arun Sadasivan, MDS, Periodontist, Trivandrum, Kerala, India. Reproduced with permission of Dr. Arun Sadasivan.)

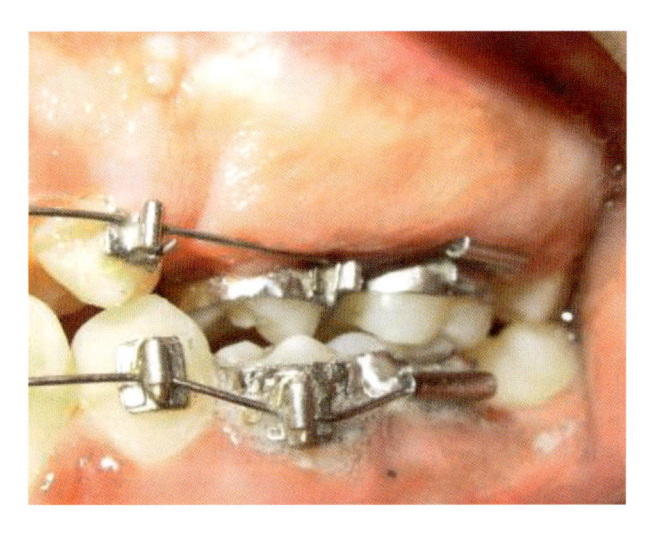

Figure 18.2 The effect of poor placement of orthodontic bands. The first molar and the second premolars were banded. Note the amount of gingival enlargement around the bands. (Source: Dr. Vinod Krishnan.)

sudden remission of this hyperplastic response within 48 hours of appliance removal (Kloehn and Pfeifer, 1974).

Gingival recession is defined as "the exposure of the root surface by an apical shift in the position of gingiva" (Gorman, 1967). Geiger (1980) reported that the incidence of gingival recession with fixed orthodontic appliances ranges from 1.3 to 10%. Dorfman (1978) suggested that mandibular incisors may be more prone to recession than any other teeth (Figure 18.3). The predisposing factors making the teeth prone to this process include:

- a thin or nonexistent labial plate of bone;
- an inadequate or absent keratinized gingiva;
- labial prominence of teeth;
- patients with chronic or marginal gingivitis;
- expansion mechanics;
- anterior thrust by Class II elastics.

The effects of gingival recession can be summarized as being associated with the development of:

- poor esthetics;
- susceptibility to root caries;
- root sensitivity;

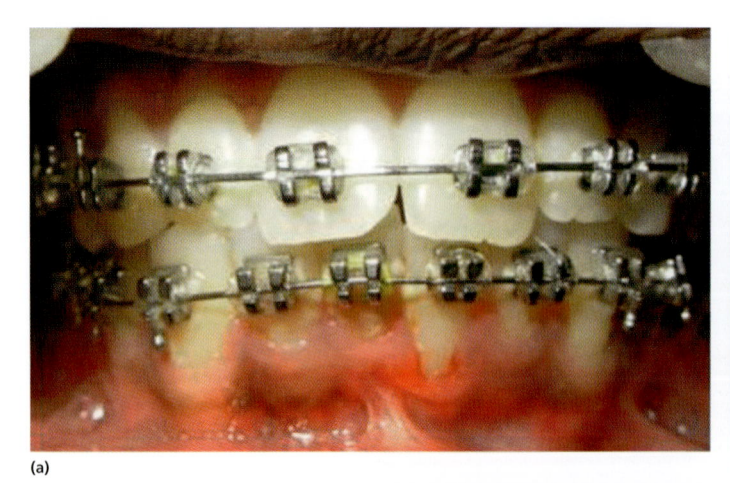

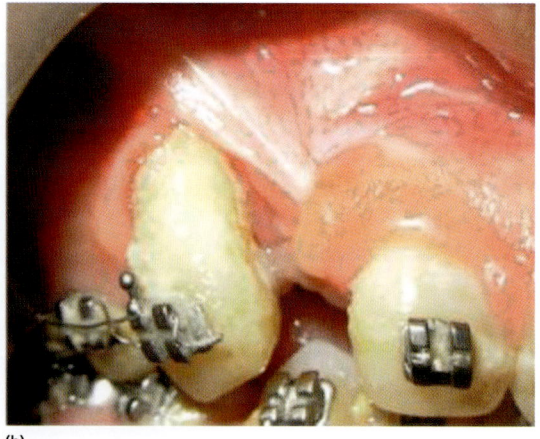

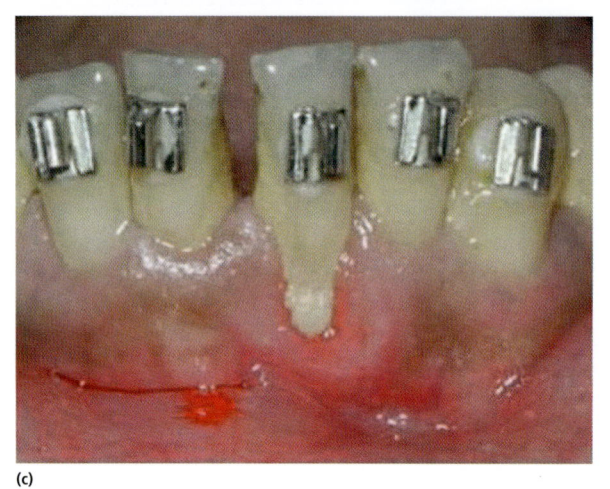

Figure 18.3 Gingival recession associated with orthodontic treatment. (a) Recession in the mandibular incisor region due to round tripping of the teeth resulting from the use of a round wire for retraction. (b) A poorly compliant patient treated with canine distraction. Due to lack of care, the sutures placed after corticotomy cuts were lost, which led to a severe gingival recession. (c) An example of poorly executed orthodontic mechanics. Note the amount of adhesive remaining below the bracket bases, promoting gingival inflammation and recession. (Source: Dr. Arun Sadasivan, MDS, Periodontist, Trivandrum, Kerala, India. Reproduced with permission of Dr. Arun Sadasivan.)

- loss of periodontal support;
- difficulty in oral hygiene maintenance.

It was suggested by Wennstrom and Prini Prato (2003) that, if the teeth are within their alveolar bone envelope, the risk of harmful effects to the gingival tissue is minimal. A systematic review by Joss-Vassalli *et al.* (2010) reported lack of high-quality animal or clinical studies on the topic. They concluded that the movement of the incisors out of the osseous envelope promotes a higher tendency for gingival recessions. In concordance, Antonarakis *et al.* (2017) has reported that orthodontic or surgical proclination of lower incisors beyond a 10° limit increases the risk of inducing lingual gingival recessions. In a long-term assessment, Morris *et al.* (2017) reported that only 5.8% of teeth exhibited recession at the end of orthodontic treatment out of which only 0.6% had a recession >1 mm. After retention, 41.7% of the teeth showed recession, but the severity was limited (only 7.0% >1 mm). Interestingly, incisors that finished treatment angulated (incisor mandibular plane angle; IMPA) at 95° or greater did not show significantly more recession than did those that finished less than 95°. Renkema *et al.* (2013) reported the prevalence of gingival recessions steadily increasing after orthodontic treatment – 7% at end of treatment to 20% at 2 years after treatment, and to 38% at 5 years after treatment. They also concluded that patients younger than 16 years of age at the end of treatment were less likely to develop recessions than patients over 16 years, at the end of treatment (Figure 18.4). The same researchers (Renkema *et al.*, 2015) also reported that gingival recession was more pronounced in nonproclined sites (12.3%) than in proclined incisors (11.7%) after 5 years of orthodontic treatment. The vulnerability of mandibular incisors, mandibular and maxillary first premolars, and maxillary first molars to gingival recession and its increase over the observation period of 7 years post-treatment was reported recently by Mijuskovic *et al.* (2018).

However, recent randomized cohort studies and systematic reviews in this regard have concluded that there is no strong scientific evidence concluding that proclination of incisors by means of fixed orthodontic appliances can affect periodontal health (Gebistorf *et al*, 2018; Tepedino *et al.*, 2018; Bahar *et al.*, 2020). Pernet *et al.* (2019) could find no association between the width of the alveolar bone process at the apex, at the level of the crest and at mid of the root, and the vertical skeletal pattern and the onset of buccal or lingual recessions. However, there is some evidence that increased symphyseal height, and the ratio between the symphysis height and

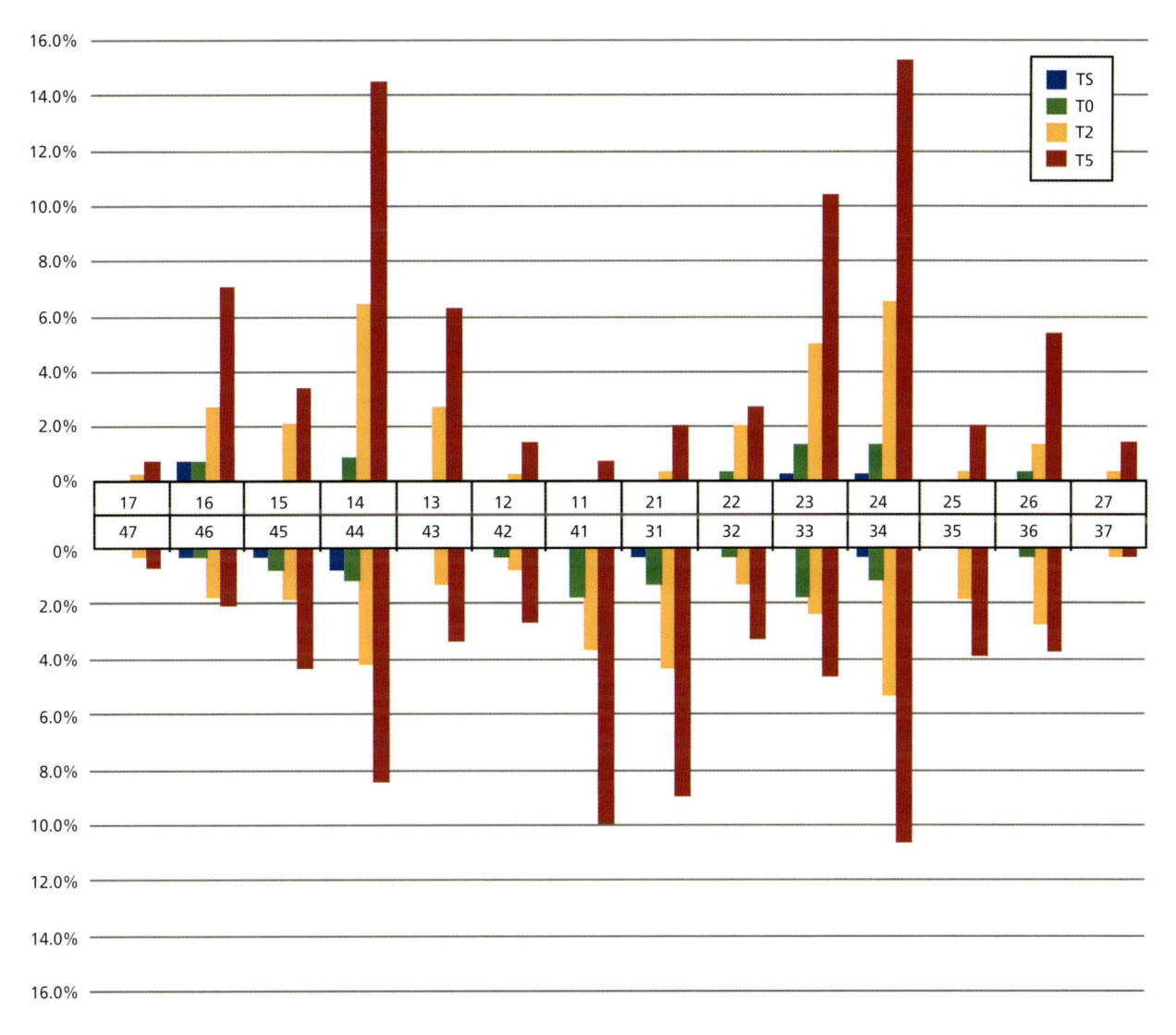

Figure 18.4 Frequencies (%) of gingival recessions per tooth at four times: TS, pretreatment; T0, end of treatment; T2, 2 years after the end of treatment; T5, 5 years after the end of treatment. (Source: Renkema *et al.*, 2013. Reproduced with permission of Elsevier.)

the width at the crest level to be associated with this. An American Academy of Periodontology best evidence review published recently (Wang *et al.* 2020) suggested phenotypic modification therapy (PhMT) involving hard tissue augmentation (PhMT-b) via particulate bone grafting together with corticotomy-assisted orthodontic therapy (CAOT) may provide clinical benefits such as modifying periodontal phenotype, maintaining or enhancing facial bone thickness, and accelerating tooth movement, expanding the scope of safe tooth movement for patients undergoing orthodontic tooth movement (OTM). They also pointed out the need for higher quality randomized controlled trials or case-control studies with longer follow-up to investigate the effects of different grafting materials.

Histological and microbiologic changes

The histological sections of orthodontically treated tissues characteristically reveal increased numbers of mononuclear infiltrates, along with hyperplasia and proliferation of pocket epithelium and dense accumulation of chronic inflammatory cells occupying large areas of connective tissue (Zachrisson and Zachrisson, 1972; Kurol *et al.*, 1982; van de Velde *et al.*, 1988). Mártha *et al.* (2013), with the help of usual histological evaluation, revealed the presence of hyperplastic chronic inflammatory changes from mild to moderate severity in gingival specimens obtained from patients undergoing fixed appliance treatment. Upon longitudinal evaluation, Kurol *et al.* (1982) stated that orthodontic forces are prone to produce permanent damage to gingival tissues in young humans. It is clear from the research report by Zanatta *et al.* (2012) that the anterior gingival enlargement seems to influence the oral health-related quality of life in subjects receiving orthodontic treatment.

Gingival invagination, defined as superficial changes in the shape of the gingiva, which arise after moving teeth in order to close spaces created by tooth extractions, is yet another common side effect of orthodontic treatment. This side effect may lead to compromised oral hygiene, jeopardizing the space closure and the long-term stability of the treatment outcome. This finding appears as a "pseudopocket," which can be probed both horizontally and vertically, and is found in 35% of cases after extraction space closure procedures. Histological and histochemical examinations of tissue specimens taken from sites of gingival invagination showed hypertrophy in the epithelium and the connective tissues, and sometimes, loss of

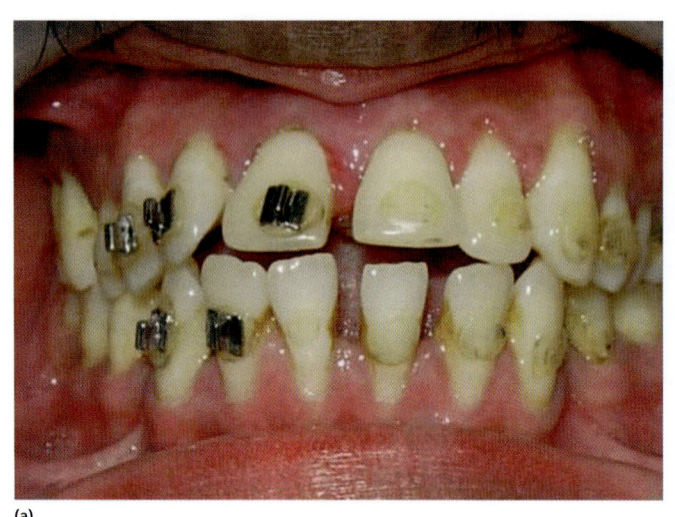

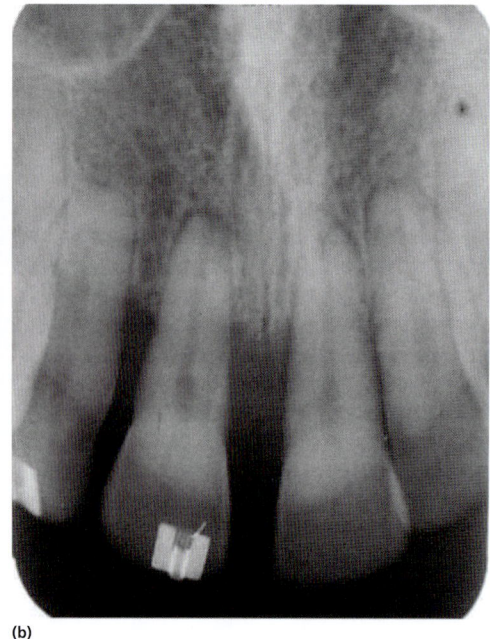

Figure 18.5 The effect of poor orthodontic mechanics: (a) the clinical picture and (b) the periapical radiograph of the teeth, showing alveolar bone loss and apical root resorption caused with these mechanics. (Source: Dr. Arun Sadasivan, MDS, Periodontist, Trivandrum, Kerala, India. Reproduced with permission of Dr. Arun Sadasivan.)

gingival collagen (Kurol *et al.*, 1982). A study by Rivera Circuns and Tulloch (1983) indicated an extremely high incidence of invaginations forming during extraction-space closure, which were more frequent, complex, and severe in the mandibular arch than in the maxillary arch. They could observe a general trend toward resolution of these defects with time but observed many to persist years after retention was discontinued. They stated that the presence and severity of gingival invaginations were related consistently to a reduction in gingival health in that area.

Along with the increase in the amount of supra- and subgingival plaque (Corbett *et al.*, 1981; Huser *et al.*, 1990), orthodontic appliances seem to offer an opportunity to shift plaque composition from a predominance of aerobic Gram-positive cocci to more destructive putative pathogens, consisting mainly of facultative and strictly anaerobic Gram-negative species. Readers are referred to Chapter 10 for detailed discussion on microbiologic changes associated with orthodontic treatment.

Periodontal changes and alveolar bone loss

The main effects, which are categorized as periodontal destruction following orthodontic mechanics, are loss of attachment and bone loss. It is very difficult for gingival inflammation to progress into periodontitis. This inability is due to the restriction of plaque-induced inflammatory reaction in the supra alveolar connective tissue (Cadarapoli and Gaveglio, 2007). However, development of destructive periodontal disease might result in formation of supra bony pockets with inflamed connective tissue and dentogingival epithelium located coronal to the alveolar crest (Waerhaug, 1979). This situation might lead to disintegration of collagen fibers attaching marginal periodontal tissue to the root surface. When the structural connection between cementum and surrounding tissue is lost, the road is open for proliferation of dentogingival epithelium beyond the cemento-enamel junction (CEJ), creating a pathologically deepened

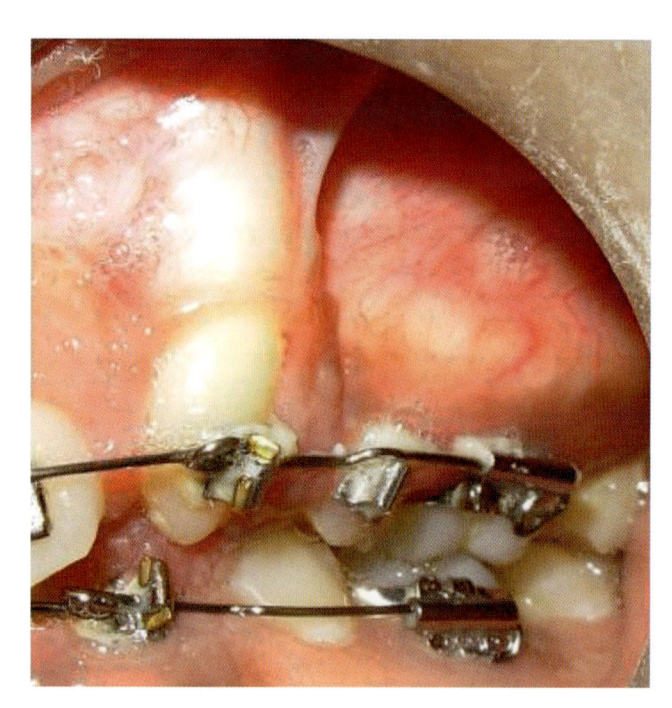

Figure 18.6 The effect of improper orthodontic mechanics, which leads to canine root prominence. Alveolar bone loss (dehiscence) is severe in this case. (Source: Dr. Vinod Krishnan.)

pocket. The most reliable clinical expression of the degree of severity of periodontal breakdown is measuring the distance from the CEJ to the bottom of the clinical pocket. This distance is termed "loss of attachment." The loss of attachment is intimately associated with a reduction in the dentoalveolar height (Figures 18.5, 18.6, and 18.7).

The initiation, progression, and recurrence of periodontitis are determined by the amount of bacterial plaque in the gingival and/

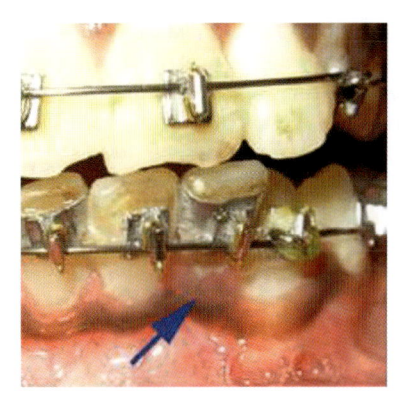

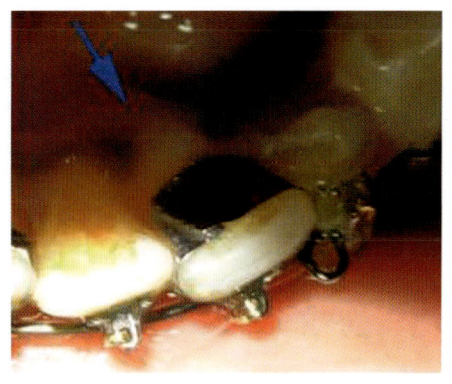

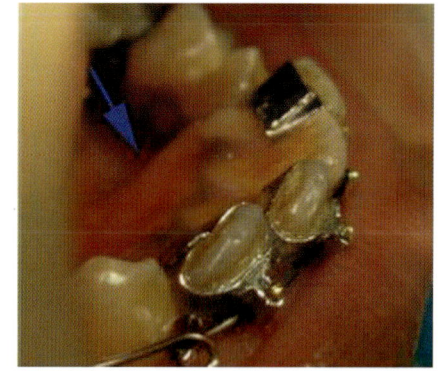

Figure 18.7 The effect of faulty orthodontic mechanics, which led to uncontrolled tipping (round-tripping) and root prominence in the mandibular incisor region (arrow). (Source: Dr. Vinod Krishnan.)

Table 18.2 Modified guidelines for periodontal follow-up during orthodontic care in adolescents and young adults. (Source: Levin et al., 2012. Reproduced with permission of *Journal of Applied Oral Science*.)

	Before orthodontic treatment	During orthodontic treatment	Follow-up after orthodontic treatment (once per year)
Plaque control	✓	✓	✓
Periodontal probing	✓	✓	✓
Intraoral periapical radiographs and bitewing radiographs	If periodontal problem is suspected and bleeding on probing is visible – localized radiographic evaluation is recommended	If periodontal problem is suspected and bleeding on probing is visible – localized radiographic evaluation is recommended (once every 6 months)	If periodontal pathologies are suspected
Referral to periodontist		In case of suspected periodontal pathologies If there is clear evidence of periodontal pockets, bleeding on probing, and radiographic evidence of bone loss (vertical and horizontal)	

or periodontal pockets. Fixed orthodontic appliances increase the number of plaque-retaining areas along with additional risk of mechanical irritation. Morais *et al.* (2018) reported that nonextraction alignment with self-ligating brackets led to arch expansion associated with tipping of teeth resulting in horizontal and vertical bone loss at the incisors and mesiobuccal root of the first molars. This is aggravated in patients with thinner bone and more severe crowding before treatment. Zacchrisson (1972) emphasized the importance of the proper maintenance of oral hygiene during orthodontic treatment, in order to reduce the risk of periodontal breakdown. According to him, 90% of patients acquired little or no periodontal breakdown with repeated motivation and instruction on oral hygiene. Suggesting guidelines for periodontal care and follow-up during orthodontic treatment in adolescents and young adults, Levin *et al.* (2012) outlined the importance of guidelines as a routine protocol for periodontal examination before, during, and following orthodontic treatment, and have also outlined the actions required if there is increased probing pocket depth, gingival recession, and root resorption (Tables 18.2 and 18.3).

Tooth-related changes

Teeth consisting of enamel, dentin, pulp, and cementum are frequently affected by the orthodontic force, as well as by the mechanics. Inappropriate mechanics and forces result in trauma to tooth tissues, and improper oral hygiene measures led to enamel damage.

Enamel decalcification and trauma

Tooth enamel is the most mineralized tissue of the human body, with the composition of 96 wt% inorganic material and 4 wt% organic material and water. Potential physical damage to tooth enamel associated with orthodontic treatment may include (Arhun and Arman, 2007):
- cleaning with abrasive materials prior to etching;
- loss of surface enamel with acid etching;
- intentional enamel reduction or stripping;
- demineralization and white-spot lesions (WSL) associated with bacterial action from dental plaque;
- enamel loss due to parafunctional activity and contact with metallic or ceramic brackets;
- enamel fractures during bracket debonding;
- mechanical removal of composite remnants with rotary instruments.

Cleaning of the enamel surface with a bristle brush for 10–15 seconds per tooth may abrade away as much as 10 μm of enamel, whereas about 5 μm may be lost when a rubber cup is used

Table 18.3 Actions required following different periodontal findings (PD, pocket depth; BL, radiographic bone loss). (Source: Levin *et al.*, 2012. Reproduced with permission of *Journal of Applied Oral Science*.).

Periodontal findings	Action required
PD > 5 mm with no BL	Oral hygiene reinforcement Shorten interval between maintenance appointments to 4–6 weeks
PD > 5 mm with BL	Pause active orthodontic treatment Refer to a periodontist Only after resolution of the periodontal disease, continue the orthodontic treatment with special care and follow-up
Gingival recession > 2 mm	Avoid facial tooth movements Consider shortening treatment time
Root resorption > 3 mm apparent in radiographs	Radiographic follow-up every 6 months

(Thompson and Way, 1981). An acid-etching procedure with 30–50% phosphoric acid for 15–60 seconds causes selective dissolution of either enamel prism cores or boundaries, creating microporosity of the enamel surface, ranging in depth from 5 to 50 μm. Van Waes et al. (1997), using a computerized three-dimensional scanner to measure enamel loss caused by orthodontic bonding and debonding after phosphoric acid etching, reported an average of 7.4 μm enamel loss. Twesme et al. (1994) concluded that, with interdental stripping, it is safe to remove 0.3–0.4 mm of enamel without rendering it prone to dissolution. Studies showing that stripping can increase the susceptibility of proximal enamel surfaces to demineralization and also led to greater plaque retention increasing the risk of secondary caries, attributed these effects to the residual furrows on the enamel surface, compared with untreated teeth (Joseph et al., 1992; Twesme et al., 1994). The results provided by Arhun and Arman (2007) demonstrated that polishing enamel after the application of stripping techniques, in order to achieve similar morphological characteristics as intact enamel, was not possible (Figure 18.8).

The components of the orthodontic appliance and the bonding materials promote plaque accumulation and bacterial colonization, especially *Streptococcus mutans* and lactobacilli, with subsequent

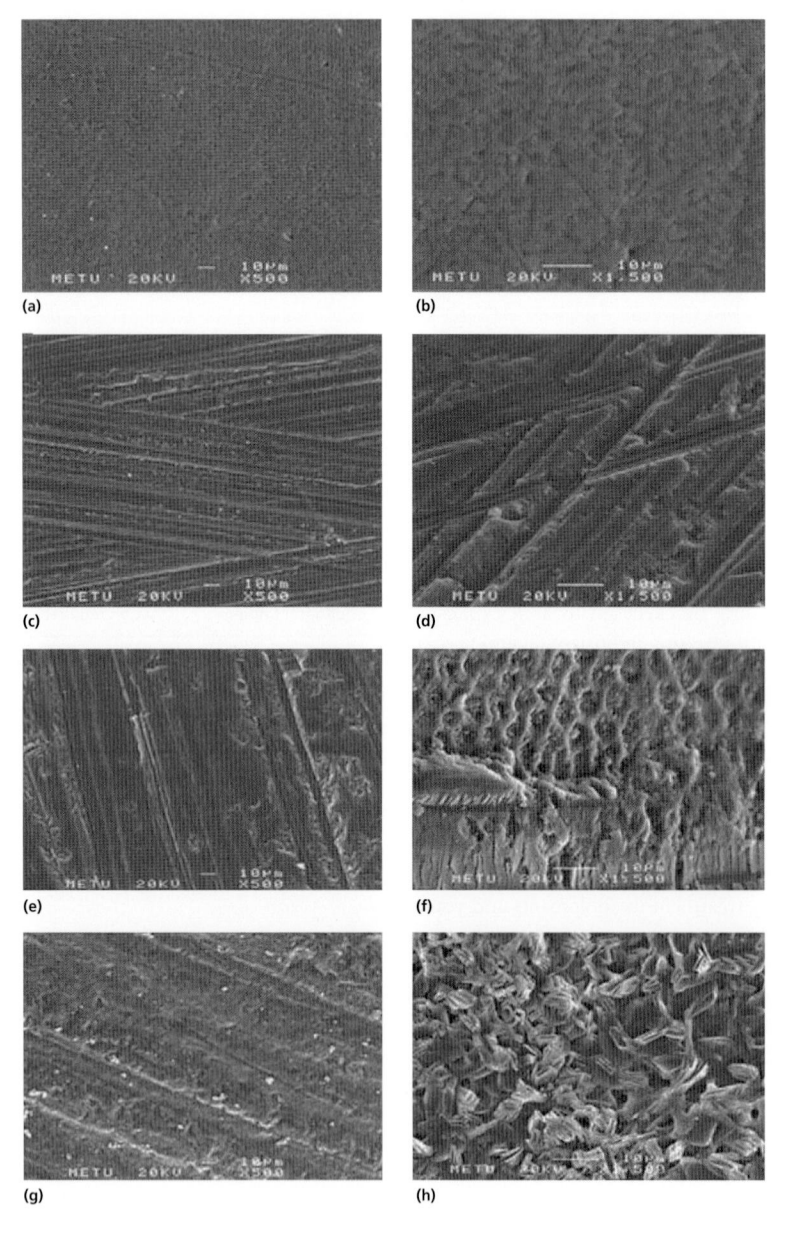

Figure 18.8 Enamel surface damage caused by various interproximal stripping methods. The evaluation was performed by scanning electron microscopy. (a) Intact undisturbed enamel (× 500). (b) Intact undisturbed enamel (× 1500). (c) Teeth stripped with a stripping disk (Komet, GebrBrasseler, Lemgo, Germany) (× 500). (d) Teeth stripped with a stripping disk (× 1500). (e) Teeth stripped with a stripping diamond coated metal strip (Dentaurum, Ispringen, Germany) (× 500). (f) Teeth stripped with a stripping diamond-coated metal strip (× 1500). (g) Chemical stripping. A diamond-coated metal strip (Dentaurum) was used (20 strokes) with 37% orthophosphoric acid (3M-ESPE) gel applied on the enamel surface. After the procedure, the acid was rinsed thoroughly with air-water spray (× 500). (h) Chemical stripping (× 1500). (Source: Arman, et al. (2006). Reproduced with permission of American Association of Orthodontists.)

acid production leading to decalcification (Fournier *et al.*, 1998; Brusca *et al.*, 2007) (Figure 18.9). This effect is often manifested as WSL on the enamel surface, the incidence rate of which ranges from 2% to 96%. It is mainly the result of a change in the pH of the oral environment, favoring diffusion of calcium and phosphate ions out of the enamel (Mitchell, 1992), and leading to a 10% reduction in the mineral content (Øgaard, 2001). Visible white lesions, which might develop within 4 weeks of appliance placement, have obvious aesthetic implications, highlighting the need for caries rate assessment. In severe cases, frank cavitations are seen, requiring restorative intervention. It was reported by Geiger *et al.* (1988) that any tooth in the mouth can be affected by this process, with the highest incidence occurring in maxillary lateral incisors, maxillary canines, and mandibular premolars and is directly correlated with duration of orthodontic treatment (Pinto *et al.*, 2018). The main procedure performed to prevent demineralization is promoting formation of fluorapatite crystals (Mellberg and Mallon, 1984). Although reports exist regarding beneficial effects of MI Paste (GC America, Alsip, Ill, USA) containing casein phosphopeptide-amorphous calcium phosphate (Robertson *et al.*, 2011) and 1.23% acidulated phosphate fluoride (APF) gel (Jiang *et al.*, 2013) in reducing the incidence of WSL and casein phosphopeptide-amorphous calcium phosphate (CPP-ACP)-containing products (Pithon *et al.*, 2019), systematic reviews in this regard found no evidence to substantiate this claim (Höchli *et al.*, 2017; Sonesson *et al.*, 2017; Fernández-Ferrer *et al.*, 2018). Recent systematic reviews in this regard have pointed

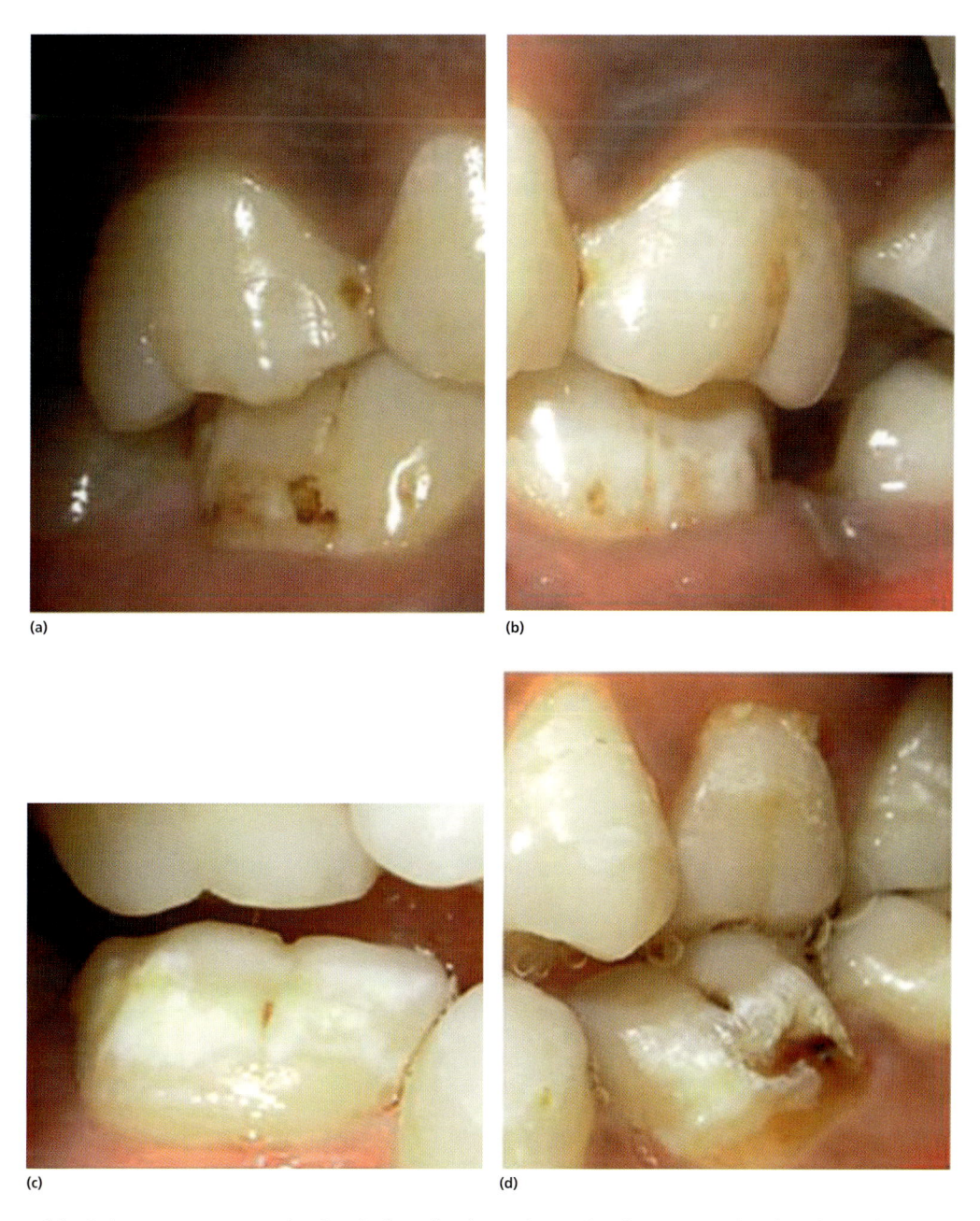

Figure 18.9 Enamel decalcification areas associated with orthodontic banding with zinc phosphate cement. The released acid, along with plaque accumulation, often leads to enamel demineralization. (a), (b), and (c) show that decalcification occurred around maxillary and mandibular first molar bands, and (d) shows the cavitation caused by enamel decalcification. (Source: Dr. Vinod Krishnan.)

out the benefits of topical fluoride application – either by patients or professionals – in reducing the burden of WSL (Benson et al., 2019; Sardana et al., 2019a, b; Tasios et al., 2019).

Attrition of enamel surfaces can occur when teeth contact either metallic or ceramic brackets. It is commonly seen on upper canine tips, as the cusp tip hits the lower canine brackets during retraction, which can be prevented by delaying the placement of brackets. Any sort of enamel erosion must be noted prior to treatment to provide proper dietary advice, which will help to minimize further tooth substance loss. Carbonated drinks and pure juices are the commonest causes of erosion and should be avoided in patients with fixed appliances (Arhun and Arman, 2007).

The process of debonding a bracket with a force level exceeding the enamel strength may result in fracture and grazing. Martin and Garcia-Godoy (1994) suggested using a weaker adhesive with a lower strength, so that failure while debonding occurs at the resin–enamel interface. It is reported that loss of enamel was more pronounced with ceramic brackets (31.9%) compared with metal brackets (13.3%) (Cochrane et al., 2017). Enamel trauma can also be the result of clumsy instrumentation, and care is required when working on a heavily restored tooth, which can result in fracture of unsupported cusps. Performing adhesive removal procedures may remove up to 55.6 μm of surface enamel (Fitzpatrick and Way, 1997). Although various methods have been introduced for efficient and safe removal of resin adhesive, such as hand scalers, tungsten carbide burs, sof-lex discs, carbon dioxide laser, and air abrasion, the enigma of enamel abrasion still persists (Figures 18.10 and 18.11). In addition, inefficient use of these techniques might result in adverse effects on pulpal tissues, especially if the heat generated is not dissipated properly with appropriate coolants (Arhun and Arman, 2007). A recent systematic review in this regard has clearly stated that the process of orthodontic debonding increases the number of enamel microcracks, but there is weak evidence indicating that the length and width of enamel microcracks increase following bracket removal (Dumbryte et al., 2018).

Pulpal reactions

The effects of orthodontic forces on the dentin–pulp complex have not yet been significantly investigated. Research reports demonstrate conflicting results concerning adverse pulpal effects. Kvinnsland et al. (1989) have found a mild inflammatory response in the dental pulp that has been subjected to orthodontic forces. Various reports have demonstrated an initial decrease in blood flow (for up to 32 hours) followed by an increase, lasting 48 hours (McDonald and Pitt Ford, 1989; Wong et al., 1999; Santamaria et al., 2006). Jiggling forces, which tend to move the tooth out of the alveolar bone envelope, severing associated blood vessels, are considered the main culprits for this reaction (Yamaguchi and Kasai, 2007).

Histologic observations by Mostafa et al. (1991) demonstrated congested and dilated blood vessels, along with edema of pulpal tissue. An experiment on rats revealed apoptosis of the dental pulp (Rana et al., 2001), and in a similar study, release of aspartate aminotransferase (an enzyme released extracellularly upon cell death) was observed (Perinetti et al., 2004). Histological studies on humans with intrusive force application to teeth resulted in vasodilatation and circulatory disturbances, local hemorrhage, and brown hemosiderin deposits from red blood cell degradation (Stenvik and Mjor, 1970). An interesting finding by Kucukkeles and Okar (1994) was resorption cavities in the inner root surface of the pulp, as the teeth are subjected to intrusive forces. Root and dentin resorption,

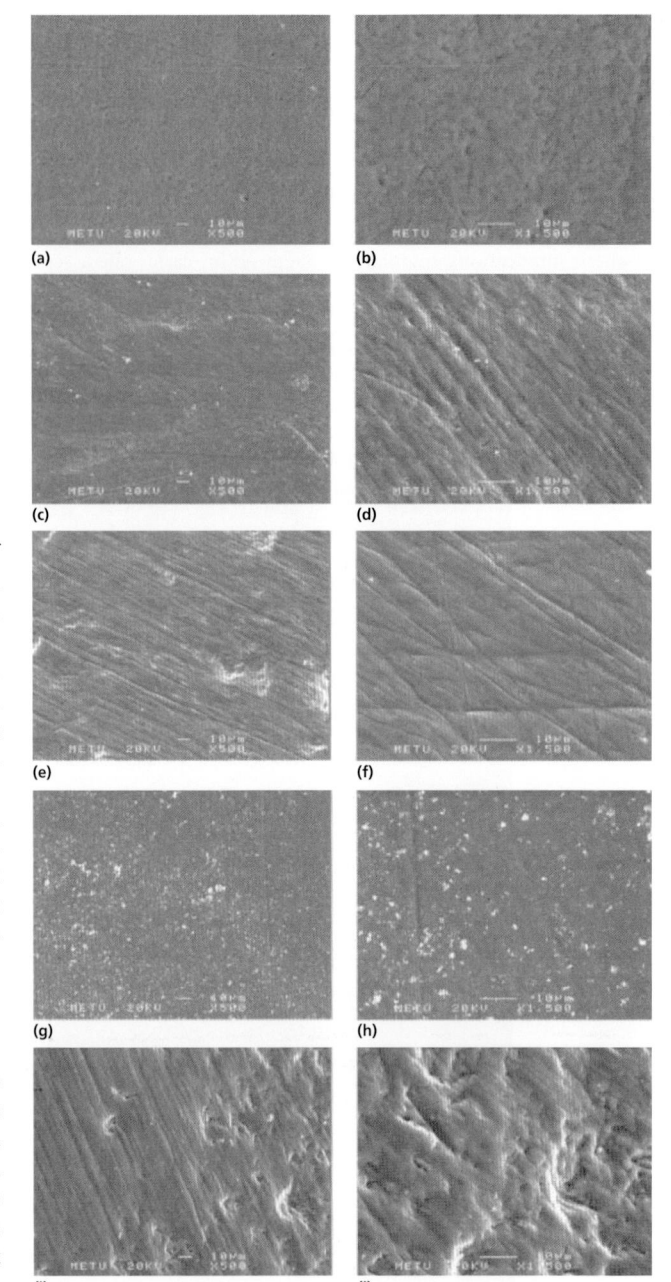

Figure 18.10 Surface damage resulting from various enamel clean-up methods after debonding. The evaluation was performed by scanning electron microscopy. (a) Intact undisturbed enamel (× 500). (b) Intact undisturbed enamel (× 1500). (c) Clean up with eight bladed low-speed tungsten carbide bur (× 500). (d) Clean up with low-speed eight-bladed tungsten carbide bur (× 1500). (e) Clean up with high-speed eight-bladed tungsten carbide bur (× 500). (f) Clean up with high-speed eight-bladed tungsten carbide bur (× 1500). (g) After using soft-lex discs (× 500). (h) After using soft-lex discs (× 1500). (i) The tooth surfaces were held approximately 5 mm from the tip of the microetcher and cleaned with 50 μm aluminum oxide particles under an enclosed ventilated hood (× 500). (j) After using microetchant and aluminum oxide particles (× 1500). (Source: Dr. Neslihan Arhun, Associate Professor, Department of Conservative Dentistry, Faculty of Dentistry, Baskent University, Ankara, Turkey.)

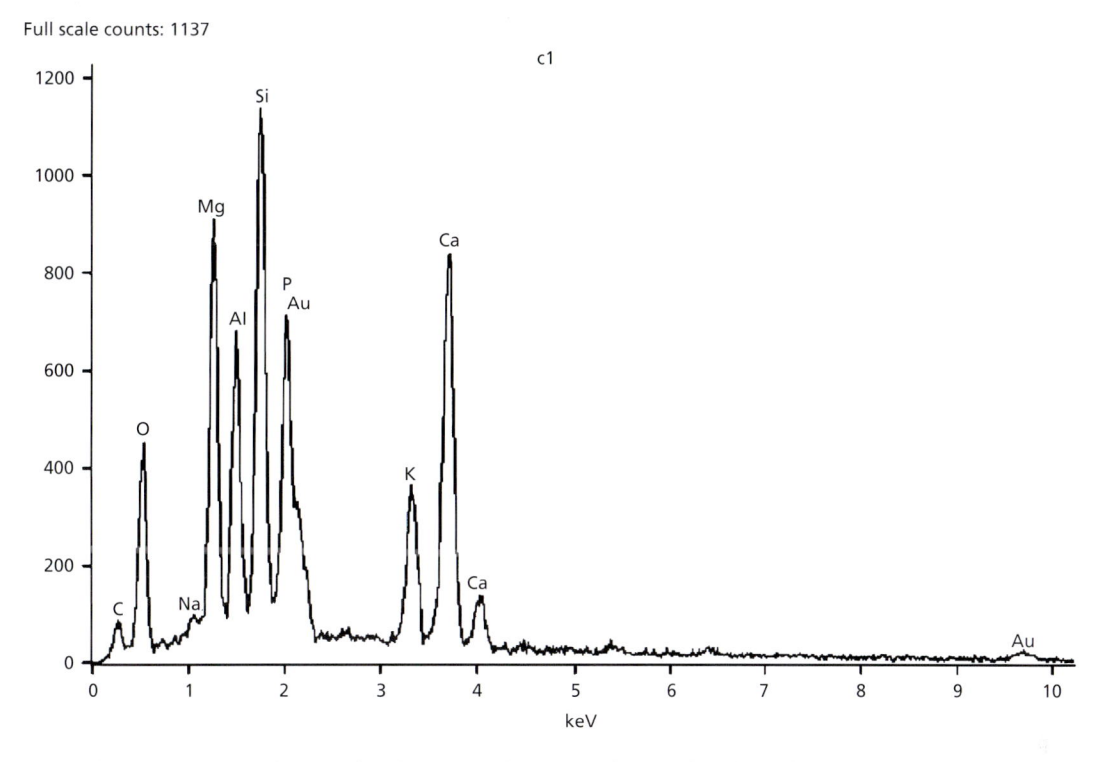

Figure 18.11 Energy dispersive spectrum (device used to characterize the opaque substances from the surface of any object) from enamel surface after clean-up with soft lex discs. Note the graph showing high traces of silicon, magnesium, and aluminum (may be the remnants of discs from the clean-up procedure). (Source: Dr. Neslihan Arhun, Associate Professor, Department of Conservative Dentistry, Faculty of Dentistry, Baskent University, Ankara, Turkey.)

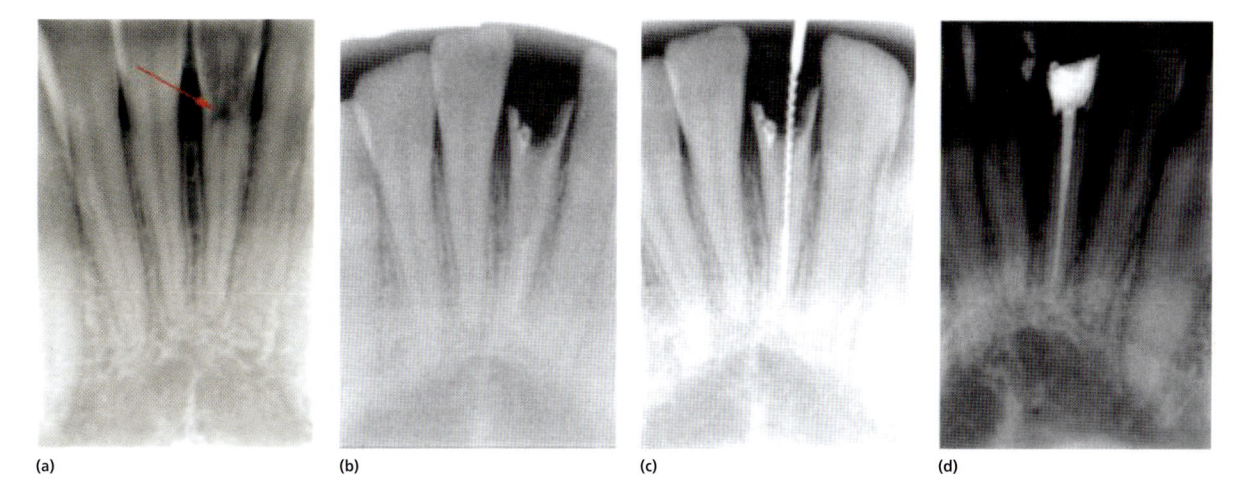

Figure 18.12 Extreme hyperreaction of the dental pulp after 40 months of orthodontic treatment. (a) Internal root resorption seen in the mandibular left central incisor (arrow). The teeth became pink and root canal treatment was planned. (b) Tooth fractured while being prepared for endodontic treatment. (c) and (d) Tooth structure reinforced with post and core restoration. This step was followed by a fixed partial denture for the mandibular incisor (jacket crown) (not shown). (Source: Dr. Vinod Krishnan.)

along with a reduction in predentin width were observed in the teeth subjected to orthodontic force, suggestive of a degenerative change in the dental pulp. Briefly, orthodontic forces are capable of inducing neurogenic inflammation, followed by release of proinflammatory cytokines, leading to pulpitis and hyperemia. If the applied forces are excessive, the pulpal respiration rate becomes abnormal, altering the blood flow rate, creating iatrogenic damage, ranging from simple necrosis to internal root resorption (Yamaguchi and Kasai, 2007) (Figure 18.12). Ma et al. (1997) found that if the temperature rises above 46–50°C for at least 39 seconds, there is a chance of developing thrombosis and curtailing circulation. It is, therefore, always important to use water or air as a coolant during clean-up procedures.

A systematic review by Von Böhl et al. (2012) and a later one by Javed et al. (2015), however, concluded that because of a lack of high-quality studies there is no conclusive scientific evidence for a relation between force level and dental pulp tissue reaction in humans. Consolaro and Consolaro (2018) also reported that

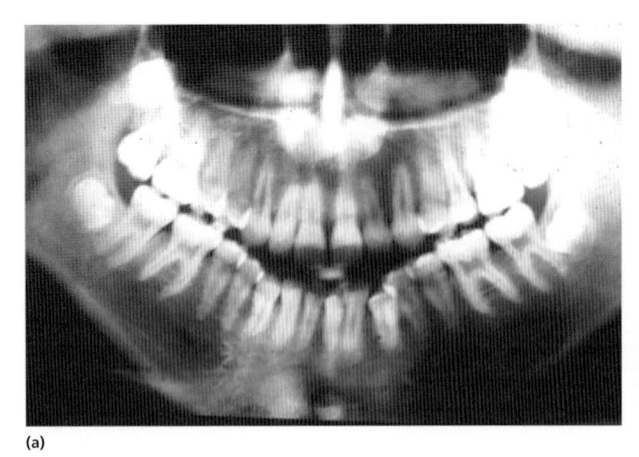

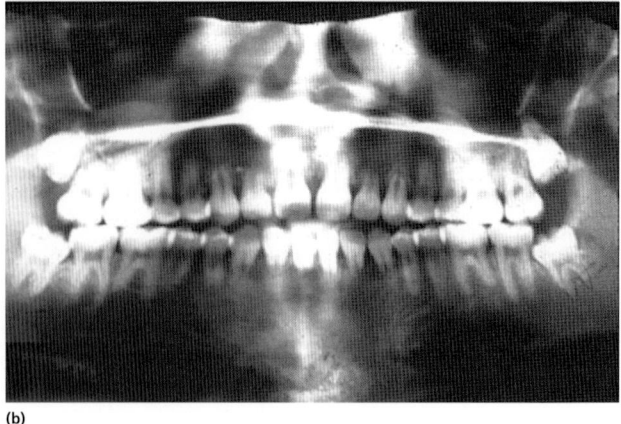

Figure 18.13 (a) A panoramic pretreatment radiograph of patient's dentition at age 16 years, prior to the onset of orthodontic treatment aimed at closing the open bite. The open bite extended from the second molars on the left side to the second molars on the right side. (b) The orthopantomogram of the patient after 3.5 years of orthodontic treatment. The radiograph shows that despite the long effort, the bite was not entirely closed, and that multiple teeth in both jaws have been substantially shortened by root resorption. (Source: Dr. Vinod Krishnan.)

orthodontic movement does not induce pulp necrosis or calcific metamorphosis of the pulp and there exists no literature or experimental and clinical models that support pulp alterations induced by orthodontic movement.

Root resorption

External apical root resorption (EARR) entails a permanent shortening of dental roots, and formation of large lacunae that erode the roots laterally. Some of these changes in root morphology may be detected radiographically (Figure 18.13) and have led to numerous lawsuits by concerned patients. Ottolengui (1914) and Ketcham (1927) were the first to report severe root resorption associated with OTM. Several studies have revealed that the maxillary central incisors are the most prone to the process, followed by the maxillary molars and canines (Krishnan, 2005). In approximately one out of 20 patients undergoing orthodontic treatment, up to 5 mm of tooth root loss can occur, potentially endangering the longevity of the tooth (Abass and Hartsfield, 2007).

When orthodontic forces are applied over a long period of time (weeks or months), local necrosis (hyalinization) of the compressed PDL may develop. Necrotic cells and extracellular matrix are removed by macrophages that accumulate in the area by chemotaxis (Feller et al., 2016). Two types of macrophages are distinguished. Type 1 macrophages are important for the development of root resorption. These macrophages express a large number of cytokines and growth factors such as NO, TNFα, PGE_2, IL1β and IL6 (Matsumoto et al., 2017; Shapouri-Moghaddam et al., 2018). Thus, the macrophages remove the necrotic periodontal tissue, differentiate and attach osteoclasts to the tooth surface, and cause root resorption (Brudvik and Rygh, 1993, 1994a, b; Iglesias-Linares and Hartsfield, 2017).

Microscopically, small resorption lacunae on the root surface are visible at the early stages of OTM, much earlier than the time when it is possible to detect it radiologically. Resorption is mostly observed radiographically in the apical region of the root because (Abass and Hartsfield, 2007):
- the apical third is covered with cellular cementum, which depends on active cells, and has more supporting vasculature, making it vulnerable to trauma and cell injury-related reactions. It is reported that blood vessels occupy 47% of the PDL space in the apical region, compared with 4% in the cervical end of the root (Blaushild et al., 1992);
- there is a decrease in the hardness and elastic modulus of the cementum, from the cervical to the apical regions, making apical areas prone to resorption (Chutimanutskul et al., 2006);
- the fulcrum of tooth movement (center of rotation) is occlusal to the apical half of the root in tipping. This fact, along with the differences in the direction of the periodontal fibers, could result in increased possibilities of trauma to the apical and middle thirds of the root (Abass and Hartsfield, 2007).

Brezniak and Wasserstein (2002) classified root resorption by its severity. Accordingly, it is possible to identify:
- cemental, or surface resorption – where only the outer layers are resorbed, to be fully regenerated or remodeled later;
- dentinal resorption with repair – where the cementum and the outer layers of dentine are resorbed and repaired along with morphological alterations;
- circumferential root resorption – where a full resorption of the hard tissue components of the root apex occurs resulting in root shortening.

Jarabak and Fizzell (1972) concluded that the magnitude of an orthodontic force, as well as rigid fixation of the archwire to the brackets, along with jiggling forces and round tripping of the moving teeth due to the mechanotherapy, can be considered to be the most important factors predisposing a tooth to the root-resorptive process. Of the possible various OTMs, tipping, intrusion, and torquing make a tooth root prone to resorption (Krishnan, 2005; Abass and Hartsfield, 2007). Tapered roots, in comparison with the blunted type, exhibit more resorption. A previous history of dentofacial trauma, pre-existing root resorption, hypofunctional PDL associated with nonoccluding teeth, drug consumption (corticosteroids and alcohol), and systemic diseases, such as asthma and allergy, have been identified as paramount factors promoting root resorption. Fernandes et al. (2019) reported that EARR was 70% higher in orthodontic treatment with maxillary premolar extraction, 58% higher in patients with increased overjet and interestingly 41% lower in two-phase orthodontic treatment, and 33% lower in patients with deep bite. They also reported that dilacerated roots were 2.26 times more likely to develop EARR, and for each additional millimeter of root length, the risk of EARR increased by 29%. There also seems to be a racial predilection, with Asians showing less resorption than Whites and Hispanics (Krishnan, 2005; Krishnan and Davidovitch, 2006; Abass and Hartsfield, 2007), and the incidence is more common in adults than in children (Tian *et al.*, 2013). Sondeijker *et al.* (2020) concluded that except for age and gender (for which they could elicit a moderate level of evidence), no other patient-related factors such as pre-existing trauma, endodontic treatment, root morphology, overjet, overbite, habits, early treatment, duration of treatment, extraction vs. non-extraction, use of Class II elastics and the like showed adequate evidence to associate with EARR. More studies in this regard are warranted.

Although familial clustering of EARR has been performed, no single specific pattern of inheritance could be observed. The pattern appears to be polygenic, with a complicated interaction of several proteins coded for by a number of genes that interact with environmental factors, such as orthodontic forces. Candidate genes associated with the resorptive process have been identified, such as IL-1β, osteoprotegerin (OPG), and RANKL, to name a few. Recently it was reported that no significant association for RANKL genetic polymorphisms except for rs3102724 was observed with EARR. A pooled meta-analysis of seven studies revealed a negative association and led the authors to discuss the prevailing confusion as to whether a real association exists between IL-1β polymorphism and predisposition to EARR. They also pointed towards the significant heterogeneity that exists among study results, warranting more studies with a significant increase in sample size and proper methodology (Nowrin *et al.*, 2018). Recently, through a multivariate analysis, de Castilhos *et al.* (2019) concluded that the initial root length, rapid maxillary expansion, and polymorphisms of the OPG gene were associated with EARR. It is likely that differential expressions of molecules that govern osteoclast/odontoclast function play a role in determining the susceptibility to root resorption during orthodontic treatment. Thus, certain individuals might react with an exaggerated response, leading to EARR (Abass and Hartsfield, 2007).

Comparison with the pretreatment radiographs still forms the mainstay of assessment along with grading systems and scoring criteria. Progress periapical and panoramic radiographs form a useful aid in detecting mid-treatment resorptive processes. Considering the fact that the degree of EARR present after 6–12 months of orthodontic treatment with fixed appliances can be closely related to that at the end of the treatment (Årtun *et al.*, 2009), it is suggested that a panoramic radiograph should be taken at 6–12 months after placement of the fixed appliance, which can also be used to check bracket position at the end of alignment stage (Sondeijker *et al.*, 2020).

There is insufficient evidence on further orthodontic management when EARR occurs during orthodontic treatment (Sondeijker *et al.*, 2020). When such an incidence occurs, it is always better to reevaluate the remaining treatment objectives and determine further treatment strategies by the practitioner together with the patient. Evaluation should include risks of continuing treatment and balance it with the risks of ending treatment. Malocclusions, which have long-term influences on oral health-related quality of life such as deep bite or traumatic occlusion should be considered for continuing treatment. Apart from this, excluding teeth affected by EARR from active treatment should also be considered as a choice while continuing treatment in such situations (Sondeijker *et al.*, 2020). Whenever root resorption is detected, a temporary halt in treatment for a minimum of 3–6 months is advised, which may help prevent further resorption (Currell *et al.*, 2019; Sondeijker *et al.*, 2020).

Some repair processes also occur, such as smoothing and remodeling of cemental surfaces with restoration of the normal width of the PDL. Even though original root contours are never established, the function of the dental apparatus is not severely affected by the loss of root length. When treatment is initiated after this rest period, an incredibly careful approach is required and it is recommended that the progress of root resorption is assessed with radiographs every 6 months (Sondeijker *et al.*, 2020).

Experiments have demonstrated several ways to slow down the rate of root resorption during mechanotherapy, such as drugs, hormones, and the use of low-intensity pulsed ultrasound (Krishnan, 2005) and even low-level laser treatment (Ng *et al.*, 2018).

EARR will stop once active treatment is over, but it is mandatory to prevent active tooth moving forces in these teeth with retention appliances and it should remain passive. It is to be understood that a tooth with less than 10 mm of remaining root length might display higher than normal mobility and mobility might increase over time and when periodontal breakdown occurs. Therefore, the family dentist should be informed about more than 2 mm of root resorption and routine screening and measures to control periodontal disease should be emphasized in these patients (Sondeijker *et al.*, 2020).

Soft tissue irritation

Lacerations or irritations to oral mucosal tissues are a common clinical observation in the orthodontic office. They often occur during treatment, mainly because of:
- ulceration from brackets, especially hooks in the initial stages;
- acid burn from etching;
- thermal burn from hot instruments;
- clumsy instrumentation:
  - ulceration from archwires;
  - distal ends;
  - long spans;
  - displacement of headgear inner bow and intermaxillary Class II correction springs.

These encounters may result in ulceration, hyperplastic reactions (Figure 18.14), and/or even deep wounds. Excessive muscular

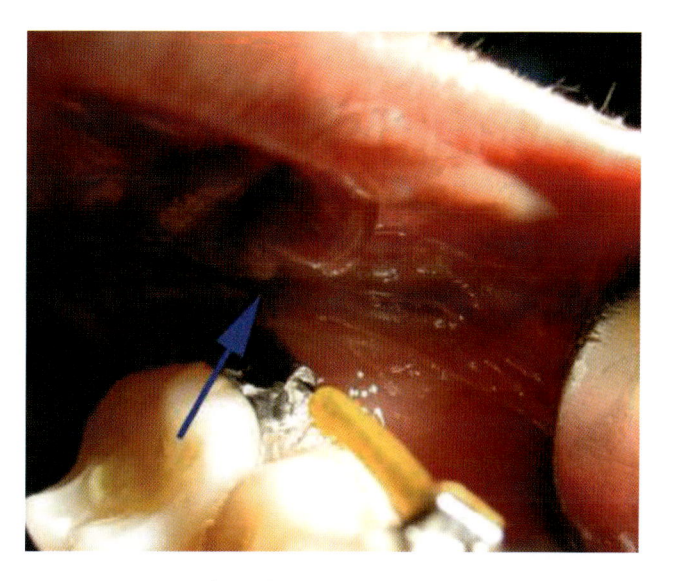

Figure 18.14 Extreme hyperplastic reaction in the cheek mucosa caused by an orthodontic appliance (arrow). (Source: Dr. Vinod Krishnan.)

activity of the cheek and tongue may act as triggers for the process (McGuinness, 1992). Careful rounding of sharp edges is one way to manage the condition. The use of dental wax over the bracket and use of an archwire sleeve over unsupported archwire spans is a great help in reducing patient discomfort.

Allergy or sensitivity reactions may occur with alloying components such as nickel, chromium, and cobalt, which are often incorporated in orthodontic attachments and archwires (Bass et al., 1993). The components or chemical catalysts used in bonding materials (Hutchinson, 1994; Connolly et al., 2006), latex elastics (Nattrass et al., 1999), and monomer/polymer used in fabrication of removable appliances, also may evoke sensitivity reactions. It is interesting to note that even though there is leaching of components of fixed appliances, reports of allergy to these materials are very rare. There are few reports on latex allergy, either with elastomerics or operator gloves (Hain et al., 2007; Pandis et al., 2007). The main signs are itching, pruritic rashes, and in severe cases ulcerations, especially in the corners of the mouth. The use of synthetic nonlatex elastics and gloves is considered a remedy in managing the problem. The use of patch testing to identify the at-risk patients, and avoidance of sensitizing agents as much as possible, are considered useful preventive measures.

Cytotoxicity and allergic reactions

A cytotoxic effect is caused by a primary irritant, which should be present in sufficient concentrations for an adequate length of time. Clinical manifestations are mainly like allergic reactions – mucosal inflammation – but can vary from erythema to necrosis, depending upon toxicity, concentration, and exposure time to the primary irritant. Some of the orthodontic appliance components are suggested to have a capacity to leach out the corrosion products and cause local cytotoxic effects. The effect is usually seen as gingival/mucosal inflammation with toxic etiology.

With this viewpoint, Grimsdottir et al. (1992) conducted cytotoxic evaluation of orthodontic appliance components. It was concluded that nickel, even though not very toxic, can induce intraoral allergic reactions. Among face bows, molar bands, brackets and archwires, a large amount of nickel and chromium release was observed from face bows containing considerable amounts of silver solder. This release may occur due to a galvanic couple, which is initiated by the silver solder, facilitating release of nickel and other metals from brackets and archwires. In a longitudinal study, Hafez et al. (2011) found that fixed orthodontic appliances have the capability of decreasing cellular viability, inducing DNA damage, and increasing the nickel and chromium contents in the buccal mucosa cells. This finding was further supported by Pazzini et al. (2011) and Retamoso et al. (2012). Amini et al. (2016) has reported that 6 months of fixed orthodontic treatment might intensify the levels of nickel (up to 510% compared with 150% at 1 month) and chromium (700% vs. 200% at 1 month) in the gingival crevicular fluid as well as gingival inflammation. It was interesting to note that placing orthodontic appliances actually reduced nickel sensitivity, as evidenced by the population-based study conducted by Fors et al. (2012). These researchers have pointed out the importance of conducting long-term studies to assess the role of dental materials in the development of immunological tolerance.

The protein content of latex elastics is a known allergen, and it was reported that, approximately, fewer than 1% of the general population, 5–15% of healthcare workers and 24–60% of patients with spina bifida are sensitive to it (Hain et al., 2007). Dos Santos (2010) compared latex and nonlatex separating elastics for their cytotoxic characteristics through cell lysis experiments and concluded that all elastics are capable of inducing cell lysis, but that nonlatex elastics were comparably less harmful. They have also stated that, overall, the amounts of cell lysis were very small, and that all the elastics, both latex and nonlatex, can be graded as biocompatible.

The detrimental biologic effects in cell cultures produced by plasticizers, polymerization initiators, and inhibitors have been evaluated through in vitro studies. Tell et al. (1988) concluded that paste–paste systems are toxic in comparison with a one-to-one agent, which led to the withdrawal of these mutagenic agents from the market. Because leaching of resins decreases with increasing filler contents, liquid resins have the highest leaching potential, followed by liquid–paste and paste–paste systems. Comparing the effect of no-mix adhesives and visible-light cured adhesives, a moderate cytostatic effect was observed in human gingival fibroblasts in vitro. TEGDMA (triethylene glycol dimethacrylate), at the millimolar level, was the culprit in provoking cytotoxicity with the help of glutathione depletion, leading to production of reactive oxygen species. Although saliva can wash away some of the leached products, long-term contact of this material with oral mucosal tissues should be looked upon with caution. Interestingly, monomers from bonding adhesives can be absorbed by the digestive tract, then can be subjected to degradation, and then form bis-phenol A (BPA), which in turn acts like a steroid hormone. This synthetic molecule will compete with natural hormones to occupy hormone-binding sites. Although BPA has serious biologic consequences, inducing premature puberty in young girls, the evidence to support this hypothesis is lacking in the orthodontic literature (Eliades et al., 2007). A systematic review on the topic by Kloukos et al. (2013) concluded that the BPA release from orthodontic bonding resins was between 0.85 and 20.88 ng/mL in vivo, and from traces to 65.67 ppm in vitro. Bis-GMA and TEGDMA leaching in vitro reached levels of 64 and 174 mg/10 μL, respectively. Deviot et al. (2018) concluded, based on the gas chromatography/mass spectrometry (GC/MS) and liquid chromatography/mass spectrometry (LC/MS), that the risk of BPA release after orthodontic bonding would be more than 42,000 times lower than the TDI for a 30-kg child.

In view of all these findings, a patch test must be undertaken in all patients with previous history of allergic reactions. It is always better to keep the sensitizing agents away while performing orthodontic treatment, to avoid serious complications.

Extraoral iatrogenic effects

Allergy

The most commonly observed extraoral side effect of orthodontic treatment is allergy. This is mainly prompted by the metallic components (headgear strap or whisker), which contains known allergens such as nickel, chromium, and cobalt or nonmetallic components (elastomerics and latex gloves). Both metallic and non-metallic components are low-molecular weight in nature, and act as haptens in the induction or elicitation of delayed hypersensitivity reactions (Jacobsen and Hensten-Pettersen, 2003). The dermal reactions usually consist of redness, irritation, itchy eczema, soreness, fissuring, and desquamation. It can appear in any part of the face and neck, including corners of the mouth, earlobes, dorsal and lateral aspects of the neck, cheek, chin, and scalp. The irritant component of these reactions may be explained by friction between skin and/or mucosa, and parts of orthodontic appliances. According to the report by Jensen *et al.* (2003), out of the 1% of the patients experiencing contact dermatitis to zippers, 3% claimed to have skin rashes with orthodontic appliances. In order to prevent the occurrence of allergic reactions, it is advised to use sticking plaster (band aid) over the area of contact with the skin, or a tape can be placed around the exposed metal of the headgear. If the allergic reactions are severe, it is always advisable to stop treatment and remove the appliance without creating further complications.

Extraoral injuries

Through an editorial (Dewel, 1975), the American Association of Orthodontists has cautioned practitioners to be aware of possible extraoral injuries from traction appliances, and to follow guidelines, in order to prevent accidental disengagement of the face bow from the buccal tube. The possible causes for facial and eye injury with headgear components include:

- accidental disengagement while playing;
- incorrect handling;
- disengagement by another child;
- unintentional disengagement while asleep.

It was reported in a survey that about 63% of injuries with extraoral appliances occur during night-time and 37% during daytime (Samuels, 1996). The presence of oral microorganisms on the outer bow at the time of injury poses serious complications. If not managed properly with antibiotics, the infection in the eye can spread very fast, leading to loss of sight. With injury to one eye, there is always a possibility for loss of sight in the other eye because of contralateral endopthalmitis. It is to be noted that penetrating eye injuries may be relatively asymptomatic, delaying the patient from seeking treatment, leading to disastrous consequences (Postlethwaite, 1990; Blum-Hareuveni *et al.*, 2004). With the introduction of intraoral absolute anchorage, in the form of mini screws, the incidence of these injuries has declined to a very minimal level due to a marked reduction in the use of headgears.

In order to prevent these injuries, a number of safety products have been marketed, such as safety bows, rigid neck straps, and snap release products, capable of preventing the inner bow from disengaging from the molar tube, or to perform like a projectile (Samuels and Brezniak, 2002). Apart from using these accessories, it should be emphasized that the head gear:

- should not be worn while playing;
- should not be grabbed by another person by holding on to the face bow;
- should be removed only after removing the strap.

Burns

There are anecdotal reports of burns, either of a chemical or physical nature, in orthodontic offices. It can happen either intraorally or extraorally. Chemical burns always result from acids used for etching teeth prior to bonding of attachments. Physical injuries are often of a thermal nature, resulting from overheated hand instruments, which have not cooled down, or from electrothermal debonding instruments. These side effects can be prevented if extra care is observed while operating on patients (McGuinness, 1992).

Systemic risks

Cross infection

A protective health component for the operator, assistant, and patient, should be an integral part of the dental practice infection control protocol (Mastaj *et al.*, 1994; Saglam and Sarikaya, 2004). Healthcare professionals working in an institutional or clinical setting are responsible for their own health status. Those who have acute or chronic medical conditions that render them susceptible to opportunistic infections should discuss with their personal physicians their ability to work in such an area. If the physician approves, they should be restricted to working on patients while taking strict precautions to prevent chances of cross infection or further spread of the disease. Great emphasis has been placed recently on exposure to blood-borne viruses, the infection of which largely depends on susceptibility of individuals, inoculation size, and route of exposure. The most attended viruses are HBV, HCV, and HIV. Avoiding occupational exposure to blood is the primary way to prevent transmission of these viruses. Standard precautions include the use of personal protection equipment (PPE) such as gloves, mask, protective eye wear or face shield, and gowns, to prevent skin and mucus membrane exposure. Other protective equipment, such as finger guards, might help to reduce injuries during dental and orthodontic procedures. It is to be noted that hand hygiene (washing, antisepsis, and scrubbing) reduces potential pathogens on the hands, and is considered the single most critical measure for reducing the risk of transmitting organisms to patients, as well as to other healthcare professionals.

Patient care items (instruments, devices, and equipment) are categorized as being critical, semicritical and noncritical, depending on the potential risk for infection associated with their intended use, and should be managed according to the recommended protocol. If exposure occurs, the postexposure management protocol should be administered to prevent the spread of the infection. Occupational blood exposure should be managed with appropriate first-aid procedures as quickly as possible, and at the same time documentation detailing the exposure must be prepared. Recommended management protocol, according to the infecting agent, should be administered without any delay.

The 2020 coronavirus disease (COVID-19) pandemic poses new challenges for the orthodontic profession. Orthodontists working in close contact with patients and being exposed to aerosol and droplets from the patients' oral cavity are at a higher risk of getting infected and potentially spreading it to their peers, families, and other patients. Postpandemic, along with the increased importance of teledentistry and virtual visits, we should envision a dental environment wherein all clinicians are wearing disposable gowns, face shields, face masks, gloves, and any new Occupational Safety and Health Administration (OSHA) PPE recommendations that modify existing guidelines (Krishnan, 2020). Interested readers are referred to a detailed description of the documentation of infection control protocols in dental offices, available at the Center for Disease Control and Prevention (http://www.cdc.gov/).

Pain

Pain, which includes sensations evoked by and reactions to noxious stimuli, often accompanies orthodontic appointments. Surveys have proven this reaction to be a major deterrent to orthodontic treatment and a major reason for discontinuing treatment. It is clear from the existing literature that all orthodontic procedures, such as separator placement, band placement and fitting, archwire placement and activations, orthopedic force application, and debonding, produce pain. The chemicals released as part of the inflammatory orthodontic reaction are the key elements eliciting the hyperalgesic response. Nonlinear relationships exist between age, gender, psychological state, and cultural background in pain perception following placement of orthodontic appliances. The literature supports the notion that orthodontic pain has a definite influence on patient compliance and daily activities, because of functional and esthetic impairment engendered by the appliance.

Presently, NSAIDs form the major tools to reduce the intensity of orthodontic pain, along with other methods, such as chewing gum, anesthetic gel, vibratory stimulation, TENS, low-level laser treatment (Krishnan, 2007) and the use of pre-emptive/preoperative analgesics, 1 hour before every orthodontic procedure (Steen Law et al., 2000; Polat et al., 2005). Monk et al. (2018), through a Cochrane review, has pointed out that analgesics are more effective at reducing pain following orthodontic treatment than placebo or no treatment. There exists no difference in effectiveness between systemic NSAIDs compared with paracetamol, or topical NSAIDs compared with local anaesthetic. Interestingly, a combination of verbal and written information on orthodontic pain after placement of fixed appliances reduced patients' self-reported pain in the early stages (Montebugnoli et al., 2019).

Swallowing or inhalation of small parts

The very small metallic attachments used as part of orthodontic appliances pose a risk of being swallowed. Umesan et al. (2012) discussed in detail the way a piece of archwire that became impacted in the larynx was successfully retrieved.

Conclusions

Iatrogenic damage due to orthodontic treatment can occur in several ways during the entire course of therapy. Unwanted side effects can involve every aspect of treatment, from the composition of the appliance to the response of each of the involved tissues. In order to reduce or minimize the risks, the orthodontist should be thoroughly familiar with every possible side effect, its causes, the latest ways to avoid causing such deleterious developments, and the means to repair the damage once it occurs. At the end, treatment should be rendered with an appliance designed based on biomechanical principles most suitable for each individual patient, in a proper physical and psychological environment. Without doubt, all patients should be properly informed prior to the start of the orthodontic treatment about the risks and limitations of the treatment. The informed consent of the American Association of Orthodontists, which is frequently updated, serves this goal (AAO-informed consent, 2020).

References

AAO Informed Consent for the Orthodontic Patient, *American Association of Orthodontists* (2020) https://www1.aaoinfo.org/aao-updates-informed-consent-form/ Accessed September 13, 2020.

Abass, K. S. and Hartsfield, J. K. (2007) Orthodontics and external apical root resorption. *Seminars in Orthodontics* 13, 246–256.

Amini, F., Shariati, M., Sobouti, F. and Rakhshan, V. (2016) Effects of fixed orthodontic treatment on nickel and chromium levels in gingival crevicular fluid as a novel systemic biomarker of trace elements: a longitudinal study. *American Journal of Orthodontics and Dentofacial Orthopedics* 149(5), 666–672.

Anderson, G. B., Bowden, J., Morrison, E. C. and Caffesse, R. G. (1997) Clinical effects of chlorhexidine mouthwashes on patients undergoing orthodontic treatment. *American Journal of Orthodontics and Dentofacial Orthopedics* 111, 606–612.

Antonarakis, G. S., Joss, C. U., Triaca, A. et al. (2017) Gingival recessions of lower incisors after proclination by orthodontics alone or in combination with anterior mandibular alveolar process distraction osteogenesis. *Clinical Oral Investigations* 21(8), 2569–2579.

Arhun, N. and Arman, A. (2007) How damaging is orthodontic mechanics to tooth enamel. *Seminars in Orthodontics* 13, 281–291.

Arman, A., Cehreli, S.B., Ozel, E. et al. (2006) Qualitative and quantitative evaluation of enamel after various stripping methods. *American Journal of Orthodontics and Dentofacial Orthopedics* 130(2), 131.e7–131.e14.

Årtun, J., Van't Hullenaar, R., Doppel, D. and Kuijpers-Jagtman, A. M. (2009) Identification of orthodontic patients at risk of severe apical root resorption. *American Journal of Orthodontics and Dentofacial Orthopedics* 135(4), 448–455.

Bahar, B. S. B., Alkhalidy, S. R., Kaklamanos, E. G. and Athanasiou, A. E. (2020) Do orthodontic patients develop more gingival recession in anterior teeth compared to untreated individuals? A systematic review of controlled studies. *International Orthodontics* 18, 1–9.

Bass, J. K., Fine, H. and Cisneros, G. J. (1993) Nickel hypersensitivity in the orthodontic patient. *American Journal of Orthodontics and Dentofacial Orthopedics* 103, 280–285.

Behrents, R. G. (1996) Iatrogenics in orthodontics. *American Journal of Orthodontics and Dentofacial Orthopedics* 110, 235–238.

Benson, P. E., Parkin, N., Dyer, F. et al. (2019) Fluorides for preventing early tooth decay (demineralised lesions) during fixed brace treatment. *Cochrane Database of Systematic Reviews* 2019(11), CD003809.

Blaushild, N., Michaeli, Y. and Steigman, S. (1992) Histomorphometric study of the periodontal vasculature of the rat incisor. *Journal of Dental Research* 71, 1908–1912.

Blum-Hareuveni, T., Rehany, U. and Rumelt, S. (2004) Blinding endophthalmitis from orthodontic headgear. *New England Journal of Medicine* 351, 2774–2775.

Brezniak, N. and Wasserstein, A. (2002) Orthodontically induced inflammatory root resorption – Part II: clinical aspects. *The Angle Orthodontist* 72, 180–184.

Brudvik, P. and Rygh, P. (1993) The initial phase of orthodontic root resorption incident to local compression of the periodontal ligament. *European Journal of Orthodontics* 15, 249–263.

Brudvik, P. and Rygh, P. (1994a) Root resorption beneath the main hyalinized zone. *European Journal of Orthodontics* 16, 249–263.

Brudvik, P. and Rygh, P. (1994b) Multi-nucleated cells remove the main hyalinized tissue and start resorption of adjacent root surfaces. *European Journal of Orthodontics* 16, 265–273.

Brusca, M. I., Chara, O., Sterin-Borda, L. and Rosa, A. C. (2007) Influence of different orthodontic brackets on adherence of microorganisms in vitro. *The Angle Orthodontist* 77, 331–336.

Cadarapoli, D. and Gaveglio, L. (2007) The influence of orthodontic tooth movement on periodontal tissue levels. *Seminars in Orthodontics* 13, 234–245.

Chutimanutskul, W., Ali Darendeliler, M., Shen, G. et al. (2006) Changes in the physical properties of human premolar cementum after application of four weeks of controlled orthodontic forces. *European Journal of Orthodontics* 28, 313–318.

Cochrane, N. J., Lo, T. W., Adams, G. G. and Schneider, P. M. (2017) Quantitative analysis of enamel on debonded orthodontic brackets. *American Journal of Orthodontics and Dentofacial Orthopedics* 152(3), 312–319.

Connolly, M., Shaw, L., Hutchinson, I. et al. (2006) Allergic contact dermatitis from bisphenol-A-glycidyldimethacrylate during application of orthodontic fixed appliance. *Contact Dermatitis* 55, 367–368.

Consolaro, A. and Consolaro, R. B. (2018) There is no pulp necrosis or calcific metamorphosis of pulp induced by orthodontic treatment: biological basis. *Dental Press Journal of Orthodontics* 23(4), 36–42.

Corbett, J. A., Brown, L. R., Keene, H. J. and Horton, I. M. (1981) Comparison of Streptococcus mutans concentrations in non-banded and banded orthodontic patients. *Journal of Dental Research* 60, 1936–1942.

Currell, S. D., Liaw, A., Grant, P. D. B. et al. (2019) Orthodontic mechanotherapies and their influence on external root resorption: a systematic review. *American Journal of Orthodontics and Dentofacial Orthopedics* 155(3), 313–329.

de Castilhos, B. B., de Souza, C. M., Fontana, M. L. S. S. N. et al. (2019) Association of clinical variables and polymorphisms in RANKL, RANK, and OPG genes with external apical root resorption. *American Journal of Orthodontics and Dentofacial Orthopedics* 155(4), 529–542.

Deviot, M., Lachaise, I., Högg, C. et al. (2018) Bisphenol A release from an orthodontic resin composite: A GC/MS and LC/MS study. *Dental Materials* 34(2), 341–354.

Dewel, B. F. (1975) Editorial: AAO issues special bulletin on extra oral appliance care. *American Journal of Orthodontics* 68, 457.

Dorfman, H. S. (1978) Mucogingival changes resulting from mandibular incisor movement. *American Journal of Orthodontics* 74, 286–297.

dos Santos, R. L., Pithon, M. M., Martins, F. O. et al. (2010) Evaluation of the cytotoxicity of latex and non-latex orthodontic separating elastics. *Orthodontics and Craniofacial Research* 13, 28–33.

Dumbryte, I., Vebriene, J., Linkeviciene, L. and Malinauskas, M. (2018) Enamel microcracks in the form of tooth damage during orthodontic debonding: a systematic review and meta-analysis of in vitro studies. *European Journal of Orthodontics* **40**(6), 636–648.

Eliades, T., Hiskia, A., Eliades, G. and Athanasiou, A. E. (2007) Assessment of bisphenol-A release from orthodontic adhesives. *American Journal of Orthodontics and Dentofacial Orthopedics* **131**, 72–75.

Feller, L., Khammissa, R. A., Thomadakis, G. et al. (2016) Apical external root resorption and repair in orthodontic tooth movement: biological events. *BioMed Research International* **2016**, 4864195.

Fernandes, L. Q. P., Figueiredo, N. C., Montalvany Antonucci, C. C. et al. (2019) Predisposing factors for external apical root resorption associated with orthodontic treatment. *Korean Journal of Orthodontics* **49**(5), 310–318.

Fernández-Ferrer, L., Vicente-Ruiz, M., Garcia-Sanz, V. et al. (2018) Enamel remineralization therapies for treating postorthodontic white-spot lesions: a systematic review. *Journal of the American Dental Association* **149**(9), 778–786.

Fitzpatrick, D. A. and Way, D. C. (1997) The effects of wear, acid etching, and bond removal on human enamel. *American Journal of Orthodontics and Dentofacial Orthopedics* **72**, 671–681.

Fors, R., Stenberg, B., Stenlund, H. and Persson, M. (2012) Nickel allergy in relation to piercing and orthodontic appliances – a population study. *Contact Dermatitis* **67**, 342–350.

Fournier, A., Payant, L. and Bouchin, R. (1998) Adherence of Streptococcus mutans to orthodontic brackets. *American Journal of Orthodontics and Dentofacial Orthopedics* **14**, 414–417.

Gebistorf, M., Mijuskovic, M., Pandis, N. et al. (2018) Gingival recession in orthodontic patients 10 to 15 years posttreatment: a retrospective cohort study. *American Journal of Orthodontics and Dentofacial Orthopedics* **153**(5), 645–655.

Geiger, A. M. (1980) Mucogingival problems and the movement of mandibular incisors – a clinical review. *American Journal of Orthodontics* **78**, 511–527.

Geiger, A. M., Gorelick, L., Gwinnett, A. J. and Griswold, P. G. (1988) The effect of a fluoride program on white spot formation during orthodontic treatment. *American Journal of Orthodontics and Dentofacial Orthopedics* **93**, 29–37.

Gorman, W. J. (1967) Prevalence and etiology of gingival recession. *Journal of Periodontology* **38**, 316–322.

Grimsdottir, M. R., Gjerdet, N. R. and Hensten-Pettersen, A. (1992) Composition and in vitro corrosion of orthodontic appliances. *American Journal of Orthodontics and Dentofacial Orthopedics* **101**, 525–532.

Hafez, H. S., Selim, E. M., KamelEid, F. H. et al. (2011) Cytotoxicity, genotoxicity, and metal release in patients with fixed orthodontic appliances: a longitudinal in-vivo study. *American Journal of Orthodontics and Dentofacial Orthopedics* **140**, 298–308.

Hain, M. A., Longman, L. P., Field, E. A. and Harrison, J. E. (2007) Natural rubber latex allergy: implications for the orthodontist. *Journal of Orthodontics* **34**, 6–11.

Höchli, D., Hersberger-Zurfluh, M., Papageorgiou, S. N. and Eliades, T. (2016) Interventions for orthodontically induced white spot lesions: a systematic review and meta-analysis. *European Journal of Orthodontics* **39**(2), 122–133.

Huser, M. C., Baehni, P. C. and Lang, R. (1990) Effects of orthodontic bands on microbiologic and clinical parameters. *American Journal of Orthodontics and Dentofacial Orthopedics* **97**, 213–218.

Hutchinson, I. (1994) Hypersensitivity to an orthodontic bonding agent. A case report. *British Journal of Orthodontics* **21**, 331–333.

Iglesias-Linares, A. and Hartsfield Jr, J. K. (2017) Cellular and molecular pathways leading to external root resorption. *Journal of Dental Research* **96**(2), 145–152.

Jacobsen, N. and Hensten-Pettersen, A. (2003) Changes in occupational health problems and adverse patient reactions in orthodontics from 1987 to 2000. *European Journal of Orthodontics* **25**, 591–598.

Jarabak, J. R. and Fizzell, J.A. (1972) *Technique and Treatment with Light Wire Edgewise Appliance*. CV Mosby, St. Louis, MO.

Javed, F., Al-Kheraif, A. A., Romanos, E. B. and Romanos, G. E. (2015) Influence of orthodontic forces on human dental pulp: a systematic review. *Archives of Oral Biology* **60**(2), 347–356.

Jensen, C. S., Lisby, S., Baadsgaard, O. et al. (2003) Release of nickel ions from stainless steel alloys used in dental braces and their patch test reactivity in nickel-sensitive individuals. *Contact Dermatitis* **48**, 300–304.

Jiang, H., Hua, F., Yao, L. et al. (2013) Effect of 1.23% acidulated phosphate fluoride foam on white spot lesions in orthodontic patients: a randomized trial. *Pediatric Dentistry* **35**, 275–278.

Joseph, V. P., Rossouw, P. E. and Basson, N. J. (1992) Orthodontic microabrasive reproximation. *American Journal of Orthodontics and Dentofacial Orthopedics* **102**, 351–359.

Joss-Vassalli, I., Grebenstein, C., Topouzelis, N. et al. (2010) Orthodontic therapy and gingival recession: a systematic review. *Orthodontics and Craniofacial Research* **13**, 127–141.

Ketcham, A. H. (1927) A preliminary report of an investigation of apical root resorption of vital permanent teeth. *International Journal of Orthodontics* **13**, 97–127.

Kloehn, J. S. and Pfeifer, J. S. (1974) The effect of orthodontic treatment on periodontium. *The Angle Orthodontist* **44**, 127–134.

Kloukos, D., Pandis, N. and Eliades, T. (2013) Bisphenol-A and residual monomer leaching from orthodontic adhesive resins and polycarbonate brackets: a systematic review. *American Journal of Orthodontics and Dentofacial Orthopedics* **143**, S104–S112.e2.

Krishnan, V. (2005) Critical issues concerning root resorption: a contemporary review. *World Journal of Orthodontics* **6**, 30–40.

Krishnan, V. (2007) Orthodontic pain: from causes to management – a review. *European Journal of Orthodontics* **29**, 170–179.

Krishnan V. (2020) Editorial: Coping with COVID-19 – the life changing pandemic. *Journal of the World Federation of Orthodontists* **9**(2): 1–2

Krishnan, V. and Davidovitch, Z. (2006) Cellular, molecular and tissue level reactions to orthodontic force. *American Journal of Orthodontics and Dentofacial Orthopedics* **129**, 469.e1–32.

Kucukkeles, N. and Okar, I. (1994) Root resorption and pulpal changes due to intrusive force. *Journal of Marmara University Dental Faculty* **2**, 404–408.

Kurol, J., Ronnetman, A. and Heyden, G. (1982) Long-term gingival conditions after orthodontic closure of extraction sites. Histological and histochemical studies. *European Journal of Orthodontics* **4**, 87–92.

Kvinnsland, S., Heyeraas, K. and Ofjord, E. S. (1989) Effect of experimental tooth movement on periodontal and pulpal blood flow. *European Journal of Orthodontics* **11**, 200–205.

Levin, L., Einy, S., Zigdon, H. et al. (2012) Guidelines for periodontal care and follow-up during orthodontic treatment in adolescents and young adults. *Journal of Applied Oral Science* **20**, 399–403.

Ma, T., Marangoni, R. D. and Flint, W. (1997) In vitro comparison of debonding force and intrapulpal temperature changes during ceramic orthodontic bracket removal using a carbon dioxide laser. *American Journal of Orthodontics and Dentofacial Orthopedics* **111**, 203–210.

Mártha, K., Mezei, T. and Janosi, K. (2013) A histological analysis of gingival condition associated with orthodontic treatment. *Romanian Journal of Morphology and Embryology* **54**(3 Suppl.), 823–827.

Martin, S. and Garcia-Godoy, F. (1994) Shear bond strength of orthodontic brackets cemented with a zinc oxide-polivinyl cement. *American Journal of Orthodontics and Dentofacial Orthopedics* **106**, 615–620.

Mastaj, L. A., Tartakow, D. J., Borislow, A. J. and Fogel, M. S. (1994) Infection control in the dental practice with emphasis on the orthodontic practice. *Compendium* **15**, 74–80.

Matsumoto, Y., Sringkarnboriboon, S. and Ono, T. (2017) Proinflammatory mediators related to orthodontically induced periapical root resorption in rat mandibular molars. *European Journal of Orthodontics* **39**(6), 686–691.

McDonald, F. and Pitt Ford, T. R. (1994) Blood flow changes in permanent maxillary canines during retraction. *European Journal of Orthodontics* **16**, 1–9.

McGuinness, N. J. (1992) Prevention in orthodontics–a review. *Dental Update* **19**, 168–175.

Mellberg, J. R. and Mallon, D. E. (1984) Acceleration of remineralization in vitro by sodium mono fluoriphosphate and sodium fluoride. *Journal of Dental Research* **63**, 1130–1155.

Mijuskovic, M., Gebistorf, M. C., Pandis, N. et al. (2018) Tooth wear and gingival recession in 210 orthodontically treated patients: a retrospective cohort study. *European Journal of Orthodontics* **40**(4), 444–450.

Mitchell, L. (1992) Decalcification during orthodontic treatment with fixed appliances – an overview. *British Journal of Orthodontics* **19**, 199–205.

Montebugnoli, F., Incerti Parenti, S., D'antò, V. et al. (2019) Effect of verbal and written information on pain perception in patients undergoing fixed orthodontic treatment: a randomized controlled trial. *European Journal of Orthodontics*. doi: 10.1093/ejo/cjz068.

Morais, J. F., Melsen, B., de Freitas, K. M. et al. (2018) Evaluation of maxillary buccal alveolar bone before and after orthodontic alignment without extractions: a cone beam computed tomographic study. *The Angle Orthodontist* **88**(6), 748–756.

Morris, J. W., Campbell, P. M., Tadlock, L. P. et al. (2017) Prevalence of gingival recession after orthodontic tooth movements. *American Journal of Orthodontics and Dentofacial Orthopedics* **151**(5), 851–859.

Monk, A. B., Harrison, J. E., Worthington, H. V. and Teague, A. (2017) Pharmacological interventions for pain relief during orthodontic treatment. *Cochrane Database of Systematic Reviews* 11(**11**) CD003976.

Mostafa, Y. A., Iskander, K. G. and El-Mangoury, N. H. (1991) Iatrogenic pulpal reactions to orthodontic extrusion. *American Journal of Orthodontics and Dentofacial Orthopedics* **99**, 30–34.

Nattrass, C., Ireland, A. J. and Lovell, C. R. (1999) Latex allergy in an orthognathic patient and implications for clinical management. *British Journal of Oral and Maxillofacial Surgery* **37**, 11–13.

Ng, D., Chan, A. K., Papadopoulou, A. K. et al. (2017) The effect of low-level laser therapy on orthodontically induced root resorption: a pilot double blind randomized controlled trial. *European Journal of Orthodontics* **40**(3), 317–325.

Nowrin, S. A., Jaafar, S., Ab Rahman, N. et al. (2018) Association between genetic polymorphisms and external apical root resorption: a systematic review and meta-analysis. *Korean Journal of Orthodontics* **48**(6), 395–404.

Øgaard, B. (2001) Oral microbiological changes, long-term enamel alterations due to decalcification, and caries prophylactic aspects, in *Orthodontic Materials: Scientific and Clinical Aspects* (eds. W. A. Bratley and T. Eliades). Thieme, Stuttgart, p. 127.

Ottolengui, R. (1914) The physiological and pathological resorption of tooth roots. *Item of Interest* **36**, 332–362.

Pandis, N., Pandis, B. D., Pandis, V. and Eliades, T. (2007) Occupational hazards in orthodontics: a review of risks and associated pathology. *American Journal of Orthodontics and Dentofacial Orthopedics* **132**, 280–292.

Pazzini, C. A., Pereira, L. J., Carlos, R. G. et al. (2011) Nickel: periodontal status and blood parameters in allergic orthodontic patients. *American Journal of Orthodontics and Dentofacial Orthopedics* **139**, 55–59.

Pernet, F., Vento, C., Pandis, N. and Kiliaridis, S. (2019) Long-term evaluation of lower incisors gingival recessions after orthodontic treatment. *European Journal of Orthodontics* **41**(6), 559–564.

Perinetti, G., Varvara, G., Festa, F. and Esposito, P. (2004) Aspartate aminotransferase activity in pulp of orthodontically treated teeth. *American Journal of Orthodontics and Dentofacial Orthopedics* **125**, 88–92.

Pithon, M. M., Baião, F. S., Sant'Anna, L. I. et al. (2019) Effectiveness of casein phosphopeptide-amorphous calcium phosphate-containing products in the prevention and treatment of white spot lesions in orthodontic patients: a systematic review. *Journal of Investigative and Clinical Dentistry* **10**(2), e12391.

Pinto, A. S., Alves, L. S., Maltz, M. et al. (2018) Does the duration of fixed orthodontic treatment affect caries activity among adolescents and young adults? *Caries Research* **52**(6), 463–467.

Polat, O., Karaman, A. I. and Durmus, E. (2005) Effects of preoperative ibuprofen and naproxen sodium on orthodontic pain. *The Angle Orthodontist* **75**, 791–796.

Postlethwaite, K. M. (1990) Headgear safety – dare we ignore it? *Dental Update* **17**, 278–284.

Rana, M. W., Pothisiri, V., Killiany, D. M. and Xu, X. M. (2001) Detection of apoptosis during orthodontic tooth movement in rats. *American Journal of Orthodontics and Dentofacial Orthopedics* **119**, 516–521.

Renkema, A. M., Fudalej, P. S., Renkema, A. et al. (2013) Development of labial gingival recessions in orthodontically treated patients. *American Journal of Orthodontics and Dentofacial Orthopedics* **143**, 206–212.

Renkema, A. M., Navratilova, Z., Mazurova, K. et al. (2015) Gingival labial recessions and the post-treatment proclination of mandibular incisors. *European Journal of Orthodontics* **37**(5), 508–513.

Retamoso, L. B., Luz, T. B., Marinowic, D. R. et al. (2012) Cytotoxicity of esthetic, metallic, and nickel-free orthodontic brackets: cellular behavior and viability. *American Journal of Orthodontics and Dentofacial Orthopedics* **142**, 70–74.

Rivera Circuns, A. L. and Camilla Tulloch, J. F. (1983) Gingival invagination in extraction sites of orthodontic patients: their incidence, effects on periodontal health, and orthodontic treatment. *American Journal of Orthodontics* **83**, 469–476.

Robertson, M. A., Kau, C. H., English, J. D. et al. (2011) MI Paste Plus to prevent demineralization in orthodontic patients: a prospective randomized controlled trial. *American Journal of Orthodontics and Dentofacial Orthopedics* **140**, 660–668.

Saglam, A. M. and Sarikaya, N. (2004) Evaluation of infection-control practices by orthodontists in Turkey. *Quintessence International* **35**, 61–66.

Sardana, D., Zhang, J., Ekambaram, M. et al. (2019a) Effectiveness of professional fluorides against enamel white spot lesions during fixed orthodontic treatment: a systematic review and meta-analysis, *Journal of Dentistry* **82**, 1–10.

Sardana, D., Manchanda, S., Ekambaram, M. et al. (2019b) Effectiveness of self-applied topical fluorides against enamel white spot lesions from multi-bracketed fixed orthodontic treatment: a systematic review. *European Journal of Orthodontics* **41**, 661–668

Samuels, R. H. (1996) A review of orthodontic face-bow injuries and safety equipment. *American Journal of Orthodontics and Dentofacial Orthopedics* **110**, 269–272.

Samuels, R. H. and Brezniak, N. (2002) Orthodontic facebows: safety issues and current management. *Journal of Orthodontics* **29**, 101–107.

Santamaria, M. Jr, Milagres, D., Stuani, A. S. et al. (2006) Initial changes in pulpal microvasculature during orthodontic tooth movement: a stereological study. *European Journal of Orthodontics* **28**, 217–220.

Shapouri-Moghaddam, A., Mohammadian, S., Vazini, H. et al. (2018) Macrophage plasticity, polarization, and function in health and disease. *Journal Of Cellular Physiology* **233**(9), 6425–6440.

Shaw, W. C., O'Brien, K. D., Richmond, S. and Brook, P. (1991) Quality control in orthodontics: risk/benefit considerations. *British Dental Journal* **170**, 33–37.

Sondeijker, C., Lamberts, A. A., Beckmann, S. H. et al. (2020) Development of a clinical practice guideline for orthodontically induced external apical root resorption. *European Journal of Orthodontics* **42**(2), 115–124.

Sonesson, M., Bergstrand, F., Gizani, S. and Twetman, S. (2017) Management of post-orthodontic white spot lesions: an updated systematic review. *European Journal of Orthodontics* **39**(2), 116–121.

Steen Law, S. L., Southard, K. A., Law, A. S. et al. (2000) An evaluation of preoperative ibuprofen for treatment of pain associated with orthodontic separator placement. *American Journal of Orthodontics and Dentofacial Orthopedics* **118**, 629–635.

Stenvik, A. and Mjor, I. A. (1970) Pulp and dentine reactions to experimental tooth intrusion. A histologic study of the initial changes. *American Journal of Orthodontics* **57**, 370–385.

Tasios, T., Papageorgiou, S. N., Papadopoulos, M. A. et al. (2019) Prevention of orthodontic enamel demineralization: a systematic review with meta-analyses. *Orthodontics and Craniofacial Research* **22**(4), 225–235.

Tepedino, M., Franchi, L., Fabbro, O. and Chimenti, C. (2018) Post-orthodontic lower incisor inclination and gingival recession – a systematic review. *Progress in Orthodontics* **19**(1), 17.

Tell, R. T., Sydiskis, R. J., Isaacs, R. D. and Davidson, W. M. (1988) Long-term cytotoxicity of orthodontic direct-bonding adhesives. *American Journal of Orthodontics and Dentofacial Orthopedics* **93**, 419–422.

Thompson, R. E. and Way, D. C. (1981) Enamel loss due to prophylaxis and multiple bonding/debonding of an orthodontic attachment. *American Journal of Orthodontics* **79**, 282–295.

Tian, Y. L., Wang, K., Wang, J. et al. (2013) Root resorption after orthodontic treatment: A study of age factor and prevalence in anterior teeth. *Shanghai Kou Qiang Yi Xue* **22**, 224–227.

Travess, H., Roberts-Harry, D. and Sandy, J. (2004) Orthodontics. Part 6: Risks in orthodontic treatment. *British Dental Journal* **196**, 71–77.

Twesme, D. A., Firestone, A. R., Heaven, T. J. et al. (1994) Air-rotor stripping and enamel demineralization in vitro. *American Journal of Orthodontics and Dentofacial Orthopedics* **105**, 142–152.

Umesan, U. K., Ahmad, W. and Balakrishnan, P. (2012) Laryngeal impaction of an archwire segment after accidental ingestion during orthodontic adjustment. *American Journal of Orthodontics and Dentofacial Orthopedics* **142**, 264–268.

van de Velde, J. P. V., Kuiter, R. B. and van Ginkel, F. C. (1988) Histologic reactions in gingival and alveolar tooth movement in rabbits. *European Journal of Orthodontics* **10**, 87–92.

van Waes, H., Matter, T. and Krejci, I. (1997) Three-dimensional measurement of enamel loss caused by bonding and debonding of orthodontic brackets. *American Journal of Orthodontics and Dentofacial Orthopedics* **112**, 666–669.

Von Böhl, M., Ren, Y., Fudalej, P. S. and Kuijpers-Jagtman, A. M. (2012) Pulpal reactions to orthodontic force application in humans: a systematic review. *Journal of Endodontics* **38**, 1463–1469.

Waerhaug, J. (1979) The infra bony pocket and its relationship to trauma from occlusion and subgingival plaque. *Journal of Periodontology* **50**, 355–365.

Wang, C. W., Yu, S. H., Mandelaris, G. A. and Wang, H. L. (2020) Is periodontal phenotypic modification therapy beneficial for patients receiving orthodontic treatment? An American Academy of periodontology best evidence review. *Journal of Periodontology* **91**, 299–310.

Wennstrom, J. L. and Pini Prato, G. P. (2003) Mucogingival therapy – periodontal plastic surgery, in *Clinical Periodontology and Implant Dentistry* (eds. J. Lindhe, T. Karring and N. P. Lang), 4th edn. Blackwell, Oxford, p. 583.

Wong, V. S., Freer, T. J., Joseph, B. K. and Daley, T. J. (1999) Tooth movement and vascularity of the dental pulp: a pilot study. *Australian Orthodontic Journal* **15**, 246–250.

Yamaguchi, M. and Kasai, K. (2007) The effects of orthodontic mechanics on dental pulp. *Seminars in Orthodontics* **13**, 272–280.

Zachrisson, B. U. (1972) Gingival condition associated with orthodontic treatment II. Histologic findings. *The Angle Orthodontist* **42**, 352–357.

Zachrisson, B. U. and Alnaes, L. (1973) Periodontal condition in orthodontically treated and untreated individuals – I. Loss of attachment, gingival pocket depth and clinical crown height. *The Angle Orthodontist* **43**, 402–411.

Zachrisson, S. and Zachrisson, B. U. (1972) Gingival condition associated with orthodontic treatment. *The Angle Orthodontist* **42**, 26–34.

Zanatta, F. B., Ardenghi, T. M., Antoniazzi, R. P. et al. (2012) Association between gingival bleeding and gingival enlargement and oral health-related quality of life (OHRQoL) of subjects under fixed orthodontic treatment: a cross-sectional study. *BMC Oral Health* **27**(12), 53.

CHAPTER 19
The Biological Background of Relapse of Orthodontic Tooth Movement

Jaap C. Maltha, Vaska Vandevska-Radunovic, and Anne Marie Kuijpers-Jagtman

> **SUMMARY**
>
> Recent years have shown increased interest and research activity in retention procedures, and a number of clinical trials have tested retainer wear and effectiveness. In contrast, published data on the biological basis of relapse after a successful course of orthodontic treatment are still scarce. The majority of the studies on this issue are descriptive and led to the hypothesis that relapse is caused by the fibrous structures within the supporting tissues of the teeth. That would suggest that retention is needed until these structures are completely reorganized. However, there is considerable evidence that the rate of collagen turnover in the periodontal ligament is extremely fast, and that the gingival fibers, and especially the transseptal fibers, are remodeled rapidly. Therefore, it is concluded that collagen turnover is probably not the important factor in the etiology of relapse, and other extracellular matrix components may contribute significantly to this process. There is a definite need for more experimental and well-designed clinical studies to elucidate the biological basis of relapse. This process will be time consuming, but only if the etiology has been unraveled, we will be able to design evidence-based retention strategies.

Introduction

Post-treatment changes are a fact of life for orthodontists. Patients, however, quite often have other expectations, as they expect stability for many years, if not for life, after investing so much time, effort, and money in their orthodontic treatment during childhood and early adolescence. But craniofacial growth does not cease at the time of completion of orthodontic treatment, and we know now that craniofacial changes continue until as late as the sixth decade of life (Behrents, 1985). Follow-up studies suggest that orthodontic treatment results tend to relapse to a certain extent with aging (Al Yami *et al.*, 1999; Renkema *et al.*, 2011). However, physiological craniofacial changes in individuals who were never treated orthodontically should also be taken into consideration when evaluating orthodontic long-term results as relevant but unpredictable changes have been found in individual cases in longitudinal studies of untreated subjects (Al Yami *et al.*, 1998; Zinad *et al.*, 2016). This suggests that orthodontic corrections have to persist in a dynamic environment of continuing skeletal changes, functional demands, and compensatory adaptations of the dentition.

Bondemark *et al.* (2007) performed a systematic review on long-term stability of orthodontic treatment at least 5 years after treatment. From this review it was concluded that treatment of crowding resulted in successful dental alignment. However, mandibular arch length and width gradually decreased, and crowding of the lower anterior teeth reoccurred after retention. These findings were unpredictable at the individual level. Treatment of Angle Class II division 1 malocclusion with the Herbst appliance normalized the occlusion, but relapse happened and, again, it could not be predicted at the individual level. The scientific evidence was insufficient for conclusions on treatment of cross-bite, Angle Class III, open bite, and various other malocclusions. In contrast, a recent systematic review focusing on mandibular alignment concluded that post-treatment mandibular irregularity changes were limited, but the systematic analysis of the literature was hampered by a lack of high-quality evidence (Swidi *et al.*, 2019). Unfortunately, despite the importance of such systematic reviews, they cannot answer any questions on the etiology of post-treatment changes.

Relapse, physiologic recovery, or aging?

A wide variety of etiological factors for post-treatment changes have been discussed in the literature, but little sound scientific evidence is available from randomized controlled trials. Basically,

---

Biological Mechanisms of Tooth Movement, Third Edition. Edited by Vinod Krishnan, Anne Marie Kuijpers-Jagtman and Ze'ev Davidovitch.
© 2021 John Wiley & Sons Ltd. Published 2021 by John Wiley & Sons Ltd.

there are four sources of post-treatment changes (Maltha et al., 2017):

- continuous reorganization of the dental supporting tissues of the teeth in their new position and physiological tooth movement;
- (neuro) muscular imbalance due to the new potentially unstable situation;
- continued facial growth and aging after orthodontic treatment;
- lasting unfavorable oral habits

Studies on the long-term effect of orthodontic treatment of a variety of malocclusions consistently show that 40–90% of the patients have dental irregularities 10–20 years post-treatment but with large individual and unpredictable variations (Little et al., 1988; Kahl-Nieke et al., 1995; Al Yami et al., 1999; Thilander, 2000a,b; Bondemark et al., 2007; Dyer et al., 2012; Bjering et al., 2017). Overall, the maxillary and mandibular arches become shorter and narrower with age, resulting in crowding. The individuals' growth status at the end of treatment and the postorthodontic craniofacial changes that come with aging may be the most significant factors (Behrents, 1985; Nanda and Nanda, 1992; Harris et al., 1999; Ormiston et al., 2005; Pecora et al., 2008). Shorter dental arch perimeter, decreased mandibular intercanine distance, and increased anterior crowding, especially in the mandible, are typical findings in untreated adult individuals in their 30s and 40s (Bondevik, 1998, 2012; Thilander, 2009; Tsiopas et al., 2013). Furthermore, a significant increase in palatal and lower face height has also been demonstrated, which is attributed not only to the skeletal remodeling but also to continuous tooth eruption (Thilander, 2009). These natural changes must be taken into consideration when long-term orthodontic stability is evaluated, and they indicate that a sharper definition of the term "relapse" after orthodontic treatment is needed.

Usually, orthodontic relapse is defined as a return toward the pre-treatment condition, and the term is used, perhaps erroneously, for all post-treatment changes including real relapse of tooth movement, physiologic recovery, and developmental changes (Rossouw, 1999). Orthodontic tooth movement (OTM) requires remodeling of the gingival and periodontal tissues. These processes also play an important role in relapse. Resultant changes in the position of individual teeth will be seen early in the post-treatment phase and should be distinguished from changes due to aging. Vaden et al. (1997) showed that the rate of change decreased with time, supporting the contention that real "relapse" occurs soon after treatment, while continued change generally cannot be distinguished from normal aging processes. Orthodontic relapse therefore should better be defined as the post-treatment changes that are induced by the withdrawal of orthodontic forces (Maltha et al., 2017).

This chapter only deals with this orthodontic relapse and it will be considered from a biological point of view. First, we will describe the process of relapse of tooth position after releasing a mechanical force from a tooth that has been moved orthodontically, and the role of retention. Secondly, the biological tissue response will be discussed, with special emphasis on tissue reactions of the gingiva and the periodontal ligament (PDL).

The process of relapse

Amount, rate, and duration

Understanding the process of relapse is essential for deciding on optimal clinical measures to overcome it. The accurate description of the process on a macroscopic level is a first prerequisite. Reitan (1960, 1967) was the first to describe the process of relapse after experimental tipping movement of teeth in a more or less quantitative way. His studies in dogs and humans showed that relapse after tipping movement started immediately after withdrawal of the force. Already after 2 hours the tooth had regained a more upright position. Apparently, this was due to its movement within the socket, and no cellular response was evident. In most cases, relapse proceeded for a short period, ranging from 1 to 4 days, at a decreasing rate, and then it came to a standstill, probably because of hyalinization of the PDL. If the tooth was observed for a longer period, it was found that undermining resorption took place and relapse restarted. Finally, it might become stable after 18 days, when the amount of relapse was between 40% and 85% of the distance the crown had moved during active treatment. In some individuals, more relapse occurred than in others, and apparently the amount of relapse was individually determined (Reitan, 1960).

Recent studies in rats confirm these findings (Franzen et al., 2013, 2014, 2015). Maxillary rat molars were moved mesially by means of closed coil springs for 10 days. After appliance removal, relapse occurred rapidly. The first day, molars relapsed more than 60% of the active movement. By the third day, relapse slowed down and appeared to have stabilized by 3 weeks. At this time, the rate of relapse approached the rate of physiological tooth drift, and the total amount of relapse was between 80% and 90% of the achieved movement. Earlier studies showed a comparable relapse pattern. Yoshida et al. (1999) also described immediate relapse after tipping tooth movement induced by insertion of an elastic band between two molars. After removal of the elastics, the initial relapse rate can be estimated to be $100\,\mu m/day$ or more. After a few days it slowed down and a more or less stable situation was achieved. The total relapse for both groups amounted to approximately 90% of the active tooth movement. This amount of relapse compares to the study of Kim et al. (1999) in which the same method was used and a relapse of 87% of the initial movement was found by day 10. King et al. (1997) moved rat molars in a mesial direction by a spring between the first molar and the incisors for 16 days and immediate relapse was allowed thereafter. In the first day, relapse was about $250\,\mu m$ and subsequent further relapse showed a constant rate of approximately $14\,\mu m/day$ over a period of 2 weeks, leading to a total relapse of approximately $500\,\mu m$. However, about one-third of this relapse was in fact physiological distal drift of $5\,\mu m/day$, as was measured at the control sides in the same period.

Summarizing the data on relapse after tipping movement it can be concluded that after release of the orthodontic force a rapid relapse occurs, which slows down after a few days. The total relapse amounts to 40–90% of the initial movement after 10–20 days.

The first accurate description of immediate relapse after bodily OTM was given by van Leeuwen et al. (2003). Standardized bodily tooth movement was performed in dogs using continuous forces of 10 or 25 cN for 4 months. Immediate relapse was then allowed, and tooth positions were measured twice a week. Initial relapse rate was approximately $40\,\mu m/day$. It gradually decreased and stabilized after about 65 days. This pattern was independent of the force level used during active movement or the total amount of active tooth movement. However, the total amount of relapse showed large individual variation, varying from 30% to 50% of the active movement. A significant positive correlation was found between the amount of active movement and the amount of relapse ($R^2 = 0.823$) (Figure 19.1). If the amount of active movement was set at 100%, logarithmic curve fitting of the relapse data over time showed an R^2 of 0.784 (Figure 19.2), indicating that such a model adequately

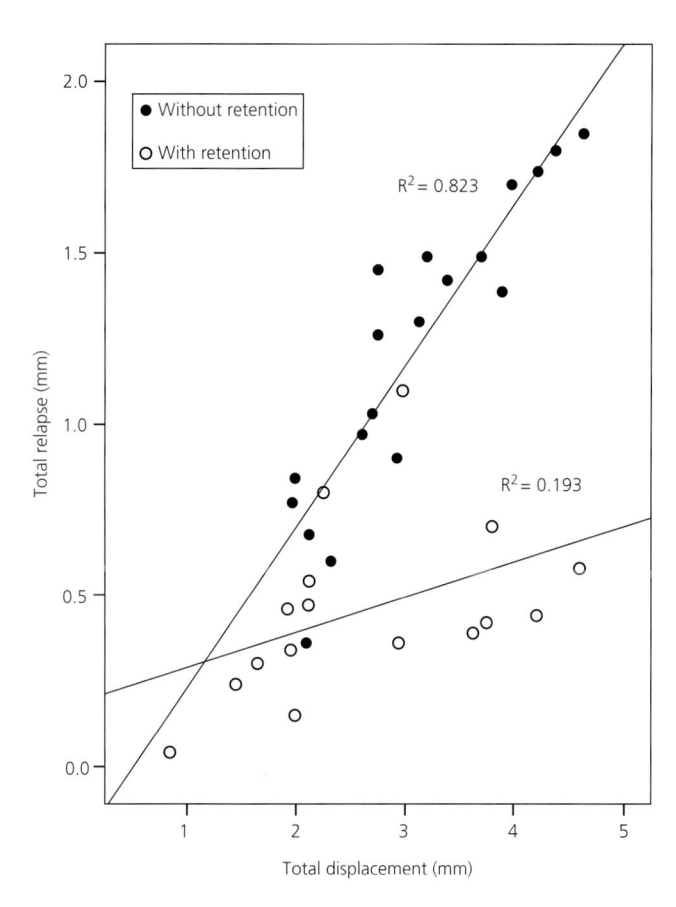

Figure 19.1 Relation between the total amount of experimental tooth movement and the total amount of relapse after a retention period of 3 months or without retention (Source: Based on data from Van Leeuwen et al., 2003).

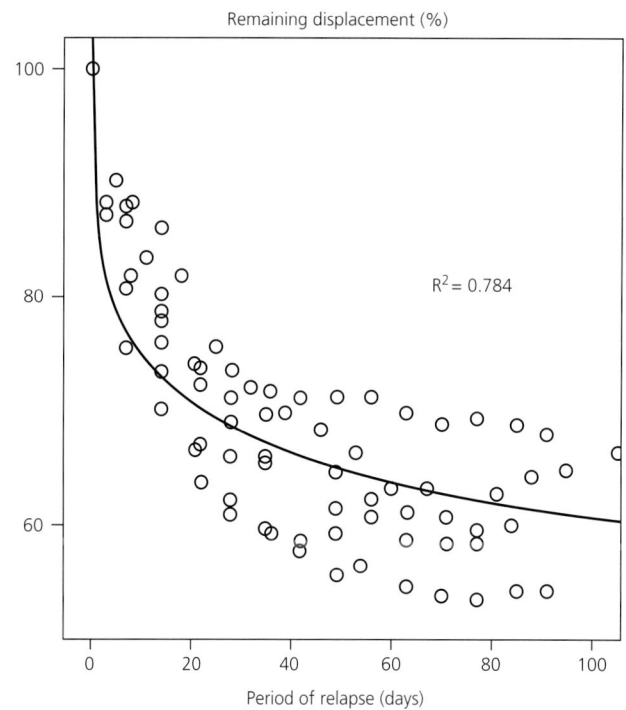

Figure 19.2 Individual data describing the relapse over time expressed as the remaining percentage of the initial active tooth movement if no retention was applied. (Source: Jaap Maltha.)

describes the process. It can be explained as a gradual fading away of the cause for relapse over time.

Besides relapse after translational movement of teeth, rotational relapse is also a well-known phenomenon in orthodontics. Immediate relapse after rotation of incisors in dogs has been shown by Edwards (1968), but the amount was not quantified. He reported that the gingiva moved with the tooth during active rotation, as shown by tattoo points, and that it slightly "re-rotated" together with a backward movement of the gingiva in a subsequent 2-week period without retention. Salehi et al. (2015) described a relapse percentage of 74% of a dog's incisor 3 months after removal of a rotational force. Ahrens et al. (1981) and more recently, Miresmaeili et al. (2019) evaluated relapse after lower incisor derotation in humans. Both studies concluded that after 1 month, relapse without retention was greater in the control groups than in the groups with supracrestal fiberotomy. As the number of patients was very small, and as the observation period was short, it is difficult to draw any definite conclusions.

Effect of retention

Another point that needs to be addressed is the effect of retention on the relapse tendency, and the question that should be answered is whether duration and type of retention have an effect on the amount of relapse.

Absence of retention in the short term negatively affects tooth alignment and interproximal contacts (Lyotard et al., 2010). This confirms the need for immediate retention after orthodontic treatment. Recent retrospective nonrandomized studies on retention duration indicate that longer retention periods, particularly in the mandible, lead to better tooth alignment than shorter ones (Bjering and Vandevska-Radunovic, 2018; Schutz-Fransson et al., 2019). Furthermore, longer retention periods are beneficial in cases with large treatment changes (Bjering et al., 2017; Bjering and Vandevska-Radunovic, 2018).

In 2016 the updated Cochrane systematic review of Littlewood and co-workers on orthodontic retention procedures was published (Littlewood et al., 2016). The only conclusion that could be drawn was that there is no evidence that full-time wearing of (thermoplastic) retainers provides greater stability than wearing them part-time. Other questions pertaining to the duration of retention and type of fixed retainers and the amount of relapse could not be answered. A recent search of the Cochrane Central Register of Controlled Trials revealed a few more randomized controlled trials after 2016 but again no additional evidence could be found for those relevant questions (Wouters et al., 2019).

Despite increasing clinical data on retention procedures since the last edition of this book, animal experiments remain a valuable source of information that cannot be clinically obtained, mainly due to ethical limitations. So, what can be learned from animal experiments?

Van Leeuwen et al. (2003) studied the effect of retention on relapse after bodily tooth movement in young adult dogs. After a standardized active movement by forces of 10 or 25 cN for 4 months, retention was applied for 3 months. Individual cases showed a decreasing rate of relapse thereafter, which stabilized again after approximately 65 days (Figure 19.3). The total amount of relapse was decreased by approximately 65%. However, the effect of retention on the amount of relapse was dependent of the amount of active tooth movement (Figure 19.1).

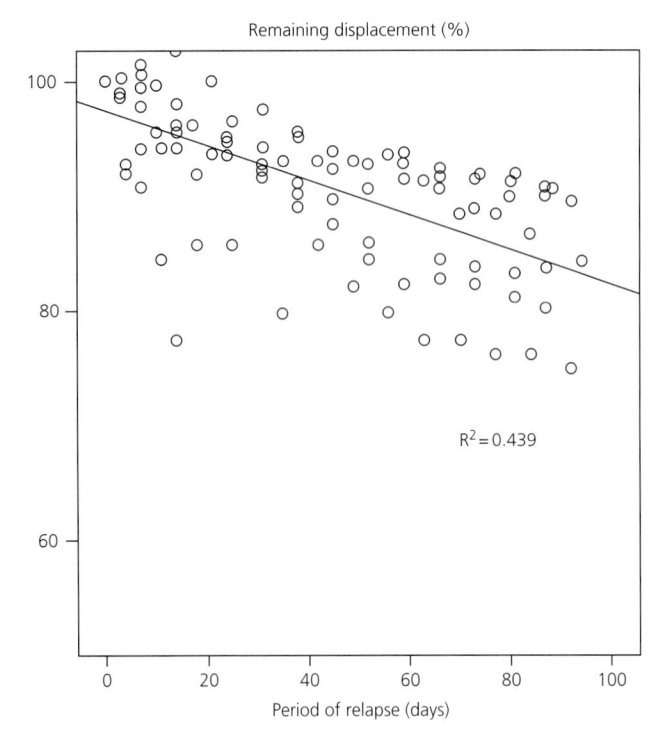

Figure 19.3 Individual data describing the relapse over time expressed as the remaining percentage of the initial active tooth movement if retention was applied for 3 months. (Source: Jaap Maltha.)

Low-level laser therapy (LLLT) has been described as a method to control relapse (Swidi et al., 2019), but did not seem very effective in rat experiments (Franzen et al., 2015). As an adjunct to conventional retention, LLLT has been shown to be more effective in facilitating collagen synthesis in the PDL of rat incisors 7 days after removal of the orthodontic appliance. However, the mRNA expression of matrix metalloproteinases showed no significant differences between the "lasered and retained" and the "only lasered" group (Kim et al., 2013). The authors suggest initiation of clinical studies to test the hypothesis that a combined laser and retainer protocol can shorten the retention period after orthodontic treatment. A similar investigation has previously been carried out where LLLT has been used after closure of a median diastema and the patients were provided with a removable retainer. There was a tendency for less diastema opening in the lasered group 1.5 years after debonding, but the clinical differences were not significant (Zahra et al., 2009).

Several authors have performed animal studies on the effect of retention on rotational relapse. Reitan (1960, 1967) reported on an experiment in dogs, in which incisors were rotated and subsequently retention was applied for 110 days. He observed that in the subsequent 22 days "some relapse" occurred. In a more recent dog study, a relapse of about 24% was found after rotation of the lower first premolars by 56 ± 13°, followed by a relapse of the released teeth by 12 ± 4° in 8 weeks (Lovatt et al., 2008). Boese (1969) performed rotations of incisors and second premolars in monkeys for 15–16 weeks, which resulted in a rotation between 35° and 124°. After a retention period of 4, 8, or 9 weeks, relapse was allowed for another 4 or 8 weeks. After 8 weeks of retention, the relapse was 0–23% of the initial rotation, and apparently, it was not yet finished.

From the available data we conclude that retention is necessary immediately after removal of the orthodontic appliances. The effect of retention on the relapse process and the effect of different retention protocols have attracted more attention in the last years and hopefully the trend will continue.

Histological changes during relapse

In his classical description of the histology during and after OTM, Reitan (1967) reported that the gingival fiber bundles were not that readily rearranged as those of the PDL. He described that the PDL fibers in the middle and apical regions are rearranged after a "fairly short" retention period, but that the strain in the gingival fibers persists even after a retention period of 232 days. Erikson et al. (1945) described some histological observations in human material after the closure of extraction diastemas and subsequent retention for 5 or 11 months. In both cases, transseptal fibers were present, even if the PDL and alveolar bone were destroyed due to periodontitis. Both studies suggested that transseptal fibers are continuously built as others are destroyed. According to Redlich et al. (1996) the gingival fibers of dog incisors became torn, ripped, and disorganized during rotation, which was supposed to be incompatible with stretching. Furthermore, the number of elastic fibers in the area increased. Unfortunately, none of the abovementioned authors addressed the histological changes during relapse itself.

Our own unpublished pilot studies have led to some initial conclusions on this subject. The data were derived from a limited number of dogs, and histology was performed after 3, 11, 13, and 15 weeks of relapse. This protocol cannot determine an accurate sequence of biological events that may occur during relapse but it suggests that this post-treatment process is dependent upon distinctive interactions between physical and biological factors.

The side that was the tension side of the PDL throughout the force-activated tooth movement can be considered as the pressure side during relapse. At this relapse-pressure side, the PDL remodels within 18 days (Figure 19.4). The normal structure of the PDL, in which principal collagen type I fibers are responsible for the anchorage of the tooth to the alveolar bone, has completely disappeared. Collagen fibers no longer attach the tooth to the alveolar bone. The PDL now consists of loose connective tissue, with mainly collagen type III fibers without clear orientation. Blood vessels and fibroblasts are present as usual in loose connective tissue. Direct resorption of the cancellous bone that had been laid down during active tooth movement is evident in most cases. In some cases, however, local areas of hyalinization were seen in the PDL (Figure 19.5). This situation will probably lead to an interruption of the relapse process until the hyalinized tissue is removed. This pattern has already been suggested by Reitan, (1960, 1967), on clinical observations. In rats, at the pressure side of actively moving teeth, removal of the hyalinized tissue by macrophages is associated with the onset of root resorption, as has been shown by the extensive work of Brudvik and Rygh (1993a, b, 1994a, b). The same process probably takes place during relapse, where root resorption in the middle part of the root can be found within 10 weeks of relapse. In most cases this development is not very serious, as it barely extends into the dentin (Figure 19.6), but in some cases almost half of the dentin appears to have been resorbed (Figure 19.7).

The side that used to be the pressure side during active tooth movement can be considered as the tension side during relapse. During active tooth movement, the normal structure of the PDL has been replaced by thin type III collagen fibers without a clear orientation. After relapse is allowed, these fibers are rapidly remodeled, and

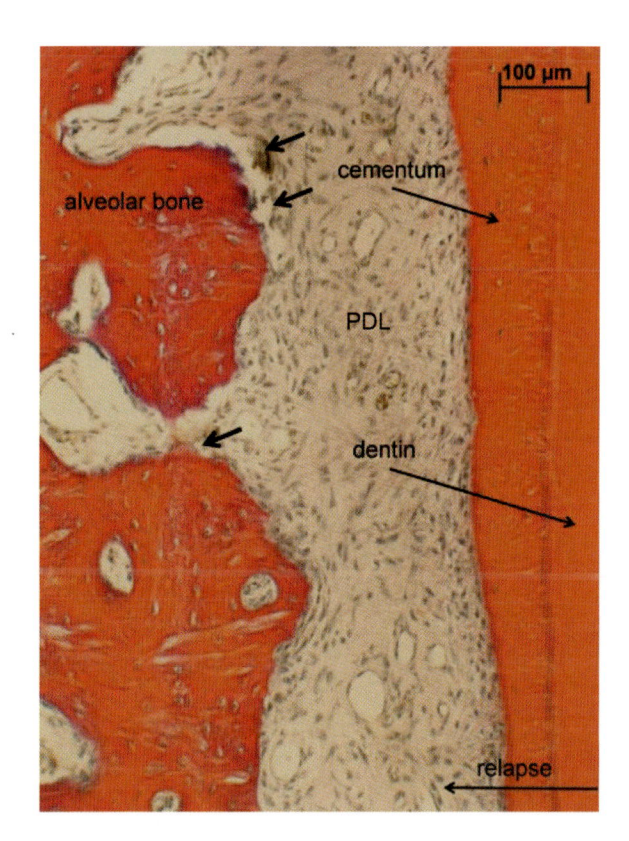

Figure 19.4 Pressure side of a dog premolar after relapse for 18 days. Loss of normal PDL structures. Arrows indicate osteoclasts. Herovici staining. (Source: Jaap Maltha.)

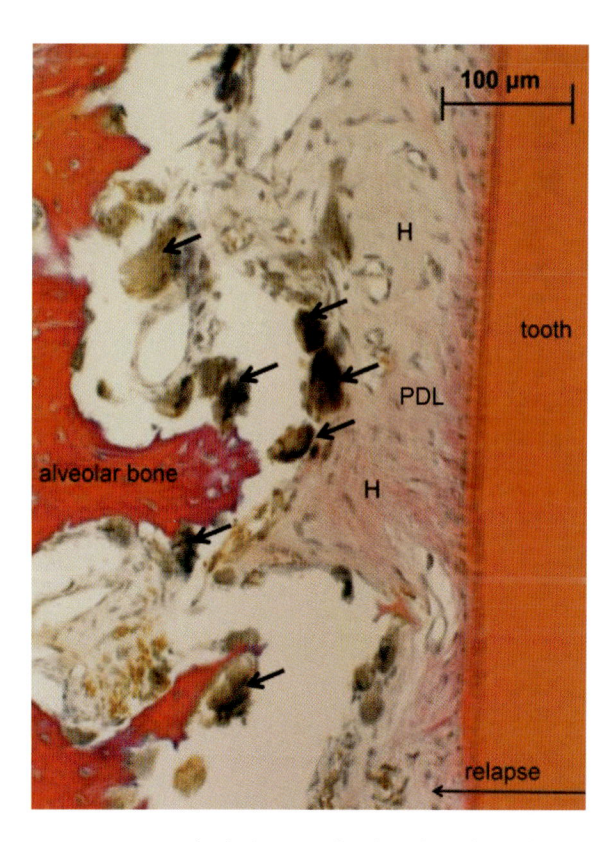

Figure 19.5 Pressure side of a dog premolar after relapse for 18 days. Loss of normal PDL structures. H, Hyalinized PDL. Bold arrows indicate osteoclasts. Herovici staining. (Source: Jaap Maltha.)

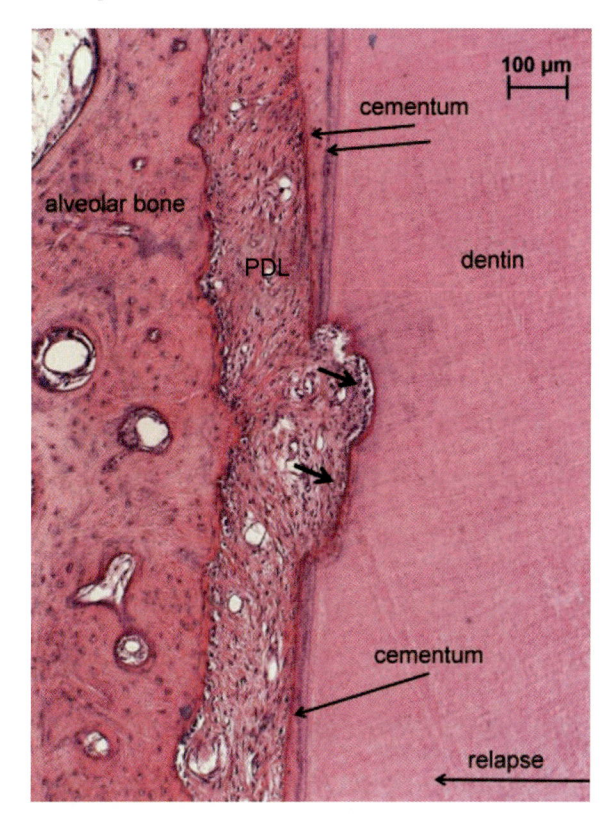

Figure 19.6 Pressure side of a dog premolar after relapse for 66 days. Localized areas of root resorption into the dentin (bold arrows). H & E staining. (Source: Jaap Maltha.)

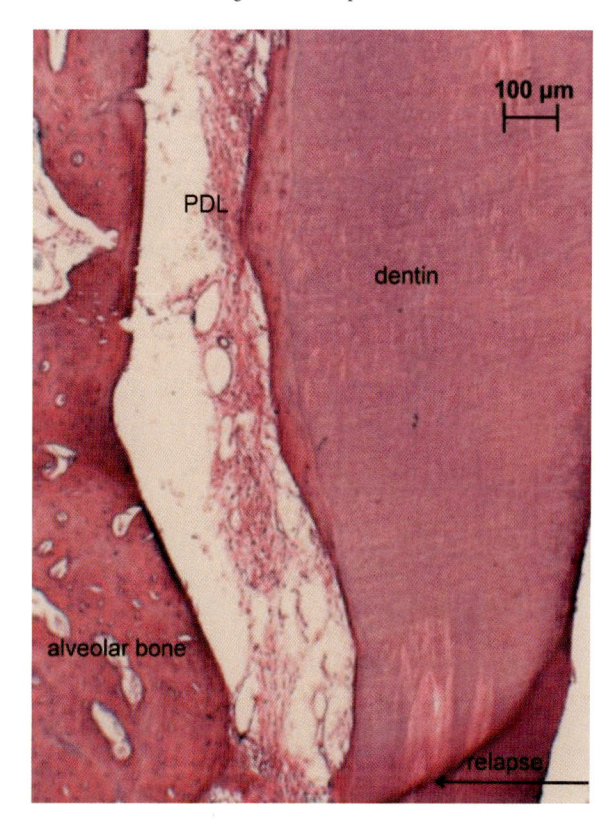

Figure 19.7 Pressure side of a dog premolar after relapse for 90 days. Complete loss of normal PDL structures. Severe generalized root resorption. H & E staining. (Source: Jaap Maltha.)

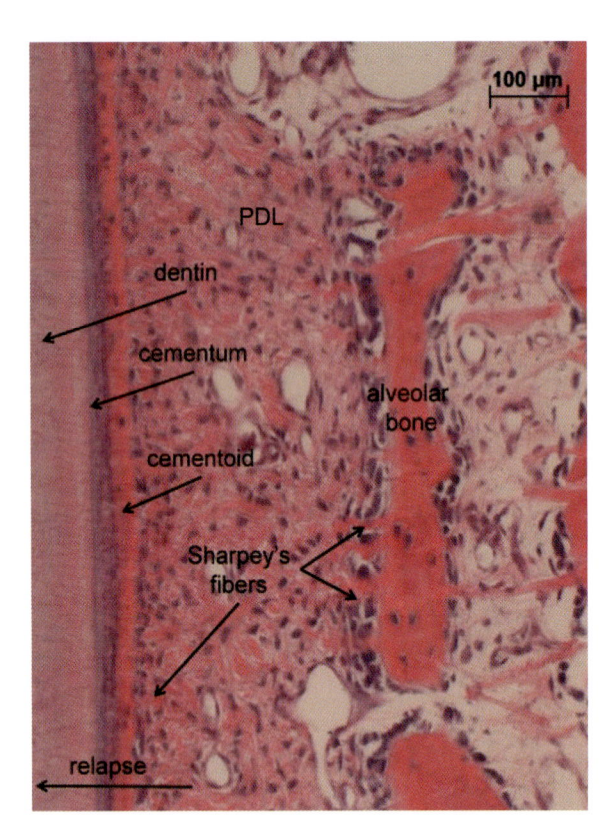

Figure 19.8 Tension side of a dog premolar after relapse for 18 days. Recovery of normal PDL structures. Sharpey's fibers inserting in newly deposited bone and cementoid. H & E staining. (Source: Jaap Maltha.)

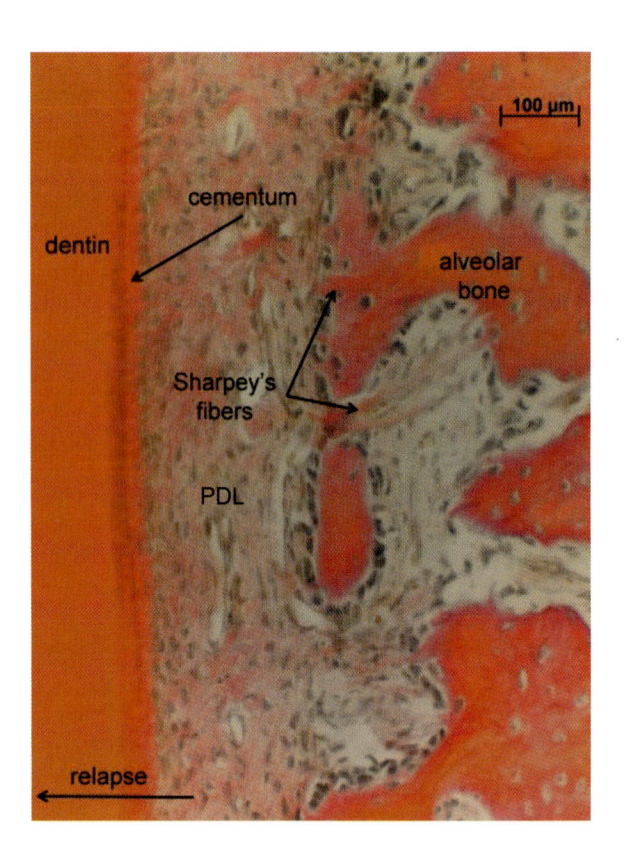

Figure 19.9 Tension side of a dog premolar after relapse for 18 days. Recovery of normal PDL structures. Sharpey's fibers inserting in newly deposited bone and cementoid. Herovici staining. (Source: Jaap Maltha.)

within 3 weeks a normal PDL structure is formed again (Figures 19.8 and 19.9). This structure consists mainly of collagen type-I fibers that cross the periodontal space and anchor the tooth to the alveolar bone by means of Sharpey's fibers that become embedded in the newly deposited bone and cementum. Furthermore, a normal distribution of fibroblasts and blood vessels is present. If no root resorption has taken place, just an additional layer of cementum is formed to allow anchorage of the Sharpey's fibers. The number of PDL fibers increases during the following weeks (Figure 19.10). If root resorption was present before relapse was allowed, reparative cementum is found to replace the resorbed cementum or dentin but without a complete restoration of the root outline (Figures 19.11 and 19.12).

These histological findings suggest that the biological processes occurring during immediate relapse are identical to those taking place during active tooth movement. The results from a study in rats fully support this concept (Franzen et al., 2013). During relapse, changes in the PDL width, redistribution of osteoclasts in the direction of relapse, and bone formation on the opposite side of the roots are consistent with experimental tooth movement. Furthermore, data from the same group show that gene expression of bone-formation markers such as collagen-I, alkaline phosphatase and osteocalcin gradually increase on the former pressure side, while bone resorption markers decrease with the onset of relapse (Franzen et al., 2014). The results from these studies clearly suggest that, at the cellular and molecular level, the periodontal and bone activity during OTM and relapse are identical.

Consequently, comparable changes in gingival crevicular fluid composition may be found during active tooth movement and relapse. Although no experimental data are available to describe

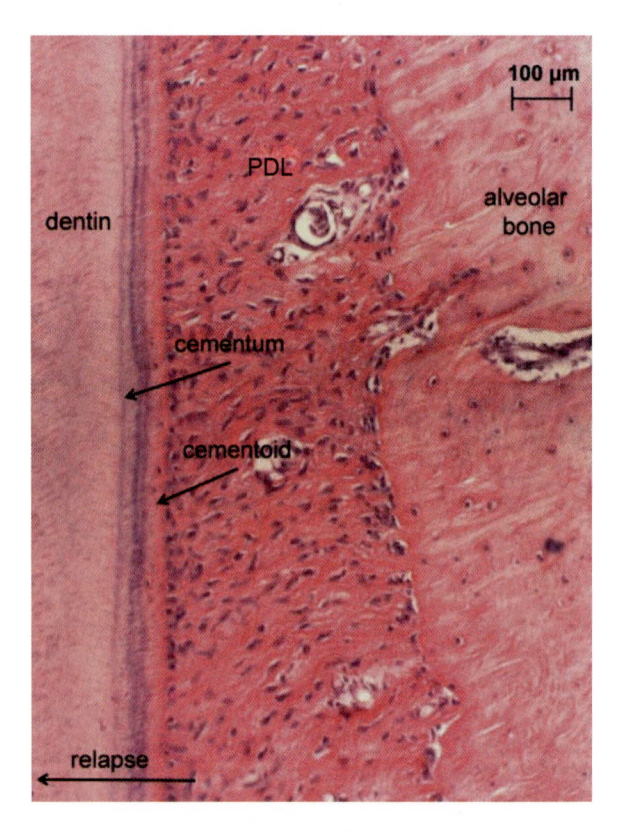

Figure 19.10 Tension side of a dog premolar after relapse for 66 days. Normal PDL structures. H & E staining. (Source: Jaap Maltha.)

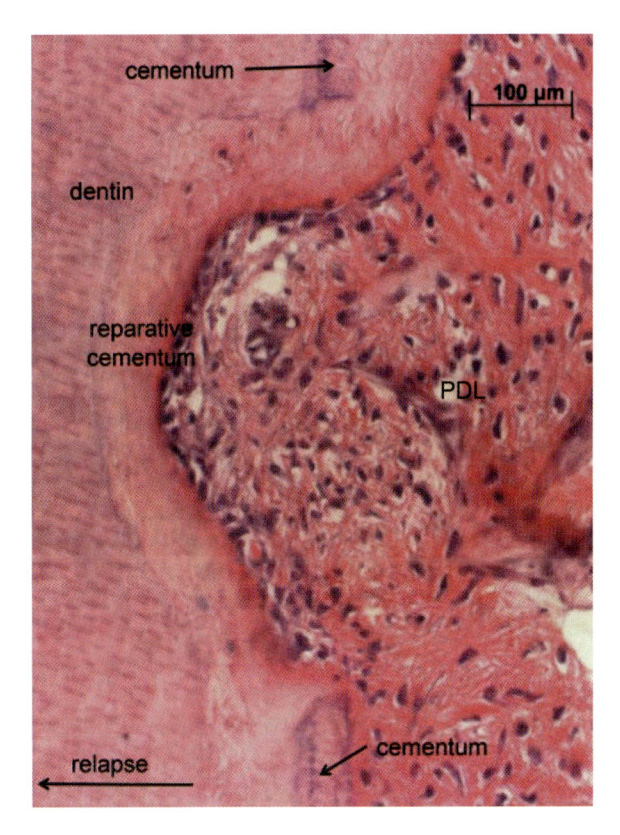

Figure 19.11 Tension side of a dog premolar after relapse for 66 days. Localized resorption area filling up with reparative cementum. H & E staining. (Source: Jaap Maltha.)

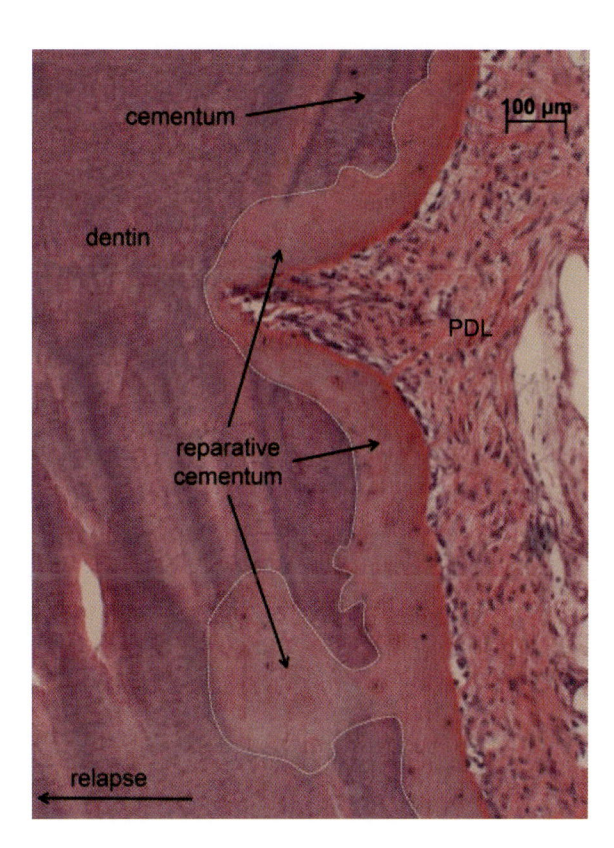

Figure 19.12 Tension side of a dog premolar after relapse for 90 days. Generalized root resorption area filled up with reparative cementum. H & E staining. (Source: Jaap Maltha.)

these changes during relapse, it is tempting to speculate on the possible use of a variety of growth factors, cytokines, colony-stimulating factors, and enzymes to detect local and temporal changes reflecting the biological activity in the PDL during relapse (Kavadia-Tsatala *et al.*, 2002; Ren and Vissink, 2008).

Collagen fibers of the periodontium and relapse

Terminology
The terminology used in literature pertaining to the periodontal fiber systems involved in the attachment of a tooth in the jaw is rather confusing. For the sake of clarity, we will use the nomenclature according to Lindhe *et al.* (2015) in this chapter. The fibers involved are divided into two major groups, the *gingival fibers* and the *PDL fibers*.

The gingival fibers, in turn, can be subdivided into four groups:
- Circular fibers, which encircle the cervical part of the tooth.
- Dentogingival fibers, which are embedded in the supra-alveolar root cementum and that fan out into the free gingival tissue of the facial, lingual, and interproximal surfaces.
- Dentoperiosteal fibers, which are also embedded in the supra-alveolar cementum, but run over the alveolar bone crest and then apically to terminate in the attached gingiva.
- Transseptal fibers, which extend between the supra-alveolar root cementum of approximating teeth. They run straight across the interdental septum and are embedded in cementum of adjacent teeth.

The other major group consists of the PDL fibers. These fibers run from the root cementum to the alveolar bone. They are also subdivided into four groups according to their orientation:
- Alveolar crest fibers, which run obliquely in an apical direction from the cervical root cementum to the top of the alveolar bone.
- Horizontal fibers, which are located apical to the alveolar crest fibers, and mainly have a horizontal orientation.
- Oblique fibers, which run obliquely into the cervical direction from the root cementum to the alveolar bone.
- Apical fibers, which are orientated more or less perpendicular to the root surface in the apical area.

Collagen fibers and relapse after translational tooth movement
The principal PDL fibers have been held responsible by several authors for relapse after OTM. During active tooth movement the fibers at the tension side are stretched by the force application and become embedded in the newly deposited bone. According to Reitan (1960, 1967), these fibers are more or less permanently elongated, and the rearrangement of the fibers and the alveolar bone after withdrawal of the force would lead to relapse. Boese (1969) agreed that relapse in the first 4 weeks is caused, to a large extent, by the PDL fibers. Gingival fibers, however, would be the most important cause of relapse thereafter. During OTM, PDL fibers at the tension side only develop in the direction of the movement. As long as no new bone is deposited between these fibers, they may be able to stimulate immediate relapse after force withdrawal (Thilander, 2000a, b). The role of retention would thus be to facilitate functional rearrangement and relaxation of these fibers.

In contrast to these ideas, Yoshida et al. (1999) are of the opinion that immediate relapse after force withdrawal is not caused by the elongated fibers, but rather by the rapid remodeling of the PDL and the surrounding alveolar bone. In recent years, several studies have provided information to support this notion. Administration of bone inductive proteins in sheep (Hassan et al., 2010) and of simvastatin and osteoprotegerin gene in rats (Han et al., 2010; Hudson et al., 2012; Zhao et al., 2012; Schneider et al., 2015; Dolci et al., 2017) have shown stimulation of bone formation and reduction of relapse in all experimental animals. The consistency of these results draws attention to the remodeling of the alveolar bone as an important but may be a neglected factor during relapse and calls for more research in this area.

Not only PDL fibers, but also the gingival fibers may be involved in relapse after translational tooth movement. The dentogingival fibers and other gingival fibers are interlaced, and, according to Reitan (1960), these fiber bundles are not as readily rearranged as those in the PDL, leading to a more persistent effect from the gingival fibers than from the PDL fibers on relapse after OTM. Also, Thilander (2000a, b) is of the opinion that the PDL fibers and the gingival fibers have different effects on relapse after translational tooth movement. The cause for this difference is that, in contrast to the PDL fibers, the gingival fibers are not embedded in alveolar bone, have a lower turnover rate than the PDL fibers and, therefore, remain stretched and unremodeled for months after experimental tooth movement. This opinion is in agreement with that of Boese (1969) who concluded that initial relapse is caused mainly by principal fibers of the PDL, and that after about a month the gingival fiber systems become most important for continuing relapse. A special function is ascribed to the transseptal fibers that connect neighboring teeth. These fibers protect the teeth from separating forces and maintain the contacts between adjacent teeth. If these contacts are changed by orthodontic means, the transseptal fibers are stretched and may generate forces that lead to relapse and reestablishment of the pre-existing situation (Tenshin et al., 1995; Thilander, 2000a, b).

The periodontal and gingival fibers are not alone in playing a role in relapse after translational tooth movement. Fukui et al. (2003) moved rat molars by putting an elastic band between the molars for 4 days, and subsequently retained them for 8 days. It was found that mechanical characteristics of the PDL, such as maximal shear load and failure strain energy density were disturbed during tooth movement. These features recovered during the retention period, but the recovery of the organization of the PDL was not yet complete. The data suggest that other factors, such as proteoglycans, may contribute to the mechanical characteristics of the PDL and in this way play a role in relapse. These findings are in line with Redlich et al. (1999), who also stressed the importance of extracellular matrix components such as proteoglycans and glycosaminoglycans for the biomechanics of the PDL.

It can be concluded that retention is needed to prevent relapse after translational tooth movement. The period during which it is applied should be long enough to allow complete remodeling or rearrangement of the fiber systems, and recovery of the biomechanical properties of the tissue.

Collagen fibers and relapse after rotational tooth movement

Studies on the stability of teeth after rotational tooth movement focus mainly on the role of the gingival fibers, which are anchored in the cervical region of the rotated tooth. These fibers remain attached to the teeth and become stretched during rotation. This stretching leads to the development of tension in the fiber system (Reitan, 1967). In addition, the whole gingiva is displaced and deformed (Edwards, 1968). According to these authors, the PDL fibers and the dentoperiosteal fibers are rapidly reorganized during and after rotation, but transseptal and other gingival fibers are persistent in remaining stretched. Such an imbalance is present for at least 5 months (Reitan, 1967; Edwards, 1968). This finding means that the tendency for relapse persists for several months, as confirmed by Boese (1969), in his study on tooth rotations in monkeys.

Contradictory findings on the persistence of transseptal fibers have been reported by Redlich et al. (1996), who showed that during rotation of dog incisors the gingival fibers became torn and disorganized, which seems to be incompatible with stretching. Furthermore, the number of elastic fibers in the area had increased. Fiberotomy, aiming at prevention of relapse, resulted in remodeling of the transseptal and other gingival fibers during postsurgical wound healing. The outcome of this remodeling process was that the fibers regained a spatial organization resembling that in the controls, providing a new anchorage by which the position of the teeth is stabilized. Fiberotomy has recently been shown to accelerate experimental tooth movement and diminish relapse in a rat model (Young et al., 2013). The authors conclude that detachment of the marginal gingiva from the root surfaces enhances bone remodeling and this is the reason for the observed results. This suggests that the mediated alveolar bone activity, and not the fiberotomy per se, are responsible for increased tooth movement and reduced relapse.

It can be concluded that the persistence of stretched transseptal and other gingival fibers has long been considered the main cause for relapse after rotational tooth movement. However, the findings of Redlich et al. (1996), that these fibers are not stretched and that the number of elastic fibers was increased after rotation, suggest that changes in the mechanical properties of the gingival tissues, more than the stretching of the fibers, are important factors for relapse after orthodontic tooth rotations.

Collagen fibers and relapse after closure of extraction space or midline diastema

A special situation seems to exist when an extraction space or diastema is closed. After completion of orthodontic treatment, extraction spaces tend to reopen. It is likely that, once brought together, both teeth will become separated after removal of the mechanical retaining device, by the action of the compressed transseptal fibers (Erikson et al., 1945). This tissue persists for a long period and its removal reduces relapse in humans, even if the transseptal fibers were not severed, indicating that in these circumstances the transseptal fibers have been remodeled or that these fibers are not necessarily involved in relapse (Edwards, 1971; McCollum and Preston, 1980). It has also been shown that compressed gingival tissues in a closed extraction site may lead to an epithelial fold, especially in a first premolar extraction site. In the invagination area, deep proliferations of the oral epithelium into the connective tissue were found with high levels of oxidative enzyme activity in the hyperplastic basal cell layers (Ronnerman et al., 1980). These epithelial folds might lead to reopening of the extraction site even in cases in which crowding in the anterior region was present (Golz et al., 2011). Alternative explanations are that the mechanical properties of the tissues change because the amount of glycosaminoglycans in the connective tissue increases, as is described by Ronnerman et al. (1980) and/or that the numbers of elastic or oxytalan fibers in the gingiva increase after extraction and space closure (Franchi et al., 1989; Redlich et al., 1999). Histological studies have shown that extraction leads to disruption of transseptal and other gingival fibers, but that these fibers are restored in the diastema during healing. This might lead to the conclusion that relapse after closure of an extraction diastema is probably associated with the presence of an elastic, gelatinous, and hyperplastic gingival tissue that would favor relapse (Redlich et al., 1999).

Turnover of collagen in the periodontium

Most research on relapse focuses on the role of the periodontal fiber systems in this process. To avoid relapse, it is assumed that teeth must be retained in their corrected positions until a total remodeling and rearrangement of all tissues involved has occurred. One of the main problems with this concept, which has drawn considerable attention, is the rate of turnover or renewal of the periodontal fiber system.

Carneiro and de Moraes (1965) were the first to study the rate of collagen synthesis in the PDL in mice by autoradiography, after a single injection of ^{3}H-proline. It was found that the uptake of label in osteoblasts and cementoblasts was highest in the apical region, followed by the middle region, and lowest in the cervical region of the PDL. The uptake in the extracellular matrix was also highest in the apical region followed by the cervical region and lowest in the middle region of the PDL. In the 1960s and 1970s many studies have focused on the half-lives of collagen in the different PDL regions. The results were rather variable, due to differences in methodology, but the main conclusions were that the half-lives of collagen in the PDL were very short in comparison to those in skin and bone. The half-life for mature collagen in the PDL was approximately 24 hours, and in the attached gingiva it was 5 days (Sodek, 1976, 1977).

Minkoff and Engstrom (1979) determined the half-lives by autoradiography of ^{3}H-proline in 40-day-old mice for different subgroups of gingival and PDL fibers,. The initial incorporation was highest in the oblique PDL fibers, second in the transseptal fibers, and far lower in the dentogingival fibers. This order corresponds with the half-lives, which were determined as 5.7 days for the oblique PDL fibers, 8.4 days for the transseptal, and 25 days for the dentogingival fibers. In young mice (18 days old) the ratio for the initial incorporation was more or less the same as in adult mice, but the half-lives in these young animals were shorter, namely 2.5 days for the oblique PDL fibers, 3.8 days for the transseptal, and 7.8 days for the dentogingival fibers. This age-related effect on the duration of collagen turnover in the mouse gingival fibers and PDL was confirmed by Tonna et al. (1980), who found a decrease in turnover of collagen in all regions with age.

More recently, Henneman et al. (2012) performed a study in young rats, which were injected twice a week, from 14 to 35 days of age, to ensure labeling of all periodontal fibers. After autoradiography, they found that the half-life for the supra-alveolar fibers was 9.6 days, for the oblique fibers 5.5 days, and in the apical region 4.3 days. The shortest half-life was reported for the interradicular fibers, where it was 1.4 days.

The role of the transseptal fibers in relapse has been questioned by Row and Johnson, (1990), who found in rats that transseptal fibers adjust their length by rapid remodeling in regions experiencing tensile forces. This remodeling appeared to be fastest in the middle region of these fibers. Moreover, Redlich et al. (1999) reported that transseptal fibers have a turnover rate that is as fast as that of the PDL fibers.

From these studies, a general trend can be established. Collagen turnover in the PDL is faster than in the gingival fibers, and within the PDL the turnover rate is fastest in the apical or the interradicular region of the root, while being slowest in the cervical or the supra-alveolar region. There is evidently a decreasing gradient from the apical to the cervical region. Among the gingival fibers, the transseptal fibers show the fastest collagen turnover rate, and, according to Redlich et al. (1999) it is as fast as in the PDL fibers.

Comparing collagen turnover rates in the PDL, gingival fibers, and skin, Henneman et al. (2012) found that the half-life of the collagen in rat skin was 9.9 days, which is comparable with the supra-alveolar fibers, and two to three times slower than the PDL fibers. Altogether, the data indicate that collagen turnover in the PDL is extremely fast, and that the gingival and transseptal fibers remodel slower but still faster than skin fibers. Thus, the turnover rate of collagen in the soft tissues surrounding the teeth is far greater than the rate found in other tissues, and the experimental data strongly suggest that the periodontal as well as the gingival fiber systems are completely remodeled in the course of orthodontic treatment. If this is true, it becomes very unlikely that these fiber systems are important causal factors for relapse. Retention, then, could be considered as a tool to provide a morphologically stable situation that allows re-establishment of normal periodontal structures after OTM.

Biological techniques affecting orthodontic relapse

Over the last few years, the role of biological factors in the process of OTM has been elucidated to a large extent. The notion that similar processes are involved in relapse has led to research aiming at the possibility of using such biological factors to inhibit postorthodontic relapse. Since bone remodeling and collagen turnover are most important, the research focusses on the effect of agents related to these processes.

In a recent review, Swidi et al. (2019) elaborated on different factors that could be promising in diminishing relapse: (i) factors involved in collagen and bone turnover, such as osteoprotegerin, bone morphogenetic proteins, and the hormone relaxin; (ii) medications used for the treatment of osteoporosis such as bisphosphonates, and a human monoclonal antibody against RANKL, namely denosumab, and (iii) the effect of cholesterol-lowering drugs such as statins. Their conclusion is that all these factors need further investigation to establish their clinical applicability, and that probably denosumab holds the greatest potential.

Swidi et al. (2019) also include the effect of physical interventions, such as LLLT and vibration devices to decrease or prevent relapse. However, they conclude that for these interventions insufficient evidence is available.

Oxytalan fibers

Fullmer (1963) was the first to describe oxytalan fibers in the PDL of humans and animals. These fibers show a well-defined anatomical arrangement in the PDL, inserting into the root cementum at one end while the other end is always close to the periodontal blood vessels (Sims, 1976).

The number of oxytalan fibers changes during experimental tooth movement, both in monkeys and dogs (Edwards, 1968; Boese, 1969). The role of these fibers is unclear but Boese (1969) suggested that it might be related to relapse. Sims conducted extensive research on oxytalan fibers, studying in detail the changes in the oxytalan fiber system in the PDL of human premolars after tipping with different forces over periods of time ranging from 3 to 28 days (Sims, 1976).

He found that, in the early phase of tooth movement, the oxytalan fibers remained visible and were associated with the moving tooth. However, in the mid-part of the root they tended to disappear. This pattern was probably related to the hyalinization of the PDL that is frequently found in that region. In the areas where oxytalan fibers persisted, they were always associated with blood vessels. In the areas under tension, the oxytalan fibers were less clearly organized, and where the blood vessels became incorporated in newly deposited alveolar bone the oxytalan fibers disappeared. In general, their numbers did not increase after the cessation of treatment, but the fibers were reorganized. This behavioral pattern indicates that the oxytalan fibers are not stretched by OTM, and thus do not contribute to relapse. These findings are in agreement with Jonas and Riede (1980) who described a clear increase in length of the fibers by fiberplasia, not by stretching, in the tension areas during tipping movements of human premolars.

In vitro studies have shown that cyclic loading of PDL fibroblasts stimulates the synthesis of oxytalan fibers. This suggests that indeed these fibers play a role in the adaptation of the PDL to mechanical changes (Nakashima *et al*., 2009; Tsuruga *et al*., 2009; Strydom *et al*., 2012). However, although the oxytalan fiber system changes during OTM, up to now, there are no indications that it plays any role in the relapse of teeth following the completion of orthodontic treatment.

Conclusions

In recent years, there has been increased interest and research activity in retention procedures and several clinical trials have tested retainer wear and effectiveness. In contrast, published data on the biological basis of relapse after a successful course of orthodontic treatment are still scarce. Most of the studies on this issue are descriptive, suggesting that relapse is caused by the fibrous structures within the supporting tissues of the teeth. This hypothesis has led to the suggestion that retention is needed until these structures are completely reorganized during the post-treatment period. This tissue reorganization phase would last at least several months, especially after rotations were corrected. However, there is considerable evidence that the rate of collagen turnover in the PDL is extremely fast, and that the gingival fibers, and especially the transseptal fibers, are remodeled rapidly. Therefore, it is concluded that collagen turnover is probably not the important factor in the etiology of relapse, and other extracellular matrix components may contribute significantly to this process.

There is a definite need for more experimental and well-designed clinical studies to elucidate the biological basis of relapse. This process will be time consuming, but only if the etiology has been unraveled, we will be able to design evidence-based clinical measures to prevent relapse.

References

Ahrens, D. G., Shapira, Y. and Kuftinec, M. M. (1981) An approach to rotational relapse. *American Journal of Orthodontics* **80**, 83–91.

Al Yami, E. A., Kuijpers-Jagtman, A. M. and Van 'T Hof, M. A. (1998) Assessment of biological changes in a nonorthodontic sample using the PAR index. *American Journal of Orthodontics and Dentofacial Orthopedics* **114**, 224–228.

Al Yami, E. A., Kuijpers-Jagtman, A. M. and Van 'T Hof, M. A. (1999) Stability of orthodontic treatment outcome: follow-up until 10 years postretention. *American Journal of Orthodontics and Dentofacial Orthopedics* **115**, 300–304.

Behrents, R. G. (1985) *Growth in the Aging Craniofacial Skeleton*. Center for Human Growth and Development, Ann Arbor, MI.

Bjering, R., Sandvik, L., Midtbo, M. and Vandevska-Radunovic, V. (2017) Stability of anterior tooth alignment 10 years out of retention. *Journal of Orofacial Orthopedics* **78**, 275–283.

Bjering, R. and Vandevska-Radunovic, V. (2018) Occlusal changes during a 10-year posttreatment period and the effect of fixed retention on anterior tooth alignment. *American Journal of Orthodontics and Dentofacial Orthopedics* **154**, 487–494.

Boese, L. R. (1969) Increased stability of orthodontically rotated teeth following gingivectomy in Macaca nemestrina. *American Journal of Orthodontics* **56**, 273–290.

Bondemark, L., Holm, A. K., Hansen, K. *et al*. (2007) Long-term stability of orthodontic treatment and patient satisfaction. A systematic review. *The Angle Orthodontist* **77**, 181–191.

Bondevik, O. (1998) Changes in occlusion between 23 and 34 years. *The Angle Orthodontist* **68**, 75–80.

Bondevik, O. (2012) Dentofacial changes in adults: a longitudinal cephalometric study in 22–33 and 33–43 year olds. *Journal of Orofacial Orthopedics* **73**, 277–288.

Brudvik, P. and Rygh, P. (1993a) The initial phase of orthodontic root resorption incident to local compression of the periodontal ligament. *European Journal of Orthodontics* **15**, 249–263.

Brudvik, P. and Rygh, P. (1993b) Non-clast cells start orthodontic root resorption in the periphery of hyalinized zones. *European Journal of Orthodontics* **15**, 467–480.

Brudvik, P. and Rygh, P. (1994a) Multi-nucleated cells remove the main hyalinized tissue and start resorption of adjacent root surfaces. *European Journal of Orthodontics* **16**, 265–273.

Brudvik, P. and Rygh, P. (1994b) Root resorption beneath the main hyalinized zone. *European Journal of Orthodontics* **16**, 249–263.

Carneiro, J. and De Moraes, F. F. (1965) Radioautographic visualization of collagen metabolism in the periodontal tissues of the mouse. *Archives of Oral Biology* **10**, 833–848.

Dolci, G. S., Portela, L. V., Onofre De Souza, D. and Medeiros Fossati, A. C. (2017) Atorvastatin-induced osteoclast inhibition reduces orthodontic relapse. *American Journal of Orthodontics and Dentofacial Orthopedics* **151**, 528–538.

Dyer, K. C., Vaden, J. L. and Harris, E. F. (2012) Relapse revisited – again. *American Journal of Orthodontics and Dentofacial Orthopedics* **142**, 221–227.

Edwards, J. G. (1968) A study of the periodontium during orthodontic rotation of teeth. *American Journal of Orthodontics* **54**, 441–461.

Edwards, J. G. (1971) The prevention of relapse in extraction cases. *American Journal of Orthodontics* **60**, 128–144.

Erikson, B. E., Kaplan, H. and Aisenberg, M. S. (1945) Orthodontics and transseptal fibers. A histological interpretation of repair phenomena following removal of first premolars with retraction of the anterior segment. *American Journal of Orthodontics and Oral Surgery* **31**, 1–20.

Franchi, M., D'Aloya, U., De Pasquale, V. *et al*. (1989) Ultrastructural changes of collagen and elastin in human gingiva during orthodontic tooth movement. *Bulletin du Group International pour la Recherche Scientifique en Stomatologie et Odontologie* **32**, 139–143.

Franzen, T. J., Brudvik, P. and Vandevska-Radunovic, V. (2013) Periodontal tissue reaction during orthodontic relapse in rat molars. *European Journal of Orthodontics* **35**, 152–159.

Franzen, T. J., Monjo, M., Rubert, M. and Vandevska-Radunovic, V. (2014) Expression of bone markers and micro-CT analysis of alveolar bone during orthodontic relapse. *Orthodontic and Craniofacial Research* **17**, 249–258.

Franzen, T. J., Zahra, S. E., El-Kadi, A. and Vandevska-Radunovic, V. (2015) The influence of low-level laser on orthodontic relapse in rats. *European Journal of Orthodontics* **37**, 111–117.

Fukui, T., Yamane, A., Komatsu, K. and Chiba, M. (2003) Restoration of mechanical strength and morphological features of the periodontal ligament following orthodontic retention in the rat mandibular first molar. *European Journal of Orthodontics* **25**, 167–174.

Fullmer, H. M. (1963) The oxytalan connective tissue fiber in health and disease. *Annals d'Histochimie* **8**, 51–54.

Golz, L., Reichert, C. and Jager, A. (2011) Gingival invagination – a systematic review. *Journal of Orofacial Orthopedics* **72**, 409–420.

Han, G., Chen, Y., Hou, J. *et al*. (2010) Effects of simvastatin on relapse and remodeling of periodontal tissues after tooth movement in rats. *American Journal of Orthodontics and Dentofacial Orthopedics* **138**, 550.e1–7; discussion 550–551.

Harris, E. H., Gardner, R. Z. and Vaden, J. L. (1999) A longitudinal cephalometric study of postorthodontic craniofacial changes. *American Journal of Orthodontics and Dentofacial Orthopedics* **115**, 77–82.

Hassan, A. H., Al-Hubail, A. and Al-Fraidi, A. A. (2010) Bone inductive proteins to enhance postorthodontic stability. *The Angle Orthodontist* **80**, 1051–1060.

Henneman, S., Reijers, R. R., Maltha, J. C. and Von Den Hoff, J. W. (2012) Local variations in turnover of periodontal collagen fibers in rats. *Journal of Periodontal Research* **47**, 383–388.

Hudson, J. B., Hatch, N., Hayami, T. et al. (2012) Local delivery of recombinant osteoprotegerin enhances postorthodontic tooth stability. *Calcified Tissue International* **90**, 330–342.

Jonas, I. E. and Riede, U. N. (1980) Reaction of oxytalan fibers in human periodontium to mechanical stress. A combined histochemical and morphometric analysis. *Journal of Histochemistry and Cytochemistry* **28**, 211–216.

Kahl-Nieke, B., Fischbach, H. and Schwarze, C. W. (1995) Post-retention crowding and incisor irregularity: a long-term follow-up evaluation of stability and relapse. *British Journal of Orthodontics* **22**, 249–257.

Kavadia-Tsatala, S., Kaklamanos, E. G. and Tsalikis, L. (2002) Effects of orthodontic treatment on gingival crevicular fluid flow rate and composition: clinical implications and applications. *International Journal of Adult Orthodontic and Orthognathic Surgery* **17**, 191–205.

Kim, S. J., Kang, Y. G., Park, J. H. et al. (2013) Effects of low-intensity laser therapy on periodontal tissue remodeling during relapse and retention of orthodontically moved teeth. *Lasers in Medical Science* **28**, 325–333.

Kim, T. W., Yoshida, Y., Yokoya, K. and Sasaki, T. (1999) An ultrastructural study of the effects of bisphosphonate administration on osteoclastic bone resorption during relapse of experimentally moved rat molars. *American Journal of Orthodontics and Dentofacial Orthopedics* **115**, 645–653.

King, G. J., Latta, L., Rutenberg, J. et al. (1997) Alveolar bone turnover and tooth movement in male rats after removal of orthodontic appliances. *American Journal of Orthodontics and Dentofacial Orthopedics* **111**, 266–275.

Lindhe, J., Karring, T. and Araúo, M. (2015) Anatomy of periodontal tissues, in *Clinical Periodontology and Implant Dentistry* (eds. J. Lindhe and N. P. Lang). Wiley Blackwell, Oxford.

Little, R. M., Riedel, R. A. and Artun, J. (1988) An evaluation of changes in mandibular anterior alignment from 10 to 20 years postretention. *American Journal of Orthodontics and Dentofacial Orthopedics* **93**, 423–428.

Littlewood, S. J., Millett, D. T., Doubleday, B. et al. (2016) Retention procedures for stabilising tooth position after treatment with orthodontic braces. *Cochrane Database Systemic Review* CD002283.

Lovatt, R., Goonewardenet, M. and Tennant, M. (2008) Relapse following orthodontic rotation of teeth in dogs. *Australian Orthodontic Journal* **24**, 5–9.

Lyotard, N., Hans, M., Nelson, S. and Valiathan, M. (2010) Short-term postorthodontic changes in the absence of retention. *The Angle Orthodontist* **80**, 1045–1050.

Maltha, J. C., Kuijpers-Jagtman, A. M., Von Den Hoff, J. W. and Onkosowito, E. M. (2017) Relapse revisited – animal studies and its translational application to the orthodontic office *Seminars in Orthodontic* **23**, 390–398.

McCollum, A. G. and Preston, C. B. (1980) Maxillary canine retraction, periodontal surgery, and relapse. *American Journal of Orthodontics* **78**, 610–622.

Minkoff, R. and Engstrom, T. G. (1979) A long-term comparison of protein turnover in subcrestal vs supracrestal fibre tracts in the mouse periodontium. *Archives of Oral Biology* **24**, 817–824.

Miresmaeili, A., Shokri, A., Salemi, F. et al. (2019) Morphology of maxilla in patients with palatally displaced canines. *International Orthodontics* **17**, 130–135.

Nakashima, K., Tsuruga, E., Hisanaga, Y. et al. (2009) Stretching stimulates fibulin-5 expression and controls microfibril bundles in human periodontal ligament cells. *Journal of Periodontal Research* **44**, 622–627.

Nanda, R. S. and Nanda, S. K. (1992) Considerations of dentofacial growth in long-term retention and stability: is active retention needed? *American Journal of Orthodontics and Dentofacial Orthopedics* **101**, 297–302.

Ormiston, J. P., Huang, G. J., Little, R. M. et al. (2005) Retrospective analysis of long-term stable and unstable orthodontic treatment outcomes. *American Journal of Orthodontics and Dentofacial Orthopedics* **128**, 568–574; quiz 669.

Pecora, N. G., Baccetti, T. and McNamara, J. A., JR. (2008) The aging craniofacial complex: a longitudinal cephalometric study from late adolescence to late adulthood. *American Journal of Orthodontics and Dentofacial Orthopedics* **134**, 496–505.

Redlich, M., Rahamim, E., Gaft, A. and Shoshan, S. (1996) The response of supraalveolar gingival collagen to orthodontic rotation movement in dogs. *American Journal of Orthodontics and Dentofacial Orthopedics* **110**, 247–255.

Redlich, M., Shoshan, S. and Palmon, A. (1999) Gingival response to orthodontic force. *American Journal of Orthodontics and Dentofacial Orthopedics* **116**, 152–158.

Reitan, K. (1960) Tissue behavior during orthodontic tooth movement. *American Journal of Orthodontics* **46**, 881–900.

Reitan, K. (1967) Clinical and histologic observations on tooth movement during and after orthodontic treatment. *American Journal of Orthodontics* **53**, 721–745.

Ren, Y. and Vissink, A. (2008) Cytokines in crevicular fluid and orthodontic tooth movement. *European Journal of Oral Science* **116**, 89–97.

Renkema, A. M., Renkema, A., Bronkhorst, E. and Katsaros, C. (2011) Long-term effectiveness of canine-to-canine bonded flexible spiral wire lingual retainers. *American Journal of Orthodontics and Dentofacial Orthopedics* **139**, 614–621.

Ronnerman, A., Thilander, B. and Heyden, G. (1980) Gingival tissue reactions to orthodontic closure of extraction sites. Histologic and histochemical studies. *American Journal of Orthodontics* **77**, 620–625.

Rossouw, P. E. (1999) Terminology: semantics of postorthodontic treatment changes in the dentition. *Seminars in Orthodontics* **5**, 138–141.

Row, K. L. and Johnson, R. B. (1990) Distribution of 3H-proline within transseptal fibers of the rat following release of orthodontic forces. *American Journal of Anatomy* **189**, 179–188.

Salehi, P., Heidari, S., Tanideh, N. and Torkan, S. (2015) Effect of low-level laser irradiation on the rate and short-term stability of rotational tooth movement in dogs. *American Journal of Orthodontics and Dentofacial Orthopedics* **147**, 578–586.

Schneider, D. A., Smith, S. M., Campbell, C. et al. (2015) Locally limited inhibition of bone resorption and orthodontic relapse by recombinant osteoprotegerin protein. *Orthodontic and Craniofacial Research* **18**(Suppl. 1), 187–195.

Schutz-Fransson, U., Lindsten, R., Bjerklin, K. and Bondemark, L. (2019) Mandibular incisor alignment in untreated subjects compared with long-term changes after orthodontic treatment with or without retainers. *American Journal of Orthodontics and Dentofacial Orthopedics* **155**, 234–242.

Sims, M. R. (1976) Reconstitution of the human oxytalan system during orthodontic tooth movement. *American Journal of Orthodontics* **70**, 38–58.

Sodek, J. (1976) A new approach to assessing collagen turnover by using a micro-assay. A highly efficient and rapid turnover of collagen in rat periodontal tissues. *Biochemical Journal* **160**, 243–246.

Sodek, J. (1977) A comparison of the rates of synthesis and turnover of collagen and non-collagen proteins in adult rat periodontal tissues and skin using a microassay. *Archives of Oral Biology* **22**, 655–665.

Strydom, H., Maltha, J. C., Kuijpers-Jagtman, A. M. and Von Den Hoff, J. W. (2012) The oxytalan fibre network in the periodontium and its possible mechanical function. *Archives of Oral Biology* **57**, 1003–1011.

Swidi, A. J., Griffin, A. E. and Buschang, P. H. (2019) Mandibular alignment changes after full-fixed orthodontic treatment: a systematic review and meta-analysis. *European Journal of Orthodontics* **41**, 609–621.

Tenshin, S., Tuchihashi, M., Sou, K. et al. (1995) Remodeling mechanisms of transseptal fibers during and after tooth movement. *The Angle Orthodontist* **65**, 141–150.

Thilander, B. (2000a) Biological basis for orthodontic relapse. *Seminars in Orthodontics* **6**, 195–205.

Thilander, B. (2000b) Orthodontic relapse versus natural development. *American Journal of Orthodontics and Dentofacial Orthopedics* **117**, 562–523.

Thilander, B. (2009) Dentoalveolar development in subjects with normal occlusion. A longitudinal study between the ages of 5 and 31 years. *European Journal of Orthodontics* **31**, 109–120.

Tonna, E. A., Stahl, S. S. and Asiedu, S. (1980) A study of the reformation of severed gingival fibers in aging mice using 3H-proline autoradiography. *Journal of Periodontal Research* **15**, 43–52.

Tsiopas, N., Nilner, M., Bondemark, L. and Bjerklin, K. (2013) A 40 years follow-up of dental arch dimensions and incisor irregularity in adults. *European Journal of Orthodontics* **35**, 230–235.

Tsuruga, E., Nakashima, K., Ishikawa, H. et al. (2009) Stretching modulates oxytalan fibers in human periodontal ligament cells. *Journal of Periodontal Research* **44**, 170–174.

Vaden, J. L., Harris, E. F. and Gardner, R. L. (1997) Relapse revisited. *American Journal of Orthodontics and Dentofacial Orthopedics* **111**, 543–553.

Van Leeuwen, E. J., Maltha, J. C., Kuijpers-Jagtman, A. M. and Van 'T Hof, M. A. (2003) The effect of retention on orthodontic relapse after the use of small continuous or discontinuous forces. An experimental study in beagle dogs. *European Journal of Oral Science* **111**, 111–116.

Wouters, C., Lamberts, T. A., Kuijpers-Jagtman, A. M. and Renkema, A. M. (2019) Development of a clinical practice guideline for orthodontic retention. *Orthodontic and Craniofacial Research* **22**, 69–80.

Yoshida, Y., Sasaki, T., Yokoya, K. et al. (1999) Cellular roles in relapse processes of experimentally-moved rat molars. *Journal of Electron Microscopy (Tokyo)* **48**, 147–157.

Young, L., Binderman, I., Yaffe, A. et al. (2013) Fiberotomy enhances orthodontic tooth movement and diminishes relapse in a rat model. *Orthodontic and Craniofacial Research* **16**, 161–168.

Zahra, S. E., Elkasi, A. A., Eldin, M. S. and Vandevska-Radunovic, V. (2009) The effect of low level laser therapy (LLLT) on bone remodeling after median diastema closure: A one year and half follow-up study. *Orthodontic Waves* **68**, 116–122.

Zhao, N., Lin, J., Kanzaki, H. et al. (2012) Local osteoprotegerin gene transfer inhibits relapse of orthodontic tooth movement. *American Journal of Orthodontics and Dentofacial Orthopedics* **141**, 30–40.

Zinad, K., Schols, A. M. and Schols, J. G. (2016) Another way of looking at treatment stability. *The Angle Orthodontist* **86**, 721–726.

PART 7

Tooth-movement Research

CHAPTER 20
Planning and Executing Tooth-movement Research

Vinod Krishnan, Ze'ev Davidovitch, and Rajesh Ramachandran

> **Summary**
>
> Orthodontic research at the biological level embraces human subjects, animals, tissues, cells, and cell components. This research has a number of goals: to elucidate further the details of the biological response to applied exogenous mechanical forces, to extrapolate the results to the clinical environment, and to improve the ability of the orthodontist to craft personalized diagnostic procedures and treatment planning. Biological basic research offers an increasing number of investigative tools to orthodontic researchers. This list includes light and electron microscopy, immunohistochemistry, immunocytochemistry, flow cytometry, cytoplasmic level studies, genomic assessments, DNA microarrays, and toxicology studies. Such investigations can be conducted *in vitro* and/or *in vivo*. Exploiting these techniques and other available study methods leads to the development of new, sophisticated investigative procedures that will help to improve our clinical performance.

Introduction

The term "biology," which is derived from the Greek words "bio" (life) and "logy" (study of), is defined as "the scientific study of living things." The main research direction in biology is to study the whole organism through the changes happening in its cells, organs, and tissues. Basic scientific research is defined as fundamental theoretical or experimental investigative research to advance knowledge, without a specifically envisaged or immediately practical application (de la Pena et al., 2004). It is simply stated as the quest to know the unknown and explore various possibilities to improve a particular situation. The development of any specialty, be it in medicine or dentistry, depends on findings derived from basic science research, and their proper application in a clinical situation. Orthodontics is no exception. Great innovations are rarely possible without prior generation of new knowledge through basic scientific research. Failure to become familiar with the constant stream of new scientific information may lead to stagnation of clinical advancements. In reality, both basic and clinical research are closely intertwined.

Orthodontics, a specialty that relies upon biological reactions to applied mechanical energy, has witnessed revolutionary changes through the 120 years of its existence. The pioneers in this field, who laid the foundation to "dentistry's first specialty," have prompted the formulation of hypotheses, explaining many of the biological details of this clinical phenomenon. The importance attributed to biology in the study of orthodontics by Angle, the "father of modern orthodontics," is exemplified by the inclusion of basic medical subjects in his orthodontic curriculum. Although his vision of considering orthodontics as part of the medical profession was not fulfilled, he made it an integral and important part of dentistry. Sadly, the main focus in orthodontics, from the earlier days, has been mainly on mechanical force application to the teeth and jaws. Appliances have been designed to address many types of malocclusion, based upon the empirical observation that orofacial tissues remodel under the influence of the applied forces, enabling the teeth to be moved to new positions. What worsened the situation was the use of typodonts (Figure 20.1) to demonstrate, as well as to educate, about the way orthodontic mechanics and appliances work, creating an illusion that teeth behave like free bodies in space, and that judicious, controlled forces are all that is needed to produce a favorable clinical response. This approach leaves little room for accommodation of the biological diversity that exists between all patients, which ultimately dictates the outcome of any treatment modality.

In contrast to the typical *modus operandi* of orthodontics, medicine and all its specialties pay extremely close attention to all advancements made in basic biological sciences in order to improve their diagnostic and therapeutic skills. This pattern of practice, while keeping constant track of recent progress in a widespread

---

Biological Mechanisms of Tooth Movement, Third Edition. Edited by Vinod Krishnan, Anne Marie Kuijpers-Jagtman and Ze'ev Davidovitch.
© 2021 John Wiley & Sons Ltd. Published 2021 by John Wiley & Sons Ltd.

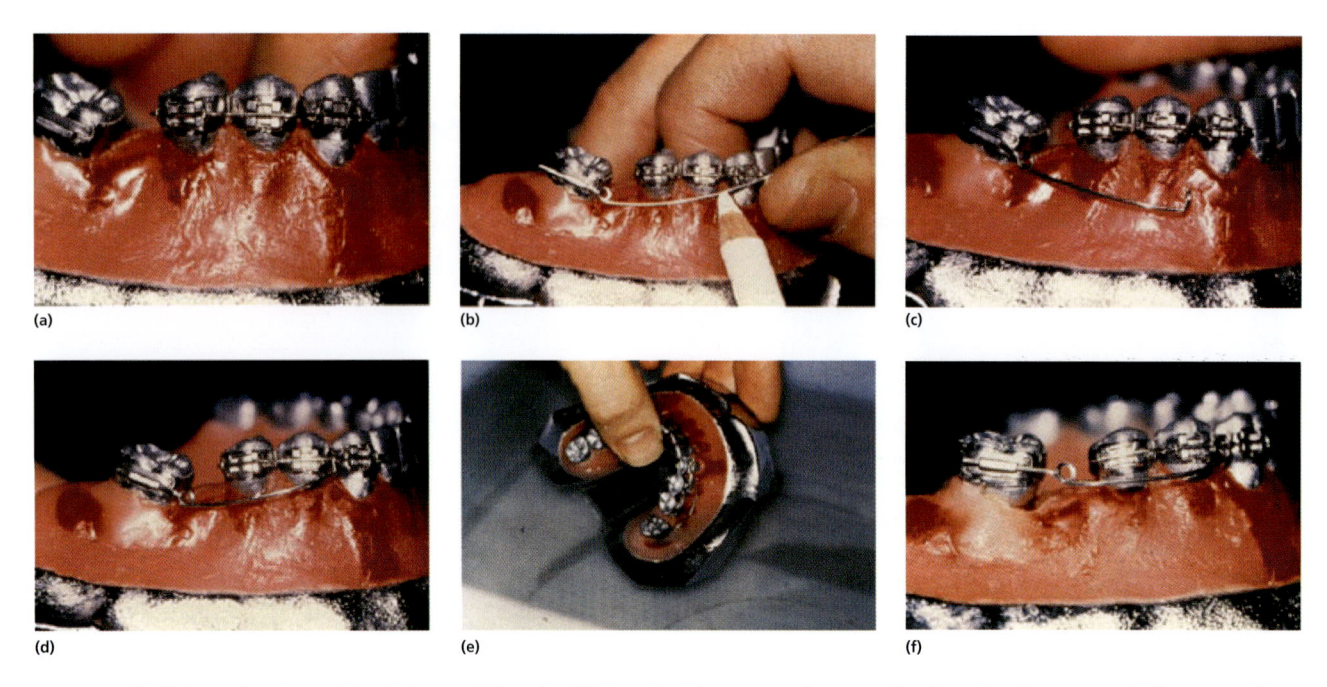

Figure 20.1 (a–f) A typodont is a training device consisting of artificial teeth, with crowns and roots, made of metal or plastic material. The roots of these teeth become embedded in dental wax, which hardens at room temperature, enabling the user to "freeze" the teeth in normal, as well as in many abnormal positions. In the latter case, one can then bond or cement orthodontic attachments to the dental crowns and fabricate a simulated orthodontic appliance. Once the appliance is fixed to the teeth, the typodont is dipped into warm water, the wax softens up, and the roots of the teeth that had been subjected to mechanical forces move with ease through the soft wax.

field of basic research, enables physicians to utilize newly acquired information to their patients' benefit. Physicians routinely bridge the gap between basic biological research and the clinical environment. They are keenly aware that organs and tissue systems are frequently exposed to pathological processes of their own, or which occur elsewhere in the body. They recognize the fact that a cellular function observed in a test tube may not be the same or may even be totally different when encountered in an actual clinical situation. Orthodontics, on the other hand, has failed to perform in a similar fashion. It is disheartening to admit that there is still a wide gap between basic biologic research and clinical orthodontics. Both areas are moving forward in parallel, but apparently with little collaboration between the two.

Many pioneer pathfinders like Sandstedt, Farrar, Ketcham, Oppenheim, Schwarz, Reitan, and Baumrind – to name a few – have been focusing on biological mechanisms behind orthodontic mechanotherapy through their research, and were instrumental in laying down a scientific foundation to the specialty. Their research succeeded in outlining the biological mechanism of tooth movement at the molecular, cellular, tissue, and organ levels. This research has also helped us to understand the reasons for overreactions by the paradental tissues, as well as for iatrogenic damages produced by orthodontic mechanics. However, regretfully, once the dental crowns are brought to an aesthetically and functionally pleasing position, both the patients and the orthodontists become satisfied, paying little attention to events that may be happening in and around the dental roots, which are powerful determinants of the final outcome of treatment. Any tissue damage discovered later, such as root resorption and alveolar bone loss, is viewed as unavoidable and unpredictable. This has led to a growing realization among teachers, researchers, and clinicians that biology is an important part of orthodontic practice and is now clearly reflected in the curricula of postgraduate orthodontic programs worldwide. Graduates of these programs have a more solid foundation for treating patients with malocclusions. The foundation of a sound biological background is critical for the well-educated clinician in order to ensure the best possible evidence-based treatment plan and treatment.

This chapter provides readers with an overview of the experimental methods that can be followed in basic biological research in orthodontics. This is not an exhaustive review and readers who are interested are encouraged to consult the available literature for more practical applications of the methodologies described. This chapter also briefly looks at the various future orthodontic research areas in tooth-movement biology so that novices and new researchers in the field are made aware of the existing void in the literature and clinical practice.

The scientific method

The scientific method is nothing but the rational and logical steps followed by every scientist to reach conclusions about the questions they have formulated. A methodological approach helps to organize thoughts and procedures, which can lead to unbiased observations, hypotheses, and deductions, to formulate proper conclusions. This process consists of four main steps: (i) observation; (ii) hypothesis; (iii) experimentation; and (iv) conclusions.

Observation of the problem requires thorough understanding of the existing literature to point out voids, which when filled might complete the process and make it clinically applicable. It can also be carried out with the unaided eye, a microscope, a volume meter, or any apparatus suitable for detecting the phenomenon. The key element of any scientific experiment is that it must be observable and reproducible. After the problem is identified by observation, the next step will be formulation of a *hypothesis*, with alternative thinking. This is always written in the form "If . . . then . . . ." After "If " we will identify the independent variable, which depicts the way we are going to solve the question, and the blank after "then" is the dependent variable, denoting what will happen when you do something to the independent variable. For example: "If I use prostaglandins [independent variable], then tooth movement will be accelerated [dependent variable]."

Experimentation involves the methodology required to analyze the hypothesis, in which *in vitro*, *ex vivo*, *in vivo*, and *in silico* experiments can be conducted to check whether the hypothesis formulated is true or not. The data generated through experimentation have to be organized properly, tabulated or interpreted, and the results should be presented in a way that even a novice in orthodontics could understand. A synthesis of all the data and discussing it in the context of the existing literature will generate proper *conclusions*, which denote what all the results mean and whether a proposed hypothesis is acceptable.

Evidence generation

Any data that provides proof concerning the matter in question can be called as evidence. There are four types of evidence, defined as (i) direct or experimental evidence, (ii) anecdotal, correlational or circumstantial evidence, (iii) argumentative evidence, and (iv) testimonial evidence. Of these, direct or experimental evidence is acceptable, as far as scientific research is concerned, which means that the evidence can be directly observed, tested, and is reproducible. Scientific research is conducted in the laboratory, on animals, or in human subjects before the molecule is marketed or released for patient use on a large scale. Laboratory studies can be either *in vitro* or *ex vivo*, while animal or human studies are categorized as *in vivo*. *In silico* research relates to the use of modeling, simulation, and visualization of biological processes in a virtual environment. This broad classification is used below to identify the type of studies conducted in biological research pertaining to orthodontic tooth movement. A brief review of instrumentation is also provided so that readers will become familiar with the newer methodologies to enable them to formulate their experimental protocols.

Laboratory studies in orthodontic biologic research – *in vitro* versus *ex vivo* studies

In vitro experiments are those that use cell lines, developed through primary culture some time ago for experimentation, while *ex vivo* means that something is experimented on or investigated outside its natural *in vivo* environment. *Ex vivo* experiments are performed in cells or tissues, which are isolated from an intact organism, and are still functional. Briefly, the cell lines available through purchase can be used for study (*in vitro*) or we can collect periodontal ligament (PDL) fibroblasts through scrapings obtained from extracted teeth; they are cultured before being subjected to mechanical stimulation (*ex vivo*). In an orthodontic context, the typical example is the study of fibroblast mechanical stimulation and its effect on either cytokine release or genetic (mRNA) or protein expression, which can either be performed on commercially available fibroblast cultures or on material that is retrieved from orthodontic patients after mechanical force application.

Cell culture methods

Ever since the advent of L929, the first "transformed cell line" derived from mouse connective tissue (Earle, 1943), cell lines became an inevitable part of research associated with cell biology. A decade later the first human transformed cell line, HeLa, was established by Gey *et al.* (1952), which revealed new insights into molecular mechanisms, pathophysiology, and regulation/signal transduction of human cells. Later, cell lines were identified as a potent source for production of monoclonal antibodies, which facilitated more research and development in primary and continuous cell lines (Persidis, 1999). Even though cell cultures can be classified based on the source of cells (organ explants/tissue) and how they adhere to the surface of the culturing flask (adherent/suspension), the division that is most popular is primary culture and cell lines.

Primary culture describes the separation and growing of cells from normal explants, which are dissociated by physical or enzymatic methods (e.g., trypsin, dispase, collagenase), which separate the cells from extracellular matrix. These cells are further grown on suitable media and the major advantage is that they mimic the natural response of cells but with only limited life span. In dentistry, dental stem cells (DSC) serve as the major primary cells and can be isolated from exfoliated deciduous teeth, from the apical papilla, and also from human PDL (Shilpa *et al.*, 2013). *Cell lines*, otherwise called immortalized cells, are described as those cells that can grow indefinitely in cultures when provided with nutrition and optimal conditions. Cell lines can be derived from cancer cells (for example, HeLa cells derived from cervical cancer) and normal cells transformed by a virus (e.g., human embryonic kidney cells – HEK 293 immortalized by incorporation of an adenovirus). Dental research mostly utilizes murine fibroblast cells (L929 cells) for toxicity assessment as per ISO 10993, and the FDA blue book memorandum. Other cell lines in use in dentistry include KB (human oral epithelial cells), and OSC (oral squamous cell carcinoma-derived cell lines), which are used in the study of oral carcinoma metastasis and the role of oncogenes.

Media preparation, trypsinization, and cell culturing

A completely aseptic, state-of-the art laboratory facility should be maintained for cell culturing, with good laboratory practice (GLP). The primary requirements for cell culturing include a biosafety cabinet, CO_2 incubator, a phase contrast microscope for analysis of cells, reagents of a high standard, and treated culture flasks and well plates for growth (Figure 20.2). Medium preparation is one of the

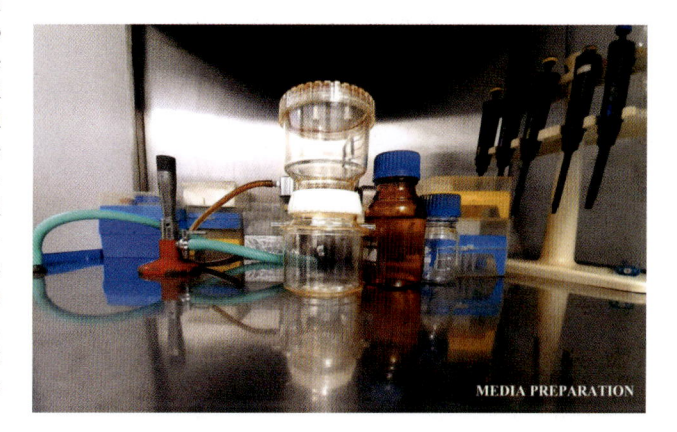

Figure 20.2 Media preparation of cell culture. *In vitro* studies require aseptic conditions for media preparation including a biosafety cabinet, vacuum manifold, filtration apparatus with a 0.2 µM pore size. (Source: Rajesh Ramachandran.)

most important segments of cell culture, which operates under pressure using a vacuum manifold. Since tissue culture media contains protein materials, heat sterilization is replaced by membrane filtration across a membrane of 0.2 μM pore size. The cell culture medias can be classified as: (i) natural media (Biological fluids [plasma, serum, lymph, human placental cord serum, amniotic fluid], tissue extracts [extract of liver, spleen, tumors, leucocytes and bone marrow, extract of the bovine embryo and chick embryo] and clots [coagulants or plasma clots]) and (ii) artificial media (balanced salt solutions [PBS, DPBS, HBSS, EBSS], basal media [MEM, DMEM], and complex media [RPMI-1640, IMDM]). Out of these, the most commonly used include MEM (minimal essential media), DMEM (Dulbecco's modified Eagle medium) and RPMI 1640 (Roswell Park Memorial Institute), which basically contains essential amino acids (which cannot be produced by cells), vitamins, inorganic ion supplements, carbohydrates (mainly glucose for energy source), glutamine (an amino acid for energy production), sodium chloride (for maintaining osmolality), and heat-inactivated fetal bovine serum (serves as a source for hormones and growth factors). Different cell types have highly specific growth requirements and, therefore, the most suitable media for each cell type must be determined experimentally. The commonly used cell lines as well as media for culture are summarized in Table 20.1. The medium is mixed with appropriate antibiotics such as penicillin and streptomycin to check the growth of unwanted microorganisms. Major applications of cell lines in dentistry include toxicity evaluation with MTT (mitochondrial tetrazolium testing, which uses the reduction of chromogen by mitochondrial succinate dehydrogenase enzyme; detailed below), NRU (neutral red uptake assay, which uses the membrane integrity of lysosomes), and LDH (lactate dehydrogenase leakage assay measuring spectrophotometrically the membrane damage induced by materials on cells).

Animal models

Although the appearance of humans and animals is different, there exists a similarity between both, on the anatomic and physiological levels. The closest animal to humans in terms of DNA similarities is the chimpanzee (99%), and next in line are mice (98%) (CBRA, n.d.). Moreover, the short lifespan of most animals makes it easy to study a disease process throughout their lifespan or between generations. Many types of animals are used in orthodontic research, including rats, mice, rabbits, guinea pigs, dogs, cats, and monkeys. When using animals as models for research purposes, it is possible to induce a disease process by altering their genomic structure through a variety of techniques, such as large-scale mutation screens, transgenesis (by injecting foreign DNA directly or through a viral vector), single gene knock-outs or knock-ins, conditioned gene modification, and chromosomal rearrangement. The advantage of using animal models is the insight into the interactive effects and response at various levels available from these studies rather than isolated results from either tissue or cellular cultures, or computerized modelling. Moreover, these approaches help to identify unwanted side effects on the molecular level, followed by explorations in animals, and finally investigating the phenomena in humans.

Research on flies (*Drosophilia*) or worms (*Caenorhabditis elegans*) does not seem to have attracted any orthodontic investigators, but even these creatures' function is governed by genes, thus sharing a common pattern of genetic control with humans. Animal research in orthodontics is usually conducted in rodents (mice, rats, and guinea pigs). About 40% of the mammal species are rodents, and their typical dentition consists of one incisor and three molars in each quadrant. The main similar oral features they share with humans are the presence of a gingival sulcus and attachment of the junctional epithelium to the tooth surface. As part of aging, the migratory path of rat molars follows an occlusal-distal-buccal direction, in comparison to the occlusal-mesial drift observed in humans. Most used rats in orthodontic research are Wistar or Sprague Dawley, while White Lobound are rarely used. Ren *et al.* (2004) has outlined the shortcomings of the rat model for orthodontic research in a review published in the *European Journal of Orthodontics*. Rats do not have osteons and marrow spaces, and the alveolar bone is thicker, so extrapolating research findings to clinical situations is difficult. Moreover, the anatomical structures of the periodontium and histopathological features of periodontal disease differ between rodents and humans (Jordan, 1971). Despite these facts, the rat is still commonly used because it is inexpensive, the preparation of histologic sections is easier, and antibodies are available exclusively for mice and rats. However, the size of mice makes it difficult to place orthodontic appliances.

The rabbit's skeletal remodeling rate makes it a suitable animal model to study tooth movement. Moreover, the animal is very docile and nonaggressive, and has very short vital cycles (gestation, lactation, and puberty). The main advantage of this animal model is its size (Mapara *et al.*, 2012). Moreover, they are considered phylogenetically closer to primates than rodents, and fill an important niche between laboratory mice and large farm mammals (Bősze and Houdebine, 2003). A PubMed search has revealed more than 300 studies in orthodontics performed on rabbits on various aspects such as mini-implant placement, functional appliances, orthopedic treatment, and drug effects, to name a few. This suggests that rabbits are suitable for conducting good quality, controlled, and safe clinical trials.

Another group of mammals that are phylogenetically related to humans are canines (cats and dogs). The main advantage is the size and availability of these animals, making them most popular as

Table 20.1 Common cell lines and recommended growth media. (Source: Adapted from Arora, 2013.)

Cell line	Morphology	Species	Medium	Applications
He La B	Epithelial	Human	MEM + 2mM glutamine + 10% fetal bovine serum (FBS) + 1% non-essential amino acids (NEAA)	Tumorigenicity and virus studies
HL60	Lymphoblast	Human	RPMI 1640 + 2mM glutamine + 10–20% FBS	Differentiation studies
3T3 clone A3	Fibroblast	Mouse	DMEM + 2mM glutamine +5% newborn calf serum (NBCS) + 5% FBS	Tumorigenicity and virus studies
COS-7	Fibroblast	Monkey	DMEM+ 2mM glutamine + 10% FBS	Gene expression and viral replication studies
CHO	Epithelial	Hamster	Ham's F12 + 2mM glutamine + 10% FBS	Nutritional and gene expression studies
HEK 293	Epithelial	Human	EMEM (EBSS) + 2mM glutamine + 1% NEAA + 10% FBS	Transformation studies
HUVEC	Endothelial	Human	F-12 K + 10% FBS + 100μg/mL heparin	Angiogenesis studies
Jurkat	Lymphoblast	Human	RPMI-1640 + 10% FBS	Signaling studies

candidates for medical and surgical explorations. Their acute hearing, excellent eyesight, and highly developed balance and spatial awareness, make them a suitable animal model to study sensory systems and neuroscience. In orthodontics, the canine model is mainly used to explore various methods to accelerate tooth movement. A recent PubMed search revealed more than 70 studies on cats and 400 on dogs. Beagle dogs are commonly used due to their convenient size and docile nature, whereas the larger Labradors are used in orthopedic research. It was concluded by Dannan and Alkattan (2007) that dogs were mostly used as animal models to study periodontal disease, due to the identical etiologic factors they share with humans. Furthermore, all periodontal tissues and size of the teeth in beagles are common to that of humans. Dogs have no occlusal contacts at the premolars, which facilitates tooth-movement experiments, and there are open contacts between teeth. The dog model has been utilized in orthodontics to study various aspects of accelerated tooth movement, force levels, mini-implants, bone density, periodontal response, and relapse, to name a few.

The most suitable animal model for the study of tooth movement is the monkey (macaques, baboons, chimpanzees), which is phylogenetically similar to humans (Struilllou et al., 2010). Their dental formula is identical to humans. Although smaller in size, the anatomy of their dental crowns and roots is similar to that of humans. However, for ethical reasons monkeys are rarely used in orthodontic research.

Other groups of animals, such as guinea pigs, sheep, hamsters, and ferrets have been used for various orthodontic research purposes.

A critical review published recently on accelerated tooth-movement experiments in animal models concluded that the rodent model can be used to understand the initial phases of tooth movement, while the dog model might be useful to understand prolonged adaptation in response to bodily tooth movement (Ibrahim et al., 2017).

When animals are being used for research purposes it is mandatory to obtain ethical clearance from the appropriate authorities. The animal housing facility should also be approved by the appropriate authorities. The Animal Welfare Act standards require "provisions to address the social needs of non-human primates of species known to exist in social groups in nature." Cages for animals should be built with ample access, space for living, as well as ease of cleaning in mind. Difficulty in housing has shown depressive attitudes in all animals, such as withdrawal, frustration, self-biting, hair pulling, rocking, and other psychotic behaviors (Rommeck et al., 2009). Moreover, these animals should be fed according to the guidelines prevailing in specific countries, and their health should be taken care of with proper veterinary assistance. However, above all, the guiding principles for the use of animals in scientific research are the so-called three R's, i.e., **R**eplace the use of animals with alternative techniques, or avoid the use of animals at all; **R**educe the number of animals to a minimum, to obtain information from fewer animals or more information from the same number of animals; and **R**efine the way experiments are carried out, to make sure animals suffer as little as possible (Balls and Parascandola, 2019; Smith and Lilley, 2019).

Studies in humans

Research projects involving human subjects are often categorized as: (i) no greater than minimal risk; (ii) minimal risk; and (iii) greater than minimal risk. They can be either observational studies (certain outcomes are measured or observed in individuals) or clinical trials, defined as the prospective accrual of patients where an intervention (for example, a drug, a device, a biologic or surgical procedure or the like) is tested on human subjects for a measurable outcome in terms of exploratory information, safety, effectiveness, and/or efficacy. Clinical trials on humans, before a product is marketed, comprise four phases, in which the numbers of participants are progressively increased from phase I to IV (Figure 20.3). Some literature discusses "Phase 0," in which preclinical data are generated, to determine proper dosage, involving very few subjects, with no therapeutic or diagnostic end.

Observational studies can be categorized as: (i) correlative studies, defined as prospective or retrospective collection of human anatomical substances (for example, tissues, blood, crevicular fluid, saliva, nail clippings, bone marrow, behavioral documentation and the like) to be used in research to answer a question regarding the

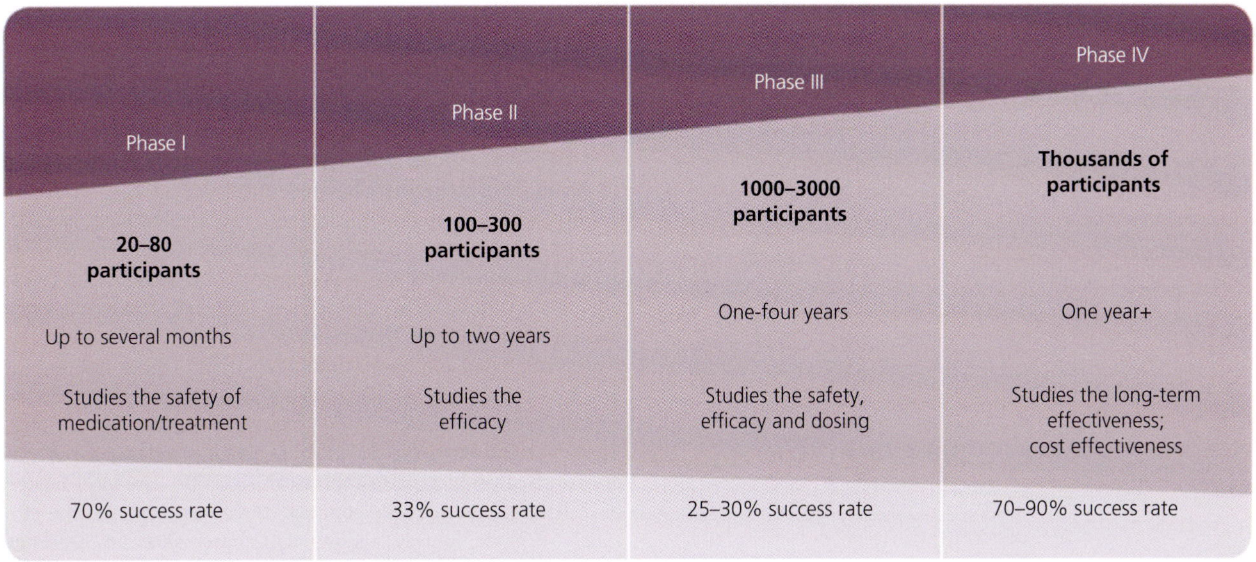

Phase I	Phase II	Phase III	Phase IV
20–80 participants	100–300 participants	1000–3000 participants	Thousands of participants
Up to several months	Up to two years	One-four years	One year+
Studies the safety of medication/treatment	Studies the efficacy	Studies the safety, efficacy and dosing	Studies the long-term effectiveness; cost effectiveness
70% success rate	33% success rate	25–30% success rate	70–90% success rate

Figure 20.3 Four phases of clinical trials in humans. (Source: Immunity Project. Reproduced with permission of Immunity Project.)

disease, injury or condition, and/or intervention; or (ii) epidemiological studies (examining the distribution of disease, injury, or condition with respect to a defined population). These are further divided into cohort studies (comparison of exposed versus nonexposed persons to a specific agent) and case-controlled studies (comparison of participants with disease, injury or condition versus participants without the disease, injury, or condition with respect to a specific agent). Human studies as part of biological research in orthodontics are mainly observational in nature, with collection of either crevicular fluid or saliva to identify biomarkers of bone, PDL, and cementum remodeling. Clinical reports on accelerated orthodontics and various treatment modalities prevail, but (randomized) controlled clinical trials are lacking in biological research related to orthodontic tooth movement. Many molecules that can accelerate tooth movement have been tried in humans (see Chapter 15 for details), but the experimental methods are largely limited in their ability to reach a proper conclusion or perform a systematic review.

Methodologies for tooth-movement research

The research question determines the design of the study and, depending on the design, the use of an appropriate methodology is the key to success in any research. Orthodontic tooth-movement research projects related to biological reactions have used a wide array of methodologies, making it difficult to describe each one comprehensively in the limited space provided for this chapter. The methodologies followed in the laboratory for studies at the tissue, cellular, and molecular levels are classified in Table 20.2. A brief overview of the techniques utilized follows, as a guide for new researchers in the field, so that they can choose their appropriate method and refer to the pertinent literature for a complete picture.

Tissue level/cellular level studies
Histological studies

After being subjected to mechanical force application, most of the animal models used will be sacrificed to obtain tissue sections, which are viewed in a microscope after proper staining. This methodology is characterized as a histologic study, which is defined as the study of cells and tissues, and their arrangement in the constitution of an organ. After the thin sections are cut from the tissue samples with a microtome, they are processed through five sequential steps:

1. Fixation. Tissue specimens obtained are preserved through fixation, which eliminates artefacts due to tissue degradation, and at the same time hardens the soft tissues. Fixatives are stabilizing or cross-linking agents and commonly used chemicals are either formalin, a 37% aqueous solution of formaldehyde, or glutaraldehyde.
2. Dehydration and clearing. To remove the water content in the tissues and to properly embed it in paraffin, the tissue is bathed through increasing concentrations of ethanol. Following this, xylene, an organic solvent, is used to remove the alcohol content,
3. Infiltration and embedding. Paraffin infiltration is the process through which paraffin infiltrates into the microscopic spaces present throughout the tissue and involves bathing the tissue in warm paraffin to form a solid block when cooled.
4. Sectioning. The paraffin block containing tissue is sliced or sectioned with a microtome and will be 4–10 μm thick. The sections are then floated on water and mounted on glass slides.
5. Staining. Tissues and cells must usually be stained for proper visualization. Most of the stains are acidic (eosin, acid fuchsin) or basic (hematoxylin, toluidine blue, methylene blue). The most used stains are eosin and hematoxylin in combination. Hematoxylin, a purple dye, stains basophilic structures like nucleus and rough endoplasmic reticulum. Sometimes glycosaminoglycan-rich ground substance in some connective tissues will stain pale purple. On the other hand, eosin stains acidophilic structures, like the cytoplasm, in pink. Collagen type I fibers are acidophilic and usually stain bright pink with eosin. Stained sections are always viewed through a light microscope, in which the light beam passed through the specimen will allow proper visualization of cells and will facilitate counting numbers, studying morphology, and cellular changes in architecture. An example of a histologic section of a tooth, its PDL, and alveolar bone, is presented in Figure 20.4. This low magnification micrograph provides an overview of the tissues, which are the most affected by orthodontic treatment. Figure 20.5 provides a close look at an osteoclast resorbing alveolar bone, in a histologic section stained for tartrate resistant acid phosphatase (TRAP). This high magnification micrograph enables the viewer to identify details of this multinucleated cell, seated in a Howship's lacuna, during the active phase of bone resorption.

There are other microscopic methods used in life science research to obtain high-resolution images, for example inverted microscopy, fluorescence microscopy, confocal microscopy, and electron (scanning or transmission) microscopy. Live-cell imaging gained immense acceptance with the introduction of the inverted microscope with setup for phase-contrast analysis. This simplified the procedures with little need for dyes and extensive staining protocols which normally take hours of valuable laboratory time. Morphological variations arising in toxicology studies can easily be documented using a phase contrast microscope. The introduction of differential interference contrast (DIC) has increased the efficiency of phase contrast analysis. DIC mode generates a pseudo three-dimensional relief shading with excellent contrast. Biocompatibility and cytotoxicity studies of dental materials can

Table 20.2 Research methods in tooth-movement biology.

Tissue/cellular-level studies	Histological studies
	• Light microscopy with H & E staining
	• Fluorescence microscopy
	• Confocal microscopy
	• Electron microscopy – transmission, scanning, reflection, and scanning transmission
	Immunohistochemistry
	Immunocytochemistry
	Flow cytometry
Genomic studies	DNA microarray
	ChIP assay
	Electrophoretic mobility shift assay (EMSA)
Proteomic analysis	Enzyme-linked immunosorbent assay (ELISA)
	Western-blot analysis
	Protein microarray
Toxicology studies	MTT assay
	Micronucleus assay
	Single-cell gel electrophoresis (COMET assay)
	DNA laddering
Mechanobiology studies	Micropipette aspiration
	Atomic force microscopy
	Magnetic twisting cytometry
	Magnetic pulling cytometry
	Laser tracking microrheology
	Microfabrication
	Microfluidics

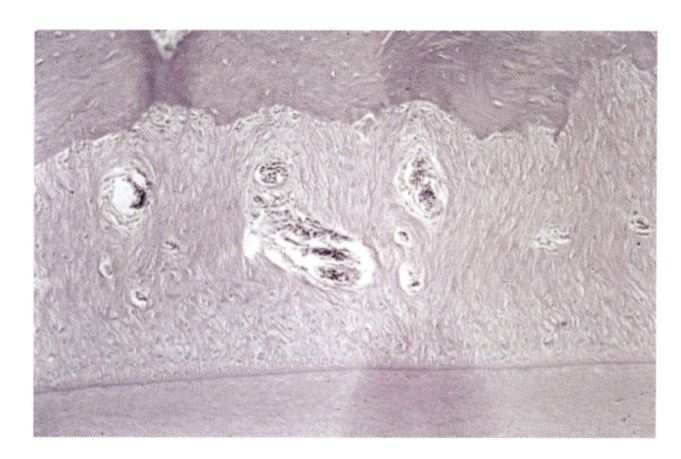

Figure 20.4 Tissue section of a maxillary canine of a 1-year-old female cat, stained with H & E. This 6 μm thick section shows the dental root of the canine, the alveolar bone, and the PDL fibers and cells. The root surface appears smooth, while the alveolar bone surface is wavy, indicating that the bone surface is remodeling, while the root does not remodel.

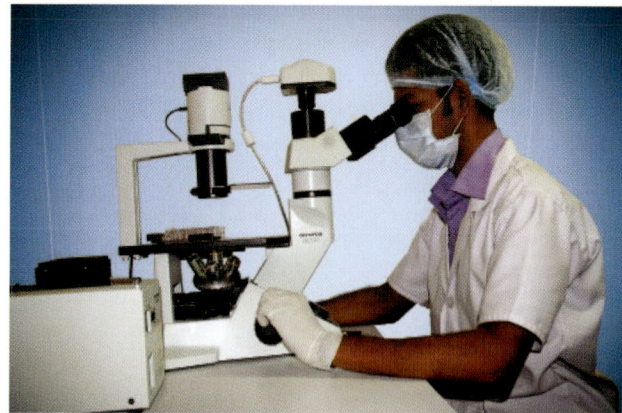

Figure 20.6 Inverted phase contrast fluorescent microscope involves the combination of inverted and fluorescent microscopes. The bigger workspace permits use of flasks and well plates, which provides an opportunity for live staining without fixing and multiple washing.

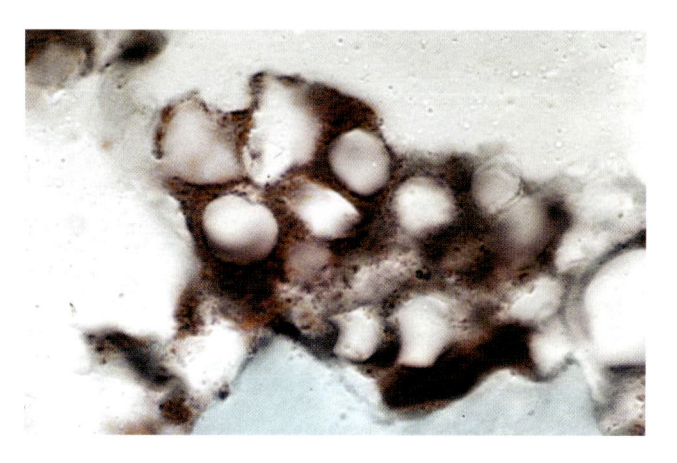

Figure 20.5 Tissue section of alveolar bone of a 3-month-old kitten, 6 μm thick, stained histochemically for tartrate resistant acid phosphatase (TRAP). An osteoclast, seated in a Howship's lacuna in the alveolar bone of the erupting mandibular second premolar, displays intense TRAP staining in the cytoplasm, while the multiple nuclei are devoid of the stain.

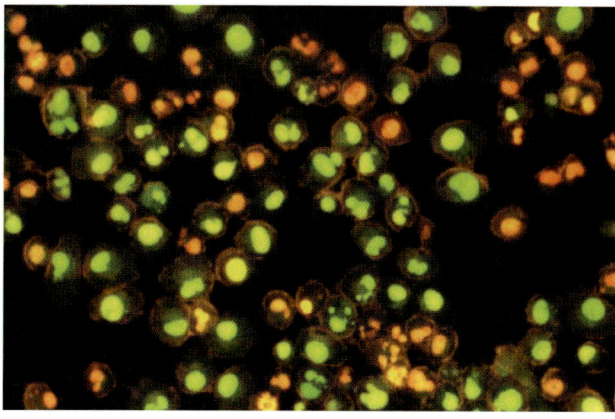

Figure 20.7 Live/dead assay – application of fluorescent staining in cell research. Staining with ethidium bromide and acridine orange offers an easy and cheaper method to study apoptosis induced by chemicals/materials on cells. The figure depicts the effect of silver nanoparticles on L929 cells. Green, live cells; orange stained cells, early apoptotic; dark red nuclei, dead cells.

use DIC analysis for determining the mechanisms of toxic action of materials/compounds on the target cells

Fluorescence microscopy refers to any microscope that uses fluorescence to generate the image (Figure 20.6), which is created with the help of fluorescent labeling (Hoechst or DAPI for nucleic acid staining) or through expression of a fluorescent protein (fluorophores or fluorochromes such as fluorescein), especially in biologic samples (Figure 20.7). It is considered as a valuable aid in detecting the distribution of proteins with the help of illuminating the specimen with light of specific wavelength, which is absorbed by fluorophores emitting light of longer wavelengths. Most of the fluorescence microscopes in use are of epifluorescence design, wherein excitation of fluorophore and detection of fluorescence are done through the same light path.

Confocal microscopy was introduced as a method to overcome limitations of fluorescence microscopy, wherein the entire specimen is illuminated from the light source and all specimens in the optical path are illuminated, resulting in fluorescence detected with a large unfocused background. Confocal microscopy is used to increase optical resolution and contrast of a micrograph using point illumination and a spatial pinhole to eliminate unfocused light in specimens that are thicker than in the focal plane. Confocal microscopes employ nonionizing radiation; hence they are increasingly being used to study living cells and tissue preparations. The main advantage is the crisp and rich detail in images, which are free of defocus blur. In addition, this allows three-dimensional reconstructions of microscopic features.

Electron microscopes are microscopes that use an electron beam to illuminate the specimen and produce a magnified image (up to 10,000,000 ×), which is of higher resolution than a light microscope. These are very commonly used to study the ultrastructure of various biological and inorganic specimens, such as biopsy materials, cells, microorganisms, as well as large molecules. There are different types of electron microscopes, such as transmission electron

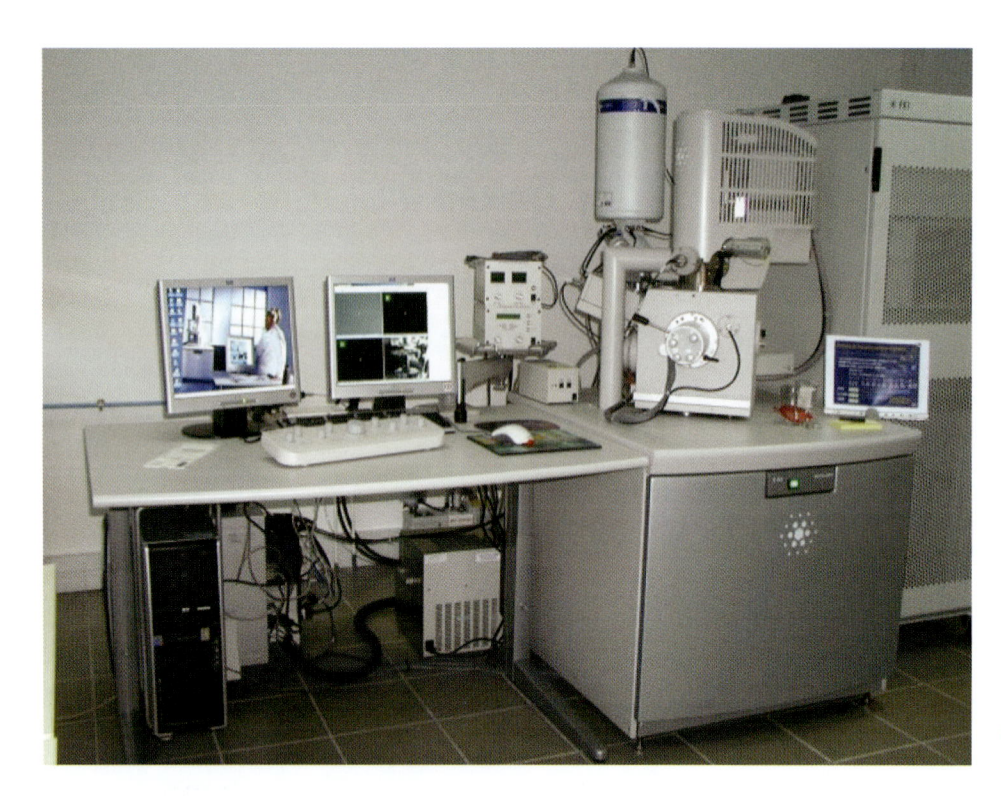

Figure 20.8 Environmental scanning electron microscope (ESEM).

microscopes (TEM), scanning electron microscopes (SEM), reflection electron microscopes (REM), and scanning transmission electron microscopes (STEM).

The original form of electron microscope is the TEM, which uses a high-voltage beam to create an image. When the beam emerges through the specimen, it carries information about the structure of the specimen, which is magnified by the objective lens system. The major disadvantage of the system is the requirement for very thin sections (about 100 nm) and that biological specimens must be chemically fixed, dehydrated, and embedded in resin to allow this thin sectioning.

SEM produces an image by probing the specimen with the focused electron beam that is scanned across the rectangular area (raster scanning). The topography and composition of the specimen is studied with the help of lost energy, which happens while the beam interacts with the specimen. The lost energy is converted to alternative forms, such as heat, secondary electrons, backscattered electrons, light or X-ray emissions. The image-generation process in SEM uses these signals. The image generated in SEM is poorer than TEM as it relies only on surface process and involves no transmission. One variant of SEM, environmental scanning electron microscopy (ESEM; Figure 20.8) can produce images of sufficient quality and resolution and is mainly used to study biologic samples.

REM use a reflected beam of elastically scattered electrons, which is detected for image creation. This technique combines reflection, high-energy electron diffraction, and reflection high-energy loss spectroscopy. Scanning transmission electron microscopy is another type of TEM in which electrons are passed through a sufficiently thin specimen but focused into a narrow spot, which is scanned over the sample in a raster. This rastering of the beam across the sample makes these microscopes suitable for integrating with analytical techniques such as energy dispersive X-ray spectroscopy (EDX), electron energy loss spectroscopy (EELS), and dark-field imaging (which is commonly used to study structural problems in biological specimens, without any need for special staining).

Immunohistochemistry

Immunohistochemistry (IHC) is localization of antigens or proteins in tissue sections by using labeled antibodies to generate an antigen–antibody reaction, which is visualized by a marker such as fluorescent dye, enzyme, or colloidal gold. Tissues retrieved for IHC are usually fixed with 4% paraformaldehyde in a 0.1 M phosphate buffer or 2% paraformaldehyde with 0.2% picric acid in 0.1 M phosphate buffer. It is mandatory that the sections obtained be kept frozen at −20°C or lower until fixation is done. It is again passed through the same phenomenon described above – paraffin embedding and sectioning. Antigen retrieval is the next step in IHC, by an antigen retrieval agent, which breaks the cross-linking of proteins formed by formalin fixation, revealing hidden antigen sites. There are basically two methods for this: heat-induced epitome retrieval (which uses a microwave, pressure cooker, or steamer along with a citrate buffer of pH 6.0 or Tris-EDTA of pH 9.0 as retrieval solutions) and proteolytic induced epitome retrieval (using proteinase K, trypsin, chymotrypsin, etc.).

There are many ways to stain IHC sections, such as the direct method, indirect method, peroxidase–antiperoxidase method, avidin–biotin complex method (ABC method; most commonly used), and the labeled streptavidin biotin method. In addition, the main advantage is the possibility of multiple labeling for more than one antigen with specific antibodies in one single section. In the indirect method, an unlabeled primary antibody, which reacts with tissue antigen and a labelled secondary antibody, is used to react with the primary antibody. This second layer antibody can be visualized by either the immunofluorescence method (using fluorescent dyes such as fluorescein isothiocyanate [FITC], rhodamine, or Texas red), using the fluorescence or confocal microscope, or the indirect

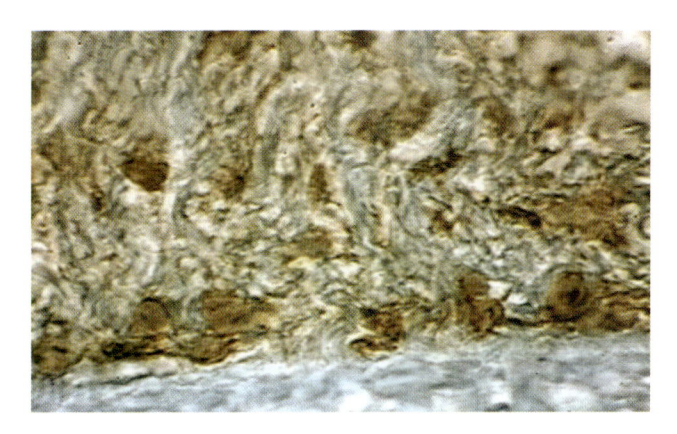

Figure 20.9 A horizontal section, 6 μm thick, of a maxillary canine of a 1-year-old female cat, stained immunohistochemically for cAMP. The cat was injected with PTH, 30 IU/kg, 3 hours before being euthanized. The cementoblasts on the root surface and the adjacent PDL fibroblasts are stained lightly with diaminobenzidine (DAB), denoting a low concentration of cAMP.

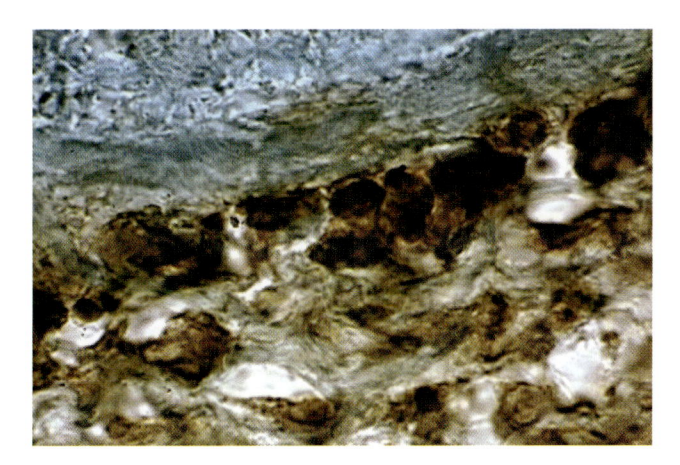

Figure 20.10 A view of the alveolar bone osteoblasts and adjacent PDL fibroblasts across the PDL from the site shown in Figure 20.9. The cells are darkly stained by diaminobenzidine (DAB), indicating a high concentration of cAMP, particularly in the bone surface cells, in response to the PTH injection.

immunoenzyme method (peroxidase, alkaline phosphatase, or glucose oxidase), viewed through the light microscope.

An example of an immunohistochemical staining of tissue sections derived from frozen, unfixed, nondemineralized cat jaws is shown in Figures 20.9 and 20.10. In this method, the jaws are removed immediately after euthanasia and frozen in liquid nitrogen. Each half jaw is embedded in a 2% solution of carboxymethyl cellulose, frozen again in liquid nitrogen, and kept overnight in a freezer, to allow the block temperature to rise to −25°C. At this temperature, the jaw is sectioned sagittally in a sledge cryostat microtome, and each section, 6 μm thick, is collected on a strip of adhesive tape and freeze dried. Afterwards, serial sections of the jaw are subjected to a routine immunohistochemical procedure, involving sequential incubations with antibodies against the tissue antigen of choice, culminating in incubation with diaminobenzidine (DAB), which stains the antigen–antibody complex brown. The degree of cellular staining intensity can be measured in the light microscope and is indicative of the antigen content of each stained cell. Figure 20.9 shows staining for cyclic AMP in cementoblasts and PDL cells of a maxillary canine of a 1-year-old female cat, which had received an injection of 30 IU/kg of PTH, 3 hours prior to euthanasia. The PDL and root surface cells are stained lightly for cAMP. In contrast, the cells shown in Figure 20.10, which are located on the alveolar bone surface opposite the cells shown in Figure 20.9, are stained darkly with DAB, indicating that the alveolar bone surface cells are more responsive to PTH than root surface cells.

Immunocytochemistry

The term immunocytochemistry (ICC) is often used interchangeably with IHC, as both techniques are similar in many aspects. The main difference between these two is the nature of specimen used. In IHC, tissues are stained whereas in ICC, most of the extracellular and stromal components are removed, leaving only whole cells to staining or primary/cell lines grown on culture dishes pretreated as per experiment requirement. Thus ICC can utilize even blood smears, swabs, aspirates, gingival crevicular fluid (GCF), or saliva as specimens. Moreover, ICC needs a special permeabilization step for antibodies to reach intracellular targets. Once these processes are done, similar staining and visualization processes are followed for ICC as in IHC.

Flow cytometry

Flow cytometry is mainly used to measure and analyze the multiple physical characteristics on a cell-by-cell basis simultaneously, as they flow in a fluid stream through a beam of light. The flow cytometer used for this purpose consists of three main systems, which are fluidics (transfers particles in the stream to the laser beam), optics system (lasers, to illuminate the particles in the stream and filters to direct light signals to appropriate detectors), and an electronics system. The electronics system in flow cytometry converts the detected light signals into electronic signals that can be processed by the computer.

Flow cytometry has major applications in microbiology, hematology, immunology, oncology, and virtually all other areas of cell and molecular biology. The ability of monoclonal antibodies to detect and bind to numerous antigens can aid in assessing cell proliferation, differentiation, function, and in putative stem cells for clinical therapy. Since its introduction, high quality publications have reported the use of flow cytometry for evaluating cellular responses to biomaterial formulations and this has now become the gold standard for determination of "biocompatibility."

Flow cytometry is usually used in biological research for cell-cycle analysis (Figure 20.11), which can be performed in three ways: (i) single time point (snap shot) cell measurement, which reveals the percentage of cells in G1 vs. S vs. G2/M, but does not provide information on cellular kinetics; (ii) time-lapse measurements of cell populations synchronized in the cycle or the action of any agent on the whole process by inhibition at some specific point of time; (iii) methods based on detection of thymidine analogue 5′-bromo-2′-deoxyuridine (BrdU) combined with DNA content measurement. In orthodontics, flow cytometry studies are mainly performed to analyze the toxic nature of adhesives, archwires, and brackets.

Techniques for genomic studies

The role of genetics in dentofacial characteristics and craniofacial anomalies has led to increased interest in genetic analysis as part of the orthodontic diagnosis. Techniques like polymerase chain reaction (PCR) and reverse-transcriptase (RT) or real-time (q) PCR are used for this purpose as is done for the determination of microbial contamination around implants even in minor loads.

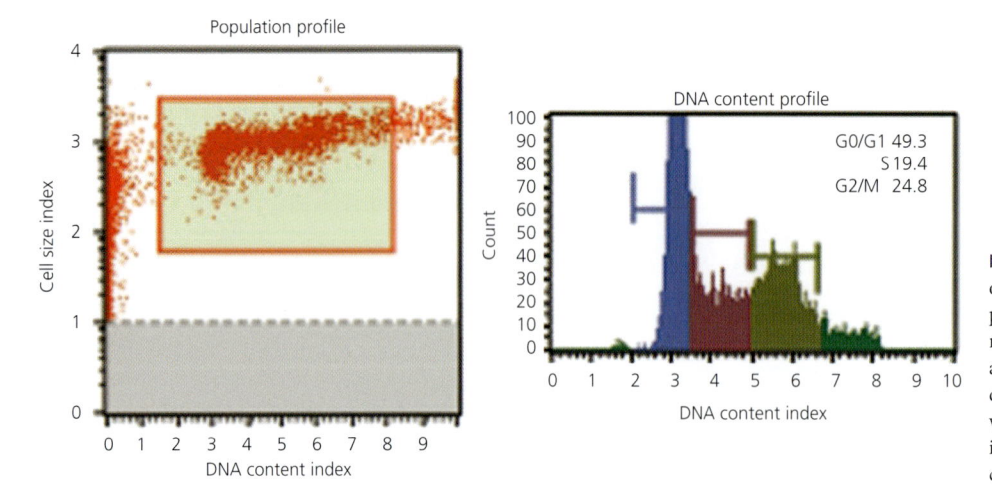

Figure 20.11 Flow cytometry analysis of cell cycle. Flow cytometry offers a precise method for analysis of cellular response at individual cells. Cell cycle analysis (DNA content profile) determines any phase arrest of cell, which is quite significant in determining the anticancer activity of compounds.

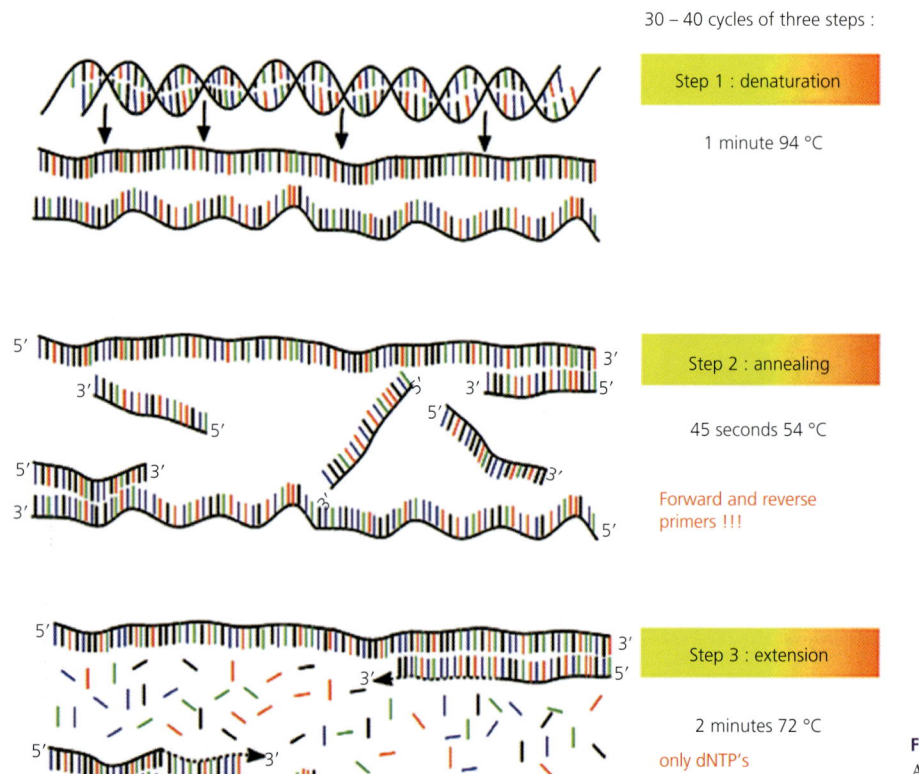

Figure 20.12 The steps in PCR. (Source: Andy Vierstraete, University of Ghent, Belgium. Reproduced with permission of Andy Vierstraete.)

Polymerase chain reaction

Developed by Kary Mullis in 1983, PCR uses DNA polymerase to synthesize and add new strands of DNA onto the specific region of the template sequence the researchers want to amplify. The basic PCR setup contains a DNA template (sample DNA containing target sequence), DNA polymerase (enzyme used to synthesize new strands of complementary DNA), nucleotides (single units of adenine, thymine, guanine, and cytosine function as building blocks for new DNA strands), and primers (short pieces of single-stranded DNA). The procedure comprises of 20–40 repeated temperature changes, called cycles, and consists of different steps: initialization, denaturation, annealing, extension/elongation, final elongation, and final hold, of which the second, third, and fourth are major steps (Figure 20.12). This procedure is mainly used to isolate selective DNA, amplification and quantification of DNA, and in the diagnosis of various diseases.

RT-PCR versus qPCR

The PCR thermal cycler gained another giant leap with the introduction of real-time PCR (qPCR), which made it possible to detect amplification-associated fluorescence at each cycle during PCR. In comparison with end-point PCR (RT-PCR; reverse transcriptase PCR), qPCR (quantitative real-time polymerase chain reaction) has increased sensitivity, precision, and easiness. This makes it a more accurate method for the detection of the amount of gene expression, virus infection, mutation studies, and the efficiency of drugs in therapeutics.

DNA microarray

Commonly known as DNA chip or biochip, it is used to measure the expression levels of a large number of genes simultaneously. This is a collection of microscopic DNA spots attached to the solid surface, each one containing picomoles (10^{-12} moles) of specific DNA sequence known as probes. Probe-target hybridization is usually detected and quantified by detection of fluorophore, silver or chemiluminescence labelled targets, to determine relative abundance of nucleic acid sequences in the target. This technique is used to measure changes in expression levels of large numbers of genes simultaneously or to genotype multiple regions of a genome. In orthodontic research, this technique has been used, for example, to analyze gene expression profiles in 3D-cultured PDL cells under static compression which simulates the biological behavior of human PDL in orthodontic tooth movement (Li *et al.*, 2013).

ChIP assay

Chromatin immunoprecipitation (ChIP) assay is often used to study interactions between protein and DNA in the cell. It helps in determining the association of a specific protein to specific genome regions, such as transcription factors or other DNA binding sites. There are two types of ChIP: cross-linked ChIP, which uses reversible crosslinked chromatin, and native ChIP, using native chromatin sheared by micrococcal nuclease digestion. This will also help to determine the specific location of a genome that various histone modifications are associated with.

Electrophoretic mobility shift assay (EMSA)

This is commonly referred to as gel-shift assay, aiming to study protein–DNA or protein–RNA interactions. This is a common affinity electrophoresis technique, which can determine whether a protein or mixture of proteins are capable of binding to a given DNA or RNA sequence and is visualized after labeling with a fluorescent, radioactive, or biotin label.

Proteomic analysis/cytoplasm-level studies
Enzyme-linked immunosorbent assay (ELISA)

This test is employed to check the presence of and quantify a particular protein that is present in a biological sample, be it GCF, saliva, or blood. This test can be performed by measuring the amount of antibody bound to the sample or checking the amount of protein bound to a particular antibody. It is performed in a 96 well plate, in which the samples with an unknown amount of antigens are immobilized and a detection antibody is added. The detection antibody can be covalently linked to the enzyme or can itself be detected by a secondary antibody that is linked to the enzyme through bioconjugation. Finally, the plate is added with an enzymatic substrate to produce visible signals denoting the amount of antigens in the sample. There are basically four types of ELISA (i) indirect ELISA; (ii) sandwich ELISA; (iii) competitive ELISA; and (iv) multiple and portable ELISA. In orthodontic research, ELISA is mainly performed for analyzing the amount of inflammatory cytokines, root resorption markers, toxicity evaluations with GCF, and salivary samples.

Western-blot analysis

Western blotting offers researchers the ability to identify specific proteins from a complex mixture of proteins extracted from cells (Figure 20.13). The technique proceeds through three steps namely:
1. Separation of proteins based on size.
2. Transfer of all proteins to a solid surface.
3. Detection of target protein using primary and secondary antibodies.

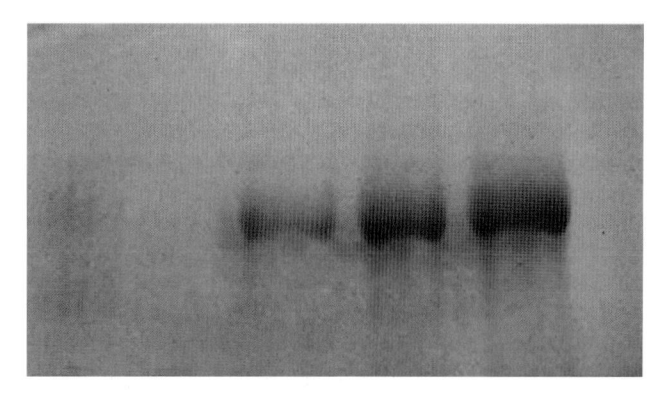

Figure 20.13 Western blot analysis of COX 2 (cyclooxygenase 2) expression in inflammation. The increase in band intensity confirms increased expression of COX 2.

Gel electrophoresis, which is part of Western blotting, makes use of two different types of polyacrylamide gels; the higher stacking gel is slightly acidic and has a lower acrylamide concentration, making it highly porous, which poorly separates proteins but allows bands to be formed, while the lower separating gel is basic (pH 8.8) with a high polyacrylamide concentration making pores narrower allowing separation of proteins.

After separating the proteins, blotting is done to either nitrocellulose membrane (high affinity for proteins but brittle in nature) or polyvinylidene fluoride (PVDF) (this provides better mechanical support and allows reprobing of the blot). Next, the most important of the steps is washing and blocking with 5% bovine serum albumin (BSA) or nonfat dried milk diluted in tris-buffered saline and tween 20 (TBST) which prevents nonspecific binding of antibodies. Because of the relative comparison of protein levels used in the system, Western blotting is often considered semiquantitative in nature. For more details on the technique, readers are referred to the article by Mahmood and Yang (2012) which was published in the *North American Journal of Medical Sciences*. In orthodontics, Western blot analysis is performed to identify various proteins released associated with inflammation and mechanotransduction pathways.

Protein microarray

Otherwise known as the protein chip, this allows the interactions and activities of a large number of proteins to be tracked simultaneously. The chip used for this purpose consist of a glass slide, nitrocellulose membrane, and a bead or microtitre plate, to which an array of captured proteins is bound. The molecules to be probed are labeled with a fluorescent dye, and added to the array, emitting fluorescent signals once a reaction is initiated, which is read with a laser scanner. There are mainly three types of protein microarrays:
1. *Analytical (capture) arrays,* using a library of antibodies to capture molecules and used mainly for comparison of protein expression in different solutions.
2. *Functional protein microarrays*, used to identify protein–protein, protein–DNA, protein–RNA and protein–phospholipid interactions. These tests are used in studying biochemical activities of an entire proteome in a single experiment.
3. *Reverse phase protein microarray,* involving cells isolated and lysed from tissue samples. The lysate is arrayed and probed with antibodies, which are detected using chemiluminescent, fluorescent, or colorimetric assays. The advantages of protein microar-

rays are that it is rapid, automated, economical, and highly sensitive and consumes only small quantities of samples and reagents. In orthodontics, protein microarrays are used to study differential expression of proteins, mainly heat shock proteins (HSP), in response to orthodontic force application (Arai et al., 2010).

Toxicology studies
MTT assay
This is the most frequently used colorimetric assay to assess cell viability (Figure 20.14). Cellular oxidoreductase enzymes dependent on NADPH (nicotinamide adenine dinucleotide phosphate-oxidase) might reflect the number of viable cells present in a culture, and these enzymes are capable of reducing tetrazolium dye MTT 3-(4,5-dimethylthiazol-2-yl)-2,5-diphenyltetrazolium bromide to its insoluble formazan, which has a purple color. The absorbance of this colored solution can be quantified by measuring a certain wavelength (between 500 and 600 nm) by a spectrophotometer. Rapidly dividing cells exhibit high rates of MTT reduction. These types of studies are usually done to assess cytotoxicity (loss of viable cells) or cytostatic activity (shift from proliferative to resting status).

Micronucleus assay
Micronucleus is the third or erratic nucleus formed during the anaphase of mitosis or meiosis and has a portion of acentric chromosome or whole chromosome, which was not carried to opposite poles during the anaphase. This test is usually used to assess genotoxicity of newly developed compounds or molecules.

Single cell gel electrophoresis (comet assay)
An uncomplicated and sensitive test to detect DNA damage, it received its name, "comet assay," due to the pattern of DNA migration through the electrophoresis gel. After embedding the cells in agarose gel and lysing it with detergent and high salt, the break in DNA strands can be measured. This forms nucleoid-containing supercoiled loops of DNA linked to the nuclear matrix, which are visualized with fluorescence microscopy. The intensity of the comet tail relative to the head reflects the number of DNA breaks and the images are scored either manually or automatically with imaging software such as comet score™ or Comet Assay IV™. A representative image from a comet assay analyzing the effect of orthodontic force on cultured PDL fibroblast is provided in Figure 20.15

DNA laddering
This is a distinctive feature of DNA degraded by caspase-activated DNase (CAD), which is a key event during apoptosis (Figure 20.16). CAD cleaves genomic DNA at internucleosomal linker regions, resulting in DNA fragments that are multiples of 180–185 base pairs in length. Separation of fragments by agarose gel electrophoresis and subsequent visualization by staining (ethidium bromide) results in a characteristic ladder pattern. It has been established as a reliable method to distinguish between apoptosis and necrosis (Yeung, 2002).

Studying mechanobiology
Mechanical force applied to cells, be it tension, pressure, or fluid shear, will influence gene expression, protein production, and the production and release of inflammatory mediators. In addition, there exists an internal mechanical force generation system, cell

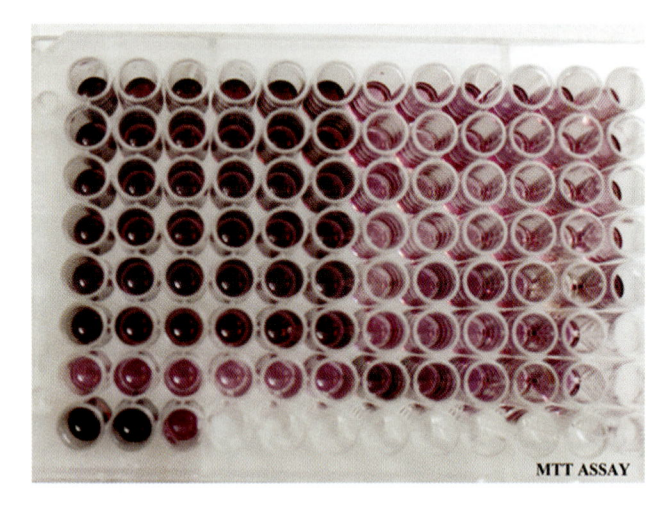

Figure 20.14 MTT assay is considered to be the most accurate method for assessing cell viability. The experiment is based on the principle of mitochondrial reduction of a tetrazolium dye, which is used in testing cytocompatibility of dental materials, polymers, and new drugs and molecules prior to human/animal use. (Source: Rajesh Ramachandran.)

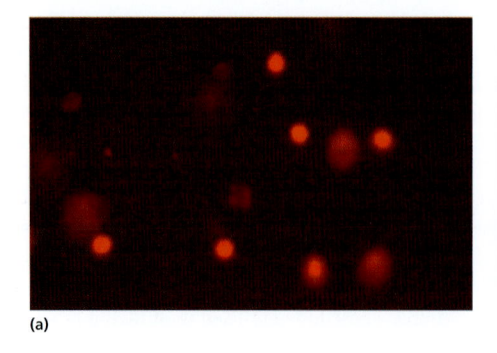

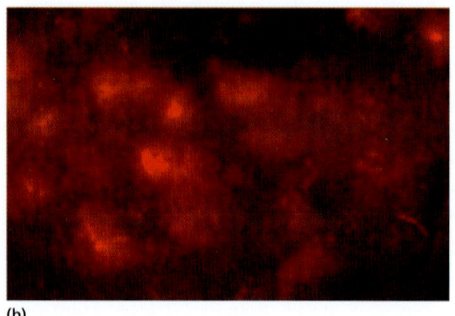

Figure 20.15 Representative images obtained through comet assay. A, Control group. B, Experimental group. Please note round nuclear shape in A, and elongated appearance of the nucleus in B portraying the tail lengthening characteristic of nuclear damage. (Source: Vinod Krishnan.)

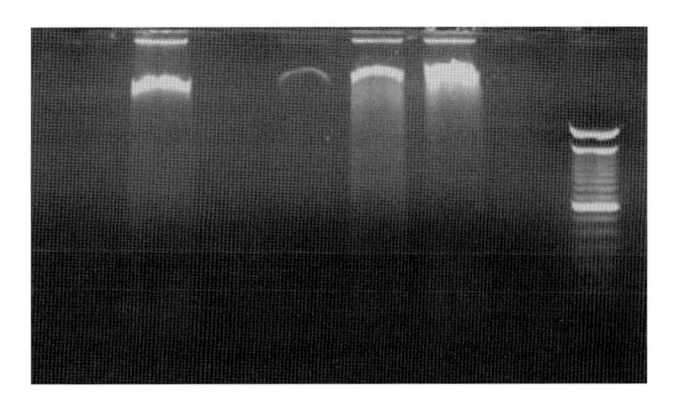

Figure 20.16 DNA fragmentation analysis: the experiment gives the opportunity to determine genotoxicity of biomaterials. More fragmentation confirms DNA damage.

traction forces developed through actin–myosin interactions, which helps maintain cell shape and integrity, at the same time influencing many processes such as wound healing and angiogenesis (Wang and Thampatty, 2008). As there are numerous types of cells in our body, the responses to load depends on cell type (e.g. osteoblast, fibroblast), cell source, developmental stage, cellular microenvironment, and mainly loading conditions, such as type, magnitude, frequency, and duration of loading (Grinnell, 2003).

Various *in vitro* systems have been developed over the years to study the cellular responses to mechanical forces, which take into account *in vivo* loading conditions of various cell types (Friedrich *et al.*, 2017). Mechanical stress in tissues and on cells can be complex and multiaxial. Therefore, in recent years devices have been developed based on elastomeric membranes that apply bi- or multiaxial stretch to 3D-embedded cells (Friedrich *et al.*, 2019). Deformable elastic substrates made up of silicon are mainly used for fibroblasts, epithelial cells, and smooth muscle cells, which will be coated with extracellular matrix for proper adhesion. Flow chambers for applying fluid shear stress are utilized for endothelial cells, and compression and hydrostatic pressure applying models were developed for chondrocytes. These systems allow proper control over loading parameters, and at the same time allow surface modifications, if required.

When the substrate is stretched, the cells will experience mechanical forces and the stretching can be done either uni-, bi-, or multiaxially. The type of stretching compatible with ligament cells is uniaxial in nature, wherein the substrate is lengthened in its stretching direction, while being compressed in its perpendicular direction. The main disadvantage of uniaxial loading is reorientation of cells cultured on the substrate while being stretched to a direction where there is minimal substrate deformation. To overcome this problem, microgrooved substrates were developed, which can orient the cells to these microgrooves while stretching and maintaining an elongated shape to give out a proper response. In addition, a biaxial system of stretching exists, wherein substrate is stretched in two mutually perpendicular directions, either equibiaxial (substrate strains are equal in all directions) or nonequibiaxial (substrate strain varies with stretching directions). Input force quantification, loading parameter controls, and homogenous deformation of cell populations are additional advantages of biaxial systems. The main disadvantages are that the force strain measurement is on the loading system (clamp to clamp) or that the substrate strain is not actually the cell strain, and because of differential adhesion of cells, only part of the force applied to the substrate is experienced by the cells.

Rheology is the science dealing with the study of deformability of soft materials, such as gels, polymer solutions, and colloidal suspensions, under conditions of mechanical stress, deformation, or flow (Hoffman and Crocker, 2009). In order to make easily interpretable measurements, many experimental techniques exist to study whole-cell deformation (parallel plates as described above, micropipette aspiration and torsional pendulum), smaller mechanical probes of cells (microneedles, atomic force microscopy [AFM]), magnetic forces (optical magnetic twisting cytometry [MTC], magnetic pulling cytometry), optical methods (laser tracking microrheology), micropatterning, and microfluidics. Figure 20.17 is a schematic of most of the rheology techniques (adapted from Holeček *et al.*, 2011).

Atomic force microscopy

Otherwise known as scanning probe microscopy, atomic force microscopy (AFM) uses a vertical microcantilever to deform the cell and measure interaction forces between sample surface and the micron scale probe fixed to the cantilever. The probe is based on silicon or silicon nitride, with the tip radius of curvature on the order of nanometers (Figure 20.17a). AFM is derived from an interaction force between the tip and the sample, requiring no special staining or fixation, and it can perfectly capture dynamic processes in living cells. The sample is mounted on a piezoelectric scanner, which translates it in the horizontal and vertical directions relative to the probe. Interaction between tip and the sample deflects the cantilever, whose position is tracked by a laser spot reflected into an array of photodiodes. The data acquired through AFM are images and force measurements. AFM is used to measure force-dependent unfolding of extracellular matrix (ECM) proteins and cell–ECM adhesion proteins, to study the path of mechanochemical conversion in the mechanotransduction mechanism. Figure 20.18 is a representative image of PDL fibroblast as observed under AFM.

Magnetic twisting cytometry

Magnetic twisting cytometry (MTC) uses ferromagnetic beads of 1–10 μm diameter, to apply shear stresses or twisting forces to specific receptors on the surface membrane of living cells (Figure 20.17b). Carboxylated ferromagnetic beads are coated with ligands such as ECM molecules, which are then added to cells in serum free chemically defined medium, and incubated for 10 minutes at 37°C, followed by a gentle wash with phosphate buffer solution (PBS) to remove the unbound beads. Using a horizontal Helmholtz coil, a strong (1000 g) but very brief (10 μs) magnetic pulse is applied to the beads and bound receptors. After a few seconds, a weaker (0–80 g) but sustained magnetic field is applied to the beads in a perpendicular direction, inducing a twist, leading to application of shearing force, which is measured using an in-line magnetometer. This procedure can analyze the mechanical behavior of integrins linked to the cytoskeleton, by measuring the stress–strain responses as well as analyzing the creep and elastic recoil behavior. It can also determine how different transmembrane adhesion receptors (integrins, cadherins, selectins, and urokinase receptors) differ in their ability to support transmembrane mechanical coupling to the cytoskeleton (Lele *et al.*, 2007).

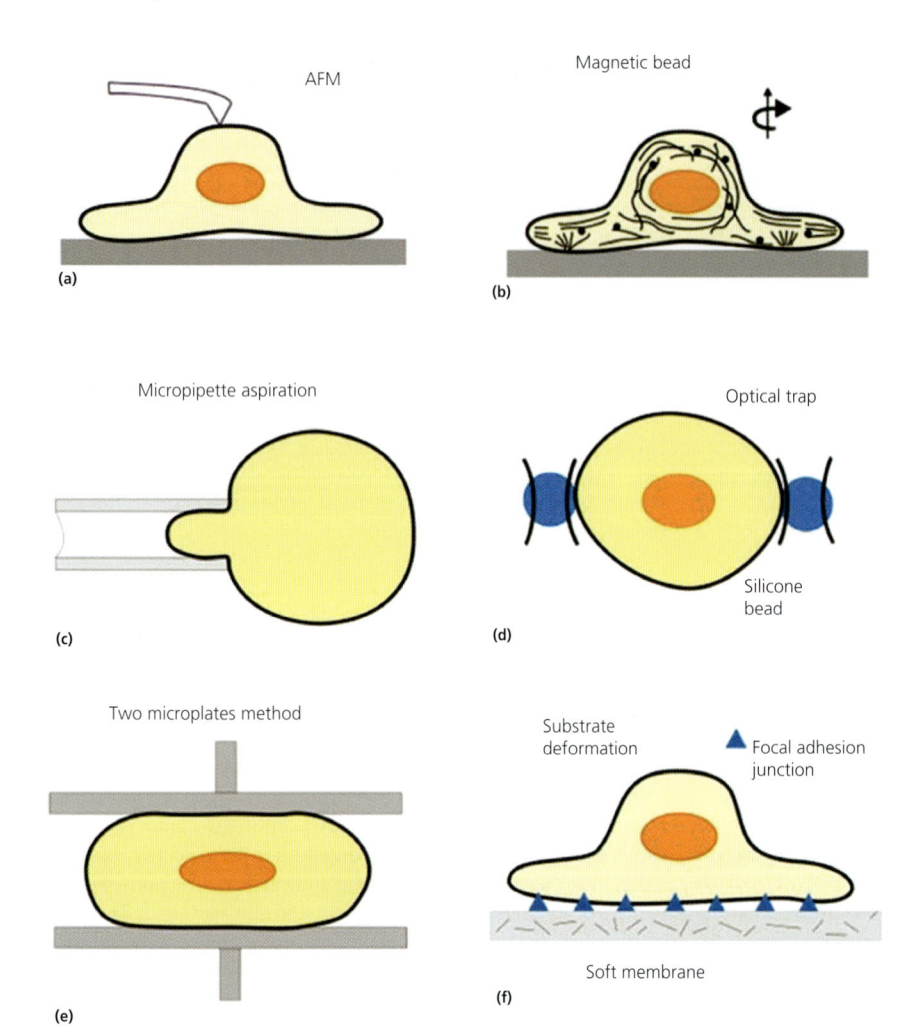

Figure 20.17 Experimental methods currently used for measuring mechanical properties at the cellular level. These include atomic force microscopy (AFM) (a), magnetic twisting and pulling cytometry (b), micropipette aspiration (c), optical particle trapping and optical tweezers (d), the two microplates method (e), and traction force microscopy (f). (Source: Holeček et al., 2011. Licensed under creative common license 3.0.)

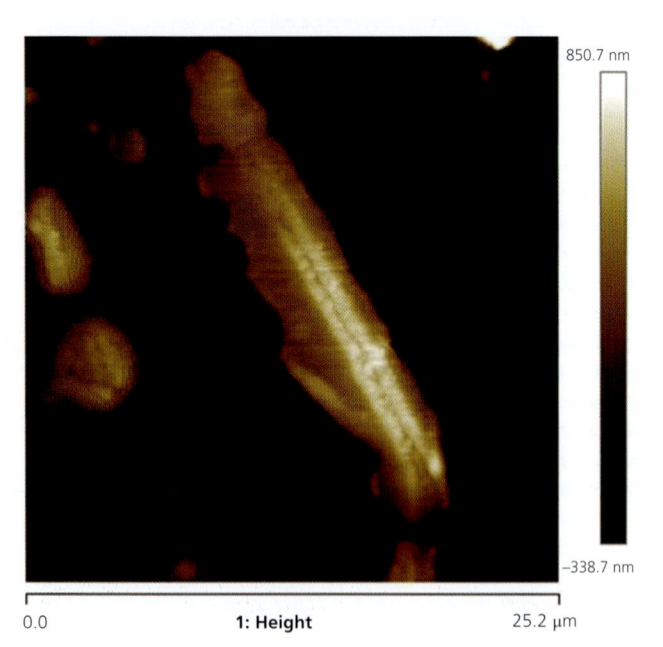

Figure 20.18 Representative image of a PDL fibroblast as observed under atomic force microscopy. (Source: Vinod Krishnan.)

Magnetic pulling cytometry

Magnetic pulling cytometry (MPC) is also known as "magnetic tweezers." It can operate through bound ligand-coated microbeads in order to measure local cell rheology (Figure 20.17b). In this technique, super paramagnetic beads are used, instead of ferromagnetic beads in MTC and a magnetic needle is used to apply tensional forces (Friedrich et al., 2017). As large-scale distortions in cells can be studied with MPC, this technique is well suited to study force-induced changes at focal adhesions or other receptor mediated anchoring complexes in single living cells (Lele et al., 2007).

Micropipette aspiration

This technique was introduced with the concept that cells are pouches with fluid interiors and continue to stay as one unit. This technique is used to measure mechanical behavior of whole cells, as well as cell-membrane mechanical properties. A micropipette is a rigid tube that tapers to the diameter of several micrometers at the tip. This hollow tube will be brought to the proximity of a cell, while suction is being applied either by mouth or by connecting the pipette to tubing that runs to a water-filled reservoir, which has a controllable height (Figure 20.17c). Once the cell is drawn to the tube, the morphology of the cell can be divided into three regimens:

(i) length of protrusion of the cell is less than radius of the pipette; (ii) protrusion length is equal to pipette radius; and (iii) protrusion is cylindrical, with a hemispherical cap. The results of micropipette aspiration can be interpreted using a liquid drop model (cellular interior is assumed to be a Newtonian viscous fluid and the surrounding membrane is assumed to be a thin layer under a constant surface tension and without any bending resistance). The analysis of the results can be done with the law of Laplace, which relates the difference in pressure between the inside and outside of a thin-walled pressure vessel, with the surface tension within the vessel wall. With this technique, we can measure the properties of membranes by applying a wide range of forces.

Laser-tracking microrheology

Laser-tracking microrheology is a fast technique that can measure the full mechanical complexity of living cytoplasm and quantifies the viscoelastic phase angle, which demonstrates solid versus liquid behavior. For this purpose, the cells are labeled with fluorescent dyes, so that actin can be identified easily. The extracted actin is then polymerized in the presence of carboxylated polystyrene particles, and a focused low-power laser beam is used to track the particle by monitoring its forward-scattered light with a quadrant photodiode detector. Any off-axis motion of the particle deflects energy away from the optical axis and produces imbalance between signals from photodiode quadrants (Figure 20.19). The laser powers used are very low (0.13 mW, λ = 670 nm) and the movement of the particle is recorded using a quadrant photodiode detector fitted into an Axiovert 100TV microscope and the images will be captured (Yamada et al., 2000; Kim et al., 2009).

Traction force microscopy

Traction force microscopy (TFM), introduced by Harris *et al.* (1980), yields spatial images of the stress exerted by cells on relatively soft elastic gel substrates such as flexible silicone substrates and provides us with an idea about mechanical forces that cells generate. Today it is used worldwide to study cell biology and soft matter physics. TFM requires three distinct procedures:

1. Cells are plated on an elastic substrate containing fiducial markers allowing gel deformation to be quantified visually, for instance fluorescent beads or quantum dots. The deformations caused by adherent cells are recorded by taking images of the gel before and after removing the cell.
2. A discrete gel displacement field u is calculated by tracking the markers. The most common techniques for tracking are particle tracking velocimetry (PTV) and particle image velocimetry (PIV).
3. Finally, the traction force field f is calculated from the displacement field u by making use of a mechanical model of the elastic substrate. A variety of methods exist for this purpose, including finite element methods, boundary element methods, and methods operating in Fourier space (Huang et al., 2019).

Basically, these techniques allow the analysis of acto-myosin-mediated cell contractility transmitted to the extracellular environment at the level of integrin adhesion points, the focal adhesions (Mulligan et al., 2018; Kechagia et al., 2019).

Microfabrication

This technology has helped to generate devices that range in size from submicrometer scale to those measuring in the tens of micrometers, corresponding well with the size of a single cell, and assists in the study of cell mechanics. Briefly, microfabrication is a technique used to manufacture various products, including integrated circuits and biological sensors. Soft lithography is one such technique, in which the final configuration formed serves as a mold to create beds for studying cellular mechanics, which can be materialized by microcontact printing, capillary lithography, and nanoimprint lithography. One more advantage is that the column nature of microfabricated structures allows study of cell deflections using beam-bending equations, making it a real time approach in studying cellular mechanics in constrained and unconstrained environments (Kumar and LeDuc, 2009).

Microfluidics

The advantage of this system is the spatiotemporal control it has over the chemical nature of living cells, by exploiting the unique properties and characteristics of low Reynolds-number flow (Kumar and LeDuc, 2009). This is a fast-developing area with many valuable applications, such as: (i) DNA transport, hybridization or separation; (ii) proteomic applications, such as protein isolation and purification, and studying protein kinetics and thermodynamics; (iii) cell biology studies with a microfluidic device after exposing cells to gradient stream of chemicals, such as hormones, cytokines, growth factors, or chemo-attractants, and measuring the responses, and also for cell culture studies; and (iv) medical device fabrication for either direct drug delivery with cellular scale precision and less pain, fabrication of biosensors, and miniaturized biomedical devices (Das and Chakraborty, 2009). The current most

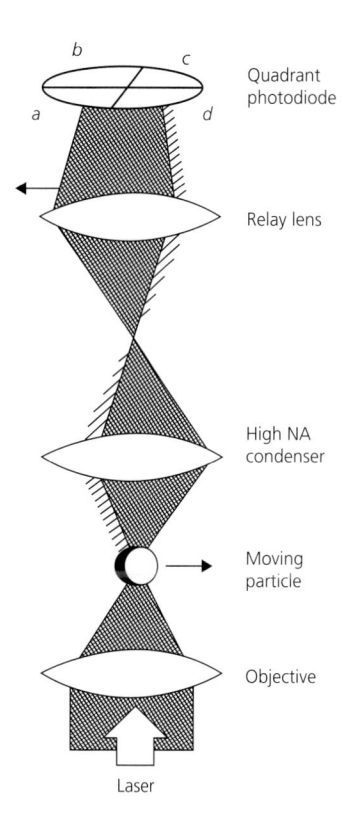

Figure 20.19 Principle of laser deflection particle tracking. A particle at the laser's focus causes far-field scatter, and its off-axis motions cause net energy to be deflected from the optical axis. A quadrant photodetector monitors the deflected energy, and position signals are generated from the difference in photocurrents between opposing pairs of quadrant elements. (Source: Yamada et al., 2000. Reproduced with permission of Elsevier.)

popular technology for the fabrication of microfluidic devices for cell biological application is based on the soft lithography of poly-di-methyl siloxane (PDMS). Microfluidic biosensors (MFB) are recommended as point-of-care diagnostic portable devices (PoC) in the monitoring of cytokine expression in a clinical setting (Kumar et al., 2013) and even has potential for use in orthodontic office settings. Moreover, microfluidic assays have been useful in saliva-based immunoassay, assisting in clinical diagnostic research (Herr et al., 2007). A full description of this developing field is beyond the scope of this chapter, and readers are encouraged to consult the available literature, so that such a potent technology is brought to the field of dentistry, particularly orthodontics.

Conclusions

At first sight, orthodontics appears to be a very narrow field. However, biological orthodontic research involves the biological response of cells and tissues to applied exogenous mechanical forces and the translation of the results to the clinical environment so that personalized treatment procedures may be applied. Mechanobiology encompasses many disciplines and has a wide application in the medical field. Basic biological research offers an increasing number of investigative tools to orthodontic researchers. The developing field of orthodontic research is undoubtedly multidisciplinary, as reflected in the methods that have been described in this chapter. Research in clinical orthodontics will benefit greatly from collaborations with researchers who have different biological and bioinformatics backgrounds.

References

Arai, C., Nomura, Y., Ishikawa, M. et al. (2010) HSPA1A is upregulated in periodontal ligament at early stage of tooth movement in rats. *Histochemistry and Cell Biology* **134**, 337–343.

Arora, M. (2013) Cell culture media: a review. *Materials Methods* **3**, 175.

Balls, M. and Parascandola, J. (2019) The emergence and early fate of the three Rs concept. *Alternatives to Laboratory Animals* **47**(5–6), 214–220.

Bősze, Z. S. and Houdebine, L. M. (2003) Application of rabbits in biomedical research: a review. *World Rabbit Science* **14**, 1–14.

CBRA (n.d.) Why Are Animals Necessary in Biomedical Research? http://ca-biomed.org/csbr/pdf/fs-whynecessary.pdf (accessed September 17, 2020).

Dannan, S. and Alkattan, F. (2007) Animal models in periodontal research: a mini review of the literature. *The Internet Journal of Veterinary Medicine* **5**(1), 5.

Das, T. and Chakraborty, S. (2009) Biomicrofluidics: recent trends and future challenges. *Sadhana* **34**, 573–590.

de la Pena, J. A., Berlucchi, G., Boksenberg, A. et al. (2004) The Value of Basic Scientific Research, https://council.science/wp-content/uploads/2017/04/Annual-Report-2004.pdf (accessed September 18, 2020).

Earle, W. R. (1943) Production of malignancy in vitro. IV. The mouse fibroblast cultures and changes seen in the living cells. *Journal of National Cancer Institute* **4**, 165–212.

Friedrich, O., Schneidereit, D., Nikolaev, Y. A. et al. (2017) Adding dimension to cellular mechanotransduction: advances in biomedical engineering of multiaxial cell-stretch systems and their application to cardiovascular biomechanics and mechano-signaling. *Progress in Biophysics and Molecular Biology* **130**(Pt B), 170–191.

Friedrich, O., Merten, A. L., Schneidereit, D. et al. (2019) Stretch in Focus: 2D inplane cell stretch systems for studies of cardiac mechano-signaling. *Frontiers in Bioengineering and Biotechnology* **7**, 55.

Gey, G. O., Coffman, W. D. and Kubicek, M. T. (1952) Tissue culture studies of the proliferative capacity of cervical carcinoma and normal epithelium. *Cancer Research* **12**, 264–265.

Grinnell, F. (2003) Fibroblast biology in three-dimensional collagen matrices. *Trends in Cell Biology* **13**, 264–269.

Harris, A. K., Wild, P. and Stopak, D. (1980) Silicone rubber substrata: a new wrinkle in the study of cell locomotion. *Science* **208**(4440), 177–179.

Herr, A. E., Hatch, A. V., Throckmorton, D. J. et al. (2007) Microfluidic immunoassays as rapid saliva-based clinical diagnostics. *Proceedings of the National Academy of Sciences* **104**(13), 5268–5273.

Hoffman, B. D. and Crocker, J. C. (2009) Cell mechanics: dissecting the physical responses of cells to force. *Annual Review of Biomedical Engineering* **11**, 259–288.

Holeček, M., Kochová, P. and Tonar, Z. (2011) Mechanical properties of living cells and tissues related to thermodynamics, experiments and quantitative morphology – a review, in *Theoretical Biomechanics* (ed. V. Klika) https://www.intechopen.com/books/theoretical-biomechanics/mechanical-properties-of-living-cells-and-tissues-related-to-thermodynamics-experiments-and-quantita (accessed September 18, 2020).

Huang, Y., Schell, C., Huber, T. B. et al. (2019) Traction force microscopy with optimized regularization and automated Bayesian parameter selection for comparing cells. *Scientific Reports* **9**(1), 1–16.

Ibrahim, A. Y., Gudhimella, S., Pandruvada, S. N. and Huja, S. S. (2017) Resolving differences between animal models for expedited orthodontic tooth movement. *Orthodontics and Craniofacial Research* **20**, 72–76.

Jordan, H. V. (1971) Rodent model systems in periodontal disease research. *Journal of Dental Research* **50**, 236–242.

Kechagia, J. Z., Ivaska, J. and Roca-Cusachs, P. (2019) Integrins as biomechanical sensors of the microenvironment. *Nature Reviews Molecular Cell Biology* **20**(8), 457–473.

Kim, D. H., Wong, P. K., Park, J. et al. (2009) Microengineered platforms for cell mechanobiology. *Annual Review of Biomedical Engineering*, **11**, 203–233.

Kumar, S. and LeDuc, P. R. (2009) Dissecting the molecular basis of the mechanics of living cells. *Experimental Mechanics* **49**, 11–23.

Kumar, S., Kumar, S., Ali, M. A. et al. (2013) Microfluidic-integrated biosensors: prospects for point-of-care diagnostics. *Biotechnology Journal* **8**(11), 1267–1279.

Lele, T. P., Sero, J. E., Matthews, B. D. et al. (2007) Tools to study cell mechanics and mechanotransduction, *Methods in Cell Biology* **83**, 443–472.

Li, Y., Li, M., Tan, L. et al. (2013) Analysis of time-course gene expression profiles of a periodontal ligament tissue model under compression. *Archives of Oral Biology* **58**(5), 511–522.

Mahmood, T. and Yang, P. C. (2012) Western blot – technique, theory and trouble shooting. *North American Journal of Medical Sciences* **4**, 429–434.

Mapara, M., Thomas, B. S. and Bhat, K. M. (2012) Rabbit as an animal model for experimental research. *Dental Research Journal (Isfahan)* **9**, 111–118.

Mulligan, J. A., Bordeleau, F., Reinhart-King, C. A. and Adie, S. G. (2018) Traction force microscopy for noninvasive imaging of cell forces. *Advances in Experimental Medicine and Biology* **1092**, 319–349.

Persidis, A. (1999) Tissue engineering. *Nature Biotechnology* **17**, 508–510.

Ren, Y., Maltha, J. C. and Kuijpers Jagtman, A. M. (2004) The rat as a model for orthodontic tooth movement – a critical review and a proposed solution. *European Journal of Orthodontics* **26**, 483–490.

Rommeck, I., Anderson, K., Heagerty, A. et al. (2009) Risk factors and remediation of self-injurious and self-abuse behavior in rhesus macaques. *Journal of Applied Animal Welfare Science* **12**, 61–72.

Shilpa, P. S., Kaul, R., Sultana, N. and Bhat, S. (2013) Stem cells: boon to dentistry and medicine. *Dental Research Journal* **10**(2), 149–154.

Smith, A. J. and Lilley, E. (2019) The role of the three rs in improving the planning and reproducibility of animal experiments. *Animals* **9**(11), 975.

Struillou, X., Boutigny, H., Soueidan, A. and Layrolle, P. (2010) Experimental animal models in periodontology: a review. *The Open Dentistry Journal* **4**, 37–47.

Wang, J. H. and Thampatty, B. P. (2008) Mechanobiology of adult and stem cells. *International Review of Cell and Molecular Biology* **271**, 301–346.

Yamada, S., Wirtz, D. and Kuo, S. C. (2000) Mechanics of living cells measured by laser tracking microrheology. *Biophysics Journal* **78**(4), 1736–1747.

Yeung, M. C. (2002) Accelerated apoptotic DNA laddering protocol. *BioTechniques* **33**, 734–736.

CHAPTER 21
Controversies and Research Directions in Tooth-movement Research

Vinod Krishnan, Anne Marie Kuijpers-Jagtman, and Ze'ev Davidovitch

> **Summary**
>
> Despite the considerable experience in mechanical force-induced tooth movement, there still exist several persisting controversies and conflicting opinions about issues crucial for the attainment of excellent results within a reasonable time period for most or all patients. Such controversies embrace the features of (optimal) orthodontic force, its best magnitude and duration, the biology of tooth movement (inflammation and mechanotransduction), biomarkers in oral fluids, best methods for acceleration of tooth movement, and long-term (deleterious) effects of orthodontic treatment. Scientists are discovering that medical care is proving to be as individualized as faces. Each of us is defined by a unique genetic and molecular makeup. This realization is modifying the way diseases are defined and treated and is the basis of a growing movement toward precision medicine, whereby diagnosis and treatment plans are tailored according to a patient's individual needs. Orthodontists are keenly cognizant of the individual variability of their patients, at least functionally and morphologically, and have begun discovering molecular, genetic, and environmental factors that appear to affect the outcome of mechanotherapy. Thus, the way ahead in terms of identifying the biological determinants of tooth movement is clear.

Introduction

Controversies in science are disagreements among researchers and/or clinicians about the validity of a theory/hypothesis, or a new or prevalent concept. The debate and the following comprehensive research into the topic are often considered essential for the progress of the science, as they lead to the formulation of evidence-based answers and/or new hypotheses. The scientific basis of orthodontics is no exception to this rule, witnessing through the years a variety of controversies on topics such as craniofacial growth modification, treatment of temporomandibular disorders, one-phase or two-phase orthodontic treatment and the rationale for clinical techniques for enhancement of the rate of tooth movement.

For example, an old controversy that still lingers is the debate between Charles Tweed and Calvin Case in the 1920s regarding the issue of extraction versus nonextraction treatment. As Lysle Johnston (2005) pointed out, orthodontic controversies persist for a long time because nobody seems to be interested in finding a solution. The statement holds true even now that "researchers often seem reluctant to ask questions that might put an end to some venerable controversy and thereby kill the goose that lays the golden research egg."

Like general orthodontics, the area of biological research also holds some controversial issues, which are still being investigated by research groups around the world seeking to reach consensus and evidence-based answers. Some have been solved in this manner, while others remain controversial.

This chapter presents some updated information on controversial topics in biological research into orthodontic tooth movement (OTM) and tries to find some evidence-based answers.

The optimal orthodontic force concept

The optimal orthodontic force is defined as the amount of force exerted on the alveolar bone through the periodontal ligament (PDL) that produces a rapid rate of tooth movement by overcoming friction within the appliance system, without discomfort and pain to the patient or ensuing tissue damage, such as hyalinization resulting in root resorption (Burstone, 1962). Nikolai (1975) emphasized considering (i) root surface area and shape, (ii) type of desired tooth movement, (iii) magnitude and time pattern (continuous or interrupted) of the applied force system, and (iv) individual biology or tissue response, before reaching conclusions regarding optimal force theory.

Biological Mechanisms of Tooth Movement, Third Edition. Edited by Vinod Krishnan, Anne Marie Kuijpers-Jagtman and Ze'ev Davidovitch.
© 2021 John Wiley & Sons Ltd. Published 2021 by John Wiley & Sons Ltd.

The concept of optimal orthodontic force started with Schwarz (1932), who experimented with a spring on mandibular teeth of a young dog, which delivered three magnitudes of force (3.5 g, 17 g and 67 g respectively). He concluded that, biologically, the most favorable force was about 20–26 g/cm² of root surface area because then blood capillaries in the PDL would not be blocked. For the next six decades researchers explored the dilemma of light versus heavy orthodontic force and the concept of the optimal force further mainly based on the pressure–tension theory of OTM (see Chapters 1 and 2). Literature mainly focused on the relationship between force level and rate of OTM during active treatment. Quinn and Yoshikawa (1985) proposed four different hypotheses for this relationship (Figure 21.1).

Model A (Figure 21.1A) assumes an on/off switch that is switched on at a certain force level. All forces above this threshold will lead to the same rate of tooth movement. In the second model (Figure 21.1B), a force threshold is also assumed but forces above the threshold, show a linear dose–response relationship. In the third model (Figure 21.1C), forces above the threshold induce tooth movement. A dose–response relationship exists in the lower force ranges up to a certain level. Then a plateau is reached, and a further increase of force leads to a decrease in the rate of tooth movement, until it stops completely. Finally, model D (Figure 21.1D) is comparable to model C except for the decreasing part of the curve in the higher force levels meaning when a certain force level is reached the rate of tooth movement remains the same whatever the force level applied.

Investigating the four different tooth movement models, Quinn and Yoshikawa (1985) concluded that the relationship between these two variables follows a linear pattern up to a point, after which no appreciable tooth movement is observed, even though stress is increased. They concluded that 100–200 g is the force magnitude that can be used for maximally efficient canine retraction. Assuming one half of the root to be under compressive stress, this force level will yield approximately 70–140 g/cm² for an average canine root. A study conducted on rats by King et al. (1991) generated results supporting the concept that overloading does not increase the rate of tooth movement. Rather, overloading will affect all three classic phases (initial, lag, and postlag) of tooth movement as proposed by Burstone (1962). In contrast, Owman-Moll et al. (1995, 1996) concluded that, whereas there was no difference in the rate of tooth movement between a 50 cN and a 100 cN force, there was a 50% increase in tooth movement with a 200 cN force. Contrary to this finding, Pilon et al. (1996) reported that the magnitude of force (50, 100, and 200 cN) does not determine the rate of tooth movement. Surprisingly, both the studies stressed individual characteristics, such as bone density and metabolism, as well as turnover of the PDL, for determining the rate of tooth movement. Emphasizing the importance of the duration of force application rather than its magnitude was the experimental result of van Leeuwen et al. (1999). Attracting attention to the use of light continuous forces, and their ability to eliminate or reduce the lag phase, Iwasaki et al. (2000) concluded that the average velocity of 0.87 and 1.27 mm/month of canine retraction was observed with forces of 18 g and 60 cN, respectively.

The first systematic review on optimal orthodontic force was conducted by Ren et al. (2003) but failed to find any solid evidence from the existing literature. The main problems they encountered were the disparity in the studies regarding calculation of distribution of stresses and strains in the PDL, and a failure to identify the precise nature of tooth movement such as tipping, bodily movement, and the like. Based on data from studies on Beagle dogs included in this systematic review the same investigators (Ren et al., 2004) developed a mathematical model to describe the relationship between stress levels and rate of OTM. This model was then applied to the human data from the same systematic review. Figure 21.2 shows the force–velocity curve for the human data which shows there is a plateau for the force between 132 and 462 cN. There is a tendency for the tooth movement to slow with higher force levels, but it should be noted that the model for the tail of the curve (Figure 21.2, gray area) is less reliable as little human data in the high force range were available to fit the model. Therefore, it remains unclear at which force the movement will cease completely, as is predicted by model C of Quinn and Yoshikawa (1985). Recently, investigators from the same laboratory updated the 2003 systematic review, only including human data (Theodorou et al., 2019). They concluded that forces between 50 cN and 250 cN produced a similar OTM rate, while forces >250 cN yielded a slightly higher rate but were accompanied by adverse effects. The amount of apical root resorption was a secondary outcome in this systematic review, but the strength of evidence was considered weak as the number of included articles reporting on external apical root resorption was insufficient. According to them, forces between 50 cN and 100 cN seem optimal for OTM, patient comfort, and potentially exhibit fewer side effects.

Challenging the existence of hyalinization only during the lag period (Burstone, 1962), and bringing in more controversy to either use light or heavy forces, was the publication by von Böhl et al. (2004a). They stated that both light (25 cN) and heavy forces (300 cN) moved teeth at the same pace. Further, hyalinization was found with both force levels, with its incidence slightly higher in the 300 cN group, and it could appear any time (from 24 hours to 80 days). Even though necrotic tissue formation depends on the force magnitude, the rate of tooth movement does not, as bone remodeling is independent of it. They further emphasized the findings of Owman-Moll et al. (1995, 1996) and Pilon et al. (1996), and stated that individual characteristics such as genetic factors, bone morphology, and density play a large role in

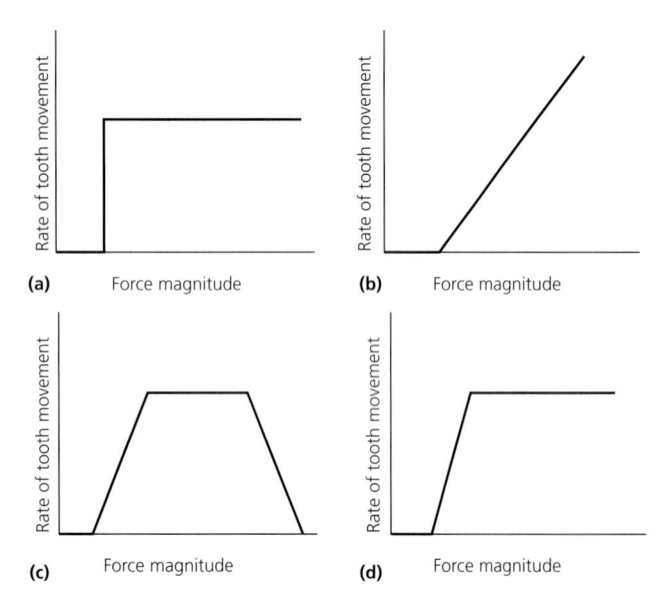

Figure 21.1 Models for the relationship between force magnitude and the rate of tooth movement, modified from Quinn and Yoshikawa (1985). (Source: Ren et al., 2004. Reproduced with permission of Elsevier.)

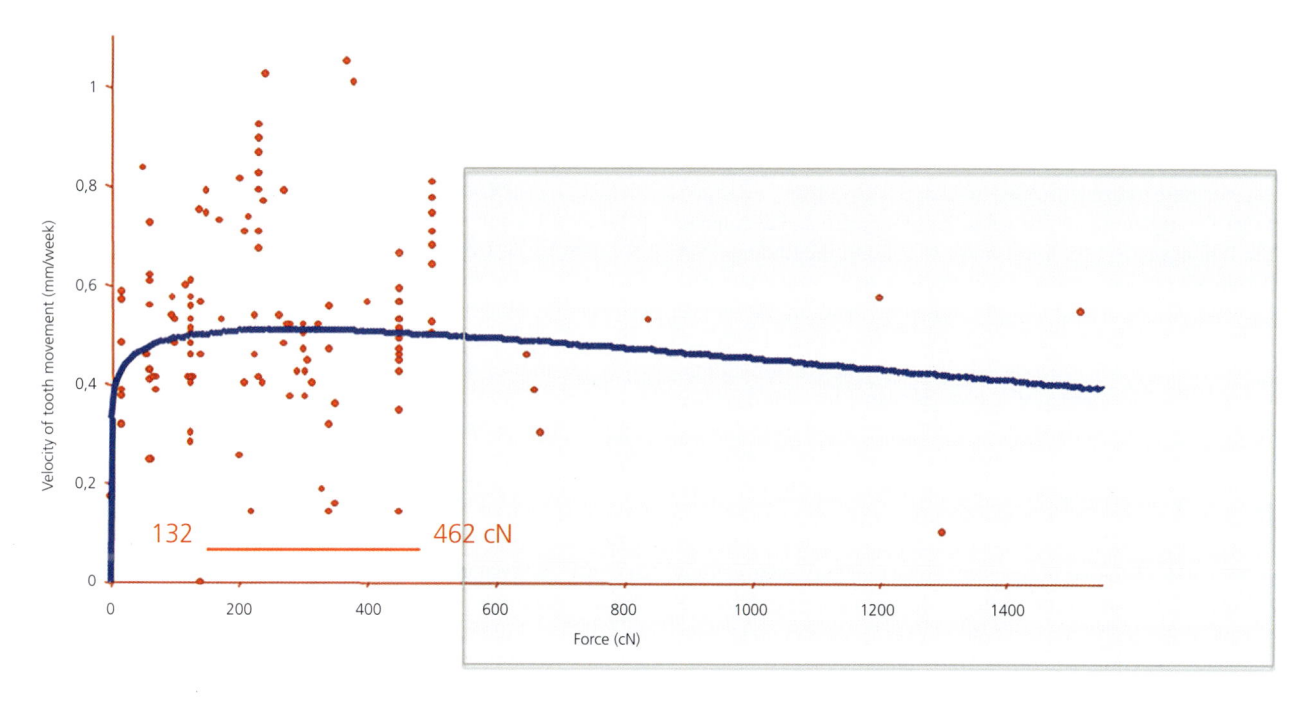

Figure 21.2 Force–velocity curve calculated for human data derived from a mathematical model for Beagle dog data (Ren *et al.*, 2003, 2004). Red dots are individual or group human data. (Sources: Ren *et al.*, 2003, 2004. Courtesy Dr. J. C. Maltha, Radboud University Nijmegen, The Netherlands.)

determining the tooth-movement pace with any applied force. In view of this controversy on existence of hyalinization reactions, Von Böhl and Kuijpers-Jagtman (2009) conducted a systematic review. However, a clear relationship between force level, timing, and extent of hyalinization could not be established. An interesting finding from a rat study, however, is that an initially light and gradually increasing force resulted in less hyalinization than a higher initial force that increased to the same final force level (Tomizuka *et al.*, 2007).

The search for an optimal orthodontic force continues. Applying heavy (300 g) and light (50 g) forces, Yee *et al.* (2009) have reached the same conclusions as other contemporary investigators. They suggested that initial tooth movement will benefit from light forces, while heavy forces tend to increase the rate of canine retraction but increase the risk for deleterious side effects. One such side effect was detected by Kilic *et al.* (2011), who observed a mean increase of 0.8 mm of tooth movement in heavy force application (60 g) in comparison with light forces (20 g), but with greater amount of relapse in the former compared with the latter. Li *et al.* (2016) evaluated effects on the cellular level after applying static compressive forces of 0, 5, 15, and 25 g/cm² on three-dimensionally cultured human PDL fibroblasts for 6, 24, and 72 hours. They reported no significant difference between force levels in the long run but they observed inhibition in proliferation of fibroblasts in a magnitude-dependent manner. Moreover, heavier forces upregulated expression of the osteoclastogenesis inducers, including receptor activator of NF-κB ligand (RANKL), COX-2, PTHrP, and IL-11, more rapidly. With the help of finite element modeling, Wu *et al.*, (2018) identified optimal force levels to be applied to maxillary canine for tipping (40–44 g for distal-direction and 28–32 g for labial-direction), and translation (130–137 g for distal-direction and 110–124 g for labial-direction). The systematic review mentioned earlier (Theodorou *et al.*, 2019) identified forces between 50 cN and 250 cN to produce a similar OTM rate.

Finite element modelling has helped us to improve our theoretical understanding of tissue reaction to an applied force of one individual at one time point, but a finite element model is as good as its biological input data. Here we still miss basic data, especially regarding the behavior of the PDL under stress. In addition, we lack quantitative three-dimensional data of the force–moment (F/M) system exerted on each individual tooth, preferably coupled with biomarkers for tooth movement and root resorption from the gingival crevicular fluid (GCF) or saliva. A start was made by Lapatki *et al.* (2007) at the University of Ulm in Germany with the development of a life-size 'smart' bracket with F/M sensors integrated in the bracket base for *in vitro* 3D measurement of the forces delivered by the appliance, but this system does not seem to have made it to application in the oral environment (Rues *et al*, 2011), and further research in this regard would be interesting.

Overall, the controversy about the identity and features of the best or the optimal orthodontic force continues to promote new research. Past investigations have taught us that our main weapon against malocclusions, mechanical force, should be on the light side most of the time, because heavy forces are frequently associated with the appearance of unwanted side effects. Another recent development on the path to the ideal force is the exploration of molecular markers in oral fluids as a reflection of cellular response to therapeutic forces. In Chapter 11 an overview is given of potential markers of paradental tissue remodeling in the GCF and saliva. Other research findings reveal that the magnitude, direction, and duration of an applied force are dictated by genetic, anatomic, physiologic, and pathologic conditions unique for every individual. In view of this situation, it appears evident that future diagnostic and therapeutic plans in clinical orthodontics will need to be custom made, as the biological response of the patient is highly individual. The ultimate goal is to predict the expected velocity of OTM prior to the start of treatment. Currently, the progress in this area has been limited.

Is tooth movement inflammatory or a mechanotransduction process?

With the findings of an increase in inflammatory infiltrates, necrotic tissues, and resolution with migration of multinucleated giant cells to the area, OTM was labelled as inflammatory in nature, leading to more research directed towards this aspect. It was pointed out that anti-inflammatory drugs such as ibuprofen and diclofenac might inhibit the pace of tooth movement. With the findings that drugs do not influence tooth movement pace to the extent that had been expected, researchers started thinking about an alternative hypothesis, which led to the formulation of the mechanotransduction hypothesis, which views the biological response to orthodontic forces as a transformation of a physical signal to a biochemical response.

Meikle (2006), trying to differentiate between the two phenomena, stated that "describing OTM as an inflammatory process marks it as a pathological event, whereas in reality, it can be considered as an exaggerated form of normal physiologic turnover combined with foci of tissue repair leading to remodeling of cementum and alveolar bone." However, this opinion disregards the fact that the application of orthodontic forces to teeth is accompanied by pain and reduced function, two of the cardinal signs of inflammation. The inflammatory process is the mechanism whereby the body tries to return an injured area to normal. In orthodontics, inflammation repairs the damage caused by mechanical forces.

The idea of labeling OTM as an inflammatory response started with findings by Storey (1955), whose experiments were carried out with heavy force application leading to tissue injury. The concept of inflammatory reaction was further reinforced with experiments on cats by Davidovitch et al. (1988), which demonstrated a significant increase in cytokines such as interleukin (IL), tumor necrosis factor (TNF), and second messengers such as cyclic adenosine monophosphate (cAMP). Further, through a review proposing a biomechanical model for tooth movement, Sandy and Farndale (1991) confirmed the role played by second messengers such as cAMP, cGMP, and inositol phosphate in effecting tooth movement. Alhashimi et al. (2001) conducted a detailed analysis regarding release of inflammatory mediators by looking at their mRNA level expression and provided conclusive evidence for IL-1β and IL-6 expression but failed to substantiate TNF-α expression. This finding has been confirmed by Yang et al. (2013), who pointed out a major role for IL-8 too. A review of literature has revealed that most of the inflammatory reactions occur on the leading side, where more tissue injury is taking place. The reactions are characterized by vasodilatation and migration of leucocytes out of capillaries, the classic inflammatory reactions. Chae et al. (2011) stated that these reactions are initiated by cytokines (IL-1β, IL-6, IL-8, and TNF-α) and growth factors (VEGF), whose expression is increased by mechanical strain-induced hypoxia. There is an immense amount of literature in orthodontics supporting the increase in cytokines and growth factors as well as neurotransmitters such as substance P and vasoactive intestinal polypeptide, which are common mediators of inflammation (see also Chapter 4).

The observation of chemokines at the site of OTM also supports the role of inflammation. The role of chemokines is mainly to promote chemotaxis, differentiation, and activation of osteoclasts favoring bone resorption. The role of the CCR2–CCL2 axis as well as CCL3 and CCR1 was demonstrated and confirmed through rat experiments by Taddei et al. (2012, 2013). Apart from that, the role of RANKL expression for the purpose of osteoclast differentiation with continuous force application in rats was demonstrated earlier by Kim et al. (2007). All these studies point to the fact that inflammation of an aseptic nature exists due to tissue injury with orthodontic force application. As rightly pointed out by Melsen et al. (2007), tooth movement happens while the repair process of the injury is carried out in the paradental tissues. The role played by inflammation in tooth movement is shown in Figure 21.3. Further to these, researchers identified the crucial role played by T-lymphocytes through significant elevation of type 1 T helper cell (Th1) cytokines TNF-α and interferon-γ (IFN-γ) around periodontal tissue in wild type mice (Yan et al., 2015) and M1-like macrophage polarization promoting alveolar bone resorption (He et al., 2015) with orthodontic force application.

The attention given to the responses created by orthodontic forces led to more research on cellular signaling mechanisms incident to mechanical forces, which included mechanosensing, transduction, and response. Harell et al. (1977) and Sandy (1998) have demonstrated the release of prostaglandins and second messengers as primary responses from any cell type incident to mechanical strain. According to the research by Ingber (1991), it was clear that integrins (the main cell adhesion molecule) are mainly responsible for the signal-transduction events. Research by Wang et al. (1993) and Clarke and Brugge (1995) outlined the role of integrins in playing key roles in cell migration, proliferation and differentiation, and function as both cell adhesion molecule and intracellular signaling receptor (Meikle, 2006). The role of mechanical coupling (conversion of mechanical energy into a form that can be detected by the cells) in OTM was reviewed by Dolce et al. (2002). He concentrated on bone remodeling, and outlined the role of streaming potentials, stretch-activated ion channels, and the importance of extracellular matrix in the whole event. Masella and Meister (2006), through their review, outlined the genetic control of osteoblast and osteoclast differentiation and the roles of genes in the bone remodeling process. They stated that the osteoblast generation from stem cells requires 10 hours postforce application and it is a five-generation process (Figure 21.4) with active involvement of cbfa1 and osterix. They could outline at least 24 genes and 60 proteins implicated in positive and negative regulation of osteoclastogenesis and osteoclast function. They concluded that orthodontic force causes physical distortion of PDL and alveolar bone cells and the extracellular matrix, triggering many biochemical cascades that affect the PDL and alveolar bone extracellular matrix, cell membrane, cytoskeleton, matrix of nuclear proteins, and genome.

Following this, Henneman et al. (2008) proposed a theoretical model based on mechanobiology to explain tooth movement, consisting of four stages: (i) matrix strain and fluid flow, (ii) cell strain, (iii) cell activation and differentiation, and (iv) remodeling (Figure 21.5). This model was widely accepted and research laboratories around the world have begun researching on each aspect proposed by them. Krishnan and Davidovitch (2009), favoring the mechanotransduction hypothesis of OTM, were successful in outlining a pathway, which included all paradental tissue reactions to orthodontic force. Chen et al. (2010) evaluated mechanoregulation of bone further, and stated that it involves a very complex process, the specific areas of which are poorly researched or elucidated. He could outline a schematic diagram of sensors, signaling pathways, and responses in osteocyte mechanobiology, regulating osteoblast

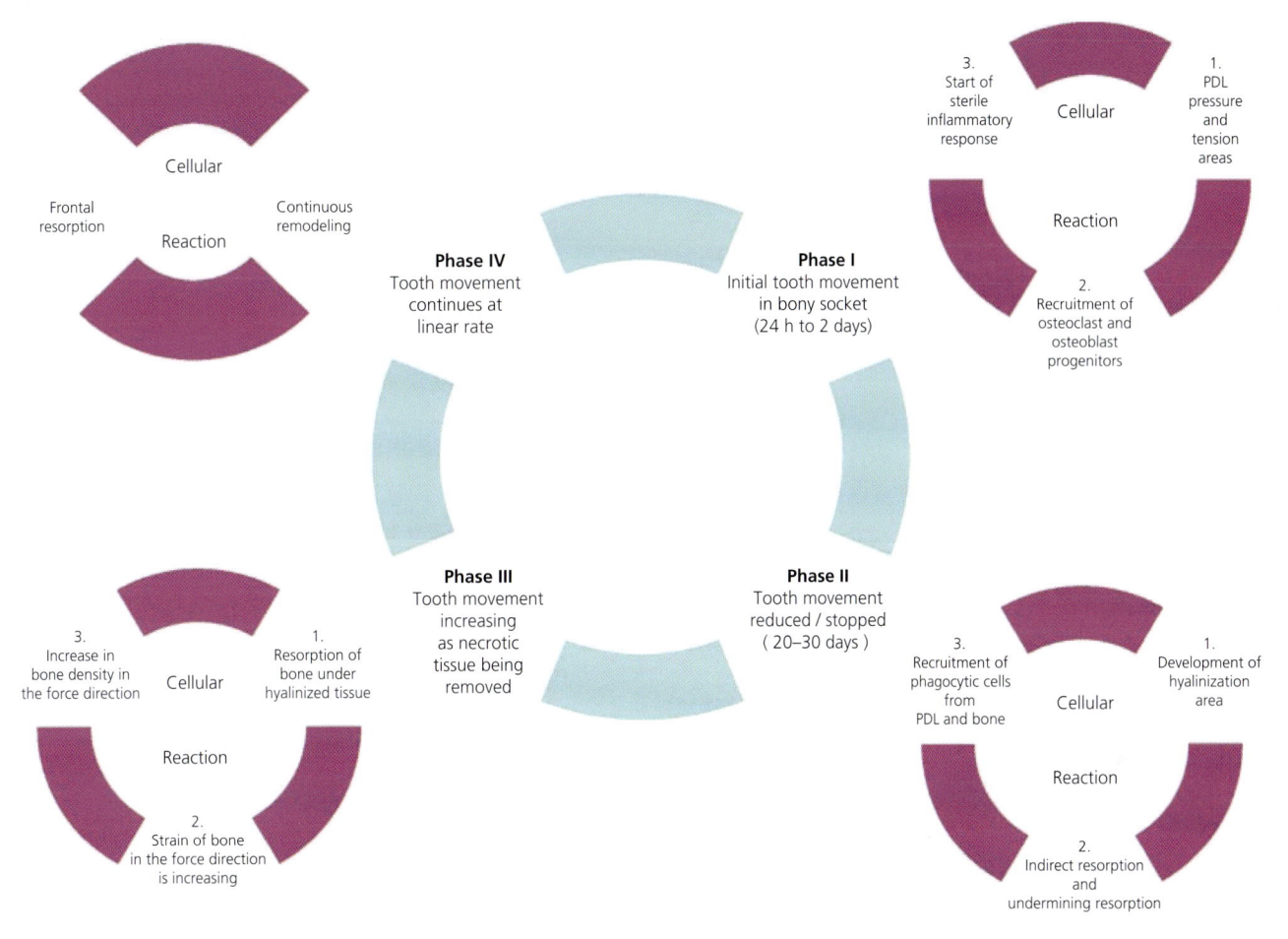

Figure 21.3 The cellular reactions related to the different stages of OTM. (Source: Melsen et al., 2007. Reproduced with permission of Elsevier.)

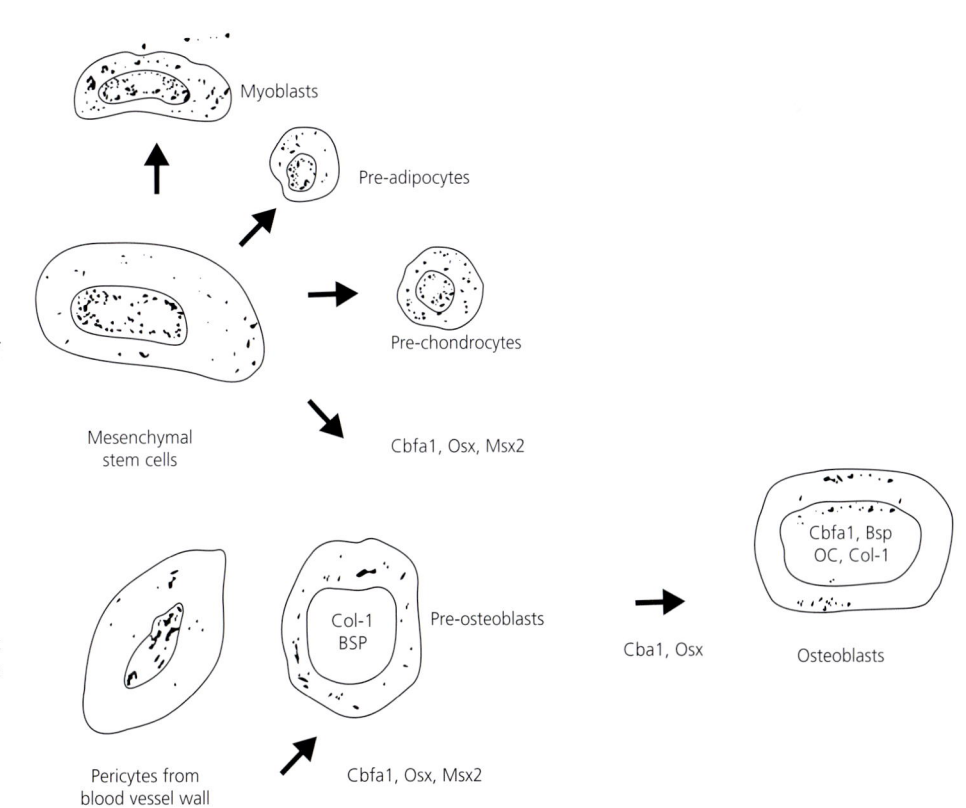

Phase I Initial tooth movement in bony socket (24 h to 2 days)
- Cellular Reaction:
  1. PDL pressure and tension areas
  2. Recruitment of osteoclast and osteoblast progenitors
  3. Start of sterile inflammatory response

Phase II Tooth movement reduced / stopped (20–30 days)
- Cellular Reaction:
  1. Development of hyalinization area
  2. Indirect resorption and undermining resorption
  3. Recruitment of phagocytic cells from PDL and bone

Phase III Tooth movement increasing as necrotic tissue being removed
- Cellular Reaction:
  1. Resorption of bone under hyalinized tissue
  2. Strain of bone in the force direction is increasing
  3. Increase in bone density in the force direction

Phase IV Tooth movement continues at linear rate
- Cellular Reaction:
  - Frontal resorption
  - Continuous remodeling

Figure 21.4 Transcriptional control of osteoblastic differentiation and progeny of pleuripotent mesenchymal stem cells (MSC). Pre-osteoblasts are derived from two sources: MSC and pericytes from blood vessel walls. Transcription factor (TF) Cbfa1 is an early promoter of osteoblast differentiation. Osterix is a late-differentiation TF that induces mature osteoblasts capable of expressing osteocalcin, a TF-inhibiting osteoblast differentiation. Bsp, bone sialoprotein; Col-1, type 1 collagen; OC, osteocalcin; Osx, osterix; Msx2, homeobox gene. (Source: Masella and Meister, 2006. Reproduced with permission of Elsevier.)

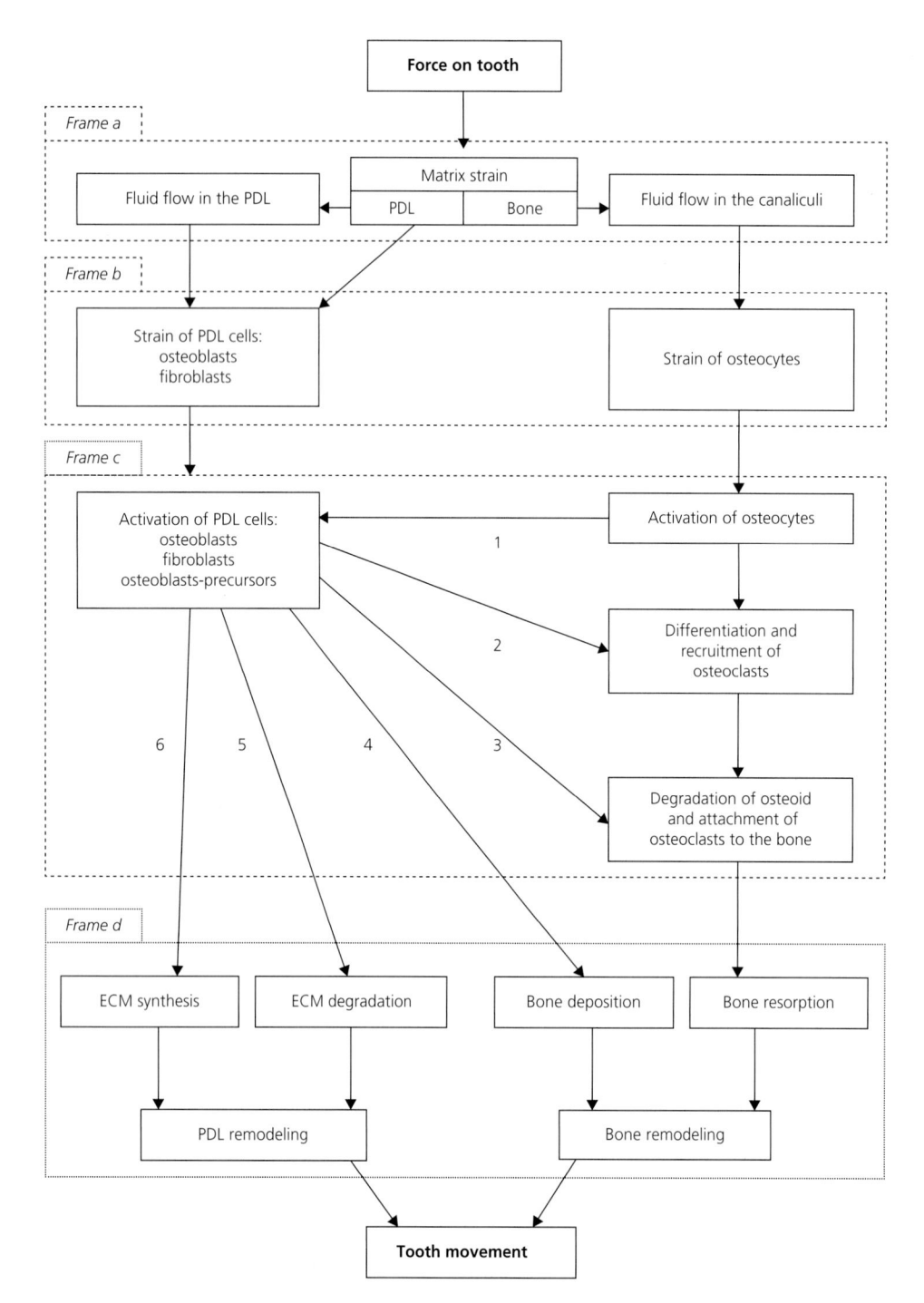

Figure 21.5 Theoretical model for tooth movement proposed by Henneman et al. (2008) which describes the four different stages such as matrix strain and fluid flow, cell strain, cell activation and differentiation, and remodeling of PDL and bone. ECM, extracellular matrix. (Source: Henneman et al., 2008. Reproduced with permission of Oxford University Press.)

and osteoclast formation, as well as bone remodeling (Figure 21.6). Liu et al. (2012) reported that with cyclic stretch of 24 hours, they could observe upregulation of 21 osteogenic-related genes from PDL cells, which included 10 growth factor-related genes, 10 extracellular matrix genes, and one cell-adhesion molecule (Figure 21.7).

Based on the mechanobiological model of OTM of Henneman et al. (2008) (Figure 21.5), Vansant et al. (2018) recently summarized the available literature on biological mediators in relation to OTM in a comprehensive systematic review. Their study provides a timeline of the role of different proteins during OTM based on both in vitro and in vivo studies (Figure 21.8). The authors investigated 139 different proteins but only about 10% of them were studied in at least 10 studies, which means that more research is needed.

Recent experiments by various researchers could outline numerous pathways through which mechanical force is converted to molecular level signals such as activation of sclerostin/sclerostin gene (Scl/SOST) independent of the RANKL-osteoprotegerin (OPG) mechanism in osteocytes (Odagaki et al., 2018), cytoskeleton

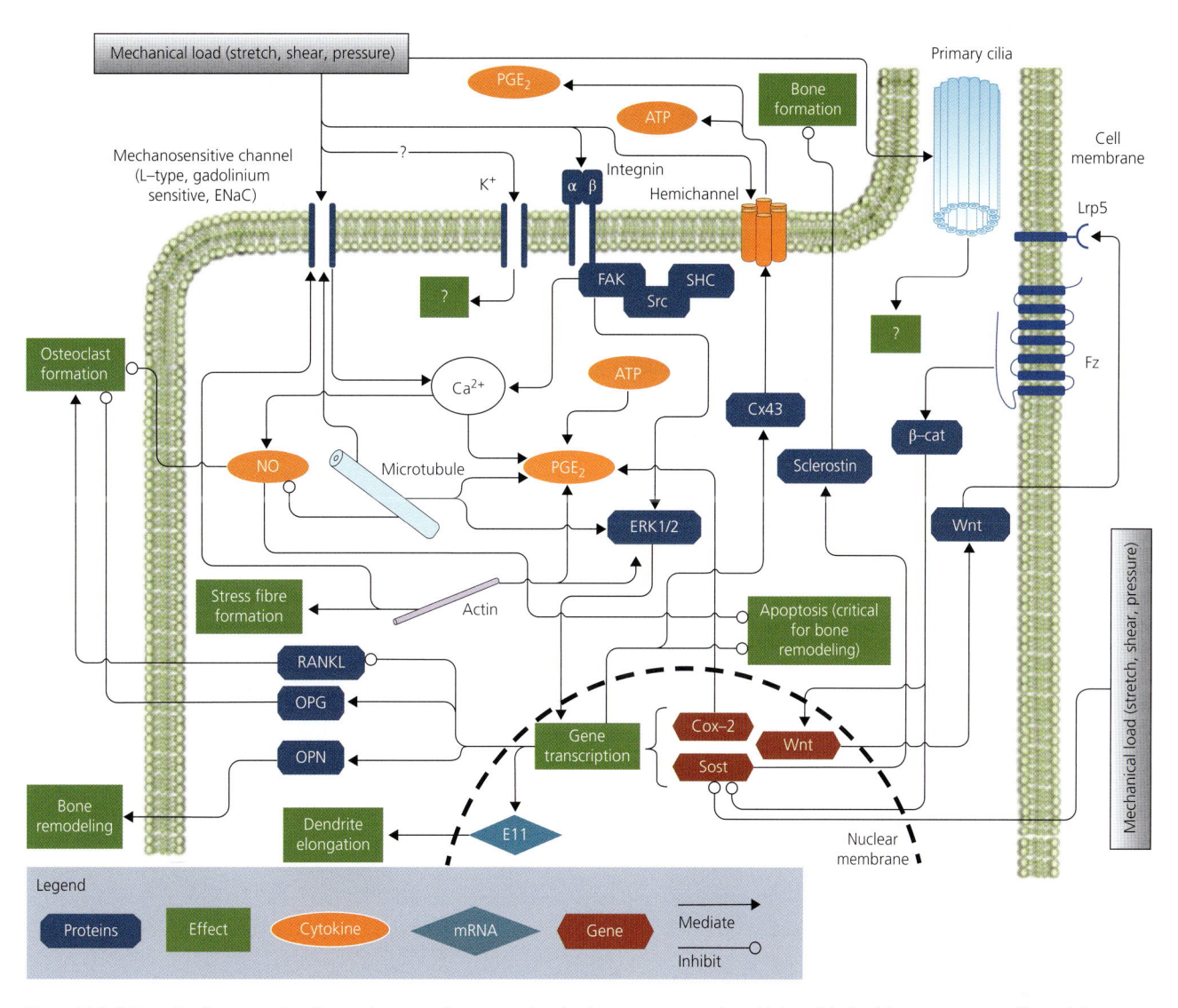

Figure 21.6 Schematic of sensors, signaling pathways, and responses involved in osteocyte mechanobiology. Much of the current state of knowledge regarding osteocyte mechanobiology is represented in the schematic but the detailed signaling mechanisms involved in osteoprogenitor mechanobiology are poorly defined. While osteoprogenitor cells appear to use many of the same sensors (e.g., integrins, ion channels, gap junctions, and primary cilia) and pathways (e.g., ERK1/2 and other MAPKs, Ca^{2+}, and Wnt) as osteocytes, their responses to distinct mechanical stimuli often differ and are not as well defined. (Source: Chen *et al.*, 2010. Reproduced with permission of Elsevier.)

remodeling-induced activation of Yes- associated protein (YAP) signaling pathway in PDL cells (Yang *et al.*, 2018), the importance of Wnt signalling point to the necessity of Wnt/Lrp5 and its localization to osteocytes for proper mechanotransduction in bone (Bullock *et al.*, 2019), the role of augmented mechanical stress-mediated [Ca^{2+}]$_i$ oscillations in hPDL fibroblasts enhancing the production and release of bone regulatory signals *via* RANKL-OPG and the canonical Wnt/β-catenin pathway (Ei Hsu Hlaing *et al.*, 2019), and increased expression of HIF-1α, COX-2, PGE$_2$, VEGF, COL1A2, collagen and ALPL, and the RANKL/OPG ratios at the mRNA/protein levels during PDL-fibroblast-mediated osteoclastogenesis along with establishment of no role played by hypoxia (Ullrich *et al.*, 2019). All these reports suggest that mechanotransduction plays a pertinent role in effecting tooth movement.

These data point to the fact that the tooth-movement process cannot be labeled as either inflammatory, genetic, or mechanotransduction in nature. All the factors have well-defined roles in the process. Initial reactions to orthodontic forces are inflammatory in nature, as evidenced by the release of cytokines and other inflammatory mediators, and this helps in cellular stimulation and initiation of signaling events. Proper mechanotransduction events are essential for a cellular response, which is genetic expression and protein synthesis. All the events must occur in concert for better response to the mechanical forces that we apply.

How far are biomarkers useful in validating OTM?

Another controversial subject as far as tooth movement research is concerned is the role of biomarkers in assessing and predicting the nature of tooth movement. The findings of elevated levels of cytokines, mRNA, proteins, and other inflammatory markers such as growth factors in GCF has generated great interest in this aspect. The current trend is the evaluation of these molecular markers in

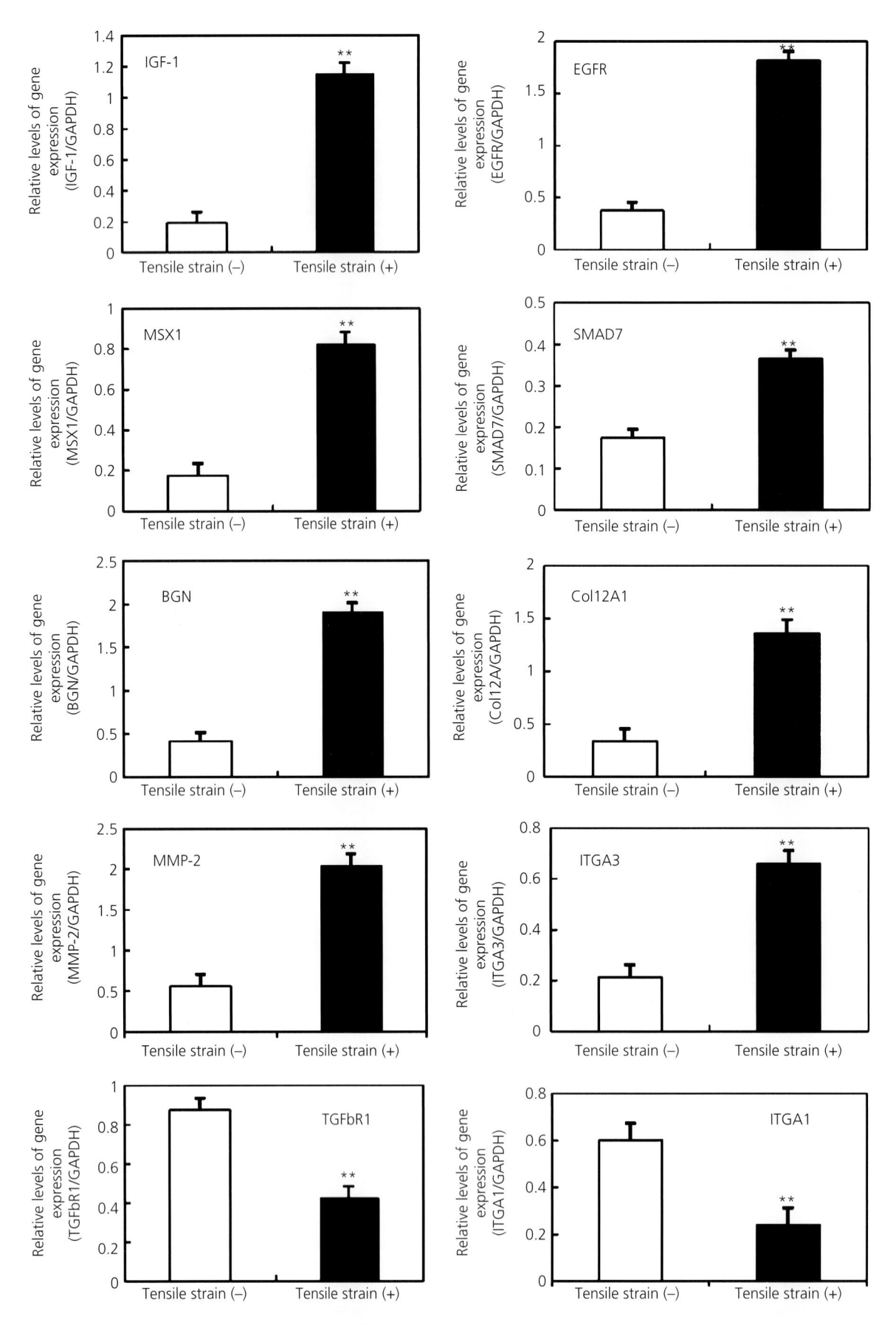

Figure 21.7 Real-time RT-PCR analysis of 10 genes differentially expressed in cyclic stretch-loaded HPDLCs as compared with control samples. Normalized transcript levels of IGF-1, EGFR, MSX1, SMAD7, BGN, Col12A1, MMP-2, and ITGA3 are identified as upregulated, and those of TGFbR1 and ITGA1 are shown to be downregulated. (Source: Liu *et al.*, 2012. Reproduced with permission of Elsevier.)

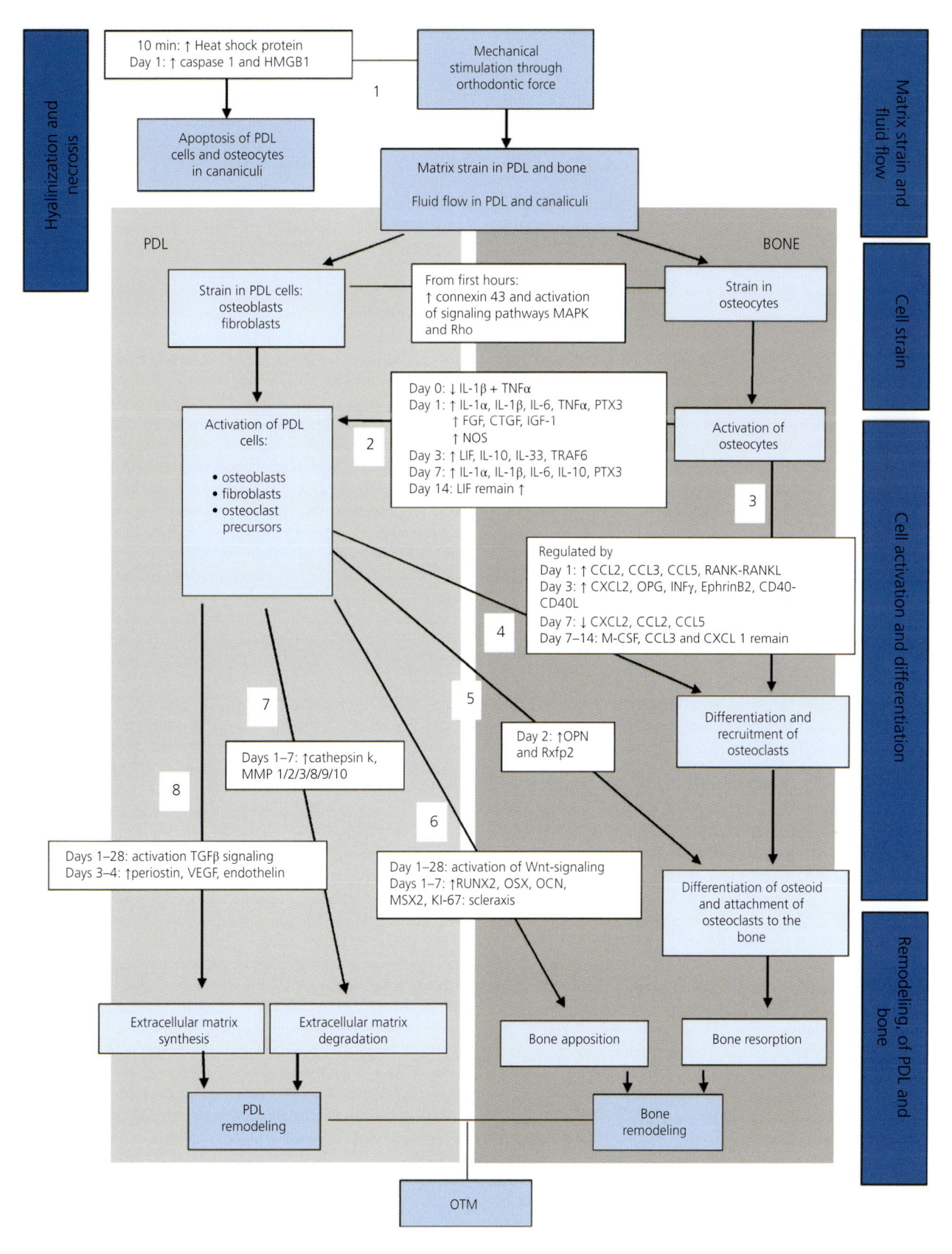

Figure 21.8 Theoretical model of OTM from the systematic review of Vansant *et al.* (2018) based on the model by Henneman *et al.* (2008) to illustrate the role of different proteins throughout the OTM process. (Source: Vansant *et al.*, 2018. Reproduced with permission of Elsevier.)

salivary samples, suggesting that noninvasive collection can also predict tooth movement pace. The reader is referred to Chapter 11 which presents an overview of the study of markers in oral fluids during OTM. The controversy exists in two dimensions, such as whether (i) biomarkers can predict the nature of tooth movement, and (ii) if yes, which is better, GCF or saliva?

GCF, a transudate from interstitial tissues produced by an osmotic gradient, consists of a complex mixture of serum, cells, oral bacteria, and many mediators and enzymes of gingival inflammation (Uitto, 2003). Iwasaki and Nickel (2009), in a review, provided a detailed list of all markers in the GCF, and categorized them as metabolic products of paradental remodeling, inflammatory mediators, enzymes, and enzyme inhibitors. Increased or elevated levels of prostaglandin E_2 (PGE_2) and IL-1β following mechanical force application were initially described by Saito et al. (1991) and Grieve et al. (1994). Subsequently, there has been a myriad of publications describing the elevated status of biomolecules in GCF with mechanical force application through orthodontic appliances. Capelli Jr. et al. (2011) observed a statistically significant elevation for MMP-3, MMP-9, and MMP-13 on the compression side of tooth movement after 1 hour of force application, but found it decreasing sharply over the following 24 hours. They attributed this finding to an immediate consumption of enzymes related to the degradation of collagen. From 24 hours to 80 days, they observed a progressive increase in MMP levels. The findings of Alfaqeeh and Sukumaran (2011) confirmed this progressive increase in collagen degradation with orthodontic force application and documented an elevation in levels of N-telopeptide, a type I collagen degradation product, incident to application of orthodontic forces. A study could even identify the presence of the secretory miRNA-29 family (the marker of periodontal remodeling) in GCF, the expression profiles of which are found to increase during tooth movement in humans (Atsawasuwan et al., 2018).

The breakthrough in GCF research was the discovery of root resorption markers through which the incidence of iatrogenic effect can be quantified. The presence of dentin degradation products in GCF was confirmed by various researchers (Mah and Prasad, 2004; Balducci et al., 2007; Zuo et al., 2011). Even though the orthodontic literature contains numerous reports on increased elevation of biomarkers in the GCF following the application of orthodontic forces, the difficulty in sample collection, its quantification and localization of molecules, interpretation of data and more importantly, its use in a clinical setting, as well as clinical validity of the results, remain questionable. Drummond et al. (2012), in a longitudinal randomized split mouth study, confirmed that the GCF volume, measured with the help of the Periotron, comparing samples from test tooth as well as control tooth at baseline (immediately before placing the orthodontic appliance), and after 1 hour, 24 hours, and 7, 14, and 21 days, cannot be taken as a reliable marker for OTM, and its volume is basically determined by subclinical inflammation. Canavarro et al. (2013) could not observe any statistically significant difference between test and control group GCF samples for MMPs as in tension and pressure sites. They stated that even though MMPs were released in sufficient quantities, their levels did not confirm GCF sampling because of the small sample volume (less than 0.5 μL) that can be obtained from healthy sites. This small volume limits studies with traditional ELISA methods and warrants use of newer methodologies such as multianalyte microsphere assays. A recent systematic review by Tarallo et al. (2019) concluded dentine phosphoprotein (DPP) as a relatively useful marker for root resorption, while the presence of other reported root resorption markers such as dentinal sialoprotein, inflammatory cytokines (pro- and antiresorption), osteopontin, OPG, RANKL, and alkaline phosphatase cannot be considered as specific enough to detect the process. The result, that GCF volume is not a reliable marker, suggests that a new, noninvasive and more reliable procedure needs to be developed for analyzing and evaluating OTM, which will facilitate the standardization of the sampling, analysis, and clinical utilization as a powerful diagnostic tool.

The serum components of saliva, which are derived primarily from the local vasculature, originating from the carotid arteries, have resulted in saliva being a prodigious fluid source of many molecules found in the systemic circulation, making it a potentially valuable aid in the diagnosis of various systemic diseases (Miller et al., 2010). Because of the rapid, noninvasive, and easy acquisition methods of saliva, which requires less manpower and materials than GCF, it is frequently being utilized for diagnosis of periodontal disease. Moreover, it represents a pooled sample from all periodontal sites, in contrast with GCF. With current advancements in this field of research, the elevation or decrease of all host-derived biomarkers, such as cytokines, chemokines, enzymes, and immunoglobulins, which were previously identified from GCF, can be identified through salivary diagnostics. Periodontal research has used saliva's potential to identify all the biomarkers such as: inflammatory mediators (β-glucoronidase, c-reactive protein, IL-1β, IL-6, TNFα, and macrophage inflammatory protein-1α), molecules of connective tissue destruction (α2-macroglobulin, matrix metalloproteinases, tissue inhibitors of matrix metalloproteinases, aminotransferases, cathepsin, and elastase), bone remodeling biomarkers (alkaline phosphatase, C-terminal cross-linking telo-peptide of type I collagen [βCTX], pyridinoline crosslinked carboxyterminal telopeptide domains of type I collagen [ICTP], RANKL and OPG, hepatocyte growth factors, osteocalcin and osteonectin) for diagnosis of various stages of disease processes (Miller et al., 2010).

The first attempt to use saliva as a diagnostic tool in orthodontics was by Burke et al. (2002) who demonstrated a significant difference in cAMP-dependent protein kinase subunit (RII) after orthodontic separator placement. Hussain and Ghaib (2005) reported a statistically significant decrease in the mean total protein concentration in males and an insignificant increase in the mean total protein concentration in females, while evaluating molecular weight of salivary proteins measured with SDS–PAGE (sodium dodecyl sulfate–polyacrylamide gel electrophoresis) in unstimulated whole saliva from 50 patients under orthodontic treatment. Following this research, Marcaccini et al. (2010) could observe the same level of increase in myeloperoxidase activity, both in saliva as well as GCF, suggesting that when most teeth are subjected to orthodontic force, evaluation of biomarkers in either of the fluids makes no difference. The use of saliva as an evaluating tool was further reinforced by Zhang et al. (2012) through their peptidome profiling with the help of matrix-assisted laser desorption/ionization time of flight mass spectroscopy (MALDI-TOF MS). Following this, Flórez-Moreno et al. (2013) observed time-related variations in salivary RANKL and OPG and linked it to different phases of tooth movement.

Root resorption research has also utilized salivary samples to evaluate the role of antidentine antibodies and the role of autoimmune mechanisms. De Paula Ramos et al. (2011) analyzed serum IgG levels and salivary secretory IgA (sIgA) levels and showed increased sIgA levels in saliva at the beginning of orthodontic therapy in patients who later showed moderate to severe resorption after 6 months of treatment. Kaczor-Urbanowicz et al. (2017), with the help of two-dimensional-gel-electrophoresis and quantitative mass spectrometry (qMS), reported differential expression of proteins in the moderate-to-severe OIIRR group from whole saliva. They could even identify and relate differential pathogenetic mechanisms behind root resorption in young (to actin cytoskeleton regulation and Fc gamma R-mediated phagocytosis) and adult (to focal adhesion) subjects. Through a recent systematic review, Allen *et al.* (2019) evaluated salivary protein changes in relation to orthodontic treatment. They included both targeting and nontargeting studies. The targeting studies used known biomarkers such as nuclear factor kappa B ligand (sRANKL), OPG, and leptin (evaluated through ELISA) and myeloperoxidase (MPO) which used enzymatic assay (Bradley-Bozeman modified technique). The nontargeting studies utilized proteomic methods such as mass spectrometry to identify target protein masses and identities. According to them, salivary proteomes have high intersubject variability. This requires a preanalysis depletion assay to be performed to remove highly abundant proteins in saliva such as amylase, immunoglobulins, and albumin so that cytokines or any proteins directly related to bone metabolism, which are present in low quantity, can be identified. Further, the secretion of these biomarkers may be temporal, composed of contributions from food, oral mucosa, respiratory tract, as well as microorganisms, and these biomarkers may disappear too fast to be detected.

Even though the research is replete with data on elevated levels of biomarkers in both saliva and GCF, no technique has been developed yet that can be used at the point of care. Moreover, as Umesan *et al.* (2013) have rightly pointed out, ELISA techniques used to quantify these biomarkers are not sensitive enough to detect changes. Furthering the controversy, they stated that GCF can be more accurate as most of the molecules analyzed have a site-specific nature, making it better than salivary samples. Complicating the issues further, there exists no standard range for any of the molecules analyzed, whether in GCF or saliva, for proper comparison, and the ranges considered normal differ from one study to other.

Development of point-of-care testing devices for analyzing the initiation and pace of tooth movement is needed, but evidence-based research cannot yet substantiate their utility in the clinical scenario.

At the same time, we should not ignore the fact that as an informative signal, biomarkers with more specificity and sensitivity will only become useful in diagnosing a condition or predicting its progress. An effective biomarker should be available in accessible body fluid such as serum, saliva, or GCF. Such a biomarker has yet to be found in orthodontics, and research should be directed towards this rather than arguing whether saliva or GCF is best for sampling.

Can we accelerate tooth movement by any means?

There has been much heated controversy in recent times related to accelerating tooth movement with various corticotomies, and the debate that appeared in the point–counterpoint section of the *American Journal of Orthodontics and Dentofacial Orthopedics* (Mathews and Kokich, 2013; Wilcko and Wilcko, 2013) has attracted much attention. The fundamental principle behind efforts to enhance the velocity of tooth movement is the concept, emanating from laboratory experiments, that has demonstrated that cells and tissues in culture can respond to more than one stimulus at the same time. The cellular response to simultaneous stimuli can be inhibitory, additive, or synergistic. In the case of mechanical force-induced tooth movement, the assumption is that the addition of an agent known to stimulate bone–cell activities, will enhance the velocity of tooth movement. Consequently, attempts to shorten orthodontic treatment time have attracted increasing interest in recent years. This topic is discussed in Chapters 15 to 17.

Jheon *et al.* (2017) distinguish four different approaches to modulate the rate of OTM: (i) by appliance-based variables such as intermittent or continuous force types, and customized wires and appliances; (ii) by physical/mechanical stimuli to teeth and bone such as photobiomodulation and vibrational forces; (iii) with surgically facilitated orthodontic treatment procedures that result in the regional acceleratory phenomenon (RAP); and (iv) local application of bioactive mediators (Figure 21.9).

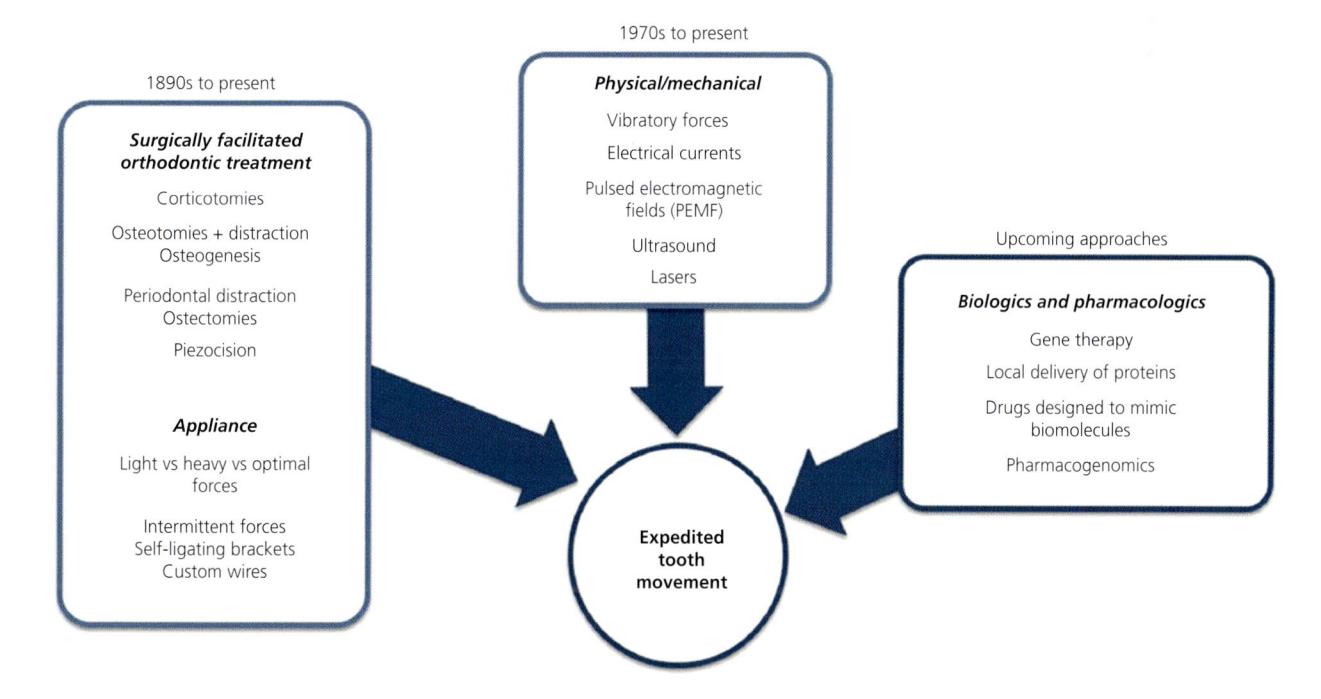

Figure 21.9 Current and upcoming approaches to modulate OTM. (Source: From Jheon *et al.*, 2017. Reprinted with permission from John Wiley & Sons.).

In the point–counterpoint section of the *American Journal of Orthodontics and Dentofacial Orthopedics*, it was stated that corticotomy surgery facilitates local reaction due to demineralization and tooth movement and occurs only close to corticotomized teeth. This helps in creating anchorage due to differential rate of tooth movement experienced by corticotomized and noncorticotomized teeth. Moreover, the alveolar volume can be increased by bone grafting procedures, and this procedure can help in correcting preexisting dehiscences and fenestrations when there is an exposure of a vital root surface (Wilcko and Wilcko, 2013). However, those arguing against this surgical procedure (Mathews and Kokich, 2013) were of the opinion that because of the short period of the existence of RAP, the effect of corticotomies will only last for 4 months, after which the tooth movement will return to its normal rate. Moreover, the additional expenses incurred by the patient, if there is no clear decrease in treatment time, are also not justifiable.

In recent times, 58 systematic reviews have been published (PubMed, accessed 20 June 2020) evaluating efficacy of various surgical interventions to accelerate OTM such as corticotomies (Fernandez-Ferrer et al., 2016; Patterson et al., 2016), piezocision (Yi et al., 2017; Mheissen et al., 2020), micro-osteo-perforations (Hoffmann et al., 2017; Sivarajan et al., 2020), and selective alveolar decortication (Fau et al., 2017). All point to the weak evidence to support these procedures as routine clinical methods to accelerate tooth movement. Emphasizing the need to conduct high quality randomized control trials, Patterson et al. (2016), supported by Fernandez-Ferrer et al. (2016) and Fau et al. (2017), concluded that corticotomies can produce statistically and clinically meaningful temporary increases in the rate of OTM with minimal side effects.

The literature on accelerating tooth movement provides weak evidence that orthodontic treatment can be accelerated by a combined application of mechanical force and another stimulatory agent – physical, chemical, or surgical. Two Cochrane reviews were conducted separately to evaluate the efficacy of both surgical (Fleming et al., 2015) and nonsurgical methods (El-Angbawi et al., 2015) of accelerating tooth movement only to conclude that there is limited research concerning the effectiveness of both methods to accelerate orthodontic treatment. The available evidence is of low quality, which indicates that further research is likely to change the estimate of the effect. Systematic reviews conducted evaluating the efficacy of nonsurgical methods of accelerating tooth movement concluded that there is a lack of meaningful evidence for vibratory stimulus (Elmotaleb et al., 2019) but controversial results with photobiomodulation with laser. From four identified systematic reviews, two favored low-level laser treatment (Ge et al., 2015; Imani et al., 2018), while two reported lack of proper evidence (Sonesson et al., 2017; Al-Shahrani et al., 2019).

A systematic review of systematic reviews conducted by Yi et al., (2017) concluded that the evidence present is of low quality for short-term (1–3 months) effects of low-level laser therapy (5 and 8 J/cm) and corticotomy, very low quality to prove the efficacy of photobiomodulation, pulsed electromagnetic field, interseptal bone reduction, two vibrational devices (Tooth Masseuse and Orthoaccel) and electrical current, and relaxin injections and extracorporeal shock waves have no impact on OTM.

Research is continuing, and the prize remains the discovery of a practical way to correct malocclusions in a short time, efficiently, and without creating undesirable side effects. Future research should move away from these indirect rather crude and invasive approaches to modulate bone turnover and should target local modification of biological processes using patient-specific biological and pharmacological interventions to ultimately bring precision orthodontics to our patients.

Alveolar bone density and shape of the alveolar wall

The use of cone beam computed tomography (CBCT) and microtomography (micro-CT) in orthodontic research has provided great insights into alveolar bone density changes incident to tooth-moving forces. With the help of three-dimensional computer models generated out of CBCT images, Chang et al. (2012) demonstrated maximum bone-density reduction towards the side of toothmovement. Contradictory results with micro-CT analysis were obtained by Zhuang et al. (2011), who found that the bone fraction increased significantly after orthodontic force was applied for 2 weeks, and trabecular separation decreased significantly with a higher orthodontic force (100 g). The results of Zhuang et al. (2011) suggested that the microarchitecture of the alveolar trabecular bone becomes denser, so it can adapt to greater mechanical stresses. This finding was in concordance with previous findings by Garat et al. (2005) in periodontitis patients, which demonstrated that, once periodontal infection is controlled, orthodontic force application results in increased bone volume with improved quality. Yu et al. (2016), using CBCT data from eight patients at three time points, concluded that a significant reduction in bone density can be seen after 7 months of active treatment in comparison to pretreatment values (23.36 ± 10.33%); but a significant increase was observed from this time period to approximately 25 months post-treatment (31.81 ± 23.80%). This clearly indicates recovery of reduced bone density during the post-treatment period to its previous state from before the orthodontic treatment.

All these results indicate the still inconclusive data on how alveolar bone behaves in response to orthodontic force application, indicating the need for well-controlled research producing evidence-based data which is especially important to provide input data for finite element models. In this respect the shape of the alveolar wall is also important, as discussed in Chapter 9, because when considering the stresses on the alveolar wall exerted by a moving tooth, the surface of the alveolus is usually assumed to be smooth. However, micro-CT-scanning has shown that the bony surface of the alveolus is not smooth, with thin bony spicules protruding into the PDL space (see Figures 9.9 and 9.10). It has been shown that these spicules contain osteocyte lacunae (Dalstra et al., 2015) and as such will register even minor local deformation. This complies with the results of the studies of von Böhl et al. (2004a, b) that showed small patches of hyalinization at the bony spicules probably delaying OTM, not only in the initial phase of OTM, but also in the later phases. These small focal hyalinizations might be a factor that could explain individual differences in the rate of tooth movement (von Böhl et al., 2009). If so, then preventing these hyalinization patches would be another step towards faster OTM.

Gingival recession

A conference of the Angle Society of Europe discussed the controversial issue of the association between orthodontic treatment and gingival recession (Johal et al., 2013). The basis of this discussion was the systematic review by Joss-Vassalli et al. (2010), which concluded that there are conflicting opinions in this matter, and a lack of high-quality animal or clinical studies that would clarify this dilemma. In the opinion of the panelists, movement of incisors outside the osseous envelope might create gingival recession and, consequently highlighted the need to undertake risk assessment and appropriate consent prior to commencement of treatment. Renkema et al. (2013) concluded that orthodontically treated lower incisors are at a great risk for development of labial gingival recession when retained with bonded lingual retainers. However, Morris et al. (2017) concluded that orthodontic treatment is not a major risk factor for the development of gingival recession after evaluating pre- and post-treatment lateral cephalograms and dental models of 205 orthodontic patients in which mandibular incisor proclination and maxillary arch widths were measured. They could observe 5.8% of teeth exhibiting recession at the end of orthodontic treatment, but the prevalence increased to 41.7% after retention with less severity (only 7.0% >1 mm). This finding of post-treatment increase in the incidence of recession was further confirmed through the long-term study conducted by Gebistorf et al. (2018). According to them, 98.9% of the orthodontically treated participants had at least one labial/buccal recession, and 85.2% of the patients had at least one lingual/palatal recession 10–15 years post-treatment. Interestingly, the prevalence of labial/buccal gingival recession were similar in the orthodontically treated patients 10–15 years post-treatment and the untreated controls.

Preventing excessive lower incisor proclination during orthodontic treatment, avoiding the risk of a bone dehiscence, and thus the risk of gingival recession, has been a dogma in orthodontic treatment planning for many years. However, nowadays there is a trend to arch expansion and proclining incisors to gain space as an alternative to extraction therapy. Tepedino et al. (2018), through a recent systematic review, concluded that there is no strong scientific evidence that proclination of incisors following orthodontic treatment with a fixed appliance increases the risk of gingival recession. The main reason was a lack of randomized controlled trials. However, it is ethically questionable to randomize patients to procline or not to procline lower incisors. Therefore, prospective or well-designed retrospective long-term cohort studies or case control studies are needed to solve the dilemma of lower incisor inclination.

Periodontal health

The systematic review by Bollen (2008) pointed out the contradictory findings existing in the literature regarding periodontal and OTM. Van Gastel et al. (2011) conducted a longitudinal study to evaluate microbiological and clinical parameters from bracket bonding to 3 months post-treatment, and concluded that placement of fixed appliances will alter microbiologic and clinical periodontal parameters, which will show a significant increase (worse) at the time of debonding. The changes were partly reversible, as the supragingival colony forming units (CFU) normalized at 3 months but subgingival CFU remained elevated. A 2-year post-treatment evaluation of periodontal parameters was published by Ghijselings et al. (2014), which supported the findings of van Gastel et al. (2011). They stated that even after 2 years of treatment, the subgingival microbiota remained altered when compared with pretreatment levels, indicating that some changes in periodontal parameters are irreversible in the long term. The study revealed that the normalization of clinical variables, such as probing pocket depth and bleeding on probing happened by 2 years, except in areas where banding was performed. In contrast, Verrusio et al. (2018), through a systematic review, concluded that an increase of periodontal parameters after orthodontic treatment associated with the accumulation and composition of the subgingival microbiota exists, which subsequently induces more inflammation and higher bleeding on probing. Jiang et al. (2018) pointed out the advantage that clear aligners hold in this aspect and stated that the parameters such as plaque index, gingival index and probing depth showed better values than with fixed appliances. However, they admitted the level of the evidence was downgraded because of the risk of bias and inconsistency in the studies included in the review. All these data point to the existing controversy regarding the subject and the need for systematic long-term evaluation to provide us with evidence-based results so that this matter can be brought to a conclusion.

Conclusions

Malocclusions have been treated for millennia by mechanical forces, which guide the malposed teeth to better positions in the dental arches. However, despite this long history, there are still several persisting controversies regarding the fundamental assumptions that comprise orthodontic mechanotherapy and its short- and long-term effects. Scientists are discovering that medical care is proving to be as individualized as faces. Each of us is defined by a unique genetic and molecular makeup. This realization is modifying the way diseases are defined and treated and is the basis of a growing movement toward precision medicine, whereby diagnosis and treatment plans are tailored according to a patient's individual needs (see Chapter 13 for a detailed review). Orthodontists are keenly cognizant of the individual variability of their patients, at least functionally and morphologically, and have begun discovering molecular, genetic, and environmental factors that appear to affect the outcome of mechanotherapy. Thus, the way ahead in terms of identifying the biological determinants of tooth movement is clear.

However, it seems as if orthodontists are satisfied knowing that mechanical force, of almost any reasonable magnitude, will move teeth. Moreover, why worry about deleterious effects of orthodontic force, such as root resorption? Why not simply put the blame on the patient's shoulders? The controversies about issues that are apparently the central core of orthodontics – including the nature of the force, tissue biomarkers in oral fluids, methods to accelerate tooth movement, and the long-term effects of orthodontic treatment on the longevity of the dentition and the patient's wellbeing – are reflections of the lack of credible published data, emanating from well-planned and performed experiments. Evidently, future research should aim at filling the voids in our knowledge about important issues related to biological basic science and clinical procedures, which compose the events of tooth movement. One meaningful goal is to explore and identify new means for enhancing the orthodontist's ability to provide precision orthodontics. The leading specialists in this drive are the oncologists, who utilize genetic and genomic investigations of individual patients so that they can choose the right medication for the specific type of cancer. In orthodontics, it would be helpful to identify the genes responsible for bone growth and remodeling, and to expose biomarkers that accurately reflect the degree of involvement of systems such as the nervous, vascular, immune, and skeletal, in the individual response to orthodontic therapy. Future research should embrace the ongoing vast improvements in technology and bioengineering, and the parallel advancements in medicine. This research should assist the orthodontist in identifying and selecting the most suitable method of orthodontic therapy for each patient.

References

Al-Shahrani, I., Togoo, R. A. and Hosmani, J. (2019) Photobiomodulation in acceleration of orthodontic tooth movement: a systematic review and meta analysis. *Complementary Therapies in Medicine* 102220.

Alfaqeeh, S. A. and Sukumaran, A. (2011) Osteocalcin and N-telopeptides of type I collagen marker levels in gingival crevicular fluid during different stages of orthodontic tooth movement. *American Journal of Orthodontics and Dentofacial Orthopedics* **139**, e553–559.

Alhashimi, N., Frithiof, L., Brudvik, P. and Bakhiet, M. (2001) Orthodontic tooth movement and de novo synthesis of proinflammatory cytokines *American Journal of Orthodontics and Dentofacial Orthopedics* **119**, 307–312.

Allen, R. K., Edelmann, A. R., Abdulmajeed, A. and Bencharit, S. (2019) Salivary protein biomarkers associated with orthodontic tooth movement: a systematic review. *Orthodontics and Craniofacial Research* **22**, 14–20.

Atsawasuwan, P., Lazari, P., Chen, Y. et al. (2018) Secretory microRNA-29 expression in gingival crevicular fluid during orthodontic tooth movement. *PloS One* **13**(3).

Balducci, L., Ramachandran, A., Hao, J. et al. (2007) Biological markers for evaluation of root resorption. *Archives in Oral Biology* **52**, 203–208.

Bollen, A. M. (2008) Effects of malocclusions and orthodontics on periodontal health: evidence from a systematic review. *Journal of Dental Education* **72**, 912–918.

Bullock, W. A., Pavalko, F. M. and Robling, A. G. (2019) Osteocytes and mechanical loading: the Wnt connection. *Orthodontics and Craniofacial Research* **22**, 175–179.

Burke, J. C., Evans, C. A., Crosby, T. R. and Mednieks, M. I. (2002) Expression of secretory proteins in oral fluid after orthodontic tooth movement. *American Journal of Orthodontics and Dentofacial Orthopedics* **121**, 310–315.

Burstone, C. J. (1962) The biomechanics of tooth movement, in *Vistas in Orthodontics* (eds. B. S. Kraus and R. A. Riedel). Lea & Febiger, Philadelphia, PA, pp. 197–213.

Canavarro, C., Teles, R. P. and Capelli Júnior, J. (2013) Matrix metalloproteinases -1, -2, -3, -7, -8, -12, and -13 in gingival crevicular fluid during orthodontic tooth movement: a longitudinal randomized split-mouth study, *European Journal of Orthodontics* **35**, 652–658.

Capelli, Jr J., Kantarci, A., Haffajee, A. et al. (2011) Matrix metalloproteinases and chemokines in the gingival crevicular fluid during orthodontic tooth movement. *European Journal of Orthodontics* **33**, 705–711.

Chae, H. S., Park, H. J., Hwang, H. R. et al. (2011) The effect of antioxidants on the production of pro-inflammatory cytokines and orthodontic tooth movement. *Molecules and Cells* **32**, 189–196.

Chang, H. W., Huang, H. L., Yu, J. H. et al. (2012) Effects of orthodontic tooth movement on alveolar bone density. *Clinical Oral Investigations* **16**, 679–688.

Chen, J. H., Liu, C., You, L. and Simmons, C. A. (2010) Boning up on Wolff's Law: mechanical regulation of the cells that make and maintain bone. *Journal of Biomechanics* **43**, 108–118.

Clarke, E. A. and Brugge, J. S. (1995) Integrins and signal transduction pathways: the road taken. *Science* **268**, 233–239.

Dalstra, M., Cattaneo, P. M., Laursen, M. G. et al. (2015) Multi-level synchrotron radiation-based microtomography of the dental alveolus and its consequences for orthodontics. *Journal of Biomechanics* **48**(5), 801–806.

Davidovitch, Z., Nicolay, O. F., Ngan, P. W. and Shanfeld, J. L. (1988) Neurotransmitters, cytokines, and the control of alveolar bone remodeling in orthodontics. *Dental Clinics of North America* **32**, 411–435.

de Paula Ramos, S., Ortolan, G. O., Dos Santos, L. M. et al. (2011) Anti-dentine antibodies with root resorption during orthodontic treatment. *European Journal of Orthodontics* **33**, 584–591.

Dolce, C., Malone, J. S. and Wheeler, T. T. (2002) Current concepts in the biology of orthodontic tooth movement. *Seminars in Orthodontics* **8**(1), 6–12.

Drummond, S., Canavarro, C., Perinetti, G. et al. (2012) The monitoring of gingival crevicular fluid volume during orthodontic treatment: a longitudinal randomized split-mouth study. *European Journal of Orthodontics* **34**(1), 109–113.

Ei Hsu Hlaing, E., Ishihara, Y., Wang, Z. et al. (2019) Role of intracellular Ca2+–based mechanotransduction of human periodontal ligament fibroblasts. *The FASEB Journal* **33**(9), 10409–10424.

El-Angbawi, A., McIntyre, G. T., Fleming, P. S. and Bearn, D. R. (2015) Non-surgical adjunctive interventions for accelerating tooth movement in patients undergoing fixed orthodontic treatment. *Cochrane Database of Systematic Reviews* **2015**(11), CD010887.

Elmotaleb, M. A. A., Elnamrawy, M. M., Sharaby, F. et al. (2019) Effectiveness of using a vibrating device in accelerating orthodontic tooth movement: a systematic review and meta-analysis. *Journal of International Society of Preventive and Community Dentistry* **9**(1), 5.

Fau, V., Diep, D., Bader, G. et al. (2017) Effectiveness of selective alveolar decortication in accelerating orthodontic treatment: a systematic review. *L'Orthodontie Francaise* **88**(2), 165–178.

Fernandez-Ferrer, L., Montiel-Company, J. M., Candel-Marti, E. et al. (2016) Corticotomies as a surgical procedure to accelerate tooth movement during orthodontic treatment: A systematic review. *Medicina Oral, Patologia Oral y Cirugia Bucal* **21**(6), e703.

Fleming, P. S., Fedorowicz, Z., Johal, A. et al. (2015) Surgical adjunctive procedures for accelerating orthodontic treatment. *Cochrane Database of Systematic Reviews* **2015**(6), CD010572.

Flórez-Moreno, G. A., Isaza-Guzmán, D. M. and Tobón-Arroyave, S. I. (2013) Time-related changes in salivary levels of the osteotropic factors sRANKL and OPG through orthodontic tooth movement. *American Journal of Orthodontics and Dentofacial Orthopedics* **143**, 92–100.

Garat, J. A., Gordillo, M. E. and Ubios, A. M. (2005) Bone response to different strength orthodontic forces in animals with periodontitis. *Journal of Periodontal Research* **40**, 441–445.

Ge, M. K., He, W. L., Chen, J. et al. (2015) Efficacy of low-level laser therapy for accelerating tooth movement during orthodontic treatment: a systematic review and meta-analysis. *Lasers in Medical Science* **30**(5), 1609–1618.

Gebistorf, M., Mijuskovic, M., Pandis, N. et al. (2018) Gingival recession in orthodontic patients 10 to 15 years posttreatment: a retrospective cohort study. *American Journal of Orthodontics and Dentofacial Orthopedics* **153**(5), 645–655.

Ghijselings, E., Coucke, W., Verdonck, A. et al. (2014) Long-term changes in microbiology and clinical periodontal variables after completion of fixed orthodontic appliances. *Orthodontics and Craniofacial Research* **17**, 49–59.

Grieve, W. G., Johnson, G. K., Moore, R. N. et al. (1994) Prostaglandin E (PGE) and interleukin-1β (IL-1β) levels in gingival crevicular fluid during human orthodontic tooth movement. *American Journal of Orthodontics and Dentofacial Orthopedics* **105**, 369–374.

Harell, A., Dekel, S. and Binderman, I. (1977) Biochemical effect of mechanical stress on cultured bone cells. *Calcified Tissue Research* (suppl.) **22**, 202–207.

He, D., Kou, X., Yang, R. et al. (2015) M1-like macrophage polarization promotes orthodontic tooth movement. *Journal of Dental Research* **94**(9), 1286–1294.

Henneman, S., Von den Hoff, J. W. and Maltha, J. C. (2008) Mechanobiology of tooth movement. *European Journal of Orthodontics* **30**, 299–306.

Hoffmann, S., Papadopoulos, N., Visel, D. et al. (2017) Influence of piezotomy and osteoperforation of the alveolar process on the rate of orthodontic tooth movement: a systematic review. *Journal of Orofacial Orthopedics/Fortschritte der Kieferorthopädie* **78**(4), 301–311

Hussain, S. F. and Ghaib, N. H. (2005) Expression of secretary proteins in whole unstimulated saliva before and after placement of orthodontic elastic separators in Iraqi samples (clinical study). *Iraqi Orthodontic Journal* **1**(1), xxi–xxii.

Imani, M. M., Golshah, A., Safari-Faramani, R. and Sadeghi, M. (2018) Effect of low-level laser therapy on orthodontic movement of human canine: a systematic review and meta-analysis of randomized clinical trials. *Acta Informatica Medica* **26**(2), 139.

Ingber, D. E. (1991) Integrins as mechanochemical transducers. *Current Opinion in Cell Biology* **3**, 841–848.

Iwasaki, L. R., Haack, J. E., Nickel, J. C. and Morton, J. (2000) Human tooth movement in response to continuous stress of low magnitude. *American Journal of Orthodontics and Dentofacial Orthopedics* **117**, 175–183.

Iwasaki, L. R. and Nickel, J. C. (2009) Markers of paradental tissue remodeling in the gingival crevicular fluid of orthodontic patients, in *Biological Mechanisms of Tooth Movement* (eds. V. Krishnan and Z. Davidovitch). Wiley-Blackwell, Oxford, pp. 123–142.

Jheon, A. H., Oberoi, S., Solem, R. C. and Kapila, S. (2017) Moving towards precision orthodontics: An evolving paradigm shift in the planning and delivery of customized orthodontic therapy. *Orthodontics and Craniofacial Research* **20**, 106–113.

Jiang, Q., Li, J., Mei, L., Du, J. et al. (2018) Periodontal health during orthodontic treatment with clear aligners and fixed appliances: *a meta-analysis. Journal of the American Dental Association* **149**(8), 712–720.

Johal, A., Katsaros, C., Kiliaridis, S. et al. (2013) State of the science on controversial topics: orthodontic therapy and gingival recession (a report of the Angle Society of Europe 2013 meeting). *Progress in Orthodontics* **14**, 16.

Johnston, L. E. (2005) The anatomy of controversy: a few random comments. *Seminars in Orthodontics* **11**, 59–61.

Joss-Vassalli, I., Grebenstein, C., Topouzelis, N. et al. (2010) Orthodontic therapy and gingival recession: a systematic review. *Orthodontics and Craniofacial Research* **13**, 127–141.

Kaczor-Urbanowicz, K. E., Deutsch, O., Zaks, B. et al. (2017) Identification of salivary protein biomarkers for orthodontically induced inflammatory root resorption. *PROTEOMICS–Clinical Applications* **11**(9–10), 1600119.

Kilic, N., Oktay, H. and Ersoz, M. (2011) Effects of force magnitude on relapse: an experimental study in rabbits. *American Journal of Orthodontics and Dentofacial Orthopedics* **140**, 44–50.

Kim, T., Handa, A., Iida, J. and Yoshida, S. (2007) RANKL expression in rat periodontal ligament subjected to a continuous orthodontic force. *Archives in Oral Biology* **52**, 244–250.

King, G. J., Keeling, S. D., McCoy, E. A. and Ward, T. H. (1991) Measuring dental drift and orthodontic tooth movement in response to various initial forces in adult rats. *American Journal of Orthodontics and Dentofacial Orthopedics* **99**(5), 456–465.

Krishnan, V. and Davidovitch, Z. (2009) On a path to unfolding the biological mechanisms of orthodontic tooth movement. *Journal of Dental Research* **88**, 597–608.

Lapatki, B. G., Bartholomeyczik, J., Ruther, P. et al. (2007) Smart bracket for multidimensional force and moment measurement. *Journal of Dental Research* **86**(1), 73–78.

Li, M., Yi, J., Yang, Y., Zheng, W. et al. (2016) Investigation of optimal orthodontic force at the cellular level through three-dimensionally cultured periodontal ligament cells. *European Journal of Orthodontics* **38**(4), 366–372.

Liu, M., Dai, J., Lin, Y. et al. (2012) Effect of the cyclic stretch on the expression of osteogenesis genes in human periodontal ligament cells. *Gene* **491**, 187–193.

Mah, J. and Prasad, N. (2004) Dentine phosphoproteins in gingival crevicular fluid during root resorption. *European Journal of Orthodontics* **26**, 25–30.

Marcaccini, A. M., Amato, P. A., Leão, F. V. et al. (2010) Myeloperoxidase activity is increased in gingival crevicular fluid and whole saliva after fixed orthodontic appliance activation. *American Journal of Orthodontics and Dentofacial Orthopedics* **138**, 613–616.

Masella, R. S. and Meister, M. (2006) Current concepts in the biology of orthodontic tooth movement. *American Journal of Orthodontics and Dentofacial Orthopedics* **129**, 458–468.

Mathews, D. P. and Kokich, V. G. (2013) Accelerating tooth movement: the case against corticotomy-induced orthodontics. *American Journal of Orthodontics and Dentofacial Orthopedics* **144**, 5–13.

Meikle, M. C. (2006) The tissue, cellular and molecular regulation of orthodontic tooth movement: 100 years after Carl Sandstedt. *European Journal of Orthodontics* **28**, 221–240.

Melsen, B., Cattaneo, P. M., Dalstra, M. and Kraft, D. C. (2007) The importance of force levels in relation to tooth movement. *Seminars in Orthodontics* **13**(4), 220–233.

Mheissen, S., Khan, H. and Samawi, S. (2020) Is piezocision effective in accelerating orthodontic tooth movement: a systematic review and meta-analysis. *PloS One* **15**(4), e0231492.

Miller, C. S., Foley, J. D., Bailey, A. L. et al. (2010) Current developments in salivary diagnostics. *Biomarkers in Medicine* **4**, 171–189.

Morris, J. W., Campbell, P. M., Tadlock, L. P. et al. (2017) Prevalence of gingival recession after orthodontic tooth movements. *American Journal of Orthodontics and Dentofacial Orthopedics* **151**(5), 851–859.

Nikolai, R. J. (1975) On optimum orthodontic force theory as applied to canine retraction. *American Journal of Orthodontics* **68**, 290–302.

Odagaki, N., Ishihara, Y., Wang, Z. et al. (2018) Role of osteocyte-PDL crosstalk in tooth movement via SOST/sclerostin. *Journal of Dental Research* **97**(12), 1374–1382.

Owman-Moll, P., Kurol, J. and Lundgren, D. (1995) Continuous versus interrupted continuous orthodontic force related to early tooth movement and root resorption. *The Angle Orthodontist* **65**(6), 395–401.

Owman-Moll, P., Kurol, J. and Lundgren, D. (1996) Effects of a doubled orthodontic force magnitude on tooth movement and root resorptions. An inter-individual study in adolescents. *European Journal of Orthodontics* **18**, 141–150.

Patterson, B. M., Dalci, O., Darendeliler, M. A. and Papadopoulou, A. K. (2016) Corticotomies and orthodontic tooth movement: a systematic review. *Journal of Oral and Maxillofacial Surgery* **74**(3), 453–473.

Pilon, J. J., Kuijpers-Jagtman, A. M. and Maltha, J. C. (1996) Magnitude of orthodontic forces and rate of bodily tooth movement: an experimental study in beagle dogs. *American Journal of Orthodontics and Dentofacial Orthopedics* **110**, 16–23.

Quinn, R. S. and Yoshikawa, D. K. (1985) A reassessment of force magnitude in orthodontics. *American Journal of Orthodontics* **88**, 252–260.

Ren, Y., Maltha, J. C. and Kuijpers-Jagtman, A. M. (2003) Optimum force magnitude to orthodontic tooth movement – a systematic review. *The Angle Orthodontist* **73**, 86–92.

Ren, Y., Maltha, J. C., Van't Hof, M. A. and Kuijpers-Jagtman, A. M. (2004) Optimum force magnitude for orthodontic tooth movement: a mathematic model. *American Journal of Orthodontics and Dentofacial Orthopedics* **125**, 71–77.

Renkema, A. M., Fudalej, P. S., Renkema, A. A. et al. (2013) Gingival labial recessions in orthodontically treated and untreated individuals: a case – control study. *Journal of Clinical Periodontology* **40**, 631–637.

Rues, S., Panchaphongsaphak, B., Gieschke, P. et al. (2011) An analysis of the measurement principle of smart brackets for 3D force and moment monitoring in orthodontics. *Journal of Biomechanics* **44**(10), 1892–1900.

Saito, M., Saito, S., Ngan, P. W. et al. (1991) Interleukin 1 beta and prostaglandin E are involved in the response of periodontal cells to mechanical stress *in vivo* and *in vitro*. *American Journal of Orthodontics and Dentofacial Orthopedics* **99**, 226–240.

Sandy, J. R. (1998) Signal transduction. *British Journal of Orthodontics* **25**, 269–274.

Sandy, J. R. and Farndale, R. W. (1991) Second messengers: regulators of mechanically-induced tissue remodelling. *European Journal of Orthodontics* **13**, 271–278.

Schwarz, A. M. (1932) Tissue changes incidental to orthodontic tooth movement. *International Journal of Orthodontia, Oral Surgery and Radiography* **18**(4), 331–352.

Sivarajan, S., Ringgingon, L. P., Fayed, M. and Wey, M. C. (2020) The effect of micro-osteoperforations on the rate of orthodontic tooth movement: a systematic review and meta-analysis. *American Journal of Orthodontics and Dentofacial Orthopedics* **157**(3), 290–304.

Sonesson, M., De Geer, E., Subraian, J. and Petrén, S. (2017) Efficacy of low-level laser therapy in accelerating tooth movement, preventing relapse and managing acute pain during orthodontic treatment in humans: a systematic review. *BMC Oral Health* **17**(1), 11.

Storey, E. (1955) Bone changes associated with tooth movement. A histological study of the effect of force for varying durations in the rabbit, guinea pig and rat. *Australian Dental Journal* **59**, 209–219.

Taddei, S. R., Andrade, I. Jr, Queiroz-Junior, C. M. et al. (2012) Role of CCR2 in orthodontic tooth movement *American Journal of Orthodontics and Dentofacial Orthopedics* **141**, 153–160.

Taddei, S. R., Queiroz-Junior, C. M., Moura, A. P. et al. (2013) The effect of CCL3 and CCR1 in bone remodeling induced by mechanical loading during orthodontic tooth movement in mice. *Bone* **52**, 259–267.

Tarallo, F., Chimenti, C., Paiella, G. et al. (2019) Biomarkers in the gingival crevicular fluid used to detect root resorption in patients undergoing orthodontic treatment: a systematic review. *Orthodontics and Craniofacial Research* **22**(4), 236–247.

Tepedino, M., Franchi, L., Fabbro, O. and Chimenti, C. (2018) Post-orthodontic lower incisor inclination and gingival recession – a systematic review. *Progress in Orthodontics* **19**(1), 17.

Theodorou, C. I., Kuijpers-Jagtman, A. M., Bronkhorst, E. M. and Wagener, F. A. (2019) Optimal force magnitude for bodily orthodontic tooth movement with fixed appliances: a systematic review. *American Journal of Orthodontics and Dentofacial Orthopedics* **156**(5), 582–592.

Tomizuka, R., Shimizu, Y., Kanetaka, H. et al. (2007) Histological evaluation of the effects of initially light and gradually increasing force on orthodontic tooth movement. *The Angle Orthodontist* **77**, 410–416.

Uitto, V. J. (2003) Gingival crevice fluid – an introduction. *Periodontology 2000* **31**, 9–11.

Ullrich, N., Schröder, A., Jantsch, J. et al. (2019) The role of mechanotransduction versus hypoxia during simulated orthodontic compressive strain – an in vitro study of human periodontal ligament fibroblasts. *International Journal of Oral Science* **11**(4), 1–10.

Umesan, U. K., Chua, K. L. and Krishnan, V. (2013) Assessing salivary biomarkers for analyzing orthodontic tooth movement. *American Journal of Orthodontics and Dentofacial Orthopedics* **143**, 446–447.

van Gastel, J., Quirynen, M., Teughels, W. et al. (2011) Longitudinal changes in microbiology and clinical periodontal parameters after removal of fixed orthodontic appliances. *European Journal of Orthodontics* **33**, 15–21.

van Leeuwen, E. J., Maltha, J. C. and Kuijpers-Jagtman, A. M. (1999) Tooth movement with light continuous and discontinuous forces in beagle dogs. *European Journal of Oral Sciences* **107**, 468–474.

Vansant, L., Cadenas De Llano-Pérula, M., Verdonck, A. and Willems, G. (2018) Expression of biological mediators during orthodontic tooth movement: a systematic review. *Archives of Oral Biology* **95**, 170–186.

Verrusio, C., Iorio-Siciliano, V., Blasi, A. et al. (2018) The effect of orthodontic treatment on periodontal tissue inflammation: a systematic review. *Quintessence International* **49**(1).

von Böhl, M., Maltha, J., Von den Hoff, H. and Kuijpers-Jagtman, A. M. (2004a) Changes in the periodontal ligament after experimental tooth movement using high and low continuous forces in beagle dogs. *The Angle Orthodontist* **74**, 16–25.

von Böhl, M., Maltha, J. C., Von Den Hoff, J. W. and Kuijpers-Jagtman, A. M. (2004b) Focal hyalinization during experimental tooth movement in beagle dogs. *American Journal of Orthodontics and Dentofacial Orthopedics* **125**(5), 615–623.

von Böhl, M. and Kuijpers-Jagtman, A. M. (2009) Hyalinization during orthodontic tooth movement: a systematic review on tissue reactions. *European Journal of Orthodontics* **31**(1), 30–36.

Wang, N., Butler, J. P. and Ingber, D. E. (1993) Mechanotransduction across the cell surface and through the cytoskeleton. *Science* **269**, 1124–1127.

Wilcko, W. and Wilcko, M. T. (2013) Accelerating tooth movement: the case for corticotomy-induced orthodontics. *American Journal of Orthodontics and Dentofacial Orthopedics* **144**, 4–12.

Wu, J. L., Liu, Y. F., Peng, W. et al. (2018) A biomechanical case study on the optimal orthodontic force on the maxillary canine tooth based on finite element analysis. *Journal of Zhejiang University-SCIENCE B* **19**(7), 535–546.

Yang, Y., Wang, B. K., Chang, M. L. et al. (2018) Cyclic stretch enhances osteogenic differentiation of human periodontal ligament cells via YAP activation. *BioMed Research International* **2018**, 2174824

Yan, Y., Liu, F., Kou, X. et al. (2015) T cells are required for orthodontic tooth movement. *Journal of Dental Research* **94**(10), 1463–1470.

Yang, J. H., Li, Z. C., Kong, W. D. et al. (2013) Effect of orthodontic force on inflammatory periodontal tissue remodeling and expression of IL-6 and IL-8 in rats. *Asian Pacific Journal of Tropical Medicine* **6**, 757–761.

Yee, J. A., Türk, T., Elekdağ-Türk, S. et al. (2009) Rate of tooth movement under heavy and light continuous orthodontic forces. *American Journal of Orthodontics and Dentofacial Orthopedics* **136**, 150.e1–9.

Yi, J., Xiao, J., Li, Y. et al. (2017) Efficacy of piezocision on accelerating orthodontic tooth movement: a systematic review. *The Angle Orthodontist* **87**(4), 491–498.

Yi, J., Xiao, J., Li, H. et al. (2017) Effectiveness of adjunctive interventions for accelerating orthodontic tooth movement: a systematic review of systematic reviews. *Journal of Oral Rehabilitation* **44**(8), 636–654.

Yu, J. H., Huang, H. L., Liu, C. F. et al. (2016) Does orthodontic treatment affect the alveolar bone density?. *Medicine* **95**(10), e3080.

Zhang, J., Zhou, S., Li, R. et al. (2012) Magnetic bead-based salivary peptidome profiling for periodontal-orthodontic treatment. *Proteome Science* **10**, 63.

Zhuang, L., Bai, Y. and Meng, X. (2011) Three-dimensional morphology of root and alveolar trabecular bone during tooth movement using micro-computed tomography. *The Angle Orthodontist* **81**, 420–425.

Zuo, Z. G., Hu, M., Jiang, H. and Tian, L. (2011) Relationship between orthodontics root resorption following experimental tooth movement and the level of dentin sialophosphoprotein and dentin sialoprotein in gingival crevicular fluid. *Hua Xi Kou Qiang Yi Xue Za Zhi* **29**, 294–298.

Index

Page locators in **bold** indicate tables. Page locators in *italics* indicate figures. This index uses letter-by-letter alphabetization.

AAOMS *see* American Association of Oral and Maxillofacial Surgeons
ACMG *see* American College of Medical Genetics and Genomics
Actinomyces spp., 143–144, 146, 148, 152–153
actins, 72
activator protein-1 (AP-1), 50
adenosine triphosphate (ATP), 68, 70, 74–75
AFM *see* atomic force microscopy
age of patient, 118
Aggregatibacter spp., 146, 148
alcohol use, 211
alkaline phosphatase (ALP)
   genetic influences, 172–173, 176, 179
   load-induced modeling, 111
allergy/allergic reactions, 292–293
all-*trans*-retinoic acid (ATRA), 108
ALP *see* alkaline phosphatase
alveolar bone
   cellular and molecular biology, 35–36, *36*
   evolution of hypotheses and concepts, 20–21, *21–22*
   genetic influences, 171, 177–180, *178*
   iatrogenic injuries in orthodontics, 282, 284–285, *284–285*, **285**
   inflammatory response, 49–51, **50**, *51*
   mechanical loading on hard and soft tissues, 68, 70–72, 75
   precision accelerated orthodontics, 265–267
   tooth-movement research, 327–329, 338
alveolar corticotomy *see* corticotomy
alveolar wall
   tissue reaction to orthodontic force systems, 133–135, *133–135*
   tooth-movement research, 338
Alzheimer disease, 196
American Association of Oral and Maxillofacial Surgeons (AAOMS), 203–204
American College of Medical Genetics and Genomics (ACMG), 192
angiogenesis, 60
Angle, Edward H., 19
angular synchondrosis (AS), 82, *82*
anticholinergic drugs, 207
antihistamines, 206
antiresorptive agents, 202–204
AP-1 *see* activator protein-1
apolipoprotein E (APOE), 196
apoptosis

genetic influences, 173
iatrogenic injuries in orthodontics, 288–289
inflammatory response, 58
load-induced modeling, 113
tissue reaction to orthodontic force systems, 131, *131*
arachidonic acid cascade
   cellular and molecular biology, 39
   drugs, medications, and supplements, 200, 202, 210–211
   genetic influences, 180
   inflammatory response, 52
   load-induced modeling, 108, *109*
   mechanical loading on hard and soft tissues, 69
Arnold, Jim, 83
AS *see* angular synchondrosis
asthma medications, 204–205
atomic force microscopy (AFM), 323, *324*
ATP *see* adenosine triphosphate
ATRA *see* all-*trans*-retinoic acid
atrophic bone, 271

bandeau, 5–6, *6*
Baumrind, Sheldon, 11, 25–26, *26*
Bien, S. M., 24–25
bioelectric signals, 26–30, *27–29*
biological anchorage, 271
biological orthodontics, 219–237
   accelerating tooth movement, 219–231, *220*, *225–226*, *228–232*
   concepts and definitions, 219
   decelerating tooth movement, 231–234, **232**, *233–234*
   early attempts to accelerate tooth movement, 219–220, *220*
   pharmacological approaches, 221–224, *222–223*, 231–234, **232**, *233–234*
   physical stimuli, 224–227, *225–226*, *228–230*
   surgical approaches, 227–230, *231–232*
biphasic theory of tooth movement
   concepts and definitions, 265–267, *276–277*
   micro-osteo-perforations, 268–271, *269–271*
   vibration, 271–273, *272–273*
bisphenol A (BPA), 292
bisphosphonates (BP), 202–204
BMD *see* bone mineral density
BMP *see* bone morphogenetic proteins
BMU *see* bone multicellular unit

bone-bending hypothesis, 11, 25–26, *26*
bone grafts, 246–248, *248–249*, **248**
bone growth and metabolism, 77–99
   calcium metabolism and tooth movement, 95
   cellular and molecular biology, 86, *87*
   concepts and definitions, 77–84
   cortical bone remodeling, 90
   dental facial orthopedics and bone modeling, 94–95
   determinants of overall craniofacial growth, 85
   endochondral ossification, 78–80, *79*
   factors influencing bone modeling and remodeling, 87–90, *89*
   genetic mechanisms for environment adaptation, 84–86, *85*, *87*
   growth and development of facial bones, 90–92, *91–92*
   inflammatory response, 86
   intramembranous ossification, 78, *79*, 80–82, *81*
   primary growth centers and sites in facial bones, 80–82, *81–82*
   temperomandibular joint development and mature adaptation, 92–93, *92*
   tooth movement and bone modeling, 93–94, *93–94*
   trabecular bone remodeling, 88, 90, *90–91*
   vascular invasion, 79, *79*, 85–86, *85*
   see also bone modeling and remodeling
bone histomorphometric analysis
   dynamic histomorphometric bone labeling, 82–83, *82–84*
   load-induced modeling, 113
bone marrow, 100
bone mineral density (BMD), 206
bone modeling and remodeling
   cellular and molecular biology, 42–45, *42–44*
   concepts and definitions, 82–84, *82–84*
   cortical bone remodeling, 90
   coupling of bone formation to resorption, 87
   dental facial orthopedics and bone modeling, 94–95
   genetic influences, 179–180
   inflammatory response, 49–51, **50**, *51*
   load-induced modeling, 100–116
   mechanical aspects, 88–89, *89*
   mechanical control, 88
   mechanical loading on hard and soft tissues, 70, 74–75

Biological Mechanisms of Tooth Movement, Third Edition. Edited by Vinod Krishnan, Anne Marie Kuijpers-Jagtman and Ze'ev Davidovitch.
© 2021 John Wiley & Sons Ltd. Published 2021 by John Wiley & Sons Ltd.

bone modeling and remodeling (Cont'd)
  metabolic control, 87–88
  microtrauma-triggered bone remodeling, 268
  tooth movement and bone modeling, 93–94, *93–94*
  tooth movement and external apical root resorption, 89–90
  trabecular bone remodeling, 88, 90, *90–91*
bone morphogenetic proteins (BMP), 79, 178–179
bone multicellular unit (BMU)
  load-induced modeling, 101, 105
  surgically assisted tooth movement, 239, 244
bone resorption
  drugs, medications, and supplements, 202–205, 210
  evolution of hypotheses and concepts, 20–21, *21–22*
  mechanical loading on hard and soft tissues, 71–72
  precision accelerated orthodontics, 267
bone sialoprotein (BSP), 176, 179, 183
bone tissue, 69–70
Borgens, R. B., 28–29
BP *see* bisphosphonates
BPA *see* bisphenol A
brown spot lesions, 144, *144*
bruxism, 130
BSP *see* bone sialoprotein
burns, 293
Burstone and Pryputniewicz curve, 241–242, *241*

calcitonin gene-related peptide (CGRP)
  cellular and molecular biology, 36
  genetic influences, 176–177
  inflammatory response, 50–51, 58–60
calcium homeostasis
  bone growth and metabolism, 87–88, 95
  drugs, medications, and supplements, 210
  mechanical loading on hard and soft tissues, 74
cAMP *see* cyclic adenosine monophosphate
Candida spp., 145–146, 147, 150
Ca/P ratio, 62
carboxy-linked collagen crosslinks (CTX), 102
cardiac neural crest, 78
cartilage, 78–82, *79*, *82*
CBCT *see* cone beam computed tomography
CBT *see* cognitive behavioral therapy
cell culture, 313–314, *313*, **314**
cellular and molecular biology, 35–48
  biomechanical characteristics of the PDL, 38, *38*
  bone growth and metabolism, 86, *87*
  cell–cell interactions, 38–39
  cell–matrix interactions, 39–40, *39–40*
  cell types, 37–38, *37*
  concepts and definitions, 35
  effects of orthodontic force application, 40–45, *41–44*
  extracellular matrix, 35–45, *36*
  general regulatory mechanisms, 38–40, *39–40*
  genetic influences, 172
  important entities for tooth movement, 35–38
  inflammatory response, 58
  initial phase processes and hyalinization, 41–42

  load-induced modeling, 100–105
  mechanical loading on hard and soft tissues, 69–70, *71*
  phases of orthodontic tooth movement, 40–41, *40–42*
  real tooth movement processes, 42–45, *42–44*
  relapse and retention, 45
  theoretical model of orthodontic tooth movement, 45, *46*
  tooth-movement research, 330–333, *331–335*
Celsus, Aulus Corneliu (25 BCE–50 CE), 5, *5*
cementoblasts, 38
cemento-enamel junction (CEJ), 284–285
cementum
  cellular and molecular biology, 35–36, *36*
  inflammatory response, 62
  mechanical loading on hard and soft tissues, 68
  relapse and retention, 302, *303*
center of resistance (CR)
  precision accelerated orthodontics, 270
  surgically assisted tooth movement, 240–241
  tissue reaction to orthodontic force systems, 129–130, *130*, 133–136
cGMP *see* cyclic guanosine monophosphate
CGRP *see* calcitonin gene-related peptide
chemical burns, 293
chemokines, 50, 55–57, 330
chromatin immunoprecipitation (ChIP) assay, 321
CNC *see* cranial neural crest
cognitive behavioral therapy (CBT), 61
collagen
  bone growth and metabolism, 79
  cellular and molecular biology, 35–36, *36*, 43
  closure of extraction space or midline diastema, 304–305
  genetic influences, 173
  load-induced modeling, 102
  relapse and retention, 300–305
  rotational tooth movement, 304
  techniques affecting relapse, 305
  terminology, 303
  translational tooth movement, 303–304
  turnover in the periodontium, 305
comet assay, 322, *322*
composite/ceramic brackets, 148–149
computed tomography (CT)
  surgically assisted tooth movement, 252–253, *252–261*
  temporary anchorage devices, 119–121, *119*
  tissue reaction to orthodontic force systems, 131–135, *132–135*
  tooth-movement research, 338
condroitin sulfate, 36
condylar secondary cartilage (CSC), 82, *82*
cone beam computed tomography (CBCT)
  surgically assisted tooth movement, 252–253, *252–261*
  temporary anchorage devices, 119
  tooth-movement research, 338
confocal microscopy, 317
connective tissue growth factor (CTGF), 178–180
conventional brackets, 148
copper, 210
cortical bone of the canine (CVC), 242

cortical bone remodeling, 90
cortical bone thickness, 120–121, *121*
corticision, 230–231, *232*
corticosteroids, 205, 224
corticotomy
  accelerating tooth movement, 227–231, *231–232*
  biological principles and biomechanical considerations, 239–242, *240–242*
  clinical examples, 250–258, *251–261*
  iatrogenic injuries in orthodontics, 283
  rules for effective alveolar corticotomy, 242–250
    facilitating orthodontic tooth movement, 243–244, *244*
    flapless corticotomy protocol, **246**, 249–250, *249–250*
    limited effect in time, 244
    limited effects in space, 244–245, *245–246*
    open flap corticotomy and grafting protocol, 245–248, *246*, *247–249*, **248**
    patient selection, 250
    postsurgical orthodontic management, 250
COX *see* cyclooxygenases
CR *see* center of resistance
cranial neural crest (CNC), 78, *78*
cross infection, 293
CSC *see* condylar secondary cartilage
CT *see* computed tomography
CTGF *see* connective tissue growth factor
CTX *see* carboxy-linked collagen crosslinks
CVC *see* cortical bone of the canine
cyclic adenosine monophosphate (cAMP)
  evolution of hypotheses and concepts, 28–29
  genetic influences, 176
  history of orthodontics, 11, *12*
  inflammatory response, 50, 52–53
  mechanical loading on hard and soft tissues, 69–71
  tooth-movement research, 319, *319*, 330
cyclic guanosine monophosphate (cGMP), 52–53, 330
cyclooxygenases (COX)
  biological orthodontics, 221
  drugs, medications, and supplements, 200–202, 211
  genetic influences, 180
  inflammatory response, 52, 61
  load-induced modeling, 108, *109*
cyclosporine A, 206–207
cytochrome P450, 191–192, 194
cytokines
  biological orthodontics, 221
  cellular and molecular biology, 38–39
  iatrogenic injuries in orthodontics, 290
  inflammatory response, 49–50, 53
  oral fluid markers of paradental tissue remodeling, 161–163, *161*, *163*
  tooth-movement research, 330
cytoskeleton, 40, *40*
cytotoxicity, 292

damage associated molecular pattern proteins (DAMP), 49–52
debonding trauma, 288, *288–289*
denosumab (DN), 202–204
dental caries

oral microbiology, 143–147, *144*, *147*, 149–150
  precision orthodontics, 192–193
dental facial orthopedics, 77, 89, 94–95
dental pulp
  genetic influences, 180–181, *181*
  iatrogenic injuries in orthodontics, 288–290, *289*
  inflammatory response, 58–60, **60**
dentin, 300–302
dentine phosphoprotein (DPP), 336
dentoalveolar distraction, 229–230
dermatan sulfate, 36
diabetes mellitus (DM), 171
diet and nutrition *see* drugs, medications, and supplements
direct electric current stimuli, 224–225
DM *see* diabetes mellitus
DN *see* denosumab
DNA laddering/fragmentation analysis, 323, *323*
DPP *see* dentine phosphoprotein
drugs, medications, and supplements, 199–215
  anticholinergic drugs, 207
  antihistamines, 206
  antiresorptive agents, 202–204
  asthma medications, 204–205
  biological orthodontics, 221–224, *222–223*, 231–234, **232**, *233–234*
  conclusions and recommendations, 211–212
  corticosteroids, 205
  fluoride, 210
  gingival enlargement, 206–207
  hormonal influences on tooth movement, 207–209
  lipids, 210–211
  minerals, 210
  nonsteroidal anti-inflammatory drugs, 200–202
  prostaglandins and analogues, 200, *201*
  psychiatric drugs, 207
  statins, 206
  substance abuse, 211
  United States context, 199–200
  vitamins, 209–210
dynamic histomorphometric bone labeling, 82–83, *82–84*

EARR *see* external apical root resorption
ECM *see* extracellular matrix
EGF *see* epidermal growth factor
eicosanoids, 39
elastin, 36
electrokinetic phenomena, 27–30
Electronic Medical Records and Genomics (eMERGE) network, 195
electrophoretic mobility shift assay (EMSA), 321
ELISA *see* enzyme-linked immunosorbent assay
eMERGE *see* Electronic Medical Records and Genomics
EMMPRIN, 45
EMSA *see* electrophoretic mobility shift assay
enamel decalcification and trauma, 285–288, *286–289*
endochondral ossification, 78–80, *79*
endothelins (ET), 173–176
environmental scanning electron microscopy (ESEM), 318, *318*
enzyme-linked immunosorbent assay (ELISA), 164, 321

epidermal growth factor (EGF), 180–181
eruption failure, 181–182, 194–195
ESEM *see* environmental scanning electron microscopy
estrogen therapy, 206–207, 208, 233–234
ET *see* endothelins
external apical root resorption (EARR)
  bone growth and metabolism, 77, 86, 89–90
  genetic influences, 183–184
  iatrogenic injuries in orthodontics, 290–291, *290*
  inflammatory response, 61–62
  precision orthodontics, 194
extracellular matrix (ECM)
  biological orthodontics, 219
  cellular and molecular biology, 35–45, *36*
  genetic influences, 172
  mechanical loading on hard and soft tissues, 68–70, 72–73
extraoral injuries, 293

Farrar, John Nutting, 7, *7*
Fauchard, Pierre (1678–1761), 5–6, *6*
FEA/FEM *see* finite element analysis/models
FGF *see* fibroblast growth factor
FGFR2/3, 80
fibrillins, 36
fibroblast growth factors (FGF)
  bone growth and metabolism, 79–80
  cellular and molecular biology, 43–45
  genetic influences, 180–181
  load-induced modeling, 101, 103
fibroblasts
  cellular and molecular biology, 42–43, *43*
  mechanical loading on hard and soft tissues, 71
  tooth-movement research, 300–306, 313, *319*, 323, 329, 333
fibrocartilage, 78–81, *79*
finite element analysis/models (FEA/FEM)
  surgically assisted tooth movement, 240–242, *241–242*
  temporary anchorage devices, 120–124, *121–123*
  tissue reaction to orthodontic force systems, 130–138, *132–138*
  tooth-movement research, 329
Fitch, Samuel, 7
flapless corticotomy protocol, **246**, 249–250, *249–250*
flow cytometry, 319, *320*
fluid dynamic hypothesis, 24–25, *25*
fluorescence microscopy, 317, *317*
fluorescent microsphere assays, 164
fluoride, 210
F/M *see* force–moment
focal adhesion complex, 39–40, *39*
force–moment (F/M) sensors, 329
force–velocity curve, 328, *329*
Frizzled, 102, 108
Frost, Harold, 82–83, 88, *89*
fungi, 145–146, *147*, 150

GAG *see* glycosaminoglycans
Galen (131–201), 5
GBI *see* gingival bleeding index
GCF *see* gingival crevicular fluid

genetic influences
  bone growth and metabolism, 80, 84–86, *85*, *87*
  cellular agents, 86, *87*
  complications of orthodontic tooth movement, 181–184, *182*
  determinants of overall craniofacial growth, 85
  eruption failure/primary failure of eruption, 181–182
  inflammatory response, 86
  personalized diagnosis and treatment, 171–188
  tissue reactions to mechanical forces, 172–180
    alveolar bone, 177–180, *178*
    neural tissues, 176–177, *176*
    periodontal ligament, 172–176, *173*, **174–175**
    pulp tissues, 180–181, *181*
    tooth relapse, 182
    tooth resorption, 182–184, *182*
    translational applications, 181, *182*
    vascular invasion, 85–86, *85*
genome-wide association studies (GWAS), 191
genomic studies, 319–321, *320*
gingival bleeding index (GBI), 149
gingival crevicular fluid (GCF)
  genetic influences, 172
  oral fluid markers of paradental tissue remodeling, 159–164, *161–163*, **161**
  precision accelerated orthodontics, 266, 268
  relapse and retention, 302–303
  tooth-movement research, 329, 333–337
gingival enlargement
  drugs, medications, and supplements, 206–207
  iatrogenic injuries in orthodontics, 280–281, *281*
gingival fibers, 303
gingival invagination, 283–284
gingival recession
  iatrogenic injuries in orthodontics, 281–283, *282–283*
  tooth-movement research, 338–339
glycoproteins, 36
glycosaminoglycans (GAG), 36, 304–305
grafting protocols, 246–248, *248–249*, **248**
growth factors
  biological orthodontics, 222–223, 225
  bone growth and metabolism, 79, 85–86
  cellular and molecular biology, 38–39, 43–45
  genetic influences, 177–181
  iatrogenic injuries in orthodontics, 290
  inflammatory response, 57–58
  load-induced modeling, 101–104, 111
  surgically assisted tooth movement, 248, *249*
  tooth-movement research, 330
growth hormone, 208
GWAS *see* genome-wide association studies

Harris, Chappin, 8
heat shock proteins (HSP), 52, 322
hedgehog proteins, 79
heparan sulfate, 36
HIF *see* hypoxia inducible factor
high mobility group box protein 1 (HMGB1), 51, 173

Hippocrates of Cos (460–377 BCE), 5
histology
    evolution of hypotheses and concepts, 17–19, *18–22*, 23, *24*
    history of orthodontics, 8–11, *8–12*
    iatrogenic injuries in orthodontics, 283–284, 288–289
    relapse and retention, 300–303, *301–303*
    surgically assisted tooth movement, *240*
    temporary anchorage devices, 124–126, *125–126*
    tooth-movement research, 316–318, *317–318*
history of orthodontics, 3–15
    bioelectric signals in orthodontic tooth movement, 26–30, *27–29*
    bone-bending hypothesis, 11, 25–26, *26*
    cellular and molecular biology era, 11–13
    conclusions and future directions, 13–14
    early attempts to accelerate tooth movement, 219–220, *220*
    early history of orthodontics, 4–5, *5*
    evolution of hypotheses and concepts, 16–31
    fluid dynamic hypothesis, 24–25, *25*
    histochemical evaluation of tissue response to applied mechanical loads, 11, *12*
    histological studies of paradental tissues, 8–11, *8–11*
    hypotheses about biological nature of OTM, 17–26
    industrial revolution, 5–7, *6–7*
    Oppenheim's transformation hypothesis, 19–20, *20*
    origins of orthodontics, 3–4, *4*
    pressure–tension hypothesis, 20–23, *21–24*
    surgically assisted tooth movement, 243
    tooth-movement research, 311–312, *312*, 327
    twentieth and twenty-first centuries, 8–13, *8–12*
    Walkhoff's hypothesis, 17–19, *18–19*
HMGB1 *see* high mobility group box protein 1
Howship's lacuna, 37, 44
HPA *see* hypothalamic–pituitary–adrenal
HSP *see* heat shock proteins
Human Genome Project, 190–191
Human Phenotype Ontology project, 191
Hunter, John (1728–1793), 6
hyaline cartilage, 78–81, *79*
hyalinization
    cellular and molecular biology, 41–42
    evolution of hypotheses and concepts, 22–23, *23*
    relapse and retention, 298, 300, 306
    tissue reaction to orthodontic force systems, 130–131, *131*
    tooth-movement research, 328–329, 338
hyaluronic acid, 36
hydroxyapatite, 210–211
hyperlocalized inflammation, 268–269
hyperplastic reactions, 291–292, *291*
hypertrophic chondrocytes, 79
hypothalamic–pituitary–adrenal (HPA) axis, 207
hypoxia inducible factor (HIF), 58

iatrogenic injuries in orthodontics
    concepts and definitions, 279–280, **280**
    cytotoxicity and allergic reactions, 292
    enamel decalcification and trauma, 285–288, *286–289*

    extraoral effects, 292–293
    gingival effects, 280–284, *281–283*
    intraoral effects, 280
    mechanical and biological determinants, 279–296
    periodontal changes and alveolar bone loss, 284–285, *284–285*, **285**
    pulpal reactions, 288–290, *289*
    root resorption, 289–290, 290–291
    soft tissue irritation, 291–292, *291*
    swallowing or inhalation of small parts, 294
    systemic risks, 293–294
    tooth-related changes, 285–291, *286–290*
ICC *see* immunocytochemistry
IEG *see* immediate early genes
IFN *see* interferons
IgE *see* immunoglobulin E
IGF *see* insulin-like growth factor
IHC *see* immunohistochemistry
IL *see* interleukins
immediate early genes (IEG), 50
immunocytochemistry (ICC), 319
immunoglobulin E (IgE), 204–205
immunohistochemistry (IHC)
    biological orthodontics, *228–230*, 233
    history of orthodontics, 11, *12*
    inflammatory response, *54*, 56, 59
    tooth-movement research, 318–319, *319*
impacted teeth, 152, *153*
indirect resorption, 131, *131*
inflammatory response, 49–67
    activation, apoptosis, and cell cycles, 58
    bone growth and metabolism, 86
    cellular and molecular biology, 41–42
    cementum, 62
    chemokines, 50, 55–57
    concepts and definitions, 49–50
    cytokines, 49–50, 53
    damage associated molecular pattern proteins, 49–52
    dental pulp, 58–60, **60**
    growth factors, 57–58
    iatrogenic injuries in orthodontics, 280–284
    inflammation during tooth movement, 50–51, **50**, *51*
    interleukins, 49–50, 53–54, *54*, 58–59, 61–62
    matrix metalloproteinases, 57
    mediators in orthodontic tooth movement, 51–58, **51**
    micro-osteo-perforations, 268–271, *269–271*
    neuropeptides/neurotransmitters, 50–51, 57–60
    oral fluid markers of paradental tissue remodeling, 159–167
    oral microbiology, 141–158
    orthodontic pain, 60–61
    periodontal ligament, 49–58, **50**, *51*
    precision accelerated orthodontics, 266–273, *269–274*
    prostaglandins, 49, 52
    root resorption, 61–62, *63*
    second-messenger system, 52–53
    temporary anchorage devices, 126
    TNF and the RANK/RANKL/OPG system, 49–50, 53–55, *56*, 61–62
    tooth-movement research, 330–333, *331–335*
    vasodilation and angiogenesis, 60

    vibration, 271–273, *272–273*
    inhalation risks, 294
inositol triphosphate (IP3), 50
insulin-like growth factor (IGF)
    biological orthodontics, 222–223
    bone growth and metabolism, 79
    genetic influences, 180
    load-induced modeling, 102, 104, 108, *109*
integrins, 39–40, *39*
interferons (IFN), 86
interleukins (IL)
    biological orthodontics, 220, 225
    bone growth and metabolism, 86
    cellular and molecular biology, 43–45
    drugs, medications, and supplements, 205
    genetic influences, 173, 179–184
    history of orthodontics, 11, *12*
    inflammatory response, 49–50, 53–54, *54*, 58–59, 61–62
    load-induced modeling, 113–114
    oral fluid markers of paradental tissue remodeling, 161–163, *163*
    tooth-movement research, 330, 336
intramembranous ossification, 78, *79*, 80–82, *81*
IP3 *see* inositol triphosphate

JAK/STAT pathway, 227

Ketcham, Albert (1870–1955), 9, *9*
Kingsley, Norman William (1829–1913), 7, *7*, 17

lacerations, 291–292, *291*
Lactobacillus spp., 143, 145–146, 148–152, 286–288
laser-tracking microrheology, 325, *325*
LED *see* light-emitting diode
light-emitting diode (LED) therapy, 225, 227, *228–230*
lingual brackets, 148, *148*
lipids, 210–211
LLLT *see* low-level laser therapy
lncRNA *see* long noncoding RNAs
load-induced modeling, 100–116
    anabolic response and vitamin A, 108
    concepts and definitions, 100–101
    musculoskeletal system functions, 100, *101*
    osteoblast and osteocyte responses to, 107–108, *109*
    osteoblast differentiation and function, 101–103, *103*
    osteoclast differentiation and function, 104–105, *104*
    osteoclast response to, 109–110, *110*
    osteocyte function, 103–104
    role of sex hormones in orthodontic tooth movement, 111–114, **113**
    role of sex hormones in osteogenic effect of loading, 110–111, *112*
    sex-hormones and their receptors, 100–101, 105–108, *106–107*
long noncoding RNAs (lncRNA), 177
loss of attachment, 284
low-level laser therapy (LLLT)
    biological orthodontics, 225–227, *228–230*
    orthodontic pain, 61
    relapse and retention, 300
LRP5, 102, 179

macrophage colony-stimulating factor (M-CSF)
  biological orthodontics, 227, *228*
  cellular and molecular biology, 43
  genetic influences, 177, 180
  load-induced modeling, 104
macrophages
  bone growth and metabolism, 89–90
  cellular and molecular biology, 38
  iatrogenic injuries in orthodontics, 290
  relapse and retention, 300
magnetic pulling cytometry (MPC), 324, *324*
magnetic twisting cytometry (MTC), 323–324, *324*
mandible
  bone growth and metabolism, 81, *82*
  temporary anchorage devices, 119, *119*
MAR *see* mineral apposition rate
marginal gingiva, 68, 71–75, *72*
mass spectroscopy, 164
matrix metalloproteinases (MMP)
  biological orthodontics, 233
  cellular and molecular biology, 42–45, *44*
  drugs, medications, and supplements, 209
  genetic influences, 172–173, 180–181, 183
  inflammatory response, 57
  load-induced modeling, 103, 109–110
  mechanical loading on hard and soft tissues, 71, *71*, *73*
  oral fluid markers of paradental tissue remodeling, 162
  relapse and retention, 300
  tooth-movement research, 336
maxilla
  bone growth and metabolism, 81, *81*
  temporary anchorage devices, 119
maximum insertion torque (MIT), 119
maximum removal torque (MRT), 119
M-CSF *see* macrophage colony-stimulating factor
mechanical loading on hard and soft tissues, 68–76
  ATP-purinoreceptors as mechanosensors in marginal gingiva, 74–75
  cellular and molecular biology, 69–70, *71*
  concepts and definitions, 68
  load-induced modeling, 100–116
  marginal gingiva as periodontal mechanosensor, 72–74, *72*
  mechanobiology, 69
  mechanotransduction in bone tissue, 69–70
  mechanotransduction in periodontal tissues, 70–71
  role of marginal gingiva in orthodontic tooth movement, 71–72
mechanotransduction hypothesis, 69–71, 330–333, *331–335*
Meckel's cartilage, 81
mesenchymal stem cells (MSC), 178
messenger RNA (mRNA), 173, 176–179
metallic brackets, 148–149
metastatic bone cancers, 202
M/F *see* moment-to-force
microarrays
  DNA microarray, 321
  oral fluid markers of paradental tissue remodeling, 164
  protein microarrays, 321–322

microfabrication, 325
microfibril bundles, 36
microfilaments, 72
microfluidics, 325–326
micronucleus assay, 322
micro-osteo-perforations (MOP)
  clinical considerations, 269–271
  hyperlocalized inflammation, 268–269
  precision accelerated orthodontics, 268–271, *269–271*
  surgically assisted tooth movement, 239, **246**, 249–250, *250*, *256*
micropipette aspiration, *324*, 325
microtomography, 338
microtrauma-triggered bone remodeling, 268
microtubules, 72
midline synchondrosis (MS), 82, *82*
mineral apposition rate (MAR), 111
minerals, 210
mini-implants, 152–154, *154*
miniscrews/miniplates *see* temporary anchorage devices
MIT *see* maximum insertion torque
MMP *see* matrix metalloproteinases
mobility, 120
moment-to-force (M/F) ratio, 241–242, *241–242*
MOP *see* micro-osteo-perforation
MPC *see* magnetic pulling cytometry
mRNA *see* messenger RNA
MRT *see* maximum removal torque
MS *see* midline synchondrosis
MSC *see* mesenchymal stem cells
MTC *see* magnetic twisting cytometry
MTT assay, 322, *322*
music therapy, 61

Nance appliance, 271
necrosis
  cellular and molecular biology, 41–42
  tissue reaction to orthodontic force systems, 131, *131*
neural crest/neural plate, 78, *78*
neural tissues, 176–177, *176*
neurokinin A (NKA), 57, 59–60
neuronal growth factor (NGF), genetic influences, 177
neuropeptides/neurotransmitters
  bone growth and metabolism, 88
  cellular and molecular biology, 36
  genetic influences, 176–177, *176*
  inflammatory response, 50–51, 57–60
neuropeptide Y (NPY), 58
next-generation sequencing (NGS), 191, 195, *195*
NF *see* nuclear factor
NGF *see* neuronal growth factor
NGS *see* next-generation sequencing
nicotine use, 211
nifedipine, 206–207
nitric oxide
  bone growth and metabolism, 88
  inflammatory response, 50
  load-induced modeling, 108–111, *109*
nitric oxide synthase (NOS), 179–180
NKA *see* neurokinin A
nod-like receptors (NLR), 51–52
nonsteroidal anti-inflammatory drugs (NSAID), 60–61, 200–202, 294

NOS *see* nitric oxide synthase
NPY *see* neuropeptide Y
NSAID *see* nonsteroidal anti-inflammatory drugs
nuclear factor (NF)-kappaB, 57, 227

omega 3,6 fatty acids, 211
open flap corticotomy and grafting protocol, 245–248, **246**, *247–249*, **248**
OPG *see* RANK/RANKL/OPG system
OPN *see* osteopontin
Oppenheim, Albin (1875–1945), 8, 17–20, *20*, 22–23, *23*
optimal orthodontic force concept, 327–329, *328–329*
oral fluid markers
  collection and analysis of GCF samples, 162–164, *163*
  conclusions and future directions, 164–165
  diagnostic trials, 162
  genetic influences, 172
  paradental tissue remodeling, 159–167
  relapse and retention, 302–303
  saliva, 159–160, 172, 329, 333–337
  study findings, 160–162
  tooth-movement research, 319, 321, 329, 333–337
  see also gingival crevicular fluid
oral microbiology, 141–158
  concepts and definitions, 141–144
  dental caries, 143–147, *144*, *147*, 149–150
  effects by orthodontic bracket type, 148–149, *148*
  fixed orthodontics, 146–147, *146–147*
  fungi, 145–146, 147, 150
  iatrogenic injuries in orthodontics, 286–288
  impacted teeth, 152
  importance of oral hygiene, 150–152, *151–152*
  mini-implants, 152–154, *154*
  normal oral flora and conditions, 141–142
  orthodontic retainers, 149–150, *151*
  orthognathic surgery, 154, *155*
  periodontal disease, 143–146, *146*, 150
  removable orthodontics, 144–146, *145*
  tooth-movement research, 338–339
orthodontia, 194
orthognathic surgery, 154, *155*
osseointegration, 124
ossification *see* bone growth and metabolism
osteoblasts
  as bone-forming cells, 102, *103*
  as regulators of osteoclast formation, 102–103
  biological orthodontics, 232
  bone growth and metabolism, 90
  cellular and molecular biology, 37
  differentiation, 101–102
  evolution of hypotheses and concepts, *29*
  genetic influences, 176, 178–179
  osteoclast factors important for osteoblast stimulation, 105
  precision accelerated orthodontics, 267
  responses to load-induced modeling, 100–101, 107–108, *109*
osteoclasts
  biological orthodontics, 221, *222*, 231–232
  bone growth and metabolism, 86, 90
  cellular and molecular biology, 37–38, 43–44, *43–44*

osteoclasts (Cont'd)
  differentiation and function, 104–105, *104*
  evolution of hypotheses and concepts, 22, *23*, *29*
  factors important for osteoblast stimulation, 105
  genetic influences, 177, *178*
  mechanical loading on hard and soft tissues, 71, 73
  osteoblasts as regulators of osteoclast formation, 102–103
  precision accelerated orthodontics, 265–267
  relapse and retention, 301
  response to load-induced modeling, 100–101, 109–110, *110*
osteocytes
  as bone-remodeling cells, 103
  as mechano-sensory cells, 103–104
  bone growth and metabolism, 90
  cellular and molecular biology, 37
  genetic influences, 178–179
  responses to load-induced modeling, 100–101, 107–108, *109*
osteoimmune interplay, 100
osteonecrosis, 203
osteophytes, 22, *22*
osteopontin (OPN), 173, 176, 179–180
osteoporesis, 203, 205, 208
osteoprotegerin (OPG) *see* RANK/RANKL/OPG system
over-the-counter (OTC) medications, 199
oxytalan fibers, 36, *36*, 305–306

P2X7 receptor, 183–184
pain and pain management, 60–61, 293–294
PAOO *see* periodontally accelerated osteogenic orthodontics
paradental tissue remodeling
  collection and analysis of GCF samples, 162–164, *163*
  conclusions and future directions, 164–165
  diagnostic trials, 162
  gingival crevicular fluid, 159–164, *161–163*, **161**
  oral fluid markers, 159–167
  saliva, 159–160
  study findings, 160–162
parathyroid hormone 1 receptor (*PTH1R*) gene, 195
parathyroid hormone (PTH)
  biological orthodontics, 220, 221–223, *223*
  bone growth and metabolism, 88, 90–92, 95
  drugs, medications, and supplements, 208
parathyroid hormone-related protein (PTHrP), 79
pattern recognition receptors (PRR), 52
PCR *see* polymerase chain reaction
PDGF *see* platelet-derived growth factor
PDL *see* periodontal ligament
pelican forceps, 5, 6
PEMF *see* pulsed electromagnetic field
pentraxin-related protein (PTX3), 43
peri-miniscrew implant crevicular fluid (PMICF), 126
periodontal disease
  iatrogenic injuries in orthodontics, 284–285, *284–285*, **285**

oral microbiology, 143–146, *146*, 150
precision orthodontics, 192–193
tooth-movement research, 338–339
periodontal ligament (PDL)
  biological orthodontics, 220, *220*
  biomechanical characteristics of the PDL, 38, *38*
  bone growth and metabolism, 80, 90, 93–94, *93–94*
  cellular and molecular biology, 35–45, *36*
  drugs, medications, and supplements, 200–202, *201*, 205, 209
  evolution of hypotheses and concepts, 16–30, *18–24*
  genetic influences, 171–176, *173*, **174–175**, 181
  history of orthodontics, 8–13, *9–10*, *12*
  iatrogenic injuries in orthodontics, 290
  inflammatory response, 49–58, *50*, *51*
  mechanical loading on hard and soft tissues, 68, 70–75
  precision accelerated orthodontics, 265–266
  relapse and retention, 45, 298, 300–306, *301–303*
  surgically assisted tooth movement, 241–242, *242*, 245
  temporary anchorage devices, 121
  tissue reaction to orthodontic force systems, 130–136, *131–132*, *135–138*
  tooth-movement research, 319, *319*, 327–329
periodontally accelerated osteogenic orthodontics (PAOO), 73
periostin, 176
personal protection equipment (PPE), 293
PFE *see* primary failure of eruption
PG *see* prostaglandins
PGP *see* protein gene product
phenotypic modification therapy (PhMT), 283
phenytoin, 206–207
PhMT *see* phenotypic modification therapy
phosphorus homeostasis, 103, 210
photobiomodulation, 225–226
photomicrography
  bone growth and metabolism, *82*
  cellular and molecular biology, *36–37*, *41–42*
physical therapy, 61
piezocision, 230–231, 239, *249*
piezoelectric hypothesis, 26–30
piezosurgery, 245–248
platelet-derived growth factor (PDGF), 180–181
platelet-rich fibrin (PRF), 248, *248*
platelet-rich growth factor (PRGF), 248, *249*
PMICF *see* peri-miniscrew implant crevicular fluid
polymerase chain reaction (PCR), 320, *320*
Porphyromonas spp., 143, 153
positional physical memory of dentition (PPMD), 73
PPE *see* personal protection equipment
PPMD *see* positional physical memory of dentition
precision accelerated orthodontics, 265–275
  biphasic theory of tooth movement, 265–267, *276–277*
  concepts and definitions, 265
  conclusions and recommendations, 273, *274*
  micro-osteo-perforations, 268–271, *269–271*

saturation of the biological response, 267–268, *268*
vibration, 271–273, *272–273*
precision orthodontics, 189–198
  application in medical practice, 191–192
  Class III malocclusion, 194
  concepts and definitions, 189, *190*
  education and training, 196
  efficacy of risk prediction of Mendelian versus complex traits, 192
  eruption failure/primary failure of eruption, 194–195
  evidence-based practice versus precision medicine practice, 189–190
  external apical root resorption concurrent with orthodontia, 194
  from personalized to precision orthodontics, 193–195, *193*
  genome-wide association studies, 191
  Human Genome Project, 190–191
  Human Phenotype Ontology project, 191
  impacts of progression in DNA analysis technology, 190–192
  next-generation sequencing, 191, 195, *195*
  precision oral healthcare, 192–193
  sagittal facial growth during puberty, 194
pressure–tension hypothesis
  evolution of hypotheses and concepts, 20–23, *21–24*
  precision accelerated orthodontics, 265–266
  tissue reaction to orthodontic force systems, 130–131, *131*
PRF *see* platelet-rich fibrin
PRGF *see* platelet-rich growth factor
primary failure of eruption (PFE), 181–182, 194–195
procollagen, 35
prostaglandins (PG)
  biological orthodontics, 220–221, *220*
  bone growth and metabolism, 88
  drugs, medications, and supplements, 200, *201*, 210–211
  history of orthodontics, 11, *12*
  inflammatory response, 49, 52
  load-induced modeling, 108, *109*, 113–114
  mechanical loading on hard and soft tissues, 69, 74
  oral fluid markers of paradental tissue remodeling, 161
protein gene product (PGP) 9.5, 176–177
proteoglycans, 36, 304–305
proteomic analysis, 321–322, *321*
PRR *see* pattern recognition receptors
psychiatric drugs, 207
PTH1R, 195
PTH *see* parathyroid hormone
PTHrP *see* parathyroid hormone-related protein
PTX3 *see* pentraxin-related protein
pulsed electromagnetic field (PEMF), 224–225
purinoreceptors, 74–75

radiography
  iatrogenic injuries in orthodontics, *284*, 289–290
  surgically assisted tooth movement, *251*
  see also computed tomography
raloxifene, 208

Raman spectroscopy, 164
RANK/RANKL/OPG system
    biological orthodontics, 221–223, *222–223*, 225–227, *226*, *229–230*, 233–234, *234*
    bone growth and metabolism, 86–88, *87*, 90–91
    cellular and molecular biology, 43, *43*, 45
    drugs, medications, and supplements, 208, 211
    genetic influences, 172–173, 176–179, 181–184
    history of orthodontics, 13
    iatrogenic injuries in orthodontics, 291
    inflammatory response, 49, 53–55, *56*, 61–62
    load-induced modeling, 102–105, 109–110
    oral fluid markers of paradental tissue remodeling, 161–162
    precision accelerated orthodontics, 266
    temporary anchorage devices, 126
    tooth-movement research, 330, 332–333, 336–337
RAP *see* regional accelaratory phenomenon
rapid orthodontics
    biological orthodontics, 219–237
    precision accelerated orthodontics, 265–275
    surgically assisted tooth movement, 238–264
    tooth-movement research, 337–338, *337*
RAR *see* retinoic acid receptors
receptor activator of nuclear factor kappa B ligand (RANKL) *see* RANK/RANKL/OPG system
reflection electron microscopy (REM), 318
regional accelaratory phenomenon (RAP)
    biological orthodontics, 227–229, 231
    bone growth and metabolism, 83
    evolution of hypotheses and concepts, 26
    mechanical loading on hard and soft tissues, 71, 73
    surgically assisted tooth movement, 239–245, *240*, *245–246*
    tooth-movement research, 337
Reitan, Kaare (1903–2000), 9–10, *9*, 23, *24*
relapse and retention
    amount, rate, and duration, 298–299, *299*
    biological background of relapse, 297–307
    cellular and molecular biology, 45
    closure of extraction space or midline diastema, 304–305
    collagen fibers of the periodontum, 303–305
    concepts and definitions, 297–298
    effect of retention, 299–300, *299–300*
    genetic influences, 182
    histological changes during relapse, 300–303, *301–303*
    oral microbiology, 149–150, *151*
    oxytalan fibers, 305–306
    process of relapse, 298–303
    rotational tooth movement, 304
    techniques affecting relapse, 305
    translational tooth movement, 303–304
    turnover of collagen in the periodontium, 305
relaxin, 209, 224
REM *see* reflection electron microscopy
renal deficiency, 95
retainers *see* relapse and retention
retinoic acid receptors (RAR), 108

retinoic X receptors (RXR), 108
retinoids, 79
root resorption
    cementum, 62
    drugs, medications, and supplements, 203–204
    evolution of hypotheses and concepts, 20–21
    iatrogenic injuries in orthodontics, *289–290*, 290–291
    inflammatory response, 61–62, *63*
    precision accelerated orthodontics, 271
    relapse and retention, 300–302, *301*, *303*
    tooth-movement research, 336–337
ruffled border, 37, 44
RUNX2, 37, 80, 102, 178–179
RXR *see* retinoic X receptors

sagittal facial growth during puberty, 194
salivary biomarkers
    genetic influences, 172
    oral fluid markers of paradental tissue remodeling, 159–160
    tooth-movement research, 329, 333–337
Sandstedt, Carl (1860–1904), 8, *8*, 17–18, *17–19*, 22–23
scanning electron microscopy (SEM)
    iatrogenic injuries in orthodontics, *286*, 288
    tooth-movement research, 318, *318*
Schwalbe–Flourens pressure hypothesis, 17
Schwarz, A. M., 20–23, *21–24*
second-messenger system, 52–53
self-ligating brackets, 148
SEM *see* scanning electron microscopy
sensitivity reactions, 292
sex-hormones and their receptors
    biological orthodontics, 224
    drugs, medications, and supplements, 208–209
    genomic signaling in bone, 106, *107*
    load-induced modeling, 100–101, 105–108, *106–107*
    non-genomic signaling, 106–107, *107*
    osteoblast and osteocyte responses to load-induced modeling, 107–108, *109*
    role in orthodontic tooth movement, 111–114, **113**
    role in osteogenic effect of loading, 110–111, *112*
Sharpey's fibers, 302, *302*
single cell gel electrophoresis, 322, *322*
single nucleotide polymorphisms (SNP), 190–191
sleep apnea, 196
SNP *see* single nucleotide polymorphisms
soft tissue grafts, 248, *248–249*
soft tissue irritation, 291–292, *291*
SOST, 102
squeeze film effect, 10–11, *11*
statins, 206
streaming potentials, 27–30
Streptococcus spp., 142–153, 286–288
substance abuse, 211
substance P
    cellular and molecular biology, 36
    genetic influences, 176–177
    inflammatory response, 50–51, 57, 59–60
surgically assisted tooth movement, 238–264

    biological principles and biomechanical considerations, 239–242, *240–242*
    clinical examples, 250–258, *251–261*
    concepts and definitions, 238–239
    conclusions and recommendations, 259–261, **261**
    finite element analysis/models, 240–242, *241–242*
    historical background, 243
    regional accelaratory phenomenon, 239–245, *240*, *245–246*
    rules for effective alveolar corticotomy, 242–250
        facilitating orthodontic tooth movement, 243–244, *244*
        flapless corticotomy protocol, **246**, 249–250, *249–250*
        limited effect in time, 244
        limited effects in space, 244–245, *245–246*
        open flap corticotomy and grafting protocol, 245–248, **246**, *247–249*, **248**
        patient selection, 250
        postsurgical orthodontic management, 250
swallowing risks, 294

TAD *see* temporary anchorage devices
Talbot, Eugene, 7
tartrate resistant acid phosphatase (TRAP)
    cellular and molecular biology, 43, 45
    inflammatory response, *56*
    tooth-movement research, *317*
TEGDMA *see* triethylene glycol dimethacrylate
TEM *see* transmission electron microscopy
temperomandibular joint (TMJ), 80, 89, 91–93, *92*
temporary anchorage devices (TAD), 117–128
    age of patient, 118
    clinical factors in success of, 118–120, *119*, 126, *126*
    concepts and definitions, 117, *118*
    cortical bone thickness, 120–121, *121*
    diameter ratio of pilot hole to miniscrew, 125
    exposed length, 124
    histological reactions, 124–126, *125–126*
    immediate loading of orthodontic miniscrews, 124–125
    implantation site, 119, *119*
    implant diameter and length, 119–120
    inflammatory responses, 126
    insertion angulations, 121–122, *122*
    insertion torque, 119
    loading time point, 118, 125
    mechanical analysis using finite element models, 120–124, *121–123*
    mobility, 120
    osseointegration process, 124
    surgically assisted tooth movement, 244
    thread location, properties, and mechanical anistropy, 122–124, *123*
temporomandibular muscle and joint disorders (TMD), 192
tetracyclins, 231–232, *233*
TFM *see* traction force microscopy
TGF *see* transforming growth factor
thyroid hormones, 207–208
time–displacement curve, 40–41, *40*

tissue inhibitors of matrix metalloproteinases (TIMP)
  cellular and molecular biology, 43–45, *44*
  genetic influences, 172–173
  inflammatory response, 57
  oral fluid markers of paradental tissue remodeling, 162
tissue reaction to orthodontic force systems, 129–138
  centre of resistance, 129–130, *130*, 133–136
  concepts and definitions, 129–130
  conclusions and future directions, 136–138
  finite element analysis/models, 130–138, *132–138*
  influence of alveolar wall morphology, 133–135, *133–135*
  influence of force level, 135–136, *136–137*
  influence of interaction with occlusion, 136, *138*
  influence of material properties, 131–133, *132*
  pressure–tension hypothesis, 130–131, *131*
TLR *see* toll-like receptors
TMD *see* temporomandibular muscle and joint disorders
TMJ *see* temporomandibular joint
TNFα *see* tumor necrosis factor
toll-like receptors (TLR), 51–52
tooth-movement research
  accelerating tooth movement, 337–338, *337*
  alveolar bone density and shape of alveolar wall, 338
  animal models, 314–315
  cell culture, 313–314, *313*, **314**
  concepts and definitions, 311–312
  controversies and research directions, 327–342
  evidence generation, 313–316
  flow cytometry, 319, *320*
  genomic studies, 319–321, *320*
  gingival recession, 338–339
  histology, 316–318, *317–318*
  history of orthodontics, 311–312, *312*, 327
  immunocytochemistry, 319
  immunohistochemistry, 318–319, *319*
  inflammation versus mechanotransduction, 330–333, *331–335*

  in vitro versus *ex vitro* studies, 313
  methodologies, 316–323, **316**
  optimal orthodontic force concept, 327–329, *328–329*
  oral fluid markers, 329, 333–337
  periodontal disease, 338–339
  planning and execution of, 311–326
  proteomic analysis/cytoplasm-level studies, 321–322, *321*
  scientific method, 312–313
  studies in humans, 315–316, *315*
  studying mechanobiology, 323–326, *324–325*
  tissue level/cellular level studies, 316–319, *317–320*
  toxicology studies, 322–323, *322–323*
tooth resorption, 182–184, *182*
torque ratio, 119
toxicology studies, 322–323, *322–323*
TPA *see* transpalatal arch
trabecular bone remodeling, 88, 90, *90–91*
traction force microscopy (TFM), *324*, 325
transcription factors, 178
transformation hypothesis, 19–20, *20*
transforming growth factor (TGF)
  genetic influences, 179–181
  inflammatory response, 57
  load-induced modeling, 102, 111
  surgically assisted tooth movement, 248
transmission electron microscopy (TEM), 10, 317–318
transpalatal arch (TPA), 271
TRAP *see* tartrate resistant acid phosphatase
triethylene glycol dimethacrylate (TEGDMA), 292
trunk neural crest, 78
tumor necrosis factor (TNFα)
  bone growth and metabolism, 86
  cellular and molecular biology, 43
  genetic influences, 173, 179, 182–184
  inflammatory response, 49–50, 54–55
  load-induced modeling, 113–114
  tooth-movement research, 330
typodonts, 311, *312*

uncoordinated-like (UNCL), 176

undermineralized thin sectioning method, 83, *83–84*

valproic acid, 206–207
vascular endothelial growth factor (VEGF)
  bone growth and metabolism, 79, 85–86
  cellular and molecular biology, 43–45
  genetic influences, 177, 181
  inflammatory response, 58
vascular invasion, 79, *79*, 85–86, *85*
vascular systems, 36
vasoactive intestinal polypeptide (VIP), 50, 58, 176
vasodilation, 60
VEGF *see* vascular endothelial growth factor
Vesalius (1514–1564), 5
vibration
  biological orthodontics, 225, *225–226*
  biphasic theory of tooth movement, 271–273, *272–273*
Vickers hardness, 62
VIP *see* vasoactive intestinal polypeptide
viral infection, 293
visible plaque index (VPI), 149
vitamin A, 108, 210
vitamin C, 209
vitamin D
  biological orthodontics, 223–224
  bone growth and metabolism, 95
  supplementation, 209–210
von Mises stresses, 120–122, *121–122*
VPI *see* visible plaque index

Walkhoff's hypothesis, 17–19, *18–19*
weightlifting, 130
Western blot analysis, 321, *321*
white spot lesions (WSL), 144, *144*, 287–288
Wnt/β-catenin signaling pathway
  bone growth and metabolism, 79
  drugs, medications, and supplements, 211
  load-induced modeling, 102, *103*, 107–108, *109*
WSL *see* white spot lesions

zeta potential, 27
zoledronic acid, 203–204